QUICK LOOK DRUG BOOK

2000

Leonard L. Lance, RPh
Senior Editor
Pharmacist
Lexi-Comp Inc.
Hudson, Ohio

Charles Lacy, RPh, PharmD
Editor
Drug Information Pharmacist
Cedars-Sinai Medical Center
Los Angeles, California

Morton P. Goldman, PharmD
Associate Editor
Infectious Diseases Pharmacist
Cleveland Clinic Foundation
Cleveland, Ohio

Lora L. Armstrong, RPh, BSPharm, BCPS
Clinical Pharmacist
Clinical Development and Information Resources
Prescription Services Division
Caremark Rx, Inc.
Northbrook, Illinois

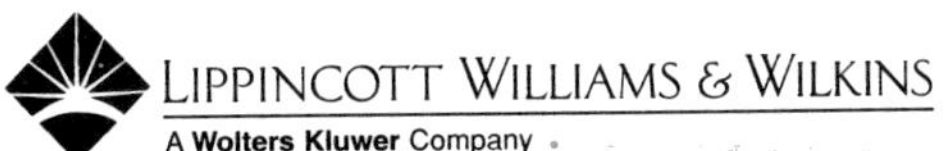

Philadelphia • Baltimore • New York • London
Buenos Aires • Hong Kong • Sydney • Tokyo

QUICK LOOK DRUG BOOK

2000

Leonard L. Lance, RPh, BSPharm
Senior Editor
Pharmacist
Lexi-Comp Inc.
Hudson, Ohio

Charles F. Lacy, RPh, PharmD, FCSHP
Editor
Drug Information Pharmacist
Cedars-Sinai Medical Center
Los Angeles, California

Morton P. Goldman, PharmD, BCPS
Associate Editor
Assistant Director, Pharmacotherapy Services
Department of Pharmacy
Cleveland Clinic Foundation
Cleveland, Ohio

Lora L. Armstrong, RPh, BSPharm, BCPS
Associate Editor
Clinical Pharmacist
Caremark Pharmaceutical Group
Northbrook, Illinois

NOTICE

This handbook is intended to serve the user as a handy quick reference and not as a complete drug information resource. It does not include information on every therapeutic agent available. The publication covers 1570 commonly used drugs and is specifically designed to present certain important aspects of drug data in a more concise format than is generally found in medical literature or product material supplied by manufacturers.

Although great care was taken to ensure the accuracy of the handbook's content when it went to press, the editors, contributors, and publisher cannot be responsible for the continued accuracy of the supplied information due to ongoing research and new developments in the field. Further, the *Quick Look Drug Book* is not offered as a guide to dosing. The reader, herewith, is advised that information shown under the heading **Usual Dosage** is provided only as an indication of the amount of the drug typically given or taken during therapy. Actual dosing amount for any specific drug should be based on an in-depth evaluation of the individual patient's therapy requirement and strong consideration given to such issues as contraindications, warnings, precautions, adverse reactions, along with the interaction of other drugs. The manufacturers most current product information or other standard recognized references should always be consulted for such detailed information prior to drug use.

The editors and contributors have written this book in their private capacities. No official support or endorsement by any federal agency or pharmaceutical company is intended or inferred.

This manual was produced using the FormuLex™ Program —
a complete publishing service of Lexi-Comp Inc.

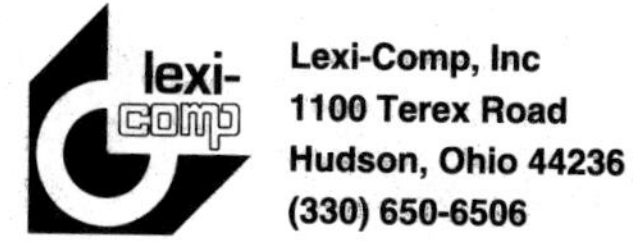

Lexi-Comp, Inc
1100 Terex Road
Hudson, Ohio 44236
(330) 650-6506

TABLE OF CONTENTS

ABOUT THE AUTHORS

Leonard L. Lance, RPh, BSPharm

Leonard L. (Bud) Lance has been directly involved in the pharmaceutical industry since receiving his bachelor's degree in pharmacy from Ohio Northern University in 1970. Upon graduation from ONU, Mr Lance spent four years as a navy pharmacist in various military assignments and was instrumental in the development and operation of the first whole hospital I.V. admixture program in a military (Portsmouth Naval Hospital) facility.

After completing his military service, he entered the retail pharmacy field and has managed both an independent and a home I.V. franchise pharmacy operation. Since the late 1970s, Mr Lance has focused much of his interest on using computers to improve pharmacy service and to advance the dissemination of drug information to practitioners and other health care professionals.

As a result of his strong publishing interest, he serves in the capacity of pharmacy editor and technical advisor as well as pharmacy (information) database coordinator for Lexi-Comp. Along with the *Quick Look Drug Book*, he provides technical support to Lexi-Comp's *Drug Information Handbook for the Allied Health Professional*, and many other titles published by Lexi-Comp, Inc. Mr Lance has also assisted approximately 120 major hospitals in producing their own formulary (pharmacy) publications through Lexi-Comp's custom publishing service.

Mr Lance is a member and past president (1984) of the Summit Pharmaceutical Association (SPA). He is also a member of the Ohio Pharmacists Association (OPA), the American Pharmaceutical Association (APhA), and the American Society of Health-System Pharmacists (ASHP).

Charles F. Lacy, RPh, PharmD, FCSHP

Dr Lacy received his doctorate from the University of Southern California School of Pharmacy. With over 18 years of clinical experience at one of the nation's largest teaching hospitals, he has developed a reputation as an acknowledged expert in drug information and critical care drug therapy.

In his current capacity as Coordinator of Drug Information Services at Cedar-Sinai Health System in Los Angeles, Dr Lacy plays an active role in the education and training of the medical, pharmacy, and nursing staff. He coordinates the Drug Information Center, the Medical Center's Intern Pharmacist Clinical Training Program, the Department's Continuing Education Program for pharmacists; maintains the Medical Center formulary program; and is editor of the Medical Center's *Drug Formulary Handbook* and the drug information newsletter *Prescription*.

Presently, Dr Lacy holds teaching affiliations with the University of Southern California School of Pharmacy, the University of California at San Francisco School of Pharmacy, the University of the Pacific School of Pharmacy, and the University of Alberta at Edmonton, School of Pharmacy and Health Sciences. Additionally, Dr Lacy is the current Director of the Center for International Health Care Practitioners at Western University of Health Sciences, where he plays a leading role in the advanced training of postgraduate pharmacists from areas throughout the Pacific rim, including Japan, Hong Kong, New Zealand, and Korea.

Dr Lacy is an active member of numerous professional associations including the American Society of Health-System Pharmacists (ASHP), the California Society of Hospital Pharmacists (CSHP), the American Society of Consultant Pharmacists (ASCP), and the American College of Clinical Pharmacy (ACCP).

Morton P. Goldman, PharmD, BCPS

Dr Goldman received his bachelor's degree in pharmacy from the University of Pittsburgh, College of Pharmacy and his Doctor of Pharmacy degree from the University of Cincinnati, Division of Graduate Studies and Research. He completed his concurrent 2-year hospital pharmacy residency at the V.A. Medical Center in Cincinnati. Dr Goldman is presently the Assistant Director of Pharmacotherapy Services for the Department of Pharmacy at the Cleveland Clinic Foundation (CCF) after having spent over 3 years at CCF as an Infectious Disease pharmacist and 4 years as Clinical Manager. He holds faculty appointments from Case Western Reserve University, College of Medicine; The University of Toledo, College of Pharmacy; and The University of Cincinnati, College of Pharmacy. Dr Goldman is a board-certified Pharmacotherapy Specialist.

In his capacity as Assistant Director of Pharmacotherapy Services at CCF, Dr Goldman remains actively involved in patient care and clinical research with the Department of Infectious Disease, as well as the continuing education of the medical and pharmacy staff. He is an editor of CCF's *Guidelines for Antibiotic Use* and coordinates their annual Antimicrobial Review retreat. He is a member of the Pharmacy and Therapeutics Committee and many of its subcommittees. Dr Goldman has authored numerous journal articles and lectures locally and nationally on infectious diseases topics and current drug therapies. He is currently a reviewer for the *Annals of Pharmacotherapy* and the *Journal of the American Medical Association*, an editorial board member of the *Journal of Infectious Disease Pharmacotherapy*, and coauthor of the *Drug Information Handbook* and the *Drug Information Handbook for the Allied Health Professional* produced by Lexi-Comp, Inc. He also provides technical support to Lexi-Comp's Clinical Reference Library™ publications.

Dr Goldman is an active member of Cleveland's local clinical pharmacy society, the Ohio College of Clinical Pharmacy, the Society of Infectious Disease Pharmacists, the American College of Clinical Pharmacy, and the American Society of Health-System Pharmacists.

Lora L. Armstrong, RPh, BSPharm, BCPS

Lora L. Armstrong received her bachelor's degree in pharmacy from Ferris State University. She has been a Board Certified Pharmacotherapy Specialist (BCPS) since 1994.

During her 17 years of clinical experience at one of the nation's most prominent teaching institutions, Ms Armstrong developed a reputation as an acknowledged expert in drug information. Ms Armstrong served as the Director of Drug Information Services at the University of Chicago Hospitals. Her interests included the areas of critical care, hematology, oncology, infectious disease, and pharmacokinetics. Ms Armstrong also played an active role in the education and training of medical, pharmacy, and nursing staff. She coordinated the Drug Information Center, the medical center's Adverse Drug Reaction Monitoring Program, and the Continuing Education Program for pharmacists. Ms Armstrong maintained the hospital's strict formulary program and was editor of the University of Chicago Hospitals *Formulary of Accepted Drugs* and the drug information monthly newsletter *Topics in Drug Therapy*.

In her current position, Ms Armstrong serves as clinical pharmacist in Clinical Development and Information Resources at Caremark Rx, Inc, Prescription Services Division. Ms Armstrong is responsible for development and enhancement of clinical management programs, physician and staff education, and formulary management. She participates in the development and evaluation of clinical programs that include

Formulary Management, Concurrent Interventions, Retrospective Case Management, Physician Profiling, and Utilization Review Pharmacy Management. Ms Armstrong also provides support for Caremark Rx, Inc's National Pharmacy and Therapeutics Committee activities.

Ms Armstrong is an active member of the Academy of Managed Care Pharmacy (AMCP), the American Society of Health-System Pharmacists (ASHP), the American Pharmaceutical Association (APhA), the American College of Clinical Pharmacy (ACCP), and the Society of Critical Care Medicine (SCCM). Ms Armstrong also serves on the Editorial Advisory Board of the Journal of the American Pharmaceutical Association.

EDITORIAL ADVISORY PANEL

EDITORIAL ADVISORY PANEL

PREFACE

Working with clinical pharmacists, hospital pharmacy and therapeutics committees, and hospital drug information centers, the editors of this handbook have directly assisted in the development and production of hospital-specific formulary documentation for several hundred major medical institutions in the United States and Canada. The resultant documentation provides pertinent detail concerning use of medications within the hospital and other clinical settings. The most current information on medications has been extracted, reviewed, coalesced, and cross-referenced by the editors to create this *Quick Look Drug Book*.

Thus, this handbook gives the user quick access to data on 1570 medications with cross referencing to 4749 U.S. and Canadian brand or trade names. Selection of the included medications was based on the analysis of those medications offered in a wide range of hospital formularies. The concise standardized format for data used in this handbook was developed to ensure a consistent presentation of information for all medications.

All generic drug names and synonyms appear in lower case, whereas brand or trade names appear in upper/lower case with the proper trademark information. These three items appear as individual entries in the alphabetical listing of drugs and, thus, there is no requirement for an alphabetical index of drugs.

Two new features for this edition of the *Quick Look Drug Book* are the inclusion of Canadian drug names and a listing of Pharmaceutical Manufacturers and Drug Distributors with their mailing and WEB site addresses.

The Indication/Therapeutic Category Index is an expedient mechanism for locating the medication of choice along with its classification. This index will help the user, with knowledge of the disease state, to identify medications which are most commonly used in treatment. All disease states are cross-referenced to a varying number of medications with the most frequently used medication(s) noted.

— L.L. Lance

ACKNOWLEDGMENTS

The *Quick Look Drug Book* exists in its present form as the result of the concerted efforts of the following individuals: Robert D. Kerscher, publisher and president of Lexi-Comp, Inc; Lynn D. Coppinger, managing editor; Barbara F. Kerscher, production manager; David C. Marcus, director of information systems; and Julian I. Graubart, American Pharmaceutical Association (APhA), Director of Books and Electronic Products.

Other members of the Lexi-Comp staff whose contributions deserve special mention include Jeanne E. Wilson, production/systems liaison; Ginger S. Conner, Leslie J. Ruggles, and Kathleen E. Schleicher, reference publishing project managers; Stacey L. Hurd, Julie A. Katzen, Jennifer L. Rocky, and Linda L. Taylor, custom project managers; Alexandra J. Hart, composition specialist; Kathy Smith, production assistant; Tracey J. Reinecke, graphic designer; Liz Tomsik, PharmD, pharmacotherapy specialist; Cynthia A. Bell, CPhT, imaging product manager; Edmund A. Harbart, vice-president, custom publishing division; Jack L. Stones, vice-president, reference publishing division; Jay L. Katzen, director of marketing and business development; Jerry M. Reeves, Marc L. Long, and Patrick T. Grubb, regional sales managers; Brad F. Bolinski, Kristin M. Thompson, Matthew C. Kerscher, Tina L. Collins, and Kelene A. Gluntz, sales and marketing representatives; Paul A. Rhine and Jason M. Buchwald, academic account managers; Kenneth J. Hughes, manager of authoring systems; Sean M. Conrad, James M. Stacey, and Matthew J. Houser, system analysts; Thury L. O'Connor, vice-president of technology; David J. Wasserbauer, vice-president, finance and administration; Elizabeth M. Conlon, Rebecca A. Dryhurst, and Leslie G. Rodia, accounting; Marta Pacur, receptionist; and Frederick C. Kerscher, inventory and fulfillment manager.

USE OF THE HANDBOOK

The *Quick Look Drug Book* is organized into a drug information section, an appendix, and an indication/therapeutic category index.

The drug information section of the handbook, wherein all drugs are listed alphabetically, details information pertinent to each drug. Extensive cross referencing is provided by brand name and synonyms.

Drug information is presented in a consistent format and for quick reference will provide the following:

Generic Name	U.S. Adopted Name (USAN) or International Nonproprietary Name (INN) If a drug product is only available in Canada, a ***(Canada only)*** will be attached to that product and will appear with every occurrence of that drug throughout the book
Pronunciation Guide	
Synonyms	
U.S./Canadian Brand Names	Common trade names used in the United States and Canada (Can)
Therapeutic Category	
Controlled Substance	Drug Enforcement Agency (DEA) classification for federally scheduled controlled substances
Use	Information pertaining to appropriate use of the drug
Usual Dosage	The amount of the drug to be typically given or taken during therapy
Dosage Forms	Information with regard to form, strength and availability of the drug

Appendix

The appendix offers a compilation of tables, guidelines, and conversion information that can often be helpful when considering patient care.

Indication/Therapeutic Category Index

This index provides a listing of accepted drugs for various disease states thus focusing attention on selection of medications most frequently prescribed in relation to a clinical diagnosis. Diseases may have other nonofficial drugs for their treatment and this indication/therapeutic category index should not be used by itself to determine the appropriateness of a particular therapy. The listed indications may encompass varying degrees of severity and, since certain medications may not be appropriate for a given degree of severity, it should not be assumed that the agents listed for specific indications are interchangeable. Also included as a valuable reference is each medication's therapeutic category.

SAFE WRITING

Health professionals and their support personnel frequently produce handwritten copies of information they see in print; therefore, such information is subjected to even greater possibilities for error or misinterpretation on the part of others. Thus, particular care must be given to how drug names and strengths are expressed when creating written health care documents.

The following are a few examples of safe writing rules suggested by the Institute for Safe Medication Practices, Inc.*

1. There should be a space between a number and its units as it is easier to read. There should be no periods after the abbreviations mg or mL.

Correct	**Incorrect**
10 mg	10mg
100 mg	100mg

2. Never place a decimal and a zero after a whole number (2 mg is correct and 2.0 mg is incorrect). If the decimal point is not seen because it falls on a line or because individuals are working from copies where the decimal point is not seen, this causes a tenfold overdose.
3. Just the opposite is true for numbers less than one. Always place a zero before a naked decimal (0.5 mL is correct, .5 mL is **in**correct).
4. Never abbreviate the word "unit." The handwritten U or u, looks like a 0 (zero), and may cause a tenfold overdose error to be made.
5. IU is not a safe abbreviation for international units. The handwritten IU looks like IV. Write out international units or use int. units.
6. Q.D. is not a safe abbreviation for once daily, as when the Q is followed by a sloppy dot, it looks like QID which means four times daily.
7. O.D. is not a safe abbreviation for once daily, as it is properly interpreted as meaning "right eye" and has caused liquid medications such as saturated solution of potassium iodide and lugol's solution to be administered incorrectly. There is no safe abbreviation for once daily. It must be written out in full.
8. Do not use chemical names such as 6-mercaptopurine or 6-thioguanine, as 6 fold overdoses have been given when these were not recognized as chemical names. The proper names of these drugs are mercaptopurine or thioguanine.
9. Do not abbreviate drug names (5FC, 6MP, 5-ASA, MTX, HCTZ CPZ, PBZ, etc) as they are misinterpreted and cause error.
10. Do not use the apothecary system or symbols.
11. Do not abbreviate microgram as µg; instead use mcg as there is less likelihood of misinterpretation.

---

*From "Safe Writing" by Davis NM, PharmD and Cohen MR, MS, Lecturers and Consultants for Safe Medication Practices, 1143 Wright Drive, Huntingdon Valley, PA 19006. Phone: (215) 947-7566.

12. When writing an outpatient prescription, write a complete prescription. A complete prescription can prevent the prescriber, the pharmacist, and/or the patient from making a mistake and can eliminate the need for further clarification. The legible prescriptions should contain:

    a. patient's full name

    b. for pediatric or geriatric patients: their age (or weight where applicable)

    c. drug name, dosage form and strength; if a drug is new or rarely prescribed, print this information

    d. number or amount to be dispensed

    e. complete instructions for the patient, including the purpose of the medication

    f. when there are recognized contraindications for a prescribed drug, indicate to the pharmacist that you are aware of this fact (ie, when prescribing a potassium salt for a patient receiving an ACE inhibitor, write "K serum leveling being monitored")

ALPHABETICAL LISTING OF DRUGS

A-200™ Shampoo [OTC] *see* pyrethrins *on page 489*

A and D™ Ointment [OTC] *see* vitamin A and vitamin D *on page 603*

abacavir (a BAK a veer)

U.S./Canadian Brand Names Ziagen™

Therapeutic Category Nucleoside Analog Reverse Transcriptase Inhibitor

Use Treatment of HIV infections in combination with other antiretroviral agents

Usual Dosage Oral:

Children: 3 months to 16 years: 8 mg/kg body weight twice daily (maximum: 300 mg twice daily) in combination with other antiretroviral agents

Adults: 300 mg twice daily in combination with other antiretroviral agents

Dosage Forms Tablet: 300 mg

Abbokinase® *see* urokinase *on page 592*

ABCD *see* amphotericin B cholesteryl sulfate complex *on page 33*

abciximab (ab SIK si mab)

Synonyms c7E3

U.S./Canadian Brand Names ReoPro®

Therapeutic Category Platelet Aggregation Inhibitor

Use Adjunct to percutaneous transluminal coronary angioplasty or atherectomy (PTCA) for the prevention of acute cardiac ischemic complications; prevent cardiac ischemic complications in a wider range of percutaneous coronary interventions (PCIs), including balloon angioplasty and stent placement, and without qualification of high risk for abrupt vessel closure; unstable angina that does not respond to conventional therapy when PCI is planned with 24 hours

Usual Dosage I.V.: 0.25 mg/kg bolus followed by an infusion of 10 mcg/minute for 12 hours

Dosage Forms Injection: 2 mg/mL (5 mL)

Abelcet™ *see* amphotericin B (lipid complex) *on page 34*

Abenol® (Can) *see* acetaminophen *on next page*

Abitrate® (Can) *see* clofibrate *on page 138*

ABLC *see* amphotericin B (lipid complex) *on page 34*

absorbable cotton *see* cellulose, oxidized *on page 110*

absorbable gelatin sponge *see* gelatin, absorbable *on page 258*

Absorbine® Antifungal [OTC] *see* tolnaftate *on page 571*

Absorbine® Antifungal Foot Powder [OTC] *see* miconazole *on page 373*

Absorbine® Jock Itch [OTC] *see* tolnaftate *on page 571*

Absorbine Jr.® Antifungal [OTC] *see* tolnaftate *on page 571*

acarbose (AY car bose)

U.S./Canadian Brand Names Precose®

Therapeutic Category Antidiabetic Agent, Oral

Use Treatment of noninsulin-dependent diabetes mellitus (NIDDM); as monotherapy or in combination with a sulfonylurea when diet plus acarbose or a sulfonylurea does not result in adequate glycemic control; also used with insulin or metformin in patients with noninsulin-dependent diabetes mellitus (NIDDM)

Usual Dosage Adults: Oral: Dosage must be individualized on the basis of effectiveness and tolerance while not exceeding the maximum recommended dose of 100 mg 3 times/day

Initial dose: 25 mg 3 times/day with the first bite of each main meal

Maintenance dose: Should be adjusted at 4- to 8-week intervals based on 1-hour postprandial glucose levels and tolerance. Dosage may be increased from 25 mg 3 times/

day to 50 mg 3 times/day; some patients may benefit from increasing the dose to 100 mg 3 times/day; maintenance dose ranges: 50-100 mg 3 times/day.

Maximum dose:

≤60 kg: 50 mg 3 times/day

>60 kg: 100 mg 3 times/day

Dosage Forms Tablet: 50 mg, 100 mg

Accolate® *see* zafirlukast *on page 609*

Accupril® *see* quinapril *on page 492*

Accuretic® (Can) *see* quinapril and hydrochlorothiazide *(Canada only)* *on page 492*

Accutane® *see* isotretinoin *on page 316*

acebutolol (a se BYOO toe lole)

U.S./Canadian Brand Names Monitan® (Can); Rhotral® (Can); Sectral®

Therapeutic Category Antiarrhythmic Agent, Class II; Beta-Adrenergic Blocker

Use Treatment of hypertension; ventricular arrhythmias; angina

Usual Dosage Adults: Oral: 400-800 mg/day in 2 divided doses

Dosage Forms Capsule, as hydrochloride: 200 mg, 400 mg

Acel-Imune® *see* diphtheria, tetanus toxoids, and acellular pertussis vaccine *on page 187*

Aceon® *see* perindopril erbumine *on page 440*

Acephen® [OTC] *see* acetaminophen *on this page*

Aceta® [OTC] *see* acetaminophen *on this page*

acetaminophen (a seet a MIN oh fen)

Synonyms APAP; n-acetyl-p-aminophenol; paracetamol

U.S./Canadian Brand Names Abenol® (Can); Acephen® [OTC]; Aceta® [OTC]; AF® (Can); Apacet® [OTC]; Atasol® (Can); Dapa® [OTC]; Dapacin® [OTC]; Dorcol® [OTC]; Feverall™ [OTC]; Genapap® [OTC]; Genebs® [OTC]; Liquiprin® [OTC]; Mapap® [OTC]; Maranox® [OTC]; Meda-Cap® [OTC]; Meda® Tab [OTC]; Myapap® [OTC]; Neopap® [OTC]; Panadol® [OTC]; Pediatrix® (Can); Redutemp® [OTC]; Ridenol® [OTC]; Silapap® [OTC]; Snaplets-FR® Granules [OTC]; Tantaphen® (Can); Tapanol® [OTC]; Tempra® [OTC]; Tylenol® [OTC]; Ty-Pap [OTC]; Uni-Ace® [OTC]

Therapeutic Category Analgesic, Non-narcotic; Antipyretic

Use Treatment of mild to moderate pain and fever; does not have antirheumatic or systemic anti-inflammatory effects

Usual Dosage Oral, rectal (if fever not controlled with acetaminophen alone, administer with full doses of aspirin on an every 4- to 6-hour schedule, if aspirin is not otherwise contraindicated):

Children <12 years: 10-15 mg/kg/dose every 4-6 hours as needed; do **not** exceed 5 doses (2.6 g) in 24 hours

Adults: 325-650 mg every 4-6 hours or 1000 mg 3-4 times/day; do **not** exceed 4 g/day

Dosage Forms

Caplet: 160 mg, 325 mg, 500 mg

Extended: 650 mg

Capsule: 80 mg

Drops: 48 mg/mL (15 mL); 60 mg/0.6 mL (15 mL); 80 mg/0.8 mL (15 mL); 100 mg/mL (15 mL, 30 mL)

Elixir: 80 mg/5 mL, 120 mg/5 mL, 160 mg/5 mL, 167 mg/5 mL, 325 mg/5 mL

Liquid, oral: 160 mg/5 mL, 500 mg/15 mL

Solution: 100 mg/mL (15 mL); 120 mg/2.5 mL

Suppository, rectal: 80 mg, 120 mg, 125 mg, 300 mg, 325 mg, 650 mg

Suspension, oral: 160 mg/5 mL

Oral drops: 80 mg/0.8 mL

Tablet: 325 mg, 500 mg, 650 mg

(Continued)

acetaminophen *(Continued)*

Chewable: 80 mg, 160 mg

acetaminophen and butalbital compound *see* butalbital compound and acetaminophen *on page 85*

acetaminophen and codeine (a seet a MIN oh fen & KOE deen)

Synonyms codeine and acetaminophen

U.S./Canadian Brand Names Atasol® 8, 15, 30 W/ Caffeine (Can); Capital® and Codeine; Empracet®-30, -60 (Can); Emtec-30® (Can); Lenoltec® No.1, 2, 3, 4 (Can); Novo-Gesic-C8® (Can); Novo-Gesic-C15® (Can); Novo-Gesic-C30® (Can); Tylenol® With Codeine

Therapeutic Category Analgesic, Narcotic

Controlled Substance C-III; C-V

Use Relief of mild to moderate pain

Usual Dosage Doses should be adjusted according to severity of pain and response of the patient. Adult doses ≥60 mg codeine fail to give commensurate relief of pain but merely prolong analgesia and are associated with an appreciably increased incidence of side effects. Oral:

Children:
- Analgesic: 0.5-1 mg codeine/kg/dose every 4-6 hours
- Acetaminophen: 10-15 mg/kg/dose every 4 hours up to a maximum of 2.6 g/24 hours for children <12 years
  - 3-6 years: 5 mL 3-4 times/day as needed of elixir
  - 7-12 years: 10 mL 3-4 times/day as needed of elixir
  - >12 years: 15 mL every 4 hours as needed of elixir

Adults:
- Antitussive: Based on codeine (15-30 mg/dose) every 4-6 hours
- Analgesic: Based on codeine (30-60 mg/dose) every 4-6 hours
  - 1-2 tablets every 4 hours to a maximum of 12 tablets/24 hours

Dosage Forms

Capsule:
- #2: Acetaminophen 325 mg and codeine phosphate 15 mg (C-III)
- #3: Acetaminophen 325 mg and codeine phosphate 30 mg (C-III)
- #4: Acetaminophen 325 mg and codeine phosphate 60 mg (C-III)

Elixir: Acetaminophen 120 mg and codeine phosphate 12 mg per 5 mL with alcohol 7% (C-V)

Suspension, oral, alcohol free: Acetaminophen 120 mg and codeine phosphate 12 mg per 5 mL (C-V)

Tablet: Acetaminophen 500 mg and codeine phosphate 30 mg (C-III); acetaminophen 650 mg and codeine phosphate 30 mg (C-III)

Tablet:
- #1: Acetaminophen 300 mg and codeine phosphate 7.5 mg (C-III)
- #2: Acetaminophen 300 mg and codeine phosphate 15 mg (C-III)
- #3: Acetaminophen 300 mg and codeine phosphate 30 mg (C-III)
- #4: Acetaminophen 300 mg and codeine phosphate 60 mg (C-III)

acetaminophen and dextromethorphan

(a seet a MIN oh fen & dex troe meth OR fan)

U.S./Canadian Brand Names Bayer® Select® Chest Cold Caplets [OTC]; Drixoral® Cough & Sore Throat Liquid Caps [OTC]

Therapeutic Category Antitussive/Analgesic

Use Treatment of mild to moderate pain; symptomatic relief of coughs caused by minor viral upper respiratory tract infections or inhaled irritants; most effective for a chronic nonproductive cough

Usual Dosage Oral:

Children: 10-15 mg/kg/dose every 4-6 hours as needed; do **not** exceed 5 doses in 24 hours

Adults: 325-650 mg every 4-6 hours or 1000 mg 3-4 times/day; do **not** exceed 4 g/day

Dosage Forms

Caplet: Acetaminophen 500 and dextromethorphan hydrobromide 15 mg

Capsule: Acetaminophen 325 and dextromethorphan hydrobromide 15 mg

acetaminophen and diphenhydramine

(a seet a MIN oh fen & dye fen HYE dra meen)

U.S./Canadian Brand Names Excedrin® P.M. [OTC]; Midol® PM [OTC]

Therapeutic Category Analgesic, Non-narcotic

Use Relief of mild to moderate pain or sinus headache

Usual Dosage Oral:

Children <12 years: Not recommended

Adults: 2 caplets or 5 mL of liquid at bedtime or as directed by physician; do not exceed recommended dosage

Dosage Forms

Caplet:

Excedrin® P.M.: Acetaminophen 500 mg and diphenhydramine citrate 30 mg

Midol® PM: Acetaminophen 500 mg and diphenhydramine 25 mg

Liquid (wild berry flavor) (Excedrin® P.M.): Acetaminophen 1000 mg and diphenhydramine hydrochloride 50 mg per 30 mL (180 mL)

acetaminophen and hydrocodone *see* hydrocodone and acetaminophen *on page 287*

acetaminophen and oxycodone *see* oxycodone and acetaminophen *on page 422*

acetaminophen and phenyltoloxamine

(a seet a MIN oh fen & fen il to LOKS a meen)

U.S./Canadian Brand Names Percogesic® [OTC]

Therapeutic Category Analgesic, Non-narcotic

Use Relief of mild to moderate pain

Usual Dosage Adults: Oral: 1-2 tablets every 4 hours

Dosage Forms Tablet: Acetaminophen 325 mg and phenyltoloxamine citrate 30 mg

acetaminophen and propoxyphene *see* propoxyphene and acetaminophen *on page 482*

acetaminophen and pseudoephedrine

(a seet a MIN oh fen & soo doe e FED rin)

Synonyms pseudoephedrine and acetaminophen

U.S./Canadian Brand Names Allerest® No Drowsiness [OTC]; Bayer® Select® Head Cold Caplets [OTC]; Coldrine® [OTC]; Dristan® Cold Caplets [OTC]; Dynafed®, Maximum Strength [OTC]; Ornex® No Drowsiness [OTC]; Sinarest®, No Drowsiness [OTC]; Sine-Aid®, Maximum Strength [OTC]; Sine-Off® Maximum Strength No Drowsiness Formula [OTC]; Sinus Excedrin® Extra Strength [OTC]; Sinus-Relief® [OTC]; Sinutab® Without Drowsiness [OTC]; Tylenol® Sinus, Maximum Strength [OTC]

Therapeutic Category Decongestant/Analgesic

Use Symptomatic relief of congestion, fever, and aches/pain of colds/flu

Usual Dosage Adults: Oral: 2 tablets every 4-6 hours

Dosage Forms Tablet:

Allerest® No Drowsiness; Coldrine®, Tylenol® Sinus, Maximum Strength; Ornex® No Drowsiness, Sinus-Relief®: Acetaminophen 325 mg and pseudoephedrine hydrochloride 30 mg

Bayer® Select Head Cold; Dristan® Cold; Dynafed®, Maximum Strength; Sinarest®, No Drowsiness; Sine-Aid®, Maximum Strength; Sine-Off® Maximum Strength No Drowsiness Formula; Sinus Excedrin® Extra Strength; Sinutab® Without Drowsiness; Tylenol® Sinus, Maximum Strength: Acetaminophen 500 mg and pseudoephedrine hydrochloride 30 mg

acetaminophen, aspirin, and caffeine

(a seet a MIN oh fen, AS pir in, & KAF een)

U.S./Canadian Brand Names Excedrin®, Extra Strength [OTC]; Gelpirin® [OTC]; Goody's® Headache Powders

Therapeutic Category Analgesic, Non-narcotic

Use Relief of mild to moderate pain or fever

Usual Dosage Adults: Oral: 1-2 tablets or powders every 2-6 hours as needed for pain

Dosage Forms

Geltab: Acetaminophen 250 mg, aspirin 250 mg, and caffeine 65 mg

Powder: Acetaminophen 250 mg, aspirin 520 mg, and caffeine 32.5 mg per dose

Tablet: Acetaminophen 125 mg, aspirin 240 mg, and caffeine 32 mg; acetaminophen 250 mg, aspirin 250 mg, and caffeine 65 mg

acetaminophen, caffeine, hydrocodone, chlorpheniramine, and phenylephrine *see* hydrocodone, chlorpheniramine, phenylephrine, acetaminophen, and caffeine *on page 290*

acetaminophen, chlorpheniramine, and pseudoephedrine

(a seet a MIN oh fen, klor fen IR a meen, & soo doe e FED rin)

U.S./Canadian Brand Names Alka-Seltzer® Plus Cold Liqui-Gels® [OTC]; Aspirin-Free Bayer® Select® Allergy Sinus Caplets [OTC]; Co-Hist® [OTC]; Sinutab® Tablets [OTC]

Therapeutic Category Antihistamine/Decongestant/Analgesic

Use Temporary relief of sinus symptoms

Usual Dosage Adults: Oral: 2 caplets/capsules/tablets every 6 hours

Dosage Forms

Caplet: Acetaminophen 500 mg, chlorpheniramine maleate 2 mg, and pseudoephedrine hydrochloride 30 mg

Capsule: Acetaminophen 250 mg, chlorpheniramine maleate 2 mg, and pseudoephedrine hydrochloride 30 mg

Tablet: Acetaminophen 325 mg, chlorpheniramine maleate 2 mg, and pseudoephedrine hydrochloride 30 mg

acetaminophen, dextromethorphan, and pseudoephedrine

(a seet a MIN oh fen, deks troe meth OR fan, & soo doe e FED rin)

Synonyms dextromethorphan, acetaminophen, and pseudoephedrine; pseudoephedrine, acetaminophen, and dextromethorphan; pseudoephedrine, dextromethorphan, and acetaminophen

U.S./Canadian Brand Names Alka-Seltzer® Plus Flu & Body Aches Non-Drowsy Liqui-Gels® [OTC]; Comtrex® Maximum Strength Non-Drowsy [OTC]; Sudafed® Severe Cold [OTC]; Theraflu® Non-Drowsy Formula Maximum Strength [OTC]; Tylenol® Cold No Drowsiness [OTC]; Tylenol® Flu Maximum Strength [OTC]

Therapeutic Category Cold Preparation

Use Symptomatic relief of congestion, fever, cough, and aches/pain of colds/flu

Usual Dosage Adults: Oral: 2 tablets every 6 hours

Dosage Forms Tablet:

Alka-Seltzer® Plus Flu & Body Aches Non-Drowsy: Acetaminophen 500 mg, dextromethorphan hydrobromide 10 mg, and pseudoephedrine hydrochloride 30 mg

Comtrex® Maximum Strength Non-Drowsy; Sudafed® Severe Cold; Theraflu® Non-Drowsy Formula Maximum Strength; Tylenol® Flu Maximum Strength: Acetaminophen 500 mg, dextromethorphan hydrobromide 15 mg, and pseudoephedrine hydrochloride 30 mg

Tylenol® Cold No Drowsiness: Acetaminophen 325 mg, dextromethorphan hydrobromide 15 mg, and pseudoephedrine hydrochloride 30 mg

acetaminophen, isometheptene, and dichloralphenazone

(a seet a MIN oh fen, eye soe me THEP teen, & dye KLOR al FEN a zone)

U.S./Canadian Brand Names Isocom®; Isopap®; Midchlor®; Midrin®; Migratine®

Therapeutic Category Analgesic, Non-narcotic

Use Relief of migraine and tension headache

Usual Dosage Adults: Oral: 2 capsules at first sign of headache, followed by 1 capsule every 60 minutes until relieved, up to 5 capsules in a 12-hour period

Dosage Forms Capsule: Acetaminophen 325 mg, isometheptene mucate 65 mg, dichloralphenazone 100 mg

Acetasol® HC Otic *see* acetic acid, propylene glycol diacetate, and hydrocortisone *on next page*

Acetazolam® (Can) *see* acetazolamide *on this page*

acetazolamide (a set a ZOLE a mide)

U.S./Canadian Brand Names Acetazolam® (Can); Apo®-Acetazolamide (Can); Diamox®; Diamox Sequels®; Novo-Zolamide® (Can)

Therapeutic Category Anticonvulsant; Carbonic Anhydrase Inhibitor

Use Reduce elevated intraocular pressure in glaucoma, a diuretic, an adjunct to the treatment of refractory seizures and acute altitude sickness; centrencephalic epilepsies

Usual Dosage

Children:

Glaucoma:

Oral: 8-30 mg/kg/day divided every 6-8 hours

I.M., I.V.: 20-40 mg/kg/day divided every 6 hours

Edema: Oral, I.M., I.V.: 5 mg/kg or 150 mg/m^2 once every day or every other day

Epilepsy: Oral: 8-30 mg/kg/day in 2-4 divided doses, not to exceed 1 g/day

Adults:

Glaucoma:

Oral: 250 mg 1-4 times/day or 500 mg sustained release capsule twice daily

I.M., I.V.: 250-500 mg, may repeat in 2-4 hours

Edema: Oral, I.M., I.V.: 250-375 mg once daily

Epilepsy: Oral: 8-30 mg/kg/day in 1-4 divided doses

Altitude sickness: Oral: 250 mg every 8-12 hours

Dosage Forms

Capsule, sustained release: 500 mg

Injection: 500 mg

Tablet: 125 mg, 250 mg

acetic acid (a SEE tik AS id)

Synonyms ethanoic acid

U.S./Canadian Brand Names Aci-jel® Vaginal; VōSol® Otic

Therapeutic Category Antibacterial, Otic; Antibacterial, Topical

Use Continuous or intermittent irrigation of the bladder; treatment of superficial bacterial infections of the external auditory canal and vagina

Usual Dosage

Irrigation: For continuous irrigation of the urinary bladder with 0.25% acetic acid irrigation, the rate of administration will approximate the rate of urine flow; usually 500-1500 mL/24 hours; for periodic irrigation of an indwelling urinary catheter to maintain patency, approximately 50 mL of 0.25% acetic acid irrigation is required. (Note: Dosage of an irrigating solution depends on the capacity or surface area of the structure being irrigated.)

Otic: Insert saturated wick, keep moist 24 hours; remove wick and instill 5 drops 3-4 times/day

Vaginal: One applicatorful morning and evening

Dosage Forms

Jelly, vaginal (Aci-jel®): 0.921% with oxyquinolone sulfate 0.025%, ricinoleic acid 0.7%, and glycerin 5% (85 g)

Solution:

Irrigation: 0.25% (1000 mL)

Otic (VōSol®): Acetic acid 2% in propylene glycol (15 mL, 30 mL, 60 mL)

acetic acid and aluminum acetate otic *see* aluminum acetate and acetic acid *on page 21*

acetic acid, propylene glycol diacetate, and hydrocortisone

(a SEE tik AS id, PRO pa leen GLY kole dye AS e tate, & hye droe KOR ti sone)

U.S./Canadian Brand Names Acetasol® HC Otic; VōSol® HC Otic

Therapeutic Category Antibiotic/Corticosteroid, Otic

Use Treatment of superficial infections of the external auditory canal caused by organisms susceptible to the action of the antimicrobial, complicated by inflammation

Usual Dosage Adults: Otic: Instill 4 drops in ear(s) 3-4 times/day

Dosage Forms Solution, otic: Acetic acid 2%, propylene glycol diacetate 3%, and hydrocortisone 1% (10 mL)

acetohexamide (a set oh HEKS a mide)

U.S./Canadian Brand Names Dymelor®

Therapeutic Category Antidiabetic Agent, Oral

Use Adjunct to diet for the management of mild to moderately severe, stable, noninsulin-dependent (type II) diabetes mellitus

Usual Dosage Adults: Oral: 250 mg to 1.5 g/day in 1-2 divided doses

Dosage Forms Tablet: 250 mg, 500 mg

acetohydroxamic acid (a SEE toe hye droks am ik AS id)

Synonyms AHA

U.S./Canadian Brand Names Lithostat®

Therapeutic Category Urinary Tract Product

Use Adjunctive therapy in chronic urea-splitting urinary infection

Usual Dosage Oral:

Children: Initial: 10 mg/kg/day

Adults: 250 mg 3-4 times/day for a total daily dose of 10-15 mg/kg/day

Dosage Forms Tablet: 250 mg

acetophenazine (a set oh FEN a zeen)

Therapeutic Category Phenothiazine Derivative

Use Management of manifestations of psychotic disorders

Usual Dosage Adults: Oral: 20 mg 3 times/day up to 40-80 mg/day

Hospitalized schizophrenic patients may require doses as high as 400-600 mg/day

Dosage Forms Tablet, as maleate: 20 mg

Acetoxyl® (Can) *see* benzoyl peroxide *on page 68*

acetoxymethylprogesterone *see* medroxyprogesterone acetate *on page 352*

acetylcholine (a se teel KOE leen)

U.S./Canadian Brand Names Miochol-E®

Therapeutic Category Cholinergic Agent

Use Produces complete miosis in cataract surgery, keratoplasty, iridectomy and other anterior segment surgery where rapid miosis is required

Usual Dosage Adults: Intraocular: 0.5-2 mL of 1% injection (5-20 mg) instilled into anterior chamber before or after securing one or more sutures

Dosage Forms Powder, intraocular, as chloride: 1:100 [10 mg/mL] (2 mL, 15 mL)

acetylcysteine (a se teel SIS teen)

Synonyms mercapturic acid; NAC; *N*-acetylcysteine; *N*-acetyl-L-cysteine

U.S./Canadian Brand Names Mucomyst®; Mucosil™; Parvolex® (Can)

Therapeutic Category Mucolytic Agent

Use Adjunctive therapy in patients with abnormal or viscid mucous secretions in broncho-pulmonary diseases, pulmonary complications of surgery, and cystic fibrosis; diagnostic bronchial studies; antidote for acute acetaminophen toxicity; enema to treat bowel obstruction due to meconium ileus or its equivalent

Usual Dosage

Acetaminophen poisoning: Children and Adults: Oral: 140 mg/kg; followed by 17 doses of 70 mg/kg every 4 hours; repeat dose if emesis occurs within 1 hour of administration; therapy should continue until all doses are administered even though the acetaminophen plasma level has dropped below the toxic range

Inhalation: Acetylcysteine 10% and 20% solution (Mucomyst®) (dilute 20% solution with sodium chloride or sterile water for inhalation); 10% solution may be used undiluted

Infants: 1-2 mL of 20% solution or 2-4 mL 10% solution until nebulized administered 3-4 times/day

Children: 3-5 mL of 20% solution or 6-10 mL of 10% solution until nebulized administered 3-4 times/day

Adolescents: 5-10 mL of 10% to 20% solution until nebulized administered 3-4 times/day

Note: Patients should receive an aerosolized bronchodilator 10-15 minutes prior to acetylcysteine

Meconium ileus equivalent: Children and Adults: 100-300 mL of 4% to 10% solution by irrigation or orally

Dosage Forms Solution, as sodium: 10% [100 mg/mL] (4 mL, 10 mL, 30 mL); 20% [200 mg/mL] (4 mL, 10 mL, 30 mL, 100 mL)

acetylsalicylic acid *see* aspirin *on page 49*

Aches-N-Pain® [OTC] *see* ibuprofen *on page 300*

Achromycin® Ophthalmic *see* tetracycline *on page 555*

Achromycin® Parenteral *(Discontinued)* *see page 700*

Achromycin® Topical *see* tetracycline *on page 555*

Achromycin® V Capsule *(Discontinued)* *see page 700*

Achromycin® V Oral Suspension *(Discontinued)* *see page 700*

aciclovir *see* acyclovir *on page 11*

Aci-jel® Vaginal *see* acetic acid *on page 7*

Acilac (Can) *see* lactulose *on page 325*

Aciphex™ *see* rabeprazole *on page 494*

acitretin (a si TRE tin)

U.S./Canadian Brand Names Soriatane™

Therapeutic Category Retinoid-like Compound

Use Treatment of severe psoriasis (includes erythrodermic and pustular types) and other disorders of keratinization

Usual Dosage Adults: Oral: Individualization of dosage is required to achieve maximum therapeutic response while minimizing side effects

Initial: Therapy should be initiated at 25 mg/day, given as a single dose with the main meal; if by 4 weeks the response is unsatisfactory, and in the absence of toxicity, the daily dose may be gradually increased to a maximum of 75 mg/day; the dose may be reduced if necessary to minimize side effects

Maintenance: Doses of 25 to 50 mg/day may be given after initial response to treatment; the maintenance dose should be based on clinical efficacy and tolerability; it may be necessary in some cases to increase the dose to a maximum of 75 mg/day

Dosage Forms Capsule: 10 mg, 25 mg

Aclovate® Topical *see* alclometasone *on page 16*

Acnex® (Can) *see* salicylic acid *on page 513*

Acnomel® B.P.5 (Can) *see* benzoyl peroxide *on page 68*

Acnomel® (Can) *see* salicylic acid *on page 513*

acrivastine and pseudoephedrine (AK ri vas teen & soo doe e FED rin)

Synonyms pseudoephedrine and acrivastine

U.S./Canadian Brand Names Semprex®-D

Therapeutic Category Antihistamine/Decongestant Combination

Use Temporary relief of nasal congestion, decongest sinus openings, running nose, itching of nose or throat, and itchy, watery eyes due to hay fever or other upper respiratory allergies

Usual Dosage Adults: 1 capsule 3-4 times/day

Dosage Forms Capsule: Acrivastine 8 mg and pseudoephedrine hydrochloride 60 mg

ACT *see* dactinomycin *on page 157*

ACT® [OTC] *see* fluoride *on page 244*

Actagen-C® *see* triprolidine, pseudoephedrine, and codeine *on page 585*

Actagen® Syrup [OTC] *see* triprolidine and pseudoephedrine *on page 584*

Actagen® Tablet [OTC] *see* triprolidine and pseudoephedrine *on page 584*

ACTH *see* corticotropin *on page 148*

ACTH-40® ***(Discontinued)*** *see page 700*

Acthar® *see* corticotropin *on page 148*

Acti-B_{12}® (Can) *see* hydroxocobalamin *on page 294*

Acticin® Cream *see* permethrin *on page 440*

Acticort® Topical *see* hydrocortisone (topical) *on page 292*

Actidil® ***(Discontinued)*** *see page 700*

Actidose-Aqua® [OTC] *see* charcoal *on page 114*

Actidose® With Sorbitol [OTC] *see* charcoal *on page 114*

Actifed® Allergy Tablet (Day) [OTC] *see* pseudoephedrine *on page 486*

Actifed® Allergy Tablet (Night) [OTC] *see* diphenhydramine and pseudoephedrine *on page 185*

Actifed® Syrup ***(Discontinued)*** *see page 700*

Actifed® With Codeine ***(Discontinued)*** *see page 700*

Actigall™ *see* ursodiol *on page 593*

Actimmune® *see* interferon gamma-1b *on page 310*

Actinex® Topical *see* masoprocol *on page 348*

actinomycin D *see* dactinomycin *on page 157*

Actiprofen® (Can) *see* ibuprofen *on page 300*

Actiq® Oral Transmucosal *see* fentanyl *on page 235*

Activase® *see* alteplase *on page 21*

activated carbon *see* charcoal *on page 114*

activated dimethicone *see* simethicone *on page 522*

activated ergosterol *see* ergocalciferol *on page 212*

activated methylpolysiloxane *see* simethicone *on page 522*

Activelle™ *see* estradiol and norethindrone *on page 218*

Actonel® *see* risedronate *on page 507*

Actos™ *see* pioglitazone *on page 453*

Actron® [OTC] *see* ketoprofen *on page 321*

ACU-dyne® [OTC] *see* povidone-iodine *on page 467*

Acular® Ophthalmic *see* ketorolac tromethamine *on page 321*

Acutrim® 16 Hours [OTC] *see* phenylpropanolamine *on page 447*

Acutrim® II, Maximum Strength [OTC] *see* phenylpropanolamine *on page 447*

Acutrim® Late Day [OTC] *see* phenylpropanolamine *on page 447*

ACV *see* acyclovir *on this page*

acycloguanosine *see* acyclovir *on this page*

acyclovir (ay SYE kloe veer)

Synonyms aciclovir; ACV; acycloguanosine

U.S./Canadian Brand Names Avirax™ (Can); Zovirax®

Therapeutic Category Antiviral Agent

Use Treatment of initial and prophylaxis of recurrent mucosal and cutaneous herpes simplex (HSV-1 and HSV-2) infections; herpes simplex encephalitis; herpes zoster infections; varicella-zoster infections in healthy, nonpregnant persons >13 years of age, children >12 months of age who have a chronic skin or lung disorder or are receiving long-term aspirin therapy, and immunocompromised patients

Usual Dosage

Children and Adults: I.V.:

- Mucocutaneous HSV infection: 750 mg/m^2/day divided every 8 hours or 15 mg/kg/day divided every 8 hours for 5-10 days
- HSV encephalitis: 1500 mg/m^2/day divided every 8 hours or 30 mg/kg/day divided every 8 hours for 10 days
- Varicella-zoster virus infection: 1500 mg/m^2/day divided every 8 hours or 30 mg/kg/day divided every 8 hours for 5-10 days

Adults:

- Oral: Initial: 200 mg every 4 hours while awake (5 times/day); prophylaxis: 200 mg 3-4 times/day or 400 mg twice daily. Prophylaxis of varicella or herpes zoster in HIV positive patients: 400 mg 5 times/day
- Topical: ½" ribbon of ointment every 3 hours (6 times/day)

Herpes zoster in immunocompromised patients:

- Children: Oral: 250-600 mg/m^2/dose 4-5 times/day
- Adults: Oral: 800 mg every 4 hours (5 times/day) for 7-10 days
- Children and Adults: I.V.: 7.5 mg/kg/dose every 8 hours

Varicella-zoster infections: Oral:

- Children: 10-20 mg/kg/dose (up to 800 mg) 4 times/day
- Adults: 600-800 mg/dose 5 times/day for 7-10 days or 1000 mg every 6 hours for 5 days

Prophylaxis of bone marrow transplant recipients: Children and Adults: I.V.:

- Autologous patients who are HSV seropositive: 150 mg/m^2/dose every 12 hours; with clinical symptoms of herpes simplex: 150 mg/m^2/dose every 8 hours
- Autologous patients who are CMV seropositive: 500 mg/m^2/dose every 8 hours; for clinically symptomatic CMV infection, ganciclovir should be used in place of acyclovir

Dosage Forms

Capsule: 200 mg

Ointment, topical: 5% [50 mg/g] (3 g, 15 g)

Powder for Injection: 500 mg (10 mL); 1000 mg (20 mL)

Suspension, oral (banana flavor): 200 mg/5 mL

Tablet: 400 mg, 800 mg

Adagen™ *see* pegademase (bovine) *on page 432*

Adalat® *see* nifedipine *on page 402*

Adalat® CC *see* nifedipine *on page 402*

Adalat PA® (Can) *see* nifedipine *on page 402*

adamantanamine *see* amantadine *on page 24*

adapalene (a DAP a leen)

U.S./Canadian Brand Names Differin®

Therapeutic Category Acne Products

Use Topical treatment of acne vulgaris

(Continued)

adapalene *(Continued)*

Usual Dosage Adults: Topical: Apply once daily, before retiring, in a thin film to affected areas after washing; not recommended in children

Dosage Forms Gel, topical (alcohol free): 0.1% (15 g, 45 g)

Adapin® Oral *see* doxepin *on page 195*

Adderall® *see* dextroamphetamine and amphetamine *on page 171*

Adeflor® *see* vitamin, multiple (pediatric) *on page 606*

adefovir (a DEF o veer)

U.S./Canadian Brand Names Preveon®

Therapeutic Category Reverse Transcriptase Inhibitor

Use Treatment of HIV infections in combination with at least two other antiretroviral agents; also has some activity against hepatitis B virus and herpes viruses

Usual Dosage Oral:

HIV: 125 mg once daily

Hepatitis B: 125 mg once daily

ADEKs® Pediatric Drops *see* vitamin, multiple (pediatric) *on page 606*

adenine arabinoside *see* vidarabine *on page 600*

Adenocard® *see* adenosine *on this page*

adenosine (a DEN oh seen)

Synonyms 9-beta-D-ribofuranosyladenine

U.S./Canadian Brand Names Adenocard®

Therapeutic Category Antiarrhythmic Agent, Miscellaneous

Use Treatment of paroxysmal supraventricular tachycardia (PSVT)

Usual Dosage

Children: Initial: Rapid I.V.: 0.05 mg/kg; if not effective within 2 minutes, increase dose in 0.05 mg/kg increments every 2 minutes to a maximum dose of 0.25 mg/kg or until termination of PSVT; median dose required: 0.15 mg/kg; do not exceed adult doses

Adults: Rapid I.V. push: 6 mg, if the dose is not effective within 1-2 minutes, a rapid I.V. dose of 12 mg may be administered; may repeat 12 mg bolus if needed

Dosage Forms Injection, preservative free: 3 mg/mL (2 mL)

Adipex-P® ***(Discontinued)*** *see page 700*

Adipost® ***(Discontinued)*** *see page 700*

Adlone® Injection *see* methylprednisolone *on page 368*

Adphen® ***(Discontinued)*** *see page 700*

ADR *see* doxorubicin *on page 196*

Adrenalin® Chloride *see* epinephrine *on page 209*

adrenaline *see* epinephrine *on page 209*

adrenocorticotropic hormone *see* corticotropin *on page 148*

Adriamycin PFS™ *see* doxorubicin *on page 196*

Adriamycin RDF® *see* doxorubicin *on page 196*

Adrin® ***(Discontinued)*** *see page 700*

Adrucil® Injection *see* fluorouracil *on page 246*

Adsorbocarpine® Ophthalmic *see* pilocarpine *on page 451*

Adsorbonac® Ophthalmic [OTC] *see* sodium chloride *on page 526*

Adsorbotear® Ophthalmic Solution [OTC] *see* artificial tears *on page 47*

Advanced Formula Oxy® Sensitive Gel [OTC] *see* benzoyl peroxide *on page 68*

Advil® [OTC] *see* ibuprofen *on page 300*

Advil® Cold & Sinus Caplets [OTC] *see* pseudoephedrine and ibuprofen *on page 487*

Aeroaid® [OTC] *see* thimerosal *on page 561*

AeroBid®-M Oral Aerosol Inhaler *see* flunisolide *on page 243*

AeroBid® Oral Aerosol Inhaler *see* flunisolide *on page 243*

Aerodine® [OTC] *see* povidone-iodine *on page 467*

Aerolate III® *see* theophylline *on page 557*

Aerolate JR® *see* theophylline *on page 557*

Aerolate® Oral Solution *(Discontinued)* *see page 700*

Aerolate SR® *see* theophylline *on page 557*

Aeroseb-Dex® *see* dexamethasone (topical) *on page 168*

Aeroseb-HC® Topical *see* hydrocortisone (topical) *on page 292*

Aerosporin® Injection *(Discontinued)* *see page 700*

AeroZoin® [OTC] *see* benzoin *on page 68*

AF® (Can) *see* acetaminophen *on page 3*

Afrin® Children's Nose Drops [OTC] *see* oxymetazoline *on page 423*

Afrin® Nasal Solution [OTC] *see* oxymetazoline *on page 423*

Afrinol® [OTC] *see* pseudoephedrine *on page 486*

Afrin® Saline Mist [OTC] *see* sodium chloride *on page 526*

Aftate® [OTC] *see* tolnaftate *on page 571*

Agenerase™ *see* amprenavir *on page 35*

Aggrastat® *see* tirofiban *on page 568*

$AgNO_3$ *see* silver nitrate *on page 521*

Agoral® Plain *(Discontinued)* *see page 700*

Agrylin™ *see* anagrelide *on page 36*

AHA *see* acetohydroxamic acid *on page 8*

AHF *see* antihemophilic factor (human) *on page 39*

A-hydroCort® Injection *see* hydrocortisone (systemic) *on page 291*

Airet® *see* albuterol *on page 15*

Akarpine® Ophthalmic *see* pilocarpine *on page 451*

AKBeta® Ophthalmic *see* levobunolol *on page 330*

AK-Chlor® Ophthalmic *see* chloramphenicol *on page 116*

AK-Cide® Ophthalmic *see* sulfacetamide and prednisolone *on page 540*

AK-Con® Ophthalmic *see* naphazoline *on page 390*

AK-Dex® Ophthalmic *see* dexamethasone (ophthalmic) *on page 167*

AK-Dilate® Ophthalmic Solution *see* phenylephrine *on page 445*

AK-Fluor Injection *see* fluorescein sodium *on page 244*

AK-Homatropine® Ophthalmic *see* homatropine *on page 282*

Akineton® *see* biperiden *on page 74*

AK-Mycin® *see* erythromycin (systemic) *on page 215*

AK-NaCl® [OTC] *see* sodium chloride *on page 526*

AK-Nefrin® Ophthalmic Solution *see* phenylephrine *on page 445*

Akne-Mycin® Topical *see* erythromycin (ophthalmic/topical) *on page 214*

AK-Neo-Dex® Ophthalmic *see* neomycin and dexamethasone *on page 395*

Agestin

Aggrenox 200 • 25 mg

Akoline® C.B. Tablet *(Discontinued)* *see page 700*

AK-Pentolate® *see* cyclopentolate *on page 153*

AK-Poly-Bac® Ophthalmic *see* bacitracin and polymyxin B *on page 58*

AK-Pred® Ophthalmic *see* prednisolone (ophthalmic) *on page 471*

AK-Spore® H.C. Ophthalmic Ointment *see* bacitracin, neomycin, polymyxin B, and hydrocortisone *on page 59*

AK-Spore® H.C. Ophthalmic Suspension *see* neomycin, polymyxin B, and hydrocortisone *on page 396*

AK-Spore® H.C. Otic *see* neomycin, polymyxin B, and hydrocortisone *on page 396*

AK-Spore® Ophthalmic Ointment *see* bacitracin, neomycin, and polymyxin B *on page 59*

AK-Spore® Ophthalmic Solution *see* neomycin, polymyxin B, and gramicidin *on page 396*

AK-Sulf® *see* sulfacetamide *on page 540*

AK-Taine® *see* proparacaine *on page 481*

AKTob® Ophthalmic *see* tobramycin *on page 569*

AK-Tracin® Ophthalmic *see* bacitracin *on page 58*

AK-Trol® *see* neomycin, polymyxin B, and dexamethasone *on page 396*

Akwa Tears® Solution [OTC] *see* artificial tears *on page 47*

AK-Zol® Tablet *(Discontinued)* *see page 700*

Ala-Cort® Topical *see* hydrocortisone (topical) *on page 292*

Ala-Scalp® Topical *see* hydrocortisone (topical) *on page 292*

Ala-Tet® *(Discontinued)* *see page 700*

alatrofloxacin *see* trovafloxacin *on page 587*

Alazide® *see* hydrochlorothiazide and spironolactone *on page 286*

Albalon-A® Ophthalmic *see* naphazoline and antazoline *on page 391*

Albalon® Liquifilm® Ophthalmic *see* naphazoline *on page 390*

albendazole (al BEN da zole)

U.S./Canadian Brand Names Albenza®

Therapeutic Category Anthelmintic

Use Treatment of parenchymal neurocysticercosis and cystic hydatid disease of the liver, lung, and peritoneum; albendazole may also be useful in the treatment of ascariasis, trichuriasis, enterobiasis, hook worm, strongyloidiasis, giardiasis, and microsporidiosis in AIDS

Usual Dosage Oral:

Children ≤2 years:

Neurocysticercosis: 15 mg/kg for 8 days; repeat as necessary

Hookworm, pinworm, roundworm: 200 mg as a single dose; may be repeated in 3 weeks

Strongyloidiasis and tapeworm: 200 mg/day for 3 days; may repeat in 3 weeks

Children >2 years and Adults:

Hydatid cyst: 400 mg twice daily with meals for 3 cycles (each cycle consists of 28 days of dosing followed by a 14-day albendazole-free interval)

Neurocysticercosis: 400 mg twice daily for 8-30 days

Roundworm, pinworm, hookworm: 400 mg as a single dose; treatment may be repeated in 3 weeks

Giardiasis: Strongyloidiasis and tapeworm: 400 mg/day for 3 days; treatment may be repeated in 3 weeks (giardiasis is a single course)

Dosage Forms Tablet: 200 mg

Albenza® *see* albendazole *on this page*

Albert® Docusate (Can) *see* docusate *on page 191*

Albert® Glyburide (Can) *see* glyburide *on page 263*

albumin (al BYOO min)

Synonyms albumin (human)

U.S./Canadian Brand Names Albuminar®; Albumisol®; Albunex®; Albutein®; Buminate®; Plasbumin®

Therapeutic Category Blood Product Derivative

Use Treatment of hypovolemia; plasma volume expansion and maintenance of cardiac output in the treatment of certain types of shock or impending shock; hypoproteinemia resulting in generalized edema or decreased intravascular volume (eg, hypoproteinemia associated with acute nephrotic syndrome, premature infants)

Usual Dosage 5% should be used in hypovolemic patients; 25% should be used in patients in whom fluid and sodium intake must be minimized

Children:
- Emergency initial dose: 25 g
- Nonemergencies: 25% to 50% of the adult dose

Adults: Dosage depends on the condition of patient, usual adult dose is 25 g; no more than 250 g should be administered within 48 hours
- Hypoproteinemia: I.V.: 0.5-1 g/kg/dose; repeat every 1-2 days as calculated to replace ongoing losses
- Hypovolemia: I.V.: 0.5-1 g/kg/dose; repeat as needed; maximum dose: 6 g/kg/day

Dosage Forms Injection, as human: 5% [50 mg/mL] (50 mL, 250 mL, 500 mL, 1000 mL); 25% [250 mg/mL] (10 mL, 20 mL, 50 mL, 100 mL)

Albuminar® *see* albumin *on this page*

albumin (human) *see* albumin *on this page*

Albumisol® *see* albumin *on this page*

Albunex® *see* albumin *on this page*

Albutein® *see* albumin *on this page*

albuterol (al BYOO ter ole)

Synonyms salbutamol

U.S./Canadian Brand Names Airet®; Apo®-Salvent (Can); Novo-Salmol® (Can); Proventil®; Proventil® HFA; Sabulin® (Can); Ventolin®; Ventolin® Rotocaps®; Volmax® (Can)

Therapeutic Category Adrenergic Agonist Agent

Use Bronchodilator in reversible airway obstruction due to asthma or COPD

Usual Dosage

Oral:
- 2-6 years: 0.1-0.2 mg/kg/dose 3 times/day; maximum dose not to exceed 12 mg/day (divided doses)
- 6-12 years: 2 mg/dose 3-4 times/day; maximum dose not to exceed 24 mg/day (divided doses)
- >12 years: 2-4 mg/dose 3-4 times/day; maximum dose not to exceed 32 mg/day (divided doses)

Inhalation:
- MDI: 90 mcg/spray:
  - <12 years: 1-2 inhalations 4 times/day using a tube spacer
  - ≥12 years: 1-2 inhalations every 4-6 hours
  - Exercise-induced bronchospasm: 2 inhalations 15 minutes before exercising
- Nebulization: 2.5 mg = 0.5 mL of the 0.5% inhalation solution to be diluted in 1-2.5 mL of NS
  - <5 years: 1.25-2.5 mg every 4-6 hours as needed
  - >5 years: 2.5-5 mg every 4-6 hours

Dosage Forms

Aerosol: 90 mcg/dose (17 g) [200 doses]

(Continued)

albuterol *(Continued)*

Proventil®, Ventolin®: 90 mcg/dose (17 g) [200 doses]
Chlorofluorocarbon free (Proventil® HFA): 90 mcg/dose (17 g)
Capsule for oral inhalation (Ventolin® Rotocaps®): 200 mcg [to be used with Rotahaler® inhalation device]
Solution, inhalation: 0.083% (3 mL); 0.5% (20 mL)
Airet®: 0.083%
Proventil®: 0.083% (3 mL); 0.5% (20 mL)
Ventolin®: 0.5% (20 mL)
Syrup, as sulfate: 2 mg/5 mL (480 mL)
Proventil®, Ventolin®: 2 mg/5 mL (480 mL)
Tablet, as sulfate: 2 mg, 4 mg
Proventil®, Ventolin®: 2 mg, 4 mg
Tablet, extended release:
Proventil® Repetabs®: 4 mg
Volmax®: 4 mg, 8 mg

Alcaine® *see* proparacaine *on page 481*

alclometasone (al kloe MET a sone)

U.S./Canadian Brand Names Aclovate® Topical
Therapeutic Category Corticosteroid, Topical
Use Inflammation of corticosteroid-responsive dermatosis
Usual Dosage Topical: Apply a thin film to the affected area 2-3 times/day
Dosage Forms Alclometasone dipropionate:
Cream: 0.05% (15 g, 45 g, 60 g)
Ointment, topical: 0.05% (15 g, 45 g, 60 g)

alcohol, ethyl (AL koe hol, ETH il)

Synonyms ethanol
U.S./Canadian Brand Names Lavacol® [OTC]
Therapeutic Category Intravenous Nutritional Therapy; Pharmaceutical Aid
Use Topical anti-infective; pharmaceutical aid; an antidote for ethylene glycol overdose; an antidote for methanol overdose
Usual Dosage
I.V.: Doses of 100-125 mg/kg/hour to maintain blood levels of 100 mg/dL are recommended after a loading dose of 0.6 g/kg; maximum dose: 400 mL of a 5% solution within 1 hour
Topical: Use as needed
Dosage Forms
Injection, absolute: 2 mL
Liquid, topical, denatured: 70% (473 mL)
Solution, inhalation: 20%, 40%

Alconefrin® Nasal Solution [OTC] *see* phenylephrine *on page 445*

Aldactazide® *see* hydrochlorothiazide and spironolactone *on page 286*

Aldactone® *see* spironolactone *on page 534*

Aldara™ *see* imiquimod *on page 303*

aldesleukin (al des LOO kin)

Synonyms interleukin-2
U.S./Canadian Brand Names Proleukin®
Therapeutic Category Biological Response Modulator
Use Primarily investigated in tumors known to have a response to immunotherapy, such as melanoma and renal cell carcinoma; has been used in conjunction with LAK cells, TIL cells, IL-1, and interferon

Usual Dosage All orders should be written in million International units (million int. units) (refer to individual protocols)

Adults: Metastatic renal cell carcinoma:

Treatment consists of two 5-day treatment cycles separated by a rest period. 600,000 int. units/kg (0.037 mg/kg)/dose administered every 8 hours by a 15-minute I.V. infusion for a total of 14 doses; following 9 days of rest, the schedule is repeated for another 14 doses, for a maximum of 28 doses per course.

Investigational regimen: I.V. continuous infusion: 4.5 million int. units/m^2/day in 250-1000 mL of D_5W for 5 days

Dose modification: Hold or interrupt a dose rather than reducing dose; refer to protocol

Retreatment: Patients should be evaluated for response ~4 weeks after completion of a course of therapy and again immediately prior to the scheduled start of the next treatment course. Additional courses of treatment may be administered to patients only if there is some tumor shrinkage following the last course and retreatment is not contraindicated. Each treatment course should be separated by a rest period of at least 7 weeks from the date of hospital discharge. Tumors have continued to regress up to 12 months following the initiation of therapy.

Dosage Forms Powder for injection, lyophilized: 22 x 10^6 int. units [18 million int. units/mL = 1.1 mg/mL when reconstituted]

Aldoclor® *see* chlorothiazide and methyldopa *on page 119*

Aldomet® *see* methyldopa *on page 367*

Aldoril® *see* methyldopa and hydrochlorothiazide *on page 367*

alendronate (a LEN droe nate)

U.S./Canadian Brand Names Fosamax®

Therapeutic Category Bisphosphonate Derivative

Use Symptomatic treatment of Paget's disease and heterotopic ossification due to spinal cord injury or after total hip replacement, hypercalcemia associated with malignancy

Usual Dosage Oral:

Adults: Patients with osteoporosis or Paget's disease should receive supplemental calcium and vitamin D if dietary intake is inadequate

Osteoporosis in postmenopausal women: 10 mg once daily. Safety of treatment for >4 years has not been studied (extension studies are ongoing).

Paget's disease of bone: 40 mg once daily for 6 months

Retreatment: Relapses during the 12 months following therapy occurred in 9% of patients who responded to treatment. Specific retreatment data are not available. Retreatment with alendronate may be considered, following a 6-month post-treatment evaluation period, in patients who have relapsed based on increases in serum alkaline phosphatase, which should be measured periodically. Retreatment may also be considered in those who failed to normalize their serum alkaline phosphatase.

Elderly: No dosage adjustment is necessary

Dosage Forms Tablet, as sodium: 5 mg, 10 mg, 40 mg

Alesse™ *see* ethinyl estradiol and levonorgestrel *on page 223*

Aleve® [OTC] *see* naproxen *on page 391*

Alfenta® *see* alfentanil *on this page*

alfentanil (al FEN ta nil)

U.S./Canadian Brand Names Alfenta®

Therapeutic Category Analgesic, Narcotic; General Anesthetic

Controlled Substance C-II

Use Analgesia; analgesia adjunct; anesthetic agent

Usual Dosage Doses should be titrated to appropriate effects; wide range of doses is dependent upon desired degree of analgesia/anesthesia

Children <12 years: Dose not established

(Continued)

alfentanil *(Continued)*

Adults: Anesthesia of ≤30 minutes: Initial (induction): 8-20 mcg/kg, then 3-5 mcg/kg/dose or 0.5-1 mcg/kg/minute for maintenance; total dose: 8-40 mcg/kg; higher doses used for longer anesthesia required procedures

Dosage Forms Injection, preservative free, as hydrochloride: 500 mcg/mL (2 mL, 5 mL, 10 mL, 20 mL)

Alferon® N *see* interferon alfa-n3 *on page 309*

alglucerase (al GLOO ser ase)

Synonyms glucocerebrosidase

U.S./Canadian Brand Names Ceredase®

Therapeutic Category Enzyme

Use Long-term enzyme replacement in patients with confirmed Type I Gaucher's disease who exhibit one or more of the following conditions: Moderate to severe anemia; thrombocytopenia and bleeding tendencies; bone disease; hepatomegaly or splenomegaly

Usual Dosage I.V. infusion: Administer 20-60 units/kg with a frequency ranging from 3 times/week to once every 2 weeks

Dosage Forms Injection: 10 units/mL (5 mL); 80 units/mL (5 mL)

alitretinoin (a li TRET i noyn)

U.S./Canadian Brand Names Panretin™

Therapeutic Category Antineoplastic Agent, Miscellaneous; Retinoic Acid Derivative

Use Topical treatment of cutaneous lesions in AIDS-related Kaposi's sarcoma; not indicated when systemic therapy for Kaposi's sarcoma is indicated

Usual Dosage Topical: Apply gel twice daily to cutaneous Kaposi's sarcoma lesions

Dosage Forms Gel: 0.1% (60 g)

Alkaban-AQ® *see* vinblastine *on page 600*

Alka-Mints® [OTC] *see* calcium carbonate *on page 89*

Alka-Seltzer® Plus Cold Liqui-Gels® [OTC] *see* acetaminophen, chlorpheniramine, and pseudoephedrine *on page 6*

Alka-Seltzer® Plus Flu & Body Aches Non-Drowsy Liqui-Gels® [OTC] *see* acetaminophen, dextromethorphan, and pseudoephedrine *on page 6*

Alkeran® *see* melphalan *on page 354*

Allbee® With C [OTC] *see* vitamin B complex with vitamin C *on page 603*

Allegra® *see* fexofenadine *on page 239*

Allegra-D™ *see* fexofenadine and pseudoephedrine *on page 239*

Aller-Chlor® Oral [OTC] *see* chlorpheniramine *on page 120*

Allercon® Tablet [OTC] *see* triprolidine and pseudoephedrine *on page 584*

Allerdryl® (Can) *see* diphenhydramine *on page 185*

Allerest® 12 Hour Capsule [OTC] *see* chlorpheniramine and phenylpropanolamine *on page 122*

Allerest® 12 Hour Nasal Solution [OTC] *see* oxymetazoline *on page 423*

Allerest® Eye Drops [OTC] *see* naphazoline *on page 390*

Allerest® Maximum Strength [OTC] *see* chlorpheniramine and pseudoephedrine *on page 122*

Allerest® No Drowsiness [OTC] *see* acetaminophen and pseudoephedrine *on page 5*

Allerfrin® Syrup [OTC] *see* triprolidine and pseudoephedrine *on page 584*

Allerfrin® Tablet [OTC] *see* triprolidine and pseudoephedrine *on page 584*

Allerfrin® w/Codeine *see* triprolidine, pseudoephedrine, and codeine *on page 585*

Allergan® Ear Drops *see* antipyrine and benzocaine *on page 41*

AllerMax® Oral [OTC] *see* diphenhydramine *on page 185*

Allernix® (Can) *see* diphenhydramine *on page 185*

Allerphed® Syrup [OTC] *see* triprolidine and pseudoephedrine *on page 584*

allopurinol (al oh PURE i nole)

U.S./Canadian Brand Names Apo®-Allopurinol (Can); Novo-purol® (Can); Purinol® (Can); Zyloprim®

Therapeutic Category Xanthine Oxidase Inhibitor

Use Prevention of attacks of gouty arthritis and nephropathy; also used to treat secondary hyperuricemia which may occur during treatment of tumors or leukemia; prevent recurrent calcium oxalate calculi

Usual Dosage Oral:

Children: 10 mg/kg/day in 2-3 divided doses or 200-300 mg/m^2/day in 2-4 divided doses, maximum: 600 mg/24 hours

Alternative:

<6 years: 150 mg/day in 3 divided doses

6-10 years: 300 mg/day in 2-3 divided doses

Children >10 years and Adults: Daily doses >300 mg should be administered in divided doses

Myeloproliferative neoplastic disorders: 600-800 mg/day in 2-3 divided doses for prevention of acute uric acid nephropathy for 2-3 days starting 1-2 days before chemotherapy

Gout: 200-300 mg/day (mild); 400-600 mg/day (severe)

Maximum dose: 800 mg/day

Dosage Forms Tablet: 100 mg, 300 mg

all-*trans*-retinoic acid *see* tretinoin (oral) *on page 575*

Alomide® Ophthalmic *see* lodoxamide tromethamine *on page 338*

Alor® 5/500 *see* hydrocodone and aspirin *on page 288*

Alora® Transdermal *see* estradiol *on page 217*

alpha$_1$-PI *see* alpha$_1$-proteinase inhibitor *on this page*

alpha$_1$-proteinase inhibitor (al fa won PRO tee in ase in HI bi tor)

Synonyms alpha$_1$-PI

U.S./Canadian Brand Names Prolastin®

Therapeutic Category Antitrypsin Deficiency Agent

Use Congenital alpha$_1$-antitrypsin deficiency

Usual Dosage Adults: I.V.: 60 mg/kg once weekly

Dosage Forms Injection (human): 500 mg alpha$_1$-PI (20 mL diluent); 1000 mg alpha $_1$-PI (40 mL diluent)

Alpha-Baclofen® (Can) *see* baclofen *on page 59*

Alphagan® *see* brimonidine *on page 79*

Alphamul® [OTC] *see* castor oil *on page 103*

AlphaNine® SD *see* factor IX complex (human) *on page 230*

Alpha-Tamoxifen® (Can) *see* tamoxifen *on page 547*

Alphatrex® Topical *see* betamethasone (topical) *on page 72*

alprazolam (al PRAY zoe lam)

U.S./Canadian Brand Names Apo®-Alpraz (Can); Novo-Alprazol® (Can); Nu-Alprax® (Can); Xanax®

Therapeutic Category Benzodiazepine

Controlled Substance C-IV

(Continued)

alprazolam *(Continued)*

Use Treatment of anxiety; adjunct in the treatment of depression; management of panic attacks

Usual Dosage Oral:

Children <18 years: Dose not established

Adults: 0.25-0.5 mg 2-3 times/day, titrate dose upward; maximum: 4 mg/day (anxiety); 10 mg/day (panic attacks)

Dosage Forms Tablet: 0.25 mg, 0.5 mg, 1 mg, 2 mg

alprostadil (al PROS ta dill)

Synonyms PGE_1; prostaglandin E_1

U.S./Canadian Brand Names Caverject® Injection; Edex® Injection; Muse® Pellet; Prostin VR Pediatric® Injection

Therapeutic Category Prostaglandin

Use Temporary maintenance of patency of ductus arteriosus in neonates with ductal-dependent congenital cyanotic or acyanotic heart disease until surgery can be performed; these defects include cyanotic (eg, pulmonary atresia, pulmonary stenosis, tricuspid atresia, Fallot's tetralogy, transposition of the great vessels) and acyanotic (eg, interruption of aortic arch, coarctation of aorta, hypoplastic left ventricle) heart disease. Alprostadil has also been used investigationally for the treatment of pulmonary hypertension in infants and children with congenital heart defects with left-to-right shunts and primary graft nonfunction following liver transplant. Used in penile erectile dysfunction

Usual Dosage

Patent ductus arteriosus (Prostin VR Pediatric®):

I.V. continuous infusion into a large vein, or alternatively through an umbilical artery catheter placed at the ductal opening: 0.05-0.1 mcg/kg/minute with therapeutic response, rate is reduced to lowest effective dosage; with unsatisfactory response, rate is increased gradually; maintenance: 0.01-0.4 mcg/kg/minute

PGE_1 is usually given at an infusion rate of 0.1 mcg/kg/minute, but it is often possible to reduce the dosage to 1/2 or even 1/10 without losing the therapeutic effect. The mixing schedule is shown in the table.

Alprostadil

Add 1 Ampul (500 mcg) to:	Concentration (mcg/mL)	Infusion Rate	
		mL/min/kg Needed to Infuse 0.1 mcg/kg/min	mL/kg/24 h
250 mL	2	0.05	72
100 mL	5	0.02	28.8
50 mL	10	0.01	14.4
25 mL	20	0.005	7.2

Therapeutic response is indicated by increased pH in those with acidosis or by an increase in oxygenation (pO_2) usually evident within 30 minutes

Erectile dysfunction:

Caverject®:

Vasculogenic, psychogenic, or mixed etiology: Individualize dose by careful titration; usual dose: 2.5-60 mcg (doses >60 mcg are not recommended); initiate dosage titration at 2.5 mcg, increasing by 2.5 mcg to a dose of 5 mcg and then in increments of 5-10 mcg depending on the erectile response until the dose produces an erection suitable for intercourse, not lasting >1 hour; if there is absolutely no response to initial 2.5 mcg dose, the second dose may increased to 7.5 mcg, followed by increments of 5-10 mcg

Neurogenic etiology (eg, spinal cord injury): Initiate dosage titration at 1.25 mcg, increasing to a doses of 2.5 mcg and then 5 mcg; increase further in increments 5 mcg until the dose is reached that produces an erection suitable for intercourse, not lasting >1 hour

Note: Patient must stay in the physician's office until complete detumescence occurs; if there is no response, then the next higher dose may be given within 1 hour; if there is still no response, a 1-day interval before giving the next dose is recommended; increasing the dose or concentration in the treatment of impotence results in increasing pain and discomfort

Muse® Pellet: Intraurethral: Administer as needed to achieve an erection; duration of action: ~30-60 minutes; use only two systems per 24-hour period

Dosage Forms

Injection:

Caverject®: 5 mcg, 10 mcg, 20 mcg

Edex® Injection: 5 mcg, 10 mcg, 20 mcg, 40 mcg

Prostin VR Pediatric®: 500 mcg/mL (1 mL)

Pellet, urethral: 125 mcg, 250 mcg, 500 mcg, 1000 mcg

Alrex™ *see* loteprednol *on page 341*

AL-Rr® Oral [OTC] *see* chlorpheniramine *on page 120*

Altace™ *see* ramipril *on page 497*

alteplase (AL te plase)

Synonyms alteplase, recombinant; tissue plasminogen activator, recombinant; t-PA

U.S./Canadian Brand Names Activase®; Lysatec-rt-PA® (Can)

Therapeutic Category Thrombolytic Agent

Use Management of acute myocardial infarction for the lysis of thrombi in coronary arteries; management of acute massive pulmonary embolism (PE) in adults

Usual Dosage

Coronary artery thrombi: I.V.: Front loading dose: Total dose is 100 mg over 1.5 hours (for patients who weigh <65 kg, use 1.25 mg/kg/total dose). Add this dose to a 100 mL bag of 0.9% sodium chloride for a total volume of 200 mL. Infuse 15 mg (30 mL) over 1-2 minutes; infuse 50 mg (100 mL) over 30 minutes. Begin heparin 5000-10,000 unit bolus followed by continuous infusion of 1000 units/hour. Infuse 35 mg/hour (70 mL) for next 2 hours.

Acute pulmonary embolism: 100 mg over 2 hours

Dosage Forms Powder for injection, lyophilized (recombinant): 20 mg [11.6 million units] (20 mL); 50 mg [29 million units] (50 mL); 100 mg [58 million units] (100 mL)

alteplase, recombinant *see* alteplase *on this page*

ALternaGEL® [OTC] *see* aluminum hydroxide *on next page*

altretamine (al TRET a meen)

Synonyms hexamethylmelamine

U.S./Canadian Brand Names Hexalen®

Therapeutic Category Antineoplastic Agent

Use Palliative treatment of persistent or recurrent ovarian cancer

Usual Dosage Adults: Oral (refer to protocol): 4-12 mg/kg/day in 3-4 divided doses for 21-90 days

Alternatively: 240-320 mg/m²/day in 3-4 divided doses for 21 days, repeated every 6 weeks

Alternatively: 260 mg/m²/day for 14-21 days of a 28-day cycle in 4 divided doses

Dosage Forms Capsule: 50 mg

Alu-Cap® [OTC] *see* aluminum hydroxide *on next page*

Aludrox® [OTC] *see* aluminum hydroxide and magnesium hydroxide *on page 23*

aluminum acetate and acetic acid

(a LOO mi num AS e tate & a SEE tik AS id)

Synonyms acetic acid and aluminum acetate otic; Burow's otic

U.S./Canadian Brand Names Otic Domeboro®

(Continued)

aluminum acetate and acetic acid *(Continued)*

Therapeutic Category Otic Agent, Anti-infective

Use Treatment of superficial infections of the external auditory canal

Usual Dosage Otic: Instill 4-6 drops in ear(s) every 2-3 hours

Dosage Forms Solution, otic: Aluminum acetate 10% and acetic acid 2% (60 mL)

aluminum acetate and calcium acetate

(a LOO mi num SUL fate & KAL see um AS e tate)

U.S./Canadian Brand Names Bluboro® [OTC]; Boropak® [OTC]; Domeboro® Topical [OTC]; Pedi-Boro® [OTC]

Therapeutic Category Topical Skin Product

Use Astringent wet dressing for relief of inflammatory conditions of the skin and to reduce weeping that may occur in dermatitis

Usual Dosage Topical: Soak affected area in the solution 2-4 times/day for 15-30 minutes or apply wet dressing soaked in the solution 2-4 times/day for 30-minute treatment periods; rewet dressing with solution every few minutes to keep it moist

Dosage Forms

Powder, to make topical solution: 1 packet/pint of water [1:40 solution]

Tablet, effervescent: 1 tablet/pint [1:40 dilution]

aluminum carbonate (a LOO mi num KAR bun ate)

U.S./Canadian Brand Names Basaljel® [OTC]

Therapeutic Category Antacid

Use Hyperacidity; hyperphosphatemia

Usual Dosage Adults: Oral:

Antacid: 2 tablets/capsules or 10 mL of suspension every 2 hours, up to 12 times/day

Hyperphosphatemia: 2 tablets/capsules or 12 mL of suspension with meals

Dosage Forms

Capsule: Equivalent to 500 mg aluminum hydroxide

Suspension: Equivalent to 400 mg/5 mL aluminum hydroxide

Tablet: Equivalent to 500 mg aluminum hydroxide

aluminum chloride hexahydrate

(a LOO mi num KLOR ide heks a HYE drate)

U.S./Canadian Brand Names Drysol™

Therapeutic Category Topical Skin Product

Use Astringent in the management of hyperhidrosis

Usual Dosage Adults: Topical: Apply at bedtime

Dosage Forms Solution, topical: 20% in SD alcohol 40 (35 mL, 37.5 mL)

aluminum hydroxide (a LOO mi num hye DROKS ide)

U.S./Canadian Brand Names ALternaGEL® [OTC]; Alu-Cap® [OTC]; Alu-Tab® [OTC]; Amphojel® [OTC]; Dialume® [OTC]; Nephrox Suspension [OTC]

Therapeutic Category Antacid

Use Hyperacidity; hyperphosphatemia

Usual Dosage Oral:

Peptic ulcer disease:

Children: 5-15 mL/dose every 3-6 hours or 1 and 3 hours after meals and at bedtime

Adults: 15-45 mL every 3-6 hours or 1 and 3 hours after meals and at bedtime

Prophylaxis against gastrointestinal bleeding:

Infants: 2-5 mL/dose every 1-2 hours

Children: 5-15 mL/dose every 1-2 hours

Adults: 30-60 mL/dose every hour

Titrate to maintain the gastric pH >5

Hyperphosphatemia:

Children: 50 mg to 150 mg/kg/24 hours in divided doses every 4-6 hours, titrate dosage to maintain serum phosphorus within normal range

Adults: 500-1800 mg, 3-6 times/day, between meals and at bedtime
Antacid: Adults: 30 mL 1 and 3 hours postprandial and at bedtime

Dosage Forms
Capsule:
Alu-Cap®: 400 mg
Dialume®: 500 mg
Liquid: 600 mg/5 mL
ALternaGEL®: 600 mg/5 mL
Suspension, oral: 320 mg/5 mL; 450 mg/5 mL; 675 mg/5 mL
Amphojel®: 320 mg/5 mL
Tablet:
Amphojel®: 300 mg, 600 mg
Alu-Tab®: 500 mg

aluminum hydroxide and magnesium carbonate

(a LOO mi num hye DROKS ide & mag NEE zhum KAR bun nate)

U.S./Canadian Brand Names Gaviscon® Liquid [OTC]

Therapeutic Category Antacid

Use Temporary relief of symptoms associated with gastric acidity

Usual Dosage Adults: Oral: 15-30 mL 4 times/day after meals and at bedtime

Dosage Forms Liquid: Aluminum hydroxide 95 mg and magnesium carbonate 358 mg per 15 mL

aluminum hydroxide and magnesium hydroxide

(a LOO mi num hye DROKS ide & mag NEE zhum hye DROK side)

Synonyms magnesium hydroxide and aluminum hydroxide

U.S./Canadian Brand Names Aludrox® [OTC]; Maalox® [OTC]; Maalox® Therapeutic Concentrate [OTC]

Therapeutic Category Antacid

Use Antacid, hyperphosphatemia in renal failure

Usual Dosage Adults: Oral: 5-10 mL or 1-2 tablets 4-6 times/day, between meals and at bedtime; may be used every hour for severe symptoms

Dosage Forms
Suspension:
Aludrox®: Aluminum hydroxide 307 mg and magnesium hydroxide 103 mg per 5 mL
Maalox®: Aluminum hydroxide 225 mg and magnesium hydroxide 200 mg per 5 mL
High potency (Maalox® TC): Aluminum hydroxide 600 mg and magnesium hydroxide 300 mg per 5 mL
Tablet, chewable (Maalox®): Aluminum hydroxide 600 mg and magnesium hydroxide 300 mg

aluminum hydroxide and magnesium trisilicate

(a LOO mi num hye DROKS ide & mag NEE zhum trye SIL i kate)

U.S./Canadian Brand Names Gaviscon®-2 Tablet [OTC]; Gaviscon® Tablet [OTC]

Therapeutic Category Antacid

Use Temporary relief of hyperacidity

Usual Dosage Adults: Oral: Chew 2-4 tablets 4 times/day or as directed by physician

Dosage Forms Tablet, chewable:
Gaviscon®: Aluminum hydroxide 80 mg and magnesium trisilicate 20 mg
Gaviscon®-2: Aluminum hydroxide 160 mg and magnesium trisilicate 40 mg

aluminum hydroxide, magnesium hydroxide, and simethicone

(a LOO mi num hye DROKS ide, mag NEE zhum hye DROKS ide, & sye METH i kone)

U.S./Canadian Brand Names Di-Gel® [OTC]; Gas-Ban DS® [OTC]; Maalox® Plus [OTC]; Magalox Plus® [OTC]; Mylanta® [OTC]; Mylanta®-II [OTC]

Therapeutic Category Antacid; Antiflatulent

(Continued)

aluminum hydroxide, magnesium hydroxide, and simethicone *(Continued)*

Use Temporary relief of hyperacidity associated with gas; may also be used for indications associated with other antacids

Usual Dosage Adults: Oral: 15-30 mL or 2-4 tablets 4-6 times/day between meals and at bedtime; may be used every hour for severe symptoms

Dosage Forms

Liquid:

Mylanta®: Aluminum hydroxide 200 mg, magnesium hydroxide, 200 mg, and simethicone 20 mg per 5 mL

Maalox® Plus: Aluminum hydroxide 225 mg, magnesium hydroxide 200 mg, and simethicone 25 mg per 5 mL (30 mL, 180 mL)

Mylanta®-II: Aluminum hydroxide 400 mg, magnesium hydroxide 400 mg, and simethicone 40 mg per 5 mL (150 mL, 360 mL)

Tablet, chewable:

Magalox Plus®: Aluminum hydroxide 200 mg, magnesium hydroxide 200 mg, and simethicone 25 mg

Mylanta®: Aluminum hydroxide 200 mg, magnesium hydroxide 200 mg, and simethicone 20 mg

Gas-Ban DS®, Mylanta®-II: Aluminum hydroxide 400 mg, magnesium hydroxide 400 mg, and simethicone 40 mg

aluminum sucrose sulfate, basic *see* sucralfate *on page 538*

Alupent® *see* metaproterenol *on page 359*

Alu-Tab® [OTC] *see* aluminum hydroxide *on page 22*

amantadine (a MAN ta deen)

Synonyms adamantanamine

U.S./Canadian Brand Names Endantadine™ (Can); PMS-Amantadine (Can); Symadine®; Symmetrel® Syrup

Therapeutic Category Anti-Parkinson's Agent; Antiviral Agent

Use Prophylaxis and treatment of influenza A viral infection; symptomatic and adjunct treatment of parkinsonism

Usual Dosage Oral:

Children:

1-9 years: 4.4-8.8 mg/kg/day in 1-2 divided doses to a maximum of 150 mg/day

9-12 years: 100-200 mg/day in 1-2 divided doses

After first influenza A virus vaccine dose, amantadine prophylaxis may be administered for up to 6 weeks or until 2 weeks after the second dose of vaccine

Adults:

Parkinson's disease: 100 mg twice daily

Influenza A viral infection: 200 mg/day in 1-2 divided doses

Prophylaxis: Minimum 10-day course of therapy following exposure or continue for 2-3 weeks after influenza A virus vaccine is administered

Elderly patients should administer the drug in 2 daily doses rather than a single dose to avoid adverse neurologic reactions

Dosage Forms Amantadine hydrochloride:

Capsule: 100 mg

Syrup: 50 mg/5 mL (480 mL)

Amaphen® *see* butalbital compound and acetaminophen *on page 85*

Amaryl® *see* glimepiride *on page 261*

ambenonium (am be NOE nee um)

U.S./Canadian Brand Names Mytelase® Caplets®

Therapeutic Category Cholinergic Agent

Use Treatment of myasthenia gravis

Usual Dosage Adults: Oral: 5-25 mg 3-4 times/day
Dosage Forms Tablet, as chloride: 10 mg

Ambenyl® Cough Syrup *see* bromodiphenhydramine and codeine *on page 80*

Ambi 10® [OTC] *see* benzoyl peroxide *on page 68*

Ambien™ *see* zolpidem *on page 613*

Ambi® Skin Tone [OTC] *see* hydroquinone *on page 294*

AmBisome® *see* amphotericin B (liposomal) *on page 34*

amcinonide (am SIN oh nide)

U.S./Canadian Brand Names Cyclocort® Topical
Therapeutic Category Corticosteroid, Topical
Use Relief of the inflammatory and pruritic manifestations of corticosteroid-responsive dermatoses
Usual Dosage Adults: Topical: Apply in a thin film 2-3 times/day
Dosage Forms
Cream: 0.1% (15 g, 30 g, 60 g)
Lotion: 0.1% (20 mL, 60 mL)
Ointment, topical: 0.1% (15 g, 30 g, 60 g)

Amcort® Injection *see* triamcinolone (systemic) *on page 577*

Amen® Oral *see* medroxyprogesterone acetate *on page 352*

Amerge® *see* naratriptan *on page 392*

Americaine® [OTC] *see* benzocaine *on page 66*

A-methaPred® Injection *see* methylprednisolone *on page 368*

amethocaine *see* tetracaine *on page 555*

amethopterin *see* methotrexate *on page 364*

amfepramone *see* diethylpropion *on page 178*

Amgenal® Cough Syrup *see* bromodiphenhydramine and codeine *on page 80*

Amicar® *see* aminocaproic acid *on next page*

Amidate® *see* etomidate *on page 228*

amifostine (am i FOS teen)

Synonyms ethiofos; gammaphos
U.S./Canadian Brand Names Ethyol®
Therapeutic Category Antidote
Use Protection against cisplatin-induced nephrotoxicity in advanced ovarian cancer patients; it may also provide protection from cisplatin-induced peripheral neuropathy
Usual Dosage I.V.: 910 mg/m^2 beginning 30 minutes before starting chemotherapy; dose adjustment is recommended for subsequent doses if the previous dose was interrupted, and not able to be resumed; secondary to hypotension, the recommended dose for subsequent administration is 740 mg/m^2
Dosage Forms Injection: 500 mg

amikacin (am i KAY sin)

U.S./Canadian Brand Names Amikin®
Therapeutic Category Aminoglycoside (Antibiotic)
Use Treatment of documented gram-negative enteric infection resistant to gentamicin and tobramycin; documented infection of mycobacterial organisms susceptible to amikacin
Usual Dosage I.M., I.V.:
Infants and Children: 15-20 mg/kg/day divided every 8 hours
Adults: 15 mg/kg/day divided every 8-12 hours
Dosage Forms Injection, as sulfate: 50 mg/mL (2 mL, 4 mL); 250 mg/mL (2 mL, 4 mL)

Amikin® *see* amikacin *on previous page*

amiloride (a MIL oh ride)

U.S./Canadian Brand Names Midamor®

Therapeutic Category Diuretic, Potassium Sparing

Use Counteract potassium loss induced by other diuretics in the treatment of hypertension or edematous conditions including CHF, hepatic cirrhosis and hypoaldosteronism; usually used in conjunction with a more potent diuretic such as thiazides or loop diuretics

Usual Dosage Oral:

Children: Although safety and efficacy have not been established by the FDA in children, a dosage of 0.625 mg/kg/day has been used in children weighing 6-20 kg

Adults: 5-10 mg/day (up to 20 mg)

Dosage Forms Tablet, as hydrochloride: 5 mg

amiloride and hydrochlorothiazide

(a MIL oh ride & hye droe klor oh THYE a zide)

Synonyms hydrochlorothiazide and amiloride

U.S./Canadian Brand Names Moduretic®

Therapeutic Category Diuretic, Combination

Use Antikaliuretic diuretic, antihypertensive

Usual Dosage Adults: Oral: Start with 1 tablet/day, then may be increased to 2 tablets/day if needed; usually administered in a single dose

Dosage Forms Tablet: Amiloride hydrochloride 5 mg and hydrochlorothiazide 50 mg

Amin-Aid® ***(Discontinued)*** *see page 700*

2-amino-6-mercaptopurine *see* thioguanine *on page 561*

2-amino-6-trifluoromethoxy-benzothiazole *see* riluzole *on page 506*

aminobenzylpenicillin *see* ampicillin *on page 34*

aminocaproic acid (a mee noe ka PROE ik AS id)

U.S./Canadian Brand Names Amicar®

Therapeutic Category Hemostatic Agent

Use Treatment of excessive bleeding resulting from systemic hyperfibrinolysis and urinary fibrinolysis

Usual Dosage In the management of acute bleeding syndromes, oral dosage regimens are the same as the I.V. dosage regimens in adults and children

Chronic bleeding: Oral, I.V.: 5-30 g/day in divided doses at 3- to 6-hour intervals

Acute bleeding syndrome:

Children: Oral, I.V.: 100 mg/kg or 3 g/m^2 during the first hour, followed by continuous infusion at the rate of 33.3 mg/kg/hour or 1 g/m^2/hour; total dosage should not exceed 18 g/m^2/24 hours

Adults:

Oral: For elevated fibrinolytic activity, administer 5 g during first hour, followed by 1-1.25 g/hour for approximately 8 hours or until bleeding stops

I.V.: Administer 4-5 g in 250 mL of diluent during first hour followed by continuous infusion at the rate of 1-1.25 g/hour in 50 mL of diluent, continue for 8 hours or until bleeding stops

Dosage Forms

Injection: 250 mg/mL (20 mL, 96 mL, 100 mL)

Syrup: 1.25 g/5 mL (480 mL)

Tablet: 500 mg

Amino-Cerv™ Vaginal Cream *see* urea *on page 591*

aminoglutethimide (a mee noe gloo TETH i mide)

U.S./Canadian Brand Names Cytadren®

Therapeutic Category Antineoplastic Agent

Use Suppression of adrenal function in selected patients with Cushing's syndrome; also used successfully in postmenopausal patients with advanced breast carcinoma and in patients with metastatic prostate carcinoma

Usual Dosage Adults: Oral: 250 mg every 6 hours, may be increased at 1- to 2-week intervals to a total of 2 g/day; administer in divided doses 2-3 times/day to reduce incidence of nausea and vomiting

Dosage Forms Tablet, scored: 250 mg

Amino-Opti-E® [OTC] *see* vitamin E *on page 604*

aminophylline (am in OFF i lin)

Synonyms theophylline ethylenediamine

U.S./Canadian Brand Names Phyllocontin®; Truphylline®

Therapeutic Category Theophylline Derivative

Use Bronchodilator in reversible airway obstruction due to asthma or COPD; increase diaphragmatic contractility; neonatal idiopathic apnea of prematurity

Usual Dosage

Neonates: Apnea of prematurity:

Loading dose: 5 mg/kg for one dose

Maintenance: I.V.:

0-24 days: Begin at 2 mg/kg/day divided every 12 hours and titrate to desired levels and effects

>24 days: 3 mg/kg/day divided every 12 hours; increased dosages may be indicated as liver metabolism matures (usually >30 days of life); monitor serum levels to determine appropriate dosages

Theophylline levels should be initially drawn after 3 days of therapy; repeat levels are indicated 3 days after each increase in dosage or weekly if on a stabilized dosage

Treatment of acute bronchospasm:

Loading dose (in patients not currently receiving aminophylline or theophylline): 6 mg/kg (based on aminophylline) administered I.V. over 20-30 minutes; administration rate should not exceed 25 mg/minute (aminophylline)

Approximate I.V. maintenance dosages are based upon **continuous infusions**; bolus dosing (often used in children <6 months of age) may be determined by multiplying the hourly infusion rate by 24 hours and dividing by the desired number of doses/day

6 weeks to 6 months: 0.5 mg/kg/hour

6 months to 1 year: 0.6-0.7 mg/kg/hour

1-9 years: 1-1.2 mg/kg/hour

9-12 years and young adult smokers: 0.9 mg/kg/hour

12-16 years: 0.7 mg/kg/hour

Adults (healthy, nonsmoking): 0.7 mg/kg/hour

Older patients and patients with cor pulmonale, patients with congestive heart failure or liver failure: 0.25 mg/kg/hour

Dosage should be adjusted according to serum level measurements during the first 12- to 24-hour period; avoid using suppositories due to erratic, unreliable absorption.

Rectal: Adults: 500 mg 3 times/day

Dosage Forms

Injection, I.V.: 25 mg/mL (10 mL, 20 mL)

Liquid, oral: 105 mg/5 mL (240 mL)

Suppository, rectal (Truphylline®): 250 mg, 500 mg

Tablet: 100 mg, 200 mg

Controlled release [12 hours] (Phyllocontin®): 225 mg

aminophylline, amobarbital, and ephedrine

(am in OFF i lin, am oh BAR bi tal, & e FED rin)

Therapeutic Category Theophylline Derivative

Use Symptomatic relief of asthma

Usual Dosage Adults: Oral: 1 capsule every 6 hours

(Continued)

aminophylline, amobarbital, and ephedrine *(Continued)*

Dosage Forms Capsule: Aminophylline 130 mg, amobarbital 24 mg, and ephedrine sulfate 24 mg

aminosalicylate sodium (a MEE noe sa LIS i late SOW dee um)

Synonyms PAS

U.S./Canadian Brand Names Tubasal® (Can)

Therapeutic Category Nonsteroidal Anti-inflammatory Drug (NSAID)

Use Treatment of tuberculosis with combination drugs

Usual Dosage Oral:

Children: 150-300 mg/kg/day in 3-4 equally divided doses

Adults: 150 mg/kg/day in 2-3 equally divided doses (usually 12-14 g/day)

Dosage Forms Tablet: 500 mg

5-aminosalicylic acid *see* mesalamine *on page 358*

amiodarone (a MEE oh da rone)

U.S./Canadian Brand Names Cordarone®; Pacerone®

Therapeutic Category Antiarrhythmic Agent, Class III

Use Management of resistant, life-threatening ventricular arrhythmias unresponsive to conventional therapy with less toxic agents; also used for treatment of supraventricular arrhythmias unresponsive to conventional therapy; injectable available from manufacturer via orphan drug status or compassionate use for acute treatment and prophylaxis of life-threatening ventricular tachycardia or ventricular fibrillation (see Dosage Forms)

Usual Dosage Children <1 year should be dosed as calculated by body surface area

Children: Loading dose: 10-15 mg/kg/day or 600-800 mg/1.73 m^2/day for 4-14 days or until adequate control of arrhythmia or prominent adverse effects occur (this loading dose may be administered in 1-2 divided doses/day); dosage should then be reduced to 5 mg/kg/day or 200-400 mg/1.73 m^2/day administered once daily for several weeks; if arrhythmia does not recur reduce to lowest effective dosage possible; usual daily minimal dose: 2.5 mg/kg; maintenance doses may be administered for 5 of 7 days/week

Adults: Ventricular arrhythmias: 800-1600 mg/day in 1-2 doses for 1-3 weeks, then 600-800 mg/day in 1-2 doses for 1 month; maintenance: 400 mg/day; lower doses are recommended for supraventricular arrhythmias, usually 100-400 mg/day

Dosage Forms Amiodarone hydrochloride:

Injection: 50 mg/mL with benzyl alcohol (3 mL)

Tablet, scored: 200 mg

Amipaque® *see* radiological/contrast media (non-ionic) *on page 496*

Ami-Tex LA® *see* guaifenesin and phenylpropanolamine *on page 270*

Amitone® [OTC] *see* calcium carbonate *on page 89*

amitriptyline (a mee TRIP ti leen)

U.S./Canadian Brand Names Apo®-Amitriptyline (Can); Elavil®; Emitrip®; Endep®; Enovil®; Levate® (Can); Novo-Tryptin® (Can)

Therapeutic Category Antidepressant, Tricyclic (Tertiary Amine)

Use Treatment of various forms of depression, often in conjunction with psychotherapy; analgesic for certain chronic and neuropathic pain; migraine prophylaxis

Usual Dosage

Children <12 years: Not recommended

Adolescents: Oral: Initial: 25-50 mg/day; may administer in divided doses; increase gradually to 100 mg/day in divided doses

Adults:

Oral: 30-100 mg/day single dose at bedtime or in divided doses; dose may be gradually increased up to 300 mg/day; once symptoms are controlled, decrease gradually to lowest effective dose

I.M.: 20-30 mg 4 times/day

Dosage Forms Amitriptyline hydrochloride:
Injection: 10 mg/mL (10 mL)
Tablet: 10 mg, 25 mg, 50 mg, 75 mg, 100 mg, 150 mg

amitriptyline and chlordiazepoxide

(a mee TRIP ti leen & klor dye az e POKS ide)

Synonyms chlordiazepoxide and amitriptyline
U.S./Canadian Brand Names Limbitrol® DS 10-25
Therapeutic Category Antidepressant, Tricyclic (Tertiary Amine)
Controlled Substance C-IV
Use Treatment of moderate to severe anxiety and/or agitation and depression
Usual Dosage Oral: Initial: 3-4 tablets in divided doses; this may be increased to 6 tablets/day as required; some patients respond to smaller doses and can be maintained on 2 tablets
Dosage Forms Tablet:
5-12.5: Amitriptyline hydrochloride 12.5 mg and chlordiazepoxide 5 mg
10-25: Amitriptyline hydrochloride 25 mg and chlordiazepoxide 10 mg

amitriptyline and perphenazine (a mee TRIP ti leen & per FEN a zeen)

Synonyms perphenazine and amitriptyline
U.S./Canadian Brand Names Etrafon®; Triavil®
Therapeutic Category Antidepressant/Phenothiazine
Use Treatment of patients with moderate to severe anxiety and depression
Usual Dosage Oral: 1 tablet 2-4 times/day
Dosage Forms Tablet:
2-10: Amitriptyline hydrochloride 10 mg and perphenazine 2 mg
4-10: Amitriptyline hydrochloride 10 mg and perphenazine 4 mg
2-25: Amitriptyline hydrochloride 25 mg and perphenazine 2 mg
4-25: Amitriptyline hydrochloride 25 mg and perphenazine 4 mg
4-50: Amitriptyline hydrochloride 50 mg and perphenazine 4 mg

amlexanox (am LEKS an oks)

U.S./Canadian Brand Names Aphthasol™
Therapeutic Category Anti-inflammatory Agent, Locally Applied
Use Treating signs and symptoms of canker sores (minor aphthous ulcers)
Usual Dosage Administer directly on ulcers 4 times/day following oral hygiene, after meals, and before going to bed
Dosage Forms Cream: 5% (5 g)

amlodipine (am LOE di peen)

U.S./Canadian Brand Names Norvasc®
Therapeutic Category Calcium Channel Blocker
Use Treatment of hypertension alone or in combination with antihypertensives; chronic stable angina alone or with other antianginal agents; vasospastic angina alone or in combination with other agents
Usual Dosage Oral:
Adults: 2.5-10 mg once daily
Elderly: 2.5 mg once daily; increase by 2.5 mg increments at 7- to 14-day intervals; maximum recommended dose: 10 mg/day
Dosage Forms Tablet: 2.5 mg, 5 mg, 10 mg

amlodipine and benazepril (am LOE di peen & ben AY ze pril)

Synonyms benazepril and amlodipine
U.S./Canadian Brand Names Lotrel®
Therapeutic Category Antihypertensive Agent, Combination
Use Treatment of hypertension
Usual Dosage Adults: Oral: 1 capsule daily
(Continued)

amlodipine and benazepril *(Continued)*

Dosage Forms Capsule:
- Amlodipine 2.5 mg and benazepril hydrochloride 10 mg
- Amlodipine 5 mg and benazepril hydrochloride 10 mg
- Amlodipine 5 mg and benazepril hydrochloride 20 mg

ammonapse *see* sodium phenylbutyrate *on page 528*

ammonia spirit, aromatic (a MOE nee ah SPEAR it, air oh MAT ik)

Synonyms smelling salts

U.S./Canadian Brand Names Aromatic Ammonia Aspirols®

Therapeutic Category Respiratory Stimulant

Use Respiratory and circulatory stimulant; treatment of fainting

Usual Dosage "Smelling salts" to treat or prevent fainting

Dosage Forms
- Inhalant, crushable glass perles: 0.33 mL, 0.4 mL
- Solution: 30 mL, 60 mL, 120 mL

ammonium chloride (a MOE nee um KLOR ide)

Therapeutic Category Electrolyte Supplement, Oral

Use Diuretic or systemic and urinary acidifying agent; treatment of hypochloremic states

Usual Dosage
- Children: Oral, I.V.: 75 mg/kg/day in 4 divided doses for urinary acidification; maximum daily dose: 6 g
- Adults:
  - Oral: 2-3 g every 6 hours
  - I.V.: 1.5 g/dose every 6 hours

Dosage Forms
- Injection: 26.75% [5 mEq/mL] (20 mL)
- Tablet: 500 mg
- Tablet, enteric coated: 500 mg

ammonium lactate *see* lactic acid with ammonium hydroxide *on page 324*

amobarbital (am oh BAR bi tal)

Synonyms amylobarbitone

U.S./Canadian Brand Names Amobarbital® (Can); Amytal®

Therapeutic Category Barbiturate

Controlled Substance C-II

Use
- Oral: Hypnotic in short-term treatment of insomnia, to reduce anxiety and provide sedation preoperatively
- I.M., I.V.: Used to control status epilepticus or acute seizure episodes; also used in catatonic, negativistic, or manic reactions and in "Amytal® Interviewing" for narcoanalysis

Usual Dosage
- Children: Oral:
  - Insomnia: 2 mg/kg or 70 mg/m^2/day in 4 equally divided doses
  - Hypnotic: 2-3 mg/kg
- Adults:
  - Insomnia: Oral: 65-200 mg at bedtime
  - Sedation: Oral: 30-50 mg 2-3 times/day
  - Preanesthetic: Oral: 200 mg 1-2 hours before surgery
  - Hypnotic:
    - Oral: 65-200 mg at bedtime
    - I.M.: 65-500 mg, should not exceed 500 mg
    - I.V.: 65-500 mg, should not exceed 1000 mg

Dosage Forms Amobarbital sodium:

Capsule: 65 mg, 200 mg
Injection: 250 mg, 500 mg
Tablet: 30 mg, 50 mg, 100 mg

amobarbital and secobarbital (am oh BAR bi tal & see koe BAR bi tal)

Synonyms secobarbital and amobarbital

U.S./Canadian Brand Names Tuinal®

Therapeutic Category Barbiturate

Controlled Substance C-II

Use Short-term treatment of insomnia

Usual Dosage Adults: Oral: 1-2 capsules at bedtime

Dosage Forms Capsule:

100: Amobarbital sodium 50 mg and secobarbital sodium 50 mg
200: Amobarbital sodium 100 mg and secobarbital sodium 100 mg

Amobarbital® (Can) *see* amobarbital *on previous page*

Amonidrin® Tablet *(Discontinued)* *see page 700*

AMO Vitrax® *see* sodium hyaluronate *on page 527*

amoxapine (a MOKS a peen)

U.S./Canadian Brand Names Asendin®

Therapeutic Category Antidepressant, Tricyclic (Secondary Amine)

Use Treatment of neurotic and endogenous depression and mixed symptoms of anxiety and depression

Usual Dosage Oral (once symptoms are controlled, decrease gradually to lowest effective dose):

Children <16 years: Dose not established

Adolescents: Initial: 25-50 mg/day; increase gradually to 100 mg/day; may administer as divided doses or as a single dose at bedtime

Adults: Initial: 25 mg 2-3 times/day, if tolerated, dosage may be increased to 100 mg 2-3 times/day; may be administered in a single bedtime dose when dosage <300 mg/day

Maximum daily dose:
Outpatient: 400 mg
Inpatient: 600 mg

Dosage Forms Tablet: 25 mg, 50 mg, 100 mg, 150 mg

amoxicillin (a moks i SIL in)

Synonyms amoxycillin; *p*-hydroxyampicillin

U.S./Canadian Brand Names Amoxil®; Apo-Amoxi® (Can); Novamoxin® (Can); Nu-Amoxi (Can); Pro-Amox® (Can); Trimox®; Wymox®

Therapeutic Category Penicillin

Use Treatment of otitis media, sinusitis, and infections involving the respiratory tract, skin, and urinary tract due to susceptible *H. influenzae, N. gonorrhoeae, E. coli, P. mirabilis, E. faecalis*, streptococci, and nonpenicillinase-producing staphylococci; prophylaxis of bacterial endocarditis

Usual Dosage Oral:

Children: 25-50 mg/kg/day in divided doses every 8 hours

Uncomplicated gonorrhea: ≥2 years: 50 mg/kg plus probenecid 25 mg/kg in a single dose; do not use this regimen in children <2 years of age, probenecid is contraindicated in this age group

SBE prophylaxis: 50 mg/kg 1 hour before procedure and 25 mg/kg 6 hours later; not to exceed adult dosage

Adults: 250-500 mg every 8 hours or 500-875 mg twice daily; maximum dose: 2-3 g/day

Uncomplicated gonorrhea: 3 g plus probenecid 1 g in a single dose

Endocarditis prophylaxis: 3 g 1 hour before procedure and 1.5 g 6 hours later

(Continued)

amoxicillin *(Continued)*

Dosage Forms
Capsule, as trihydrate: 250 mg, 500 mg
Powder for oral suspension, as trihydrate: 125 mg/5 mL (5 mL, 80 mL, 100 mL, 150 mL, 200 mL); 250 mg/5 mL (5 mL, 80 mL, 100 mL, 150 mL, 200 mL)
Powder for oral suspension, drops, as trihydrate: 50 mg/mL (15 mL, 30 mL)
Tablet:
Chewable, as trihydrate: 125 mg, 250 mg
Film coated: 500 mg, 875 mg

amoxicillin and clavulanate potassium

(a moks i SIL in & klav yoo LAN ate poe TASS ee um)

Synonyms amoxicillin and clavulanic acid; clavulanate potassium and amoxicillin
U.S./Canadian Brand Names Augmentin®; Clavulin® (Can)
Therapeutic Category Penicillin
Use Infections caused by susceptible organisms involving the lower respiratory tract, otitis media, sinusitis, skin and skin structure, and urinary tract; spectrum same as amoxicillin in addition to beta-lactamase-producing *B. catarrhalis, H. influenzae, N. gonorrhoeae,* and *S. aureus* (not MRSA)
Usual Dosage Oral:
Children ≤40 kg: 20-40 mg (amoxicillin)/kg/day in divided doses every 8 hours
Children >40 kg and Adults: 250-500 mg every 8 hours or 875 mg every 12 hours
Dosage Forms
Suspension, oral:
125 (banana flavor): Amoxicillin trihydrate 125 mg and clavulanate potassium 31.25 mg per 5 mL (75 mL, 150 mL)
200: Amoxicillin 200 mg and clavulanate potassium 28.5 mg per 5 mL (50 mL, 75 mL, 100 mL)
250 (orange flavor): Amoxicillin trihydrate 250 mg and clavulanate potassium 62.5 mg per 5 mL (75 mL, 150 mL)
400: Amoxicillin 400 mg and clavulanate potassium 57 mg per 5 mL (50 mL, 75 mL, 100 mL)
Tablet:
250: Amoxicillin trihydrate 250 mg and clavulanate potassium 125 mg
500: Amoxicillin trihydrate 500 mg and clavulanate potassium 125 mg
875: Amoxicillin trihydrate 875 mg and clavulanate potassium 125 mg
Tablet, chewable:
125: Amoxicillin trihydrate 125 mg and clavulanate potassium 31.25 mg
250: Amoxicillin trihydrate 250 mg and clavulanate potassium 62.5 mg

amoxicillin and clavulanic acid *see* amoxicillin and clavulanate potassium *on this page*

Amoxil® *see* amoxicillin *on previous page*

amoxycillin *see* amoxicillin *on previous page*

amphetamine (am FET a meen)

Therapeutic Category Amphetamine
Controlled Substance C-II
Use Narcolepsy; exogenous obesity; abnormal behavioral syndrome in children (minimal brain dysfunction); attention-deficit hyperactivity disorder (ADHD)
Usual Dosage Oral:
Narcolepsy:
Children:
6-12 years: 5 mg/day, increase by 5 mg at weekly intervals
>12 years: 10 mg/day, increase by 10 mg at weekly intervals
Adults: 5-60 mg/day in divided doses
Minimal brain dysfunction: Children:
3-5 years: 2.5 mg/day, increase by 2.5 mg at weekly intervals

>6 years: 5 mg/day, increase by 5 mg at weekly intervals

Short-term adjunct to exogenous obesity: Children >12 years and Adults: 10 mg or 15 mg long-acting capsule daily, up to 30 mg/day; or 5-30 mg/day in divided doses (immediate release tablets only)

Dosage Forms Tablet, as sulfate: 5 mg, 10 mg

Amphojel® [OTC] *see* aluminum hydroxide *on page 22*

Amphotec® *see* amphotericin B cholesteryl sulfate complex *on this page*

amphotericin B cholesteryl sulfate complex

(am foe TER i sin bee kole LES te ril SUL fate KOM plecks)

Synonyms ABCD; amphotericin B colloidal dispersion

U.S./Canadian Brand Names Amphotec®

Therapeutic Category Antifungal Agent

Use Effective in the treatment of invasive mycoses in patient refractory to or intolerant of conventional amphotericin B

Usual Dosage Children and Adults: 3-4 mg/kg/day I.V. (infusion of 1 mg/kg/hour); maximum: 7.5 mg/kg/day; duration of therapy is often <6 weeks

Dosage Forms Suspension for injection: 5 mg/mL (20 mL)

amphotericin B colloidal dispersion *see* amphotericin B cholesteryl sulfate complex *on this page*

amphotericin B (conventional) (am foe TER i sin bee)

U.S./Canadian Brand Names Fungizone®

Therapeutic Category Antifungal Agent

Use Treatment of severe systemic infections and meningitis caused by susceptible fungi such as *Candida* species, *Histoplasma capsulatum*, *Cryptococcus neoformans*, *Aspergillus* species, *Blastomyces dermatitidis*, *Torulopsis glabrata*, and *Coccidioides immitis*; fungal peritonitis; irrigant for bladder fungal infections; and topically for cutaneous and mucocutaneous candidal infections

Usual Dosage

I.V.:

Infants and Children:

Test dose (not required): I.V.: 0.1 mg/kg/dose to a maximum of 1 mg; infuse over 30-60 minutes

Initial therapeutic dose: 0.25 mg/kg gradually increased, usually in 0.25 mg/kg increments on each subsequent day, until the desired daily dose is reached

Maintenance dose: 0.25-1 mg/kg/day given once daily; infuse over 2-6 hours. Once therapy has been established, amphotericin B can be administered on an every other day basis at 1-1.5 mg/kg/dose; cumulative dose: 1.5-2 g over 6-10 week

Adults:

Test dose (not required): 1 mg infused over 20-30 minutes

Initial dose: 0.25 mg/kg administered over 2-6 hours, gradually increased on subsequent days to the desired level by 0.25 mg/kg increments per day; in critically ill patients, may initiate with 1-1.5 mg/kg/day with close observation

Maintenance dose: 0.25-1 mg/kg/day or 1.5 mg/kg over 4-6 hours every other day; do not exceed 1.5 mg/kg/day; cumulative dose: 1-4 g over 4-10 weeks

Duration of therapy varies with nature of infection: histoplasmosis, *Cryptococcus*, or blastomycosis may be treated with total dose of 2-4 g

I.T.:

Children.: 25-100 mcg every 48-72 hours; increase to 500 mcg as tolerated

Adults: 25-300 mcg every 48-72 hours; increase to 500 mcg to 1 mg as tolerated

Oral: 1 mL (100 mg) 4 times daily

Topical: Apply to affected areas 2-4 times/day for 1-4 weeks of therapy depending on nature and severity of infection

(Continued)

amphotericin B (conventional) *(Continued)*

Administration in dialysate: Children and Adults: 1-2 mg/L of peritoneal dialysis fluid either with or without low-dose I.V. amphotericin B (a total dose of 2-10 mg/kg given over 7-14 days)

Administration via bladder irrigation: Children and Adults: 50 mg/day in 1 L of sterile water irrigation solution instilled over 24 hours for 2-7 days or until cultures are clear

Dosage Forms

Cream: 3% (20 g)
Lotion: 3% (30 mL)
Ointment, topical: 3% (20 g)
Powder for injection, lyophilized: 50 mg
Suspension, oral: 100 mg/mL (24 mL with dropper)

amphotericin B (lipid complex) (am foe TER i sin bee LIP id KOM pleks)

Synonyms ABLC

U.S./Canadian Brand Names Abelcet™

Therapeutic Category Antifungal Agent

Use Treatment of aspergillosis in patients who are refractory to or intolerant of conventional amphotericin B therapy. This indication is based on results obtained primarily from emergency use studies for the treatment of aspergillosis; orphan drug status for cryptococcal meningitis

Usual Dosage Children and Adults: I.V.: 2.5-5 mg/kg/day as a single infusion **Note:** Significantly higher dose of ABLC are tolerated; it appears that attaining higher doses with ABLC produce more rapid fungicidal activity *in vivo* than standard amphotericin B preparations

Dosage Forms Injection: 5 mg/mL (20 mL)

amphotericin B (liposomal) (am foe TER i sin bee lye po SO mal)

Synonyms L-AmB

U.S./Canadian Brand Names AmBisome®

Therapeutic Category Antifungal Agent, Systemic

Use Empirical therapy for presumed fungal infection in febrile, neutropenic patients. Treatment of patients with *Aspergillus* species, *Candida* species and/or *Cryptococcus* species infections refractory to amphotericin B deoxycholate, or in patients where renal impairment or unacceptable toxicity precludes the use of amphotericin B deoxycholate. Treatment of visceral leishmaniasis. In immunocompromised patients with visceral leishmaniasis treated with AmBisome, relapse rates were high following initial clearance of parasites

Usual Dosage Children and Adults: I.V.:

Empirical therapy: Recommended initial dose of 3 mg/kg/day

Systemic fungal infections (*Aspergillus*, *Candida*, *Cryptococcus*): Recommended initial dose of 3-5 mg/kg/day

Treatment of visceral leishmaniasis: AmBisome® achieved high rates of acute parasite clearance in immunocompetent patients when total doses of 12-30 mg/kg were administered. Most of these immunocompetent patients remained relapse-free during follow-up periods of 6 months or longer. While acute parasite clearance was achieved in most of the immunocompromised patients who received total doses of 30-40 mg/kg, the majority of these patients were observed to relapse in the 6 months following the completion of therapy.

Dosage Forms Injection: 50 mg

ampicillin (am pi SIL in)

Synonyms aminobenzylpenicillin

U.S./Canadian Brand Names Ampicin® (Can); Apo-Ampi® (Can); Jaa Amp® (Can); Marcillin®; Nu-Ampi (Can); Omnipen®; Omnipen®-N; Principen®; Pro-Ampi® (Can); Taro-Ampicillin® (Can); Totacillin®

Therapeutic Category Penicillin

Use Treatment of susceptible bacterial infections caused by streptococci, pneumococci, nonpenicillinase-producing staphylococci, *Listeria*, meningococci; some strains of *H. influenzae*, *Salmonella*, *Shigella*, *E. coli*, *Enterobacter*, and *Klebsiella*

Usual Dosage

Infants and Children:

Oral: 50-100 mg/kg/day divided every 6 hours; maximum dose: 2-3 g/day

I.M., I.V.: 100-200 mg/kg/day in 4-6 divided doses; meningitis: 200-400 mg/kg/day in 4-6 divided doses; maximum dose: 12 g/day

Adults:

Oral: 250-500 mg every 6 hours

I.M., I.V.: 8-12 g/day in 4-6 divided doses

Dosage Forms

Ampicillin anhydrous: Capsule: 250 mg, 500 mg

Ampicillin sodium: Powder for injection: 125 mg, 250 mg, 500 mg, 1 g, 2 g, 10 g

Ampicillin trihydrate:

Capsule: 250 mg, 500 mg

Powder for oral suspension: 125 mg/5 mL (5 mL unit dose, 80 mL, 100 mL, 150 mL, 200 mL); 250 mg/5 mL (5 mL unit dose, 80 mL, 100 mL, 150 mL, 200 mL); 500 mg/5 mL (5 mL unit dose, 100 mL)

Powder for oral suspension, drops: 100 mg/mL (20 mL)

ampicillin and sulbactam (am pi SIL in & SUL bak tam)

Synonyms sulbactam and ampicillin

U.S./Canadian Brand Names Unasyn®

Therapeutic Category Penicillin

Use Treatment of susceptible bacterial infections involved with skin and skin structure, intra-abdominal infections, gynecological infections; spectrum is that of ampicillin plus organisms producing beta-lactamases such as *S. aureus*, *H. influenzae*, *E. coli*, *Klebsiella*, *Acinetobacter*, *Enterobacter* and anaerobes

Usual Dosage Unasyn® (ampicillin/sulbactam) is a combination product. Each 3 g vial contains 2 g of ampicillin and 1 g of sulbactam. Sulbactam has very little antibacterial activity by itself, but effectively extends the spectrum of ampicillin to include beta-lactamase-producing strains that are resistant to ampicillin alone. Therefore, dosage recommendations for Unasyn® are based on the ampicillin component.

I.M., I.V.:

Children: 100-200 mg ampicillin/kg/day (150-300 mg Unasyn®) divided every 6 hours; maximum dose: 8 g ampicillin/day (12 g Unasyn®)

Adults: 1-2 g ampicillin (1.5-3 g Unasyn®) every 6-8 hours; maximum dose: 8 g ampicillin/day (12 g Unasyn®)

Dosage Forms Powder for injection: 1.5 g [ampicillin sodium 1 g and sulbactam sodium 0.5 g]; 3 g [ampicillin sodium 2 g and sulbactam sodium 1 g]

Ampicin® (Can) *see* ampicillin *on previous page*

amprenavir (am PRE na veer)

U.S./Canadian Brand Names Agenerase™

Therapeutic Category Protease Inhibitor

Use Treatment of HIV infections in combination with at least two other antiretroviral agents

Usual Dosage Adults: Oral: 1200 mg twice daily

Dosage Forms

Capsule: 50 mg, 150 mg

Solution, oral: 15 mg/mL (240 mL)

AMPT *see* metyrosine *on page 373*

amrinone (AM ri none)

U.S./Canadian Brand Names Inocor®

Therapeutic Category Adrenergic Agonist Agent

(Continued)

amrinone *(Continued)*

Use Treatment of low cardiac output states (sepsis, congestive heart failure); adjunctive therapy of pulmonary hypertension

Usual Dosage Dosage is based on clinical response. **Note:** Dose should not exceed 10 mg/kg/24 hours.

Children: 0.75 mg/kg I.V. bolus over 2-3 minutes followed by maintenance infusion 5-10 mcg/kg/minute; I.V. bolus may need to be repeated in 30 minutes

Adults: 0.75 mg/kg I.V. bolus over 2-3 minutes followed by maintenance infusion of 5-10 mcg/kg/minute

Dosage Forms Injection, as lactate: 5 mg/mL (20 mL)

Amvisc® *see* sodium hyaluronate *on page 527*

Amvisc® Plus *see* sodium hyaluronate *on page 527*

Amyl Nitrate Vaporole® *see* amyl nitrite *on this page*

amyl nitrite (AM il NYE trite)

Synonyms isoamyl nitrite

U.S./Canadian Brand Names Amyl Nitrate Vaporole®; Amyl Nitrite Aspirols®

Therapeutic Category Vasodilator

Use Coronary vasodilator in angina pectoris; an adjunct in treatment of cyanide poisoning; also used to produce changes in the intensity of heart murmurs

Usual Dosage 1-6 inhalations from 1 capsule are usually sufficient to produce the desired effect

Dosage Forms Inhalant, crushable glass perles: 0.18 mL, 0.3 mL

Amyl Nitrite Aspirols® *see* amyl nitrite *on this page*

amylobarbitone *see* amobarbital *on page 30*

Amytal® *see* amobarbital *on page 30*

Anabolin® *see* nandrolone *on page 390*

Anacin® [OTC] *see* aspirin *on page 49*

Anacin-3® (all Products) ***(Discontinued)*** *see page 700*

Anadrol® *see* oxymetholone *on page 424*

Anafranil® *see* clomipramine *on page 138*

anagrelide (an AG gre lide)

U.S./Canadian Brand Names Agrylin™

Therapeutic Category Platelet Aggregation Inhibitor

Use Agent for essential thrombocythemia (ET)

Usual Dosage Adults: Oral: 0.5 mg 4 times/day or 1 mg twice daily, maintain for ≥1 week, then adjust to the lowest effective dose to reduce and maintain platelet count <600,000 µL ideally to the normal range

Dosage Forms Capsule, as hydrochloride: 0.5 mg, 1 mg

Anaids® Tablet ***(Discontinued)*** *see page 700*

Ana-Kit® *see* insect sting kit *on page 306*

Anamine® Syrup [OTC] *see* chlorpheniramine and pseudoephedrine *on page 122*

Anandron® (Can) *see* nilutamide *on page 402*

Anaplex® Liquid [OTC] *see* chlorpheniramine and pseudoephedrine *on page 122*

Anapolon® (Can) *see* oxymetholone *on page 424*

Anaprox® *see* naproxen *on page 391*

Anaspaz® *see* hyoscyamine *on page 297*

anastrozole (an AS troe zole)

U.S./Canadian Brand Names Arimidex®

Therapeutic Category Antineoplastic Agent

Use Treatment of advanced breast cancer in postmenopausal women with disease progression following tamoxifen therapy. Patients with ER-negative disease and patients who did not respond to tamoxifen therapy rarely responded to anastrozole.

Usual Dosage Breast cancer: Adults: Oral (refer to individual protocols): 1 mg once daily

Dosage Forms Tablet: 1 mg

Anatrast® *see* radiological/contrast media (ionic) *on page 495*

Anatuss® [OTC] *see* guaifenesin, phenylpropanolamine, and dextromethorphan *on page 271*

Anatuss® DM [OTC] *see* guaifenesin, pseudoephedrine, and dextromethorphan *on page 273*

Anbesol® [OTC] *see* benzocaine *on page 66*

Anbesol® Maximum Strength [OTC] *see* benzocaine *on page 66*

Ancef® *see* cefazolin *on page 105*

Ancobon® *see* flucytosine *on page 242*

Ancotil® (Can) *see* flucytosine *on page 242*

ancrod (AN krod)

U.S./Canadian Brand Names Viprinex® (Can)

Therapeutic Category Anticoagulant

Use Safe for anticoagulation of patients with heparin induced thrombocytopenia (HIT syndrome); to establish and maintain anticoagulation in herparin-intolerant patients undergoing cardiopulmonary bypass; drug derived from the venom of Malaysian pit vipers that appears to be effective in increasing recovery rates from stroke (U.S. orphan drug)

Usual Dosage Adults: I.V:

Bolus: 1-2 int. units/kg over 8-12 hours

Maintenance dose: 0.5-1 int. units/kg over 6-24 hours to maintain fibrinogen levels 0.2-0.7 g/L; may be given as intermittent I.V. injections every 12 hours or as continuous infusion; should not be given I.M. as it may induce antibody formation

Dosage Forms Injection: 70 int. units/mL (1 mL)

Androcur® (Can) *see* cyproterone *(Canada only) on page 155*

Androcur® Depot (Can) *see* cyproterone *(Canada only) on page 155*

Androderm® Transdermal System *see* testosterone *on page 552*

Andro/Fem® *see* estradiol and testosterone *on page 218*

Android® *see* methyltestosterone *on page 369*

Andro-L.A.® Injection *see* testosterone *on page 552*

Androlone® *see* nandrolone *on page 390*

Androlone®-D *see* nandrolone *on page 390*

Andropository® Injection *see* testosterone *on page 552*

Anectine® Chloride *see* succinylcholine *on page 537*

Anectine® Flo-Pack® *see* succinylcholine *on page 537*

Anergan® 25 Injection *(Discontinued)* *see page 700*

Anestacon® Topical Solution *see* lidocaine *on page 333*

aneurine *see* thiamine *on page 561*

Anexate® (Can) *see* flumazenil *on page 242*

Anexsia® *see* hydrocodone and acetaminophen *on page 287*

Angio Conray® *see* radiological/contrast media (ionic) *on page 495*

Angiovist® *see* radiological/contrast media (ionic) *on page 495*

anisotropine (an iss oh TROE peen)

U.S./Canadian Brand Names Miradon® (Can)

Therapeutic Category Anticholinergic Agent

Use Adjunctive treatment of peptic ulcer

Usual Dosage Adults: Oral: 50 mg 3 times/day

Dosage Forms Tablet, as methylbromide: 50 mg

anisoylated plasminogen streptokinase activator complex *see* anistreplase *on this page*

anistreplase (a NISS tre plase)

Synonyms anisoylated plasminogen streptokinase activator complex; APSAC

U.S./Canadian Brand Names Eminase®

Therapeutic Category Thrombolytic Agent

Use Management of acute myocardial infarction (AMI) in adults; lysis of thrombi obstructing coronary arteries, reduction of infarct size; and reduction of mortality associated with AMI

Usual Dosage Adults: I.V.: 30 units injected over 2-5 minutes as soon as possible after onset of symptoms

Dosage Forms Powder for injection, lyophilized: 30 units

Anodynos-DHC® *see* hydrocodone and acetaminophen *on page 287*

Anoquan® *see* butalbital compound and acetaminophen *on page 85*

Anoxine-AM® Capsule *(Discontinued)* *see page 700*

Ansaid® Oral *see* flurbiprofen *on page 248*

ansamycin *see* rifabutin *on page 504*

Antabuse® *see* disulfiram *on page 189*

Antagon™ *see* ganirelix *on page 257*

Antazoline-V® Ophthalmic *see* naphazoline and antazoline *on page 391*

Antazone® (Can) *see* sulfinpyrazone *on page 543*

Anthra-Derm® *see* anthralin *on this page*

Anthraforte® (Can) *see* anthralin *on this page*

anthralin (AN thra lin)

Synonyms dithranol

U.S./Canadian Brand Names Anthra-Derm®; Anthraforte® (Can); Anthranol® (Can); Anthrascalp® (Can); Drithocreme®; Drithocreme® HP 1%; Dritho-Scalp®; Micanol® Cream

Therapeutic Category Keratolytic Agent

Use Treatment of psoriasis

Usual Dosage Adults: Topical: Generally, apply once daily or as directed. The irritant potential of anthralin is directly related to the strength being used and each patient's individual tolerance. Always commence treatment for at least one week using the lowest strength possible.

Skin application: Apply sparingly only to psoriatic lesions and rub gently and carefully into the skin until absorbed. Avoid applying an excessive quantity which may cause unnecessary soiling and staining of the clothing or bed linen.

Scalp application: Comb hair to remove scalar debris and, after suitably parting, rub cream well into the lesions, taking care to prevent the cream from spreading onto the forehead

Remove by washing or showering; optimal period of contact will vary according to the strength used and the patient's response to treatment. Continue treatment until the skin is entirely clear (ie, when there is nothing to feel with the fingers and the texture is normal)

Dosage Forms

Cream: 0.1% (50 g, 65 g); 0.2% (65 g); 0.25% (50 g); 0.4% (65 g); 0.5% (50 g); 1% (50 g, 65 g)

Ointment, topical: 0.1% (42.5 g); 0.25% (42.5 g); 0.4% (60 g); 0.5% (42.5 g); 1% (42.5 g)

Anthranol® (Can) *see* anthralin *on previous page*

Anthrascalp® (Can) *see* anthralin *on previous page*

anthrax vaccine, adsorbed (AN thraks vak SEEN ad SORBED)

Therapeutic Category Vaccine

Use Recommended for individuals who may come in contact with animal products which come from anthrax endemic areas and may be contaminated with *Bacillus anthracis* spores; recommended for high-risk persons such as veterinarians and other handling potentially infected animals. Routine immunization for the general population is not recommended.

The Department of Defense is implementing an anthrax vaccination program against the biological warfare agent anthrax, which will be administered to all active duty and reserve personnel.

Usual Dosage

Primary immunization: S.C.: Three injections of 0.5 mL each given 2 weeks apart followed by three additional S.C. injections given at 6, 12, and 18 months

Subsequent booster injections: 0.5 mL at 1-year intervals are recommended for immunity to be maintained

Dosage Forms Injection: 5 mL (10 doses)

AntibiOtic® Otic *see* neomycin, polymyxin B, and hydrocortisone *on page 396*

anti-CD20 monoclonal antibodies *see* rituximab *on page 507*

antidigoxin Fab fragments *see* digoxin immune Fab *on page 180*

antidiuretic hormone (ADH) *see* vasopressin *on page 597*

antihemophilic factor (human) (an tee hee moe FIL ik FAK tor HYU man)

Synonyms AHF; factor VIII

U.S./Canadian Brand Names Hemofil® M; Humate-P®; Koāte®-HP; Monoclate-P®; Profilate® OSD; Profilate® SD

Therapeutic Category Blood Product Derivative

Use Management of hemophilia A in patients whom a deficiency in factor VIII has been demonstrated

Usual Dosage I.V.: Individualize dosage based on coagulation studies performed prior to and during treatment at regular intervals. One AHF unit is the activity present in 1 mL of normal pooled human plasma; dosage should be adjusted to actual vial size currently stocked in the pharmacy.

Hospitalized patients: 20-50 units/kg/dose; may be higher for special circumstances; dose can be administered every 12-24 hours and more frequently in special circumstances

Dosage Forms Injection: 10 mL, 20 mL, 30 mL

antihemophilic factor (porcine) (an tee hee moe FIL ik FAK ter POR seen)

U.S./Canadian Brand Names Hyate®:C

Therapeutic Category Antihemophilic Agent

Use Treatment of congenital hemophiliacs with antibodies to human factor VIII:C and also for previously nonhemophiliac patients with spontaneously acquired inhibitors to human factor VIII:C; patients with inhibitors who are bleeding or who are to undergo surgery

Usual Dosage Clinical response should be used to assess efficacy rather than relying upon a particular laboratory value for recovery of factor VIII:C.

(Continued)

antihemophilic factor (porcine) *(Continued)*

Initial dose:

Antibody level to human factor VIII:C <50 Bethesda units/mL: 100-150 porcine units/kg (body weight) is recommended

Antibody level to human factor VIII:C >50 Bethesda units/mL: Activity of the antibody to porcine factor VIII:C should be determined; **an antiporcine antibody level** >20 Bethesda units/mL indicates that the patient is unlikely to benefit from treatment; for lower titers, a dose of 100-150 porcine units/kg is recommended

If a patient has previously been treated with Hyate®:C, this may provide a guide to his likely response and, therefore, assist in estimation of the preliminary dose

Subsequent doses: Following administration of the initial dose, if the recovery of factor VIII:C in the patient's plasma is not sufficient, a further higher dose should be administered; if recovery after the second dose is still insufficient, a third and higher dose may prove effective

Dosage Forms Powder for injection, lyophilized: 400-700 porcine units to be reconstituted with 20 mL sterile water

antihemophilic factor (recombinant)

(an tee hee moe FIL ik FAK tor ree KOM be nant)

Synonyms factor VIII recombinant

U.S./Canadian Brand Names Bioclate®; Helixate®; Kogenate®; Recombinate®

Therapeutic Category Blood Product Derivative

Use Management of hemophilia A in patients whom a deficiency in factor VIII has been demonstrated

Usual Dosage I.V.: Individualize dosage based on coagulation studies performed prior to and during treatment at regular intervals. One AHF unit is the activity present in 1 mL of normal pooled human plasma; dosage should be adjusted to actual vial size currently stocked in the pharmacy.

Hospitalized patients: 20-50 units/kg/dose; may be higher for special circumstances; dose can be administered every 12-24 hours and more frequently in special circumstances

Dosage Forms Injection: 250 units, 500 units, 1000 units

Antihist-1® [OTC] *see* clemastine *on page 135*

Antihist-D® *see* clemastine and phenylpropanolamine *on page 136*

anti-inhibitor coagulant complex

(an tee-in HI bi tor coe AG yoo lant KOM pleks)

Synonyms coagulant complex inhibitor

U.S./Canadian Brand Names Autoplex® T; Feiba VH Immuno®

Therapeutic Category Hemophilic Agent

Use Patients with factor VIII inhibitors who are to undergo surgery or those who are bleeding

Usual Dosage Dosage range: I.V.: 25-100 factor VIII correctional units per kg depending on the severity of hemorrhage

Dosage Forms Injection:

Autoplex® T, with heparin 2 units: Each bottle is labeled with correctional units of factor VIII

Feiba VH Immuno®, heparin free: Each bottle is labeled with correctional units of factor VIII

Antilirium® *see* physostigmine *on page 450*

Antiminth® [OTC] *see* pyrantel pamoate *on page 488*

Antinea® Cream *(Discontinued)* *see page 700*

antipyrine and benzocaine (an tee PYE reen & BEN zoe kane)

Synonyms benzocaine and antipyrine

U.S./Canadian Brand Names Allergan® Ear Drops; Auralgan®; Auroto®; Otocalm® Ear

Therapeutic Category Otic Agent, Analgesic; Otic Agent, Cerumenolytic

Use Temporary relief of pain and reduction of inflammation associated with acute congestive and serous otitis media, swimmer's ear, otitis externa; facilitates ear wax removal

Usual Dosage Otic: Fill ear canal; moisten cotton pledget, place in external ear, repeat every 1-2 hours until pain and congestion is relieved; for ear wax removal instill drops 3-4 times/day for 2-3 days

Dosage Forms Solution, otic: Antipyrine 5.4% and benzocaine 1.4% (10 mL, 15 mL)

antirabies serum (equine) (an tee RAY beez SEER um EE kwine)

Synonyms ARS

Therapeutic Category Serum

Use Rabies prophylaxis

Usual Dosage I.M.: 1000 units/55 lb in a single dose, infiltrate up to 50% of dose around the wound

Dosage Forms Injection: 125 units/mL (8 mL)

Antispas® Injection *see* dicyclomine *on page 177*

antithrombin III (an tee THROM bin three)

Synonyms ATIII; heparin cofactor I

U.S./Canadian Brand Names ATnativ®; Thrombate III™

Therapeutic Category Blood Product Derivative

Use Agent for hereditary antithrombin III deficiency

Usual Dosage After first dose of antithrombin III, level should increase to 120% of normal; thereafter maintain at levels >80%. Generally, achieved by administration of maintenance doses once every 24 hours; initially and until patient is stabilized, measure antithrombin III level at least twice daily, thereafter once daily and always immediately before next infusion.

Initial dosage (units) = [desired AT-III level % - baseline AT-III level %] x body weight (kg) divided by 1%/units/kg

Measure antithrombin III preceding and 30 minutes after dose to calculate *in vivo* recovery rate; maintain level within normal range for 2-8 days depending on type of surgery or procedure

Dosage Forms Powder for injection: 500 units (50 mL)

antithymocyte globulin (equine) *see* lymphocyte immune globulin *on page 343*

antithymocyte globulin (rabbit) (an te THY moe site GLOB yu lin RAB bit)

Therapeutic Category Immunosuppressant Agent

Use Treatment of acute moderate-to-severe renal allograft rejection

Usual Dosage Adults: I.V.: Treatment of acute renal allograft rejection: 1.5 mg/kg/day for 7-14 days.

Dosage Forms Each package contains two 7 mL vials:
Vial 1: antithymocyte globulin (rabbit) 25 mg
Vial 2: Diluent (sterile water for injection) >5 mL

Anti-Tuss® Expectorant [OTC] *see* guaifenesin *on page 267*

antivenin (*Crotalidae*) polyvalent
(an tee VEN in (kroe TAL ih die) pol i VAY lent)

Synonyms crotaline antivenin, polyvalent; North and South American antisnake-bite serum; pit vipers antivenin; snake (pit vipers) antivenin

Therapeutic Category Antivenin

(Continued)

antivenin (*Crotalidae*) polyvalent *(Continued)*

Use Neutralization of venoms of North and South American crotalids: rattlesnake, copperhead, cottonmouth, tropical moccasins, fer-de-lance, bushmaster

Usual Dosage Initial intradermal sensitivity test. The entire initial dose of antivenin should be administered as soon as possible to be most effective (within 4 hours after the bite).

Children and Adults: I.V.: Minimal envenomation: 20-40 mL; moderate envenomation: 50-90 mL; severe envenomation: 100-150 mL

Additional doses of antivenin is based on clinical response to the initial dose. If swelling continues to progress, symptoms increase in severity, hypotension occurs, or decrease in hematocrit appears, an additional 10-50 mL should be administered.

For I.V. infusion: 1:1-1:10 dilution of reconstituted antivenin in normal saline or D_5W should be prepared. Infuse the initial 5-10 mL of diluted antivenin over 3-5 minutes monitoring closely for signs of sensitivity reactions.

Dosage Forms Injection: Lyophilized serum, diluent (10 mL); one vacuum vial to yield 10 mL of serum

antivenin (*Latrodectus mactans*) (an tee VEN in lak tro DUK tus MAK tans)

Synonyms black widow spider antivenin (*Latrodectus mactans*); *Latrodectus mactans* antivenin

Therapeutic Category Antivenin

Use Treat patients with symptoms of black widow spider bites

Usual Dosage

Children <12 years (severe or shock): I.V.: 2.5 mL in 10-50 mL over 15 minutes

Children and Adults: I.M.: 2.5 mL

Dosage Forms Powder for injection: 6000 antivenin units (2.5 mL)

antivenin (*Micrurus fulvius*) (an tee VEN in mye KRU rus FUL vee us)

Synonyms North American coral snake antivenin

Therapeutic Category Antivenin

Use Neutralize the venom of Eastern coral snake and Texas coral snake but does not neutralize venom of Arizona or Sonoran coral snake

Usual Dosage I.V.: 3-5 vials by slow injection

Dosage Forms Injection: One vial antivenin and one vial diluent

Antivert® *see* meclizine *on page 351*

Antivert® Chewable Tablet *(Discontinued)* *see page 700*

Antizol™ *see* fomepizole *on page 252*

Antrizine® *see* meclizine *on page 351*

Antrocol® Capsule & Tablet *(Discontinued)* *see page 700*

Anturan® (Can) *see* sulfinpyrazone *on page 543*

Anturane® *see* sulfinpyrazone *on page 543*

Anusol® HC-1 Topical [OTC] *see* hydrocortisone (topical) *on page 292*

Anusol® HC-2.5% Topical [OTC] *see* hydrocortisone (topical) *on page 292*

Anusol-HC® Suppository *see* hydrocortisone (rectal) *on page 291*

Anusol® Ointment [OTC] *see* pramoxine *on page 469*

Anxanil® Oral *see* hydroxyzine *on page 297*

Anzemet® *see* dolasetron *on page 192*

Apacet® [OTC] *see* acetaminophen *on page 3*

APAP *see* acetaminophen *on page 3*

Apatate® [OTC] *see* vitamin B complex *on page 603*

Aphrodyne™ *see* yohimbine *on page 609*

Aphthasol™ *see* amlexanox *on page 29*

A.P.L.® *see* chorionic gonadotropin *on page 130*

Aplisol® *see* tuberculin tests *on page 588*

Aplitest® *see* tuberculin tests *on page 588*

Apo®-Acetazolamide (Can) *see* acetazolamide *on page 7*

Apo®-Allopurinol (Can) *see* allopurinol *on page 19*

Apo®-Alpraz (Can) *see* alprazolam *on page 19*

Apo®-Amitriptyline (Can) *see* amitriptyline *on page 28*

Apo-Amoxi® (Can) *see* amoxicillin *on page 31*

Apo-Ampi® (Can) *see* ampicillin *on page 34*

Apo®-ASA (Can) *see* aspirin *on page 49*

Apo®-Atenol (Can) *see* atenolol *on page 51*

Apo®-Bisacodyl (Can) *see* bisacodyl *on page 74*

Apo® Bromocriptine (Can) *see* bromocriptine *on page 79*

Apo-Cal® (Can) *see* calcium carbonate *on page 89*

Apo®-Capto (Can) *see* captopril *on page 96*

Apo®-Carbamazepine (Can) *see* carbamazepine *on page 97*

Apo®-C (Can) *see* ascorbic acid *on page 48*

Apo®-Cephalex (Can) *see* cephalexin *on page 111*

Apo-Chlordiazepoxide® (Can) *see* chlordiazepoxide *on page 116*

Apo®-Chlorpromazine (Can) *see* chlorpromazine *on page 127*

Apo-Chlorpropamide® (Can) *see* chlorpropamide *on page 127*

Apo-Chlorthalidone® (Can) *see* chlorthalidone *on page 128*

Apo®-Cimetidine (Can) *see* cimetidine *on page 131*

Apo-Clomipramine® (Can) *see* clomipramine *on page 138*

Apo®-Clonidine (Can) *see* clonidine *on page 139*

Apo®-Clorazepate (Can) *see* clorazepate *on page 140*

Apo®-Cloxi (Can) *see* cloxacillin *on page 141*

Apo®-Diazepam (Can) *see* diazepam *on page 173*

Apo®-Diclo (Can) *see* diclofenac *on page 175*

Apo-Diflunisal® (Can) *see* diflunisal *on page 179*

Apo®-Diltiaz (Can) *see* diltiazem *on page 182*

Apo®-Dimenhydrinate (Can) *see* dimenhydrinate *on page 182*

Apo®-Dipyridamole FC (Can) *see* dipyridamole *on page 188*

Apo®-Dipyridamole SC (Can) *see* dipyridamole *on page 188*

Apo®-Doxepin (Can) *see* doxepin *on page 195*

Apo®-Doxy (Can) *see* doxycycline *on page 197*

Apo®-Doxy Tabs (Can) *see* doxycycline *on page 197*

Apo®-Enalapril (Can) *see* enalapril *on page 206*

Apo®-Erythro E-C (Can) *see* erythromycin (systemic) *on page 215*

Apo®-Famotidine (Can) *see* famotidine *on page 231*

Apo-Ferrous® Gluconate (Can) *see* ferrous gluconate *on page 236*

Apo-Ferrous® Sulfate (Can) *see* ferrous sulfate *on page 237*

Apo®-Fluphenazine (Can) *see* fluphenazine *on page 247*

Apo®-Flurazepam (Can) *see* flurazepam *on page 248*

Apo®-Folic (Can) *see* folic acid *on page 251*

Apo®-Furosemide (Can) *see* furosemide *on page 255*
Apo®-Gain (Can) *see* minoxidil *on page 377*
Apo-Gemfibrozil® (Can) *see* gemfibrozil *on page 259*
Apo-Glyburide® (Can) *see* glyburide *on page 263*
Apo-Guanethidine® (Can) *see* guanethidine *on page 274*
Apo®-Hydralazine (Can) *see* hydralazine *on page 284*
Apo®-Hydro (Can) *see* hydrochlorothiazide *on page 286*
Apo®-Hydroxyzine (Can) *see* hydroxyzine *on page 297*
Apo®-Ibuprofen (Can) *see* ibuprofen *on page 300*
Apo®-Imipramine (Can) *see* imipramine *on page 302*
Apo®-Indomethacin (Can) *see* indomethacin *on page 305*
Apo-ISDN® (Can) *see* isosorbide dinitrate *on page 315*
Apo-Keto-E® (Can) *see* ketoprofen *on page 321*
Apo®-Lorazepam (Can) *see* lorazepam *on page 340*
Apo-Meprobamate® (Can) *see* meprobamate *on page 356*
Apo®-Methyldopa (Can) *see* methyldopa *on page 367*
Apo®-Metoclop (Can) *see* metoclopramide *on page 370*
Apo-Metoprolol® (Can) *see* metoprolol *on page 371*
Apo®-Metronidazole (Can) *see* metronidazole *on page 372*
Apo-Minocycline® (Can) *see* minocycline *on page 377*
Apomorphine *(Discontinued)* *see page 700*
Apo®-Nadol (Can) *see* nadolol *on page 387*
Apo®-Naproxen (Can) *see* naproxen *on page 391*
Apo®-Nifed (Can) *see* nifedipine *on page 402*
Apo®-Nitrofurantoin (Can) *see* nitrofurantoin *on page 403*
Apo-Oxazepam® (Can) *see* oxazepam *on page 420*
Apo®-Pen VK (Can) *see* penicillin V potassium *on page 435*
Apo-Pindol® (Can) *see* pindolol *on page 452*
Apo®-Piroxicam (Can) *see* piroxicam *on page 454*
Apo®-Prazo (Can) *see* prazosin *on page 470*
Apo®-Prednisone (Can) *see* prednisone *on page 472*
Apo®-Primidone (Can) *see* primidone *on page 474*
Apo®-Procainamide (Can) *see* procainamide *on page 475*
Apo®-Propranolol (Can) *see* propranolol *on page 483*
Apo®-Ranitidine (Can) *see* ranitidine hydrochloride *on page 497*
Apo®-Salvent (Can) *see* albuterol *on page 15*
Apo®-Sulfamethoxazole (Can) *see* sulfamethoxazole *on page 542*
Apo®-Sulfasalazine (Can) *see* sulfasalazine *on page 542*
Apo®-Sulfatrim (Can) *see* co-trimoxazole *on page 149*
Apo-Sulfinpyrazone® (Can) *see* sulfinpyrazone *on page 543*
Apo®-Sulin (Can) *see* sulindac *on page 544*
Apo-Tamox® (Can) *see* tamoxifen *on page 547*
Apo®-Terfenadine (Can) *see* terfenadine *on page 551*
Apo®-Tetra (Can) *see* tetracycline *on page 555*
Apo®-Thioridazine (Can) *see* thioridazine *on page 563*

Apo®-Timol (Can) *see* timolol *on page 567*

Apo®-Timop (Can) *see* timolol *on page 567*

Apo-Tolbutamide® (Can) *see* tolbutamide *on page 570*

Apo-Triazide® (Can) *see* hydrochlorothiazide and triamterene *on page 287*

Apo®-Triazo (Can) *see* triazolam *on page 579*

Apo®-Trihex (Can) *see* trihexyphenidyl *on page 581*

Apo-Trimip® (Can) *see* trimipramine *on page 583*

Apo®-Verap (Can) *see* verapamil *on page 598*

Apo®-Zidovudine (Can) *see* zidovudine *on page 610*

APPG *see* penicillin G procaine *on page 435*

apraclonidine (a pra KLOE ni deen)

U.S./Canadian Brand Names Iopidine®

Therapeutic Category Alpha$_2$-Adrenergic Agonist Agent, Ophthalmic

Use 1%: Prevention and treatment of postsurgical intraocular pressure elevation; 0.5%: Short-term adjunctive therapy in patients on maximally tolerated medical therapy who require additional redirection of intraocular pressure

Usual Dosage Adults: Ophthalmic: Instill 1 drop in operative eye 1 hour prior to laser surgery, second drop in eye upon completion of procedure

Dosage Forms Solution, ophthalmic, as hydrochloride: 0.5% (5 mL); 1% (0.1 mL, 0.25 mL)

Apresazide® *see* hydralazine and hydrochlorothiazide *on page 285*

Apresoline® *see* hydralazine *on page 284*

Aprodine® Syrup [OTC] *see* triprolidine and pseudoephedrine *on page 584*

Aprodine® Tablet [OTC] *see* triprolidine and pseudoephedrine *on page 584*

Aprodine® w/C *see* triprolidine, pseudoephedrine, and codeine *on page 585*

Apro-Flurbiprofen® (Can) *see* flurbiprofen *on page 248*

aprotinin (a proe TYE nin)

U.S./Canadian Brand Names Trasylol®

Therapeutic Category Hemostatic Agent

Use Reduction or prevention of blood loss in patients undergoing coronary artery bypass surgery when a high index of suspicion of excessive bleeding potential exists; this includes open heart reoperation, pre-existing coagulopathy, operations on the great vessels, and patients whose religious beliefs prohibit blood transfusions

Usual Dosage Test dose: **All** patients should receive a 1 mL I.V. test dose at least 10 minutes prior to the loading dose to assess the potential for allergic reactions

Regimen A (standard dose):
- 2 million units (280 mg) loading dose I.V. over 20-30 minutes
- 2 million units (280 mg) into pump prime volume
- 500,000 units/hour (70 mg/hour) I.V. during operation

Regimen B (low dose):
- 1 million units (140 mg) loading dose I.V. over 20-30 minutes
- 1 million units (140 mg) into pump prime volume
- 250,000 units/hour (35 mg/hour) I.V. during operation

Dosage Forms Injection: 1.4 mg/mL [10,000 units/mL] (100 mL, 200 mL)

APSAC *see* anistreplase *on page 38*

Aquacare® Topical [OTC] *see* urea *on page 591*

Aquachloral® Supprettes® *see* chloral hydrate *on page 115*

Aquacort® (Can) *see* hydrocortisone (topical) *on page 292*

AquaMEPHYTON® Injection *see* phytonadione *on page 451*

Aquaphyllin® *see* theophylline *on page 557*

AquaSite® Ophthalmic Solution [OTC] *see* artificial tears *on next page*

Aquasol A® *see* vitamin A *on page 602*

Aquasol E® [OTC] *see* vitamin E *on page 604*

AquaTar® [OTC] *see* coal tar *on page 141*

Aquatensen® *see* methyclothiazide *on page 366*

aqueous procaine penicillin G *see* penicillin G procaine *on page 435*

aqueous testosterone *see* testosterone *on page 552*

Aquest® *see* estrone *on page 220*

ARA-A *see* vidarabine *on page 600*

arabinofuranosyladenine *see* vidarabine *on page 600*

arabinosylcytosine *see* cytarabine *on page 156*

ARA-C *see* cytarabine *on page 156*

Aralen® Phosphate *see* chloroquine phosphate *on page 119*

Aralen® Phosphate With Primaquine Phosphate *see* chloroquine and primaquine *on page 118*

Aramine® *see* metaraminol *on page 360*

Arava™ *see* leflunomide *on page 327*

Arcotinic® Tablet *(Discontinued)* *see page 700*

ardeparin (ar dee PA rin)

U.S./Canadian Brand Names Normiflo®

Therapeutic Category Anticoagulant

Use Prevention of deep vein thrombosis (DVT) which may lead to pulmonary embolism following knee replacement surgery

Usual Dosage Adults: S.C.: 50 anti-Xa units every 12 hours

Dosage Forms Injection, as sodium: Anti-Xa units 5000 (0.5 mL); anti-Xa units 10,000 (0.5 mL)

Arduan® *see* pipecuronium *on page 453*

Aredia™ *see* pamidronate *on page 426*

Argesic®-SA *see* salsalate *on page 515*

arginine (AR ji neen)

U.S./Canadian Brand Names R-Gene®

Therapeutic Category Diagnostic Agent

Use Pituitary function test (growth hormone); management of severe, uncompensated, metabolic alkalosis (pH ≥7.55) **after** optimizing therapy with sodium, potassium, or ammonium chloride supplements

Usual Dosage I.V.:

Growth hormone (pituitary function) reserve test:

- Children: 500 mg (5 mL) kg/dose administered over 30 minutes
- Adults: 30 g (300 mL) administered over 30 minutes

Metabolic alkalosis: Children and Adults: Usual dose: 10 g/hour

Acid required (mEq) =

[1] 0.2 (L/kg) x wt (kg) x [103 - serum chloride] (mEq/L) **or**

[2] 0.3 (L/kg) x wt (kg) x base excess (mEq/L) **or**

[3] 0.5 (L/kg) x wt (kg) x [serum HCO_3 - 24] (mEq/L)

Administer $^1/_2$ to $^2/_3$ of calculated dose and re-evaluate

Note: Arginine hydrochloride should never be used as an alternative to chloride supplementation but used in the patient who is unresponsive to sodium chloride or potassium chloride supplementation

Dosage Forms Injection, as hydrochloride: 10% [100 mg/mL = 950 mOsm/L] (500 mL)

8-arginine vasopressin *see* vasopressin *on page 597*

Argyrol® S.S. *(Discontinued)* *see page 700*

Aricept® *see* donepezil *on page 193*

Arimidex® *see* anastrozole *on page 37*

Aristocort® A Topical *see* triamcinolone (topical) *on page 578*

Aristocort® Forte Injection *see* triamcinolone (systemic) *on page 577*

Aristocort® Intralesional Injection *see* triamcinolone (systemic) *on page 577*

Aristocort® Oral *see* triamcinolone (systemic) *on page 577*

Aristocort® Topical *see* triamcinolone (topical) *on page 578*

Aristospan® Intra-articular Injection *see* triamcinolone (systemic) *on page 577*

Aristospan® Intralesional Injection *see* triamcinolone (systemic) *on page 577*

Arlidin® *(Discontinued)* *see page 700*

Arm-a-Med® Isoetharine *see* isoetharine *on page 313*

Arm-a-Med® Isoproterenol *see* isoproterenol *on page 314*

Arm-a-Med® Metaproterenol *see* metaproterenol *on page 359*

A.R.M.® Caplet [OTC] *see* chlorpheniramine and phenylpropanolamine *on page 122*

Armour® Thyroid *see* thyroid *on page 564*

Aromatic Ammonia Aspirols® *see* ammonia spirit, aromatic *on page 30*

Arrestin® *see* trimethobenzamide *on page 582*

ARS *see* antirabies serum (equine) *on page 41*

Artane® *see* trihexyphenidyl *on page 581*

Artha-G® *see* salsalate *on page 515*

Arthritis Foundation® Ibuprofen *(Discontinued)* *see page 700*

Arthritis Foundation® Nighttime *(Discontinued)* *see page 700*

Arthritis Foundation® Pain Reliever, Aspirin Free *(Discontinued)* *see page 700*

Arthritis Strength Bufferin® *(Discontinued)* *see page 700*

Arthropan® [OTC] *see* choline salicylate *on page 129*

Arthrotec® *see* diclofenac and misoprostol *on page 176*

Articulose-50® Injection *(Discontinued)* *see page 700*

artificial tears (ar ti FISH il tears)

Synonyms polyvinyl alcohol

U.S./Canadian Brand Names Adsorbotear® Ophthalmic Solution [OTC]; Akwa Tears® Solution [OTC]; AquaSite® Ophthalmic Solution [OTC]; Bion® Tears Solution [OTC]; Comfort® Tears Solution [OTC]; Dakrina® Ophthalmic Solution [OTC]; Dry Eye® Therapy Solution [OTC]; Dry Eyes® Solution [OTC]; Dwelle® Ophthalmic Solution [OTC]; Eye-Lube-A® Solution [OTC]; HypoTears PF Solution [OTC]; HypoTears Solution [OTC]; Isopto® Plain Solution [OTC]; Isopto® Tears Solution [OTC]; Just Tears® Solution [OTC]; Lacril® Ophthalmic Solution [OTC]; Liquifilm® Tears Solution [OTC]; Liquifilm® Forte Solution [OTC]; LubriTears® Solution [OTC]; Moisture® Ophthalmic Drops [OTC]; Murine® Solution [OTC]; Murocel® Ophthalmic Solution [OTC]; Nature's Tears® Solution [OTC]; Nu-Tears® Solution [OTC]; Nu-Tears® II Solution [OTC]; OcuCoat® Ophthalmic Solution [OTC]; OcuCoat® PF Ophthalmic Solution [OTC]; Puralube® Tears Solution [OTC]; Refresh® Ophthalmic Solution [OTC]; Refresh® Plus Ophthalmic Solution [OTC]; Tear Drop® Solution [OTC]; TearGard® Ophthalmic Solution [OTC]; Teargen® Ophthalmic Solution [OTC]; Tearisol® Solution [OTC]; Tears Naturale® Free Solution

(Continued)

artificial tears *(Continued)*

[OTC]; Tears Naturale® II Solution [OTC]; Tears Naturale® Solution [OTC]; Tears Plus® Solution [OTC]; Tears Renewed® Solution [OTC]; Ultra Tears® Solution [OTC]; Viva-Drops® Solution [OTC]

Therapeutic Category Ophthalmic Agent, Miscellaneous

Use Ophthalmic lubricant; relief of dry eyes and eye irritation

Usual Dosage Ophthalmic: Use as needed to relieve symptoms, 1-2 drops into eye(s) 3-4 times/day

Dosage Forms Solution, ophthalmic: 15 mL and 30 mL with dropper

ASA *see* aspirin *on next page*

A.S.A. [OTC] *see* aspirin *on next page*

5-ASA *see* mesalamine *on page 358*

ASA® (Can) *see* aspirin *on next page*

Asacol® Oral *see* mesalamine *on page 358*

Asaphen (Can) *see* aspirin *on next page*

Asasantine® [with Aspirin also] (Can) *see* dipyridamole *on page 188*

Asasantine® (Can) *see* dipyridamole and aspirin *(Canada only)* *on page 188*

Asbron-G® Elixir *(Discontinued)* *see page 700*

Asbron-G® Tablet *(Discontinued)* *see page 700*

Ascorbic® 500 (Can) *see* ascorbic acid *on this page*

ascorbic acid (a SKOR bik AS id)

Synonyms vitamin C

U.S./Canadian Brand Names Apo®-C (Can); Ascorbic® 500 (Can); Ascorbicap® [OTC]; C-Crystals® [OTC]; Cebid®; Cecon® [OTC]; Cevalin® [OTC]; Cevi-bid® [OTC]; Ce-Vi-Sol® [OTC]; Dull-C® [OTC]; Duo-CVP® (Can); Flavorcee® [OTC]; N'ice®; Redoxon® (Can); Revitalose C-1000® (Can); Timecelles® [OTC]; Vita-C® [OTC]; Vitamin C Drops [OTC]

Therapeutic Category Vitamin, Water Soluble

Use Prevention and treatment of scurvy; urinary acidification; dietary supplementation; prevention and reduction in the severity of colds

Usual Dosage Oral, I.M., I.V., S.C.:

Recommended daily allowance (RDA):
- <6 months: 30 mg
- 6 months to 1 year: 35 mg
- 1-3 years: 40 mg
- 4-10 years: 45 mg
- 11-14 years: 50 mg
- >14 years and Adults: 60 mg

Children:
- Scurvy: 100-300 mg/day in divided doses for at least 2 weeks
- Urinary acidification: 500 mg every 6-8 hours
- Dietary supplement: 35-100 mg/day

Adults:
- Scurvy: 100-250 mg 1-2 times/day for at least 2 weeks
- Urinary acidification: 4-12 g/day in 3-4 divided doses
- Prevention and treatment of colds: 1-3 g/day
- Dietary supplement: 50-200 mg/day

Dosage Forms

Capsule, timed release: 500 mg
Crystals: 4 g/teaspoonful (100 g, 500 g); 5 g/teaspoonful (180 g)
Injection: 250 mg/mL (2 mL, 30 mL); 500 mg/mL (2 mL, 50 mL)
Liquid, oral: 35 mg/0.6 mL (50 mL)
Lozenges: 60 mg
Powder: 4 g/teaspoonful (100 g, 500 g)

Solution, oral: 100 mg/mL (50 mL)
Syrup: 500 mg/5 mL (5 mL, 10 mL, 120 mL, 480 mL)
Tablet: 25 mg, 50 mg, 100 mg, 250 mg, 500 mg, 1000 mg
Tablet:
 Chewable: 100 mg, 250 mg, 500 mg
 Timed release: 500 mg, 1000 mg, 1500 mg

ascorbic acid and ferrous sulfate *see* ferrous salt and ascorbic acid *on page 237*

Ascorbicap® [OTC] *see* ascorbic acid *on previous page*

Ascriptin® [OTC] *see* aspirin *on this page*

Asendin® *see* amoxapine *on page 31*

Asmalix® *see* theophylline *on page 557*

asparaginase (a SPIR a ji nase)

Synonyms colaspase

U.S./Canadian Brand Names Elspar®; Kidrolase® (Can)

Therapeutic Category Antineoplastic Agent

Use Treatment of acute lymphocytic leukemia, lymphoma; used for induction therapy

Usual Dosage Refer to individual protocols; the manufacturer recommends performing intradermal sensitivity testing before the initial dose

Children and Adults:
 I.M. (preferred route): 6000 units/m^2 3 times/week for 3 weeks for combination therapy
 I.V.: 1000 units/kg/day for 10 days for combination therapy or 200 units/kg/day for 28 days if combination therapy is inappropriate

Dosage Forms Injection: 10,000 units/vial

A-Spas® S/L *see* hyoscyamine *on page 297*

Aspergum® [OTC] *see* aspirin *on this page*

aspirin (AS pir in)

Synonyms acetylsalicylic acid; ASA

U.S./Canadian Brand Names Anacin® [OTC]; Apo®-ASA (Can); A.S.A. [OTC]; ASA® (Can); Asaphen (Can); Ascriptin® [OTC]; Aspergum® [OTC]; Bayer® Aspirin [OTC]; Bufferin® [OTC]; Easprin®; Ecotrin® [OTC]; Empirin® [OTC]; Entrophen® (Can); Halfprin® [OTC]; Measurin® [OTC]; MSD® Enteric Coated ASA (Can); Novasen (Can); ZORprin®

Therapeutic Category Analgesic, Non-narcotic; Antiplatelet Agent; Antipyretic; Nonsteroidal Anti-inflammatory Drug (NSAID)

Use Treatment of mild to moderate pain, inflammation and fever; adjunctive treatment of Kawasaki disease; may be used for prophylaxis of myocardial infarction and transient ischemic attacks (TIA)

Usual Dosage

Children:
 Analgesic and antipyretic: Oral, rectal: 10-15 mg/kg/dose every 4-6 hours
 Anti-inflammatory: Oral: Initial: 60-90 mg/kg/day in divided doses; usual maintenance: 80-100 mg/kg/day divided every 6-8 hours; monitor serum concentrations
 Kawasaki disease: Oral: 100 mg/kg/day divided every 6 hours; after fever resolves: 8-10 mg/kg/day once daily; monitor serum concentrations

Adults:
 Analgesic and antipyretic: Oral, rectal: 325-1000 mg every 4-6 hours up to 4 g/day
 Anti-inflammatory: Oral: Initial: 2.4-3.6 g/day in divided doses; usual maintenance: 3.6-5.4 g/day; monitor serum concentrations
 Transient ischemic attack: Oral: 1.3 g/day in 2-4 divided doses
 Myocardial infarction prophylaxis: 160-325 mg/day

Dosage Forms

Capsule: 356.4 mg and caffeine 30 mg
(Continued)

aspirin *(Continued)*

Suppository, rectal: 60 mg, 120 mg, 125 mg, 130 mg, 195 mg, 200 mg, 300 mg, 325 mg, 600 mg, 650 mg, 1.2 g
Tablet: 65 mg, 75 mg, 81 mg, 325 mg, 500 mg
Tablet: 400 mg and caffeine 32 mg
Tablet:
Buffered: 325 mg and magnesium-aluminum hydroxide 150 mg; 325 mg, magnesium hydroxide 75 mg, aluminum hydroxide 75 mg, buffered with calcium carbonate; 325 mg and magnesium-aluminum hydroxide 75 mg
Chewable: 81 mg
Controlled release: 800 mg
Delayed release: 81 mg
Enteric coated: 81 mg, 325 mg, 500 mg, 650 mg, 975 mg
Gum: 227.5 mg
Timed release: 650 mg

aspirin and butalbital compound *see* butalbital compound and aspirin *on page 85*

aspirin and codeine (AS pir in & KOE deen)

Synonyms codeine and aspirin
U.S./Canadian Brand Names Coryphen® Codeine (Can); Empirin® With Codeine
Therapeutic Category Analgesic, Narcotic
Controlled Substance C-III
Use Relief of mild to moderate pain
Usual Dosage Oral:
Children:
Aspirin: 10 mg/kg/dose every 4 hours
Codeine: 0.5-1 mg/kg/dose every 4 hours
Adults: 1-2 tablets every 4-6 hours as needed for pain
Dosage Forms Tablet:
#2: Aspirin 325 mg and codeine phosphate 15 mg
#3: Aspirin 325 mg and codeine phosphate 30 mg
#4: Aspirin 325 mg and codeine phosphate 60 mg

aspirin and hydrocodone *see* hydrocodone and aspirin *on page 288*

aspirin and meprobamate (AS pir in & me proe BA mate)

Synonyms meprobamate and aspirin
U.S./Canadian Brand Names Equagesic®
Therapeutic Category Skeletal Muscle Relaxant
Controlled Substance C-IV
Use Adjunct to treatment of skeletal muscular disease in patients exhibiting tension and/or anxiety
Usual Dosage Oral: 1 tablet 3-4 times/day
Dosage Forms Tablet: Aspirin 325 mg and meprobamate 200 mg

aspirin and methocarbamol *see* methocarbamol and aspirin *on page 363*

aspirin and oxycodone *see* oxycodone and aspirin *on page 423*

aspirin and propoxyphene *see* propoxyphene and aspirin *on page 482*

Aspirin-Free Bayer® Select® Allergy Sinus Caplets [OTC] *see* acetaminophen, chlorpheniramine, and pseudoephedrine *on page 6*

aspirin, orphenadrine, and caffeine *see* orphenadrine, aspirin, and caffeine *on page 418*

Asproject® ***(Discontinued)*** *see page 700*

Astelin® Nasal Spray *see* azelastine *on page 56*

AsthmaHaler® Mist [OTC] *see* epinephrine *on page 209*

AsthmaNefrin® [OTC] *see* epinephrine *on page 209*

Astramorph™ PF Injection *see* morphine sulfate *on page 382*

Atabrine® Tablet *(Discontinued)* *see page 700*

Atacand™ *see* candesartan *on page 94*

Atarax® Oral *see* hydroxyzine *on page 297*

Atasol® 8, 15, 30 W/ Caffeine (Can) *see* acetaminophen and codeine *on page 4*

Atasol® (Can) *see* acetaminophen *on page 3*

atenolol (a TEN oh lole)

U.S./Canadian Brand Names Apo®-Atenol (Can); Novo-Atenol® (Can); Nu-Atenol® (Can); Taro-Atenol® (Can); Tenormin®

Therapeutic Category Beta-Adrenergic Blocker

Use Treatment of hypertension, alone or in combination with other agents; management of angina pectoris; antiarrhythmic; postmyocardial infarction patients; acute alcohol withdrawal

Usual Dosage

Oral:

Children: 1-2 mg/kg/dose administered daily

Adults:

Hypertension: 50 mg once daily, may increase to 100 mg/day; doses >100 mg are unlikely to produce any further benefit

Angina pectoris: 50 mg once daily, may increase to 100 mg/day; some patients may require 200 mg/day

Postmyocardial infarction: Follow I.V. dose with 100 mg/day or 50 mg twice daily for 6-9 days postmyocardial infarction

I.V.: Postmyocardial infarction: Early treatment: 5 mg slow I.V. over 5 minutes; may repeat in 10 minutes; if both doses are tolerated, may start oral atenolol 50 mg every 12 hours or 100 mg/day for 6-9 days postmyocardial infarction

Dosage Forms

Injection: 0.5 mg/mL (10 mL)

Tablet: 25 mg, 50 mg, 100 mg

atenolol and chlorthalidone (a TEN oh lole & klor THAL i done)

Synonyms chlorthalidone and atenolol

U.S./Canadian Brand Names Tenoretic®

Therapeutic Category Antihypertensive Agent, Combination

Use Treatment of hypertension with a cardioselective beta-blocker and a diuretic

Usual Dosage Adults: Oral: Initial: 1 tablet (50) once daily, then individualize dose until optimal dose is achieved

Dosage Forms Tablet:

50: Atenolol 50 mg and chlorthalidone 25 mg

100: Atenolol 100 mg and chlorthalidone 25 mg

ATG *see* lymphocyte immune globulin *on page 343*

Atgam® *see* lymphocyte immune globulin *on page 343*

ATIII *see* antithrombin III *on page 41*

Ativan® *see* lorazepam *on page 340*

ATnativ® *see* antithrombin III *on page 41*

Atolone® Oral *see* triamcinolone (systemic) *on page 577*

atorvastatin (a TORE va sta tin)

U.S./Canadian Brand Names Lipitor®

Therapeutic Category HMG-CoA Reductase Inhibitor

(Continued)

atorvastatin *(Continued)*

Use Adjunct to diet for the reduction of elevated total and LDL-cholesterol levels in patients with hypercholesterolemia (Type IIa, IIb, and IIc); used in hypercholesterolemic patients without clinically evident heart disease to reduce the risk of myocardial infarction, to reduce the risk for revascularization, and reduce the risk of death due to cardiovascular causes with no increase in death from noncardiovascular diseases

Usual Dosage Adults: Oral: Initial: 10 mg/day, with a range of 10-80 mg/day, administered as a single dose at any time of day, with or without food

Dosage Forms Tablet: 10 mg, 20 mg, 40 mg

atovaquone (a TOE va kwone)

U.S./Canadian Brand Names Mepron™

Therapeutic Category Antiprotozoal

Use Acute oral treatment of mild to moderate *Pneumocystis carinii* pneumonia (PCP) in patients who are intolerant to co-trimoxazole

Usual Dosage Adults: Oral: 750 mg twice daily with food for 21 days

Dosage Forms Suspension, oral (citrus flavor): 750 mg/5 mL (210 mL)

Atozine® Oral *see* hydroxyzine *on page 297*

atracurium (a tra KYOO ree um)

U.S./Canadian Brand Names Tracrium®

Therapeutic Category Skeletal Muscle Relaxant

Use Eases endotracheal intubation as an adjunct to general anesthesia and relaxes skeletal muscle during surgery or mechanical ventilation

Usual Dosage I.V.:

Children 1 month to 2 years: Initial: 0.3-0.4 mg/kg followed by maintenance doses of 0.08-0.1 mg/kg as needed to maintain neuromuscular blockade

Children >2 years to Adults: Initial: 0.4-0.5 mg/kg then 0.08-0.1 mg/kg every 20-45 minutes after initial dose to maintain neuromuscular block

Continuous infusion: 0.4-0.8 mg/kg/hour

Dosage Forms Atracurium besylate:

Injection: 10 mg/mL (5 mL, 10 mL)

Injection, preservative-free: 10 mg/mL (5 mL)

Atrohist® Plus *see* chlorpheniramine, phenylephrine, phenylpropanolamine, and belladonna alkaloids *on page 124*

Atromid-S® *see* clofibrate *on page 138*

Atropair® *see* atropine *on this page*

atropine (A troe peen)

U.S./Canadian Brand Names Atropair®; Atropine-Care®; Atropisol®; Isopto® Atropine; I-Tropine®

Therapeutic Category Anticholinergic Agent

Use Preoperative medication to inhibit salivation and secretions; treatment of sinus bradycardia; management of peptic ulcer; treatment of exercise-induced bronchospasm; antidote for organophosphate pesticide poisoning; used to produce mydriasis and cycloplegia for examination of the retina and optic disk and accurate measurement of refractive errors; treatment of uveitis

Usual Dosage

Preanesthesia: I.M., I.V., S.C.:

Infants:

<5 kg: 0.04 mg/kg/dose repeated every 4-6 hours as needed

>5 kg: 0.03 mg/kg/dose repeated every 4-6 hours as needed

Children: 0.01 mg/kg/dose up to a maximum of 0.4 mg/dose; repeat every 4-6 hours as needed

Adults: 0.5 mg/dose repeated every 4-6 hours as needed

Bronchodilation:
Children:
Oral: 0.02 mg/kg/dose 3 times/day
Inhalation: 0.03-0.05 mg/kg/dose 3-4 times/day
Adults: Inhalation: 0.025-0.05 mg/kg/dose over 10 minutes, repeated every 4-5 hours as needed
Cardiopulmonary resuscitation (bradycardia): I.T., I.V.:
Infants: 0.02-0.04 mg/kg/dose; repeat every 2-5 minutes, if needed, up to 2-3 times
Children: 0.01-0.02 mg/kg/dose; repeat every 2-5 minutes, if needed, up to 2-3 times; minimum dose should be 0.1 mg (smaller doses may cause paradoxic bradycardia); maximum total dose is 1 mg (2 mg for adolescents)
Adults: 0.5 mg/dose; repeat every 5 minutes, if needed, up to 2-3 times for a maximum total dose of 2 mg
Organophosphate or carbamate poisoning: I.V.:
Children: 0.02-0.05 mg/kg/dose every 10-20 minutes until atropine effect (dry flushed skin, tachycardia, mydriasis, fever) is observed, then every 1-4 hours to maintain atropine effect for at least 24 hours
Children >12 years and Adults: 1-2 mg/dose every 10-20 minutes until atropine effect (see above) is observed, then 1-3 mg/dose every 1-4 hours, as needed to maintain atropine effect for at least 24 hours
Neuromuscular blockade reversal: I.V.:
Before neostigmine: Administer 25-30 mcg/kg (0.025-0.03 mg/kg) 30 seconds before neostigmine (0.07-0.08 mg/kg)
Before edrophonium: 10 mcg/kg (0.01 mg/kg) 30 seconds before edrophonium (1 mg/kg)

Note: May contain benzyl alcohol as a preservative; administration of benzyl alcohol in doses ranging from 99-234 mg/kg has been associated with a fatal gasping syndrome in neonates; clinical signs of this syndrome include metabolic acidosis, hypotension, CNS depression, and cardiovascular collapse

Dosage Forms Atropine sulfate:
Injection: 0.1 mg/mL (5 mL, 10 mL); 0.3 mg/mL (1 mL, 30 mL); 0.4 mg/mL (1 mL, 20 mL, 30 mL); 0.5 mg/mL (1 mL, 5 mL, 30 mL); 0.8 mg/mL (0.5 mL, 1 mL); 1 mg/mL (1 mL, 10 mL)
Ointment, ophthalmic: 0.5%, 1% (3.5 g)
Solution, ophthalmic: 0.5% (1 mL, 5 mL); 1% (1 mL, 2 mL, 5 mL, 15 mL); 2% (1 mL, 2 mL); 3% (5 mL)
Tablet: 0.4 mg

atropine and difenoxin *see* difenoxin and atropine *on page 178*

atropine and diphenoxylate *see* diphenoxylate and atropine *on page 186*

Atropine-Care® *see* atropine *on previous page*

atropine, hyoscyamine, scopolamine, and phenobarbital *see* hyoscyamine, atropine, scopolamine, and phenobarbital *on page 298*

Atropine Soluble Tablet *(Discontinued)* *see page 700*

Atropisol® *see* atropine *on previous page*

Atrovent® *see* ipratropium *on page 311*

A/T/S® Topical *see* erythromycin (ophthalmic/topical) *on page 214*

attapulgite (at a PULL gite)

U.S./Canadian Brand Names Children's Kaopectate® [OTC]; Diasorb® [OTC]; Kaopectate® Advanced Formula [OTC]; Kaopectate® Maximum Strength Caplets; Rheaban® [OTC]

Therapeutic Category Antidiarrheal

Use Treatment of uncomplicated diarrhea

Usual Dosage Oral:
Children:
<3 years: Not recommended
(Continued)

attapulgite *(Continued)*

3-6 years: 750 mg/dose up to 2250 mg/24 hours
6-12 years: 1200-1500 mg/dose up to 4500 mg/24 hours
Adults: 1200-1500 mg after each loose bowel movement or every 2 hours; 15-30 mL up to 8 times/day, up to 9000 mg/24 hours

Dosage Forms
Liquid, oral concentrate: 600 mg/15 mL (180 mL, 240 mL, 360 mL, 480 mL); 750 mg/15 mL (120 mL)
Tablet: 750 mg
Chewable: 300 mg, 600 mg

Attenuvax® *see* measles virus vaccine, live *on page 350*
Augmentin® *see* amoxicillin and clavulanate potassium *on page 32*
Auralgan® *see* antipyrine and benzocaine *on page 41*

auranofin (au RANE oh fin)

U.S./Canadian Brand Names Ridaura®
Therapeutic Category Gold Compound
Use Management of active stage of classic or definite rheumatoid or psoriatic arthritis in patients that do not respond to or tolerate other agents
Usual Dosage Oral:
Children: Initial: 0.1 mg/kg/day divided daily; usual maintenance: 0.15 mg/kg/day in 1-2 divided doses; maximum: 0.2 mg/kg/day in 1-2 divided doses
Adults: 6 mg/day in 1-2 divided doses; after 3 months may be increased to 9 mg/day in 3 divided doses; if still no response after 3 months at 9 mg/day, discontinue drug
Dosage Forms Capsule: 3 mg [gold 29%]

Aureomycin® *(Discontinued)* *see page 700*
Auro® Ear Drops [OTC] *see* carbamide peroxide *on page 98*
Aurolate® *see* gold sodium thiomalate *on page 265*

aurothioglucose (aur oh thye oh GLOO kose)

U.S./Canadian Brand Names Solganal®
Therapeutic Category Gold Compound
Use Management of active stage of classic or definite rheumatoid or psoriatic arthritis in patients that do not respond to or tolerate other agents
Usual Dosage I.M. (doses should initially be administered at weekly intervals):
Children 6-12 years: Initial: 0.25 mg/kg/dose first week; increment at 0.25 mg/kg/dose increasing with each weekly dose; maintenance: 0.75-1 mg/kg/dose weekly not to exceed 25 mg/dose to a total of 20 doses, then every 2-4 weeks
Adults: 10 mg first week; 25 mg second and third week; then 50 mg/week until 800 mg to 1 g cumulative dose has been administered - if improvement occurs without adverse reactions, administer 25-50 mg every 2-3 weeks, then every 3-4 weeks
Dosage Forms Injection, suspension: 50 mg/mL [gold 50%] (10 mL)

Auroto® *see* antipyrine and benzocaine *on page 41*
Autoplex® T *see* anti-inhibitor coagulant complex *on page 40*
Avandia® *see* rosiglitazone *on page 510*
Avapro® *see* irbesartan *on page 312*
Avapro® HCT *see* irbesartan and hydrochlorothiazide *on page 312*
AVC™ Cream *see* sulfanilamide *on page 542*
AVC™ Suppository *see* sulfanilamide *on page 542*
Aveeno® Cleansing Bar [OTC] *see* sulfur and salicylic acid *on page 543*
Aventyl® Hydrochloride *see* nortriptyline *on page 408*

Avirax™ (Can) *see* acyclovir *on page 11*

Avitene® *see* microfibrillar collagen hemostat *on page 374*

Avlosulfon® *see* dapsone *on page 159*

Avonex™ *see* Interferon beta-1a *on page 309*

Axid® *see* nizatidine *on page 405*

Axid® AR [OTC] *see* nizatidine *on page 405*

Axocet® *see* butalbital compound and acetaminophen *on page 85*

Axotal® ***(Discontinued)*** *see page 700*

Ayercillin® (Can) *see* penicillin G procaine *on page 435*

Aygestin® *see* norethindrone *on page 406*

Ayr® Nasal [OTC] *see* sodium chloride *on page 526*

azacitidine (ay za SYE ti deen)

Synonyms AZA-CR; 5-azacytidine; 5-AZC; ladakamycin

U.S./Canadian Brand Names Mylosar®

Therapeutic Category Antineoplastic Agent

Use Refractory acute lymphocytic and myelogenous leukemia

Usual Dosage Children and Adults: I.V.: 200-300 mg/m^2/day for 5-10 days, repeated at 2- to 3-week intervals

Dosage Forms Injection: 100 mg

AZA-CR *see* azacitidine *on this page*

Azactam® *see* aztreonam *on page 57*

5-azacytidine *see* azacitidine *on this page*

azatadine (a ZA ta deen)

U.S./Canadian Brand Names Optimine®

Therapeutic Category Antihistamine

Use Treatment of perennial and seasonal allergic rhinitis and chronic urticaria

Usual Dosage Children >12 years and Adults: Oral: 1-2 mg twice daily

Dosage Forms Tablet, as maleate: 1 mg

azatadine and pseudoephedrine (a ZA ta deen & soo doe e FED rin)

Synonyms pseudoephedrine and azatadine

U.S./Canadian Brand Names Rynatan®; Trinalin®

Therapeutic Category Antihistamine/Decongestant Combination

Use Perennial and seasonal allergic rhinitis and other allergic symptoms including urticaria

Usual Dosage Adults: 1 tablet twice daily

Dosage Forms Tablet: Azatadine maleate 1 mg and pseudoephedrine sulfate 120 mg

azathioprine (ay za THYE oh preen)

U.S./Canadian Brand Names Imuran®

Therapeutic Category Immunosuppressant Agent

Use Adjunct with other agents in prevention of transplant rejection; also used as an immunosuppressant in a variety of autoimmune diseases such as systemic lupus erythematosus, severe rheumatoid arthritis unresponsive to other agents, and nephrotic syndrome

Usual Dosage

Children and Adults: Renal transplantation: Oral, I.V.: Initial: 3-5 mg/kg/day; maintenance: 1-3 mg/kg/day

Adults: Rheumatoid arthritis: Oral: 1 mg/kg/day for 6-8 weeks; increase by 0.5 mg/kg every 4 weeks until response or up to 2.5 mg/kg/day I.V. dose is equivalent to oral dose

Dosage Forms Azathioprine sodium:

Injection: 100 mg (20 mL)

(Continued)

azathioprine *(Continued)*

Tablet (scored): 50 mg

5-AZC *see* azacitidine *on previous page*

Azdone® *see* hydrocodone and aspirin *on page 288*

azelaic acid (a zeh LAY ik AS id)

U.S./Canadian Brand Names Azelex®

Therapeutic Category Topical Skin Product

Use Treatment of mild to moderate acne vulgaris

Usual Dosage Adults: Topical: After skin is thoroughly washed and patted dry, gently but thoroughly massage a thin film of azelaic acid cream into the affected areas twice daily, in the morning and evening. The duration of use can vary and depends on the severity of the acne. In the majority of patients with inflammatory lesions, improvement of the condition occurs within 4 weeks.

Dosage Forms Cream: 20% (30 g)

azelastine (a ZEL as teen)

U.S./Canadian Brand Names Astelin® Nasal Spray

Therapeutic Category Antihistamine

Use Seasonal allergic rhinitis

Usual Dosage Children ≥12 years and Adults: Nasal: 2 sprays in each nostril twice daily

Dosage Forms Spray, nasal, as hydrochloride: 137 mcg/actuation [100 actuations/bottle]

Azelex® *see* azelaic acid *on this page*

azidothymidine *see* zidovudine *on page 610*

azithromycin (az ith roe MYE sin)

U.S./Canadian Brand Names Zithromax™

Therapeutic Category Macrolide (Antibiotic)

Use

Children: Treatment of acute otitis media due to *H. influenzae*, *M. catarrhalis* or *S. pneumoniae*; pharyngitis/tonsillitis due to *S. pyogenes*

Adults:

Treatment of mild to moderate upper and lower respiratory tract infections, infections of the skin and skin structure, and sexually transmitted diseases due to susceptible strains of *C. trachomatis*, *M. catarrhalis*, *H. influenzae*, *S. aureus*, *S. pneumoniae*, *Mycoplasma pneumoniae*, and *C. psittaci*; community-acquired pneumonia, pelvic inflammatory disease (PID)

For preventing or delaying the onset of infection with *Mycobacterium avium* complex (MAC)

Usual Dosage Oral:

Children:

Acute otitis media: 10 mg/kg on day 1 (not to exceed 500 mg/day) followed by 5 mg/kg/day once daily on days 2-5 (not to exceed 250 mg/day)

Pharyngitis/tonsillitis: 12 mg/kg/day for 5 days (not to exceed 500 mg/day)

Adolescents ≥16 years and Adults:

Mild to moderate respiratory tract, skin, and soft tissue infections: 500 mg in a single dose on day 1; 250 mg in a single dose on days 2-5

Nongonococcal urethritis and cervicitis: 1 g in a single dose

Chancroid and *Chlamydia*: 1 g in a single dose

I.V.: Adults:

Community-acquired pneumonia: 500 mg as a single dose for at least 2 days, follow I.V. therapy by the oral route with a single daily dose of 500 mg to complete a 7- to 10-day course of therapy

Pelvic inflammatory disease (PID): 500 mg as a single dose for 1-2 days, follow I.V. therapy by the oral route with a single daily dose of 250 mg to complete a 7-day course of therapy

Dosage Forms Azithromycin dihydrate:

Capsule: 250 mg

Capsule (Z-PAK®): 6 capsules per package: 250 mg

Powder for oral suspension: 100 mg/5 mL (15 mL); 200 mg/5 mL (15 mL, 22.5 mL); 1 g (single-dose packet)

Tablet: 250 mg, 600 mg

Azlin® Injection *(Discontinued)* *see page 700*

Azmacort™ Oral Inhaler *see* triamcinolone (inhalation, oral) *on page 577*

Azo Gantanol® *(Discontinued)* *see page 700*

Azo Gantrisin® *(Discontinued)* *see page 700*

Azopt® *see* brinzolamide *on page 79*

Azo-Standard® *see* phenazopyridine *on page 442*

AZT *see* zidovudine *on page 610*

AZT + 3TC *see* zidovudine and lamivudine *on page 611*

azthreonam *see* aztreonam *on this page*

aztreonam (AZ tree oh nam)

Synonyms azthreonam

U.S./Canadian Brand Names Azactam®

Therapeutic Category Antibiotic, Miscellaneous

Use Treatment of patients with documented multidrug resistant aerobic gram-negative infection in which beta-lactam therapy is contraindicated; used for urinary tract infection, lower respiratory tract infections, septicemia, skin/skin structure infections, intra-abdominal infections and gynecological infections caused by susceptible *Enterobacteriaceae*, *H. influenzae*, and *P. aeruginosa*

Usual Dosage

Children >1 month: I.M., I.V.: 90-120 mg/kg/day divided every 6-8 hours

Cystic fibrosis: 50 mg/kg/dose every 6-8 hours (ie, up to 200 mg/kg/day); maximum: 6-8 g/day

Adults:

Urinary tract infection: I.M., I.V.: 500 mg to 1 g every 8-12 hours

Moderately severe systemic infections: 1 g I.V. or I.M. or 2 g I.V. every 8-12 hours

Severe systemic or life-threatening infections (especially caused by *Pseudomonas aeruginosa*): I.V.: 2 g every 6-8 hours; maximum: 8 g/day

Dosage Forms Powder for injection: 500 mg (15 mL, 100 mL); 1 g (15 mL, 100 mL); 2 g (15 mL, 100 mL)

Azulfidine® *see* sulfasalazine *on page 542*

Azulfidine® EN-tabs® *see* sulfasalazine *on page 542*

Azulfidine® Suspension *(Discontinued)* *see page 700*

Babee® Teething® [OTC] *see* benzocaine *on page 66*

BAC *see* benzalkonium chloride *on page 66*

bacampicillin (ba kam pi SIL in)

Synonyms carampicillin

U.S./Canadian Brand Names Spectrobid® Tablet

Therapeutic Category Penicillin

Use Treatment of susceptible bacterial infections involving the urinary tract, skin structure, upper and lower respiratory tract; activity is identical to that of ampicillin

Usual Dosage Oral:

Children: 25-50 mg/kg/day in divided doses every 12 hours

(Continued)

bacampicillin *(Continued)*

Adults: 400-800 mg every 12 hours

Dosage Forms Bacampicillin hydrochloride:

Tablet: 400 mg [chemically equivalent to ampicillin 280 mg]

B-A-C® *(Discontinued)* *see page 700*

Bacid® [OTC] *see* Lactobacillus *on page 324*

Baciguent® Topical [OTC] *see* bacitracin *on this page*

Baci-IM® Injection *see* bacitracin *on this page*

Bacillus Calmette-Guérin (BCG) Live *see* BCG vaccine *on page 61*

Bacimyxin (Can) *see* bacitracin and polymyxin B *on this page*

Bacitin (Can) *see* bacitracin *on this page*

bacitracin (bas i TRAY sin)

U.S./Canadian Brand Names AK-Tracin® Ophthalmic; Baciguent® Topical [OTC]; Baci-IM® Injection; Bacitin (Can)

Therapeutic Category Antibiotic, Ophthalmic; Antibiotic, Topical; Antibiotic, Miscellaneous

Use Treatment of pneumonia and emphysema caused by susceptible staphylococci; prevention or treatment of superficial skin infections or infections of the eye caused by susceptible organisms; due to its toxicity, use of bacitracin systemically or as an irrigant should be limited to situations where less toxic alternatives would not be effective; treatment of antibiotic-associated colitis

Usual Dosage I.M. recommended; **do not administer I.V.**:

Infants:

<2.5 kg: 900 units/kg/day in 2-3 divided doses

>2.5 kg: 1000 units/kg/day in 2-3 divided doses

Children: 800-1200 units/kg/day divided every 8 hours

Adults: 10,000-25,000 units/dose every 6 hours; not to exceed 100,000 units/day

Topical: Apply 1-5 times/day

Ophthalmic ointment: 1/4" to 1/2" ribbon every 3-4 hours to conjunctival sac for acute infections or 2-3 times/day for mild to moderate infections for 7-10 days

Irrigation, solution: 50-100 units/mL in normal saline, lactated Ringer's, or sterile water for irrigation; soak sponges in solution for topical compresses 1-5 times/day or as needed during surgical procedures

Dosage Forms

Injection: 50,000 units

Ointment:

Ophthalmic: 500 units/g (3.5 g, 3.75 g)

AK-Tracin®: 500 units/g (3.5 g)

Topical: 500 units/g (1.5 g, 3.75 g, 15 g, 30 g, 120 g, 454 g)

bacitracin and polymyxin B (bas i TRAY sin & pol i MIKS in bee)

Synonyms polymyxin B and bacitracin

U.S./Canadian Brand Names AK-Poly-Bac® Ophthalmic; Bacimyxin (Can); Betadine® First Aid Antibiotics + Moisturizer [OTC]; Bioderm (Can); Polysporin® Ophthalmic; Polysporin® Topical; Polytopic® (Can); Polytracin® (Can)

Therapeutic Category Antibiotic, Ophthalmic; Antibiotic, Topical

Use Treatment of superficial infections involving the conjunctiva and/or cornea caused by susceptible organisms; prevent infection in minor cuts, scrapes and burns

Usual Dosage

Ophthalmic: Apply 1/2" ribbon to the affected eye(s) every 3-4 hours

Topical: Apply to affected area 1-3 times/day; may cover with sterile bandage if needed

Dosage Forms

Ointment:

Ophthalmic: Bacitracin 500 units and polymyxin B sulfate 10,000 units per g (3.5 g)

Topical: Bacitracin 500 units and polymyxin B sulfate 10,000 units per g in white petrolatum (15 g, 30 g)

Powder: Bacitracin 500 units and polymyxin B sulfate 10,000 units per g (10 g)

bacitracin, neomycin, and polymyxin B

(bas i TRAY sin, nee oh MYE sin & pol i MIKS in bee)

Synonyms neomycin, bacitracin, and polymyxin B; polymyxin B, bacitracin, and neomycin

U.S./Canadian Brand Names AK-Spore® Ophthalmic Ointment; Medi-Quick® Topical Ointment [OTC]; Mycitracin® Topical [OTC]; Neomixin® Topical; Neosporin® Ophthalmic Ointment; Neosporin® Topical Ointment [OTC]; Neotopic® (Can); Ocutricin® Topical Ointment; Septa® Topical Ointment [OTC]; Triple Antibiotic® Topical

Therapeutic Category Antibiotic, Ophthalmic; Antibiotic, Topical

Use Help prevent infection in minor cuts, scrapes and burns; short-term treatment of superficial external ocular infections caused by susceptible organisms

Usual Dosage Children and Adults:

Ophthalmic ointment: Instill into the conjunctival sac one or more times/day every 3-4 hours for 7-10 days

Topical: Apply 1-3 times/day

Dosage Forms Ointment:

Ophthalmic: Bacitracin 400 units, neomycin sulfate 3.5 mg, and polymyxin B sulfate 10,000 units and per g

Topical: Bacitracin 400 units, neomycin sulfate 3.5 mg, and polymyxin B sulfate 5000 units per g

bacitracin, neomycin, polymyxin B, and hydrocortisone

(bas i TRAY sin, nee oh MYE sin, pol i MIKS in bee & hye droe KOR ti sone)

Synonyms hydrocortisone, bacitracin, neomycin, and polymyxin B; neomycin, bacitracin, polymyxin B, and hydrocortisone; polymyxin B, bacitracin, neomycin, and hydrocortisone

U.S./Canadian Brand Names AK-Spore® H.C. Ophthalmic Ointment; Cortisporin® Ophthalmic Ointment; Cortisporin® Topical Ointment; Neotricin HC® Ophthalmic Ointment

Therapeutic Category Antibiotic/Corticosteroid, Ophthalmic; Antibiotic/Corticosteroid, Topical

Use Prevention and treatment of susceptible superficial topical infections

Usual Dosage

Ophthalmic ointment: Apply ½" ribbon to inside of lower lid every 3-4 hours until improvement occurs

Topical: Apply sparingly 2-4 times/day

Dosage Forms Ointment:

Ophthalmic: Bacitracin 400 units, neomycin sulfate 3.5 mg, polymyxin B sulfate 10,000 units, and hydrocortisone 10 mg per g (3.5 g)

Topical: Bacitracin 400 units, neomycin sulfate 3.5 mg, polymyxin B sulfate 10,000 units, and hydrocortisone 10 mg per g (15 g)

bacitracin, neomycin, polymyxin B, and lidocaine

(bas i TRAY sin, nee oh MYE sin, pol i MIKS in bee & LYE doe kane)

U.S./Canadian Brand Names Clomycin® [OTC]

Therapeutic Category Antibiotic, Topical

Use Prevention and treatment of susceptible superficial topical infections

Usual Dosage Adults: Topical: Apply 1-4 times/day to infected areas; cover with sterile bandage if needed

Dosage Forms Ointment, topical: Bacitracin 500 units, neomycin base 3.5 g, polymyxin B sulfate 5000 units, and lidocaine 40 mg per g (28.35 g)

baclofen (BAK loe fen)

U.S./Canadian Brand Names Alpha-Baclofen® (Can); Lioresal®; PMS-Baclofen (Can)

Therapeutic Category Skeletal Muscle Relaxant

(Continued)

baclofen *(Continued)*

Use Treatment of reversible spasticity associated with multiple sclerosis or spinal cord lesions; intrathecal use for the management of spasticity in patients who are unresponsive to oral baclofen or experience intolerable CNS side effects; treatment of trigeminal neuralgia; adjunctive treatment of tardive dyskinesia

Usual Dosage

Oral:

Children:

2-7 years: Initial: 10-15 mg/24 hours divided every 8 hours; titrate dose every 3 days in increments of 5-15 mg/day to a maximum of 40 mg/day

≥8 years: Maximum: 60 mg/day in 3 divided doses

Adults: 5 mg 3 times/day, may increase 5 mg/dose every 3 days to a maximum of 80 mg/day

Intrathecal:

Test dose: 50-100 mcg, doses >50 mcg should be administered in 25 mcg increments, separated by 24 hours

Maintenance: After positive response to test dose, a maintenance intrathecal infusion can be administered via an implanted intrathecal pump. Initial dose via pump: Infusion at a 24-hourly rate dosed at twice the test dose.

Dosage Forms

Injection, intrathecal, preservative free: 500 mcg/mL (20 mL); 2000 mcg/mL (5 mL)

Tablet: 10 mg, 20 mg

Bactigras® (Chlorhexadine Acetate) (Can) *see* chlorhexidine gluconate *on page 117*

Bactine® Hydrocortisone [OTC] *see* hydrocortisone (topical) *on page 292*

Bactocill® ***(Discontinued)*** *see page 700*

BactoShield® [OTC] *see* chlorhexidine gluconate *on page 117*

Bactrim™ *see* co-trimoxazole *on page 149*

Bactrim™ DS *see* co-trimoxazole *on page 149*

Bactroban® *see* mupirocin *on page 384*

Bactroban® Nasal *see* mupirocin *on page 384*

Baker's P&S Topical [OTC] *see* phenol *on page 444*

baking soda *see* sodium bicarbonate *on page 525*

BAL *see* dimercaprol *on page 183*

balanced salt solution (BAL anced salt soe LOO shun)

U.S./Canadian Brand Names BSS® Ophthalmic

Therapeutic Category Ophthalmic Agent, Miscellaneous

Use Intraocular irrigating solution; also used to soothe and cleanse the eye in conjunction with hard contact lenses

Usual Dosage Use as needed for foreign body removal, gonioscopy, and other general ophthalmic office procedures

Dosage Forms Ophthalmic:

Drops: 15 mL

Solution, sterile: 500 mL

Baldex® *see* dexamethasone (ophthalmic) *on page 167*

BAL in Oil® *see* dimercaprol *on page 183*

Balminil® Decongestant (Can) *see* pseudoephedrine *on page 486*

Balminil®-DM, -DM Children (Can) *see* dextromethorphan *on page 171*

Balminil® Expectorant (Can) *see* guaifenesin *on page 267*

Balnetar® [OTC] *see* coal tar, lanolin, and mineral oil *on page 142*

Balnetar® (Can) *see* coal tar *on page 141*

Bancap® ***(Discontinued)*** *see page 700*

Bancap HC® *see* hydrocodone and acetaminophen *on page 287*

Banesin® ***(Discontinued)*** *see page 700*

Banophen® Decongestant Capsule [OTC] *see* diphenhydramine and pseudoephedrine *on page 185*

Banophen® Oral [OTC] *see* diphenhydramine *on page 185*

Banthine® *see* methantheline *on page 362*

Bantron® ***(Discontinued)*** *see page 700*

Bapadin® (Can) *see* bepridil *on page 70*

Barbidonna® *see* hyoscyamine, atropine, scopolamine, and phenobarbital *on page 298*

Barbilixir® (Can) *see* phenobarbital *on page 443*

Barbita® *see* phenobarbital *on page 443*

Barc™ Liquid [OTC] *see* pyrethrins *on page 489*

Baricon® *see* radiological/contrast media (ionic) *on page 495*

Baridium® *see* phenazopyridine *on page 442*

Barobag® *see* radiological/contrast media (ionic) *on page 495*

Baro-CAT® *see* radiological/contrast media (ionic) *on page 495*

Baroflave® *see* radiological/contrast media (ionic) *on page 495*

Barosperse® *see* radiological/contrast media (ionic) *on page 495*

Bar-Test® *see* radiological/contrast media (ionic) *on page 495*

Basaljel® [OTC] *see* aluminum carbonate *on page 22*

basiliximab (ba si LIKS i mab)

U.S./Canadian Brand Names Simulect®

Therapeutic Category Immunosuppressant Agent

Use Prophylaxis of acute organ rejection in renal transplantation

Usual Dosage I.V.:

Children: 12 mg/m^2 (maximum: 20 mg) within 2 hours prior to transplant surgery, followed by a second dose of 12 mg/m^2 (maximum: 20 mg) 4 days after transplantation

Adults: 20 mg within 2 hours prior to transplant surgery, followed by a second 20 mg dose 4 days after transplantation

Dosage Forms Powder for injection: 20 mg

Baycol™ *see* cerivastatin *on page 112* — hypercholesterolemia

Bayer® Aspirin [OTC] *see* aspirin *on page 49*

Bayer® Select® Chest Cold Caplets [OTC] *see* acetaminophen and dextromethorphan *on page 4*

Bayer® Select® Head Cold Caplets [OTC] *see* acetaminophen and pseudoephedrine *on page 5*

Baypress® ***(Discontinued)*** *see page 700*

BCG vaccine (bee see jee vak SEEN)

Synonyms Bacillus Calmette-Guérin (BCG) Live

U.S./Canadian Brand Names ImmuCyst® (Can); Pacis™ (Can); TheraCys®; TICE® BCG

Therapeutic Category Biological Response Modulator

Use BCG vaccine is no longer recommended for adults at high risk for tuberculosis in the United States. BCG vaccination may be considered for infants and children who are skin test-negative to 5 tuberculin units of tuberculin and who cannot be given isoniazid preventive therapy but have close contact with untreated or ineffectively treated active

(Continued)

BCG vaccine *(Continued)*

tuberculosis patients or who belong to groups which other control measures have not been successful.

In the United States, tuberculosis control efforts are directed toward early identification, treatment of cases, and preventive therapy with isoniazid.

Usual Dosage Intravesical treatment and prophylaxis for carcinoma *in situ* of the urinary bladder: Begin between 7-14 days after biopsy or transurethral resection. Administer a dose of 3 vials of BCG live intravesically under aseptic conditions once weekly for 6 weeks (induction therapy). Each dose (3 reconstituted vials) is further diluted in an additional 50 mL sterile, preservative free saline for a total of 53 mL. A urethral catheter is inserted into the bladder under aseptic conditions, the bladder is drained, and then the 53 mL suspension is instilled slowly by gravity, following which the catheter is withdrawn. If the bladder catheterization has been traumatic, BCG live should not be administered, and there must be a treatment delay of at least 1 week. Resume subsequent treatment; follow the induction therapy by one treatment administered 3, 6, 12, 18 and 24 months following the initial treatment.

Dosage Forms Freeze-dried suspension for reconstitution

Injection, intravesical: TICE BCG® 50 mg (2 mL)

Injection, intravesical: TheraCys® 81 mg (1 vial)

BCNU *see* carmustine *on page 102*

B-D Glucose® [OTC] *see* glucose, instant *on page 262*

Beben® (Can) *see* betamethasone (topical) *on page 72*

becaplermin (be KAP ler min)

U.S./Canadian Brand Names Regranex®

Therapeutic Category Topical Skin Product

Use Treatment of diabetic ulcers that occur on the lower limbs and feet

Usual Dosage Adults: Topical: Apply once daily; applied with a cotton swab or similar tool, as a coating over the ulcer

Dosage Forms Gel, topical: 0.01%

Because® [OTC] *see* nonoxynol 9 *on page 406*

Beclodisk® Diskhaler® (Can) *see* beclomethasone *on this page*

Becloforte® (Can) *see* beclomethasone *on this page*

beclomethasone (be kloe METH a sone)

U.S./Canadian Brand Names Beclodisk® Diskhaler® (Can); Becloforte® (Can); Beclovent® Oral Inhaler; Beconase AQ® Nasal Inhaler; Beconase® Nasal Inhaler; Propaderm® (Can); Vancenase® AQ 84 mcg; Vancenase® AQ Inhaler; Vancenase® Nasal Inhaler; Vanceril® 84 mcg Double Strength; Vanceril® Oral Inhaler

Therapeutic Category Adrenal Corticosteroid

Use

Oral inhalation: Treatment of bronchial asthma in patients who require chronic administration of corticosteroids

Nasal aerosol: Symptomatic treatment of seasonal or perennial rhinitis and nasal polyposis

Usual Dosage

Inhalation:

- Children 6-12 years: 1-2 inhalations 3-4 times/day, not to exceed 10 inhalations/day
- Adults: 2-4 inhalations twice daily, not to exceed 20 inhalations/day

Aerosol inhalation (nasal):

- Children 6-12 years: 1 spray each nostril 3 times/day
- Adults: 2-4 sprays each nostril twice daily

Aqueous inhalation (nasal): 1-2 sprays each nostril twice daily

Dosage Forms
Beclomethasone dipropionate:
Nasal:
Inhalation: (Beconase®, Vancenase®): 42 mcg/inhalation [200 metered doses] (16.8 g)
Spray, (Vancenase® AQ Nasal): 0.084% [120 actuations] (19 g)
Spray, aqueous, nasal, (Beconase® AQ, Vancenase® AQ): 42 mcg/inhalation [≥200 metered doses] (25 g); 84 mcg/inhalation [≥200 metered doses] (25 g)
Oral: Inhalation:
Beclovent®, Vanceril®: 42 mcg/inhalation [200 metered doses] (16.8 g)
Vanceril® Double Strength: 84 mcg/inhalation (5.4 g - 40 metered doses, 12.2 g - 120 metered doses)

Beclovent® Oral Inhaler *see* beclomethasone *on previous page*

Becomject-100® ***(Discontinued)*** *see page 700*

Beconase AQ® Nasal Inhaler *see* beclomethasone *on previous page*

Beconase® Nasal Inhaler *see* beclomethasone *on previous page*

Becotin® Pulvules® *see* vitamin, multiple (oral) *on page 604*

Beepen-VK® *see* penicillin V potassium *on page 435*

Beesix® ***(Discontinued)*** *see page 700*

Belix® Oral [OTC] *see* diphenhydramine *on page 185*

belladonna (bel a DON a)

Therapeutic Category Anticholinergic Agent
Use Decrease gastrointestinal activity in functional bowel disorders and to delay gastric emptying as well as decrease gastric secretion
Usual Dosage Tincture: Oral:
Children: 0.03 mL/kg 3 times/day
Adults: 0.6-1 mL 3-4 times/day
Dosage Forms Tincture: Belladonna alkaloids (principally hyoscyamine and atropine) 0.3 mg/mL with alcohol 65% to 70% (120 mL, 480 mL, 3780 mL)

belladonna and opium (bel a DON a & OH pee um)

Synonyms opium and belladonna
U.S./Canadian Brand Names B&O Supprettes®; PMS-Opium & Beladonna (Can)
Therapeutic Category Analgesic, Narcotic
Controlled Substance C-II
Use Relief of moderate to severe pain associated with rectal or bladder tenesmus that may occur in postoperative states and neoplastic situations; pain associated with ureteral spasms not responsive to non-narcotic analgesics and to space intervals between injections of opiates
Usual Dosage Rectal:
Children: Dose not established
Adults: 1 suppository 1-2 times/day, up to 4 doses/day
Dosage Forms Suppository:
#15 A: Belladonna extract 15 mg and opium 30 mg
#16 A: Belladonna extract 15 mg and opium 60 mg

belladonna, phenobarbital, and ergotamine tartrate

(bel a DON a, fee noe BAR bi tal, & er GOT a meen TAR trate)

Synonyms ergotamine tartrate, belladonna, and phenobarbital; phenobarbital, belladonna, and ergotamine tartrate
U.S./Canadian Brand Names Bellergal-S®; Bel-Phen-Ergot S®; Phenerbel-S®
Therapeutic Category Ergot Alkaloid and Derivative
Use Management and treatment of menopausal disorders, gastrointestinal disorders and recurrent throbbing headache
Usual Dosage Oral: 1 tablet each morning and evening
(Continued)

belladonna, phenobarbital, and ergotamine tartrate *(Continued)*

Dosage Forms Tablet, sustained release: l-alkaloids of belladonna 0.2 mg, phenobarbital 40 mg, and ergotamine tartrate 0.6 mg

Bellafoline® *(Discontinued)* *see page 700*

Bellatal® *see* hyoscyamine, atropine, scopolamine, and phenobarbital *on page 298*

Bellergal-S® *see* belladonna, phenobarbital, and ergotamine tartrate *on previous page*

Bel-Phen-Ergot S® *see* belladonna, phenobarbital, and ergotamine tartrate *on previous page*

Bemote® *(Discontinued)* *see page 700*

Bena-D® *(Discontinued)* *see page 700*

Benadryl® 50 mg Capsule *(Discontinued)* *see page 700*

Benadryl® Cold/Flu *(Discontinued)* *see page 700*

Benadryl® Decongestant Allergy Tablet [OTC] *see* diphenhydramine and pseudoephedrine *on page 185*

Benadryl® Injection *see* diphenhydramine *on page 185*

Benadryl® Oral [OTC] *see* diphenhydramine *on page 185*

Benadryl® Topical *see* diphenhydramine *on page 185*

Benahist® Injection *(Discontinued)* *see page 700*

Ben-Allergin-50® Injection *see* diphenhydramine *on page 185*

Ben-Aqua® [OTC] *see* benzoyl peroxide *on page 68*

benazepril (ben AY ze pril)

U.S./Canadian Brand Names Lotensin®

Therapeutic Category Angiotensin-Converting Enzyme (ACE) Inhibitor

Use Treatment of hypertension, either alone or in combination with other antihypertensive agents

Usual Dosage Adults: Oral: 20-40 mg/day as a single dose or 2 divided doses

Dosage Forms Tablet, as hydrochloride: 5 mg, 10 mg, 20 mg, 40 mg

benazepril and amlodipine *see* amlodipine and benazepril *on page 29*

benazepril and hydrochlorothiazide

(ben AY ze pril & hye droe klor oh THYE a zide)

Synonyms hydrochlorothiazide and benazepril

U.S./Canadian Brand Names Lotensin® HCT

Therapeutic Category Antihypertensive Agent, Combination

Use Treatment of hypertension

Usual Dosage Dose is individualized

Dosage Forms Tablet:

Benazepril 5 mg and hydrochlorothiazide 6.25 mg
Benazepril 10 mg and hydrochlorothiazide 12.5 mg
Benazepril 20 mg and hydrochlorothiazide 12.5 mg
Benazepril 20 mg and hydrochlorothiazide 25 mg

bendroflumethiazide (ben droe floo meth EYE a zide)

U.S./Canadian Brand Names Naturetin®

Therapeutic Category Diuretic, Thiazide

Use Management of mild to moderate hypertension, edema associated with congestive heart failure, pregnancy, or nephrotic syndrome; reportedly does not alter serum electrolyte concentrations appreciably at recommended doses

Usual Dosage Oral:

Children: Initial: 0.1-0.4 mg/kg in 1-2 doses; maintenance dose: 0.05-0.1 mg/kg/day in 1-2 doses

Adults: 2.5-20 mg/day or twice daily in divided doses

Dosage Forms Tablet: 5 mg, 10 mg

BeneFix™ *see* factor IX complex (human) *on page 230*

Benemid® (Can) *see* probenecid *on page 474*

Benoject® ***(Discontinued)*** *see page 700*

Benoquin® *see* monobenzone *on page 381*

Benoxyl® *see* benzoyl peroxide *on page 68*

benserazide and levodopa *(Canada only)*

(ben SER a zide & lee voe DOE pa)

U.S./Canadian Brand Names Prolopa® (Can)

Therapeutic Category Anti-Parkinson's Agent

Use Treatment of Parkinson's syndrome with exception of drug-induced parkinsonism

Usual Dosage Adult: Oral: The optimal dose for most patients is usually 4-8 capsules of 100-25 daily (400-800 mg levodopa) divided into 4-6 doses

Dosage Forms Capsule:

50-12.5: Levodopa 50 and benserazide 12.5 mg

100-25: Levodopa 100 mg and benserazide 25 mg

200-50: Levodopa 200 mg and benserazide 50 mg

bentoquatam (ben to KWA tam)

U.S./Canadian Brand Names IvyBlock®

Therapeutic Category Protectant, Topical

Use To protect the skin from rash due to exposure to poison sumac, poison ivy or poison oak

Usual Dosage Topical: Apply to exposed skin at least 15 minutes before potential contact and reapply every 4 hours

Dosage Forms Lotion: 5% (120 mL)

Bentyl® Hydrochloride Injection *see* dicyclomine *on page 177*

Bentyl® Hydrochloride Oral *see* dicyclomine *on page 177*

Bentylol® (Can) *see* dicyclomine *on page 177*

Benuryl™ (Can) *see* probenecid *on page 474*

Benylin® Cough Syrup [OTC] *see* diphenhydramine *on page 185*

Benylin DM® [OTC] *see* dextromethorphan *on page 171*

Benylin® Expectorant [OTC] *see* guaifenesin and dextromethorphan *on page 268*

Benylin® Pediatric [OTC] *see* dextromethorphan *on page 171*

Benza® [OTC] *see* benzalkonium chloride *on next page*

Benzac AC® Gel *see* benzoyl peroxide *on page 68*

Benzac AC® Wash *see* benzoyl peroxide *on page 68*

Benzac W® Gel *see* benzoyl peroxide *on page 68*

Benzac W® Wash *see* benzoyl peroxide *on page 68*

5-Benzagel® *see* benzoyl peroxide *on page 68*

10-Benzagel® *see* benzoyl peroxide *on page 68*

Benzagel® Gel (Can) *see* benzoyl peroxide *on page 68*

Benzagel® Lotion (Can) *see* benzoyl peroxide *on page 68*

Benzagel® Wash (Can) *see* benzoyl peroxide *on page 68*

benzalkonium chloride (benz al KOE nee um KLOR ide)

Synonyms BAC

U.S./Canadian Brand Names Benza® [OTC]; Zephiran® [OTC]

Therapeutic Category Antibacterial, Topical

Use Surface antiseptic and germicidal preservative

Usual Dosage Thoroughly rinse anionic detergents and soaps from the skin or other areas prior to use of solutions because they reduce the antibacterial activity of BAC; to protect metal instruments stored in BAC solution, add crushed Anti-Rust Tablets, 4 tablets per quart, to antiseptic solution, change solution at least once weekly; not to be used for storage of aluminum or zinc instruments, instruments with lenses fastened by cement, lacquered catheters or some synthetic rubber goods

Dosage Forms

Concentrate, topical: 17% (500 mL, 4000 mL)
Solution, aqueous: 1:750 (60 mL, 120 mL, 240 mL)
Tincture: 1:750 (30 mL, 960 mL)
Spray: 1:750 (30 g, 180 g)
Tissue: 1:750 (packets)

benzalkonium chloride, benzocaine, butyl aminobenzoate, tetracaine *see* benzocaine, butyl aminobenzoate, tetracaine, and benzalkonium chloride *on next page*

Benzamycin® *see* erythromycin and benzoyl peroxide *on page 214*

Benzashave® Cream *see* benzoyl peroxide *on page 68*

benzathine benzylpenicillin *see* penicillin G benzathine *on page 433*

benzathine penicillin G *see* penicillin G benzathine *on page 433*

benzazoline *see* tolazoline *on page 570*

Benzedrex® [OTC] *see* propylhexedrine *on page 484*

benzene hexachloride *see* lindane *on page 335*

benzhexol *see* trihexyphenidyl *on page 581*

benzocaine (BEN zoe kane)

Synonyms ethyl aminobenzoate

U.S./Canadian Brand Names Americaine® [OTC]; Anbesol® [OTC]; Anbesol® Maximum Strength [OTC]; Babee® Teething® [OTC]; Benzocol® [OTC]; Benzodent® [OTC]; Chiggertox® [OTC]; Cylex® [OTC]; Dermoplast® [OTC]; Foille® [OTC]; Foille® Medicated First Aid [OTC]; Hurricaine®; Lanacane® [OTC]; Maximum Strength Anbesol® [OTC]; Maximum Strength Orajel® [OTC]; Mycinettes® [OTC]; Numzitdent® [OTC]; Numzit Teething® [OTC]; Orabase®-B [OTC]; Orabase®-O [OTC]; Orajel® Brace-Aid Oral Anesthetic [OTC]; Orajel® Maximum Strength [OTC]; Orajel® Mouth-Aid [OTC]; Orasept® [OTC]; Orasol® [OTC]; Rhulicaine® [OTC]; Rid-A-Pain® [OTC]; Slim-Mint® [OTC]; Solarcaine® [OTC]; Spec-T® [OTC]; Tanac® [OTC]; Trocaine® [OTC]; Unguentine® [OTC]; Vicks Children's Chloraseptic® [OTC]; Vicks Chloraseptic® Sore Throat [OTC]; Zilactin-B® Medicated [OTC]

Therapeutic Category Local Anesthetic

Use Temporary relief of pain associated with pruritic dermatosis, pruritus, minor burns, toothache, minor sore throat pain, canker sores, hemorrhoids, rectal fissures; anesthetic lubricant for passage of catheters and endoscopic tubes

Usual Dosage

Children and Adults:

Mucous membranes: Dosage varies depending on area to be anesthetized and vascularity of tissues

Oral mouth/throat preparations: Do not administer for >2 days or in children <2 years of age, unless directed by a physician; refer to specific package labeling

Topical: Apply to affected area as needed

Adults: Nonprescription diet aid: 6-15 mg just prior to food consumption, not to exceed 45 mg/day

Dosage Forms
Topical for mucous membranes:
Gel: 6% (7.5 g); 20% (2.5 g, 3.75 g, 7.5 g, 30 g)
Liquid: 20% (3.75 mL, 9 mL, 13.3 mL, 30 mL)
Topical for skin disorders:
Aerosol, external use: 5% (92 mL, 105 g); 20% (82.5 mL, 90 mL, 92 mL, 150 mL)
Cream: (30 g, 60 g); 5% (30 g, 1 lb); 6% (28.4 g)
Lotion: (120 mL); 8% (90 mL)
Ointment: 5% (3.5 g, 28 g)
Spray: 5% (97.5 mL); 20% (20 g, 60 g, 120 g, 13.3 mL, 120 mL)
Mouth/throat preparations:
Cream: 5% (10 g)
Gel: 6.3% (7.5 g); 7.5% (7.2 g, 9.45 g, 14.1 g); 10% (6 g, 9.45 g, 10 g, 15 g); 15% (10.5 g); 20% (9.45 g, 14.1 g)
Liquid: 20% (3.7 mL); 5% (8.8 mL); 6.3% (9 mL, 22 mL, 14.79 mL); 10% (13 mL); 20% (13.3 mL)
Lotion: 0.2% (15 mL); 2.5% (15 mL)
Lozenges: 5 mg, 6 mg, 10 mg, 15 mg
Ointment: 20% (30 g)
Paste: 20% (5 g, 15 g)
Nonprescription diet aid:
Candy: 6 mg
Gum: 6 mg

benzocaine and antipyrine *see* antipyrine and benzocaine *on page 41*

benzocaine and cetylpyridinium chloride *see* cetylpyridinium and benzocaine *on page 113*

benzocaine, butyl aminobenzoate, tetracaine, and benzalkonium chloride

(BEN zoe kane, BYOO til a meen oh BENZ oh ate, TET ra kane, & benz al KOE nee um KLOR ide)

Synonyms benzalkonium chloride, benzocaine, butyl aminobenzoate, tetracaine; butyl aminobenzoate, benzocaine, tetracaine, and benzalkonium chloride; tetracaine hydrochloride, benzocaine, butyl aminobenzoate, and benzalkonium chloride

U.S./Canadian Brand Names Cetacaine®

Therapeutic Category Local Anesthetic

Use Topical anesthetic to control pain or gagging

Usual Dosage Topical: Apply to affected area for approximately 1 second or less

Dosage Forms Aerosol: Benzocaine 14%, butyl aminobenzoate 2%, tetracaine 2%, and benzalkonium chloride 0.5% (56 g)

benzocaine, gelatin, pectin, and sodium carboxymethylcellulose

(BEN zoe kane, JEL a tin, PEK tin, & SOW dee um kar box ee meth il SEL yoo lose)

U.S./Canadian Brand Names Orabase® With Benzocaine [OTC]

Therapeutic Category Local Anesthetic

Use Topical anesthetic and emollient for oral lesions

Usual Dosage Topical: Apply 2-4 times/day

Dosage Forms Paste: Benzocaine 20%, gelatin, pectin, and sodium carboxymethylcellulose (15 g, 5 g)

Benzocol® [OTC] *see* benzocaine *on previous page*

Benzodent® [OTC] *see* benzocaine *on previous page*

benzoic acid and salicylic acid (ben ZOE ik AS id & sal i SIL ik AS id)

Synonyms salicylic acid and benzoic acid

U.S./Canadian Brand Names Whitfield's Ointment [OTC]

Therapeutic Category Antifungal Agent

(Continued)

benzoic acid and salicylic acid *(Continued)*

Use Treatment of athlete's foot and ringworm of the scalp

Usual Dosage Topical: Apply 1-4 times/day

Dosage Forms

Lotion, topical:

Full strength: Benzoic acid 12% and salicylic acid 6% with isopropyl alcohol 70% (240 mL)

Half strength: Benzoic acid 6% and salicylic acid 3% with isopropyl alcohol 70% (240 mL)

Ointment, topical: Benzoic acid 12% and salicylic acid 6% in anhydrous lanolin and petrolatum (30 g, 454 g)

benzoin (BEN zoyn)

Synonyms gum benjamin

U.S./Canadian Brand Names AeroZoin® [OTC]; TinBen® [OTC]; TinCoBen® [OTC]

Therapeutic Category Pharmaceutical Aid; Protectant, Topical

Use Protective application for irritations of the skin; sometimes used in boiling water as steam inhalants for their expectorant and soothing action

Usual Dosage Topical: Apply 1-2 times/day

Dosage Forms

Spray, as compound tincture: 40% (105 mL)

Tincture: 79% (480 mL)

As compound tincture: 20% (60 mL); 25% (120 mL)

benzonatate (ben ZOE na tate)

U.S./Canadian Brand Names Tessalon® Perles

Therapeutic Category Antitussive

Use Symptomatic relief of nonproductive cough

Usual Dosage Oral:

Children <10 years: 8 mg/kg in 3-6 divided doses

Children >10 years and Adults: 100 mg 3 times/day up to 600 mg/day

Dosage Forms Capsule: 100 mg

benzoyl peroxide (BEN zoe il peer OKS ide)

U.S./Canadian Brand Names Acetoxyl® (Can); Acnomel® B.P.5 (Can); Advanced Formula Oxy® Sensitive Gel [OTC]; Ambi 10® [OTC]; Ben-Aqua® [OTC]; Benoxyl®; Benzac AC® Gel; Benzac AC® Wash; Benzac W® Gel; Benzac W® Wash; 5-Benzagel®; 10-Benzagel®; Benzagel® Gel (Can); Benzagel® Lotion (Can); Benzagel® Wash (Can); Benzashave® Cream; BlemErase® Lotion [OTC]; Brevoxyl® Gel; Clear By Design® Gel [OTC]; Clearsil® Maximum Strength [OTC]; Del Aqua-5® Gel; Del Aqua-10® Gel; Desquam-E™ Gel; Desquam-X® Gel; Desquam-X® Wash; Dryox® Gel [OTC]; Dryox® Wash [OTC]; Exact® Cream [OTC]; Fostex® 10% BPO Gel [OTC]; Fostex® 10% Wash [OTC]; Fostex® Bar [OTC]; H_2Oxyl® (Can); Loroxide® [OTC]; Neutrogena® Acne Mask [OTC]; Oxy-5® Advanced Formula for Sensitive Skin [OTC]; Oxy-5® Tinted [OTC]; Oxy-10® Advanced Formula for Sensitive Skin [OTC]; Oxy 10® Wash [OTC]; Oxyderm™ 5%, 10%, 20% (Can); PanOxyl®-AQ; PanOxyl® Bar [OTC]; Perfectoderm® Gel [OTC]; Peroxin A5®; Peroxin A10®; Persa-Gel®; Solugel® 4, 8 (Can); Theroxide® Wash [OTC]; Vanoxide® [OTC]

Therapeutic Category Acne Products

Use Adjunctive treatment of mild to moderate acne vulgaris

Usual Dosage Children and Adults:

Cleansers: Wash once or twice daily; control amount of drying or peeling by modifying dose frequency or concentration

Topical: Apply sparingly once daily; gradually increase to 2-3 times/day if needed. If excessive dryness or peeling occurs, reduce dose frequency or concentration; if excessive stinging or burning occurs, remove with mild soap and water; resume use the next day.

Dosage Forms

Bar: 5% (113 g); 10% (106 g, 113 g)

Cream: 5% (18 g, 113.4 g); 10% (18 g, 28 g, 113.4 g)

Gel: 2.5% (30 g, 42.5 g, 45 g, 57 g, 60 g, 90 g, 113 g); 5% (42.5 g, 45 g, 60 g, 80 g, 90 g, 113.4 g); 10% (30 g, 42.5 g, 45 g, 56.7 g, 60 g, 90 g, 113.4 g, 120 g); 20% (30 g, 60 g)

Liquid: 5% (120 mL, 150 mL, 240 mL); 10% (120 mL, 150 mL, 240 mL)

Lotion: 5% (25 mL, 30 mL); 5.5% (25 mL); 10% (12 mL, 29 mL, 30 mL, 60 mL)

Mask: 5% (30 mL, 60 mL, 60 g)

benzoyl peroxide and erythromycin *see* erythromycin and benzoyl peroxide *on page 214*

benzoyl peroxide and hydrocortisone

(BEN zoe il peer OKS ide & hye droe KOR ti sone)

Synonyms hydrocortisone and benzoyl peroxide

U.S./Canadian Brand Names Vanoxide-HC®

Therapeutic Category Acne Products

Use Treatment of acne vulgaris and oily skin

Usual Dosage Topical: Shake well; apply thin film 1-3 times/day, gently massage into skin

Dosage Forms Lotion: Benzoyl peroxide 5% and hydrocortisone alcohol 0.5% (25 mL)

benzphetamine (benz FET a meen)

U.S./Canadian Brand Names Didrex®

Therapeutic Category Anorexiant

Controlled Substance C-III

Use Short-term adjunct in exogenous obesity

Usual Dosage Adults: Oral: 25-50 mg 2-3 times/day, preferably twice daily, midmorning and midafternoon

Dosage Forms Tablet, as hydrochloride: 25 mg, 50 mg

benzthiazide (benz THYE a zide)

U.S./Canadian Brand Names Exna®

Therapeutic Category Diuretic, Thiazide

Use Management of mild to moderate hypertension; treatment of edema in congestive heart failure and nephrotic syndrome

Usual Dosage Adults: Oral: 50-200 mg/day

Dosage Forms Tablet: 50 mg

benztropine (BENZ troe peen)

U.S./Canadian Brand Names Cogentin®; PMS-Benztropine (Can)

Therapeutic Category Anticholinergic Agent; Anti-Parkinson's Agent

Use Adjunctive treatment of parkinsonism; also used in treatment of drug-induced extrapyramidal effects (except tardive dyskinesia) and acute dystonic reactions

Usual Dosage Titrate dose in 0.5 mg increments at 5- to 6-day intervals

Extrapyramidal reaction, drug induced: Oral, I.M., I.V.:

Children >3 years: 0.02-0.05 mg/kg/dose 1-2 times/day

Adults: 1-4 mg/dose 1-2 times/day

Parkinsonism: Oral: 0.5-6 mg/day in 1-2 divided doses; if one dose is greater, administer at bedtime

Dosage Forms Benztropine mesylate:

Injection: 1 mg/mL (2 mL)

Tablet: 0.5 mg, 1 mg, 2 mg

benzylpenicillin *see* penicillin G, parenteral, aqueous *on page 434*

benzylpenicillin benzathine *see* penicillin G benzathine *on page 433*

benzylpenicilloyl-polylysine (BEN zil pen i SIL oyl pol i LIE seen)

Synonyms penicilloyl-polylysine; PPL

U.S./Canadian Brand Names Pre-Pen®

Therapeutic Category Diagnostic Agent

Use As an adjunct in assessing the risk of administering penicillin (penicillin or benzylpenicillin) in patients with a history of clinical penicillin hypersensitivity

Usual Dosage

Use scratch technique with a 20-gauge needle to make 3-5 mm scratch on epidermis, apply a small drop of solution to scratch, rub in gently with applicator or toothpick

A positive reaction consists of a pale wheal surrounding the scratch site which develops within 10 minutes and ranges from 5-15 mm or more in diameter

If the scratch test is negative an intradermal test may be performed

Intradermal test: Use intradermal test with a tuberculin syringe with a 26- to 30-gauge short bevel needle; a dose of 0.01-0.02 mL is injected intradermally. A control of 0.9% sodium chloride should be injected at least 1½" from the PPL test site. Most skin responses to the intradermal test will develop within 5-15 minutes.

(-) = no reaction or increase in size compared to control

(±) = wheal slightly larger with or without erythematous flare and larger than control site

(+) = itching and increase in size of original bleb may exceed 20 mm in diameter

Dosage Forms Solution: 0.25 mL

bepridil (BE pri dil)

U.S./Canadian Brand Names Bapadin® (Can); Vascor®

Therapeutic Category Calcium Channel Blocker

Use Treatment of chronic stable angina; only approved indication is hypertension, but may be used for congestive heart failure; doses should not be adjusted for at least 10 days after beginning therapy

Usual Dosage Adults: Oral: Initial: 200 mg/day, then adjust dose until optimal response is achieved; maximum daily dose: 400 mg

Dosage Forms Tablet, as hydrochloride: 200 mg, 300 mg, 400 mg

beractant (ber AKT ant)

Synonyms bovine lung surfactant; natural lung surfactant

U.S./Canadian Brand Names Survanta®

Therapeutic Category Lung Surfactant

Use Prevention and treatment of respiratory distress syndrome (RDS) in premature infants

Prophylactic therapy: Infants with body weight <1250 g who are at risk for developing or with evidence of surfactant deficiency

Rescue therapy: Treatment of infants with RDS confirmed by x-ray and requiring mechanical ventilation

Usual Dosage Intratracheal:

Prophylactic treatment: Administer 4 mL/kg as soon as possible; as many as 4 doses may be administered during the first 48 hours of life, no more frequently than 6 hours apart. The need for additional doses is determined by evidence of continuing respiratory distress; if the infant is still intubated and requiring at least 30% inspired oxygen to maintain a $PaO_2 \le 80$ torr.

Rescue treatment: Administer 4 mL/kg as soon as the diagnosis of RDS is made

Dosage Forms Suspension: 200 mg (8 mL)

Berocca® *see* vitamin B complex with vitamin C and folic acid *on page 603*

Berotec® Forte Inhalation Aerosol (Can) *see* fenoterol *(Canada only) on page 234*

Berotec® Inhalation Aerosol (Can) *see* fenoterol *(Canada only) on page 234*

Berotec® Solution (Can) *see* fenoterol *(Canada only) on page 234*

Berubigen® *see* cyanocobalamin *on page 152*

Beta-2® *see* isoetharine *on page 313*

beta-carotene (BAY tah KARE oh teen)

Therapeutic Category Vitamin, Fat Soluble

Use Reduce the severity of photosensitivity reactions in patients with erythropoietic protoporphyria (EPP)

Usual Dosage Oral:
Children <14 years: 30-150 mg/day
Adults: 30-300 mg/day

Dosage Forms Capsule: 15 mg, 30 mg

Betachron® *see* propranolol *on page 483*

Betacort™ (Can) *see* betamethasone (topical) *on next page*

Betaderm (Can) *see* betamethasone (topical) *on next page*

Betadine® [OTC] *see* povidone-iodine *on page 467*

Betadine® 5% Sterile Ophthalmic Prep Solution *see* povidone-iodine *on page 467*

Betadine® First Aid Antibiotics + Moisturizer [OTC] *see* bacitracin and polymyxin B *on page 58*

9-beta-D-ribofuranosyladenine *see* adenosine *on page 12*

Betagan® [OTC] *see* povidone-iodine *on page 467*

Betagan® Liquifilm® Ophthalmic *see* levobunolol *on page 330*

betahistine *(Canada only)* (bay ta HISS teen)

U.S./Canadian Brand Names Serc® (Can)

Therapeutic Category Antihistamine

Use May be of value in the treatment of Ménière's disease

Usual Dosage Adult: Oral: 4-8 mg 3 times/day

Dosage Forms Tablet, as hydrochloride: 4 mg

betaine anhydrous (BAY tayne an HY drus)

U.S./Canadian Brand Names Cystadane®

Therapeutic Category Urinary Tract Product

Use Treatment of homocystinuria

Usual Dosage Oral: 6 g/day, usually given in two 3 g doses

Dosage Forms Powder: 1 g/1.7 mL (180 g)

Betalene® Topical *see* betamethasone (topical) *on next page*

Betalin®S *see* thiamine *on page 561*

Betaloc® (Can) *see* metoprolol *on page 371*

Betaloc Durules® (Can) *see* metoprolol *on page 371*

betamethasone and clotrimazole (bay ta METH a sone & kloe TRIM a zole)

Synonyms clotrimazole and betamethasone

U.S./Canadian Brand Names Lotrisone®

Therapeutic Category Antifungal/Corticosteroid

Use Topical treatment of various dermal fungal infections

Usual Dosage Topical: Apply twice daily

Dosage Forms Cream: Betamethasone dipropionate 0.05% and clotrimazole 1% (15 g, 45 g)

betamethasone (systemic) (bay ta METH a sone)

U.S./Canadian Brand Names Celestone® Oral; Celestone® Phosphate Injection; Celestone® Soluspan®; Cel-U-Jec® Injection; Selestoject® (Can)

Therapeutic Category Adrenal Corticosteroid

Use Anti-inflammatory; immunosuppressant agent; corticosteroid replacement therapy

(Continued)

betamethasone (systemic) *(Continued)*

Usual Dosage Children and Adults:

I.M.: Betamethasone sodium phosphate and betamethasone acetate: 0.5-9 mg/day ($^1/_3$ to $^1/_2$ of oral dose)

Intrabursal, intra-articular: 0.5-2 mL

Oral: 0.6-7.2 mg/day

Dosage Forms

Betamethasone base (Celestone®), Oral:

Syrup: 0.6 mg/5 mL (118 mL)

Tablet: 0.6 mg

Injection: Sodium phosphate (Celestone® Phosphate, Cel-U-Jec®): 4 mg betamethasone phosphate/mL (equivalent to 3 mg betamethasone/mL) (5 mL)

Injection, suspension: Sodium phosphate and acetate (Celestone® Soluspan®): 6 mg/mL (3 mg of betamethasone sodium phosphate and 3 mg of betamethasone acetate per mL) (5 mL)

betamethasone (topical) (bay ta METH a sone)

Synonyms flubenisolone

U.S./Canadian Brand Names Alphatrex® Topical; Beben® (Can); Betacort™ (Can); Betaderm (Can); Betalene® Topical; Betatrex® Topical; Beta-Val® Topical; Betnesol® (Can); Betnovate® (Can); Celestoderm®-V, -EV/2 (Can); Diprolene® AF Topical; Diprolene® Glycol (Can); Diprolene® Topical; Diprosone® Topical; Ectosone (Can); Maxivate® Topical; Occlucort® (Can); Psorion® Topical; Rhoprolene® (Can); Rhoprosone® (Can); Taro-Sone® (Can); Teladar® Topical; Topilene® (Can); Topisone® (Can); Valisone® Topical

Therapeutic Category Corticosteroid, Topical

Use Inflammatory dermatoses such as psoriasis, seborrheic or atopic dermatitis, neurodermatitis, inflammatory phase of xerosis, late phase of allergic dermatitis or irritant dermatitis

Usual Dosage Topical: Adults: Apply thin film 2-4 times/day

Dosage Forms

Betamethasone dipropionate

Aerosol: 0.1% (85 g)

Cream: 0.05% (15 g, 45 g)

Lotion: 0.05% (20 mL, 30 mL, 60 mL)

Ointment: 0.05% (15 g, 45 g)

Betamethasone dipropionate augmented

Cream: 0.05% (15 g, 45 g)

Gel: 0.05% (15 g, 45 g)

Lotion: 0.05% (30 mL, 60 mL)

Ointment, topical: 0.05% (15 g, 45 g)

Betamethasone valerate

Cream: 0.01% (15 g, 60 g); 0.1% (15 g, 45 g, 110 g, 430 g)

Lotion: 0.1% (20 mL, 60 mL)

Ointment: 0.1% (15 g, 45 g)

Betapace® *see* sotalol *on page 532*

Betapen-VK® ***(Discontinued)*** *see page 700*

Betasept® [OTC] *see* chlorhexidine gluconate *on page 117*

Betaseron® *see* interferon beta-1b *on page 310*

Beta-Tim® (Can) *see* timolol *on page 567*

Betatrex® Topical *see* betamethasone (topical) *on this page*

Beta-Val® Ointment ***(Discontinued)*** *see page 700*

Beta-Val® Topical *see* betamethasone (topical) *on this page*

Betaxin® (Can) *see* thiamine *on page 561*

betaxolol (be TAKS oh lol)

U.S./Canadian Brand Names Betoptic® Ophthalmic; Betoptic® S Ophthalmic; Kerlone® Oral

Therapeutic Category Beta-Adrenergic Blocker

Use Treatment of chronic open-angle glaucoma, ocular hypertension; management of hypertension

Usual Dosage Adults:

Ophthalmic: Instill 1 drop twice daily

Oral: 10 mg/day; may increase dose to 20 mg/day after 7-14 days if desired response is not achieved; initial dose in elderly patients: 5 mg/day

Dosage Forms Betaxolol hydrochloride:

Solution, ophthalmic, (Betoptic®): 0.5% (2.5 mL, 5 mL, 10 mL)

Suspension, ophthalmic, (Betoptic® S): 0.25% (2.5 mL, 10 mL, 15 mL)

Tablet, (Kerlone®): 10 mg, 20 mg

bethanechol (be THAN e kole)

U.S./Canadian Brand Names Duvoid®; Myotonachol™; PMS-Bethanechol Chloride (Can); Urabeth®; Urecholine®

Therapeutic Category Cholinergic Agent

Use Treatment of nonobstructive urinary retention and retention due to neurogenic bladder; gastroesophageal reflux

Usual Dosage

Children:

Oral:

Abdominal distention or urinary retention: 0.6 mg/kg/day divided 3-4 times/day

Gastroesophageal reflux: 0.1-0.2 mg/kg/dose administered 30 minutes to 1 hour before each meal to a maximum of 4 times/day

S.C.: 0.15-0.2 mg/kg/day divided 3-4 times/day

Adults:

Oral: 10-50 mg 2-4 times/day

S.C.: 2.5-5 mg 3-4 times/day, up to 7.5-10 mg every 4 hours for neurogenic bladder

Dosage Forms Bethanechol chloride:

Injection: 5 mg/mL (1 mL)

Tablet: 5 mg, 10 mg, 25 mg, 50 mg

Betnesol® (Can) *see* betamethasone (topical) *on previous page*

Betnovate® (Can) *see* betamethasone (topical) *on previous page*

Betoptic® Ophthalmic *see* betaxolol *on this page*

Betoptic® S Ophthalmic *see* betaxolol *on this page*

Bewon® (Can) *see* thiamine *on page 561*

Bexophene® *see* propoxyphene and aspirin *on page 482*

bezafibrate *(Canada only)* (be za FYE brate)

U.S./Canadian Brand Names Bezalip® (Can)

Therapeutic Category Antilipemic Agent

Use Adjunct to dietary therapy in the management of hyperlipidemias associated with high triglyceride levels (types III, IV, V); primarily lowers triglycerides and very low density lipoprotein

Usual Dosage Adult: Oral: 200 mg 3 times/day

Dosage Forms Tablet: 200 mg, 400 mg

Bezalip® (Can) *see* bezafibrate *(Canada only)* *on this page*

Biamine® Injection *(Discontinued)* *see page 700*

Biavax® II *see* rubella and mumps vaccines, combined *on page 511*

Biaxin™ *see* clarithromycin *on page 135*

bicalutamide (bye ka LOO ta mide)

U.S./Canadian Brand Names Casodex®

Therapeutic Category Androgen

Use Combination therapy with a luteinizing hormone-releasing hormone (LHRH) analog for the treatment of advanced prostate cancer

Usual Dosage Adults: Oral: 50 mg once daily (morning or evening), with or without food, in combination with a LHRH analog

Dosage Forms Tablet: 50 mg

Bicillin® C-R *see* penicillin G benzathine and procaine combined *on page 434*

Bicillin® C-R 900/300 *see* penicillin G benzathine and procaine combined *on page 434*

Bicillin® L-A *see* penicillin G benzathine *on page 433*

BiCNU® *see* carmustine *on page 102*

Bilezyme® Tablet *(Discontinued)* *see page 700*

Bilopaque® *see* radiological/contrast media (ionic) *on page 495*

Biltricide® *see* praziquantel *on page 469*

Biocef® *see* cephalexin *on page 111*

Bioclate® *see* antihemophilic factor (recombinant) *on page 40*

Bioderm (Can) *see* bacitracin and polymyxin B *on page 58*

Biodine [OTC] *see* povidone-iodine *on page 467*

Biohist-LA® *see* carbinoxamine and pseudoephedrine *on page 99*

Biomox® *(Discontinued)* *see page 700*

Bion® Tears Solution [OTC] *see* artificial tears *on page 47*

Bio-Tab® *see* doxycycline *on page 197*

Biozyme-C® *see* collagenase *on page 146*

biperiden (bye PER i den)

U.S./Canadian Brand Names Akineton®

Therapeutic Category Anticholinergic Agent; Anti-Parkinson's Agent

Use Treatment of all forms of Parkinsonism including drug-induced type (extrapyramidal symptoms)

Usual Dosage Adults:

Parkinsonism: Oral: 2 mg 3-4 times/day

Extrapyramidal:

- Oral: 2-6 mg 2-3 times/day
- I.M., I.V.: 2 mg every 30 minutes up to 4 doses or 8 mg/day

Dosage Forms

Injection, as lactate: 5 mg/mL (1 mL)

Tablet, as hydrochloride: 2 mg

Biphetamine® *(Discontinued)* *see page 700*

Biquin® Durules® (Can) *see* quinidine *on page 492*

Bisac-Evac® [OTC] *see* bisacodyl *on this page*

bisacodyl (bis a KOE dil)

U.S./Canadian Brand Names Apo®-Bisacodyl (Can); Bisac-Evac® [OTC]; Bisacodyl Uniserts®; Bisco-Lax® [OTC]; Carter's Little Pills® [OTC]; Clysodrast®; Dacodyl® [OTC]; Deficol® [OTC]; Dulcolax® [OTC]; Fleet® Laxative [OTC]; PMS-Bisacodyl (Can)

Therapeutic Category Laxative

Use Treatment of constipation; colonic evacuation prior to procedures or examination

Usual Dosage
Children:
Oral: >6 years: 5-10 mg (0.3 mg/kg) at bedtime or before breakfast
Rectal suppository:
<2 years: 5 mg as a single dose
>2 years: 10 mg
Adults:
Oral: 5-15 mg as single dose (up to 30 mg when complete evacuation of bowel is required)
Rectal suppository: 10 mg as single dose
Tannex:
Enema: 2.5 g in 1000 mL warm water
Barium enema: 2.5-5 g in 1000 mL barium suspension
Do not administer >10 g within a 72-hour period

Dosage Forms
Powder, as tannex: 2.5 g packets (50 packet/box)
Suppository, rectal: 5 mg, 10 mg
Tablet, enteric coated: 5 mg

Bisacodyl Uniserts® *see* bisacodyl *on previous page*

Bisco-Lax® [OTC] *see* bisacodyl *on previous page*

bishydroxycoumarin *see* dicumarol *on page 176*

Bismatrol® [OTC] *see* bismuth subsalicylate *on this page*

bismuth subgallate (BIZ muth sub GAL ate)

U.S./Canadian Brand Names Devrom® [OTC]
Therapeutic Category Gastrointestinal Agent, Miscellaneous
Use Symptomatic treatment of mild, nonspecific diarrhea
Usual Dosage Oral: 1-2 tablets 3 times/day with meals
Dosage Forms Tablet, chewable: 200 mg

bismuth subsalicylate (BIZ muth sub sa LIS i late)

U.S./Canadian Brand Names Bismatrol® [OTC]; Pepto-Bismol® [OTC]
Therapeutic Category Gastrointestinal Agent, Miscellaneous
Use Symptomatic treatment of mild, nonspecific diarrhea including traveler's diarrhea; chronic infantile diarrhea
Usual Dosage Oral:
Nonspecific diarrhea:
Children: Up to 8 doses/24 hours:
3-6 years: 1/3 tablet or 5 mL every 30 minutes to 1 hour as needed
6-9 years: 2/3 tablet or 10 mL every 30 minutes to 1 hour as needed
9-12 years: 1 tablet or 15 mL every 30 minutes to 1 hour as needed
Adults: 2 tablets or 30 mL every 30 minutes to 1 hour as needed up to 8 doses/24 hours
Prevention of traveler's diarrhea: 2.1 g/day or 2 tablets 4 times/day before meals and at bedtime

Dosage Forms
Caplet, swallowable: 262 mg
Liquid: 262 mg/15 mL (120 mL, 240 mL, 360 mL, 480 mL); 524 mg/15 mL (120 mL, 240 mL, 360 mL)
Tablet, chewable: 262 mg

bismuth subsalicylate, metronidazole, and tetracycline

(BIZ muth sub sa LIS i late, me troe NI da zole, & tet ra SYE kleen)
U.S./Canadian Brand Names Helidac™
Therapeutic Category Antidiarrheal
Use In combination with an H_2 antagonist, used to treat and decrease rate of recurrence of active duodenal ulcer associated with *H. pylori* infection
(Continued)

bismuth subsalicylate, metronidazole, and tetracycline *(Continued)*

Usual Dosage Adults: Chew 2 bismuth subsalicylate 262.4 mg tablets, swallow 1 metronidazole 250 mg tablet, and swallow 1 tetracycline 500 mg capsule plus an H_2 antagonist 4 times/day at meals and bedtime for 14 days; follow with 8 oz of water

Dosage Forms

Tablet:

Bismuth subsalicylate: Chewable: 262.4 mg

Metronidazole: 250 mg

Capsule: Tetracycline: 500 mg

bisoprolol (bis OH proe lol)

U.S./Canadian Brand Names Zebeta®

Therapeutic Category Beta-Adrenergic Blocker

Use Treatment of hypertension, alone or in combination with other agents

Usual Dosage Adults: Oral: 5 mg once daily, may be increased to 10 mg, and then up to 20 mg once daily, if necessary

Dosage Forms Tablet, as fumarate: 5 mg, 10 mg

bisoprolol and hydrochlorothiazide

(bis OH proe lol & hye droe klor oh THYE a zide)

Synonyms hydrochlorothiazide and bisoprolol

U.S./Canadian Brand Names Ziac™

Therapeutic Category Antihypertensive Agent, Combination

Use Treatment of hypertension

Usual Dosage Adults: Oral: Dose is individualized, administered once daily

Dosage Forms Tablet:

Bisoprolol fumarate 2.5 mg and hydrochlorothiazide 6.25 mg

Bisoprolol fumarate 5 mg and hydrochlorothiazide 6.25 mg

Bisoprolol fumarate 10 mg and hydrochlorothiazide 6.25 mg

bistropamide *see* tropicamide *on page 587*

bitolterol (bye TOLE ter ole)

U.S./Canadian Brand Names Tornalate®

Therapeutic Category Adrenergic Agonist Agent

Use Prevent and treat bronchial asthma and bronchospasm

Usual Dosage Children >12 years and Adults:

Bronchospasm: 2 inhalations at an interval of at least 1-3 minutes, followed by a third inhalation if needed

Prevention of bronchospasm: 2 inhalations every 8 hours

Dosage Forms Bitolterol mesylate:

Aerosol, oral: 0.8% [370 mcg/metered spray, 300 inhalations] (15 mL)

Solution, inhalation: 0.2% (10 mL, 30 mL, 60 mL)

Black Draught® [OTC] *see* senna *on page 518*

black widow spider antivenin (*Latrodectus mactans*) *see* antivenin (*Latrodectus mactans*) *on page 42*

Blanex® Capsule *(Discontinued)* *see page 700*

BlemErase® Lotion [OTC] *see* benzoyl peroxide *on page 68*

Blenoxane® *see* bleomycin *on this page*

bleomycin (blee oh MYE sin)

Synonyms BLM

U.S./Canadian Brand Names Blenoxane®

Therapeutic Category Antineoplastic Agent

Use Palliative treatment of squamous cell carcinoma, testicular carcinoma, germ cell tumors, and the following lymphomas: Hodgkin's, lymphosarcoma and reticulum cell sarcoma; sclerosing agent to control malignant effusions

Usual Dosage Refer to individual protocol

Children and Adults:

Test dose for lymphoma patients: I.M., I.V., S.C.: 1-2 units of bleomycin for the first 2 doses; monitor vital signs every 15 minutes; wait a minimum of 1 hour before administering remainder of dose

I.M., I.V., S.C.: 10-20 units/m^2 (0.25-0.5 units/kg) 1-2 times/week in combination regimens

I.V. continuous infusion: 15-20 units/m^2/day for 4-5 days

Adults: Intracavitary injection for pleural effusion: 15-240 units have been administered

Dosage Forms Powder for injection, as sulfate: 15 units

Bleph®-10 *see* sulfacetamide *on page 540*

Blephamide® Ophthalmic *see* sulfacetamide and prednisolone *on page 540*

BLM *see* bleomycin *on previous page*

Blocadren® Oral *see* timolol *on page 567*

Bluboro® [OTC] *see* aluminum acetate and calcium acetate *on page 22*

Bonamine® (Can) *see* meclizine *on page 351*

Bonine® [OTC] *see* meclizine *on page 351*

Bontril PDM® *see* phendimetrazine *on page 442*

Bontril® Slow-Release *see* phendimetrazine *on page 442*

boric acid (BOR ik AS id)

U.S./Canadian Brand Names Borofax® Topical [OTC]; Dri-Ear® Otic [OTC]; Swim-Ear® Otic [OTC]

Therapeutic Category Pharmaceutical Aid

Use

Ophthalmic: Mild antiseptic used for inflamed eyelids

Otic: Prophylaxis of swimmer's ear

Topical ointment: Temporary relief of chapped, chafed, or dry skin, diaper rash, abrasions, minor burns, sunburn, insect bites, and other skin irritations

Usual Dosage

Ophthalmic: Apply to lower eyelid 1-2 times/day

Otic: Place 2-4 drops in ears

Topical: Apply as needed

Dosage Forms

Ointment:

Ophthalmic: 5% (3.5 g); 10% (3.5 g)

Topical: 5% (52.5 g); 10% (28 g)

Topical (Borofax®): 5% boric acid and lanolin (1¾ oz)

Solution, otic: 2.75% with isopropyl alcohol (30 mL)

Borofax® Topical [OTC] *see* boric acid *on this page*

Boropak® [OTC] *see* aluminum acetate and calcium acetate *on page 22*

B&O Supprettes® *see* belladonna and opium *on page 63*

Botox® *see* botulinum toxin type A *on this page*

botulinum toxin type A (BOT yoo lin num TOKS in type aye)

U.S./Canadian Brand Names Botox®

Therapeutic Category Ophthalmic Agent, Toxin

Use Treatment of strabismus and blepharospasm

Usual Dosage

Strabismus: 1.25-5 units (0.05-0.15 mL) injected into any one muscle

(Continued)

botulinum toxin type A *(Continued)*

Subsequent doses for residual/recurrent strabismus: Re-examine patients 7-14 days after each injection to assess the effect of that dose. Subsequent doses for patients experiencing incomplete paralysis of the target may be increased up to two fold the previously administered dose. Maximum recommended dose as a single injection for any one muscle is 25 units.

Blepharospasm: 1.25-2.5 units (0.05-0.10 mL) injected into the orbicularis oculi muscle

Subsequent doses: Each treatment lasts approximately 3 months. At repeat treatment sessions, the dose may be increased up to twofold if the response from the initial treatment is considered insufficient (usually defined as an effect that does not last >2 months). There appears to be little benefit obtainable from injecting >5 units per site. Some tolerance may be found if treatments are administered any more frequently than every 3 months.

The cumulative dose should not exceed 200 units in a 30-day period

Dosage Forms Injection: 100 units *Clostridium botulinum* toxin type A

bovine lung surfactant *see* beractant *on page 70*

Breathe Free® [OTC] *see* sodium chloride *on page 526*

Breezee® Mist Antifungal [OTC] *see* miconazole *on page 373*

Breonesin® [OTC] *see* guaifenesin *on page 267*

Brethaire® *see* terbutaline *on page 551*

Brethine® *see* terbutaline *on page 551*

Bretylate® (Can) *see* bretylium *on this page*

bretylium (bre TIL ee um)

U.S./Canadian Brand Names Bretylate® (Can)

Therapeutic Category Antiarrhythmic Agent, Class III

Use Ventricular tachycardia or ventricular fibrillation; other serious ventricular arrhythmias resistant to lidocaine

Usual Dosage

Children:

I.M.: 2-5 mg/kg as a single dose

I.V.: Initial: 5 mg/kg, then attempt electrical defibrillation; repeat with 10 mg/kg if ventricular fibrillation persists

Maintenance dose: I.M., I.V.: 5 mg/kg every 6-8 hours

Adults:

Immediate life-threatening ventricular arrhythmias; ventricular fibrillation; unstable ventricular tachycardia. **Note**: Patients should undergo defibrillation/cardioversion before and after bretylium doses as necessary:

Initial dose: I.V.: 5 mg/kg (undiluted) over 1 minute; if arrhythmia persists, administer 10 mg/kg (undiluted) over 1 minute and repeat as necessary (usually at 15- to 30-minute intervals) up to a total dose of 30 mg/kg

Other life-threatening ventricular arrhythmias:

Initial dose: I.M., I.V.: 5-10 mg/kg, may repeat every 1-2 hours if arrhythmia persist; administer I.V. dose (diluted) over 10-30 minutes

Maintenance dose: I.M.: 5-10 mg/kg every 6-8 hours; I.V. (diluted): 5-10 mg/kg every 6 hours; I.V. infusion (diluted): 1-2 mg/minute (little experience with doses >40 mg/kg/day)

Dosage Forms Bretylium tosylate:

Infusion, premixed in D_5W: 1 mg/mL (500 mL); 2 mg/mL (250 mL); 4 mg/mL (250 mL, 500 mL)

Injection: 50 mg/mL (10 mL, 20 mL)

Bretylol® *(Discontinued)* *see page 700*

Brevibloc® *see* esmolol *on page 216*

Brevicon® *see* ethinyl estradiol and norethindrone *on page 224*

Brevital® Sodium *see* methohexital *on page 364*

Brevoxyl® Gel *see* benzoyl peroxide *on page 68*

Bricanyl® *see* terbutaline *on page 551*

Brietal Sodium® (Can) *see* methohexital *on page 364*

brimonidine (bri MOE ni deen)

U.S./Canadian Brand Names Alphagan®

Therapeutic Category $Alpha_2$-Adrenergic Agonist Agent, Ophthalmic

Use Lowering of intraocular pressure in patients with open-angle glaucoma or ocular hypertension

Usual Dosage Adults: Ophthalmic: 1 drop in affected eye(s) 3 times/day (approximately every 8 hours)

Dosage Forms Solution, ophthalmic, as tartrate: 0.2% (5 mL, 10 mL)

brinzolamide (brin ZOH la mide)

U.S./Canadian Brand Names Azopt®

Therapeutic Category Carbonic Anhydrase Inhibitor

Use Lowers intraocular pressure to treat glaucoma in patients with ocular hypertension or open-angle glaucoma

Usual Dosage Adults: Ophthalmic: Instill 1 drop in eye(s) 3 times/day

Dosage Forms Suspension, ophthalmic: 1% (2.5 mL, 5 mL, 10 mL, 15 mL)

British anti-lewisite *see* dimercaprol *on page 183*

Brofed® Elixir [OTC] *see* brompheniramine and pseudoephedrine *on page 81*

Bromaline® Elixir [OTC] *see* brompheniramine and phenylpropanolamine *on page 81*

Bromanate® DC *see* brompheniramine, phenylpropanolamine, and codeine *on page 82*

Bromanate® Elixir [OTC] *see* brompheniramine and phenylpropanolamine *on page 81*

Bromanyl® Cough Syrup *see* bromodiphenhydramine and codeine *on next page*

Bromarest® [OTC] *see* brompheniramine *on next page*

Bromatapp® [OTC] *see* brompheniramine and phenylpropanolamine *on page 81*

bromazepam *(Canada only)* (broe MA ze pam)

U.S./Canadian Brand Names Lectopam® (Can)

Therapeutic Category Benzodiazepine; Sedative

Use Short-term, symptomatic relief of manifestations of excessive anxiety in patients with anxiety nerosis

Usual Dosage Adults: Oral: 6-18 mg/day in equally divided doses. depending on the severity of symptoms and response of the patient

Dosage Forms Tablet: 1.5 mg, 3 mg, 6 mg

Brombay® [OTC] *see* brompheniramine *on next page*

Bromfed® Syrup [OTC] *see* brompheniramine and pseudoephedrine *on page 81*

Bromfed® Tablet [OTC] *see* brompheniramine and pseudoephedrine *on page 81*

Bromfenex® *see* brompheniramine and pseudoephedrine *on page 81*

Bromfenex® PD *see* brompheniramine and pseudoephedrine *on page 81*

bromocriptine (broe moe KRIP teen)

U.S./Canadian Brand Names Apo® Bromocriptine (Can); Parlodel®

Therapeutic Category Anti-Parkinson's Agent; Ergot Alkaloid and Derivative

(Continued)

bromocriptine *(Continued)*

Use Treatment of parkinsonism in patients unresponsive or allergic to levodopa; also used in conditions associated with hyperprolactinemia and to suppress lactation

Usual Dosage Oral:

Parkinsonism: 1.25 mg twice daily, increased by 2.5 mg/day in 2- to 4-week intervals (usual dose range: 30-90 mg/day in 3 divided doses)

Hyperprolactinemia and postpartum lactation: 2.5 mg 2-3 times/day

Dosage Forms Bromocriptine mesylate:

Capsule: 5 mg

Tablet: 2.5 mg

bromodiphenhydramine and codeine

(brome oh dye fen HYE dra meen & KOE deen)

Synonyms codeine and bromodiphenhydramine

U.S./Canadian Brand Names Ambenyl® Cough Syrup; Amgenal® Cough Syrup; Bromanyl® Cough Syrup; Bromotuss® w/Codeine Cough Syrup

Therapeutic Category Antihistamine/Antitussive

Controlled Substance C-V

Use Relief of upper respiratory symptoms and cough associated with allergies or common cold

Usual Dosage Oral: 5-10 mL every 4-6 hours

Dosage Forms Liquid: Bromodiphenhydramine hydrochloride 12.5 mg and codeine phosphate 10 mg per 5 mL

Bromotuss® w/Codeine Cough Syrup *see* bromodiphenhydramine and codeine *on this page*

Bromphen® [OTC] *see* brompheniramine *on this page*

Bromphen® DC w/Codeine *see* brompheniramine, phenylpropanolamine, and codeine *on page 82*

brompheniramine (brome fen IR a meen)

Synonyms parabromdylamine

U.S./Canadian Brand Names Bromarest® [OTC]; Brombay® [OTC]; Bromphen® [OTC]; Brotane® [OTC]; Chlorphed® [OTC]; Cophene-B®; Diamine T.D.® [OTC]; Dimetane® Extentabs® [OTC]; Nasahist B®; ND-Stat®

Therapeutic Category Antihistamine

Use Perennial and seasonal allergic rhinitis and other allergic symptoms including urticaria

Usual Dosage

Oral:

Children:

<6 years: 0.125 mg/kg/dose administered every 6 hours; maximum: 6-8 mg/day

6-12 years: 2-4 mg every 6-8 hours; maximum: 12-16 mg/day

Adults: 4 mg every 4-6 hours or 8 mg of sustained release form every 8-12 hours or 12 mg of sustained release every 12 hours; maximum: 24 mg/day

I.M., I.V., S.C.:

Children <12 years: 0.5 mg/kg/24 hours divided every 6-8 hours

Adults: 5-50 mg every 4-12 hours, maximum: 40 mg/24 hours

Dosage Forms Brompheniramine maleate:

Elixir: 2 mg/5 mL with 3% alcohol (120 mL, 480 mL, 4000 mL)

Injection: 10 mg/mL (10 mL)

Tablet: 4 mg, 8 mg, 12 mg

Sustained release: 8 mg, 12 mg

brompheniramine and phenylephrine

(brome fen IR a meen & fen il EF rin)

U.S./Canadian Brand Names Dimetane® Decongestant Elixir [OTC]

Therapeutic Category Antihistamine/Decongestant Combination

Use Temporary relief of symptoms of seasonal and perennial allergic rhinitis, and vasomotor rhinitis, including nasal obstruction

Usual Dosage Children >12 years and Adults: Oral: 10 mL every 4 hours

Dosage Forms Elixir: Brompheniramine maleate 4 mg and phenylephrine hydrochloride 5 mg per 5 mL

brompheniramine and phenylpropanolamine

(brome fen IR a meen & fen il proe pa NOLE a meen)

Synonyms phenylpropanolamine and brompheniramine

U.S./Canadian Brand Names Bromaline® Elixir [OTC]; Bromanate® Elixir [OTC]; Bromatapp® [OTC]; Bromphen® Tablet [OTC]; Cold & Allergy® Elixir [OTC]; Dimaphen® Elixir [OTC]; Dimaphen® Tablets [OTC]; Dimetapp® 4-Hour Liqui-Gel Capsule [OTC]; Dimetapp® Elixir [OTC]; Dimetapp® Extentabs® [OTC]; Dimetapp® Tablet [OTC]; Genatap® Elixir [OTC]; Tamine® [OTC]; Vicks® DayQuil® Allergy Relief 4 Hour Tablet [OTC]

Therapeutic Category Antihistamine/Decongestant Combination

Use Temporary relief of nasal congestion, running nose, sneezing, and itchy, watery eyes

Usual Dosage Oral:

Children:

1-6 months: 1.25 mL 3-4 times/day

7-24 months: 2.5 mL 3-4 times/day

2-4 years: 3.75 mL 3-4 times/day

4-12 years: 5 mL 3-4 times/day

Adults: 5-10 mL 3-4 times/day or regular capsule or tablet 3-4 times daily or 1 sustained release tablet twice daily

Dosage Forms

Capsule (Dimetapp® 4-Hour Liqui-Gel): Brompheniramine maleate 4 mg and phenylpropanolamine hydrochloride 25 mg

Liquid (Bromaline®, Bromanate®, Cold & Allergy®, Dimaphen®, Dimetapp®, Genatap®): Brompheniramine maleate 2 mg and phenylpropanolamine hydrochloride 12.5 mg per 5 mL

Tablet (Dimaphen®, Dimetapp®, Vicks® DayQuil® Allergy Relief 4 Hour): Brompheniramine maleate 4 mg and phenylpropanolamine hydrochloride 25 mg

Tablet, sustained release: Brompheniramine maleate 12 mg and phenylpropanolamine hydrochloride 75 mg

brompheniramine and pseudoephedrine

(brome fen IR a meen & soo doe e FED rin)

U.S./Canadian Brand Names Brofed® Elixir [OTC]; Bromfed® Syrup [OTC]; Bromfed® Tablet [OTC]; Bromfenex®; Bromfenex® PD; Drixoral® Syrup [OTC]; Iofed®; Iofed® PD

Therapeutic Category Antihistamine/Decongestant Combination

Use Temporary relief of symptoms of seasonal and perennial allergic rhinitis, and vasomotor rhinitis, including nasal obstruction

Usual Dosage Oral:

Children 6-12 years: 5-10 mL 3-4 times/day

Children >12 years and Adults: 1 or 2 capsules every 12 hours or 1 or 2 tablets 3-4 times/day or 5-10 mL 3-4 times/day

Dosage Forms

Capsule, extended release:

Bromfenex® PD, Iofed® PD: Brompheniramine maleate 6 mg and pseudoephedrine hydrochloride 60 mg

Bromfenex®, Iofed®: Brompheniramine maleate 12 mg and pseudoephedrine hydrochloride 120 mg

Elixir:

Brofed®: Brompheniramine maleate 4 mg and pseudoephedrine hydrochloride 30 mg per 5 mL

Bromfed®: Brompheniramine maleate 2 mg and pseudoephedrine hydrochloride 30 mg per 5 mL

(Continued)

brompheniramine and pseudoephedrine *(Continued)*

Drixoral®: Brompheniramine maleate 2 mg and pseudoephedrine sulfate 30 mg per 5 mL

Tablet (Bromfed®): Brompheniramine maleate 4 mg and pseudoephedrine hydrochloride 60 mg

brompheniramine, phenylpropanolamine, and codeine

(brome fen IR a meen, fen il proe pa NOLE a meen, & KOE deen)

Synonyms codeine, brompheniramine, and phenylpropanolamine; phenylpropanolamine, brompheniramine, and codeine

U.S./Canadian Brand Names Bromanate® DC; Bromphen® DC w/Codeine; Dimetane®-DC; Myphetane DC®; Poly-Histine CS®

Therapeutic Category Antihistamine/Decongestant/Antitussive

Controlled Substance C-V

Use Relief of coughs and upper respiratory symptoms, including nasal congestion, associated with allergy or the common cold

Usual Dosage Oral:

Children:

2-6 years: 2.5 mL every 4 hours

6-12 years: 5 mL every 4 hours

Children >12 years and Adults: 10 mL every 4 hours

Dosage Forms Liquid: Brompheniramine maleate 2 mg, phenylpropanolamine hydrochloride 12.5 mg, and codeine phosphate 10 mg per 5 mL with alcohol 0.95% (480 mL)

Bromphen® Tablet [OTC] *see* brompheniramine and phenylpropanolamine *on previous page*

Bronalide® (Can) *see* flunisolide *on page 243*

Bronchial® *see* theophylline and guaifenesin *on page 559*

Bronitin® Mist [OTC] *see* epinephrine *on page 209*

Bronkaid® Mist [OTC] *see* epinephrine *on page 209*

Bronkephrine® ***(Discontinued)*** *see page 700*

Bronkometer® *see* isoetharine *on page 313*

Bronkosol® *see* isoetharine *on page 313*

Brontex® Liquid *see* guaifenesin and codeine *on page 268*

Brontex® Tablet *see* guaifenesin and codeine *on page 268*

Brotane® [OTC] *see* brompheniramine *on page 80*

BSS® Ophthalmic *see* balanced salt solution *on page 60*

budesonide (byoo DES oh nide)

U.S./Canadian Brand Names Entocort® (Can); Pulmicort® Turbuhaler®; Rhinocort®; Rhinocort® Turbuhaler® (Can)

Therapeutic Category Adrenal Corticosteroid

Use

Children and Adults: Management of symptoms of seasonal or perennial rhinitis

Adults: Nonallergic perennial rhinitis

Usual Dosage Children ≥6 years and Adults: 256 mcg/day, administered as either 2 sprays in each nostril in the morning and evening or as 4 sprays in each nostril in the morning

Dosage Forms

Aerosol, nasal: 32 mcg per actuation (7 g)

Powder (dry) for inhalation: 200 mcg per metered dose

Buffered®, Tri-buffered ***(Discontinued)*** *see page 700*

Bufferin® [OTC] *see* aspirin *on page 49*

Bufferin® Arthritis Strength *(Discontinued)* *see page 700*

Bufferin® Extra Strength *(Discontinued)* *see page 700*

Buf-Puf® Acne Cleansing Bar *(Discontinued)* *see page 700*

bumetanide (byoo MET a nide)

U.S./Canadian Brand Names Bumex®; Burinex® (Can)

Therapeutic Category Diuretic, Loop

Use Management of edema secondary to congestive heart failure or hepatic or renal disease including nephrotic syndrome; may also be used alone or in combination with antihypertensives in the treatment of hypertension

Usual Dosage

Children:

<6 months: Dose not established

>6 months:

Oral: Initial: 0.015 mg/kg/dose once daily or every other day; maximum dose: 0.1 mg/kg/day

I.M., I.V.: Dose not established

Adults:

Oral: 0.5-2 mg/dose (maximum: 10 mg/day) 1-2 times/day

I.M., I.V.: 0.5-1 mg/dose (maximum: 10 mg/day)

Dosage Forms

Injection: 0.25 mg/mL (2 mL, 4 mL, 10 mL)

Tablet: 0.5 mg, 1 mg, 2 mg

Bumex® *see* bumetanide *on this page*

Buminate® *see* albumin *on page 15*

Bupap® *see* butalbital compound and acetaminophen *on page 85*

Buphenyl® *see* sodium phenylbutyrate *on page 528*

bupivacaine (byoo PIV a kane)

U.S./Canadian Brand Names Marcaine®; Sensorcaine®; Sensorcaine®-MPF

Therapeutic Category Local Anesthetic

Use Local anesthetic (injectable) for peripheral nerve block, infiltration, sympathetic block, caudal or epidural block, retrobulbar block

Usual Dosage Dose varies with procedure, depth of anesthesia, vascularity of tissues, duration of anesthesia and condition of patient

Caudal block (with or without epinephrine):

Children: 1-3.7 mg/kg

Adults: 15-30 mL of 0.25% or 0.5%

Epidural block (other than caudal block):

Children: 1.25 mg/kg/dose

Adults: 10-20 mL of 0.25% or 0.5%

Peripheral nerve block: 5 mL dose of 0.25% or 0.5% (12.5-25 mg); maximum: 2.5 mg/kg (plain); 3 mg/kg (with epinephrine); up to a maximum of 400 mg/day

Sympathetic nerve block: 20-50 mL of 0.25% (no epinephrine) solution

Dosage Forms Bupivacaine hydrochloride:

Injection: 0.25% (10 mL, 20 mL, 30 mL, 50 mL); 0.5% (10 mL, 20 mL, 30 mL, 50 mL); 0.75% (2 mL, 10 mL, 20 mL, 30 mL)

Injection with epinephrine (1:200,000): 0.25% (10 mL, 30 mL, 50 mL); 0.5% (1.8 mL, 3 mL, 5 mL, 10 mL, 30 mL, 50 mL); 0.75% (30 mL)

Buprenex® *see* buprenorphine *on this page*

buprenorphine (byoo pre NOR feen)

U.S./Canadian Brand Names Buprenex®

Therapeutic Category Analgesic, Narcotic

Controlled Substance C-V

(Continued)

buprenorphine *(Continued)*

Use Management of moderate to severe pain

Usual Dosage Adults: I.M., slow I.V.: 0.3-0.6 mg every 6 hours as needed

Dosage Forms Injection, as hydrochloride: 0.3 mg/mL (1 mL)

bupropion (byoo PROE pee on)

U.S./Canadian Brand Names Wellbutrin®; Wellbutrin® SR; Zyban™

Therapeutic Category Antidepressant, Aminoketone

Use Treatment of depression; as an aid to smoking cessation treatment

Usual Dosage Oral:

Adults:

Depression: 100 mg 3 times/day; begin at 100 mg twice daily; may increase to a maximum dose of 450 mg/day

Smoking cessation: Initiate with 150 mg once daily for 3 days; increase to 150 mg twice daily; treatment should continue for 7-12 weeks

Elderly: Depression: 50-100 mg/day, increase by 50-100 mg every 3-4 days as tolerated; there is evidence that the elderly respond at 150 mg/day in divided doses, but some may require a higher dose

Dosage Forms

Tablet: 75 mg, 100 mg

Tablet, sustained release: 100 mg, 150 mg

Tablet, sustained release (Zyban™): 150 mg

Burinex® (Can) *see* bumetanide *on previous page*

Burow's otic *see* aluminum acetate and acetic acid *on page 21*

BuSpar® *see* buspirone *on this page*

buspirone (byoo SPYE rone)

U.S./Canadian Brand Names BuSpar®

Therapeutic Category Antianxiety Agent

Use Management of anxiety

Usual Dosage Adults: Oral: 15 mg/day (5 mg 3 times/day); may increase to a maximum of 60 mg/day

Dosage Forms Tablet, as hydrochloride: 5 mg, 10 mg

busulfan (byoo SUL fan)

U.S./Canadian Brand Names Busulfex®; Myleran®

Therapeutic Category Antineoplastic Agent

Use

Injection: Use in combination with cyclophosphamide as a conditioning regimen prior to allogeneic hematopoietic progenitor cell transplantation for chronic myelogenous leukemia

Oral: Chronic myelogenous leukemia and bone marrow disorders, such as polycythemia vera and myeloid metaplasia, conditioning regimens for bone marrow transplantation

Usual Dosage

I.V.: Adult: As a component of a conditioning regimen prior to bone marrow or peripheral blood progenitor cell replacement support is 0.8 mg/kg of ideal body weight or actual body weight, whichever is lower, administered every 6 hours for 4 days (a total of 16 doses)

Oral (**refer to individual protocols**):

Children:

For remission induction of CML: 0.06-0.12 mg/kg/day **or** 1.8-4.6 mg/m^2/day; titrate dosage to maintain leukocyte count above 40,000/mm^3; reduce dosage by 50% if the leukocyte count reaches 30,000-40,000/mm^3; discontinue drug if counts fall to ≤20,000/mm^3

BMT marrow-ablative conditioning regimen: 1 mg/kg/dose (ideal body weight) every 6 hours for 16 doses

Adults:
BMT marrow-ablative conditioning regimen: 1 mg/kg/dose (ideal body weight) every 6 hours for 16 doses

Dosage Forms Tablet: 2 mg

Busulfex® *see* busulfan *on previous page*

butabarbital sodium (byoo ta BAR bi tal SOW dee um)

U.S./Canadian Brand Names Butalan®; Buticaps®; Butisol Sodium®

Therapeutic Category Barbiturate

Controlled Substance C-III

Use Sedative, hypnotic

Usual Dosage

Children: Preop: 2-6 mg/kg/dose; maximum: 100 mg
Adults:
Sedative: 15-30 mg 3-4 times/day
Hypnotic: 50-100 mg
Preop: 50-100 mg 1-1½ hours before surgery

Dosage Forms

Capsule: 15 mg, 30 mg
Elixir, with alcohol 7%: 30 mg/5 mL (480 mL, 3780 mL); 33.3 mg/5 mL (480 mL, 3780 mL)
Tablet: 15 mg, 30 mg, 50 mg, 100 mg

Butace® ***(Discontinued)*** *see page 700*

Butalan® *see* butabarbital sodium *on this page*

butalbital compound and acetaminophen

(byoo TAL bi tal KOM pound & a seet a MIN oh fen)

Synonyms acetaminophen and butalbital compound

U.S./Canadian Brand Names Amaphen®; Anoquan®; Axocet®; Bupap®; Endolor®; Esgic®; Esgic-Plus®; Femcet®; Fioricet®; G-1®; Medigesic®; Phrenilin®; Phrenilin® Forte; Repan®; Sedapap-10®; Triapin®; Two-Dyne®

Therapeutic Category Barbiturate/Analgesic

Controlled Substance C-III

Use Relief of the symptomatic complex of tension or muscle contraction headache

Usual Dosage Adults: Oral: 1-2 tablets or capsules every 4 hours; not to exceed 6/day

Dosage Forms

Capsule:
Amaphen®, Anoquan®, Endolor®, Esgic®, Femcet®, G-1®, Medigesic®, Repan®, Two-Dyne®: Butalbital 50 mg, caffeine 40 mg, and acetaminophen 325 mg
Axocet®; Phrenilin® Forte: Butalbital 50 mg and acetaminophen 650 mg
Triapin®: Butalbital 50 mg and acetaminophen 325 mg
Tablet:
Esgic®, Fioricet®, Repan®: Butalbital 50 mg, caffeine 40 mg, and acetaminophen 325 mg
Phrenilin®: Butalbital 50 mg and acetaminophen 325 mg
Sedapap-10®: Butalbital 50 mg and acetaminophen 650 mg

butalbital compound and aspirin (byoo TAL bi tal KOM pound & AS pir in)

Synonyms aspirin and butalbital compound

U.S./Canadian Brand Names Fiorgen PF®; Fiorinal®; Isollyl® Improved; Lanorinal®

Therapeutic Category Barbiturate/Analgesic

Controlled Substance C-III (Fiorinal®)

Use Relief of the symptomatic complex of tension or muscle contraction headache

Usual Dosage Adults: Oral: 1-2 tablets or capsules every 4 hours; not to exceed 6/day

(Continued)

butalbital compound and aspirin *(Continued)*

Dosage Forms

Capsule: (Fiorgen PF®, Fiorinal®, Isollyl® Improved, Lanorinal®, Marnal®): Butalbital 50 mg, caffeine 40 mg, and aspirin 325 mg

Tablet: (Fiorinal®, Isollyl® Improved, Lanorinal®, Marnal®): Butalbital 50 mg, caffeine 40 mg, and aspirin 325 mg

butalbital compound and codeine

(byoo TAL bi tal KOM pound & KOE deen)

Synonyms codeine and butalbital compound

U.S./Canadian Brand Names Fiorinal® With Codeine

Therapeutic Category Analgesic, Narcotic; Barbiturate

Controlled Substance C-III

Use Mild to moderate pain when sedation is needed

Usual Dosage Adults: Oral: 1-2 capsules every 4 hours as needed for pain; up to 6/day

Dosage Forms Capsule: Butalbital 50 mg, caffeine 40 mg, aspirin 325 mg and codeine phosphate 30 mg

butenafine (byoo TEN a fine)

U.S./Canadian Brand Names Mentax®

Therapeutic Category Antifungal Agent

Use Topical treatment of interdigital tinea pedis (athlete's foot) due to *Epidermophyton floccosum*, *Trichophyton mentagrophytes*, or *Trichophyton rubrum*

Usual Dosage Adults: Topical: Apply cream to the affected area and surrounding skin once daily for 4 weeks

Dosage Forms Cream, as hydrochloride: 1% (2 g, 15 g, 30 g)

Buticaps® *see* butabarbital sodium *on previous page*

Butisol Sodium® *see* butabarbital sodium *on previous page*

butoconazole (byoo toe KOE na zole)

Therapeutic Category Antifungal Agent

Use Local treatment of vulvovaginal candidiasis

Usual Dosage Adults:

Nonpregnant: Insert 1 applicatorful (~5 g) intravaginally at bedtime for 3 days, may extend for up to 6 days if necessary

Pregnant: **Use only during second or third trimesters**

Dosage Forms Cream, vaginal, as nitrate: 2% with applicator (28 g)

butorphanol (byoo TOR fa nole)

U.S./Canadian Brand Names Stadol®; Stadol® NS

Therapeutic Category Analgesic, Narcotic

Controlled Substance C-IV

Use Management of moderate to severe pain

Usual Dosage Adults:

I.M.: 1-4 mg every 3-4 hours as needed

I.V.: 0.5-2 mg every 3-4 hours as needed

Nasal: Initial: 1 mg (1 spray in one nostril), allow 60-90 minutes to elapse before deciding whether a second 1 mg dose is needed; this 2-dose sequence may be repeated in 3-4 hours if needed

Dosage Forms Butorphanol tartrate:

Injection: 1 mg/mL (1 mL); 2 mg/mL (1 mL, 2 mL, 10 mL)

Spray, nasal: 10 mg/mL [14-15 doses] (2.5 mL)

butyl aminobenzoate, benzocaine, tetracaine, and benzalkonium chloride *see* benzocaine, butyl aminobenzoate, tetracaine, and benzalkonium chloride *on page 67*

Byclomine® Injection *see* dicyclomine *on page 177*

Bydramine® Cough Syrup [OTC] *see* diphenhydramine *on page 185*

C2B8 monoclonal antibody *see* rituximab *on page 507*

c7E3 *see* abciximab *on page 2*

C8-CCK *see* sincalide *on page 523*

311C90 *see* zolmitriptan *on page 613*

cabergoline (ca BER go leen)

U.S./Canadian Brand Names Dostinex®

Therapeutic Category Ergot-like Derivative

Use Treatment of hyperprolactinemia

Usual Dosage Adults: Oral: 0.25 mg twice weekly; dosage may be increased by 0.25 mg twice weekly to a dose of up to 1 mg twice weekly (according to the patient's prolactin level)

Dosage Forms Tablet: 0.5 mg

Cafatine-PB® *see* ergotamine *on page 213*

Cafergot® *see* ergotamine *on page 213*

Cafetrate® *see* ergotamine *on page 213*

caffeine and sodium benzoate (KAF een & SOW dee um BEN zoe ate)

Synonyms sodium benzoate and caffeine

Therapeutic Category Diuretic, Miscellaneous

Use Emergency stimulant in acute circulatory failure; as a diuretic; and to relieve spinal puncture headache

Usual Dosage

Children: I.M., I.V., S.C.: 8 mg/kg every 4 hours as needed

Adults: I.M., I.V.: 500 mg, maximum single dose: 1 g

Dosage Forms Injection: Caffeine 125 mg and sodium benzoate 125 mg per mL (2 mL)

caffeine, citrated (KAF een, SIT rated)

Therapeutic Category Respiratory Stimulant

Use Central nervous system stimulant; used in the treatment of idiopathic apnea of prematurity

Usual Dosage Apnea of prematurity: Oral:

Loading dose: 10-20 mg/kg as caffeine citrate (5-10 mg/kg as caffeine base). If theophylline has been administered to the patient within the previous 5 days, a full or modified loading dose (50% to 75% of a loading dose) may be administered at the discretion of the physician.

Maintenance dose: 5-10 mg/kg/day as caffeine citrate (2.5-5 mg/kg/day as caffeine base) once daily starting 24 hours after the loading dose. Maintenance dose is adjusted based on patient's response, (efficacy and adverse effects), and serum caffeine concentrations.

Dosage Forms

Solution, oral: 20 mg/mL [anhydrous caffeine 10 mg/mL]

Tablet: 65 mg [anhydrous caffeine 32.5 mg]

caffeine, hydrocodone, chlorpheniramine, phenylephrine, and acetaminophen *see* hydrocodone, chlorpheniramine, phenylephrine, acetaminophen, and caffeine *on page 290*

caffeine, orphenadrine, and aspirin *see* orphenadrine, aspirin, and caffeine *on page 418*

Caladryl® Spray *(Discontinued)* *see page 700*

Calan® *see* verapamil *on page 598*

Calan® SR *see* verapamil *on page 598*

Cal Carb-HD® [OTC] *see* calcium carbonate *on next page*

Calcibind® *see* cellulose sodium phosphate *on page 110*

Calci-Chew™ [OTC] *see* calcium carbonate *on next page*

Calciday-667® [OTC] *see* calcium carbonate *on next page*

calcifediol (kal si fe DYE ole)

Synonyms 25-D_3; 25-hydroxycholecalciferol; 25-hydroxyvitamin D_3

U.S./Canadian Brand Names Calderol®

Therapeutic Category Vitamin D Analog

Use Treatment and management of metabolic bone disease associated with chronic renal failure

Usual Dosage Hepatic osteodystrophy: Oral:

Infants: 5-7 mcg/kg/day

Children and Adults: 20-100 mcg/day or every other day; titrate to obtain normal serum calcium/phosphate levels

Dosage Forms Capsule: 20 mcg, 50 mcg

Calciferol™ *see* ergocalciferol *on page 212*

Calcijex™ *see* calcitriol *on next page*

Calcilean® [HepCalium] (Can) *see* heparin *on page 278*

Calcimar® *see* calcitonin *on this page*

Calci-Mix™ [OTC] *see* calcium carbonate *on next page*

Calciparine® Injection *(Discontinued)* *see page 700*

calcipotriene (kal si POE try een)

U.S./Canadian Brand Names Dovonex®

Therapeutic Category Antipsoriatic Agent

Use Treatment of plaque psoriasis

Usual Dosage Topical: Apply to skin lesions twice daily

Dosage Forms

Cream: 0.005% (30 g, 60 g, 100 g)

Ointment, topical: 0.005% (30 g, 60 g, 100 g)

Solution, topical: 0.005%

Calcite-500 (Can) *see* calcium carbonate *on next page*

calcitonin (kal si TOE nin)

Synonyms calcitonin (human); calcitonin (salmon)

U.S./Canadian Brand Names Calcimar®; Caltine® (Can); Cibacalcin®; Miacalcin®; Miacalcin® Nasal Spray; Osteocalcin®; Salmonine®

Therapeutic Category Polypeptide Hormone

Use

Calcitonin (salmon): Treatment of Paget's disease of bone and as adjunctive therapy for hypercalcemia; also used in postmenopausal osteoporosis and osteogenesis imperfecta

Calcitonin (human): Treatment of Paget's disease of bone

Usual Dosage

Children: Dosage not established

Adults:

Paget's disease: Salmon calcitonin:

I.M., S.C.: 100 units/day to start, 50 units/day or 50-100 units every 1-3 days maintenance dose

Human calcitonin: S.C.: Initial: 0.5 mg/day (maximum: 0.5 mg twice daily); maintenance: 0.5 mg 2-3 times/week or 0.25 mg/day

Hypercalcemia: Initial: Salmon calcitonin: I.M., S.C.: 4 units/kg every 12 hours; may increase up to 8 units/kg every 12 hours to a maximum of every 6 hours

Osteogenesis imperfecta: Salmon calcitonin: I.M., S.C.: 2 units/kg 3 times/week
Postmenopausal osteoporosis: Salmon calcitonin:
I.M., S.C.: 100 units/day
Intranasal: 200 units (1 spray)/day

Dosage Forms
Injection:
Human (Cibacalcin®): 0.5 mg/vial
Salmon: 200 units/mL (2 mL)
Spray, nasal: 200 units/activation (0.09 mL/dose) (2 mL glass bottle with pump)

calcitonin (human) *see* calcitonin *on previous page*

calcitonin (salmon) *see* calcitonin *on previous page*

calcitriol (kal si TRYE ole)

Synonyms 1,25 dihydroxycholecalciferol
U.S./Canadian Brand Names Calcijex™; Rocaltrol®
Therapeutic Category Vitamin D Analog
Use Management of hypocalcemia in patients on chronic renal dialysis; reduce elevated parathyroid hormone levels
Usual Dosage Individualize dosage to maintain calcium levels of 9-10 mg/dL
Renal failure: Oral:
Children: Initial: 15 ng/kg/day; maintenance: 30-60 ng/kg/day
Adults: 0.25 mcg/day or every other day (may require 0.5-1 mcg/day)
Unlabeled dose:
Renal failure: I.V.: Adults: 0.5 mcg (0.01 mcg/kg) 3 times/week; most doses in the range of 0.5-3 mcg (0.01-0.05 mcg/kg) 3 times/week
Hypoparathyroidism/pseudohypoparathyroidism: Oral:
Children 1-5 years: 0.25-0.75 mcg/day
Children >6 years and Adults: 0.5-2 mcg/day

Dosage Forms
Capsule: 0.25 mcg, 0.5 mcg
Injection: 1 mcg/mL (1 mL); 2 mcg/mL (1 mL)

calcium acetate (KAL see um AS e tate)

U.S./Canadian Brand Names Calphron®; PhosLo®
Therapeutic Category Electrolyte Supplement, Oral
Use Control of hyperphosphatemia in end-stage renal failure and does not promote aluminum absorption
Usual Dosage Adults: Oral: 2 tablets with each meal; dosage may be increased to bring serum phosphate value to <6 mg/dL; most patients require 3-4 tablets with each meal
Dosage Forms Elemental calcium listed in brackets
Capsule (Phos-Ex® 125): 500 mg [125 mg]
Tablet:
Calphron®: 667 mg [169 mg]
PhosLo®: 667 mg [169 mg]

calcium carbonate (KAL see um KAR bun ate)

U.S./Canadian Brand Names Alka-Mints® [OTC]; Amitone® [OTC]; Apo-Cal® (Can); Cal Carb-HD® [OTC]; Calci-Chew™ [OTC]; Calciday-667® [OTC]; Calci-Mix™ [OTC]; Calcite-500 (Can); Cal-Plus® [OTC]; Calsan® (Can); Caltrate® 600 [OTC]; Caltrate, Jr.® [OTC]; Chooz® [OTC]; Dicarbosil® [OTC]; Equilet® [OTC]; Florical® [OTC]; Gencalc® 600 [OTC]; Mallamint® [OTC]; Nephro-Calci® [OTC]; Os-Cal® 500 [OTC]; Oyst-Cal 500 [OTC]; Oystercal® 500; Pharmacal® (Can); Rolaids® Calcium Rich [OTC]; Tums® [OTC]; Tums® E-X Extra Strength Tablet [OTC]; Tums® Extra Strength Liquid [OTC]
Therapeutic Category Antacid; Electrolyte Supplement, Oral
Use Treatment and prevention of calcium depletion; relief of acid indigestion, heartburn
Usual Dosage Dosage is in terms of elemental calcium
(Continued)

calcium carbonate *(Continued)*

Recommended daily allowance (RDA): Oral:
- <6 months: 360 mg/day
- 6-12 months: 540 mg/day
- 1-10 years: 800 mg/day
- 10-18 years: 1200 mg/day
- Adults: 800 mg/day

Hypocalcemia (dose depends on clinical condition and serum calcium level):
- Children: 20-65 mg/kg/day in 4 divided doses
- Adults: 1-2 g or more per day

Dosage Forms Elemental calcium listed in brackets

Capsule: 1500 mg [600 mg]
- Calci-Mix™: 1250 mg [500 mg]
- Florical®: 364 mg [145.6 mg] with sodium fluoride 8.3 mg

Liquid (Tums® Extra Strength): 1000 mg/5 mL (360 mL)

Lozenge (Mylanta® Soothing Antacids): 600 mg [240 mg]

Powder (Cal Carb-HD®): 6.5 g/packet [2.6 g]

Suspension, oral: 1250 mg/5 mL [500 mg]

Tablet: 650 mg [260 mg], 1500 mg [600 mg]
- Calciday-667®: 667 mg [267 mg]
- Os-Cal® 500, Oyst-Cal 500, Oystercal® 500: 1250 mg [500 mg]
- Cal-Plus®, Caltrate® 600, Gencalc® 600, Nephro-Calci®: 1500 mg [600 mg]
- Chewable:
  - Alka-Mints®: 850 mg [340 mg]
  - Amitone®: 350 mg [140 mg]
  - Caltrate, Jr.®: 750 mg [300 mg]
  - Calci-Chew™, Os-Cal®: 750 mg [300 mg]
  - Chooz®, Dicarbosil®, Equilet®, Tums®: 500 mg [200 mg]
  - Mallamint®: 420 mg [168 mg]
  - Rolaids® Calcium Rich: 550 mg [220 mg]
  - Tums® E-X Extra Strength: 750 mg [300 mg]
  - Tums® Ultra®: 1000 mg [400 mg]
- Florical®: 364 mg [145.6 mg]with sodium fluoride 8.3 mg

calcium carbonate and magnesium carbonate

(KAL see um KAR bun ate & mag NEE zhum KAR bun ate)

U.S./Canadian Brand Names Mylanta® Gelcaps®

Therapeutic Category Antacid

Use Hyperacidity

Usual Dosage Adults: Oral: 2-4 Gelcaps® as needed

Dosage Forms Capsule: Calcium carbonate 311 mg and magnesium carbonate 232 mg

calcium carbonate and simethicone

(KAL see um KAR bun ate & sye METH i kone)

Synonyms simethicone and calcium carbonate

U.S./Canadian Brand Names Titralac® Plus Liquid [OTC]

Therapeutic Category Antacid; Antiflatulent

Use Relief of acid indigestion, heartburn, peptic esophagitis, hiatal hernia, and gas

Usual Dosage Oral: 0.5-2 g 4-6 times/day

Dosage Forms Elemental calcium listed in brackets

Liquid: Calcium carbonate 500 mg [200 mg] and simethicone 20 mg per 5 mL

calcium chloride (KAL see um KLOR ide)

Therapeutic Category Electrolyte Supplement, Oral

Use Emergency treatment of hypocalcemic tetany; treatment of hypermagnesemia; cardiac disturbances of hyperkalemia, hypocalcemia or calcium channel blocking agent toxicity

Usual Dosage I.V.:

Cardiac arrest in the presence of hyperkalemia or hypocalcemia, magnesium toxicity, or calcium antagonist toxicity:

Infants and Children: 10-20 mg/kg; may repeat in 10 minutes if necessary

Adults: 1.5-4 mg/kg/dose or 2.5-5 mL/dose every 10 minutes

Hypocalcemia:

Infants and Children: 10-20 mg/kg/dose, repeat every 4-6 hours if needed

Adults: 500 mg to 1 g at 1- to 3-day intervals

Exchange transfusion: 0.45 mEq after each 100 mL of blood exchanged I.V.

Hypocalcemia secondary to citrated blood transfusion: Administer 0.45 mEq **elemental** calcium for each 100 mL citrated blood infused

Tetany:

Infants and Children: 10 mg/kg over 5-10 minutes; may repeat after 6 hours or follow with an infusion with a maximum dose of 200 mg/kg/day

Adults: 1 g over 10-30 minutes; may repeat after 6 hours

Dosage Forms Elemental calcium listed in brackets

Injection: 10% = 100 mg/mL [27.2 mg/mL] (10 mL)

calcium citrate (KAL see um SIT rate)

U.S./Canadian Brand Names Citracal® [OTC]

Therapeutic Category Electrolyte Supplement, Oral

Use Adjunct in prevention of postmenopausal osteoporosis, treatment and prevention of calcium depletion

Usual Dosage Oral (dosage is in terms of elemental calcium): Adults: Oral: 1-2 g/day

Recommended daily allowance (RDA):

<6 months: 360 mg/day

6-12 months: 540 mg/day

1-10 years: 800 mg/day

10-18 years: 1200 mg/day

Adults: 800 mg/day

Dosage Forms Elemental calcium listed in brackets

Tablet: 950 mg [200 mg]

Effervescent: 2376 mg [500 mg]

Calcium Disodium Versenate® *see* edetate calcium disodium *on page 203*

calcium edta *see* edetate calcium disodium *on page 203*

calcium glubionate (KAL see um gloo BYE oh nate)

U.S./Canadian Brand Names Neo-Calglucon® [OTC]

Therapeutic Category Electrolyte Supplement, Oral

Use Treatment and prevention of calcium depletion

Usual Dosage Oral (syrup is a hyperosmolar solution; dosage is in terms of calcium glubionate):

Neonatal hypocalcemia: 1200 mg/kg/day in 4-6 divided doses

Maintenance: Infants and Children: 600-2000 mg/kg/day in 4 divided doses up to a maximum of 9 g/day

Adults: 6-18 g/day in divided doses

Recommended daily allowance (RDA):

<6 months: 360 mg/day

6-12 months: 540 mg/day

1-10 years: 800 mg/day

10-18 years: 1200 mg/day

Adults: 800 mg/day

Dosage Forms Elemental calcium listed in brackets

Syrup: 1.8 g/5 mL [115 mg/5 mL] (480 mL)

calcium gluceptate (KAL see um gloo SEP tate)

Therapeutic Category Electrolyte Supplement, Oral

Use Emergency treatment of hypocalcemia; treatment of hypermagnesemia; cardiac disturbances of hyperkalemia, hypocalcemia, or calcium channel blocker toxicity

Usual Dosage I.V.:

Cardiac resuscitation in the presence of hypocalcemia, hyperkalemia, or calcium channel blocker toxicity:

Children: 110 mg/kg/dose or 0.5 mL/kg/dose every 10 minutes

Adults: 5 mL every 10 minutes

Hypocalcemia:

Children: 200-500 mg/kg/day divided every 6 hours

Adults: 500 mg to 1.1 g/dose as needed

Exchange transfusion: 0.45 mEq (0.5 mL) after each 100 mL of blood exchanged

After citrated blood administration: Children and Adults: 0.4 mEq/100 mL blood infused

Dosage Forms Elemental calcium listed in brackets

Injection: 220 mg/mL [18 mg/mL] (5 mL, 50 mL)

calcium gluconate (KAL see um GLOO koe nate)

U.S./Canadian Brand Names Kalcinate®

Therapeutic Category Electrolyte Supplement, Oral

Use Treatment and prevention of hypocalcemia, hypermagnesemia, cardiac disturbances of hyperkalemia, hypocalcemia, or calcium channel blocker toxicity

Usual Dosage Dosage is in terms of elemental calcium

Recommended daily allowance (RDA):

<6 months: 360 mg/day

6-12 months: 540 mg/day

1-10 years: 800 mg/day

10-18 years: 1200 mg/day

Adults: 800 mg/day

Calcium gluconate electrolyte requirement in newborn period:

Premature: 200-1000 mg/kg/24 hours

Term:

0-24 hours: 0-500 mg/kg/24 hours

24-48 hours: 200-500 mg/kg/24 hours

48-72 hours: 200-600 mg/kg/24 hours

>3 days: 200-800 mg/kg/24 hours

Hypocalcemia:

I.V.:

Infants and Children: 200-1000 mg/kg/day as a continuous infusion or in 4 divided doses

Adults: 2-15 g/24 hours as a continuous infusion or in divided doses

Oral:

Children: 200-500 mg/kg/day divided every 6 hours

Adults: 500 mg to 2 g 2-4 times/day

Calcium antagonist toxicity, magnesium intoxication; cardiac arrest in the presence of hyperkalemia or hypocalcemia: I.V.:

Infants and Children: 100 mg/kg/dose

Adults: 1-3 g

Tetany: I.V.: doses or as an infusion

Infants and Children: 100-200 mg/kg/dose over 5-10 minutes; may repeat after 6 hours or follow with an infusion of 500 mg/kg/day

Adults: 1-3 g may be administered until therapeutic response occurs

Cardiac resuscitation: I.V.:

Infants and Children: 100 mg/kg/dose (1 mL/kg/dose) every 10 minutes

Adults: 500-800 mg/dose (5-8 mL) every 10 minutes

Hypocalcemia secondary to citrated blood infusion; administer 0.45 mEq **elemental** calcium for each 100 mL citrated blood infused

Exchange transfusion:

Adults: 300 mg/100 mL of citrated blood exchanged

Maintenance electrolyte requirements for total parenteral nutrition: I.V.: Daily requirements: Adults: 10-20 mEq/1000 kcals/24 hours

Dosage Forms Elemental calcium listed in brackets

Injection: 10% = 100 mg/mL [9 mg/mL] (10 mL, 50 mL, 100 mL, 200 mL)

Tablet: 500 mg [45 mg], 650 mg [58.5 mg], 975 mg [87.75 mg], 1 g [90 mg]

calcium lactate (KAL see um LAK tate)

Therapeutic Category Electrolyte Supplement, Oral

Use Treatment and prevention of calcium depletion

Usual Dosage Oral:

Infants: 400-500 mg/kg/day divided every 4-6 hours

Children: 500 mg/kg/day divided every 6-8 hours; maximum daily dose: 9 g

Adults: 1.5-3 g divided every 8 hours

Dosage Forms Elemental calcium listed in brackets

Tablet: 325 mg [42.25 mg], 650 mg [84.5 mg]

calcium pantothenate *see* pantothenic acid *on page 428*

calcium phosphate, dibasic (KAL see um FOS fate dye BAY sik)

Synonyms dicalcium phosphate

U.S./Canadian Brand Names Posture® [OTC]

Therapeutic Category Electrolyte Supplement, Oral

Use Adjunct in prevention of postmenopausal osteoporosis, treatment and prevention of calcium depletion

Usual Dosage Oral:

Children: 45-65 mg/kg/day

Adults: 1-2 g/day (doses in g of elemental calcium)

Dosage Forms Elemental calcium listed in brackets

Tablet, sugar free: 1565.2 mg [600 mg]

calcium polycarbophil (KAL see um pol i KAR boe fil)

U.S./Canadian Brand Names Equalactin® Chewable Tablet [OTC]; Fiberall® Chewable Tablet [OTC]; FiberCon® Tablet [OTC]; Fiber-Lax® Tablet [OTC]; Mitrolan® Chewable Tablet [OTC]

Therapeutic Category Gastrointestinal Agent, Miscellaneous; Laxative

Use Treatment of constipation or diarrhea by restoring a more normal moisture level and providing bulk in the patient's intestinal tract; calcium polycarbophil is supplied as the approved substitute whenever a bulk-forming laxative is ordered in a tablet, capsule, wafer, or other oral solid dosage form

Usual Dosage Oral:

Children:

- 2-6 years: 500 mg 1-2 times/day, up to 1.5 g/day
- 6-12 years: 500 mg 1-3 times/day, up to 3 g/day

Adults: 1 g 4 times/day, up to 6 g/day

Dosage Forms Tablet:

Sodium free:

- Fiber-Lax®: 625 mg
- FiberCon®: 500 mg

Chewable:

- Equalactin®, Mitrolan®: 500 mg
- Equalactin®: 650 mg
- Fiberall®: 1250 mg

CaldeCort® Anti-Itch Topical Spray *see* hydrocortisone (topical) *on page 292*

CaldeCort® Topical [OTC] *see* hydrocortisone (topical) *on page 292*

Calderol® *see* calcifediol *on page 88*

Caldesene® Topical [OTC] *see* undecylenic acid and derivatives *on page 590*

calfactant (cal FAC tant)

U.S./Canadian Brand Names Infasurf®

Therapeutic Category Lung Surfactant

Use Prevention of respiratory distress syndrome (RDS) in premature infants at high risk for RDS and for the treatment ("rescue") of premature infants who develop RDS; decreases the incidence of RDS, mortality due to RDS, and air leaks associated with RDS

Usual Dosage Should be administered intratracheally through a side-port adapter into the endotracheal tube; two attendants, one to instill the suspension, the other to monitor the patient and assist in positioning, facilitate the dosing; the dose (3 mL/kg) should be administered in two aliquots of 1.5 mL/kg each; after each aliquot is instilled, the infant should be positioned with either the right or the left side dependent; administration is made while ventilation is continued over 20-30 breaths for each aliquot, with small bursts timed only during the inspiratory cycles; a pause followed by evaluation of the respiratory status and repositioning should separate the two aliquots

Dosage Forms Suspension, intratracheal: 6 mL

Calm-X® Oral [OTC] *see* dimenhydrinate *on page 182*

Calmylin Expectorant (Can) *see* guaifenesin *on page 267*

Calphron® *see* calcium acetate *on page 89*

Cal-Plus® [OTC] *see* calcium carbonate *on page 89*

Calsan® (Can) *see* calcium carbonate *on page 89*

Caltine® (Can) *see* calcitonin *on page 88*

Caltrate® 600 [OTC] *see* calcium carbonate *on page 89*

Caltrate, Jr.® [OTC] *see* calcium carbonate *on page 89*

Camalox® Suspension & Tablet *(Discontinued)* *see page 700*

Campho-Phenique® [OTC] *see* camphor and phenol *on this page*

camphor and phenol (KAM for & FEE nole)

U.S./Canadian Brand Names Campho-Phenique® [OTC]

Therapeutic Category Topical Skin Product

Use Relief of pain and for minor infections

Usual Dosage Topical: Apply as needed

Dosage Forms Liquid: Camphor 10.8% and phenol 4.7%

camphorated tincture of opium *see* paregoric *on page 429*

camphor, menthol, and phenol (KAM for, MEN thol, & FEE nole)

U.S./Canadian Brand Names Sarna [OTC]

Therapeutic Category Topical Skin Product

Use Relief of dry, itching skin

Usual Dosage Topical: Apply as needed for dry skin

Dosage Forms Lotion, topical: Camphor 0.5%, menthol 0.5%, and phenol 0.5% in emollient base (240 mL)

Camptosar® *see* irinotecan *on page 312*

642® (Can) *see* propoxyphene *on page 482*

candesartan (kan de SAR tan)

U.S./Canadian Brand Names Atacand™

Therapeutic Category Angiotensin II Antagonist

Use Treatment of hypertension; may be used alone or in combination with other antihypertensive agents

Usual Dosage Adults: Oral: Dosage must be individualized; blood pressure response is dose-related over the range of 2-32 mg; the usual recommended starting dose of 16 mg once daily when it is used as monotherapy in patients who are not volume depleted; it can be administered once or twice daily with total daily doses ranging from 8-32 mg; larger doses do not appear to have a greater effect and there is relatively little experience with such doses; most of the antihypertensive effect is present within 2 weeks and maximal blood pressure reduction is generally obtained within 4-6 weeks of treatment

Dosage Forms Tablet, as cilexetil: 4 mg, 8 mg, 16 mg, 32 mg

Candida albicans (*Monilia*) (KAN dee da AL bi kans mo NIL ya)

Synonyms *Monilia* skin test

U.S./Canadian Brand Names Dermatophytin-O

Therapeutic Category Diagnostic Agent

Use Screen for detection of nonresponsiveness to antigens in immunocompromised individuals

Usual Dosage Intradermal: 0.1 mL, examine reaction site in 24-48 hours; induration of ≥5 mm in diameter is a positive reaction

Dosage Forms Injection:

Intradermal: 1:100 (5 mL)

Scratch: 1:10 (5 mL)

Candistatin® (Can) *see* nystatin *on page 412*

Canesten® Topical (Can) Canesten® Vaginal (Can) *see* clotrimazole *on page 140*

Cantharone® ***(Discontinued)*** *see page 700*

Cantharone Plus® ***(Discontinued)*** *see page 700*

Cantil® *see* mepenzolate *on page 355*

Capastat® Sulfate *see* capreomycin *on this page*

capecitabine (kap eh SITE a bean)

U.S./Canadian Brand Names Xeloda™

Therapeutic Category Antineoplastic Agent, Antimetabolite

Use Treatment of patients with metastatic breast cancer resistant to both paclitaxel and an anthracycline-containing chemotherapy regimen or resistant to paclitaxel and for whom further anthracycline therapy is not indicated (eg, patients who have received cumulative doses of 400 mg/m² of doxorubicin or doxorubicin equivalents). Resistance is defined as progressive disease while on treatment, with or without an initial response, or relapse within 6 months of completing treatment with an anthracycline-containing adjuvant regimen.

Usual Dosage Refer to individual protocols.

2510 mg/m² days 1-14 every 3 weeks

1657 mg/m² days 1-14 every 3 weeks

1331 mg/m²/day

Dosage Forms Tablet: 150 mg, 500 mg

Capital® and Codeine *see* acetaminophen and codeine *on page 4*

Capitrol® *see* chloroxine *on page 120*

Capoten® *see* captopril *on next page*

Capozide® *see* captopril and hydrochlorothiazide *on next page*

capreomycin (kap ree oh MYE sin)

U.S./Canadian Brand Names Capastat® Sulfate

Therapeutic Category Antibiotic, Miscellaneous

Use In conjunction with at least one other antituberculosis agent in the treatment of tuberculosis

Usual Dosage Adults: I.M.: 15 mg/kg/day up to 1 g/day for 60-120 days

Dosage Forms Injection, as sulfate: 100 mg/mL (10 mL)

capsaicin (kap SAY sin)

U.S./Canadian Brand Names Capsin® [OTC]; Capzasin-P® [OTC]; Dolorac™ [OTC]; No Pain-HP® [OTC]; R-Gel® [OTC]; Zostrix® [OTC]; Zostrix®-HP [OTC]

Therapeutic Category Analgesic, Topical

Use FDA approved for the topical treatment of pain associated with postherpetic neuralgia, rheumatoid arthritis, osteoarthritis, diabetic neuropathy, and postsurgical pain

Unlabeled uses: Treatment of pain associated with psoriasis, chronic neuralgias unresponsive to other forms of therapy, and intractable pruritus

Usual Dosage Children >2 years and Adults: Topical: Apply to area up to 3-4 times/day only

Dosage Forms

Cream:

Capzasin-P®, Zostrix®: 0.025% (45 g, 90 g)

Dolorac™: 0.25% (28 g)

Zostrix®-HP: 0.075% (30 g, 60 g)

Gel (R-Gel®): 0.025% (15 g, 30 g)

Lotion (Capsin®): 0.025% (59 mL); 0.075% (59 mL)

Roll-on (No Pain-HP®): 0.075% (60 mL)

Capsin® [OTC] *see* capsaicin *on this page*

captopril (KAP toe pril)

U.S./Canadian Brand Names Apo®-Capto (Can); Capoten®; Novo-Captopril® (Can); Nu-Capto® (Can); Syn-Captopril® (Can)

Therapeutic Category Angiotensin-Converting Enzyme (ACE) Inhibitor

Use Management of hypertension and treatment of congestive heart failure; in postmyocardial infarction, improves survival in clinically stable patients with left ventricular dysfunction

Usual Dosage Note: Dosage must be titrated according to patient's response; use lowest effective dose. Oral:

Infants: Initial: 0.15-0.3 mg/kg/dose; titrate dose upward to maximum of 6 mg/kg/day in 1-4 divided doses; usual required dose: 2.5-6 mg/kg/day

Children: Initial: 0.5 mg/kg/dose; titrate upward to maximum of 6 mg/kg/day in 2-4 divided doses

Older Children: Initial: 6.25-12.5 mg/dose every 12-24 hours; titrate upward to maximum of 6 mg/kg/day

Adolescents and Adults: Initial: 12.5-25 mg/dose administered every 8-12 hours; increase by 25 mg/dose to maximum of 450 mg/day

Note: Smaller dosages administered every 8-12 hours are indicated in patients with renal dysfunction. Renal function and leukocyte count should be carefully monitored during therapy.

Dosage Forms Tablet: 12.5 mg, 25 mg, 50 mg, 100 mg

captopril and hydrochlorothiazide

(KAP toe pril & hye droe klor oh THYE a zide)

Synonyms hydrochlorothiazide and captopril

U.S./Canadian Brand Names Capozide®

Therapeutic Category Antihypertensive Agent, Combination

Use Management of hypertension and treatment of congestive heart failure

Usual Dosage Adults: Oral:

Hypertension: Initial: 25 mg 2-3 times/day; may increase at 1- to 2-week intervals up to 150 mg 3 times/day (captopril dosages)

Congestive heart failure: 6.25-25 mg 3 times/day (maximum: 450 mg/day) (captopril dosages)

Dosage Forms Tablet:

25/15: Captopril 25 mg and hydrochlorothiazide 15 mg

25/25: Captopril 25 mg and hydrochlorothiazide 25 mg

50/15: Captopril 50 mg and hydrochlorothiazide 15 mg

50/25: Captopril 50 mg and hydrochlorothiazide 25 mg

Capzasin-P® [OTC] *see* capsaicin *on previous page*

Carafate® *see* sucralfate *on page 538*

caramiphen and phenylpropanolamine

(kar AM i fen & fen il proe pa NOLE a meen)

Synonyms phenylpropanolamine and caramiphen

U.S./Canadian Brand Names Ordrine AT® Extended Release Capsule; Rescaps-D® S.R. Capsule; Tuss-Allergine® Modified T.D. Capsule; Tussogest® Extended Release Capsule

Therapeutic Category Antihistamine/Decongestant Combination

Use Symptomatic relief of cough and nasal congestion associated with the common cold

Usual Dosage Oral:

Children:

2-6 years: 1/2 teaspoonful every 4 hours

6-12 years: 1 teaspoonful every 4 hours

Children >12 years and Adults: 1 capsule every 12 hours or 2 teaspoonfuls every 4 hours

Dosage Forms

Capsule, timed release: Caramiphen edisylate 40 mg and phenylpropanolamine hydrochloride 75 mg

Liquid: Caramiphen edisylate 6.7 mg and phenylpropanolamine hydrochloride 12.5 mg per 5 mL

carampicillin *see* bacampicillin *on page 57*

carbachol (KAR ba kole)

Synonyms carbacholine; carbamylcholine chloride

U.S./Canadian Brand Names Carbastat® Ophthalmic; Carboptic® Ophthalmic; Isopto® Carbachol Ophthalmic; Miostat® Intraocular

Therapeutic Category Cholinergic Agent

Use Lower intraocular pressure in the treatment of glaucoma; to cause miosis during surgery

Usual Dosage Adults:

Intraocular: 0.5 mL instilled into anterior chamber before or after securing sutures

Ophthalmic: Instill 1-2 drops up to 4 times/day

Dosage Forms Solution:

Intraocular (Carbastat®, Miostat®): 0.01% (1.5 mL);

Topical, ophthalmic:

Carboptic®: 3% (15 mL)

Isopto® Carbachol: 0.75% (15 mL, 30 mL); 1.5% (15 mL, 30 mL); 2.25% (15 mL); 3% (15 mL, 30 mL)

carbacholine *see* carbachol *on this page*

carbamazepine (kar ba MAZ e peen)

U.S./Canadian Brand Names Apo®-Carbamazepine (Can); Epitol®; Mazepine® (Can); Novo-Carbamaz® (Can); Nu-Carbamazepine® (Can); PMS-Carbamazepine (Can); Tegretol®; Tegretol®-XR

Therapeutic Category Anticonvulsant

Use Prophylaxis of generalized tonic-clonic, partial (especially complex partial), and mixed partial or generalized seizure disorder; may be used to relieve pain in trigeminal neuralgia or diabetic neuropathy; has been used to treat bipolar disorders

Usual Dosage Oral (dosage must be adjusted according to patient's response and serum concentrations):

Children:

<6 years: Initial: 5 mg/kg/day; dosage may be increased every 5-7 days to 10 mg/kg/day; then up to 20 mg/kg/day if necessary; administer in 2-4 divided doses/day

(Continued)

carbamazepine *(Continued)*

6-12 years: Initial: 100 mg twice daily or 10 mg/kg/day in 2 divided doses; increase by 100 mg/day depending upon response; usual maintenance: 15-30 mg/kg/day in 2-4 divided doses/day; maximum: 1000 mg/24 hours

Children >12 years and Adults: 200 mg twice daily to start, increase by 200 mg/day at weekly intervals until therapeutic levels achieved; usual dose: 800-1200 mg/day in 3-4 divided doses; some patients have required up to 1.6-2.4 g/day

Dosage Forms

Suspension, oral (citrus-vanilla flavor): 100 mg/5 mL (450 mL)
Tablet: 200 mg
Tablet:
Chewable: 100 mg
Extended release: 100 mg, 200 mg, 400 mg

carbamide *see* urea *on page 591*

carbamide peroxide (KAR ba mide per OKS ide)

Synonyms urea peroxide

U.S./Canadian Brand Names Auro® Ear Drops [OTC]; Clamurid® (Can); Debrox® Otic [OTC]; E•R•O Ear [OTC]; Gly-Oxide® Oral [OTC]; Mollifene® Ear Wax Removing Formula [OTC]; Murine® Ear Drops [OTC]; Orajel® Perioseptic® [OTC]; Proxigel® Oral [OTC]

Therapeutic Category Anti-infective Agent, Oral; Otic Agent, Cerumenolytic

Use

Oral: Relief of minor inflammation of gums, oral mucosal surfaces and lips including canker sores and dental irritation; adjunct in oral hygiene

Otic: Emulsify and disperse ear wax

Usual Dosage Children >12 years and Adults:

Oral: Apply several drops undiluted to affected area of the mouth 4 times/day and at bedtime for up to 7 days, expectorate after 2-3 minutes; as an adjunct to oral hygiene after brushing, swish 10 drops for 2-3 minutes, then expectorate; gel: massage on affected area 4 times/day

Otic: Instill 5-10 drops twice daily for up to 4 days; keep drops in ear for several minutes by keeping head tilted or placing cotton in ear

Dosage Forms

Gel, oral (Proxigel®): 10% (34 g)
Solution:
Oral:
Gly-Oxide®: 10% in glycerin (15 mL, 60 mL)
Orajel® Perioseptic®: 15% in glycerin (13.3 mL)
Otic (Auro® Ear Drops, Debrox®, Mollifene® Ear Wax Removing, Murine® Ear Drops): 6.5% in glycerin (15 mL, 30 mL)

carbamylcholine chloride *see* carbachol *on previous page*

Carbastat® Ophthalmic *see* carbachol *on previous page*

carbenicillin (kar ben i SIL in)

Synonyms carindacillin

U.S./Canadian Brand Names Geocillin®; Geopen® (Can)

Therapeutic Category Penicillin

Use Treatment of urinary tract infections, asymptomatic bacteriuria, or prostatitis caused by susceptible strains of *Pseudomonas aeruginosa*, *E. coli*, indole-positive *Proteus*, and *Enterobacter*

Usual Dosage Oral:

Children: 30-50 mg/kg/day divided every 6 hours; maximum dose: 2-3 g/day
Adults: 1-2 tablets every 6 hours

Dosage Forms Tablet, film coated, as indanyl sodium ester: 382 mg [base]

carbidopa (kar bi DOE pa)

U.S./Canadian Brand Names Lodosyn®

Therapeutic Category Anti-Parkinson's Agent; Dopaminergic Agent (Anti-Parkinson's)

Use With levodopa in the treatment of parkinsonism to enable a lower dosage of the latter to be used and a more rapid response to be obtained, and to decrease side-effects; for details of administration and dosage

Usual Dosage Adults: Oral: 70-100 mg/day; maximum daily dose: 200 mg

Dosage Forms Tablet: 25 mg

carbidopa and levodopa *see* levodopa and carbidopa *on page 331*

carbinoxamine and pseudoephedrine

(kar bi NOKS a meen & soo doe e FED rin)

Synonyms pseudoephedrine and carbinoxamine

U.S./Canadian Brand Names Biohist-LA®; Carbiset® Tablet; Carbiset-TR® Tablet; Carbodec® Syrup; Carbodec® Tablet; Carbodec® TR Tablet; Cardec-S® Syrup; Rondec® Drops; Rondec® Filmtab®; Rondec® Syrup; Rondec-TR®

Therapeutic Category Antihistamine/Decongestant Combination

Use Temporary relief of nasal congestion, running nose, sneezing, itching of nose or throat, and itchy, watery eyes due to the common cold, hay fever, or other respiratory allergies

Usual Dosage Oral:

- Children:
  - Drops: 1-18 months: 0.25-1 mL 4 times/day
  - Syrup:
    - 18 months to 6 years: 2.5 mL 3-4 times/day
    - >6 years: 5 mL 2-4 times/day
- Adults:
  - Liquid: 5 mL 4 times/day
  - Tablet: 1 tablet 4 times/day

Dosage Forms

- Drops: Carbinoxamine maleate 2 mg and pseudoephedrine hydrochloride 25 mg per mL (30 mL with dropper)
- Syrup: Carbinoxamine maleate 4 mg and pseudoephedrine hydrochloride 60 mg per 5 mL (120 mL, 480 mL)
- Tablet:
  - Film-coated: Carbinoxamine maleate 4 mg and pseudoephedrine hydrochloride 60 mg
  - Sustained release: Carbinoxamine maleate 8 mg and pseudoephedrine hydrochloride 120 mg

carbinoxamine, pseudoephedrine, and dextromethorphan

(kar bi NOKS a meen, soo doe e FED rin, & deks troe meth OR fan)

U.S./Canadian Brand Names Carbodec DM®; Cardec DM®; Pseudo-Car® DM; Rondamine-DM® Drops; Rondec®-DM; Tussafed® Drops

Therapeutic Category Antihistamine/Decongestant/Antitussive

Use Relief of coughs and upper respiratory symptoms, including nasal congestion, associated with allergy or the common cold

Usual Dosage

- Infants: Drops:
  - 1-3 months: 1/4 mL 4 times/day
  - 3-6 months: 1/2 mL 4 times/day
  - 6-9 months: 3/4 mL 4 times/day
  - 9-18 months: 1 mL 4 times/day
- Children 1 1/2 to 6 years: Syrup: 2.5 mL 4 times/day
- Children >6 years and Adults: Syrup: 5 mL 4 times/day

Dosage Forms

- Drops: Carbinoxamine maleate 2 mg, pseudoephedrine hydrochloride 25 mg, and dextromethorphan hydrobromide 4 mg per mL (30 mL)

(Continued)

carbinoxamine, pseudoephedrine, and dextromethorphan *(Continued)*

Syrup: Carbinoxamine maleate 4 mg, pseudoephedrine hydrochloride 60 mg, and dextromethorphan hydrobromide 15 mg per 5 mL (120 mL, 480 mL, 4000 mL)

Carbiset® Tablet *see* carbinoxamine and pseudoephedrine *on previous page*

Carbiset-TR® Tablet *see* carbinoxamine and pseudoephedrine *on previous page*

Carbocaine® *see* mepivacaine *on page 356*

Carbodec DM® *see* carbinoxamine, pseudoephedrine, and dextromethorphan *on previous page*

Carbodec® Syrup *see* carbinoxamine and pseudoephedrine *on previous page*

Carbodec® Tablet *see* carbinoxamine and pseudoephedrine *on previous page*

Carbodec® TR Tablet *see* carbinoxamine and pseudoephedrine *on previous page*

carbol-fuchsin solution (kar bol-FOOK sin soe LOO shun)

Synonyms Castellani paint

Therapeutic Category Antifungal Agent

Use Treatment of superficial mycotic infections

Usual Dosage Topical: Apply to affected area 2-4 times/day

Dosage Forms Solution: Basic fuchsin 0.3%, boric acid 1%, phenol 4.5%, resorcinol 10%, acetone 5%, and alcohol 10%

carbolic acid *see* phenol *on page 444*

Carbolith™ (Can) *see* lithium *on page 337*

carboplatin (KAR boe pla tin)

Synonyms CBDCA

U.S./Canadian Brand Names Paraplatin®

Therapeutic Category Antineoplastic Agent

Use Palliative treatment of ovarian carcinoma; also used in the treatment of small cell lung cancer, squamous cell carcinoma of the esophagus; solid tumors of the bladder, cervix and testes; pediatric brain tumor, neuroblastoma

Usual Dosage I.V. (refer to individual protocols):

Children:

Solid tumor: 560 mg/m^2 once every 4 weeks

Brain tumor: 175 mg/m^2 once weekly for 4 weeks with a 2-week recovery period between courses; dose is then adjusted on platelet count and neutrophil count values

Adults: Single agent: 360 mg/m^2 once every 4 weeks; dose is then adjusted on platelet count and neutrophil count values

Dosage Forms Powder for injection, lyophilized: 50 mg, 150 mg, 450 mg

carboprost tromethamine (KAR boe prost tro METH a meen)

U.S./Canadian Brand Names Hemabate™

Therapeutic Category Prostaglandin

Use Termination of pregnancy

Usual Dosage I.M.: Initial: 250 mcg, then 250 mcg at 1½-hour to 3½-hour intervals depending on uterine response; a 500 mcg dose may be administered if uterine response is not adequate after several 250 mcg doses

Dosage Forms Injection: Carboprost 250 mcg and tromethamine 83 mcg per mL (1 mL)

Carboptic® Ophthalmic *see* carbachol *on page 97*

carbose d *see* carboxymethylcellulose *on next page*

carboxymethylcellulose (kar boks ee meth il SEL yoo lose)
Synonyms carbose d; carboxymethylcellulose sodium
U.S./Canadian Brand Names Cellufresh® [OTC]; Celluvisc® [OTC]
Therapeutic Category Ophthalmic Agent, Miscellaneous
Use Preservative-free artificial tear substitute
Usual Dosage Adults: Ophthalmic: Instill 1-2 drops into eye(s) 3-4 times/day
Dosage Forms Solution, ophthalmic, as sodium, preservative free: 0.5% (0.3 mL); 1% (0.3 mL)

carboxymethylcellulose sodium *see* carboxymethylcellulose *on this page*

Cardec DM® *see* carbinoxamine, pseudoephedrine, and dextromethorphan *on page 99*

Cardec-S® Syrup *see* carbinoxamine and pseudoephedrine *on page 99*

Cardene® *see* nicardipine *on page 400*

Cardene® SR *see* nicardipine *on page 400*

Cardilate® *see* erythrityl tetranitrate *on page 214*

Cardio-Green® *see* indocyanine green *on page 304*

Cardioquin® *see* quinidine *on page 492*

Cardizem® CD *see* diltiazem *on page 182*

Cardizem® Injectable *see* diltiazem *on page 182*

Cardizem® SR *see* diltiazem *on page 182*

Cardizem® Tablet *see* diltiazem *on page 182*

Cardura® *see* doxazosin *on page 195*

carindacillin *see* carbenicillin *on page 98*

carisoprodate *see* carisoprodol *on this page*

carisoprodol (kar i soe PROE dole)
Synonyms carisoprodate; isobamate
U.S./Canadian Brand Names Soma®
Therapeutic Category Skeletal Muscle Relaxant
Use Skeletal muscle relaxant
Usual Dosage Adults: Oral: 350 mg 3-4 times/day; administer last dose at bedtime; compound: 1-2 tablets 4 times/day
Dosage Forms Tablet: 350 mg

carisoprodol and aspirin (kar i soe PROE dole & AS pir in)
U.S./Canadian Brand Names Soma® Compound
Therapeutic Category Skeletal Muscle Relaxant
Use Skeletal muscle relaxant
Usual Dosage Adults: Oral: 1-2 tablets 4 times/day
Dosage Forms Tablet: Carisoprodol 200 mg and aspirin 325 mg

carisoprodol, aspirin, and codeine
(kar i soe PROE dole, AS pir in, and KOE deen)
U.S./Canadian Brand Names Soma® Compound w/Codeine
Therapeutic Category Skeletal Muscle Relaxant
Controlled Substance C-III
Use Skeletal muscle relaxant
Usual Dosage Adults: Oral: 1-2 tablets 4 times/day
Dosage Forms Tablet: Carisoprodol 200 mg, aspirin 325 mg, and codeine phosphate 16 mg

Carmol-HC® Topical *see* urea and hydrocortisone *on page 591*

Carmol® Topical [OTC] *see* urea *on page 591*

carmustine (kar MUS teen)

Synonyms BCNU

U.S./Canadian Brand Names BiCNU®

Therapeutic Category Antineoplastic Agent

Use Brain tumors, multiple myeloma, Hodgkin's disease, and non-Hodgkin's lymphomas; some activity in malignant melanoma; glioblastoma multiforme (wafer)

Usual Dosage Children and Adults:

I.V. infusion (refer to individual protocols): 75-100 mg/m²/day for 2 days or 150-200 mg/m² every 6 weeks as a single dose or divided into daily injections on 2 successive days; next dose is to be determined based on hematologic response to the previous dose

Wafer: Implant 8 wafer in resected brain cavity, if size and shape allow

Dosage Forms

Powder for injection: 100 mg/vial packaged with 3 mL of absolute alcohol for use as a sterile diluent

Wafer: 7.7 mg

Carnation Instant Breakfast® [OTC] *see* enteral nutritional products *on page 208*

Carnitor® Injection *see* levocarnitine *on page 330*

Carnitor® Oral *see* levocarnitine *on page 330*

Caroid® ***(Discontinued)*** *see page 700*

carteolol (KAR tee oh lole)

U.S./Canadian Brand Names Cartrol® Oral; Ocupress® Ophthalmic

Therapeutic Category Beta-Adrenergic Blocker

Use Management of hypertension; treatment of increased intraocular pressure

Usual Dosage Adults:

Oral: 2.5 mg as a single daily dose, maintenance dose: 2.5-5 mg once daily

Ophthalmic: 1 drop in eye(s) twice daily

Dosage Forms Carteolol hydrochloride:

Solution, ophthalmic (Ocupress®): 1% (5 mL, 10 mL)

Tablet (Cartrol®): 2.5 mg, 5 mg

Carter's Little Pills® [OTC] *see* bisacodyl *on page 74*

Cartrol® Oral *see* carteolol *on this page*

carvedilol (KAR ve dil ole)

U.S./Canadian Brand Names Coreg®

Therapeutic Category Beta-Adrenergic Blocker

Use Management of hypertension, congestive heart failure; can be used alone or in combination with other agents, especially thiazide-type diuretics

Usual Dosage Adults: Oral:

Hypertension: 6.25 mg twice daily; if tolerated, dose should be maintained for 1-2 weeks, then increased to 12.5 mg twice daily; dosage may be increased to a maximum of 25 mg twice daily after 1-2 weeks; reduce dosage if heart rate drops to <55 beats/minute

Congestive heart failure: 3.125 mg twice daily for 2 weeks; if this dose is tolerated, may increase to 6.25 mg twice daily. Double the dose every 2 weeks to the highest dose tolerated by patient. (Prior to initiating therapy, other heart failure medications should be stabilized.)

Maximum recommended dose:

<85 kg: 25 mg twice daily

>85 kg: 50 mg twice daily

Angina pectoris (unlabeled use): 25-50 mg twice daily

Idiopathic cardiomyopathy (unlabeled use): 6.25-25 mg twice daily

Dosage Forms Tablet: 3.125 mg, 6.25 mg, 12.5 mg, 25 mg

casanthranol and docusate *see* docusate and casanthranol *on page 191*

cascara sagrada (kas KAR a sah GRAH dah)

Therapeutic Category Laxative

Use Temporary relief of constipation; sometimes used with milk of magnesia ("black and white" mixture)

Usual Dosage Note: Cascara sagrada fluid extract is 5 times more potent than cascara sagrada aromatic fluid extract

Oral (aromatic fluid extract):
- Infants: 1.25 mL/day (range: 0.5-1.5 mL) as needed
- Children 2-11 years: 2.5 mL/day (range: 1-3 mL) as needed
- Children ≥12 years and Adults: 5 mL/day (range: 2-6 mL) as needed at bedtime (1 tablet as needed at bedtime)

Dosage Forms

Aromatic fluid extract: 120 mL, 473 mL

Tablet: 325 mg

Casodex® *see* bicalutamide *on page 74*

Castellani paint *see* carbol-fuchsin solution *on page 100*

castor oil (KAS tor oyl)

Synonyms oleum ricini

U.S./Canadian Brand Names Alphamul® [OTC]; Emulsoil® [OTC]; Fleet® Flavored Castor Oil [OTC]; Neoloid® [OTC]; Purge® [OTC]

Therapeutic Category Laxative

Use Preparation for rectal or bowel examination or surgery; rarely used to relieve constipation; also applied to skin as emollient and protectant

Usual Dosage Oral:

Castor oil:
- Infants <2 years: 1-5 mL or 15 mL/m^2/dose as a single dose
- Children 2-11 years: 5-15 mL as a single dose
- Children ≥12 years and Adults: 15-60 mL as a single dose

Emulsified castor oil:
- Infants: 2.5-7.5 mL/dose
- Children <2 years: 5-15 mL/dose
- Children 2-11 years: 7.5-30 mL/dose
- Children ≥12 years and Adults: 30-60 mL/dose

Dosage Forms

Emulsion, oral:
- Alphamul®: 60% (90 mL, 3780 mL)
- Emulsoil®: 95% (63 mL)
- Fleet® Flavored Castor Oil: 67% (45 mL, 90 mL)
- Neoloid®: 36.4% (118 mL)

Liquid, oral:
- 100% (60 mL, 120 mL, 480 mL)
- Purge®: 95% (30 mL, 60 mL)

Cataflam® Oral *see* diclofenac *on page 175*

Catapres® Oral *see* clonidine *on page 139*

Catapres-TTS® Transdermal *see* clonidine *on page 139*

Catarase® 1:5000 *(Discontinued)* *see page 700*

Caverject® Injection *see* alprostadil *on page 20*

CBDCA *see* carboplatin *on page 100*

CCNU *see* lomustine *on page 338*

C-Crystals® [OTC] *see* ascorbic acid *on page 48*

2-CdA *see* cladribine *on page 134*

CDDP *see* cisplatin *on page 133*

Cebid® *see* ascorbic acid *on page 48*

Ceclor® *see* cefaclor *on this page*

Ceclor® CD *see* cefaclor *on this page*

Cecon® [OTC] *see* ascorbic acid *on page 48*

Cedax® *see* ceftibuten *on page 108*

Cedilanid-D® Injection *(Discontinued)* *see page 700*

Cedocard-SR® (Can) *see* isosorbide dinitrate *on page 315*

CeeNU® *see* lomustine *on page 338*

Ceepryn® [OTC] *see* cetylpyridinium *on page 113*

cefaclor (SEF a klor)

U.S./Canadian Brand Names Ceclor®; Ceclor® CD

Therapeutic Category Cephalosporin (Second Generation)

Use Infections caused by susceptible organisms including *Staph aureus, S. pneumoniae,* and *H. influenzae*; treatment of otitis media, sinusitis, and infections involving the respiratory tract, skin and skin structure, bone and joint, and urinary tract

Usual Dosage Oral:

Children >1 month: 20-40 mg/kg/day divided every 8-12 hours; maximum dose: 2 g/day (twice daily option is for treatment of otitis media or pharyngitis)

Adults: 250-500 mg every 8 hours or daily dose can be administered in 2 divided doses

Dosage Forms

Capsule: 250 mg, 500 mg

Powder for oral suspension (strawberry flavor): 125 mg/5 mL (75 mL, 150 mL); 187 mg/5 mL (50 mL, 100 mL); 250 mg/5 mL (75 mL, 150 mL); 375 mg/5 mL (50 mL, 100 mL)

Tablet, extended release: 375 mg, 500 mg

cefadroxil (sef a DROKS il)

U.S./Canadian Brand Names Duricef®

Therapeutic Category Cephalosporin (First Generation)

Use Treatment of susceptible bacterial infections including group A beta-hemolytic streptococcal pharyngitis or tonsillitis; skin and soft tissue infections caused by streptococci or staphylococci; urinary tract infections caused by *Klebsiella, E. coli,* and *Proteus mirabilis*

Usual Dosage Oral:

Children: 30 mg/kg/day divided twice daily up to a maximum of 2 g/day

Adults: 1-2 g/day in 2 divided doses

Dosage Forms Cefadroxil monohydrate:

Capsule: 500 mg

Suspension, oral: 125 mg/5 mL, 250 mg/5 mL, 500 mg/5 mL (50 mL, 100 mL)

Tablet: 1 g

Cefadyl® *see* cephapirin *on page 112*

cefamandole (sef a MAN dole)

U.S./Canadian Brand Names Mandol®

Therapeutic Category Cephalosporin (Second Generation)

Use Treatment of susceptible bacterial infection; mainly respiratory tract, skin and skin structure, bone and joint, urinary tract and gynecologic as well as septicemia, perioperative prophylaxis

Usual Dosage I.M., I.V.:

Children: 100-150 mg/kg/day in divided doses every 4-6 hours

Adults: 4-12 g/24 hours divided every 4-6 hours 500-1000 mg every 4-8 hours

Dosage Forms Powder for injection, as nafate: 500 mg (10 mL); 1 g (10 mL, 100 mL); 2 g (20 mL, 100 mL); 10 g (100 mL)

Cefanex® *see* cephalexin *on page 111*

cefazolin (sef A zoe lin)

U.S./Canadian Brand Names Ancef®; Kefzol®; Zolicef®

Therapeutic Category Cephalosporin (First Generation)

Use Treatment of respiratory tract, skin and skin structure, urinary tract, biliary tract, bone and joint infections and septicemia due to susceptible gram-positive cocci (except enterococcus); some gram-negative bacilli including *E. coli*, *Proteus*, and *Klebsiella* may be susceptible; perioperative prophylaxis

Usual Dosage I.M., I.V.:

Infants and Children: 50-100 mg/kg/day in 3 divided doses; maximum dose: 6 g/day

Adults: 1-2 g every 8 hours

Dosage Forms Cefazolin sodium:

Infusion, premixed in D_5W (frozen) (Ancef®): 500 mg (50 mL); 1 g (50 mL)

Injection (Kefzol®): 500 mg, 1 g

Powder for injection (Ancef®, Zolicef®): 250 mg, 500 mg, 1 g, 5 g, 10 g, 20 g

cefdinir (SEF di ner)

Synonyms CFDN

U.S./Canadian Brand Names Omnicef®

Therapeutic Category Cephalosporin (Third Generation)

Use Treatment of community-acquired pneumonia, acute exacerbations of chronic bronchitis, acute bacterial otitis media, acute maxillary sinusitis, pharyngitis/tonsillitis, and uncomplicated skin and skin structure infections.

Usual Dosage Oral:

Children (otitis media with effusion): 7 mg/kg orally twice daily or 14 mg/kg orally once daily

Adolescents and Adults: 300 mg orally twice daily; an oral dose of 600 mg once daily has been used in streptococcal pharyngitis

Dosage Forms

Capsule: 300 mg

Suspension, oral: 125 mg/5 mL (60 mL, 100 mL)

cefepime (SEF e pim)

U.S./Canadian Brand Names Maxipime®

Therapeutic Category Cephalosporin (Fourth Generation)

Use Treatment of respiratory tract infections (including bronchitis and pneumonia), cellulitis and other skin and soft tissue infections, and urinary tract infections; considered a fourth generation cephalosporin because it has good gram-negative coverage similar to third generation cephalosporins, but better gram-positive coverage

Usual Dosage I.V.:

Children: Unlabeled: 50 mg/kg every 8 hours; maximum dose: 2 g

Adults:

Most infections: 1-2 g every 12 hours for 5-10 days; higher doses or more frequent administration may be required in pseudomonal infections

Urinary tract infections, uncomplicated: 500 mg every 12 hours

Dosage Forms Powder for injection, as hydrochloride: 500 mg, 1 g, 2 g

cefixime (sef IKS eem)

U.S./Canadian Brand Names Suprax®

Therapeutic Category Cephalosporin (Third Generation)

Use Treatment of urinary tract infections, otitis media, respiratory infections due to susceptible organisms including *S. pneumoniae* and *pyogenes*, *H. influenzae*, *M. catarrhalis*, and many *Enterobacteriaceae*; documented poor compliance with other oral antimicrobials; outpatient therapy of serious soft tissue or skeletal infections due to susceptible organisms; single-dose oral treatment of uncomplicated cervical/urethral gonorrhea due to *N. gonorrhoeae*; treatment of shigellosis in areas with a high rate of resistance to TMP-SMX

(Continued)

cefixime *(Continued)*

Usual Dosage Oral:
Children: 8 mg/kg/day in 1-2 divided doses; maximum dose: 400 mg/day
Children >50 kg or >12 years and Adults: 400 mg/day in 1-2 divided doses

Dosage Forms
Powder for oral suspension (strawberry flavor): 100 mg/5 mL (50 mL, 100 mL)
Tablet, film coated: 200 mg, 400 mg

Cefizox® *see* ceftizoxime *on page 108*

cefmetazole (sef MET a zole)

U.S./Canadian Brand Names Zefazone®

Therapeutic Category Cephalosporin (Second Generation)

Use Second generation cephalosporin with an antibacterial spectrum similar to cefoxitin, useful on many aerobic and anaerobic gram-positive and gram-negative bacteria

Usual Dosage Adults: I.V.:
Infections: 2 g every 6-12 hours for 5-14 days
Prophylaxis: 2 g 30-90 minutes before surgery

Dosage Forms Powder for injection, as sodium: 1 g, 2 g

Cefobid® *see* cefoperazone *on this page*

Cefol® Filmtab® *see* vitamin, multiple (oral) *on page 604*

cefonicid (se FON i sid)

U.S./Canadian Brand Names Monocid®

Therapeutic Category Cephalosporin (Second Generation)

Use Treatment of susceptible bacterial infection; mainly respiratory tract, skin and skin structure, bone and joint, urinary tract and gynecologic as well as septicemia; second generation cephalosporin

Usual Dosage Adults: I.M., I.V.: 1 g every 24 hours

Dosage Forms Powder for injection, as sodium: 500 mg, 1 g, 10 g

cefoperazone (sef oh PER a zone)

U.S./Canadian Brand Names Cefobid®

Therapeutic Category Cephalosporin (Third Generation)

Use Treatment of susceptible bacterial infections, mainly respiratory tract, skin and skin structure, urinary tract and sepsis; as a third generation cephalosporin, cefoperazone has activity against gram-negative bacilli (eg, *E. coli*, *Klebsiella*, and *Haemophilus*) but variable activity against *Streptococcus* and *Staphylococcus* species; it has activity against *Pseudomonas aeruginosa*, but less than ceftazidime

Usual Dosage I.M., I.V.:
Children: 100-150 mg/kg/day divided every 8-12 hours
Adults: 2-4 g/day in divided doses every 12 hours (up to 12 g/day)

Dosage Forms Cefoperazone sodium:
Injection, premixed (frozen): 1 g (50 mL); 2 g (50 mL)
Powder for injection: 1 g, 2 g

Cefotan® *see* cefotetan *on next page*

cefotaxime (sef oh TAKS eem)

U.S./Canadian Brand Names Claforan®

Therapeutic Category Cephalosporin (Third Generation)

Use Treatment of susceptible lower respiratory tract, skin and skin structure, bone and joint, intra-abdominal and genitourinary tract infections; treatment of a documented or suspected meningitis due to susceptible organisms such as *H. influenzae* and *N. meningitidis*; nonpseudomonal gram-negative rod infection in a patient at risk of developing aminoglycoside-induced nephrotoxicity and/or ototoxicity; infection due to an organism whose susceptibilities clearly favor cefotaxime over cefuroxime or an aminoglycoside

Usual Dosage I.M., I.V.:

Infants and Children 1 month to 12 years:

<50 kg: 100-200 mg/kg/day in 3-4 divided doses

Meningitis: 200 mg/kg/day in 4 divided doses

>50 kg: Moderate to severe infection: 1-2 g every 6-8 hours; life-threatening infection: 2 g/dose every 4 hours; maximum dose: 12 g/day

Children >12 years and Adults: 1-2 g every 6-8 hours (up to 12 g/day)

Dosage Forms Cefotaxime sodium:

Infusion, premixed in D_5W (frozen): 1 g (50 mL); 2 g (50 mL)

Powder for injection: 500 mg, 1 g, 2 g, 10 g

cefotetan (SEF oh tee tan)

U.S./Canadian Brand Names Cefotan®

Therapeutic Category Cephalosporin (Second Generation)

Use Treatment of susceptible lower respiratory tract, skin and skin structure, bone and joint, genitourinary tract, sepsis, gynecologic, and intra-abdominal infections; active against anaerobes including *Bacteroides* species of gastrointestinal tract, gram-negative enteric bacilli including *E. coli*, *Klebsiella*, and *Proteus*; active against many strains of *N. gonorrhoeae*; perioperative prophylaxis

Usual Dosage I.M., I.V.:

Children: 40-80 mg/kg/day divided every 12 hours

Adults: 1-6 g/day in divided doses every 12 hours, 1-2 g may be administered every 24 hours for urinary tract infection

Dosage Forms Powder for injection, as disodium: 1 g (10 mL, 100 mL); 2 g (20 mL, 100 mL); 10 g (100 mL)

cefoxitin (se FOKS i tin)

U.S./Canadian Brand Names Mefoxin®

Therapeutic Category Cephalosporin (Second Generation)

Use Treatment of susceptible lower respiratory tract, skin and skin structure, bone and joint, genitourinary tract, sepsis, gynecologic, and intra-abdominal infections; active against anaerobes including *Bacteroides* species of the gastrointestinal tract, gram-negative enteric bacilli including *E. coli*, *Klebsiella*, and *Proteus*; active against many strains of *N. gonorrhoeae*; perioperative prophylaxis

Usual Dosage I.M., I.V.:

Infants >3 months and Children:

Mild-moderate infection: 80-100 mg/kg/day in divided doses every 4-6 hours

Severe infection: 100-160 mg/kg/day in divided doses every 4-6 hours

Maximum dose: 12 g/day

Adults: 1-2 g every 6-8 hours (I.M. injection is painful)

Dosage Forms Cefoxitin sodium:

Infusion, premixed in D_5W (frozen): 1 g (50 mL); 2 g (50 mL)

Powder for injection: 1 g, 2 g, 10 g

cefpodoxime (sef pode OKS eem)

U.S./Canadian Brand Names Vantin®

Therapeutic Category Cephalosporin (Second Generation)

Use Treatment of susceptible acute, community-acquired pneumonia caused by *S. pneumoniae* or nonbeta-lactamase-producing *H. influenzae*; alternative regimen for acute uncomplicated gonorrhea caused by *N. gonorrhoeae*; uncomplicated skin and skin structure infections caused by *S. aureus* or *S. pyogenes*; acute otitis media caused by *S. pneumoniae*, *H. influenzae*, or *M. catarrhalis*; pharyngitis or tonsillitis; and uncomplicated urinary tract infections caused by *E. coli*, *Klebsiella*, and *Proteus*

Usual Dosage Oral:

Children >6 months to 12 years: 10 mg/kg/day divided every 12 hours for 10 days

Adults: 100-400 mg every 12 hours for 7-14 days

(Continued)

cefpodoxime *(Continued)*

Dosage Forms Cefpodoxime proxetil:

Granules for oral suspension (lemon creme flavor): 50 mg/5 mL (100 mL); 100 mg/5 mL (100 mL)

Tablet, film coated: 100 mg, 200 mg

cefprozil (sef PROE zil)

U.S./Canadian Brand Names Cefzil®

Therapeutic Category Cephalosporin (Second Generation)

Use Infections caused by susceptible organisms including *S. pneumoniae*, *H. influenzae*, *M. catarrhalis*, *S. aureus*, *S. pyogenes*; treatment of infections involving the respiratory tract, skin and skin structure, and otitis media

Usual Dosage Oral:

Infants and Children >6 months to 12 years: 15 mg/kg every 12 hours for 10 days

Children >13 years and Adults: 250-500 mg every 12-24 hours for 10 days

Dosage Forms

Powder for oral suspension, as anhydrous: 125 mg/5 mL (50 mL, 75 mL, 100 mL); 250 mg/5 mL (50 mL, 75 mL, 100 mL)

Tablet, as anhydrous: 250 mg, 500 mg

ceftazidime (SEF tay zi deem)

U.S./Canadian Brand Names Ceptaz™; Fortaz®; Tazicef®; Tazidime®

Therapeutic Category Cephalosporin (Third Generation)

Use Treatment of infections of the respiratory tract, urinary tract, skin and skin structure, intra-abdominal, osteomyelitis, sepsis, and meningitis caused by susceptible gram-negative aerobic organisms *Enterobacteriaceae pseudomonas*; pseudomonal infection in patient at risk of developing aminoglycoside-induced nephrotoxicity and/or ototoxicity; empiric therapy for febrile, granulocytopenic patients

Usual Dosage

Infants and Children 1 month to 12 years: 30-50 mg/kg/dose every 8 hours; maximum dose: 6 g/day

Adults: 1-2 g every 8-12 hours (250-500 mg every 12 hours for urinary tract infections)

Dosage Forms

Infusion, premixed (frozen) (Fortaz®): 1 g (50 mL); 2 g (50 mL)

Powder for injection: 500 mg, 1 g, 2 g, 6 g

ceftibuten (sef TYE byoo ten)

U.S./Canadian Brand Names Cedax®

Therapeutic Category Cephalosporin (Third Generation)

Use Oral cephalosporin for bronchitis, otitis media, and strep throat

Usual Dosage Oral:

Children: 9 mg/kg/day for 10 days; maximum daily dose: 400 mg

Children ≥12 years and Adults: 400 mg once daily for 10 days

Dosage Forms

Capsule: 400 mg

Powder for oral suspension (cherry flavor): 90 mg/5 mL (30 mL, 60 mL, 120 mL); 180 mg/5 mL (30 mL, 60 mL, 120 mL)

Ceftin® Oral *see* cefuroxime *on next page*

ceftizoxime (sef ti ZOKS eem)

U.S./Canadian Brand Names Cefizox®

Therapeutic Category Cephalosporin (Third Generation)

Use Treatment of susceptible bacterial infections, mainly respiratory tract, skin and skin structure, bone and joint, urinary tract and sepsis; as a third generation cephalosporin, ceftizoxime has activity against gram-negative enteric bacilli (eg, *E. coli*, *Klebsiella*), and cocci (eg, *Neisseria*), and variable activity against gram-positive cocci (*Staphylococcus* and *Streptococcus*); it has some anaerobic coverage but is less active against *B. fragilis* than cefoxitin; also indicated for *Neisseria gonorrhoeae* infections (including uncomplicated cervical and urethral gonorrhea and gonorrhea pelvic inflammatory disease), and *Haemophilus influenzae* meningitis

Usual Dosage I.M., I.V.:

Children ≥6 months: 50 mg/kg every 6-8 hours to 200 mg/kg/day to maximum of 12 g/24 hours

Adults: 1-2 g every 8-12 hours, up to 2 g every 4 hours or 4 g every 8 hours for life-threatening infections

Dosage Forms Ceftizoxime sodium:

Injection in D_5W (frozen): 1 g (50 mL); 2 g (50 mL)

Powder for injection: 500 mg, 1 g, 2 g, 10 g

ceftriaxone (sef trye AKS one)

U.S./Canadian Brand Names Rocephin®

Therapeutic Category Cephalosporin (Third Generation)

Use Treatment of sepsis, meningitis, infections of the lower respiratory tract, skin and skin structure, bone and joint, intra-abdominal and urinary tract due to susceptible organisms as a third generation cephalosporin, ceftriaxone has activity against gram-negative aerobic bacteria (ie, *H. influenzae*, Enterobacteriaceae, *Neisseria*) and variable activity against gram-positive cocci; documented or suspected infection due to susceptible organisms in home care patients and patients without I.V. line access; treatment of documented or suspected gonococcal infection or chancroid; emergency room management of patients at high risk for bacteremia, periorbital or buccal cellulitis, salmonellosis or shigellosis and pneumonia of unestablished etiology (<5 years of age)

Usual Dosage

Gonococcal ophthalmia: 25-50 mg/kg/day administered every 24 hours

Infants and Children: 50-100 mg/kg/day in 1-2 divided doses

Meningitis: 100 mg/kg/day divided every 12 hours; loading dose of 75 mg/kg may be administered at the start of therapy

Chancroid, uncomplicated gonorrhea: I.M.:

<45 kg: 125 mg as a single dose

>45 kg: 250 mg as a single dose

Adults: 1-2 g every 12-24 hours depending on the type and severity of the infection; maximum dose: 4 g/day

Dosage Forms Ceftriaxone sodium:

Infusion, premixed (frozen): 1 g in $D_{3.8}W$ (50 mL); 2 g in $D_{2.4}W$ (50 mL)

Powder for injection: 250 mg, 500 mg, 1 g, 2 g, 10 g

cefuroxime (se fyoor OKS eem)

U.S./Canadian Brand Names Ceftin® Oral; Kefurox® Injection; Zinacef® Injection

Therapeutic Category Cephalosporin (Second Generation)

Use Second generation cephalosporin useful in infections caused by susceptible staphylococci, group B streptococci, pneumococci, *H. influenzae* (type A and B), *E. coli*, *Enterobacter*, and *Klebsiella*; treatment of susceptible infections of the upper and lower respiratory tract, otitis media, urinary tract, skin and soft tissue, bone and joint, and sepsis

Usual Dosage

Children:

Oral:

<12 years: 125 mg twice daily

>12 years: 250 mg twice daily

I.M., I.V.: 75-150 mg/kg/day divided every 8 hours; maximum dose: 9 g/day

Adults:

Oral: 125-500 mg twice daily, depending on severity of infection

I.M., I.V.: 100-150 mg/kg/day in divided doses every 6-8 hours; maximum: 6 g/24 hours

Dosage Forms

Cefuroxime sodium:

Infusion, premixed (frozen) (Zinacef®): 750 mg (50 mL); 1.5 g (50 mL)

Powder for injection: 750 mg, 1.5 g, 7.5 g

(Continued)

cefuroxime *(Continued)*

Powder for injection (Kefurox®, Zinacef®): 750 mg, 1.5 g, 7.5 g

Cefuroxime axetil:

Powder for oral suspension (tutti-frutti flavor) (Ceftin®): 125 mg/5 mL (50 mL, 100 mL, 200 mL)

Tablet (Ceftin®): 125 mg, 250 mg, 500 mg

Cefzil® *see* cefprozil *on page 108*

Celebrex™ *see* celecoxib *on this page*

celecoxib (ce le COX ib)

U.S./Canadian Brand Names Celebrex™

Therapeutic Category Selective Cyclooxygenase-2 Inhibitor

Use Short-term efficacy in rheumatoid arthritis and osteoarthritis

Usual Dosage Adults: Oral:

Osteoarthritis: 200 mg once/day or 100 mg twice daily

Rheumatoid arthritis: 100-200 mg twice daily

Dosage Forms Capsule: 100 mg, 200 mg

Celestoderm®-V, -EV/2 (Can) *see* betamethasone (topical) *on page 72*

Celestone® Oral *see* betamethasone (systemic) *on page 71*

Celestone® Phosphate Injection *see* betamethasone (systemic) *on page 71*

Celestone® Soluspan® *see* betamethasone (systemic) *on page 71*

Celexa® *see* citalopram *on page 134*

CellCept® *see* mycophenolate *on page 385*

Cellufresh® [OTC] *see* carboxymethylcellulose *on page 101*

cellulose, oxidized (SEL yoo lose, OKS i dyzed)

Synonyms absorbable cotton

U.S./Canadian Brand Names Oxycel®; Surgicel®

Therapeutic Category Hemostatic Agent

Use Temporary packing for the control of capillary, venous, or small arterial hemorrhage

Usual Dosage Minimal amounts of an appropriate size are laid on the bleeding site

Dosage Forms

Pad (Oxycel®): 3" x 3", 8 ply

Pledget (Oxycel®): 2" x 1" x 1"

Strip:

Oxycel®:

18" x 2", 4 ply

5" x 1/2", 4 ply

36" x 1/2", 4 ply

Surgicel®:

2" x 14"

4" x 8"

2" x 3"

1/2" x 2"

cellulose sodium phosphate (sel yoo lose SOW dee um FOS fate)

Synonyms CSP; sodium cellulose phosphate

U.S./Canadian Brand Names Calcibind®

Therapeutic Category Urinary Tract Product

Use Adjunct to dietary restriction to reduce renal calculi formation in absorptive hypercalciuria type I

Usual Dosage Adults: Oral: 5 g 3 times/day with meals; decrease dose to 5 g with main meal and 2.5 g with each of two other meals when urinary calcium declines to <150 mg/day

Dosage Forms Powder: 2.5 g packets (90s), 300 g bulk pack

Celluvisc® [OTC] *see* carboxymethylcellulose *on page 101*

Celontin® *see* methsuximide *on page 366*

Cel-U-Jec® Injection *see* betamethasone (systemic) *on page 71*

Cenafed® [OTC] *see* pseudoephedrine *on page 486*

Cenafed® Plus Tablet [OTC] *see* triprolidine and pseudoephedrine *on page 584*

Cena-K® *see* potassium chloride *on page 464*

Cenestin™ *see* estrogens, conjugated, A (synthetic) *on page 219*

Cenocort® A-40 *(Discontinued)* *see page 700*

Cenocort® Forte *(Discontinued)* *see page 700*

Cenolate® *see* sodium ascorbate *on page 525*

Centrax Capsule & Tablet *(Discontinued)* *see page 700*

Cēpacol® Anesthetic Troches [OTC] *see* cetylpyridinium and benzocaine *on page 113*

Cēpacol® Troches [OTC] *see* cetylpyridinium *on page 113*

Cēpastat® [OTC] *see* phenol *on page 444*

cephalexin (sef a LEKS in)

U.S./Canadian Brand Names Apo®-Cephalex (Can); Biocef®; Cefanex®; Keflex®; Keftab®; Novo-Lexin® (Can); Nu-Cephalex® (Can); Zartan®

Therapeutic Category Cephalosporin (First Generation)

Use Treatment of susceptible bacterial infections, including those caused by group A beta-hemolytic *Streptococcus*, *Staphylococcus*, *Klebsiella pneumoniae*, *E. coli*, and *Proteus mirabilis*; not active against enterococci; used to treat susceptible infections of the respiratory tract, skin and skin structure, bone, genitourinary tract, and otitis media

Usual Dosage Oral:

Children: 25-50 mg/kg/day every 6 hours; severe infections: 50-100 mg/kg/day in divided doses every 6 hours; maximum: 3 g/24 hours

Adults: 250-1000 mg every 6 hours

Dosage Forms

Cephalexin monohydrate:

- Capsule: 250 mg, 500 mg
- Powder for oral suspension: 125 mg/5 mL (5 mL unit dose, 60 mL, 100 mL, 200 mL); 250 mg/5 mL (5 mL unit dose, 100 mL, 200 mL)
- Suspension, oral, pediatric: 100 mg/mL [5 mg/drop] (10 mL)
- Tablet: 250 mg, 500 mg, 1 g

Cephalexin hydrochloride: Tablet: 500 mg

cephalothin (sef A loe thin)

U.S./Canadian Brand Names Ceporacin® (Can)

Therapeutic Category Cephalosporin (First Generation)

Use Treatment of respiratory tract, skin and skin structure, urinary tract, bone and joint infections, endocarditis, and septicemia due to susceptible gram-positive cocci (except enterococcus); some gram-negative bacilli including *E. coli*, *Proteus*, and *Klebsiella* may be susceptible; perioperative prophylaxis

Usual Dosage I.M., I.V.:

Children: 75-125 mg/kg/day divided every 4-6 hours; maximum dose: 10 g in a 24-hour period

Adults: 500 mg to 2 g every 4-6 hours

Dosage Forms Cephalothin sodium:

Infusion, in D_5W (frozen): 1 g (50 mL); 2 g (50 mL)

Powder for injection: 1 g, 2 g, 20 g

cephapirin (sef a PYE rin)

U.S./Canadian Brand Names Cefadyl®

Therapeutic Category Cephalosporin (First Generation)

Use Treatment of respiratory tract, skin and skin structure, urinary tract, bone and joint infections, endocarditis and septicemia due to susceptible gram-positive cocci (except enterococcus); some gram-negative bacilli including *E. coli*, *Proteus*, and *Klebsiella*, may be susceptible; perioperative prophylaxis

Usual Dosage I.M., I.V.:

Children: 10-20 mg/kg every 6 hours up to 4 g/24 hours

Adults: 1 g every 6 hours up to 12 g/day

Dosage Forms Powder for injection, as sodium: 500 mg, 1 g, 2 g, 4 g, 20 g

cephradine (SEF ra deen)

U.S./Canadian Brand Names Velosef®

Therapeutic Category Cephalosporin (First Generation)

Use Treatment of susceptible bacterial infections, including those caused by group A beta-hemolytic *Streptococcus*

Usual Dosage Oral:

Children ≥9 months: 25-100 mg/kg/day in equally divided doses every 6-12 hours up to 4 g/day

Adults: 2-4 g/day in 4 equally divided doses up to 8 g/day

Dosage Forms

Capsule: 250 mg, 500 mg

Powder for injection: 250 mg, 500 mg, 1 g, 2 g (in ready to use infusion bottles)

Powder for oral suspension: 125 mg/5 mL (5 mL, 100 mL, 200 mL); 250 mg/5 mL (5 mL, 100 mL, 200 mL)

Cephulac® *see* lactulose *on page 325*

Ceporacin® (Can) *see* cephalothin *on previous page*

Ceptaz™ *see* ceftazidime *on page 108*

Cerebyx® *see* fosphenytoin *on page 253*

Ceredase® *see* alglucerase *on page 18*

Cerespan® ***(Discontinued)*** *see page 700*

Cerezyme® *see* imiglucerase *on page 302*

cerivastatin (se ree va STAT in)

U.S./Canadian Brand Names Baycol™

Therapeutic Category HMG-CoA Reductase Inhibitor

Use Adjunct to dietary therapy to for the reduction of elevated total and LDL cholesterol levels in patients with primary hypercholesterolemia and mixed dyslipidemia when the response to dietary restriction of saturated fat and cholesterol and other nonpharmacological measures alone has been inadequate

Usual Dosage Adults: Oral: 0.3 mg once daily in the evening; may be taken with or without food

Dosage Forms Tablet, as sodium: 0.2 mg, 0.3 mg

Cerose-DM® [OTC] *see* chlorpheniramine, phenylephrine, and dextromethorphan *on page 124*

Certiva® *see* diphtheria, tetanus toxoids, and acellular pertussis vaccine *on page 187*

Cerubidine® *see* daunorubicin hydrochloride *on page 160*

Cerumenex® Otic *see* triethanolamine polypeptide oleate-condensate *on page 580*

Cervidil® Vaginal Insert *see* dinoprostone *on page 184*

CES *see* estrogens, conjugated (equine) *on page 219*

Cesamet® *see* nabilone *on page 386*

C.E.S.™ (Can) *see* estrogens, conjugated (equine) *on page 219*

Cetacaine® *see* benzocaine, butyl aminobenzoate, tetracaine, and benzalkonium chloride *on page 67*

Cetacort® Topical *see* hydrocortisone (topical) *on page 292*

Cetamide® *see* sulfacetamide *on page 540*

Cetane® *(Discontinued)* *see page 700*

Cetapred® Ophthalmic *see* sulfacetamide and prednisolone *on page 540*

cetirizine (se TI ra zeen)

Synonyms P-071; UCB-P071

U.S./Canadian Brand Names Reactine™ (Can); Zyrtec®

Therapeutic Category Antihistamine

Use Perennial and seasonal allergic rhinitis and other allergic symptoms including urticaria

Usual Dosage Children ≥6 years and Adults: Oral: 5-10 mg once daily, depending upon symptom severity

Dosage Forms Cetirizine hydrochloride:

Syrup: 5 mg/5 mL (120 mL)

Tablet: 5 mg, 10 mg

cetylpyridinium (SEE til peer i DI nee um)

U.S./Canadian Brand Names Ceepryn® [OTC]; Cēpacol® Troches [OTC]

Therapeutic Category Local Anesthetic

Use Temporary relief of sore throat

Usual Dosage Children >6 years and Adults: Oral: Dissolve 1 lozenge in the mouth every 2 hours as needed

Dosage Forms Cetylpyridinium chloride:

Mouthwash: 0.05% and alcohol 14% (180 mL)

Troche: 1:1500 (24s)

cetylpyridinium and benzocaine (SEE til peer i DI nee um & BEN zoe kane)

Synonyms benzocaine and cetylpyridinium chloride; cetylpyridinium chloride and benzocaine

U.S./Canadian Brand Names Cēpacol® Anesthetic Troches [OTC]

Therapeutic Category Local Anesthetic

Use Symptomatic relief of sore throat

Usual Dosage Oral: Use as needed for sore throat

Dosage Forms Troche: Cetylpyridinium chloride 1:1500 and benzocaine 10 mg per troche (18s)

cetylpyridinium chloride and benzocaine *see* cetylpyridinium and benzocaine *on this page*

Cevalin® [OTC] *see* ascorbic acid *on page 48*

Cevi-bid® [OTC] *see* ascorbic acid *on page 48*

Ce-Vi-Sol® [OTC] *see* ascorbic acid *on page 48*

CFDN *see* cefdinir *on page 105*

CG *see* chorionic gonadotropin *on page 130*

Charcadole®, -Aqueous, -TFS (Can) *see* charcoal *on next page*

Charcoaid® [OTC] *see* charcoal *on next page*

charcoal (CHAR kole)

Synonyms activated carbon; liquid antidote; medicinal carbon

U.S./Canadian Brand Names Actidose-Aqua® [OTC]; Actidose® With Sorbitol [OTC]; Charcadole®, -Aqueous, -TFS (Can); Charcoaid® [OTC]; Charcocaps® [OTC]; Liqui-Char® [OTC]

Therapeutic Category Antidote

Use Emergency treatment in poisoning by drugs and chemicals; repetitive doses for gastrointestinal dialysis in drug overdose to enhance the elimination of certain drugs (eg, theophylline, phenobarbital, and aspirin) and in uremia to adsorb various waste products

Usual Dosage Oral:

Acute poisoning: Single dose: Charcoal with sorbitol:

Children 1-12 years: 1-2 g/kg/dose or 15-30 g or approximately 5-10 times the weight of the ingested poison; 1 g adsorbs 100-1000 mg of poison; the use of repeat oral charcoal with sorbitol doses is not recommended. In young children sorbitol should be repeated no more than 1-2 times/day.

Adults: 30-100 g

Charcoal in water:

Single dose:

Infants <1 year: 1 g/kg

Children 1-12 years: 15-30 g or 1-2 g/kg

Adults: 30-100 g or 1-2 g/kg

Multiple dose:

Infants <1 year: 1 g/kg every 4-6 hours

Children 1-12 years: 20-60 g or 1-2 g/kg every 2-6 hours until clinical observations and serum drug concentration have returned to a subtherapeutic range

Adults: 20-60 g or 1-2 g/kg every 2-6 hours

Gastric dialysis: Adults: 20-50 g every 6 hours for 1-2 days

Dosage Forms

Capsule (Charcocaps®): 260 mg

Liquid, activated:

Actidose-Aqua®: 12.5 g (60 mL); 25 g (120 mL)

Liqui-Char®: 12.5 g (60 mL); 15 g (75 mL); 25 g (120 mL); 30 g (120 mL); 50 g (240 mL)

Liquid, activated, with propylene glycol: 12.5 g (60 mL); 25 g (120 mL)

Liquid, activated, with sorbitol:

Actidose® With Sorbitol: 25 g (120 mL); 50 g (240 mL)

Charcoaid®: 30 g (150 mL)

Powder for suspension, activated: 15 g, 30 g, 40 g, 120 g, 240 g

Charcocaps® [OTC] *see* charcoal *on this page*

Chealamide® *see* edetate disodium *on page 203*

Chemet® *see* succimer *on page 537*

Chenix® Tablet *(Discontinued)* *see page 700*

Cheracol® *see* guaifenesin and codeine *on page 268*

Cheracol® D [OTC] *see* guaifenesin and dextromethorphan *on page 268*

Chibroxin™ Ophthalmic *see* norfloxacin *on page 407*

chicken pox vaccine *see* varicella virus vaccine *on page 596*

Chiggertox® [OTC] *see* benzocaine *on page 66*

Children's Advil® Suspension *see* ibuprofen *on page 300*

Children's Hold® [OTC] *see* dextromethorphan *on page 171*

Children's Kaopectate® [OTC] *see* attapulgite *on page 53*

Children's Motrin® Suspension [OTC] *see* ibuprofen *on page 300*

Children's Silfedrine® [OTC] *see* pseudoephedrine *on page 486*

children's vitamins *see* vitamin, multiple (pediatric) *on page 606*

Chirocaine® *see* levobupivacaine *on page 330*

Chlo-Amine® Oral [OTC] *see* chlorpheniramine *on page 120*

Chlorafed® Liquid [OTC] *see* chlorpheniramine and pseudoephedrine *on page 122*

chloral *see* chloral hydrate *on this page*

chloral hydrate (KLOR al HYE drate)

Synonyms chloral; trichloroacetaldehyde monohydrate

U.S./Canadian Brand Names Aquachloral® Supprettes®; Novo-Chlorhydrate® (Can); PMS-Chloral Hydrate (Can)

Therapeutic Category Hypnotic, Nonbarbiturate

Controlled Substance C-IV

Use Short-term sedative and hypnotic (<2 weeks), sedative/hypnotic prior to nonpainful therapeutic or diagnostic procedures (eg, EEG, CT scan, MRI, ophthalmic exam, dental procedure)

Usual Dosage

Children:

- Sedation, anxiety: Oral, rectal: 5-15 mg/kg/dose every 8 hours, maximum: 500 mg/dose
- Prior to EEG: Oral, rectal: 20-25 mg/kg/dose, 30-60 minutes prior to EEG; may repeat in 30 minutes to maximum of 100 mg/kg or 2 g total
- Hypnotic: Oral, rectal: 20-40 mg/kg/dose up to a maximum of 50 mg/kg/24 hours or 1 g/dose or 2 g/24 hours
- Sedation, nonpainful procedure: Oral: 50-75 mg/kg/dose 30-60 minutes prior to procedure; may repeat 30 minutes after initial dose if needed, to a total maximum dose of 120 mg/kg or 1 g total

Adults: Oral, rectal:

- Sedation, anxiety: 250 mg 3 times/day
- Hypnotic: 500-1000 mg at bedtime or 30 minutes prior to procedure, not to exceed 2 g/24 hours

Dosage Forms

Capsule: 250 mg, 500 mg

Suppository, rectal: 324 mg, 500 mg, 648 mg

Syrup: 250 mg/5 mL (10 mL); 500 mg/5 mL (5 mL, 10 mL, 480 mL)

chlorambucil (klor AM byoo sil)

U.S./Canadian Brand Names Leukeran®

Therapeutic Category Antineoplastic Agent

Use Management of chronic lymphocytic leukemia (CLL), Hodgkin's and non-Hodgkin's lymphoma; breast and ovarian carcinoma, testicular carcinoma, choriocarcinoma; Waldenström's macroglobulinemia, and nephrotic syndrome unresponsive to conventional therapy

Usual Dosage Children and Adults: Oral (refer to individual protocols):

- General short courses: 0.1-0.2 mg/kg/day or 4-8 mg/m^2/day for 2-3 weeks for remission induction, then adjust dose on basis of blood counts; maintenance therapy: 0.03-0.1 mg/kg/day
- Nephrotic syndrome: 0.1-0.2 mg/kg/day every day for 5-15 weeks with low-dose prednisone
- Chronic lymphocytic leukemia:
  - Biweekly regimen: Initial: 0.4 mg/kg dose is increased by 0.1 mg/kg every 2 weeks until a response occurs and/or myelosuppression occurs
  - Monthly regimen: Initial: 0.4 mg/kg, increase dose by 0.2 mg/kg every 4 weeks until a response occurs and/or myelosuppression occurs
- Malignant lymphomas:
  - Non-Hodgkins: 0.1 mg/kg/day
  - Hodgkins: 0.2 mg/kg/day

Dosage Forms Tablet, sugar coated: 2 mg

chloramphenicol (klor am FEN i kole)

U.S./Canadian Brand Names AK-Chlor® Ophthalmic; Chloromycetin® Injection; Chloroptic® Ophthalmic; Diochloram (Can); Ophthochlor® Ophthalmic; Ortho-Chloram® (Can); Pentamycetin® (Can); Sopamycetin® (Can)

Therapeutic Category Antibiotic, Ophthalmic; Antibiotic, Otic; Antibiotic, Miscellaneous

Use Treatment of serious infections due to organisms resistant to other less toxic antibiotics or when its penetrability into the site of infection is clinically superior to other antibiotics to which the organism is sensitive; useful in infections caused by *Bacteroides*, *H. influenzae*, *Neisseria meningitidis*, *S. pneumoniae*, *Salmonella*, and *Rickettsia*

Usual Dosage

I.V.:

Infants and Children: 50-75 mg/kg/day divided every 6 hours; maximum daily dose: 4 g/day

Adults: 50 mg/kg/day in divided doses every 6 hours; maximum daily dose: 4 g/day

Ophthalmic: Children and Adults: Instill 1-2 drops or small amount of ointment every 3-6 hours; increase interval between applications after 48 hours

Dosage Forms

Capsule: 250 mg

Ointment, ophthalmic: 1% [10 mg/g] (3.5 g)

AK-Chlor®, Chloroptic® S.O.P.®: 1% [10 mg/g] (3.5 g)

Powder for injection, as sodium succinate: 1 g

Solution: 0.5% [5 mg/mL] (7.5 mL, 15 mL)

Ophthalmic (AK-Chlor®, Chloroptic®): 0.5% [5 mg/mL] (2.5 mL, 7.5 mL, 15 mL)

Otic: 0.5% (15 mL)

chloramphenicol and prednisolone (klor am FEN i kole & pred NIS oh lone)

Synonyms prednisolone and chloramphenicol

U.S./Canadian Brand Names Chloroptic-P® Ophthalmic

Therapeutic Category Antibiotic/Corticosteroid, Ophthalmic

Use Topical anti-infective and corticosteroid for treatment of ocular infections

Usual Dosage Ophthalmic: Instill 1-2 drops in eye(s) 2-4 times/day

Dosage Forms Ointment, ophthalmic: Chloramphenicol 1% and prednisolone 0.5% (3.5 g)

chloramphenicol, polymyxin B, and hydrocortisone

(klor am FEN i kole, pol i MIKS in bee, & hye droe KOR ti sone)

Therapeutic Category Antibiotic/Corticosteroid, Ophthalmic

Use Topical anti-infective and corticosteroid for treatment of ocular infections

Usual Dosage Ophthalmic: Apply 1/2" ribbon every 3-4 hours until improvement occurs

Dosage Forms Solution, ophthalmic: Chloramphenicol 1%, polymyxin B sulfate 10,000 units, and hydrocortisone acetate 0.5% per g (3.75 g)

Chloraseptic® Oral [OTC] *see* phenol *on page 444*

Chlorate® Oral [OTC] *see* chlorpheniramine *on page 120*

chlordiazepoxide (klor dye az e POKS ide)

Synonyms methaminodiazepoxide

U.S./Canadian Brand Names Apo-Chlordiazepoxide® (Can); Corax® (Can); Libritabs®; Librium®; Medilium® (Can); Mitran® Oral; Novo-Poxide® (Can); Reposans-10® Oral; Solium® (Can)

Therapeutic Category Benzodiazepine

Controlled Substance C-IV

Use Management of anxiety and as a preoperative sedative, symptoms of alcohol withdrawal

Usual Dosage

Children >6 years: Anxiety: Oral, I.M.: 0.5 mg/kg/24 hours divided every 6-8 hours

Adults:
Anxiety: Oral: 15-100 mg divided 3-4 times/day
Severe anxiety: 20-25 mg 3-4 times/day
Preoperative sedation:
Oral: 5-10 mg 3-4 times/day, 1-day preop
I.M.: 50-100 mg 1-hour preop
Alcohol withdrawal symptoms: Oral, I.V.: 50-100 mg to start, dose may be repeated in 2-4 hours as necessary to a maximum of 300 mg/24 hours

Dosage Forms Chlordiazepoxide hydrochloride:
Capsule: 5 mg, 10 mg, 25 mg
Powder for injection: 100 mg
Tablet: 5 mg, 10 mg, 25 mg

chlordiazepoxide and amitriptyline *see* amitriptyline and chlordiazepoxide *on page 29*

chlordiazepoxide and clidinium *see* clidinium and chlordiazepoxide *on page 136*

Chloresium® [OTC] *see* chlorophyll *on next page*

Chlorgest-HD® Elixir *(Discontinued)* *see page 700*

chlorhexidine gluconate (klor HEKS i deen GLOO koe nate)

U.S./Canadian Brand Names Bactigras® (Chlorhexadine Acetate) (Can); BactoShield® [OTC]; Betasept® [OTC]; Dyna-Hex® [OTC]; Exidine® Scrub [OTC]; Hibiclens® [OTC]; Hibidil® 1:2000 (Can); Hibistat® [OTC]; Hibitane® Skin Cleanser (Can); Oro-Clense (Can); Peridex®; Periochip®; PerioGard®

Therapeutic Category Antibiotic, Oral Rinse; Antibiotic, Topical

Use
Dental:
Antibacterial dental rinse; chlorhexidine is active against gram-positive and gram-negative organisms, facultative anaerobes, aerobes, and yeast
Chip, for periodontal pocket insertion; indicated as an adjunct to scaling and root planing procedures for reduction of pocket depth in patients with adult periodontitis; may be used as part of a periodontal maintenance program
Medical: Skin cleanser for surgical scrub, cleanser for skin wounds, germicidal hand rinse

Usual Dosage Oral rinse (Peridex®)
Precede use of solution by flossing and brushing teeth, completely rinse toothpaste from mouth; swish 15 mL undiluted oral rinse around in mouth for 30 seconds, then expectorate. Caution patient not to swallow the medicine; avoid eating for 2-3 hours after treatment. (The cap on bottle of oral rinse is a measure for 15 mL.)
When used as a treatment of gingivitis, the regimen begins with oral prophylaxis. Patient treats mouth with 15 mL chlorhexidine; swish for 30 seconds, then expectorate; this is repeated twice daily (morning and evening). Patient should have a re-evaluation followed by a dental prophylaxis every 6 months.

Dosage Forms
Chip, for periodontal pocket insertion (PerioChip®): 2.5 mg
Foam, topical, with isopropyl alcohol 4% (BactoShield®): 4% (180 mL)
Liquid, topical, with isopropyl alcohol 4%:
Dyna-Hex® Skin Cleanser: 2% (120 mL, 240 mL, 480 mL, 960 mL, 4000 mL); 4% (120 mL, 240 mL, 480 mL, 4000 mL)
BactoShield® 2: 2% (960 mL)
BactoShield®, Betasept®, Exidine® Skin Cleanser, Hibiclens® Skin Cleanser: 4% (15 mL, 120 mL, 240 mL, 480 mL, 960 mL, 4000 mL)
Rinse:
Oral (mint flavor) (Peridex®, PerioGard®): 0.12% with alcohol 11.6% (480 mL)
Topical (Hibistat® Hand Rinse): 0.5% with isopropyl alcohol 70% (120 mL, 240 mL)
Sponge/Brush (Hibiclens®): 4% with isopropyl alcohol 4% (22 mL)
Wipes (Hibistat®): 0.5% (50s)

2-chlorodeoxyadenosine *see* cladribine *on page 134*

chloroethane *see* ethyl chloride *on page 226*

Chlorofon-A® Tablet *(Discontinued)* *see page 700*

Chloromycetin® Cream *(Discontinued)* *see page 700*

Chloromycetin® Injection *see* chloramphenicol *on page 116*

Chloromycetin® Kapseals *(Discontinued)* *see page 700*

Chloromycetin® Ophthalmic *(Discontinued)* *see page 700*

Chloromycetin® Otic *(Discontinued)* *see page 700*

Chloromycetin® Palmitate Oral Suspension *(Discontinued)* *see page 700*

chlorophylin *see* chlorophyll *on this page*

chlorophyll (KLOR oh fil)

Synonyms chlorophylin

U.S./Canadian Brand Names Chloresium® [OTC]; Derifil® [OTC]; Nullo® [OTC]; PALS® [OTC]

Therapeutic Category Gastrointestinal Agent, Miscellaneous

Use Topically promotes normal healing, relieves pain and inflammation, and reduces malodors in wounds, burns, surface ulcers, abrasions and skin irritations; used orally to control fecal and urinary odors in colostomy, ileostomy, or incontinence

Usual Dosage

Oral: 1-2 tablets/day

Topical: Apply generously and cover with gauze, linen, or other appropriate dressing; do not change dressings more often than every 48-72 hours

Dosage Forms

Ointment, topical (Chloresium®): Chlorophyllin copper complex 0.5% (30 g, 120 g)

Solution, topical, in isotonic saline (Chloresium®): Chlorophyllin copper complex 0.2% (240 mL, 946 mL)

Tablet:

Chloresium®: Chlorophyllin copper complex 14 mg

Derifil®: Water soluble chlorophyll: 100 mg

Nullo®: Chlorophyllin copper complex 33.3 mg

PALS®: Chlorophyllin copper complex 100 mg

Sodium free, sugar free: 20 mg

chloroprocaine (klor oh PROE kane)

U.S./Canadian Brand Names Nesacaine®; Nesacaine®-MPF

Therapeutic Category Local Anesthetic

Use For infiltration anesthesia and for peripheral and epidural anesthesia

Usual Dosage Dosage varies with anesthetic procedure, the area to be anesthetized, the vascularity of the tissues, depth of anesthesia required, degree of muscle relaxation required, and duration of anesthesia

Dosage Forms Chloroprocaine hydrochloride: Injection:

Preservative free (Nesacaine®-MPF): 2% (30 mL); 3% (30 mL)

With preservative (Nesacaine®): 1% (30 mL); 2% (30 mL)

Chloroptic® Ophthalmic *see* chloramphenicol *on page 116*

Chloroptic-P® Ophthalmic *see* chloramphenicol and prednisolone *on page 116*

chloroquine and primaquine (KLOR oh kwin & PRIM a kween)

Synonyms primaquine and chloroquine

U.S./Canadian Brand Names Aralen® Phosphate With Primaquine Phosphate

Therapeutic Category Aminoquinoline (Antimalarial)

Use Prophylaxis of malaria, regardless of species, in all areas where the disease is endemic

Usual Dosage Adults: Start at least 1 day before entering the endemic area; administer 1 tablet/week on the same day each week; continue for 8 weeks after leaving the endemic area

Dosage Forms Tablet: Chloroquine phosphate 500 mg [base 300 mg] and primaquine phosphate 79 mg [base 45 mg]

chloroquine phosphate (KLOR oh kwin FOS fate)

U.S./Canadian Brand Names Aralen® Phosphate

Therapeutic Category Aminoquinoline (Antimalarial)

Use Suppression or chemoprophylaxis of malaria; treatment of uncomplicated or mild-moderate malaria; extraintestinal amebiasis; rheumatoid arthritis; discoid lupus erythematosus, scleroderma, pemphigus

Usual Dosage Oral:

Malaria (excluding resistant *P. falciparum*):

Suppression or prophylaxis in endemic areas (begin 1-2 weeks prior to, and continue for 6-8 weeks after the period of potential exposure):

Children: 5 mg base/kg/dose weekly, up to a maximum of 300 mg/dose

Adults: 300 mg/dose weekly

Treatment:

Children: 10 mg base/kg/dose, up to a maximum of 600 mg base/dose one time, followed by 5 mg base/kg/dose one time after 6 hours, and then daily for 2 days (total dose of 25 mg base/kg)

Adults: 600 mg base/dose one time, followed by 300 mg base/dose one time after 6 hours, and then daily for 2 days

Extraintestinal amebiasis: Dosage expressed in mg base:

Children: 10 mg/kg once daily for 2-3 weeks (up to 300 mg base/day)

Adults: 600 mg base/day for 2 days followed by 300 mg base/day for at least 2-3 weeks

Rheumatoid arthritis: Adults: 150 mg base once daily

Melanoma treatment: Children: 10 mg/kg base/dose (maximum: 600 mg) as a single dose followed by 5 mg/kg base one time after 6 hours, then daily for 2 days

Dosage Forms Tablet: 250 mg [150 mg base]; 500 mg [300 mg base]

Chloroserpine® ***(Discontinued)*** *see page 700*

chlorothiazide (klor oh THYE a zide)

U.S./Canadian Brand Names Diurigen®; Diuril®

Therapeutic Category Diuretic, Thiazide

Use Management of mild to moderate hypertension; edema associated with congestive heart failure, pregnancy, or nephrotic syndrome

Usual Dosage I.V. has been limited in infants and children and is generally not recommended

Infants <6 months and patients with pulmonary interstitial edema:

Oral: 20-40 mg/kg/day in 2 divided doses

I.V.: 2-8 mg/kg/day in 2 divided doses

Infants >6 months and Children:

Oral: 20 mg/kg/day in 2 divided doses

I.V.: 4 mg/kg/day

Adults:

Oral: 500 mg to 2 g/day divided in 1-2 doses

I.V.: 100-500 mg/day

Dosage Forms

Powder for injection, lyophilized, as sodium: 500 mg

Suspension, oral: 250 mg/5 mL (237 mL)

Tablet: 250 mg, 500 mg

chlorothiazide and methyldopa (klor oh THYE a zide & meth il DOE pa)

Synonyms methyldopa and chlorothiazide

U.S./Canadian Brand Names Aldoclor®

(Continued)

chlorothiazide and methyldopa *(Continued)*

Therapeutic Category Antihypertensive Agent, Combination
Use Treatment of hypertension
Usual Dosage Oral: 1 tablet 2-3 times/day for first 48 hours, then adjust
Dosage Forms Tablet:
150: Chlorothiazide 150 mg and methyldopa 250 mg
250: Chlorothiazide 250 mg and methyldopa 250 mg

chlorothiazide and reserpine (klor oh THYE a zide & re SER peen)

Synonyms reserpine and chlorothiazide
Therapeutic Category Antihypertensive Agent, Combination
Use Management of hypertension
Usual Dosage Oral: 1-2 tablets 1-2 times/day
Dosage Forms Tablet:
250: Chlorothiazide 250 mg and reserpine 0.125 mg
500: Chlorothiazide 500 mg and reserpine 0.125 mg

chlorotrianisene (klor oh trye AN i seen)

U.S./Canadian Brand Names TACE®
Therapeutic Category Estrogen Derivative
Use Treat inoperable prostatic cancer; management of atrophic vaginitis, female hypogonadism, vasomotor symptoms of menopause; prevention of postpartum breast engorgement (no longer recommended because increased risk of thrombophlebitis)
Usual Dosage Adults: Oral:
Prostatic cancer: 12-25 mg/day
Atrophic vaginitis: 12-25 mg/day in 28-day cycles (21 days on and 7 days off)
Female hypogonadism: 12-25 mg for 21 days followed by I.M. progesterone 100 mg or 5 days of oral progestin; next course may begin on days of induced uterine bleeding
Menopause: 12-25 mg for 30 days
Postpartum breast engorgement: 12 mg 4 times/day for 7 days or 72 mg twice daily for 2 days
Dosage Forms Capsule: 12 mg, 25 mg

chloroxine (klor OKS een)

U.S./Canadian Brand Names Capitrol®
Therapeutic Category Antiseborrheic Agent, Topical
Use Treatment of dandruff or seborrheic dermatitis of the scalp
Usual Dosage Topical: Use twice weekly, massage into wet scalp, lather should remain on the scalp for approximately 3 minutes, then rinsed; application should be repeated and scalp rinsed thoroughly
Dosage Forms Shampoo: 2% (120 mL)

Chlorphed® [OTC] *see* bromphéniramine *on page 80*

Chlorphed®-LA Nasal Solution [OTC] *see* oxymetazoline *on page 423*

chlorphenesin (klor FEN e sin)

U.S./Canadian Brand Names Maolate®
Therapeutic Category Skeletal Muscle Relaxant
Use Adjunctive treatment of discomfort in short-term, acute, painful musculoskeletal conditions
Usual Dosage Adults: Oral: 800 mg 3 times/day, then adjusted to lowest effective dosage, usually 400 mg 4 times/day for up to a maximum of 2 months
Dosage Forms Tablet, as carbamate: 400 mg

chlorpheniramine (klor fen IR a meen)

U.S./Canadian Brand Names Aller-Chlor® Oral [OTC]; AL-Rr® Oral [OTC]; Chlo-Amine® Oral [OTC]; Chlorate® Oral [OTC]; Chlor-Pro® Injection; Chlor-Trimeton® Injection; Chlor-

Trimeton® Oral [OTC]; Chlor-Tripolon® (Can); Klorominr® Oral [OTC]; Telachlor® Oral; Teldrin® Oral [OTC]

Therapeutic Category Antihistamine

Use Perennial and seasonal allergic rhinitis and other allergic symptoms including urticaria

Usual Dosage

Children: Oral: 0.35 mg/kg/day in divided doses every 4-6 hours

2-6 years: 1 mg every 4-6 hours, not to exceed 6 mg in 24 hours

6-12 years: 2 mg every 4-6 hours, not to exceed 12 mg/day or sustained release 8 mg at bedtime

Children >12 years and Adults: Oral: 4 mg every 4-6 hours, not to exceed 24 mg/day or sustained release 8-12 mg every 8-12 hours, not to exceed 24 mg/day

Adults: Allergic reactions: I.M., I.V., S.C.: 10-20 mg as a single dose; maximum recommended dose: 40 mg/24 hours

Elderly: 4 mg once or twice daily. **Note:** Duration of action may be 36 hours or more when serum concentrations are low.

Dosage Forms Chlorpheniramine maleate:

Capsule: 12 mg

Timed release: 8 mg, 12 mg

Injection: 10 mg/mL (1 mL, 30 mL); 100 mg/mL (2 mL)

Syrup: 2 mg/5 mL (120 mL, 473 mL)

Tablet: 4 mg, 8 mg, 12 mg

Chewable: 2 mg

Timed release: 8 mg, 12 mg

chlorpheniramine and acetaminophen

(klor fen IR a meen & a seet a MIN oh fen)

U.S./Canadian Brand Names Coricidin® [OTC]

Therapeutic Category Antihistamine/Analgesic

Use Symptomatic relief of congestion, headache, aches, and pains of colds and flu

Usual Dosage Adults: Oral: 2 tablets every 4 hours, up to 20 tablets/day

Dosage Forms Tablet: Chlorpheniramine maleate 2 mg and acetaminophen 325 mg

chlorpheniramine and hydrocodone *see* hydrocodone and chlorpheniramine *on page 288*

chlorpheniramine and phenylephrine (klor fen IR a meen & fen il EF rin)

Synonyms phenylephrine and chlorpheniramine

U.S./Canadian Brand Names Dallergy-D® Syrup; Ed A-Hist® Liquid; Histatab® Plus Tablet [OTC]; Histor-D® Syrup; Rolatuss® Plain Liquid; Ru-Tuss® Liquid

Therapeutic Category Antihistamine/Decongestant Combination

Use Temporary relief of nasal congestion and eustachian tube congestion as well as runny nose, sneezing, itching of nose or throat, itchy and watery eyes

Usual Dosage Oral:

Children:

2-5 years: 2.5 mL every 4 hours

6-12 years: 5 mL every 4 hours

Adults: 10 mL every 4 hours or 1-2 regular tablets 3-4 times daily or 1 sustained release capsule every 12 hours

Dosage Forms

Capsule, sustained release: Chlorpheniramine maleate 8 mg and phenylephrine hydrochloride 20 mg

Liquid:

Dallergy-D®, Histor-D®, Rolatuss® Plain, Ru-Tuss®: Chlorpheniramine maleate 2 mg and phenylephrine hydrochloride 5 mg per 5 mL

Ed A-Hist® Liquid: Chlorpheniramine maleate 4 mg and phenylephrine hydrochloride 10 mg per 5 mL

Tablet (Histatab® Plus): Chlorpheniramine maleate 2 mg and phenylephrine hydrochloride 5 mg

chlorpheniramine and phenylpropanolamine

(klor fen IR a meen & fen il proe pa NOLE a meen)

Synonyms phenylpropanolamine and chlorpheniramine

U.S./Canadian Brand Names Allerest® 12 Hour Capsule [OTC]; A.R.M.® Caplet [OTC]; Chlor-Rest® Tablet [OTC]; Demazin® Syrup [OTC]; Genamin® Cold Syrup [OTC]; Ornade® Spansule®; Resaid®; Rescon Liquid [OTC]; Silaminic® Cold Syrup [OTC]; Temazin® Cold Syrup [OTC]; Thera-Hist® Syrup [OTC]; Triaminic® Allergy Tablet [OTC]; Triaminic® Cold Tablet [OTC]; Triaminic® Syrup [OTC]; Tri-Nefrin® Extra Strength Tablet [OTC]; Triphenyl® Syrup [OTC]

Therapeutic Category Antihistamine/Decongestant Combination

Use Symptomatic relief of nasal congestion, runny nose, sneezing, itchy nose or throat, and itchy or watery eyes due to the common cold or allergic rhinitis

Usual Dosage Oral:

Children <12 years: 5 mL every 3-4 hours

Children >12 years and Adults: 1 sustained release capsule or tablet every 12 hours or 5-10 mL every 3-4 hours or 1-2 regular tablets 3-4 times/day

Dosage Forms

Capsule, sustained release: Chlorpheniramine maleate 12 mg and phenylpropanolamine hydrochloride 75 mg

Liquid:

Triphenyl®, Genamin®: Chlorpheniramine maleate 1 mg and phenylpropanolamine hydrochloride 6.25 mg per 5 mL

Demazin®, Rescon®, Silaminic®, Temazin®, Thera-Hist®: Chlorpheniramine maleate 2 mg and phenylpropanolamine hydrochloride 12.5 mg per 5 mL

Syrup: Chlorpheniramine maleate 2 mg and phenylpropanolamine hydrochloride 12.5 mg per 5 mL

Tablet:

Triaminic® Cold: Chlorpheniramine maleate 2 mg and phenylpropanolamine hydrochloride 12.5 mg

Chlor-Rest®: Chlorpheniramine maleate 2 mg and phenylpropanolamine hydrochloride 18.7 mg

A.R.M.®, Triaminic® Allergy, Tri-Nefrin® Extra Strength: Chlorpheniramine maleate 4 mg and phenylpropanolamine hydrochloride 25 mg

Tablet, sustained release: Chlorpheniramine maleate 12 mg and phenylpropanolamine hydrochloride 75 mg

chlorpheniramine and pseudoephedrine

(klor fen IR a meen & soo doe e FED rin)

Synonyms pseudoephedrine and chlorpheniramine

U.S./Canadian Brand Names Allerest® Maximum Strength [OTC]; Anamine® Syrup [OTC]; Anaplex® Liquid [OTC]; Chlorafed® Liquid [OTC]; Chlor-Trimeton® 4 Hour Relief Tablet [OTC]; Co-Pyronil® 2 Pulvules® [OTC]; Deconamine® SR; Deconamine® Syrup [OTC]; Deconamine® Tablet [OTC]; Fedahist® Tablet [OTC]; Hayfebrol® Liquid [OTC]; Histalet® Syrup [OTC]; Klerist-D® Tablet [OTC]; Pseudo-Gest Plus® Tablet [OTC]; Rhinosyn® Liquid [OTC]; Rhinosyn-PD® Liquid [OTC]; Ryna® Liquid [OTC]; Sudafed® Plus Tablet [OTC]

Therapeutic Category Antihistamine/Decongestant Combination

Use Relief of nasal congestion associated with the common cold, hay fever, and other allergies, sinusitis, eustachian tube blockage, and vasomotor and allergic rhinitis

Usual Dosage Oral:

Capsule: 1 capsule every 12 hours

Liquid: 5 mL 3-4 times/day

Tablet: 1 tablet 3-4 times/day

Dosage Forms

Capsule:

Co-Pyronil® 2 Pulvules®: Chlorpheniramine maleate 4 mg and pseudoephedrine hydrochloride 60 mg

Capsule, sustained release: Chlorpheniramine maleate 4 mg and pseudoephedrine hydrochloride 60 mg; chlorpheniramine maleate 8 mg and pseudoephedrine hydrochloride 120 mg

Liquid:

Anamine®, Anaplex®, Chlorafed®, Deconamine®, Hayfebrol®, Rhinosyn-PD®, Ryna®: Chlorpheniramine maleate 2 mg and pseudoephedrine sulfate 30 mg per 5 mL

Rhinosyn®: Chlorpheniramine maleate 2 mg and pseudoephedrine sulfate 60 mg per 5 mL

Histalet®: Chlorpheniramine maleate 3 mg and pseudoephedrine sulfate 45 mg per 5 mL

Tablet:

Allerest® Maximum Strength: Chlorpheniramine maleate 2 mg and pseudoephedrine hydrochloride 30 mg

Deconamine®, Fedahist®, Klerist-D®, Pseudo-Gest Plus®, Sudafed® Plus: Chlorpheniramine maleate 4 mg and pseudoephedrine hydrochloride 60 mg

Chlor-Trimeton® 4 Hour Relief: Chlorpheniramine maleate 4 mg and pseudoephedrine sulfate 60 mg

chlorpheniramine, ephedrine, phenylephrine, and carbetapentane

(klor fen IR a meen, e FED rin, fen il EF rin, & kar bay ta PEN tane)

U.S./Canadian Brand Names Rentamine®; Rynatuss® Pediatric Suspension; Tri-Tannate Plus®

Therapeutic Category Antihistamine/Decongestant/Antitussive

Use Symptomatic relief of cough

Usual Dosage Children: Oral:

<2 years: Titrate dose individually

2-6 years: 2.5-5 mL every 12 hours

>6 years: 5-10 mL every 12 hours

Dosage Forms Liquid: Carbetapentane tannate 30 mg, ephedrine tannate 5 mg, phenylephrine tannate 5 mg, and chlorpheniramine tannate 4 mg per 5 mL

chlorpheniramine, hydrocodone, phenylephrine, acetaminophen, and caffeine *see* hydrocodone, chlorpheniramine, phenylephrine, acetaminophen, and caffeine *on page 290*

chlorpheniramine, phenindamine, and phenylpropanolamine

(klor fen IR a meen, fen IN dah meen, & fen il proe pa NOLE a meen)

U.S./Canadian Brand Names Nolamine®

Therapeutic Category Antihistamine/Decongestant Combination

Use Relief of upper respiratory and nasal congestion

Usual Dosage Adults: Oral: 1 tablet every 8-12 hours

Dosage Forms Tablet, timed release: Chlorpheniramine maleate 4 mg, phenindamine tartrate 24 mg, and phenylpropanolamine hydrochloride 50 mg

chlorpheniramine, phenylephrine, and codeine

(klor fen IR a meen, fen il EF rin, & KOE deen)

U.S./Canadian Brand Names Pediacof®; Pedituss®

Therapeutic Category Antihistamine/Decongestant/Antitussive

Controlled Substance C-IV

Use Symptomatic relief of rhinitis, nasal congestion, and cough due to colds or allergy

Usual Dosage Children 6 months to 12 years: Oral: 1.25-10 mL every 4-6 hours

Dosage Forms Liquid: Chlorpheniramine maleate 0.75 mg, phenylephrine hydrochloride 2.5 mg, and codeine phosphate 5 mg with potassium iodide 75 mg per 5 mL

chlorpheniramine, phenylephrine, and dextromethorphan

(klor fen IR a meen, fen il EF rin, & deks troe meth OR fan)

U.S./Canadian Brand Names Cerose-DM® [OTC]

Therapeutic Category Antihistamine/Decongestant/Antitussive

Use Temporary relief of cough due to minor throat and bronchial irritation; relief of nasal congestion, runny nose, and sneezing

Usual Dosage Adults: Oral: 5-10 mL 4 times/day

Dosage Forms Liquid: Chlorpheniramine maleate 4 mg, phenylephrine hydrochloride 10 mg, and dextromethorphan hydrobromide 15 mg per 5 mL

chlorpheniramine, phenylephrine, and methscopolamine

(klor fen IR a meen, fen il EF rin, & meth skoe POL a meen)

U.S./Canadian Brand Names D.A.II® Tablet; Dallergy®; Dura-Vent/DA®; Extendryl® SR; Histor-D® Timecelles®

Therapeutic Category Antihistamine/Decongestant/Anticholinergic

Use Relief of nasal congestion, runny nose, and sneezing

Usual Dosage Adults: Oral: 1 capsule or caplet every 12 hours or 5 mL every 4-6 hours

Dosage Forms

Caplet, sustained release: Chlorpheniramine maleate 8 mg, phenylephrine hydrochloride 20 mg, and methscopolamine nitrate 2.5 mg

Capsule, sustained release: Chlorpheniramine maleate 8 mg, phenylephrine hydrochloride 10 mg, and methscopolamine nitrate 2.5 mg

Syrup: Chlorpheniramine maleate 2 mg, phenylephrine hydrochloride 10 mg, and methscopolamine nitrate 0.625 mg per 5 mL

Tablet: Chlorpheniramine maleate 4 mg, phenylephrine hydrochloride 10 mg, and methscopolamine nitrate 1.25 mg

chlorpheniramine, phenylephrine, and phenylpropanolamine

(klor fen IR a meen, fen il EF rin, & fen il proe pa NOLE a meen)

U.S./Canadian Brand Names Hista-Vadrin® Tablet

Therapeutic Category Antihistamine/Decongestant Combination

Use Symptomatic relief of rhinitis and nasal congestion due to colds or allergy

Usual Dosage Adults: Oral: 1 tablet every 6 hours

Dosage Forms Tablet: Chlorpheniramine maleate 6 mg, phenylephrine hydrochloride 5 mg, and phenylpropanolamine hydrochloride 40 mg

chlorpheniramine, phenylephrine, and phenyltoloxamine

(klor fen IR a meen, fen il EF rin, & fen il tole LOKS a meen)

U.S./Canadian Brand Names Comhist®; Comhist® LA

Therapeutic Category Antihistamine/Decongestant Combination

Use Symptomatic relief of rhinitis and nasal congestion due to colds or allergy

Usual Dosage Oral: 1 capsule every 8-12 hours or 1-2 tablets 3 times/day

Dosage Forms

Capsule, sustained release (Comhist® LA): Chlorpheniramine maleate 4 mg, phenylephrine hydrochloride 20 mg, and phenyltoloxamine citrate 50 mg

Tablet (Comhist®): Chlorpheniramine maleate 2 mg, phenylephrine hydrochloride 10 mg, and phenyltoloxamine citrate 25 mg

chlorpheniramine, phenylephrine, phenylpropanolamine, and belladonna alkaloids

(klor fen IR a meen, fen il EF rin, fen il proe pa NOLE a meen, & bel a DON a AL ka loydz)

Synonyms phenylephrine, chlorpheniramine, phenylpropanolamine, and belladonna alkaloids; phenylpropanolamine, chlorpheniramine, phenylephrine, and belladonna alkaloids

U.S./Canadian Brand Names Atrohist® Plus; Phenahist-TR®; Phenchlor® S.H.A.; Ru-Tuss®; Stahist®

Therapeutic Category Cold Preparation

Use Relief of symptoms resulting from irritation of sinus, nasal, and upper respiratory tract tissues, including nasal congestion, watering eyes, and postnasal drip; this product contains anticholinergic agents and should be reserved for patients who do not respond to other antihistamine/decongestants

Usual Dosage Children ≥12 years and Adults: Oral: 1 tablet morning and evening, swallowed whole

Dosage Forms Tablet, sustained release: Chlorpheniramine 8 mg, phenylephrine 25 mg, phenylpropanolamine 50 mg, hyoscyamine 0.19 mg, atropine 0.04 mg, and scopolamine 0.01 mg

chlorpheniramine, phenylpropanolamine, and acetaminophen

(klor fen IR a meen, fen il proe pa NOLE a meen, & a seet a MIN oh fen)

U.S./Canadian Brand Names Congestant D® [OTC]; Coricidin D® [OTC]; Dapacin® Cold Capsule [OTC]; Duadacin® Capsule [OTC]; Tylenol® Cold Effervescent Medication Tablet [OTC]

Therapeutic Category Antihistamine/Decongestant/Analgesic

Use Symptomatic relief of nasal congestion and headache from colds/sinus congestion

Usual Dosage Adults: Oral: 2 capsules/tablets every 4 hours, up to 12/day

Dosage Forms

Capsule: Chlorpheniramine maleate 2 mg, phenylpropanolamine hydrochloride 12.5 mg, and acetaminophen 325 mg

Tablet: Chlorpheniramine maleate 2 mg, phenylpropanolamine hydrochloride 12.5 mg, and acetaminophen 325 mg

chlorpheniramine, phenylpropanolamine, and dextromethorphan

(klor fen IR a meen, fen il proe pa NOLE a meen, & deks troe meth OR fan)

U.S./Canadian Brand Names Triaminicol® Multi-Symptom Cold Syrup [OTC]

Therapeutic Category Antihistamine/Decongestant/Antitussive

Use Relief of runny nose, sneezing; cough suppressant; promote nasal and sinus drainage

Usual Dosage

Children 6-12 years: 5 mL every 4 hours

Adults: 10 mL every 4 hours

Dosage Forms Liquid: Chlorpheniramine maleate 2 mg, phenylpropanolamine hydrochloride 12.5 mg, and dextromethorphan hydrobromide 10 mg per 5 mL

chlorpheniramine, phenyltoloxamine, phenylpropanolamine, and phenylephrine

(klor fen IR a meen, fen il tole LOKS a meen, fen il proe pa NOLE a meen & fen il EF rin)

U.S./Canadian Brand Names Naldecon®; Naldelate®; Nalgest®; Nalspan®; New Decongestant®; Par Decon®; Tri-Phen-Chlor®; Uni-Decon®

Therapeutic Category Antihistamine/Decongestant Combination

Use Symptomatic treatment of nasal and eustachian tube congestion associated with sinusitis and acute upper respiratory infection; symptomatic relief of perennial and allergic rhinitis

Usual Dosage Oral:

Children:

- 3-6 months: 0.25 mL (pediatric drops) every 3-4 hours
- 6-12 months: 2.5 mL (pediatric syrup) or 0.5 mL (pediatric drops) every 3-4 hours
- 1-6 years: 5 mL (pediatric syrup) or 1 mL (pediatric drops) every 3-4 hours
- 6-12 years: 2.5 mL (syrup) or 10 mL (pediatric syrup) or 1/2 tablet every 3-4 hours

Children >12 years and 5 mL (syrup) or 1 tablet every 3-4 hours

Dosage Forms

Drops, pediatric: Chlorpheniramine maleate 0.5 mg, phenyltoloxamine citrate 2 mg, phenylpropanolamine hydrochloride 5 mg, and phenylephrine hydrochloride 1.25 mg per mL

(Continued)

chlorpheniramine, phenyltoloxamine, phenylpropanolamine, and phenylephrine *(Continued)*

Syrup: Chlorpheniramine maleate 2.5 mg, phenyltoloxamine citrate 7.5 mg, phenylpropanolamine hydrochloride 20 mg, and phenylephrine hydrochloride 5 mg per 5 mL

Syrup, pediatric: Chlorpheniramine maleate 0.5 mg, phenyltoloxamine citrate 2 mg, phenylpropanolamine hydrochloride 5 mg, and phenylephrine hydrochloride 1.25 mg per 5 mL

Tablet, sustained release: Chlorpheniramine maleate 5 mg, phenyltoloxamine citrate 15 mg, phenylpropanolamine hydrochloride 40 mg, and phenylephrine hydrochloride 10 mg

chlorpheniramine, pseudoephedrine, and codeine

(klor fen IR a meen, soo doe e FED rin, & KOE deen)

U.S./Canadian Brand Names Codehist® DH; Decohistine® DH; Dihistine® DH; Ryna-C® Liquid

Therapeutic Category Antihistamine/Decongestant/Antitussive

Controlled Substance C-V

Use Temporary relief of cough associated with minor throat or bronchial irritation; relief of nasal congestion due to common cold, allergic rhinitis, or sinusitis

Usual Dosage Oral:

Children:

25-50 lb: 1.25-2.50 mL every 4-6 hours, up to 4 doses in a 24-hour period

50-90 lb: 2.5-5 mL every 4-6 hours, up to 4 doses in a 24-hour period

Adults: 10 mL every 4-6 hours, up to 4 doses in a 24-hour period

Dosage Forms Liquid: Chlorpheniramine maleate 2 mg, pseudoephedrine hydrochloride 30 mg, and codeine phosphate 10 mg (120 mL, 480 mL)

chlorpheniramine, pyrilamine, and phenylephrine

(klor fen IR a meen, pye RIL a meen, & fen il EF rin)

U.S./Canadian Brand Names Rhinatate® Tablet; R-Tannamine® Tablet; R-Tannate® Tablet; Rynatan® Pediatric Suspension; Rynatan® Tablet; Tanoral® Tablet; Triotann® Tablet; Tri-Tannate® Tablet

Therapeutic Category Antihistamine/Decongestant Combination

Use Symptomatic relief of nasal congestion associated with upper respiratory tract condition

Usual Dosage Oral:

Children:

<2 years: Titrate dose individually

2-6 years: 2.5-5 mL every 12 hours

Children >6 years and Adults: 5-10 mL every 12 hours

Dosage Forms

Liquid: Chlorpheniramine tannate 2 mg, pyrilamine tannate 12.5 mg, and phenylephrine tannate 5 mg per 5 mL

Tablet: Chlorpheniramine tannate 8 mg, pyrilamine maleate 12.5 mg, and phenylephrine tannate 25 mg

chlorpheniramine, pyrilamine, phenylephrine, and phenylpropanolamine

(klor fen IR a meen, pye RIL a meen, fen il EF rin, & fen il proe pa NOLE a meen)

U.S./Canadian Brand Names Histalet Forte® Tablet

Therapeutic Category Antihistamine/Decongestant Combination

Use Symptomatic relief of rhinitis and nasal congestion due to colds or allergy

Usual Dosage Adults: Oral: 1 tablet 2-3 times/day

Dosage Forms Tablet: Chlorpheniramine maleate 4 mg, pyrilamine maleate 25 mg, phenylephrine hydrochloride 10 mg, and phenylpropanolamine hydrochloride 50 mg

Chlor-Pro® Injection *see* chlorpheniramine *on page 120*

Chlorpromanyl® (Can) *see* chlorpromazine *on next page*

chlorpromazine (klor PROE ma zeen)

U.S./Canadian Brand Names Apo®-Chlorpromazine (Can); Chlorpromanyl® (Can); Chlorprom® (Can); Largactil® (Can); Novo-Chlorpromazine® (Can); Ormazine®; Thorazine®

Therapeutic Category Phenothiazine Derivative

Use Treatment of nausea and vomiting; psychoses; Tourette's syndrome; mania; intractable hiccups (adults); behavioral problems (children)

Usual Dosage

Children >6 months:

Psychosis:

Oral: 0.5-1 mg/kg/dose every 4-6 hours; older children may require 200 mg/day or higher

I.M., I.V.: 0.5-1 mg/kg/dose every 6-8 hours; maximum I.M./I.V. dose for <5 years (22.7 kg): 40 mg/day; maximum I.M./I.V. for 5-12 years (22.7-45.5 kg): 75 mg/day

Nausea and vomiting:

Oral: 0.5-1 mg/kg/dose every 4-6 hours as needed

I.M., I.V.: 0.5-1 mg/kg/dose every 6-8 hours; maximum dose: Same as psychoses

Rectal: 1 mg/kg/dose every 6-8 hours as needed

Adults:

Psychosis:

Oral: Range: 30-800 mg/day in 1-4 divided doses, initiate at lower doses and titrate as needed; usual dose is 200 mg/day; some patients may require 1-2 g/day

I.M., I.V.: Initial: 25 mg, may repeat (25-50 mg) in 1-4 hours, gradually increase to a maximum of 400 mg/dose every 4-6 hours until patient controlled; usual dose: 300-800 mg/day

Nausea and vomiting:

Oral: 10-25 mg every 4-6 hours

I.M., I.V.: 25-50 mg every 4-6 hours

Rectal: 50-100 mg every 6-8 hours

Intractable hiccups: Oral, I.M.: 25-50 mg 3-4 times/day

Dosage Forms

Chlorpromazine hydrochloride:

Capsule, sustained action: 30 mg, 75 mg, 150 mg, 200 mg, 300 mg

Concentrate, oral: 30 mg/mL (120 mL); 100 mg/mL (60 mL, 240 mL)

Injection: 25 mg/mL (1 mL, 2 mL, 10 mL)

Syrup: 10 mg/5 mL (120 mL)

Tablet: 10 mg, 25 mg, 50 mg, 100 mg, 200 mg

Suppository, rectal, as base: 25 mg, 100 mg

Chlorprom® (Can) *see* chlorpromazine *on this page*

chlorpropamide (klor PROE pa mide)

U.S./Canadian Brand Names Apo-Chlorpropamide® (Can); Diabinese®; Novo-Propamide® (Can)

Therapeutic Category Antidiabetic Agent, Oral

Use Control blood sugar in adult onset, noninsulin-dependent diabetes (type II)

Usual Dosage The dosage of chlorpropamide is variable and should be individualized based upon the patient's response

Adults: Oral: 250 mg once daily; initial dose in elderly patients: 100 mg once daily; subsequent dosages may be increased or decreased by 50-125 mg/day at 3- to 5-day intervals; maximum daily dose: 750 mg

Dosage Forms Tablet: 100 mg, 250 mg

Chlor-Rest® Tablet [OTC] *see* chlorpheniramine and phenylpropanolamine *on page 122*

Chlortab® ***(Discontinued)*** *see page 700*

chlorthalidone (klor THAL i done)

U.S./Canadian Brand Names Apo-Chlorthalidone® (Can); Hygroton®; Novo-Thalidone® (Can); Thalitone®; Uridon® (Can)

Therapeutic Category Diuretic, Miscellaneous

Use Management of mild to moderate hypertension, used alone or in combination with other agents; treatment of edema associated with congestive heart failure, nephrotic syndrome, or pregnancy

Usual Dosage Oral:

Children: 2 mg/kg 3 times/week

Adults: 25-100 mg/day or 100 mg 3 times/week

Dosage Forms

Tablet: 25 mg, 50 mg, 100 mg

Hygroton®: 25 mg, 50 mg, 100 mg

Thalitone®: 15 mg, 25 mg

chlorthalidone and atenolol *see* atenolol and chlorthalidone *on page 51*

chlorthalidone and clonidine *see* clonidine and chlorthalidone *on page 139*

Chlor-Trimeton® 4 Hour Relief Tablet [OTC] *see* chlorpheniramine and pseudoephedrine *on page 122*

Chlor-Trimeton® Injection *see* chlorpheniramine *on page 120*

Chlor-Trimeton® Oral [OTC] *see* chlorpheniramine *on page 120*

Chlor-Tripolon® (Can) *see* chlorpheniramine *on page 120*

chlorzoxazone (klor ZOKS a zone)

U.S./Canadian Brand Names Flexaphen®; Paraflex®; Parafon Forte™ DSC

Therapeutic Category Skeletal Muscle Relaxant

Use Symptomatic treatment of muscle spasm and pain associated with acute musculoskeletal conditions

Usual Dosage Oral:

Children: 20 mg/kg/day or 600 mg/m^2/day in 3-4 divided doses

Adults: 250-500 mg 3-4 times/day up to 750 mg 3-4 times/day

Dosage Forms

Caplet (Parafon Forte™ DSC): 500 mg

Capsule (Flexaphen®, Mus-Lax®): 250 mg with acetaminophen 300 mg

Tablet: Paraflex®: 250 mg

Cholac® *see* lactulose *on page 325*

Cholan-HMB® *see* dehydrocholic acid *on page 162*

Cholebrine® *see* radiological/contrast media (ionic) *on page 495*

cholecalciferol (kole e kal SI fer ole)

Synonyms D_3

U.S./Canadian Brand Names Delta-D®

Therapeutic Category Vitamin D Analog

Use Dietary supplement, treatment of vitamin D deficiency or prophylaxis of deficiency

Usual Dosage Adults: Oral: 400-1000 units/day

Dosage Forms Tablet: 400 units, 1000 units

Choledyl® ***(Discontinued)*** *see page 700*

cholera vaccine (KOL er a vak SEEN)

Therapeutic Category Vaccine, Inactivated Bacteria

Use Primary immunization for cholera prophylaxis

Usual Dosage I.M., S.C.:

Children:

6 months to 4 years: 0.2 mL with same dosage schedule

5-10 years: 0.3 mL with same dosage schedule

Children >10 years and Adults: 0.5 mL in 2 doses 1 week to 1 month or more apart

Dosage Forms Injection: Suspension of killed *Vibrio cholerae* (Inaba and Ogawa types) 8 units of each serotype per mL (1.5 mL, 20 mL)

cholestyramine resin (koe LES tir a meen REZ in)

U.S./Canadian Brand Names LoCHOLEST®; LoCHOLEST® Light; PMS-Cholestyramine (Can); Prevalite®; Questran®; Questran® Light

Therapeutic Category Bile Acid Sequestrant

Use Adjunct in the management of primary hypercholesterolemia; pruritus associated with elevated levels of bile acids; diarrhea associated with excess fecal bile acids; pseudomembraneous colitis

Usual Dosage Dosages are expressed in terms of anhydrous resin. Oral:

Children: 240 mg/kg/day in 3 divided doses; need to titrate dose depending on indication

Adults: 3-4 g 3-4 times/day to a maximum of 16-32 g/day in 2-4 divided doses

Dosage Forms

Powder: 4 g of resin/9 g of powder (9 g, 378 g)

For oral suspension:

With aspartame: 4 g of resin/5 g of powder (5 g, 210 g)

With phenylalanine: 4 g of resin/5.5 g of powder (60s)

choline magnesium trisalicylate

(KOE leen mag NEE zhum trye sa LIS i late)

U.S./Canadian Brand Names Trilisate®

Therapeutic Category Analgesic, Non-narcotic; Nonsteroidal Anti-inflammatory Drug (NSAID)

Use Management of osteoarthritis, rheumatoid arthritis, and other arthritides

Usual Dosage Oral (based on total salicylate content):

Children: 30-60 mg/kg/day administered in 3-4 divided doses

Adults: 500 mg to 1.5 g 1-3 times/day

Dosage Forms

Liquid: 500 mg/5 mL [choline salicylate 293 mg and magnesium salicylate 362 mg per 5 mL] (237 mL)

Tablet:

500 mg: Choline salicylate 293 mg and magnesium salicylate 362 mg

750 mg: Choline salicylate 440 mg and magnesium salicylate 544 mg

1000 mg: Choline salicylate 587 mg and magnesium salicylate 725 mg

choline salicylate (KOE leen sa LIS i late)

U.S./Canadian Brand Names Arthropan® [OTC]; Teejel® (Can)

Therapeutic Category Analgesic, Non-narcotic; Nonsteroidal Anti-inflammatory Drug (NSAID)

Use Temporary relief of pain of rheumatoid arthritis, rheumatic fever, osteoarthritis, and other conditions for which oral salicylates are recommended; useful in patients in which there is difficulty in administering doses in a tablet or capsule dosage form, because of the liquid dosage form

Usual Dosage Adults: Oral: 5 mL every 3-4 hours, if necessary, but not more than 6 doses in 24 hours

Dosage Forms Liquid (mint flavor): 870 mg/5 mL (240 mL, 480 mL)

choline theophyllinate *see* oxtriphylline *on page 421*

Cholografin® Meglumine *see* radiological/contrast media (ionic) *on page 495*

Choloxin® *see* dextrothyroxine *on page 172*

chondroitin sulfate-sodium hyaluronate
(kon DROY tin SUL fate-SOW de um hye a loo ROE nate)

Synonyms sodium hyaluronate-chrondroitin sulfate

U.S./Canadian Brand Names Viscoat®

Therapeutic Category Ophthalmic Agent, Viscoelastic

Use Surgical aid in anterior segment procedures, protects corneal endothelium and coats intraocular lens thus protecting it

Usual Dosage Ophthalmic: Carefully introduce into anterior chamber after thoroughly cleaning the chamber with a balanced salt solution

Dosage Forms Solution: Sodium chondroitin 40 mg and sodium hyaluronate 30 mg (0.25 mL, 0.5 mL)

Chooz® [OTC] *see* calcium carbonate *on page 89*

Chorex® *see* chorionic gonadotropin *on this page*

chorionic gonadotropin (kor ee ON ik goe NAD oh troe pin)

Synonyms CG; HCG

U.S./Canadian Brand Names A.P.L.®; Chorex®; Choron®; Corgonject®; Follutein®; Glukor®; Gonic®; Pregnyl®; Profasi® HP

Therapeutic Category Gonadotropin

Use Treatment of hypogonadotropic hypogonadism, prepubertal cryptorchidism; induce ovulation

Usual Dosage Children: I.M.:

Prepubertal cryptorchidism: 1000-2000 units/m^2/dose 3 times/week for 3 weeks

Hypogonadotropic hypogonadism: 500-1000 USP units 3 times/week for 3 weeks, followed by the same dose twice weekly for 3 weeks

Dosage Forms Powder for injection: 200 units/mL (10 mL, 25 mL); 500 units/mL (10 mL); 1000 units/mL (10 mL); 2000 units/mL (10 mL)

Choron® *see* chorionic gonadotropin *on this page*

Chromagen® OB [OTC] *see* vitamin, multiple (prenatal) *on page 606*

Chroma-Pak® *see* trace metals *on page 573*

chromium injection *see* trace metals *on page 573*

Chronulac® *see* lactulose *on page 325*

Chymex® *(Discontinued)* *see page 700*

Chymodiactin® *see* chymopapain *on this page*

chymopapain (KYE moe pa pane)

U.S./Canadian Brand Names Chymodiactin®

Therapeutic Category Enzyme

Use Alternative to surgery in patients with herniated lumbar intervertebral disks

Usual Dosage 2000-4000 units/disk with a maximum cumulative dose not to exceed 8000 units for patients with multiple disk herniations

Dosage Forms Injection: 4000 units [4 nKat]; 10,000 units [10 nKat]

Cibacalcin® *see* calcitonin *on page 88*

ciclopirox (sye kloe PEER oks)

U.S./Canadian Brand Names Loprox®

Therapeutic Category Antifungal Agent

Use Treatment of tinea pedis, tinea cruris, tinea corporis, cutaneous candidiasis, tinea versicolor

Usual Dosage Children >10 years and Adults: Topical: Apply twice daily, gently massage into affected areas; safety and efficacy in children <10 years have not been established

Dosage Forms Ciclopirox olamine:

Cream, topical: 1% (15 g, 30 g, 90 g)

Gel: 1%
Lotion: 1% (30 mL)

cidofovir (si DOF o veer)

U.S./Canadian Brand Names Vistide®
Therapeutic Category Antiviral Agent
Use Treatment of CMV retinitis in patients with acquired immunodeficiency syndrome (AIDS)
Usual Dosage
Induction treatment: 5 mg/kg once weekly for 2 consecutive weeks
Maintenance treatment: 5 mg/kg administered once every 2 weeks
Probenecid must be administered orally with each dose of cidofovir
Probenecid dose: 2 g 3 hours prior to cidofovir dose, 1 g 2 hours and 8 hours after completion of the infusion; patients should also receive 1 L of normal saline intravenously prior to each infusion of cidofovir; saline should be infused over 1-2 hours
Dosage Forms Injection: 75 mg/mL (5 mL)

Cidomycin® (Can) *see* gentamicin *on page 260*

cilastatin and imipenem *see* imipenem and cilastatin *on page 302*

cilazapril *(Canada only)* (sye LAY za pril)

U.S./Canadian Brand Names Inhibace® (Can)
Therapeutic Category Angiotensin-Converting Enzyme (ACE) Inhibitor
Use Management of hypertension and treatment of congestive heart failure
Usual Dosage Adults: Oral:
Congestive heart failure: Recommended starting dose is 0.5 mg once daily, usual maintenance dose: 1-2.5 mg/day
Hypertension: 2.5-5 mg once daily
Dosage Forms Tablet: 1 mg, 2.5 mg, 5 mg

cilostazol (sil OH sta zol)

U.S./Canadian Brand Names Pletal®
Therapeutic Category Platelet Aggregation Inhibitor
Use Symptomatic management of peripheral vascular disease, primarily intermittent claudication
Usual Dosage Adults: Oral: 100 mg twice daily taken at least 30 minutes before or 2 hours after breakfast and dinner; dosage should be reduced to 50 mg twice daily during concurrent therapy with inhibitors of CYP3A4 or CYP2C19
Dosage Forms Tablet: 50 mg, 100 mg

Ciloxan™ Ophthalmic *see* ciprofloxacin *on next page*

cimetidine (sye MET i deen)

U.S./Canadian Brand Names Apo®-Cimetidine (Can); Novo-Cimetidine® (Can); Nu-Cimet® (Can); Peptol® (Can); Tagamet®; Tagamet-HB® [OTC]
Therapeutic Category Histamine H_2 Antagonist
Use Short-term treatment of active duodenal ulcers and benign gastric ulcers; long-term prophylaxis of duodenal ulcer; gastric hypersecretory states; gastroesophageal reflux
Usual Dosage Oral, I.M., I.V.:
Infants: 10-20 mg/kg/day divided every 6-12 hours
Children: 20-30 mg/kg/day in divided doses every 6 hours

Patients with an active bleed: Administer cimetidine as a continuous infusion

Adults:
Short-term treatment of active ulcers:
Oral: 300 mg 4 times/day or 800 mg at bedtime or 400 mg twice daily for up to 8 weeks
I.M., I.V.: 300 mg every 6 hours or 37.5 mg/hour by continuous infusion; I.V. dosage should be adjusted to maintain an intragastric pH of 5 or greater

(Continued)

cimetidine *(Continued)*

Duodenal ulcer prophylaxis: Oral: 400-800 mg at bedtime

Gastric hypersecretory conditions: Oral, I.M., I.V.: 300-600 mg every 6 hours; dosage not to exceed 2.4 g/day

Dosage Forms

Infusion, as hydrochloride, in NS: 300 mg (50 mL)

Injection, as hydrochloride: 150 mg/mL (2 mL, 8 mL)

Liquid, oral, as hydrochloride (mint-peach flavor): 300 mg/5 mL with alcohol 2.8% (5 mL, 240 mL)

Tablet: 200 mg, 300 mg, 400 mg, 800 mg

Cinobac® Pulvules® *see* cinoxacin *on this page*

cinoxacin (sin OKS a sin)

U.S./Canadian Brand Names Cinobac® Pulvules®

Therapeutic Category Quinolone

Use Urinary tract infections

Usual Dosage Children >12 years and Adults: Oral: 1 g/day in 2-4 doses

Dosage Forms Capsule: 250 mg, 500 mg

Cipralan® *(Discontinued)* *see page 700*

Cipro® *see* ciprofloxacin *on this page*

ciprofloxacin (sip roe FLOKS a sin)

U.S./Canadian Brand Names Ciloxan™ Ophthalmic; Cipro®

Therapeutic Category Antibiotic, Ophthalmic; Quinolone

Use Treatment of documented or suspected pseudomonal infection of the respiratory or urinary tract, acute sinusitis, skin and soft tissue, bone and joint, eye and ear; documented multidrug-resistant, aerobic gram-negative bacilli and some gram-positive staphylococci; documented infectious diarrhea due to *Campylobacter jejuni*, *Shigella*, or *Salmonella*; osteomyelitis caused by susceptible organisms in which parenteral therapy is not feasible; empiric therapy for patients with febrile neutropenia; ocular infections caused by susceptible bacterial organisms in patients with corneal ulcers or conjunctivitis

Usual Dosage

Children: Oral: 20-30 mg/kg/day in 2 divided doses; maximum dose: 1.5 g/day

Adults:

Oral: 250-750 mg every 12 hours, depending on severity of infection and susceptibility

Ophthalmic: Instill 1-2 drops in eye(s) every 2 hours while awake for 2 days and 1-2 drops every 4 hours while awake for the next 5 days

I.V.: 200-400 mg every 12 hours depending on severity of infection

Dosage Forms Ciprofloxacin hydrochloride:

Infusion in D_5W: 400 mg (200 mL)

Infusion in NS or D_5W: 200 mg (100 mL)

Injection: 200 mg (20 mL); 400 mg (40 mL)

Solution, ophthalmic: 3.5 mg/mL (2.5 mL, 5 mL)

Suspension, oral: 250 mg/5 mL (100 mL); 500 mg/5 mL (100 mL)

Tablet: 100 mg, 250 mg, 500 mg, 750 mg

ciprofloxacin and hydrocortisone

(sip roe FLOKS a sin & hye droe KOR ti sone)

U.S./Canadian Brand Names Cipro® HC Otic

Therapeutic Category Antibiotic/Corticosteroid, Otic

Use Treatment of acute otitis externa, sometimes known as "swimmer's ear"

Usual Dosage Children >1 year of age and Adults: Otic: The recommended dosage for all patients is three drops of the suspension in the affected ear twice daily for seven day; twice-daily dosing schedule is more convenient for patients than that of existing treatments with hydrocortisone, which are typically administered three or four times a day; a twice-daily dosage schedule may be especially helpful for parents and caregivers of young children

Dosage Forms Suspension, otic: Ciprofloxacin hydrochloride 0.2% and hydrocortisone 1%

Cipro® HC Otic *see* ciprofloxacin and hydrocortisone *on previous page*

cisapride (SIS a pride)

U.S./Canadian Brand Names Prepulsid® (Can); Propulsid®

Therapeutic Category Gastrointestinal Agent, Prokinetic

Use Treatment of nocturnal symptoms of gastroesophageal reflux disease (GERD), also demonstrated effectiveness for gastroparesis, refractory constipation, and nonulcer dyspepsia

Usual Dosage Adults: Oral: 10 mg 4 times/day at least 15 minutes before meals and at bedtime; in some patients the dosage will need to be increased to 20 mg to obtain a satisfactory result

Dosage Forms

Suspension, oral (cherry cream flavor): 1 mg/mL (450 mL)

Tablet, scored: 10 mg, 20 mg

cisatracurium (sis a tra KYOO ree um)

U.S./Canadian Brand Names Nimbex®

Therapeutic Category Skeletal Muscle Relaxant

Use As an adjunct to general anesthesia to facilitate endotracheal intubation and to relax skeletal muscles during surgery; to facilitate mechanical ventilation in ICU patients; does not relieve pain or produce sedation

Usual Dosage I.V.: Dose to effect; doses will vary due to interpatient variability; use ideal body weight for obese patients

Surgery:

Children 2-12 years: 0.1 mg/kg, produces clinically effective block for 28 minutes

Adults: 0.15-0.2 mg/kg, then 0.03 mg/kg 40-60 minutes after initial dose to maintain neuromuscular block, followed by repeat doses of 0.03 mg/kg at 20-minute intervals; initial dose after succinylcholine for intubation: 0.1 mg/kg

Continuous infusion: At initial signs of recovery from bolus dose, begin at 3 mcg/kg/minute, block usually maintained by a rate of 1-2 mcg/kg/minute

Pretreatment/priming: 10% of intubating dose given 3-5 minutes before initial dose

ICU: Adults: 0.1 mg/kg bolus; at initial signs of recovery begin at rate of 3 mcg/kg/minute and adjust accordingly (rates of 0.5-10 mcg/kg/minute reported)

Dosage Forms Injection, as besylate: 2 mg/mL (5 mL, 10 mL); 10 mg/mL (20 mL)

cisplatin (SIS pla tin)

Synonyms CDDP

U.S./Canadian Brand Names Platinol®; Platinol®-AQ

Therapeutic Category Antineoplastic Agent

Use Management of metastatic testicular or ovarian carcinoma, advanced bladder cancer, osteosarcoma, Hodgkin's and non-Hodgkin's lymphoma, head or neck cancer, cervical cancer, lung cancer, brain tumors, neuroblastoma; used alone or in combination with other agents

Usual Dosage Children and Adults (refer to individual protocols): I.V.:

Intermittent dosing schedule: 37-75 mg/m^2 once every 2-3 weeks or 50-120 mg/m^2 once every 3-4 weeks

Daily dosing schedule: 15-20 mg/m^2/day for 5 days every 3-4 weeks

Dosage Forms

Injection, aqueous: 1 mg/mL (50 mL, 100 mL)

Powder for injection: 10 mg, 50 mg

13-*cis*-retinoic acid *see* isotretinoin *on page 316*

citalopram (sye TAL oh pram)

Synonyms Citalopram Hydrobromide; Nitalapram

U.S./Canadian Brand Names Celexa®

Therapeutic Category Antidepressant

Use Depression

Usual Dosage Oral: 20-60 mg/day; reduce dosage in elderly or those with hepatic impairment

Dosage Forms Tablet, as hydrobromide: 20 mg, 40 mg, 60 mg

Citalopram Hydrobromide *see* citalopram *on this page*

Citanest® Forte *see* prilocaine *on page 473*

Citanest® Plain *see* prilocaine *on page 473*

Cithalith-S® Syrup *(Discontinued)* *see page 700*

Citracal® [OTC] *see* calcium citrate *on page 91*

citrate of magnesia *see* magnesium citrate *on page 344*

citric acid and d-gluconic acid irrigant *see* citric acid bladder mixture *on this page*

citric acid and potassium citrate *see* potassium citrate and citric acid *on page 465*

citric acid bladder mixture (SI trik AS id BLAD dur MIKS chur)

Synonyms citric acid and d-gluconic acid irrigant; hemiacidrin

U.S./Canadian Brand Names Renacidin®

Therapeutic Category Irrigating Solution

Use Preparing solutions for irrigating indwelling urethral catheters; to dissolve or prevent formation of calcifications

Usual Dosage 30-60 mL of 10% (sterile) solution 2-3 times/day by means of a rubber syringe

Dosage Forms

Powder for solution: Citric acid 156-171 g, magnesium hydroxycarbonate 75-87 g, d-gluconic acid 21-30 g, magnesium acid citrate 9-15 g, calcium carbonate 2-6 g (150 g, 300 g)

Solution, irrigation: Citric acid 6.602 g, magnesium hydroxycarbonate 3.177 g, glucono-delta-lactone 0.198 g and benzoic acid 0.023 g per 100 mL (500 mL)

Citrisource® (Can) *see* enteral nutritional products *on page 208*

Citro-Nesia® Solution *(Discontinued)* *see page 700*

Citrotein® [OTC] *see* enteral nutritional products *on page 208*

citrovorum factor *see* leucovorin *on page 328*

Citrucel® [OTC] *see* methylcellulose *on page 367*

CI-719 *see* gemfibrozil *on page 259*

CLA *see* clarithromycin *on next page*

cladribine (KLA dri been)

Synonyms 2-CdA; 2-chlorodeoxyadenosine

U.S./Canadian Brand Names Leustatin™

Therapeutic Category Antineoplastic Agent

Use Hairy cell and chronic lymphocytic leukemias

Usual Dosage Adults: I.V. continuous infusion: 0.09 mg/kg/day

Dosage Forms Injection, preservative free: 1 mg/mL (10 mL)

Claforan® *see* cefotaxime *on page 106*

Clamurid® (Can) *see* carbamide peroxide *on page 98*

Claripex® (Can) *see* clofibrate *on page 138*

clarithromycin (kla RITH roe mye sin)

Synonyms CLA

U.S./Canadian Brand Names Biaxin™

Therapeutic Category Macrolide (Antibiotic)

Use Treatment of upper and lower respiratory tract infections, acute otitis media, and infections of the skin and skin structure due to susceptible strains of *S. aureus*, *S. pyogenes*, *S. pneumoniae*, *H. influenzae*, *M. catarrhalis*, *Mycoplasma pneumoniae*, *C. trachomatis*, *Legionella* sp, and *M. avium*; prophylaxis of disseminated *M. avium* Complex (MAC) infections in HIV-infected patients

Usual Dosage Oral: 250-500 mg every 12 hours for 7-14 days

Upper respiratory tract: 250-500 mg every 12 hours for 10-14 days

Pharyngitis/tonsillitis: 250 mg every 12 hours for 10 days

Acute maxillary sinusitis: 500 mg every 12 hours for 14 days

Lower respiratory tract: 250-500 mg every 12 hours for 7-14 days

Acute exacerbation of chronic bronchitis due to:

S. pneumoniae: 250 mg every 12 hours for 7-14 days

M. catarrhalis: 250 mg every 12 hours for 7-14 days

H. influenzae: 500 mg every 12 hours for 7-14 days

Pneumonia due to:

S. pneumoniae: 250 mg every 12 hours for 7-14 days

M. pneumoniae: 250 mg every 12 hours for 7-14 days

Uncomplicated skin and skin structure: 250 mg every 12 hours for 7-14 days

Dosage Forms

Granules for oral suspension: 125 mg/5 mL (50 mL, 100 mL); 250 mg/5 mL (50 mL, 100 mL)

Tablet, film coated: 250 mg, 500 mg

Claritin® *see* loratadine *on page 339*

Claritin-D® *see* loratadine and pseudoephedrine *on page 339*

Claritin-D® 24-Hour *see* loratadine and pseudoephedrine *on page 339*

Claritin® RediTab® *see* loratadine *on page 339*

clavulanate potassium and amoxicillin *see* amoxicillin and clavulanate potassium *on page 32*

clavulanic acid and ticarcillin *see* ticarcillin and clavulanate potassium *on page 566*

Clavulin® (Can) *see* amoxicillin and clavulanate potassium *on page 32*

Clear Away® Disc [OTC] *see* salicylic acid *on page 513*

Clear By Design® Gel [OTC] *see* benzoyl peroxide *on page 68*

Clear Eyes® [OTC] *see* naphazoline *on page 390*

Clearsil® Maximum Strength [OTC] *see* benzoyl peroxide *on page 68*

Clear Tussin® 30 *see* guaifenesin and dextromethorphan *on page 268*

clemastine (KLEM as teen)

U.S./Canadian Brand Names Antihist-1® [OTC]; Tavist®; Tavist®-1 [OTC]

Therapeutic Category Antihistamine

Use Perennial and seasonal allergic rhinitis and other allergic symptoms including urticaria

Usual Dosage Oral:

Children:

<12 years: 0.67-1.34 mg every 8-12 hours as needed

>12 years: 1.34 mg twice daily to 2.68 mg 3 times/day; do not exceed 8.04 mg/day

Adults: 1.34 mg twice daily to 2.68 mg 3 times/day; do not exceed 8.04 mg/day

Dosage Forms Clemastine fumarate:

Syrup (citrus flavor): 0.67 mg/5 mL with alcohol 5.5% (120 mL)

Tablet: 1.34 mg, 2.68 mg

clemastine and phenylpropanolamine

KLEM as teen & fen il proe pa NOLE a meen)

U.S./Canadian Brand Names Antihist-D®; Tavist-D®

Therapeutic Category Antihistamine/Decongestant Combination

Use Symptomatic relief of allergic rhinitis; pruritus of the eyes, nose or throat, lacrimation and nasal congestion

Usual Dosage Children >12 years and Adults: Oral: 1 tablet every 12 hours

Dosage Forms Tablet: Clemastine fumarate 1.34 mg and phenylpropanolamine hydrochloride 75 mg

Cleocin HCl® Oral *see* clindamycin *on this page*

Cleocin Pediatric® Oral *see* clindamycin *on this page*

Cleocin Phosphate® Injection *see* clindamycin *on this page*

Cleocin T® Topical *see* clindamycin *on this page*

Cleocin® Vaginal *see* clindamycin *on this page*

clidinium and chlordiazepoxide (kli DI nee um & klor dye az e POKS ide)

Synonyms chlordiazepoxide and clidinium

U.S./Canadian Brand Names Clindex®; Librax®

Therapeutic Category Anticholinergic Agent

Use Adjunct treatment of peptic ulcer, treatment of irritable bowel syndrome

Usual Dosage Oral: 1-2 capsules 3-4 times/day, before meals or food and at bedtime

Dosage Forms Capsule: Clidinium bromide 2.5 mg and chlordiazepoxide hydrochloride 5 mg

Climara® Transdermal *see* estradiol *on page 217*

Clinda-Derm® Topical *see* clindamycin *on this page*

clindamycin (klin da MYE sin)

U.S./Canadian Brand Names Cleocin HCl® Oral; Cleocin Pediatric® Oral; Cleocin Phosphate® Injection; Cleocin T® Topical; Cleocin® Vaginal; Clinda-Derm® Topical; Dalacin® C Topical (Can); Dalacin® C Vaginal Cream (Can)

Therapeutic Category Acne Products; Antibiotic, Miscellaneous

Use Useful agent against most aerobic gram-positive staphylococci and streptococci (except enterococci); also useful against *Fusobacterium*, *Bacteroides* sp. and *Actinomyces* for treatment of respiratory tract infections, skin and soft tissue infections, sepsis, intra-abdominal infections, and infections of the female pelvis and genital tract; used topically in treatment of severe acne

Usual Dosage Avoid in neonates (contains benzyl alcohol)

Infants and Children:

- Oral: 10-30 mg/kg/day in 3-4 divided doses
- I.M., I.V.: 25-40 mg/kg/day in 3-4 divided doses

Children and Adults: Topical: Apply twice daily

Adults:

- Oral: 150-450 mg/dose every 6-8 hours; maximum dose: 1.8 g/day
- I.M., I.V.: 1.2-1.8 g/day in 2-4 divided doses; maximum dose: 4.8 g/day
- Vaginal: 1 full applicator (100 mg) inserted intravaginally once daily before bedtime for 7 consecutive days

Dosage Forms

Clindamycin hydrochloride:

- Capsule: 75 mg, 150 mg, 300 mg

Clindamycin palmitate:

- Granules for oral solution: 75 mg/5 mL (100 mL)

Clindamycin phosphate:

- Cream, vaginal: 2% (40 g)
- Gel, topical: 1% [10 mg/g] (7.5 g, 30 g)
- Infusion in D_5W: 300 mg (50 mL); 600 mg (50 mL)

Injection: 150 mg/mL (2 mL, 4 mL, 6 mL, 50 mL, 60 mL)
Solution, topical: 1% [10 mg/mL] (30 mL, 60 mL, 480 mL)
Lotion, topical: 1% [10 mg/mL] (60 mL)

Clindex® *see* clidinium and chlordiazepoxide *on previous page*

Clinoril® *see* sulindac *on page 544*

clioquinol (klye oh KWIN ole)

U.S./Canadian Brand Names Clioquinol® (Can); Vioform® [OTC]

Therapeutic Category Antifungal Agent

Use Treatment of tinea pedis, tinea cruris, and skin infections caused by dermatophytic fungi (ring worm)

Usual Dosage Children and Adults: Topical: Apply 2-4 times/day; do not use for >7 days

Dosage Forms
Cream: 3% (30 g)
Ointment, topical: 3% (30 g)

clioquinol and hydrocortisone (klye oh KWIN ole & hye droe KOR ti sone)

Synonyms hydrocortisone and clioquinol; iodochlorhydroxyquin and hydrocortisone

U.S./Canadian Brand Names Corque® Topical; Pedi-Cort V® Creme

Therapeutic Category Antifungal/Corticosteroid

Use Contact or atopic dermatitis; eczema; neurodermatitis; anogenital pruritus; mycotic dermatoses; moniliasis

Usual Dosage Topical: Apply in a thin film 3-4 times/day

Dosage Forms Cream: Clioquinol 3% and hydrocortisone 1% (20 g)

Clioquinol® (Can) *see* clioquinol *on this page*

Clistin® Tablet *(Discontinued)* *see page 700*

clobetasol (kloe BAY ta sol)

U.S./Canadian Brand Names Cormax® Ointment; Dermasone (Can); Dermovate® (Can); Gen-Clobetasol (Can); Novo-Clobetasol (Can); Temovate®

Therapeutic Category Corticosteroid, Topical

Use Short-term relief of inflammation of moderate to severe corticosteroid-responsive dermatosis

Usual Dosage Topical: Apply twice daily for up to 2 weeks with no more than 50 g/week

Dosage Forms Clobetasol propionate:
Cream: 0.05% (15 g, 30 g, 45 g)
Cream in emollient base: 0.05% (15 g, 30 g, 60 g)
Gel: 0.05% (15 g, 30 g, 45 g)
Ointment, topical: 0.05% (15 g, 30 g, 45 g)
Scalp application: 0.05% (25 mL, 50 mL)
Solution, topical: 0.05%

Clocort® Maximum Strength [OTC] *see* hydrocortisone (topical) *on page 292*

clocortolone (kloe KOR toe lone)

U.S./Canadian Brand Names Cloderm® Topical

Therapeutic Category Corticosteroid, Topical

Use Inflammation of corticosteroid-responsive dermatoses

Usual Dosage Topical: Apply sparingly and gently rub into affected area 1-4 times/day

Dosage Forms Cream, as pivalate: 0.1% (15 g, 45 g)

Cloderm® Topical *see* clocortolone *on this page*

clofazimine (kloe FA zi meen)

U.S./Canadian Brand Names Lamprene®

Therapeutic Category Leprostatic Agent

(Continued)

clofazimine *(Continued)*

Use Treatment of dapsone-resistant lepromatous leprosy (*Mycobacterium leprae*); multibacillary dapsone-sensitive leprosy; erythema nodosum leprosum; *Mycobacterium avium-intracellulare* (MAI) infections

Usual Dosage Oral:

Children: Leprosy: 1 mg/kg/day every 24 hours in combination with dapsone and rifampin

Adults:

Dapsone-resistant leprosy: 50-100 mg/day in combination with one or more antileprosy drugs for 2 years; then alone 50-100 mg/day

Dapsone-sensitive multibacillary leprosy: 50-100 mg/day in combination with two or more antileprosy drugs for at least 2 years and continue until negative skin smears are obtained, then institute single drug therapy with appropriate agent

Erythema nodosum leprosum: 100-200 mg/day for up to 3 months or longer then taper dose to 100 mg/day when possible

MAI: Combination therapy using clofazimine 100 mg 1 or 3 times/day in combination with other antimycobacterial agents

Dosage Forms Capsule, as palmitate: 50 mg

clofibrate (kloe FYE brate)

U.S./Canadian Brand Names Abitrate® (Can); Atromid-S®; Claripex® (Can); Novo-Fibrate® (Can)

Therapeutic Category Antihyperlipidemic Agent, Miscellaneous

Use Adjunct to dietary therapy in the management of hyperlipidemias associated with high triglyceride levels

Usual Dosage Adults: Oral: 500 mg 4 times/day

Dosage Forms Capsule: 500 mg

Clomid® *see* clomiphene *on this page*

clomiphene (KLOE mi feen)

U.S./Canadian Brand Names Clomid®; Milophene®; Serophene®

Therapeutic Category Ovulation Stimulator

Use Treatment of ovulatory failure in patients desiring pregnancy

Usual Dosage Oral: 50 mg/day for 5 days (first course); start the regimen on or about the fifth day of cycle; if ovulation occurs do not increase dosage; if not, increase next course to 100 mg/day for 5 days

Dosage Forms Tablet, as citrate: 50 mg

clomipramine (kloe MI pra meen)

U.S./Canadian Brand Names Anafranil®; Apo-Clomipramine® (Can)

Therapeutic Category Antidepressant, Tricyclic (Tertiary Amine)

Use Treatment of obsessive-compulsive disorder (OCD)

Usual Dosage Oral:

Children: Initial: 25 mg/day and gradually increase, as tolerated to a maximum of 3 mg/kg or 100 mg, whichever is smaller

Adults: Initial: 25 mg/day and gradually increase, as tolerated to 100 mg/day the first 2 weeks, may then be increased to a total of 250 mg/day

Dosage Forms Capsule, as hydrochloride: 25 mg, 50 mg, 75 mg

Clomycin® [OTC] *see* bacitracin, neomycin, polymyxin B, and lidocaine *on page 59*

clonazepam (kloe NA ze pam)

U.S./Canadian Brand Names Klonopin™; PMS-Clonazepam (Can); Rivotril® (Can)

Therapeutic Category Benzodiazepine

Controlled Substance C-IV

Use Prophylaxis of absence (petit mal), petit mal variant (Lennox-Gastaut), akinetic, and myoclonic seizures

Usual Dosage Oral:

Children <10 years or 30 kg:

Initial daily dose: 0.01-0.03 mg/kg/day (maximum: 0.05 mg/kg/day) administered in 2-3 divided doses; increase by no more than 0.5 mg every third day until seizures are controlled or adverse effects are seen

Maintenance dose: 0.1-0.2 mg/kg/day divided 3 times/day; not to exceed 0.2 mg/kg/day

Adults:

Initial daily dose not to exceed 1.5 mg administered in 3 divided doses; may increase by 0.5-1 mg every third day until seizures are controlled or adverse effects seen

Maintenance dose: 0.05-0.2 mg/kg; do not exceed 20 mg/day

Dosage Forms Tablet: 0.5 mg, 1 mg, 2 mg

clonidine (KLOE ni deen)

U.S./Canadian Brand Names Apo®-Clonidine (Can); Catapres® Oral; Catapres-TTS® Transdermal; Dixarit® (Can); Duraclon™ Injection; Novo-Clonidine® (Can); Nu-Clonidine® (Can)

Therapeutic Category Alpha-Adrenergic Agonist

Use Management of hypertension; aid in the diagnosis of pheochromocytoma and growth hormone deficiency; has orphan drug status for epidural use for pain control; used for heroin withdrawal and smoking cessation therapy in adults

Investigational use: Alternate agent for the treatment of attention-deficit/hyperactivity disorder (ADHD)

Usual Dosage

Epidural infusion (continuous): 30 mcg/hour, titrated up or down depending on pain relief

Oral:

Children: Initial: 5-10 mcg/kg/day in divided doses every 8-12 hours; increase gradually at 5- to 7-day intervals to 25 mcg/kg/day in divided doses every 6 hours; maximum: 0.9 mg/day

Clonidine tolerance test (test of growth hormone release from pituitary): 0.15 mg/m^2 or 4 mcg/kg as single dose

Adults: Initial dose: 0.1 mg twice daily, usual maintenance dose: 0.2-1.2 mg/day in 2-4 divided doses; maximum recommended dose: 2.4 mg/day

Nicotine withdrawal symptoms: 0.1 mg twice daily to maximum of 0.4 mg/day for 3-4 weeks

Elderly: Initial: 0.1 mg once daily at bedtime, increase gradually as needed

Transdermal: Apply once every 7 days; for initial therapy start with 0.1 mg and increase by 0.1 mg at 1- to 2-week intervals; dosages >0.6 mg do not improve efficacy

Dosage Forms Clonidine hydrochloride:

Injection, preservative free: 100 mcg/mL (10 mL)

Patch, transdermal: 1, 2, and 3 (0.1, 0.2, 0.3 mg/day, 7-day duration)

Tablet: 0.1 mg, 0.2 mg, 0.3 mg

clonidine and chlorthalidone (KLOE ni deen & klor THAL i done)

Synonyms chlorthalidone and clonidine

U.S./Canadian Brand Names Combipres®

Therapeutic Category Antihypertensive Agent, Combination

Use Management of mild to moderate hypertension

Usual Dosage Oral: 1 tablet 1-2 times/day

Dosage Forms Tablet:

0.1: Clonidine 0.1 mg and chlorthalidone 15 mg

0.2: Clonidine 0.2 mg and chlorthalidone 15 mg

0.3: Clonidine 0.3 mg and chlorthalidone 15 mg

clopidogrel (kloh PID oh grel)

U.S./Canadian Brand Names Plavix®

Therapeutic Category Antiplatelet Agent

(Continued)

clopidogrel *(Continued)*

Use The reduction of atherosclerotic events (myocardial infarction, stroke, vascular deaths) in patients with atherosclerosis documented by recent myocardial infarctions, recent stroke or established peripheral arterial disease

Usual Dosage Adults: Oral: 75 mg once daily

Dosage Forms Tablet, as bisulfate: 75 mg

Clopixol-Acuphase® (Can) *see* zuclopenthixol *(Canada only) on page 613*

Clopixol® (Can) *see* zuclopenthixol *(Canada only) on page 613*

Clopixol® Depot (Can) *see* zuclopenthixol *(Canada only) on page 613*

Clopra® *see* metoclopramide *on page 370*

clorazepate (klor AZ e pate)

U.S./Canadian Brand Names Apo®-Clorazepate (Can); Gen-XENE®; Novo-Clopate® (Can); Tranxene®

Therapeutic Category Anticonvulsant; Benzodiazepine

Controlled Substance C-IV

Use Treatment of generalized anxiety and panic disorders; management of alcohol withdrawal; adjunct anticonvulsant in management of partial seizures

Usual Dosage Oral:

Anticonvulsant:

Children:

<9 years: Dose not established

9-12 years: Initial: 3.75-7.5 mg/dose twice daily; increase dose by 3.75 mg at weekly intervals, not to exceed 60 mg/day in 2-3 divided doses

Children >12 years and Adults: Initial: Up to 7.5 mg/dose 2-3 times/day; increase dose by 7.5 mg at weekly intervals; usual dose: 0.5-1 mg/kg/day; not to exceed 90 mg/day (up to 3 mg/kg/day has been used)

Anxiety: Adults: 7.5-15 mg 2-4 times/day, or administered as single dose of 15-22.5 mg at bedtime

Alcohol withdrawal: Adults: Initial: 30 mg, then 15 mg 2-4 times/day on first day; maximum daily dose: 90 mg; gradually decrease dose over subsequent days

Dosage Forms Clorazepate dipotassium:

Capsule: 3.75 mg, 7.5 mg, 15 mg

Tablet: 3.75 mg, 7.5 mg, 15 mg

Tablet, single dose: 11.25 mg, 22.5 mg

Clorpactin® WCS-90 *see* oxychlorosene *on page 422*

Clorpactin® XCB Powder *(Discontinued)* *see page 700*

Clotrimaderm (Can) *see* clotrimazole *on this page*

clotrimazole (kloe TRIM a zole)

U.S./Canadian Brand Names Canesten® Topical (Can) Canesten® Vaginal (Can); Clotrimaderm (Can); Gyne-Lotrimin® Vaginal [OTC]; Lotrimin AF® Topical [OTC]; Lotrimin® Topical; Mycelex®-G Topical; Mycelex®-G Vaginal [OTC]; Mycelex® Troche; Myclo-Derm® (Can); Myclo-Gyne® (Can)

Therapeutic Category Antifungal Agent

Use Treatment of susceptible fungal infections, including oropharyngeal candidiasis, dermatophytoses, superficial mycoses, cutaneous candidiasis, as well as vulvovaginal candidiasis; limited data suggests that the use of clotrimazole troches may be effective for prophylaxis against oropharyngeal candidiasis in neutropenic patients

Usual Dosage

Children >3 years and Adults:

Oral: 10 mg troche dissolved slowly 5 times/day

Topical: Apply twice daily

Adults: Vaginal: 100 mg/day for 7 days or 200 mg/day for 3 days or 500 mg single dose or 5 g (1 applicatorful) of 1% vaginal cream daily for 7-14 days

Dosage Forms
Combination pack (Mycelex-7®): Vaginal tablet 100 mg (7's) and vaginal cream 1% (7 g)
Cream:
Topical (Lotrimin®, Lotrimin® AF, Mycelex®, Mycelex® OTC) : 1% (15 g, 30 g, 45 g, 90 g)
Vaginal (Femizole-7®, Gyne-Lotrimin®, Mycelex®-G): 1% (45 g, 90 g)
Lotion (Lotrimin®): 1% (30 mL)
Solution, topical (Fungoid®, Lotrimin®, Lotrimin® AF, Mycelex®, Mycelex® OTC): 1% (10 mL, 30 mL)
Tablet, vaginal (Gyne-Lotrimin®, Mycelex®-G): 100 mg (7s); 500 mg (1s)
Troche (Mycelex®): 10 mg
Twin pack (Mycelex®): Vaginal tablet 500 mg (1's) and vaginal cream 1% (7 g)

clotrimazole and betamethasone *see* betamethasone and clotrimazole *on page 71*

cloxacillin (kloks a SIL in)

U.S./Canadian Brand Names Apo®-Cloxi (Can); Cloxapen®; Novo-Cloxin® (Can); Nu-Cloxi® (Can); Orbenin® (Can); Taro-Cloxacillin® (Can)
Therapeutic Category Penicillin
Use Treatment of susceptible bacterial infections of the respiratory tract, skin and skin structure, bone and joint caused by penicillinase-producing staphylococci
Usual Dosage Oral:
Children >1 month: 50-100 mg/kg/day in divided doses every 6 hours; up to a maximum of 4 g/day
Adults: 250-500 mg every 6 hours
Dosage Forms Cloxacillin sodium:
Capsule: 250 mg, 500 mg
Powder for oral suspension: 125 mg/5 mL (100 mL, 200 mL)

Cloxapen® *see* cloxacillin *on this page*

clozapine (KLOE za peen)

U.S./Canadian Brand Names Clozaril®
Therapeutic Category Antipsychotic Agent, Dibenzodiazepine
Use Management of schizophrenic patients
Usual Dosage Adults: Oral: Initial: 25 mg once or twice daily, increase as tolerated to a target dose of 300-450 mg/day, may require doses as high as 600-900 mg/day
Dosage Forms Tablet: 25 mg, 100 mg

Clozaril® *see* clozapine *on this page*

Clysodrast® *see* bisacodyl *on page 74*

CMV-IGIV *see* cytomegalovirus immune globulin (intravenous-human) *on page 156*

coagulant complex inhibitor *see* anti-inhibitor coagulant complex *on page 40*

coagulation factor VIIa *see* factor VIIa, recombinant *on page 230*

coal tar (KOLE tar)

Synonyms crude coal tar; LCD; pix carbonis
U.S./Canadian Brand Names AquaTar® [OTC]; Balnetar® (Can); Denorex® [OTC]; DHS® Tar [OTC]; Duplex® T [OTC]; Estar® [OTC]; Fototar® [OTC]; Ionil-T® Plus (Can); Neutrogena® T/Derm; Pentrax® [OTC]; Polytar® [OTC]; psoriGel® [OTC]; T/Gel® [OTC]; Zetar® [OTC]
Therapeutic Category Antipsoriatic Agent; Antiseborrheic Agent, Topical
Use Topically for controlling dandruff, seborrheic dermatitis, or psoriasis
Usual Dosage
Bath: Add appropriate amount to bath water, for adults usually 60-90 mL of a 5% to 20% solution or 15-25 mL of 30% lotion; soak 5-20 minutes, then pat dry; use once daily for 3 days
(Continued)

coal tar *(Continued)*

Shampoo: Rub shampoo onto wet hair and scalp, rinse thoroughly; repeat; leave on 5 minutes; rinse thoroughly; apply twice weekly for the first 2 weeks then once weekly or more often if needed

Skin: Apply to the affected area 1-4 times/day; decrease frequency to 2-3 times/week once condition has been controlled

Scalp psoriasis: Tar oil bath or coal tar solution may be painted sparingly to the lesions 3-12 hours before each shampoo

Psoriasis of the body, arms, legs: Apply at bedtime; if thick scales are present, use product with salicylic acid and apply several times during the day

Dosage Forms

Cream: 1% to 5%

Gel: Coal tar 5%

Lotion: 2.5% to 30%

Lotion: 2%; 5%; 25%

Shampoo:

Coal tar: 0.5% to 5%

Coal tar extract 2% with salicylic acid 2% (60 mL)

Solution:

Coal tar: 2.5%, 5%, 20%

Coal tar extract: 5%

Suspension, coal tar: 30% to 33.3%

coal tar and salicylic acid (KOLE tar & sal i SIL ik AS id)

U.S./Canadian Brand Names X-seb® T [OTC]

Therapeutic Category Antipsoriatic Agent; Antiseborrheic Agent, Topical

Use Treatment of seborrheal dermatitis, dandruff

Usual Dosage Topical: Shampoo twice weekly

Dosage Forms Shampoo: Coal tar solution 10% and salicylic acid 4% (120 mL)

coal tar, lanolin, and mineral oil (KOLE tar, LAN oh lin, & MIN er al oyl)

U.S./Canadian Brand Names Balnetar® [OTC]

Therapeutic Category Antipsoriatic Agent; Antiseborrheic Agent, Topical

Use Treatment of psoriasis, seborrheal dermatitis, atopic dermatitis, eczematoid dermatitis

Usual Dosage Add to bath water, soak for 5-20 minutes then pat dry

Dosage Forms Oil, bath: Water-dispersible emollient tar 2.5%, lanolin fraction, and mineral oil (240 mL)

Cobalasine® Injection *(Discontinued)* *see page 700*

Cobex® *see* cyanocobalamin *on page 152*

cocaine (koe KANE)

Therapeutic Category Local Anesthetic

Controlled Substance C-II

Use Topical anesthesia for mucous membranes

Usual Dosage Topical: Use lowest effective dose; do not exceed 1 mg/kg; patient tolerance, anesthetic technique, vascularity of tissue and area to be anesthetized will determine dose needed

Dosage Forms Cocaine hydrochloride:

Powder: 5 g, 25 g

Solution, topical: 4% [40 mg/mL] (2 mL, 4 mL, 10 mL); 10% [100 mg/mL] (4 mL, 10 mL)

Solution, topical, viscous: 4% [40 mg/mL] (4 mL, 10 mL); 10% [100 mg/mL] (4 mL, 10 mL)

Tablet, soluble, for topical solution: 135 mg

coccidioidin skin test (koks i dee OH i din skin test)

U.S./Canadian Brand Names Spherulin®

Therapeutic Category Diagnostic Agent

Use Intradermal skin test in diagnosis of coccidioidomycosis; differential diagnosis of this disease from histoplasmosis, sarcoidosis and other mycotic and bacterial infections. The skin test may be negative in severe forms of disease (anergy) or when prolonged periods of time have passed since infection.

Usual Dosage Children and Adults: Intradermally: 0.1 mL of 1:100 or flexor surface of forearm

Positive reaction: Induration of 5 mm or more; erythema without induration is considered negative; read the test at 24 and 48 hours, since some reactions may not be noticeable after 36 hours. A positive reaction indicates present or past infection with *Coccidioides immitis.*

Negative reaction: A negative test means the individual has not been sensitized to coccidioidin or has lost sensitivity

Dosage Forms Injection: 1:10 (0.5 mL); 1:100 (1 mL)

Codafed® Expectorant *see* guaifenesin, pseudoephedrine, and codeine *on page 272*

Codamine® *see* hydrocodone and phenylpropanolamine *on page 289*

Codamine® Pediatric *see* hydrocodone and phenylpropanolamine *on page 289*

Codehist® DH *see* chlorpheniramine, pseudoephedrine, and codeine *on page 126*

codeine (KOE deen)

Synonyms methylmorphine

U.S./Canadian Brand Names Codeine Conhn® (Can); Linctus Codeine Blac (Can); Linctus With Codeine Phosphate (Can); Paveral Stanley Syrup With Codeine Phosphate (Can)

Therapeutic Category Analgesic, Narcotic; Antitussive

Controlled Substance C-II

Use Treatment of mild to moderate pain; antitussive in lower doses

Usual Dosage Doses should be titrated to appropriate analgesic effect; when changing routes of administration, note that oral dose is $^2/_3$ as effective as parenteral dose

Analgesic: Oral, I.M., S.C.:
- Children: 0.5-1 mg/kg/dose every 4-6 hours as needed; maximum: 60 mg/dose
- Adults: 30 mg/dose; range: 15-60 mg every 4-6 hours as needed

Antitussive: Oral (for nonproductive cough):
- Children: 1-1.5 mg/kg/day in divided doses every 4-6 hours as needed: Alternatively dose according to age:
  - 2-6 years: 2.5-5 mg every 4-6 hours as needed; maximum: 30 mg/day
  - 6-12 years: 5-10 mg every 4-6 hours as needed; maximum: 60 mg/day
- Adults: 10-20 mg/dose every 4-6 hours as needed; maximum: 120 mg/day

Dosage Forms

Codeine phosphate:
- Injection: 30 mg (1 mL, 2 mL); 60 mg (1 mL, 2 mL)
- Tablet, soluble: 30 mg, 60 mg

Codeine sulfate:
- Tablet: 15 mg, 30 mg, 60 mg
- Tablet, soluble: 15 mg, 30 mg, 60 mg

codeine and acetaminophen *see* acetaminophen and codeine *on page 4*

codeine and aspirin *see* aspirin and codeine *on page 50*

codeine and bromodiphenhydramine *see* bromodiphenhydramine and codeine *on page 80*

codeine and butalbital compound *see* butalbital compound and codeine *on page 86*

codeine and guaifenesin *see* guaifenesin and codeine *on page 268*

codeine and promethazine *see* promethazine and codeine *on page 479*

codeine, brompheniramine, and phenylpropanolamine *see* brompheniramine, phenylpropanolamine, and codeine *on page 82*

Codeine Conhn® (Can) *see* codeine *on previous page*

codeine, guaifenesin, and pseudoephedrine *see* guaifenesin, pseudoephedrine, and codeine *on page 272*

codeine, promethazine, and phenylephrine *see* promethazine, phenylephrine, and codeine *on page 479*

Codiclear® DH *see* hydrocodone and guaifenesin *on page 288*

Codimal-A® Injection *(Discontinued)* *see page 700*

Codimal® Expectorant *(Discontinued)* *see page 700*

cod liver oil *see* vitamin A and vitamin D *on page 603*

Codoxy® *see* oxycodone and aspirin *on page 423*

Cogentin® *see* benztropine *on page 69*

Co-Gesic® *see* hydrocodone and acetaminophen *on page 287*

Cognex® *see* tacrine *on page 546*

Co-Hist® [OTC] *see* acetaminophen, chlorpheniramine, and pseudoephedrine *on page 6*

Colace® [OTC] *see* docusate *on page 191*

colaspase *see* asparaginase *on page 49*

Co-Lav® *see* polyethylene glycol-electrolyte solution *on page 459*

Colax-C® (Can) *see* docusate *on page 191*

colchicine (KOL chi seen)

Therapeutic Category Antigout Agent

Use Treat acute gouty arthritis attacks and to prevent recurrences of such attacks; management of familial Mediterranean fever

Usual Dosage

Acute gouty arthritis:

Oral: Initial: 0.5-1.2 mg, then 0.5-0.6 mg every 1-2 hours or 1-1.2 mg every 2 hours until relief or GI side effects occur to a maximum total dose of 8 mg, wait 3 days before initiating a second course

I.V.: Initial: 1-3 mg, then 0.5 mg every 6 hours until response, not to exceed 4 mg/day; following a full course of colchicine (4 mg), wait 7 days before initiating another course of colchicine (by any route)

Prophylaxis of recurrent attacks: Oral:

<1 attack/year: 0.5 or 0.6 mg/day/dose for 3-4 days/week

>1 attack/year: 0.5 or 0.6 mg/day/dose

Severe cases: 1-1.8 mg/day

Dosage Forms

Injection: 0.5 mg/mL (2 mL)

Tablet: 0.5 mg, 0.6 mg

colchicine and probenecid (KOL chi seen & proe BEN e sid)

Synonyms probenecid and colchicine

Therapeutic Category Antigout Agent

Use Treatment of chronic gouty arthritis when complicated by frequent, recurrent acute attacks of gout

Usual Dosage Adults: Oral: 1 tablet daily for 1 week, then 1 tablet twice daily thereafter

Dosage Forms Tablet: Colchicine 0.5 mg and probenecid 0.5 g

Cold & Allergy® Elixir [OTC] *see* brompheniramine and phenylpropanolamine *on page 81*

Coldlac-LA® *see* guaifenesin and phenylpropanolamine *on page 270*

Coldloc® *see* guaifenesin, phenylpropanolamine, and phenylephrine *on page 272*

Coldrine® [OTC] *see* acetaminophen and pseudoephedrine *on page 5*

Colestid® *see* colestipol *on this page*

colestipol (koe LES ti pole)

U.S./Canadian Brand Names Colestid®

Therapeutic Category Antihyperlipidemic Agent, Miscellaneous

Use Adjunct in the management of primary hypercholesterolemia; to relieve pruritus associated with elevated levels of bile acids, possibly used to decrease plasma half-life of digoxin as an adjunct in the treatment of toxicity

Usual Dosage Oral: 15-30 g/day in divided doses 2-4 times/day

Dosage Forms Colestipol hydrochloride:

Granules: 5 g packet, 300 g, 500 g

Tablet: 1 g

colfosceril palmitate (kole FOS er il PALM i tate)

Synonyms dipalmitoylphosphatidylcholine; DPPC; synthetic lung surfactant

U.S./Canadian Brand Names Exosurf® Neonatal™

Therapeutic Category Lung Surfactant

Use Neonatal respiratory distress syndrome (RDS):

Prophylactic therapy: Infants at risk for developing RDS with body weight <1350 g; infants with evidence of pulmonary immaturity with body weight >1350 g

Rescue therapy: Treatment of infants with RDS based on respiratory distress not attributable to any other causes and chest radiographic findings consistent with RDS

Usual Dosage

Prophylactic treatment: Administer 5 mL/kg as soon as possible; the second and third doses should be administered at 12 and 24 hours later to those infants remaining on ventilators

Rescue treatment: Administer 5 mL/kg as soon as the diagnosis of RDS is made; the second 5 mL/kg dose should be administered 12 hours later

Dosage Forms Powder for injection, lyophilized: 108 mg (10 mL)

colistimethate (koe lis ti METH ate)

U.S./Canadian Brand Names Coly-Mycin® M Parenteral

Therapeutic Category Antibiotic, Miscellaneous

Use Treatment of infections due to sensitive strains of certain gram-negative bacilli

Usual Dosage Children and Adults: I.M., I.V.: 2.5-5 mg/kg/day in 2-4 divided doses

Dosage Forms Powder for injection, as sodium, lyophilized: 150 mg

colistin, neomycin, and hydrocortisone

(koe LIS tin, nee oh MYE sin & hye droe KOR ti sone)

Synonyms hydrocortisone, colistin, and neomycin; neomycin, colistin, and hydrocortisone

U.S./Canadian Brand Names Coly-Mycin® S Otic Drops; Cortisporin-TC® Otic

Therapeutic Category Antibiotic/Corticosteroid, Otic

Use Treatment of superficial and susceptible bacterial infections of the external auditory canal; for treatment of susceptible bacterial infections of mastoidectomy and fenestration cavities

Usual Dosage Otic:

Children: 3 drops in affected ear 3-4 times/day

Adults: 4 drops in affected ear 3-4 times/day

Dosage Forms Suspension, otic:

Coly-Mycin® S Otic Drops: Colistin sulfate 0.3%, neomycin sulfate 0.47%, and hydrocortisone acetate 1% (5 mL, 10 mL)

Cortisprorin-TC®: Colistin sulfate 0.3%, neomycin sulfate 0.33%, and hydrocortisone acetate 1% (5 mL, 10 mL)

collagenase (KOL la je nase)

U.S./Canadian Brand Names Biozyme-C®; Santyl®

Therapeutic Category Enzyme

Use Promote debridement of necrotic tissue in dermal ulcers and severe burns

Usual Dosage Topical: Apply daily or every other day

Dosage Forms Ointment, topical: 250 units/g (15 g, 30 g)

collagen implants (KOL a jen im PLANTS)

Therapeutic Category Ophthalmic Agent, Miscellaneous

Use Relief of dry eyes; enhance the effect of ocular medications

Usual Dosage Implants inserted by physician

Dosage Forms Implant: 0.2 mm, 0.3 mm, 0.4 mm, 0.5 mm, 0.6 mm

Collyrium Fresh® Ophthalmic [OTC] *see* tetrahydrozoline *on page 556*

Colovage® *see* polyethylene glycol-electrolyte solution *on page 459*

Coly-Mycin® M Parenteral *see* colistimethate *on previous page*

Coly-Mycin® S Oral *(Discontinued)* *see page 700*

Coly-Mycin® S Otic Drops *see* colistin, neomycin, and hydrocortisone *on previous page*

CoLyte® *see* polyethylene glycol-electrolyte solution *on page 459*

CoLyte®-Flavored *see* polyethylene glycol-electrolyte solution *on page 459*

Comalose-R (Can) *see* lactulose *on page 325*

Combantrin® (Can) *see* protirelin *on page 485*

Combipres® *see* clonidine and chlorthalidone *on page 139*

Combivent® *see* ipratropium and albuterol *on page 312*

Combivir® *see* zidovudine and lamivudine *on page 611*

Comfort® Ophthalmic [OTC] *see* naphazoline *on page 390*

Comfort® Tears Solution [OTC] *see* artificial tears *on page 47*

Comhist® *see* chlorpheniramine, phenylephrine, and phenyltoloxamine *on page 124*

Comhist® LA *see* chlorpheniramine, phenylephrine, and phenyltoloxamine *on page 124*

Compazine® *see* prochlorperazine *on page 476*

compound E *see* cortisone acetate *on page 148*

compound F *see* hydrocortisone (systemic) *on page 291*

compound S *see* zidovudine *on page 610*

Compoz® Gel Caps [OTC] *see* diphenhydramine *on page 185*

Compoz® Nighttime Sleep Aid [OTC] *see* diphenhydramine *on page 185*

Comtrex® Maximum Strength Non-Drowsy [OTC] *see* acetaminophen, dextromethorphan, and pseudoephedrine *on page 6*

Comvax® *see Haemophilus* B conjugate and hepatitis B vaccine *on page 275*

Condylox® *see* podofilox *on page 458*

Conex® [OTC] *see* guaifenesin and phenylpropanolamine *on page 270*

Congess® Jr *see* guaifenesin and pseudoephedrine *on page 270*

Congess® Sr *see* guaifenesin and pseudoephedrine *on page 270*

Congestac® *see* guaifenesin and pseudoephedrine *on page 270*

Congestant D® [OTC] *see* chlorpheniramine, phenylpropanolamine, and acetaminophen *on page 125*

Congest (Can) *see* estrogens, conjugated (equine) *on page 219*

conjugated estrogen and methyltestosterone *see* estrogens and methyltestosterone *on page 219*

conjugated estrogens *see* estrogens, conjugated (equine) *on page 219*

Conray® *see* radiological/contrast media (ionic) *on page 495*

Constant-T® Tablet *(Discontinued)* *see page 700*

Constilac® *see* lactulose *on page 325*

Constulose® *see* lactulose *on page 325*

Contac® Cough Formula Liquid [OTC] *see* guaifenesin and dextromethorphan *on page 268*

Contergan® *see* thalidomide *on page 557*

Control® [OTC] *see* phenylpropanolamine *on page 447*

Control-L® *(Discontinued)* *see page 700*

Contuss® *see* guaifenesin, phenylpropanolamine, and phenylephrine *on page 272*

Contuss® XT *see* guaifenesin and phenylpropanolamine *on page 270*

Copaxone® *see* glatiramer acetate *on page 261*

Cophene-B® *see* brompheniramine *on page 80*

Cophene XP® *see* hydrocodone, pseudoephedrine, and guaifenesin *on page 290*

copolymer-1 *see* glatiramer acetate *on page 261*

copper injection *see* trace metals *on page 573*

Coptin® (Can) *see* sulfadiazine *on page 541*

Co-Pyronil® 2 Pulvules® [OTC] *see* chlorpheniramine and pseudoephedrine *on page 122*

Coradur® (Can) *see* isosorbide dinitrate *on page 315*

Corax® (Can) *see* chlordiazepoxide *on page 116*

Cordarone® *see* amiodarone *on page 28*

Cordran® *see* flurandrenolide *on page 248*

Cordran® SP *see* flurandrenolide *on page 248*

Coreg® *see* carvedilol *on page 102*

Corgard® *see* nadolol *on page 387*

Corgonject® *see* chorionic gonadotropin *on page 130*

Coricidin® [OTC] *see* chlorpheniramine and acetaminophen *on page 121*

Coricidin D® [OTC] *see* chlorpheniramine, phenylpropanolamine, and acetaminophen *on page 125*

Corlopam® *see* fenoldopam *on page 233*

Cormax® Ointment *see* clobetasol *on page 137*

Corque® Topical *see* clioquinol and hydrocortisone *on page 137*

CortaGel® Topical [OTC] *see* hydrocortisone (topical) *on page 292*

Cortaid® Maximum Strength Topical [OTC] *see* hydrocortisone (topical) *on page 292*

Cortaid® Ointment *(Discontinued)* *see page 700*

Cortaid® with Aloe Topical [OTC] *see* hydrocortisone (topical) *on page 292*

Cortamed® (Can) *see* hydrocortisone (topical) *on page 292*

Cortate® (Can) *see* hydrocortisone (topical) *on page 292*

Cortatrigen® Otic *see* neomycin, polymyxin B, and hydrocortisone *on page 396*

Cort-Dome® Topical *see* hydrocortisone (topical) *on page 292*

Cortef® Feminine Itch Topical *see* hydrocortisone (topical) *on page 292*

Cortef® Oral *see* hydrocortisone (systemic) *on page 291*

Cortenema® Rectal *see* hydrocortisone (rectal) *on page 291*

Corticaine® Topical *see* dibucaine and hydrocortisone *on page 175*

corticotropin (kor ti koe TROE pin)

Synonyms ACTH; adrenocorticotropic hormone

U.S./Canadian Brand Names Acthar®; H.P. Acthar® Gel

Therapeutic Category Adrenal Corticosteroid

Use Infantile spasms; diagnostic aid in adrenocortical insufficiency; acute exacerbations of multiple sclerosis; severe muscle weakness in myasthenia gravis

Usual Dosage

Acute exacerbation of multiple sclerosis: I.M.: 80-120 units/day for 2-3 weeks

Diagnostic purposes:

- I.M., S.C.: 20 units 4 times/day
- I.V.: 10-25 units in 500 mL 5% dextrose in water over 8 hours

Dosage Forms

Injection, repository (H.P. Acthar® Gel): 40 units/mL (1 mL, 5 mL); 80 units/mL (1 mL, 5 mL)

Powder for injection (Acthar®): 25 units, 40 units

Corticreme® (Can) *see* hydrocortisone (topical) *on page 292*

Cortifoam® Rectal *see* hydrocortisone (rectal) *on page 291*

Cortiment® (Can) *see* hydrocortisone (topical) *on page 292*

cortisone acetate (KOR ti sone AS e tate)

Synonyms compound E

U.S./Canadian Brand Names Cortone® Acetate

Therapeutic Category Adrenal Corticosteroid

Use Management of adrenocortical insufficiency

Usual Dosage Depends upon the condition being treated and the response of the patient

Children:

- Anti-inflammatory or immunosuppressive:
  - Oral: 2.5-10 mg/kg/day or 20-300 mg/m^2/day in divided doses every 6-8 hours
  - I.M.: 1-5 mg/kg/day or 14-375 mg/m^2/day in divided doses every 12-24 hours
- Physiologic replacement:
  - Oral: 0.5-0.75 mg/kg/day in divided doses every 8 hours
  - I.M.: 0.25-0.35 mg/kg/day once daily

Stress coverage for surgery: I.M.: 1 and 2 days before preanesthesia, and 1-3 days after surgery: 50-62.5 mg/m^2/day; 4 days after surgery: 31-50 mg/m^2/day

Adults: Oral, I.M.: 20-300 mg/day

Dosage Forms Cortisone acetate:

Injection: 50 mg/mL (10 mL)

Tablet: 5 mg, 10 mg, 25 mg

Cortisporin® Ophthalmic Ointment *see* bacitracin, neomycin, polymyxin B, and hydrocortisone *on page 59*

Cortisporin® Ophthalmic Suspension *see* neomycin, polymyxin B, and hydrocortisone *on page 396*

Cortisporin® Otic *see* neomycin, polymyxin B, and hydrocortisone *on page 396*

Cortisporin-TC® Otic *see* colistin, neomycin, and hydrocortisone *on page 145*

Cortisporin®-TC Otic Suspension *see* neomycin, colistin, hydrocortisone, and thonzonium *on page 396*

Cortisporin® Topical Cream *see* neomycin, polymyxin B, and hydrocortisone *on page 396*

Cortisporin® Topical Ointment *see* bacitracin, neomycin, polymyxin B, and hydrocortisone *on page 59*

Cortizone®-5 Topical [OTC] *see* hydrocortisone (topical) *on page 292*

Cortizone®-10 Topical [OTC] *see* hydrocortisone (topical) *on page 292*

Cortoderm (Can) *see* hydrocortisone (topical) *on page 292*

Cortone® Acetate *see* cortisone acetate *on previous page*

Cortrophin-Zinc® *(Discontinued)* *see page 700*

Cortrosyn® *see* cosyntropin *on this page*

Corvert® *see* ibutilide *on page 300*

Coryphen® Codeine (Can) *see* aspirin and codeine *on page 50*

Cosmegen® *see* dactinomycin *on page 157*

Cosopt™ *see* dorzolamide and timolol *on page 194*

cosyntropin (koe sin TROE pin)

Synonyms synacthen; tetracosactide

U.S./Canadian Brand Names Cortrosyn®; Synacthen® Depot (Can)

Therapeutic Category Diagnostic Agent

Use Diagnostic test to differentiate primary adrenal from secondary (pituitary) adrenocortical insufficiency

Usual Dosage

Adrenocortical insufficiency: I.M., I.V.:

Children <2 years: 0.125 mg injected over 2 minutes

Children >2 years and Adults: 0.25 mg injected over 2 minutes

When greater cortisol stimulation is needed, an I.V. infusion may be used: I.V. infusion: 0.25 mg administered over 4-8 hours

Congenital adrenal hyperplasia evaluation: 1 mg/m²/dose up to a maximum of 1 mg

Dosage Forms Powder for injection: 0.25 mg

Cotazym® *see* pancrelipase *on page 427*

Cotazym-S® *see* pancrelipase *on page 427*

Cotrim® *see* co-trimoxazole *on this page*

Cotrim® DS *see* co-trimoxazole *on this page*

co-trimoxazole (koe trye MOKS a zole)

Synonyms SMX-TMP; sulfamethoxazole and trimethoprim; TMP-SMX; trimethoprim and sulfamethoxazole

U.S./Canadian Brand Names Apo®-Sulfatrim (Can); Bactrim™; Bactrim™ DS; Cotrim®; Cotrim® DS; Novo-Trimel® (Can); Nu-Cotrimox® (Can); Pro-Trin® (Can); Roubac® (Can); Septra®; Septra® DS; Sulfamethoprim®; Sulfatrim®; Sulfatrim® DS; Trisulfa® (Can); Trisulfa-S® (Can); Uroplus® DS; Uroplus® SS

Therapeutic Category Sulfonamide

Use Treatment of urinary tract infections caused by susceptible *E. coli*, *Klebsiella*, *Enterobacter*, *Proteus mirabilis*, *Proteus* (indole positive); acute otitis media due to amoxicillin-resistant *H. influenzae*, *S. pneumoniae*, and *M. catarrhalis*; acute exacerbations of chronic bronchitis; prophylaxis and treatment of *Pneumocystis carinii* pneumonitis (PCP); treatment of susceptible shigellosis, typhoid fever, *Nocardia asteroides* infection, and *Xanthomonas maltophilia* infection; the I.V. preparation is used for treatment of *Pneumocystis carinii* pneumonitis, *Shigella*, and severe urinary tract infections

Usual Dosage Oral, I.V. (dosage recommendations are based on the trimethoprim component):

Children >2 months:

Mild to moderate infections: 6-12 mg TMP/kg/day in divided doses every 12 hours

Serious infection/*Pneumocystis*: 15-20 mg TMP/kg/day in divided doses every 6 hours

Urinary tract infection prophylaxis: 2 mg TMP/kg/dose daily

(Continued)

co-trimoxazole *(Continued)*

Prophylaxis of *Pneumocystis*: 5-10 mg TMP/kg/day or 150 mg TMP/m^2/day in divided doses every 12 hours 3 days/week; dose should not exceed 320 mg trimethoprim and 1600 mg sulfamethoxazole 3 days/week; Mon, Tue, Wed

Adults: Urinary tract infection/chronic bronchitis: 1 double strength tablet every 12 hours for 10-14 days

Dosage Forms The 5:1 ratio (SMX to TMP) remains constant in all dosage forms:

Injection: Sulfamethoxazole 80 mg and trimethoprim 16 mg per mL (5 mL, 10 mL, 20 mL, 30 mL, 50 mL)

Suspension, oral: Sulfamethoxazole 200 mg and trimethoprim 40 mg per 5 mL (20 mL, 100 mL, 150 mL, 200 mL, 480 mL)

Tablet: Sulfamethoxazole 400 mg and trimethoprim 80 mg

Double strength: Sulfamethoxazole 800 mg and trimethoprim 160 mg

Coumadin® *see* warfarin *on page 607*

Covera-HS® *see* verapamil *on page 598*

Coversyl® (Can) *see* perindopril erbumine *on page 440*

Cozaar® *see* losartan *on page 340*

CP-99,219-27 *see* trovafloxacin *on page 587*

CPM *see* cyclophosphamide *on page 153*

Creon® *see* pancreatin *on page 426*

Creon® 10 *see* pancrelipase *on page 427*

Creon® 20 *see* pancrelipase *on page 427*

Creo-Terpin® [OTC] *see* dextromethorphan *on page 171*

Cresylate® *see* m-cresyl acetate *on page 350*

Crinone™ *see* progesterone *on page 477*

Criticare HN® [OTC] *see* enteral nutritional products *on page 208*

Crixivan® *see* indinavir *on page 304*

Crolom® *see* cromolyn sodium *on this page*

cromoglicic acid *see* cromolyn sodium *on this page*

cromolyn sodium (KROE moe lin SOW dee um)

Synonyms cromoglicic acid; disodium cromoglycate; DSCG

U.S./Canadian Brand Names Crolom®; Gastrocrom®; Intal®; Nasalcrom® [OTC]; Novo-Cromolyn® (Can); Opticrom®; PMS-Sodium Cromoglycate (Can); Rynacrom® (Can)

Therapeutic Category Mast Cell Stabilizer

Use Adjunct in the prophylaxis of allergic disorders, including rhinitis, conjunctivitis, and asthma; inhalation product may be used for prevention of exercise-induced bronchospasm

Ophthalmologic: Vernal conjunctivitis, vernal keratoconjunctivitis, and vernal keratitis

Systemic: Mastocytosis, food allergy, and treatment of inflammatory bowel disease

Usual Dosage

Children:

Inhalation: >2 years: 20 mg 4 times/day

Nebulization solution: >5 years: 2 inhalations 4 times/day by metered spray, or 20 mg 4 times/day (Spinhaler®); taper frequency to the lowest effective level

For prevention of exercise-induced bronchospasm: Single dose of 2 inhalations (aerosol) just prior to exercise

Nasal: >6 years: 1 spray in each nostril 3-4 times/day

Adults: Nasal: 1 spray in each nostril 3-4 times/day

Systemic mastocytosis: Oral:

Infants ≤2 years: 20 mg/kg/day in 4 divided doses, not to exceed 30 mg/kg/day

Children 2-12 years: 100 mg 4 times/day; not to exceed 40 mg/kg/day

Adults: 200 mg 4 times/day

Food allergy and inflammatory bowel disease: Oral:

Children: 100 mg 4 times/day 15-20 minutes before meals, not to exceed 40 mg/kg/day

Adults: 200 mg 4 times/day 15-20 minutes before meal, up to 400 mg 4 times/day

Dosage Forms

Capsule: Oral (Gastrocrom®): 100 mg

Solution:

For nebulization: 10 mg/mL (2 mL)

Intal®: 10 mg/mL (2 mL)

Nasal (Nasalcrom®): 40 mg/mL (13 mL)

Ophthalmic (Crolom®): 4% (2.5 mL, 10 mL)

crotaline antivenin, polyvalent *see* antivenin (*Crotalidae*) polyvalent *on page 41*

crotamiton (kroe TAM i tonn)

U.S./Canadian Brand Names Eurax® Topical

Therapeutic Category Scabicides/Pediculicides

Use Treatment of scabies (*Sarcoptes scabiei*) in infants and children

Usual Dosage Scabicide: Children and Adults: Topical: Wash thoroughly and scrub away loose scales, then towel dry; apply a thin layer and massage drug onto skin of the entire body from the neck to the toes (with special attention to skin folds, creases, and interdigital spaces). Repeat application in 24 hours; patient should take a cleansing bath 48 hours after the final application.

Dosage Forms

Cream: 10% (60 g)

Lotion: 10% (60 mL, 454 mL)

crude coal tar *see* coal tar *on page 141*

crystalline penicillin *see* penicillin G, parenteral, aqueous *on page 434*

Crystamine® *see* cyanocobalamin *on next page*

Crysticillin® 300 A.S. *(Discontinued)* *see page 700*

Crysticillin® 600 A.S. *(Discontinued)* *see page 700*

Crysticillin® A.S. *see* penicillin G procaine *on page 435*

Crystodigin® *see* digitoxin *on page 179*

Crystodigin® 0.05 mg & 0.15 mg Tablet *(Discontinued)* *see page 700*

CSP *see* cellulose sodium phosphate *on page 110*

CTX *see* cyclophosphamide *on page 153*

Cuprimine® *see* penicillamine *on page 433*

Curretab® Oral *see* medroxyprogesterone acetate *on page 352*

Cutivate™ *see* fluticasone (topical) *on page 250*

CYA *see* cyclosporine *on page 154*

cyanide antidote kit (SYE a nide AN tee dote kit)

Therapeutic Category Antidote

Use Treatment of cyanide poisoning

Usual Dosage Cyanide poisoning: 0.3 mL ampul of amyl nitrite is crushed every minute and vapor is inhaled for 15-30 seconds until an I.V. sodium nitrite infusion is available. Following administration of 300 mg I.V. sodium nitrite, inject 12.5 g sodium thiosulfate I.V. (over ~10 minutes), if needed; injection of both may be repeated at ½ the original dose.

Dosage Forms Kit: Sodium nitrite 300 mg/10 mL (#2); sodium thiosulfate 12.5 g/50 mL (#2); amyl nitrite 0.3 mL (#12); also disposable syringes, stomach tube, tourniquet and instructions

cyanocobalamin (sye an oh koe BAL a min)

Synonyms vitamin B_{12}

U.S./Canadian Brand Names Berubigen®; Cobex®; Crystamine®; Cyanoject®; Cyomin®; Ener-B® [OTC]; Kaybovite-1000®; Redisol®; Rubramin® (Can); Rubramin-PC®; Sytobex®

Therapeutic Category Vitamin, Water Soluble

Use Pernicious anemia; vitamin B_{12} deficiency; increased B_{12} requirements due to pregnancy, thyrotoxicosis, hemorrhage, malignancy, liver or kidney disease

Usual Dosage

Congenital pernicious anemia (if evidence of neurologic involvement): I.M.: 1000 mcg/day for at least 2 weeks; maintenance: 50 mcg/month

Vitamin B_{12} deficiency: I.M., S.C. (oral is not recommended due to poor absorption):

Children: 100 mcg/day for 10-15 days (total dose of 1-1.5 mg), then once or twice weekly for several months; may taper to 250-1000 mcg every month

Adults: 100 mcg/day for 6-7 days

Hematologic signs only:

Children: 10-50 mcg/day for 5-10 days, then maintenance: 100-250 mcg/dose every 2-4 weeks

Adults: 30 mcg/day for 5-10 days, followed by 100-200 mcg/month

Methylmalonic aciduria: I.M.: 1 mg/day

Dosage Forms

Gel, nasal:

Ener-B®: 400 mcg/0.1 mL

Nascobal®: 500 mcg/0.1 mL (5 mL)

Injection: 30 mcg/mL (30 mL); 100 mcg/mL (1 mL, 10 mL, 30 mL); 1000 mcg/mL (1 mL, 10 mL, 30 mL)

Tablet [OTC]: 25 mcg, 50 mcg, 100 mcg, 250 mcg, 500 mcg, 1000 mcg

Cyanoject® *see* cyanocobalamin *on this page*

cyclandelate (sye KLAN de late)

Therapeutic Category Vasodilator, Peripheral

Use Considered as "possibly effective" for adjunctive therapy in peripheral vascular disease and possibly senility due to cerebrovascular disease or multi-infarct dementia; migraine prophylaxis, vertigo, tinnitus, and visual disturbances secondary to cerebrovascular insufficiency and diabetic peripheral polyneuropathy

Usual Dosage Adults: Oral: Initial: 1.2-1.6 g/day in divided doses before meals and at bedtime until response; maintenance therapy: 400-800 mg/day in 2-4 divided doses; start with lowest dose in elderly due to hypotensive potential; decrease dose by 200 mg decrements to achieve minimal maintenance dose; improvement can usually be seen over weeks of therapy and prolonged use; short courses of therapy are usually ineffective and not recommended

Dosage Forms Tablet: 200 mg

cyclizine (SYE kli zeen)

U.S./Canadian Brand Names Marezine® Oral [OTC]

Therapeutic Category Antihistamine

Use Prevention and treatment of nausea, vomiting and vertigo associated with motion sickness; control of postoperative nausea and vomiting

Usual Dosage Oral:

Children 6-12 years: 25 mg up to 3 times/day

Adults: 50 mg taken 30 minutes before departure, may repeat in 4-6 hours if needed, up to 200 mg/day

Dosage Forms

Injection, as lactate: 50 mg/mL (1 mL)

Tablet, as hydrochloride: 50 mg

cyclobenzaprine (sye kloe BEN za preen)

U.S./Canadian Brand Names Flexeril®; Novo-Cycloprine® (Can)

Therapeutic Category Skeletal Muscle Relaxant

Use Treatment of muscle spasm associated with acute painful musculoskeletal conditions; supportive therapy in tetanus

Usual Dosage Oral:

Children: Dosage has not been established

Adults: 20-40 mg/day in 2-4 divided doses; maximum dose: 60 mg/day

Dosage Forms Tablet, as hydrochloride: 10 mg

Cyclocort® Topical *see* amcinonide *on page 25*

Cyclogyl® *see* cyclopentolate *on this page*

Cyclomen® (Can) *see* danazol *on page 158*

Cyclomydril® Ophthalmic *see* cyclopentolate and phenylephrine *on this page*

cyclopentolate (sye kloe PEN toe late)

U.S./Canadian Brand Names AK-Pentolate®; Cyclogyl®; I-Pentolate®

Therapeutic Category Anticholinergic Agent

Use Diagnostic procedures requiring mydriasis and cycloplegia

Usual Dosage Ophthalmic:

Infants: Instill 1 drop of 0.5% into each eye 5-10 minutes before examination

Children: Instill 1 drop of 0.5%, 1%, or 2% in eye followed by 1 drop of 0.5% or 1% in 5 minutes, if necessary

Adults: Instill 1 drop of 1% followed by another drop in 5 minutes; 2% solution in heavily pigmented iris

Dosage Forms Solution, ophthalmic, as hydrochloride: 0.5% (2 mL, 5 mL, 15 mL); 1% (2 mL, 5 mL, 15 mL); 2% (2 mL, 5 mL, 15 mL)

cyclopentolate and phenylephrine (sye kloe PEN toe late & fen il EF rin)

Synonyms phenylephrine and cyclopentolate

U.S./Canadian Brand Names Cyclomydril® Ophthalmic

Therapeutic Category Anticholinergic/Adrenergic Agonist

Use Induce mydriasis greater than that produced with cyclopentolate HCl alone

Usual Dosage Ophthalmic: Instill 1 drop every 5-10 minutes, not to exceed 3 instillations

Dosage Forms Solution, ophthalmic: Cyclopentolate hydrochloride 0.2% and phenylephrine hydrochloride 1% (2 mL, 5 mL)

cyclophosphamide (sye kloe FOS fa mide)

Synonyms CPM; CTX; CYT

U.S./Canadian Brand Names Cytoxan®; Neosar®; Procytox® (Can)

Therapeutic Category Antineoplastic Agent

Use Management of Hodgkin's disease, malignant lymphomas, multiple myeloma, leukemias, sarcomas, mycosis fungoides, neuroblastoma, ovarian carcinoma, breast carcinoma, a variety of other tumors; nephrotic syndrome, lupus erythematosus, severe rheumatoid arthritis, and rheumatoid vasculitis

Usual Dosage

Children (with no hematologic problems):

Induction:

Oral: 2-8 mg/kg/day

I.V.: 10-20 mg/kg/day divided once daily

Maintenance: Oral: 2-5 mg/kg (50-150 mg/m^2) twice weekly

Pediatric solid tumors: I.V.: 250-1800 mg/m^2 once daily for 1-5 days every 21-28 days

Adults with no hematologic problems:

Induction:

Oral: 1-5 mg/kg/day

I.V.: 40-50 mg/kg (1.5-1.8 g/m^2) in divided doses over 2-5 days

(Continued)

cyclophosphamide *(Continued)*

Maintenance:
Oral: 1-5 mg/kg/day
I.V.: 10-15 mg/kg (350-550 mg/m^2) every 7-10 days or 3-5 mg/kg (110-185 mg/m^2) twice weekly
Children and Adults: I.V.:
SLE: 500-750 mg/m^2 every month; maximum: 1 g/m^2
JRA/vasculitis: 10 mg/kg every 2 weeks
BMT conditioning regimen: I.V.: 50 mg/kg/day once daily for 3-4 days
Nephrotic syndrome: Oral: 2-3 mg/kg/day every day for up to 12 weeks when corticosteroids are unsuccessful

Dosage Forms
Powder for injection: 100 mg, 200 mg, 500 mg, 1 g, 2 g
Powder for injection, lyophilized: 100 mg, 200 mg, 500 mg, 1 g, 2 g
Tablet: 25 mg, 50 mg

cycloserine (sye kloe SER een)

U.S./Canadian Brand Names Seromycin® Pulvules®
Therapeutic Category Antibiotic, Miscellaneous
Use Adjunctive treatment in pulmonary or extrapulmonary tuberculosis; treatment of acute urinary tract infections caused by *E. coli* or *Enterobacter* sp when less toxic conventional therapy has failed or is contraindicated
Usual Dosage Oral:
Tuberculosis:
Children: 10-20 mg/kg/day in 2 divided doses up to 1000 mg/day
Adults: Initial: 250 mg every 12 hours for 14 days, then administer 500 mg to 1 g/day in 2 divided doses
Urinary tract infection: Adults: 250 mg every 12 hours for 14 days
Dosage Forms Capsule: 250 mg

Cyclospasmol® ***(Discontinued)*** *see page 700*

cyclosporin A *see* cyclosporine *on this page*

cyclosporine (SYE kloe spor een)

Synonyms CYA; cyclosporin A
U.S./Canadian Brand Names Neoral®; Sandimmune®; SangCya™
Therapeutic Category Immunosuppressant Agent
Use Immunosuppressant used with corticosteroids to prevent graft vs host disease in patients with kidney, liver, heart, and bone marrow transplants; has been used in the treatment of nephrotic syndrome in patients with documented focal glomerulosclerosis when corticosteroids and cyclophosphamide were unsuccessful; monotherapy or in combination with methotrexate for treatment of severe active rheumatoid arthritis where the disease has not adequately responded to methotrexate
Usual Dosage Children and Adults:
Oral: Initial: 14-18 mg/kg/dose daily, beginning 4-12 hours prior to organ transplantation; maintenance: 5-10 mg/kg/day
I.V.: Initial: 5-6 mg/kg/day in divided doses every 12-24 hours; patients should be switched to oral cyclosporine as soon as possible

Dosage Forms
Capsule (Sandimmune®): 25 mg, 100 mg
Soft gel (Sandimmune®): 50 mg
Soft gel for microemulsion (Neoral®): 25 mg, 100 mg
Injection (Sandimmune®): 50 mg/mL (5 mL)
Solution:
Oral (Sandimmune®): 100 mg/mL (50 mL)
Oral for microemulsion (Neoral®): 100 mg/mL (50 mL)

Cycofed® Pediatric *see* guaifenesin, pseudoephedrine, and codeine *on page 272*

Cycrin® 10 mg Tablet *(Discontinued)* *see page 700*

Cycrin® Oral *see* medroxyprogesterone acetate *on page 352*

Cyklokapron® *see* tranexamic acid *on page 574*

Cylert® *see* pemoline *on page 432*

Cylex® [OTC] *see* benzocaine *on page 66*

Cyomin® *see* cyanocobalamin *on page 152*

cyproheptadine (si proe HEP ta deen)

U.S./Canadian Brand Names Periactin®; PMS-Cyproheptadine (Can)

Therapeutic Category Antihistamine

Use Perennial and seasonal allergic rhinitis and other allergic symptoms including urticaria

Usual Dosage Oral:

Children: 0.25 mg/kg/day in 2-3 divided doses **or**

2-6 years: 2 mg every 8-12 hours (not to exceed 12 mg/day)

7-14 years: 4 mg every 8-12 hours (not to exceed 16 mg/day)

Adults: 12-16 mg/day every 8 hours (not to exceed 0.5 mg/kg/day)

Dosage Forms Cyproheptadine hydrochloride:

Syrup: 2 mg/5 mL with alcohol 5% (473 mL)

Tablet: 4 mg

cyproterone *(Canada only)* (sye PROE ter one)

U.S./Canadian Brand Names Androcur® (Can); Androcur® Depot (Can)

Therapeutic Category Antiandrogen; Progestin

Use Palliative treatment of patients with advanced prostatic carcinoma

Usual Dosage Adults:

I.M.: 300 mg (3 mL) once a week

Oral: 200-300 mg divided into 2-3 doses and taken after meals

Dosage Forms

Injection, as acetate: 100 mg/mL (3 mL)

Tablet, as acetate: 50 mg

Cystadane® *see* betaine anhydrous *on page 71*

Cystagon® *see* cysteamine *on this page*

cysteamine (sis TEE a meen)

U.S./Canadian Brand Names Cystagon®

Therapeutic Category Urinary Tract Product

Use Nephropathic cystinosis in children and adults

Usual Dosage Initiate therapy with $^1/_4$ to $^1/_8$ of maintenance dose; titrate slowly upward over 4-6 weeks

Children <12 years: Oral: Maintenance: 1.3 g/m^2/day divided into 4 doses

Children >12 years and Adults (>110 lbs): Oral: 2 g/day in 4 divided doses; dosage may in increased to 1.95 g/m^2/day if cystine levels are <1 nmol/$^1/_2$ cystine/mg protein, although intolerance and incidence of adverse events may be increased

Dosage Forms Capsule, as bitartrate: 50 mg, 150 mg

cysteine (SIS teen)

Therapeutic Category Nutritional Supplement

Use Total parenteral nutrition of infants as an additive to meet the I.V. amino acid requirements

Usual Dosage Combine 500 mg of cysteine with 12.5 g of amino acid, then dilute with 50% dextrose

Dosage Forms Injection, as hydrochloride: 50 mg/mL (10 mL)

Cystografin® *see* radiological/contrast media (ionic) *on page 495*

Cystospaz® *see* hyoscyamine *on page 297*

Cystospaz-M® *see* hyoscyamine *on page 297*

CYT *see* cyclophosphamide *on page 153*

Cytadren® *see* aminoglutethimide *on page 26*

cytarabine (sye TARE a been)

Synonyms arabinosylcytosine; ARA-C; cytosine arabinosine

U.S./Canadian Brand Names Cytosar-U®; Tarabine® PFS

Therapeutic Category Antineoplastic Agent

Use In combination regimens for the treatment of leukemias and non-Hodgkin's lymphomas

Usual Dosage Children and Adults (refer to individual protocols):

Induction remission:

I.T.: 5-75 mg/m^2 once daily for 4 days or 1 every 4 days until CNS

I.V.: 200 mg/m^2/day for 5 days at 2-week intervals; 100-200 mg/m^2/day for 5- to 10-day therapy course or every day until remission administered I.V. continuous drip, or in 2-3 divided doses findings normalize

Maintenance remission:

I.M., S.C.: 1-1.5 mg/kg single dose for maintenance at 1- to 4-week intervals

I.V.: 70-200 mg/m^2/day for 2-5 days at monthly intervals

High-dose therapies: Doses as high as 1-3 g/m^2 have been used for refractory or secondary leukemias or refractory non-Hodgkins lymphoma; dosages of 3 g/m^2 every 12 hours for up to 12 doses have been used

Dosage Forms Cytarabine hydrochloride:

Powder for injection: 100 mg, 500 mg, 1 g, 2 g

Powder for injection (Cytosar-U®): 100 mg, 500 mg, 1 g, 2 g

cytarabine (liposomal) (sye TARE a been lip po SOE mal)

U.S./Canadian Brand Names DepoCyt™

Therapeutic Category Antineoplastic Agent, Antimetabolite (Purine)

Use Intrathecal treatment of lymphomatous meningitis

Usual Dosage Adults:

Induction: 50 mg intrathecally every 14 days for a total of 2 doses (weeks 1 and 3)

Consolidation: 50 mg intrathecally every 14 days for 3 doses (weeks 5, 7, and 9), followed by an additional dose at week 13

Maintenance: 50 mg intrathecally every 28 days for 4 doses (weeks 17, 21, 25, and 29)

If drug-related neurotoxicity develops, the dose should be reduced to 25 mg; if toxicity persists, treatment with liposomal cytarabine should be discontinued

Note: Patients should be started on dexamethasone 4 mg twice daily (oral or I.V.) for 5 days, beginning on the day of liposomal cytarabine injection

Dosage Forms Injection: 10 mg/mL (5 mL)

CytoGam™ *see* cytomegalovirus immune globulin (intravenous-human) *on this page*

cytomegalovirus immune globulin (intravenous-human)

(sye toe meg a low VYE rus i MYUN GLOB yoo lin in tra VEE nus, HYU man)

Synonyms CMV-IGIV

U.S./Canadian Brand Names CytoGam™

Therapeutic Category Immune Globulin

Use Attenuation of primary CMV disease associated with kidney transplantation

Usual Dosage I.V.: Initial: Administer at 15 mg/kg/hour, then increase to 30 mg/kg/hour after 30 minutes if no untoward reactions, then increase to 60 mg/kg/hour after another 30 minutes, volume not to exceed 75 mL/hour

Dosage Forms Powder for injection, lyophilized, detergent treated: 2500 mg ± 250 mg (50 mL)

Cytomel® Oral *see* liothyronine *on page 335*

Cytosar-U® *see* cytarabine *on previous page*

cytosine arabinosine *see* cytarabine *on previous page*

Cytotec® *see* misoprostol *on page 378*

Cytovene® *see* ganciclovir *on page 257*

Cytoxan® *see* cyclophosphamide *on page 153*

D_3 *see* cholecalciferol *on page 128*

25-D_3 *see* calcifediol *on page 88*

d-3-mercaptovaline *see* penicillamine *on page 433*

d4T *see* stavudine *on page 535*

dacarbazine (da KAR ba zeen)

Synonyms DIC; imidazole carboxamide

U.S./Canadian Brand Names DTIC-Dome®

Therapeutic Category Antineoplastic Agent

Use Singly or in various combination therapy to treat malignant melanoma, Hodgkin's disease, soft-tissue sarcomas (fibrosarcomas, rhabdomyosarcoma), islet cell carcinoma, medullary carcinoma of the thyroid, and neuroblastoma

Usual Dosage Refer to individual protocols. I.V.:

Children:

Solid tumors: 200-470 mg/m²/day over 5 days every 21-28 days

Neuroblastoma: 800-900 mg/m² as a single dose every 3-4 weeks in combination therapy

Adults:

Malignant melanoma: 2-4.5 mg/kg/day for 10 days, repeat in 4 weeks or may use 250 mg/m²/day for 5 days, repeat in 3 weeks

Hodgkin's disease: 150 mg/m²/day for 5 days, repeat every 4 weeks or 375 mg/m² on day 1, repeat in 15 days of each 28-day cycle in combination with other agents

Dosage Forms Injection: 100 mg (10 mL, 20 mL); 200 mg (20 mL, 30 mL); 500 mg (50 mL)

daclizumab (da KLIK si mab)

U.S./Canadian Brand Names Zenapax®

Therapeutic Category Immunosuppressant Agent

Use In combination with an immunosuppressive regimen, including cyclosporine and corticosteroids, for prophylaxis of acute organ rejection in patients receiving renal transplants

Usual Dosage Children and Adults: IVPB: 1 mg/kg, used as part of an immunosuppressive regimen that includes cyclosporine and corticosteroids for a total of 5 doses; give the first dose ≤24 hours before transplantation. The 4 remaining doses should be administered at intervals of 14 days.

Dosage Forms Injection: 5 mg/mL (5 mL)

Dacodyl® [OTC] *see* bisacodyl *on page 74*

dactinomycin (dak ti noe MYE sin)

Synonyms ACT; actinomycin D

U.S./Canadian Brand Names Cosmegen®

Therapeutic Category Antineoplastic Agent

Use Management, either alone or in combination with other treatment modalities of Wilms' tumor, rhabdomyosarcoma, neuroblastoma, retinoblastoma, Ewing's sarcoma, trophoblastic neoplasms, testicular carcinoma, and other malignancies

Usual Dosage Refer to individual protocols; dosage should be based on body surface area in obese or edematous patients

(Continued)

dactinomycin *(Continued)*

Children >6 months and Adults: I.V.: 15 mcg/kg/day or 400-600 mcg/m^2/day for 5 days, may repeat every 3-6 weeks; or 2.5 mg/m^2 administered in divided doses over 1 week; 0.75-2 mg/m^2 as a single dose administered at intervals of 1-4 weeks have been used

Dosage Forms Powder for injection, lyophilized: 0.5 mg

D.A.II® Tablet *see* chlorpheniramine, phenylephrine, and methscopolamine *on page 124*

Dairy Ease® [OTC] *see* lactase *on page 323*

Dakin's solution *see* sodium hypochlorite solution *on page 528*

Dakrina® Ophthalmic Solution [OTC] *see* artificial tears *on page 47*

Dalacin® C Topical (Can) *see* clindamycin *on page 136*

Dalacin® C Vaginal Cream (Can) *see* clindamycin *on page 136*

Dalgan® *see* dezocine *on page 172*

Dallergy® *see* chlorpheniramine, phenylephrine, and methscopolamine *on page 124*

Dallergy-D® Syrup *see* chlorpheniramine and phenylephrine *on page 121*

Dalmane® *see* flurazepam *on page 248*

***d*-alpha tocopherol** *see* vitamin E *on page 604*

dalteparin (dal TE pa rin)

U.S./Canadian Brand Names Fragmin®

Therapeutic Category Anticoagulant

Use Prevent deep vein thrombosis following abdominal surgery

Usual Dosage Adults: S.C.: 2500 units 1-2 hours prior to surgery, then once daily for 5-10 days postoperatively

Dosage Forms Injection: Prefilled syringe: 2500 units (16 mg) in 0.2 mL

Damason-P® *see* hydrocodone and aspirin *on page 288*

D-Amp® ***(Discontinued)*** *see page 700*

danaparoid (da NAP a roid)

U.S./Canadian Brand Names Orgaran®

Therapeutic Category Anticoagulant

Use Prophylaxis of postoperative deep vein thrombosis (DVT)

Usual Dosage Adults: S.C.: 750 anti-Xa units twice daily beginning 1-4 hours preoperatively, and then not sooner than 2 hours hours after surgery

Dosage Forms Injection, as sodium: 750 anti-Xa units/0.6 mL

danazol (DA na zole)

U.S./Canadian Brand Names Cyclomen® (Can); Danocrine®

Therapeutic Category Androgen

Use Treatment of endometriosis, fibrocystic breast disease, and hereditary angioedema

Usual Dosage Adults: Oral:

Endometriosis: 100-400 mg twice daily

Fibrocystic breast disease: 50-200 mg twice daily for 2-6 months

Hereditary angioedema: 400-600 mg/day in 2-3 divided doses

Dosage Forms Capsule: 50 mg, 100 mg, 200 mg

Danex® Shampoo ***(Discontinued)*** *see page 700*

Danocrine® *see* danazol *on this page*

Dantrium® *see* dantrolene *on next page*

dantrolene (DAN troe leen)

U.S./Canadian Brand Names Dantrium®

Therapeutic Category Skeletal Muscle Relaxant

Use Treatment of spasticity associated with upper motor neuron disorders such as spinal cord injury, stroke, cerebral palsy, or multiple sclerosis; also used as treatment of malignant hyperthermia

Usual Dosage

Spasticity: Oral:

Children: Initial: 0.5 mg/kg/dose twice daily, increase frequency to 3-4 times/day at 4- to 7-day intervals, then increase dose by 0.5 mg/kg to a maximum of 3 mg/kg/dose 2-4 times/day up to 400 mg/day

Adults: 25 mg/day to start, increase frequency to 3-4 times/day, then increase dose by 25 mg every 4-7 days to a maximum of 100 mg 2-4 times/day or 400 mg/day

Hyperthermia: Children and Adults:

Oral: 4-8 mg/kg/day in 4 divided doses

I.V.: 1 mg/kg; may repeat dose up to cumulative dose of 10 mg/kg (mean effective dose: 2.5 mg/kg), then switch to oral dosage

Dosage Forms Dantrolene sodium:

Capsule: 25 mg, 50 mg, 100 mg

Powder for injection: 20 mg

Dapa® [OTC] *see* acetaminophen *on page 3*

Dapacin® [OTC] *see* acetaminophen *on page 3*

Dapacin® Cold Capsule [OTC] *see* chlorpheniramine, phenylpropanolamine, and acetaminophen *on page 125*

Dapex-37.5® ***(Discontinued)*** *see page 700*

dapiprazole (DA pi pray zole)

U.S./Canadian Brand Names Rēv-Eyes™

Therapeutic Category Alpha-Adrenergic Blocking Agent

Use Treatment of iatrogenically induced mydriasis produced by adrenergic or parasympatholytic agents

Usual Dosage Ophthalmic: Instill 2 drops followed 5 minutes later by an additional 2 drops applied to the conjunctiva

Dosage Forms Powder, lyophilized, as hydrochloride: 25 mg [0.5% solution when mixed with supplied diluent]

dapsone (DAP sone)

Synonyms DDS; diaminodiphenylsulfone

U.S./Canadian Brand Names Avlosulfon®

Therapeutic Category Sulfone

Use Treatment of leprosy due to susceptible strains of *M. leprae*; treatment of dermatitis herpetiformis; prophylaxis against *Pneumocystis carinii* in children who cannot tolerate sulfamethoxazole/trimethoprim or aerosolized pentamidine

Usual Dosage Oral:

Children: Leprosy: 1-2 mg/kg/24 hours; maximum: 100 mg/day

Adults:

Leprosy: 50-100 mg/day

Dermatitis herpetiformis: Start at 50 mg/day, increase to 300 mg/day, or higher to achieve full control, reduce dosage to minimum level as soon as possible

Dosage Forms Tablet: 25 mg, 100 mg

Daranide® *see* dichlorphenamide *on page 175*

Daraprim® *see* pyrimethamine *on page 490*

Darbid® Tablet ***(Discontinued)*** *see page 700*

Daricon® ***(Discontinued)*** *see page 700*

Darvocet-N® *see* propoxyphene and acetaminophen *on page 482*

Darvocet-N® 100 *see* propoxyphene and acetaminophen *on page 482*

Darvon® *see* propoxyphene *on page 482*

Darvon® 32 mg Capsule *(Discontinued)* *see page 700*

Darvon® Compound-65 Pulvules® *see* propoxyphene and aspirin *on page 482*

Darvon-N® *see* propoxyphene *on page 482*

Darvon-N® Oral Suspension *(Discontinued)* *see page 700*

Datril® Extra Strength *(Discontinued)* *see page 700*

daunomycin *see* daunorubicin hydrochloride *on this page*

daunorubicin citrate (liposomal)

(daw noe ROO bi sin SI trate lip po SOE mal)

U.S./Canadian Brand Names DaunoXome®

Therapeutic Category Antineoplastic Agent

Use Advanced HIV-associated Kaposi's sarcoma

Usual Dosage I.V. (refer to individual protocols):

Children:

ALL combination therapy: Remission induction: 25-45 mg/m² on day 1 every week for 4 cycles **or** 30-45 mg/m²/day for 3 days

In children <2 years or <0.5 m², daunorubicin should be based on weight (mg/kg): 1 mg/kg per protocol with frequency dependent on regimen employed

Cumulative dose should not exceed 300 mg/m² in children >2 years or 10 mg/kg in children <2 years

Adults: 30-60 mg/m²/day for 3-5 days, repeat dose in 3-4 weeks

Single agent induction for AML: 60 mg/m²/day for 3 days; repeat every 3-4 weeks

Combination therapy induction for AML: 45 mg/m²/day for 3 days of the first course of induction therapy; subsequent courses: Every day for 2 days

ALL combination therapy: 45 mg/m²/day for 3 days

Cumulative dose should not exceed 400-600 mg/m²

Dosage Forms Injection: 2 mg/mL equivalent to 50 mg daunorubicin base

daunorubicin hydrochloride (daw noe ROO bi sin hye droe KLOR ide)

Synonyms daunomycin; DNR; rubidomycin

U.S./Canadian Brand Names Cerubidine®

Therapeutic Category Antineoplastic Agent

Use In combination with other agents in the treatment of leukemias (ALL, AML)

Usual Dosage I.V.:

Children:

Combination therapy: Remission induction for ALL: 25-45 mg/m² on day 1 every week for 4 cycles

<2 years or <0.5 m²: Manufacturer recommends that the dose is based on body weight rather than body surface area

Adults: 30-60 mg/m²/day for 3-5 days, repeat dose in 3-4 weeks; total cumulative dose should not exceed 400-600 mg/m²

Single agent induction for AML: 60 mg/m²/day for 3 days; repeat every 3-4 weeks

Combination therapy induction for AML: 45 mg/m²/day for 3 days; Subsequent courses: Every day for 2 days

Combination therapy: Remission induction for ALL: 45 mg/m² on days 1, 2, and 3

Dosage Forms Powder for injection, lyophilized: 20 mg

DaunoXome® *see* daunorubicin citrate (liposomal) *on this page*

Daypro™ *see* oxaprozin *on page 420*

Dayto Himbin® *see* yohimbine *on page 609*

DC 240® Softgel® [OTC] *see* docusate *on page 191*

DCF *see* pentostatin *on page 438*

DDAVP® *see* desmopressin acetate *on page 166*

ddC *see* zalcitabine *on page 609*

ddI *see* didanosine *on page 177*

DDS *see* dapsone *on page 159*

1-deamino-8-d-arginine vasopressin *see* desmopressin acetate *on page 166*

Debrisan® [OTC] *see* dextranomer *on page 170*

Debrox® Otic [OTC] *see* carbamide peroxide *on page 98*

Decadron® 0.25 mg & 6 mg Tablets *(Discontinued)* *see page 700*

Decadron® Injection *see* dexamethasone (systemic) *on page 167*

Decadron®-LA *see* dexamethasone (systemic) *on page 167*

Decadron® Ophthalmic *see* dexamethasone (ophthalmic) *on page 167*

Decadron® Oral *see* dexamethasone (systemic) *on page 167*

Decadron® Phosphate *see* dexamethasone (topical) *on page 168*

Deca-Durabolin® *see* nandrolone *on page 390*

Decaject® *see* dexamethasone (systemic) *on page 167*

Decaject-LA® *see* dexamethasone (systemic) *on page 167*

Decaspray® *(Discontinued)* *see page 700*

Decholin® *see* dehydrocholic acid *on next page*

Declomycin® *see* demeclocycline *on page 163*

Decofed® Syrup [OTC] *see* pseudoephedrine *on page 486*

Decohistine® DH *see* chlorpheniramine, pseudoephedrine, and codeine *on page 126*

Decohistine® Expectorant *see* guaifenesin, pseudoephedrine, and codeine *on page 272*

Deconamine® SR *see* chlorpheniramine and pseudoephedrine *on page 122*

Deconamine® Syrup [OTC] *see* chlorpheniramine and pseudoephedrine *on page 122*

Deconamine® Tablet [OTC] *see* chlorpheniramine and pseudoephedrine *on page 122*

Deconsal® II *see* guaifenesin and pseudoephedrine *on page 270*

Deconsal® Sprinkle® *see* guaifenesin and phenylephrine *on page 269*

Defen-LA® *see* guaifenesin and pseudoephedrine *on page 270*

deferoxamine (de fer OKS a meen)

U.S./Canadian Brand Names Desferal® Mesylate

Therapeutic Category Antidote

Use Acute iron intoxication; chronic iron overload secondary to multiple transfusions; diagnostic test for iron overload

Investigational use: Treatment of aluminum accumulation in renal failure

Usual Dosage

Children and Adults: Acute iron toxicity: I.V. route is used when severe toxicity is evidenced by systemic symptoms (coma, shock, metabolic acidosis, or severe gastrointestinal bleeding) or potentially severe intoxications (serum iron level >500 μg/dL). When severe symptoms are not present, the I.M. route may be preferred; however, the use of deferoxamine in situations where the serum iron concentration is <500 μg/dL or when severe toxicity is not evident is a subject of some clinical debate.

Dose: 15 mg/kg/hour (although rates up to 40-50 mg/kg/hour have been given in patients with massive iron intoxication); maximum recommended dose: 6 g/day (however, doses as high as 16-37 g have been administered)

(Continued)

deferoxamine *(Continued)*

Children:
Chronic iron overload:
I.V.: 15 mg/kg/hour
S.C.: 20-40 mg/kg/day over 8-12 hours
Aluminum-induced bone disease: 20-40 mg/kg every hemodialysis treatment, frequency dependent on clinical status of the patient
Adults:
Chronic iron overload:
I.M.: 0.5-1 g every day
S.C.: 1-2 g every day over 8-24 hours

Dosage Forms Powder for injection, as mesylate: 500 mg

Deficol® [OTC] *see* bisacodyl *on page 74*

Degas® [OTC] *see* simethicone *on page 522*

Degest® 2 Ophthalmic [OTC] *see* naphazoline *on page 390*

Dehist® *(Discontinued)* *see page 700*

Dehydral™ (Can) *see* methenamine *on page 362*

dehydrocholic acid (dee hye droe KOE lik AS id)

U.S./Canadian Brand Names Cholan-HMB®; Decholin®

Therapeutic Category Laxative

Use Relief of constipation; adjunct to various biliary tract conditions

Usual Dosage Children >12 years and Adults: Oral: 250-500 mg 2-3 times/day after meals up to 1.5 g/day

Dosage Forms Tablet: 250 mg

Deladumone® *see* estradiol and testosterone *on page 218*

Del Aqua-5® Gel *see* benzoyl peroxide *on page 68*

Del Aqua-10® Gel *see* benzoyl peroxide *on page 68*

Delatest® Injection *see* testosterone *on page 552*

Delatestryl® Injection *see* testosterone *on page 552*

delavirdine (de la VIR deen)

Synonyms U-90152S

U.S./Canadian Brand Names Rescriptor®

Therapeutic Category Antiviral Agent

Use Treatment of HIV-1 infection in combination with appropriate antiretrovirals

Usual Dosage Adults: Oral: 400 mg 3 times/day

Dosage Forms Tablet: 100 mg

Delcort® Topical *see* hydrocortisone (topical) *on page 292*

Delfen® [OTC] *see* nonoxynol 9 *on page 406*

Del-Mycin® Topical *see* erythromycin (ophthalmic/topical) *on page 214*

Delsym® [OTC] *see* dextromethorphan *on page 171*

Delta-Cortef® Oral *see* prednisolone (systemic) *on page 471*

deltacortisone *see* prednisone *on page 472*

Delta-D® *see* cholecalciferol *on page 128*

deltadehydrocortisone *see* prednisone *on page 472*

deltahydrocortisone *see* prednisolone (ophthalmic) *on page 471*

deltahydrocortisone *see* prednisolone (systemic) *on page 471*

Deltalin® Capsule *(Discontinued)* *see page 700*

Deltasone® *see* prednisone *on page 472*

Delta-Tritex® Topical *see* triamcinolone (topical) *on page 578*

Del-Vi-A® *see* vitamin A *on page 602*

Demadex® *see* torsemide *on page 573*

Demazin® Syrup [OTC] *see* chlorpheniramine and phenylpropanolamine *on page 122*

demecarium (dem e KARE ee um)

U.S./Canadian Brand Names Humorsol® Ophthalmic

Therapeutic Category Cholinesterase Inhibitor

Use Management of chronic simple glaucoma, chronic and acute angle-closure glaucoma; counter effects of cycloplegics

Usual Dosage Ophthalmic:

Children: Instill 1 drop into eyes twice weekly to a maximum dosage of 1 or 2 drops twice daily for up to 4 months

Adults: Instill 1-2 drops into eyes twice weekly to a maximum dosage of 1 or 2 drops twice daily for up to 4 months

Dosage Forms Solution, ophthalmic, as bromide: 0.125% (5 mL); 0.25% (5 mL)

demeclocycline (dem e kloe SYE kleen)

Synonyms demethylchlortetracycline

U.S./Canadian Brand Names Declomycin®

Therapeutic Category Tetracycline Derivative

Use Treatment of susceptible bacterial infections (acne, gonorrhea, pertussis, chronic bronchitis, and urinary tract infections) caused by both gram-negative and gram-positive organisms; treatment of chronic syndrome of inappropriate antidiuretic hormone (SIADH) secretion

Usual Dosage Oral:

Children ≥8 years: 8-12 mg/kg/day divided every 6-12 hours

Adults: 150 mg 4 times/day or 300 mg twice daily

Uncomplicated gonorrhea: 600 mg stat, 300 mg every 12 hours for 4 days (3 g total)

SIADH: Initial: 900-1200 mg/day or 13-15 mg/kg/day divided every 6-8 hours, then decrease to 0.6-0.9 g/day

Dosage Forms Demeclocycline hydrochloride:

Capsule: 150 mg

Tablet: 150 mg, 300 mg

Demerol® *see* meperidine *on page 355*

4-demethoxydaunorubicin *see* idarubicin *on page 301*

demethylchlortetracycline *see* demeclocycline *on this page*

Demser® *see* metyrosine *on page 373*

Demulen® *see* ethinyl estradiol and ethynodiol diacetate *on page 222*

Denavir™ *see* penciclovir *on page 433*

denileukin deftitox (de ne LU kin DEFT e tox)

U.S./Canadian Brand Names Ontak®

Therapeutic Category Antineoplastic Agent, Miscellaneous

Use Treatment of patients with persistent or recurrent cutaneous T-cell lymphoma whose malignant cells express the CD25 component of the IL-2 receptor

Usual Dosage Adults: I.V.: A treatment cycle consists of 9 or 18 mcg/kg/day for 5 consecutive days administered every 21 days. The optimal duration of therapy has not been determined. Only 2% of patients who failed to demonstrate a response (at least a 25% decrease in tumor burden) prior to the fourth cycle responded to subsequent treatment.

Dosage Forms Injection: 150 mcg/mL (2 mL)

Denorex® [OTC] *see* coal tar *on page 141*

deodorized opium tincture *see* opium tincture *on page 416*

2′-deoxycoformycin *see* pentostatin *on page 438*

Depacon® *see* valproic acid and derivatives *on page 594*

Depade® *see* naltrexone *on page 390*

Depakene® *see* valproic acid and derivatives *on page 594*

Depakote® *see* valproic acid and derivatives *on page 594*

depAndrogyn® *see* estradiol and testosterone *on page 218*

depAndro® Injection *see* testosterone *on page 552*

Depen® *see* penicillamine *on page 433*

depGynogen® Injection *see* estradiol *on page 217*

depMedalone® Injection *see* methylprednisolone *on page 368*

DepoCyt™ *see* cytarabine (liposomal) *on page 156*

Depo®-Estradiol Injection *see* estradiol *on page 217*

Depogen® Injection *see* estradiol *on page 217*

Depoject® Injection *see* methylprednisolone *on page 368*

Depo-Medrol® Injection *see* methylprednisolone *on page 368*

Deponit® Patch *see* nitroglycerin *on page 404*

Depopred® Injection *see* methylprednisolone *on page 368*

Depo-Provera® 100 mg/mL *(Discontinued)* *see page 700*

Depo-Provera® Injection *see* medroxyprogesterone acetate *on page 352*

Depo-Testadiol® *see* estradiol and testosterone *on page 218*

Depotest® Injection *see* testosterone *on page 552*

Depotestogen® *see* estradiol and testosterone *on page 218*

Depo®-Testosterone Injection *see* testosterone *on page 552*

deprenyl *see* selegiline *on page 518*

Deproist® Expectorant With Codeine *see* guaifenesin, pseudoephedrine, and codeine *on page 272*

Deprol® *(Discontinued)* *see page 700*

Dequadin® (Can) *see* dequalinium *(Canada only) on this page*

dequalinium *(Canada only)* (de kwal LI ne um)

U.S./Canadian Brand Names Dequadin® (Can)

Therapeutic Category Antibacterial, Topical; Antifungal Agent, Topical

Use Treatment of mouth and throat infections

Usual Dosage Adults:

Lozenge: One lozenge sucked slowly every 2-3 hours

Oral paint: Apply freely to infected area, every 2-3 hours, or as directed by physician

Dosage Forms

Lozenge, as chloride: 0.25 mg (20s)

Oral paint, as chloride: 0.5% (25 mL)

Derifil® [OTC] *see* chlorophyll *on page 118*

Dermacort® Topical *see* hydrocortisone (topical) *on page 292*

Dermarest Dricort® Topical *see* hydrocortisone (topical) *on page 292*

Derma-Smoothe/FS® Topical *see* fluocinolone *on page 243*

Dermasone (Can) *see* clobetasol *on page 137*

Dermatop® *see* prednicarbate *on page 470*

Dermatophytin® *see Trichophyton* skin test *on page 579*

Dermatophytin-O *see Candida albicans* (*Monilia*) *on page 95*

Dermazin™ (Can) *see* silver sulfadiazine *on page 522*

Dermolate® Topical [OTC] *see* hydrocortisone (topical) *on page 292*

Dermoplast® [OTC] *see* benzocaine *on page 66*

Dermovate® (Can) *see* clobetasol *on page 137*

Dermoxyl® Gel *(Discontinued)* *see page 700*

Dermtex® HC with Aloe Topical [OTC] *see* hydrocortisone (topical) *on page 292*

DES *see* diethylstilbestrol *on page 178*

Desenex® [OTC] *see* tolnaftate *on page 571*

deserpidine and methyclothiazide *see* methyclothiazide and deserpidine *on page 366*

Desferal® Mesylate *see* deferoxamine *on page 161*

desflurane (des FLOO rane)

U.S./Canadian Brand Names Suprane®

Therapeutic Category General Anesthetic

Use Induction or maintenance of anesthesia for adults in outpatient and inpatient surgery

Usual Dosage

Children: Maintenance: Surgical levels of anesthesia may be maintained with concentrations of 5.2% to 10% desflurane, with or without nitrous oxide

Adults: Titrate dose based on individual response; see table in the product packaging for specific details; minimum alveolar concentration (MAC) should be reduced in elderly patients

Induction: Frequent starting concentration 3%; increased in 0.5% to 1% increments every 2-3 breaths; end tidal concentrations of 4% to 11% desflurane with and without nitrous oxide produce anesthesia within 2-4 minutes

Maintenance: Surgical levels of anesthesia in adults may be maintained with concentrations of 2.5% to 8.5% desflurane, with or without nitrous oxide

Note: Because of the higher vapor pressure and higher MAC of desflurane, special vaporizer canisters must be used. Equipment is **not** interchangeable with that for isoflurane.

Dosage Forms Liquid: 240 mL

desiccated thyroid *see* thyroid *on page 564*

desipramine (des IP ra meen)

Synonyms desmethylimipramine

U.S./Canadian Brand Names Norpramin®; PMS-Desipramine (Can)

Therapeutic Category Antidepressant, Tricyclic (Secondary Amine)

Use Treatment of various forms of depression, often in conjunction with psychotherapy; analgesic in chronic pain, peripheral neuropathies

Usual Dosage Oral (not recommended for use in children <12 years):

Adolescents: Initial: 25-50 mg/day; gradually increase to 100 mg/day in single or divided doses; maximum: 150 mg/day

Adults: Initial: 75 mg/day in divided doses; increase gradually to 150-200 mg/day in divided or single dose; maximum: 300 mg/day

Dosage Forms Tablet, as hydrochloride: 10 mg, 25 mg, 50 mg, 75 mg, 100 mg, 150 mg

Desitin® [OTC] *see* zinc oxide, cod liver oil, and talc *on page 612*

desmethylimipramine *see* desipramine *on this page*

desmopressin acetate (des moe PRES in AS e tate)

Synonyms 1-deamino-8-d-arginine vasopressin

U.S./Canadian Brand Names DDAVP®; Octostim® (Can); Stimate®

Therapeutic Category Vasopressin Analog, Synthetic

Use Treatment of diabetes insipidus and controlling bleeding in certain types of hemophilia

Usual Dosage

Children:

Diabetes insipidus: 3 months to 12 years: Intranasal: Initial: 5 mcg/day divided 1-2 times/day; range: 5-30 mcg/day divided 1-2 times/day

Hemophilia: >3 months: I.V.: 0.3 mcg/kg by slow infusion; may repeat dose if needed

Nocturnal enuresis: ≥6 years: Intranasal: Initial: 20 mcg at bedtime; range: 10-40 mcg

Adults:

Diabetes insipidus: I.V., S.C.: 2-4 mcg/day in 2 divided doses or $^1/_{10}$ of the maintenance intranasal dose; intranasal: 5-40 mcg/day 1-3 times/day

Hemophilia: I.V.: 0.3 mcg/kg by slow infusion

Dosage Forms Desmopressin acetate:

Injection (DDAVP®): 4 mcg/mL (1 mL)

Solution, nasal:

DDAVP®: 100 mcg/mL (2.5 mL, 5 mL)

Stimate®: 1.5 mg/mL (2.5 mL)

Tablet (DDAVP®): 0.1 mg, 0.2 mg

Desocort® (Can) *see* desonide *on this page*

Desogen® *see* ethinyl estradiol and desogestrel *on page 222*

desogestrel and ethinyl estradiol *see* ethinyl estradiol and desogestrel *on page 222*

desonide (DES oh nide)

U.S./Canadian Brand Names Desocort® (Can); DesOwen® Topical; Tridesilon® Topical

Therapeutic Category Corticosteroid, Topical

Use Adjunctive therapy for inflammation in acute and chronic corticosteroid responsive dermatosis

Usual Dosage Topical: Apply 2-4 times/day

Dosage Forms

Cream, topical: 0.05% (15 g, 60 g)

Lotion: 0.05% (60 mL, 120 mL)

Ointment, topical: 0.05% (15 g, 60 g)

DesOwen® Topical *see* desonide *on this page*

desoximetasone (des oks i MET a sone)

U.S./Canadian Brand Names Topicort®; Topicort®-LP

Therapeutic Category Corticosteroid, Topical

Use Relief of inflammation and pruritic symptoms of corticosteroid-responsive dermatosis

Usual Dosage Topical:

Children: Apply sparingly in a very thin film to affected area 1-2 times/day

Adults: Apply sparingly in a thin film twice daily

Dosage Forms

Cream, topical:

Topicort®: 0.25% (15 g, 60 g, 120 g)

Topicort®-LP: 0.05% (15 g, 60 g)

Gel, topical: 0.05% (15 g, 60 g)

Ointment, topical (Topicort®): 0.25% (15 g, 60 g)

desoxyephedrine *see* methamphetamine *on page 362*

Desoxyn® *see* methamphetamine *on page 362*

desoxyphenobarbital *see* primidone *on page 474*

Despec® Liquid *(Discontinued)* *see page 700*

Desquam-E™ Gel *see* benzoyl peroxide *on page 68*

Desquam-X® Gel *see* benzoyl peroxide *on page 68*

Desquam-X® Wash *see* benzoyl peroxide *on page 68*

Desyrel® *see* trazodone *on page 575*

Detensol® (Can) *see* propranolol *on page 483*

Detrol™ *see* tolterodine *on page 571*

Detussin® Expectorant *see* hydrocodone, pseudoephedrine, and guaifenesin *on page 290*

Detussin® Liquid *see* hydrocodone and pseudoephedrine *on page 289*

Devrom® [OTC] *see* bismuth subgallate *on page 75*

Dexacen-4® *(Discontinued)* *see page 700*

Dexacen® LA-8 *(Discontinued)* *see page 700*

Dexacidin® *see* neomycin, polymyxin B, and dexamethasone *on page 396*

Dexacort® Phosphate in Respihaler® *see* dexamethasone (oral inhalation) *on this page*

Dexacort® Phosphate Turbinaire® *see* dexamethasone (nasal) *on this page*

dexamethasone and neomycin *see* neomycin and dexamethasone *on page 395*

dexamethasone and tobramycin *see* tobramycin and dexamethasone *on page 569*

dexamethasone (nasal) (deks a METH a sone)

U.S./Canadian Brand Names Dexacort® Phosphate Turbinaire®

Therapeutic Category Adrenal Corticosteroid

Use Chronic inflammation and/or allergic conditions

Dosage Forms Dexamethasone sodium phosphate: Aerosol, nasal 84 mcg/activation [170 metered doses] (12.6 g)

dexamethasone, neomycin, and polymyxin B *see* neomycin, polymyxin B, and dexamethasone *on page 396*

dexamethasone (ophthalmic) (deks a METH a sone)

U.S./Canadian Brand Names AK-Dex® Ophthalmic; Baldex®; Decadron® Ophthalmic; Maxidex®

Therapeutic Category Adrenal Corticosteroid

Use Inflammatory or allergic conjunctivitis

Usual Dosage Ophthalmic: Instill 3-4 times/day

Dosage Forms Dexamethasone base:

Suspension, ophthalmic: 0.1% (5 mL)
Ointment, ophthalmic: 0.05% (3.5 g)
Solution, ophthalmic: 0.1% (5 mL)

dexamethasone (oral inhalation) (deks a METH a sone)

U.S./Canadian Brand Names Dexacort® Phosphate in Respihaler®

Therapeutic Category Adrenal Corticosteroid

Use Chronic inflammation or allergic conditions

Dosage Forms Aerosol, oral: 84 mcg/activation [170 metered doses] (12.6 g)

dexamethasone (systemic) (deks a METH a sone)

U.S./Canadian Brand Names Decadron® Injection; Decadron®-LA; Decadron® Oral; Decaject®; Decaject-LA®; Dexasone®; Dexasone® L.A.; Dexone®; Dexone® LA; Hexadrol®; Solurex L.A.®

(Continued)

dexamethasone (systemic) *(Continued)*

Therapeutic Category Adrenal Corticosteroid

Use Systemically for chronic inflammation, allergic, hematologic, neoplastic, and autoimmune diseases; may be used in management of cerebral edema, septic shock, and as a diagnostic agent

Usual Dosage

Children:

Antiemetic (prior to chemotherapy): 10 mg/m^2/dose for first dose then 5 mg/m^2/dose every 6 hours as needed

Physiologic replacement: Oral, I.M., I.V.: 0.03-0.15 mg/kg/day or 0.6-0.75 mg/m^2/day in divided doses every 6-12 hours

Extubation or airway edema: Oral, I.M., I.V.: 0.5-1 mg/kg/day in divided doses every 6 hours beginning 24 hours prior to extubation and continuing for 4-6 doses afterwards

Anti-inflammatory: Oral, I.M., I.V.: 0.75-9 mg/day in divided doses every 6-12 hours

Cerebral edema: I.V. 10 mg stat, 4 mg I.M./I.V. every 6 hours until response is maximized, then switch to oral regimen, then taper off if appropriate

Diagnosis for Cushing's syndrome: Oral: 1 mg at 11 PM, draw blood at 8 AM

ANLL protocol: I.V.: 2 mg/m^2/dose every 8 hours for 12 doses

Dosage Forms

Dexamethasone acetate:

Injection:

Dalalone L.A.®, Decadron®-LA, Decaject-LA®, Dexasone® L.A., Dexone® LA, Solurex L.A.®: 8 mg/mL (1 mL, 5 mL)

Dalalone D.P.®: 16 mg/mL (1 mL, 5 mL)

Dexamethasone base:

Elixir (Decadron®, Hexadrol®): 0.5 mg/5 mL (5 mL, 20 mL, 100 mL, 120 mL, 240 mL, 500 mL)

Solution, oral: 0.5 mg/5 mL (5 mL, 20 mL, 500 mL)

Solution, oral concentrate: 0.5 mg/0.5 mL (30 mL)

Tablet (Decadron®, Dexone®, Hexadrol®): 0.25 mg, 0.5 mg, 0.75 mg, 1 mg, 1.5 mg, 2 mg, 4 mg, 6 mg

Therapeutic pack: Six 1.5 mg tablets and eight 0.75 mg tablets

Injection:

Dalalone®, Decadron® Phosphate, Decaject®, Dexasone®, Hexadrol® Phosphate, Solurex®: 4 mg/mL (1 mL, 2 mL, 2.5 mL, 5 mL, 10 mL, 30 mL)

Hexadrol® Phosphate: 10 mg/mL (1 mL, 10 mL); 20 mg/mL (5 mL)

Decadron® Phosphate: 24 mg/mL (5 mL, 10 mL)

dexamethasone (topical) (deks a METH a sone)

U.S./Canadian Brand Names Aeroseb-Dex®; Decadron® Phosphate

Therapeutic Category Adrenal Corticosteroid

Use For chronic inflammation and/or allergic conditions

Usual Dosage Topical: Apply 2-4 times daily

Dosage Forms Dexamethasone base:

Aerosol, topical: 0.01% (58 g)

Cream: 0.1% (15 g, 30 g)

Dexasone® *see* dexamethasone (systemic) *on previous page*

Dexasone® L.A. *see* dexamethasone (systemic) *on previous page*

Dexasporin® *see* neomycin, polymyxin B, and dexamethasone *on page 396*

Dexatrim® Pre-Meal [OTC] *see* phenylpropanolamine *on page 447*

dexbrompheniramine and pseudoephedrine

(deks brom fen EER a meen & soo doe e FED rin)

Synonyms pseudoephedrine and dexbrompheniramine

U.S./Canadian Brand Names Disobrom® [OTC]; Disophrol® Chronotabs® [OTC]; Disophrol® Tablet [OTC]; Drixomed®; Drixoral® [OTC]

Therapeutic Category Antihistamine/Decongestant Combination

Use Relief of symptoms of upper respiratory mucosal congestion in seasonal and perennial nasal allergies, acute rhinitis, rhinosinusitis and eustachian tube blockage

Usual Dosage Children >12 years and Adults: Oral: 1 tablet every 12 hours, may require 1 tablet every 8 hours

Dosage Forms

Tablet (Disophrol®): Dexbrompheniramine maleate 2 mg and pseudoephedrine sulfate 60 mg

Timed release (Disobrom®, Disophrol® Chrontabs®, Drixomed®, Drixoral®, Histrodrix®, Resporal®): Dexbrompheniramine maleate 6 mg and pseudoephedrine sulfate 120 mg

Dexchlor® *see* dexchlorpheniramine *on this page*

dexchlorpheniramine (deks klor fen EER a meen)

U.S./Canadian Brand Names Dexchlor®; Poladex®; Polaramine®

Therapeutic Category Antihistamine

Use Perennial and seasonal allergic rhinitis and other allergic symptoms including urticaria

Usual Dosage Oral:

Children:

2-5 years: 0.5 mg every 4-6 hours

6-11 years: 1 mg every 4-6 hours or 4 mg timed release at bedtime

Adults: 2 mg every 4-6 hours or 4-6 mg timed release at bedtime or 8-10 hours

Dosage Forms Dexchlorpheniramine maleate:

Syrup (orange flavor): 2 mg/5 mL with alcohol 6% (480 mL)

Tablet: 2 mg

Tablet, sustained action: 4 mg, 6 mg

Dexedrine® *see* dextroamphetamine *on next page*

Dexedrine® Elixir *(Discontinued)* *see page 700*

Dexferrum® *see* iron dextran complex *on page 312*

Dexone® *see* dexamethasone (systemic) *on page 167*

Dexone® LA *see* dexamethasone (systemic) *on page 167*

dexpanthenol (deks PAN the nole)

Synonyms pantothenyl alcohol

U.S./Canadian Brand Names Ilopan-Choline® Oral; Ilopan® Injection; Panthoderm® Cream [OTC]

Therapeutic Category Gastrointestinal Agent, Stimulant

Use Prophylactic use to minimize paralytic ileus, treatment of postoperative distention

Usual Dosage

Children and Adults: Relief of itching and aid in skin healing: Topical: Apply to affected area 1-2 times/day

Adults:

Relief of gas retention: Oral: 2-3 tablets 3 times/day

Prevention of postoperative ileus: I.M.: 250-500 mg stat, repeat in 2 hours, followed by doses every 6 hours until danger passes

Paralyzed ileus: I.M.: 500 mg stat, repeat in 2 hours, followed by doses every 6 hours, if needed

Dosage Forms

Cream: 2% (30 g, 60 g)

Injection (Ilopan®): 250 mg/mL (2 mL, 10 mL, 30 mL)

Tablet (Ilopan-Choline®): 50 mg with choline bitartrate 25 mg

dexrazoxane (deks ray ZOKS ane)

Synonyms ICRF-187

U.S./Canadian Brand Names Zinecard®

Therapeutic Category Cardiovascular Agent, Other

(Continued)

dexrazoxane *(Continued)*

Use Prevention of cardiomyopathy associated with doxorubicin administration

Usual Dosage I.V.: 1000 mg/m^2 30 minutes before administration of doxorubicin; maximal doses in patients with and without prior treatment with nitrosoureas, respectively = 750 mg/m^2 and 120 mg/m^2; 3500 mg/m^2/day for 3 days has been maximally used in pediatric patients. The recommended dosage ratio of dexrazoxane:doxorubicin is 10:1.

Dosage Forms Powder for injection, lyophilized: 250 mg, 500 mg (10 mg/mL when reconstituted)

dextran (DEKS tran)

Synonyms dextran, high molecular weight; dextran, low molecular weight

U.S./Canadian Brand Names Gentran®; LMD®; Macrodex®; Rheomacrodex®

Therapeutic Category Plasma Volume Expander

Use Fluid replacement and blood volume expander used in the treatment of hypovolemia, shock, or near shock states

Usual Dosage I.V.:

Children: Total dose should not be >20 mL/kg during first 24 hours

Adults: 500-1000 mL at rate of 20-40 mL/minute

Dosage Forms Injection:

High molecular weight:

- 6% dextran 75 in dextrose 5% (500 mL)
- Gentran®: 6% dextran 75 in sodium chloride 0.9% (500 mL)
- Gentran®, Macrodex®: 6% dextran 70 in sodium chloride 0.9% (500 mL)
- Macrodex®: 6% dextran 70 in dextrose 5% (500 mL)

Low molecular weight: Gentran®, LMD®, Rheomacrodex®:

- 10% dextran 40 in dextrose 5% (500 mL)
- 10% dextran 40 in sodium chloride 0.9% (500 mL)

dextran 1 (DEKS tran won)

U.S./Canadian Brand Names Promit®

Therapeutic Category Plasma Volume Expander

Use Prophylaxis of serious anaphylactic reactions to I.V. infusion of dextran

Usual Dosage I.V. (time between dextran 1 and dextran solution should not exceed 15 minutes):

Children: 0.3 mL/kg 1-2 minutes before I.V. infusion of dextran

Adults: 20 mL 1-2 minutes before I.V. infusion of dextran

Dosage Forms Injection: 150 mg/mL (20 mL)

dextran, high molecular weight *see* dextran *on this page*

dextran, low molecular weight *see* dextran *on this page*

dextranomer (deks TRAN oh mer)

U.S./Canadian Brand Names Debrisan® [OTC]

Therapeutic Category Topical Skin Product

Use Clean exudative wounds; no controlled studies have found dextranomer to be more effective than conventional therapy

Usual Dosage Topical: Apply to affected area once or twice daily

Dosage Forms

Beads: 4 g, 25 g, 60 g, 120 g

Paste: 10 g foil packets

dextroamphetamine (deks troe am FET a meen)

U.S./Canadian Brand Names Dexedrine®

Therapeutic Category Amphetamine

Controlled Substance C-II

Use Adjunct in treatment of attention-deficit/hyperactivity disorder (ADHD) in children, narcolepsy, exogenous obesity

Usual Dosage Oral:

Children:

Narcolepsy: 6-12 years: Initial: 5 mg/day, may increase at 5 mg increments in weekly intervals until side effects appear; maximum dose: 60 mg/day

Attention deficit disorder:

3-5 years: Initial: 2.5 mg/day administered every morning; increase by 2.5 mg/day in weekly intervals until optimal response is obtained, usual range is 0.1-0.5 mg/kg/dose every morning with maximum of 40 mg/day

≥6 years: 5 mg once or twice daily; increase in increments of 5 mg/day at weekly intervals until optimal response is reached, usual range is 0.1-0.5 mg/kg/dose every morning (5-20 mg/day) with maximum of 40 mg/day

Adults:

Narcolepsy: Initial: 10 mg/day, may increase at 10 mg increments in weekly intervals until side effects appear; maximum: 60 mg/day

Exogenous obesity: 5-30 mg/day in divided doses of 5-10 mg 30-60 minutes before meals

Dosage Forms Dextroamphetamine sulfate:

Capsule, sustained release: 5 mg, 10 mg, 15 mg

Tablet: 5 mg, 10 mg (5 mg tablets contain tartrazine)

dextroamphetamine and amphetamine

(deks troe am FET a meen & am FET a meen)

U.S./Canadian Brand Names Adderall®

Therapeutic Category Amphetamine

Use Treatment of narcolepsy; exogenous obesity; abnormal behavioral syndrome in children (minimal brain dysfunction); attention-deficit/hyperactivity disorder (ADHD)

Usual Dosage Oral:

Narcolepsy:

Children:

6-12 years: 5 mg/day, increase by 5 mg at weekly intervals

>12 years: 10 mg/day, increase by 10 mg at weekly intervals

Adults: 5-60 mg/day in 2-3 divided doses

Attention deficit disorder: Children:

3-5 years: 2.5 mg/day, increase by 2.5 mg at weekly intervals

>6 years: 5 mg/day, increase by 5 mg at weekly intervals not to exceed 40 mg/day

Short-term adjunct to exogenous obesity: Children >12 years and Adults: 5-30 mg/day in divided doses

Dosage Forms Tablet:

10 mg [dextroamphetamine sulfate 2.5 mg, dextroamphetamine saccharate 2.5 mg and amphetamine aspartate 2.5 mg, amphetamine sulfate 2.5 mg]

30 mg [dextroamphetamine sulfate 7.5 mg, dextroamphetamine saccharate 7.5 mg and amphetamine aspartate 7.55 mg, amphetamine sulfate 7.5 mg]

dextromethorphan (deks troe meth OR fan)

U.S./Canadian Brand Names Balminil®-DM, -DM Children (Can); Benylin DM® [OTC]; Benylin® Pediatric [OTC]; Children's Hold® [OTC]; Creo-Terpin® [OTC]; Delsym® [OTC]; Drixoral® Cough Liquid Caps [OTC]; Hold® DM [OTC]; Koffex® DM, -DM Children (Can); Pertussin® CS [OTC]; Pertussin® ES [OTC]; Robitussin® Cough Calmers [OTC]; Robitussin® Pediatric [OTC]; Scot-Tussin DM® Cough Chasers [OTC]; Silphen DM® [OTC]; St. Joseph® Cough Suppressant [OTC]; Sucrets® Cough Calmers [OTC]; Suppress® [OTC]; Triaminic DM (Can); Trocal® [OTC]; Vicks Formula 44® [OTC]; Vicks Formula 44® Pediatric Formula [OTC]

Therapeutic Category Antitussive

Use Symptomatic relief of coughs caused by minor viral upper respiratory tract infections or inhaled irritants; most effective for a chronic nonproductive cough

Usual Dosage Oral:

Children:

2-5 years: 2.5-5 mg every 4 hours or 7.5 mg every 6-8 hours; extended release is 50 mg twice daily

(Continued)

dextromethorphan *(Continued)*

6-11 years: 5-10 mg every 4 hours or 15 mg every 6-8 hours; extended release is 30 mg twice daily

Adults: 10-20 mg every 4 hours or 30 mg every 6-8 hours; extended release is 60 mg twice daily

Dosage Forms

Capsule (Drixoral® Cough Liquid Caps): 30 mg

Liquid:

Creo-Terpin®: 10 mg/15 mL (120 mL)

Pertussin® CS: 3.5 mg/5 mL (120 mL)

Robitussin® Pediatric, St. Joseph® Cough Suppressant: 7.5 mg/5 mL (60 mL, 120 mL, 240 mL)

Pertussin® ES, Vicks Formula 44®: 15 mg/5 mL (120 mL, 240 mL)

Liquid, sustained release, as polistirex (Delsym®): 30 mg/5 mL (89 mL)

Lozenges:

Scot-Tussin DM® Cough Chasers: 2.5 mg

Children's Hold®, Hold® DM, Robitussin® Cough Calmers, Sucrets® Cough Calmers: 5 mg

Suppress®, Trocal®: 7.5 mg

Syrup:

Benylin® Pediatric: 7.5 mg/mL (118 mL)

Benylin DM®, Silphen DM®: 10 mg/5 mL (120 mL, 3780 mL)

Vicks Formula 44® Pediatric Formula: 15 mg/15 mL (120 mL)

dextromethorphan, acetaminophen, and pseudoephedrine *see* acetaminophen, dextromethorphan, and pseudoephedrine *on page 6*

dextromethorphan and guaifenesin *see* guaifenesin and dextromethorphan *on page 268*

dextromethorphan and promethazine *see* promethazine and dextromethorphan *on page 479*

dextromethorphan, guaifenesin, and phenylpropanolamine *see* guaifenesin, phenylpropanolamine, and dextromethorphan *on page 271*

dextromethorphan, guaifenesin, and pseudoephedrine *see* guaifenesin, pseudoephedrine, and dextromethorphan *on page 273*

dextropropoxyphene *see* propoxyphene *on page 482*

dextrose, levulose and phosphoric acid *see* phosphorated carbohydrate solution *on page 450*

dextrothyroxine (deks troe thye ROKS een)

U.S./Canadian Brand Names Choloxin®

Therapeutic Category Antihyperlipidemic Agent, Miscellaneous

Use Reduction of elevated serum cholesterol

Usual Dosage Oral:

Children: 0.1 mg/kg/day

Adults: 1-2 mg/day, up to 8 mg/day

Dosage Forms Tablet, as sodium: 2 mg, 4 mg, 6 mg

Dey-Dose® Isoproterenol *see* isoproterenol *on page 314*

Dey-Dose® Metaproterenol *see* metaproterenol *on page 359*

Dey-Drop® Ophthalmic Solution *see* silver nitrate *on page 521*

Dey-Lute® Isoetharine *see* isoetharine *on page 313*

dezocine (DEZ oh seen)

U.S./Canadian Brand Names Dalgan®

Therapeutic Category Analgesic, Narcotic

Use Relief of moderate to severe postoperative, acute renal and ureteral colic, and cancer pain

Usual Dosage Adults:

I.M.: Initial: 5-20 mg; may be repeated every 3-6 hours as needed; maximum: 120 mg/day

I.V.: Initial: 2.5-10 mg; may be repeated every 2-4 hours as needed

Dosage Forms Injection, single-dose vial: 5 mg/mL (2 mL); 10 mg/mL (2 mL); 15 mg/mL (2 mL)

DFP *see* isoflurophate *on page 314*

DHAD *see* mitoxantrone *on page 378*

DHC Plus® *see* dihydrocodeine compound *on page 180*

D.H.E. 45® Injection *see* dihydroergotamine *on page 180*

DHPG sodium *see* ganciclovir *on page 257*

DHS® Tar [OTC] *see* coal tar *on page 141*

DHS Zinc® [OTC] *see* pyrithione zinc *on page 491*

DHT™ *see* dihydrotachysterol *on page 181*

Diaβeta® *see* glyburide *on page 263*

Diabetic Tussin DM® [OTC] *see* guaifenesin and dextromethorphan *on page 268*

Diabetic Tussin® EX [OTC] *see* guaifenesin *on page 267*

Diabinese® *see* chlorpropamide *on page 127*

Dialose® Capsule *(Discontinued)* *see page 700*

Dialose® Plus Capsule [OTC] *see* docusate and casanthranol *on page 191*

Dialose® Tablet [OTC] *see* docusate *on page 191*

Dialume® [OTC] *see* aluminum hydroxide *on page 22*

Diamicron® (Can) *see* gliclazide *(Canada only)* *on page 261*

Diamine T.D.® [OTC] *see* brompheniramine *on page 80*

diaminodiphenylsulfone *see* dapsone *on page 159*

Diamox® *see* acetazolamide *on page 7*

Diamox Sequels® *see* acetazolamide *on page 7*

Diaparene® [OTC] *see* methylbenzethonium chloride *on page 366*

Diaparene® Cradol® *(Discontinued)* *see page 700*

Diapid® Nasal Spray *see* lypressin *on page 343*

Diar-aid® [OTC] *see* loperamide *on page 339*

Diasorb® [OTC] *see* attapulgite *on page 53*

Diastat® Rectal Delivery System *see* diazepam *on this page*

Diazemuls® Injection *see* diazepam *on this page*

diazepam (dye AZ e pam)

U.S./Canadian Brand Names Apo®-Diazepam (Can); Diastat® Rectal Delivery System; Diazemuls® Injection; Diazepam Intensol®; Dizac® Injectable Emulsion; E Pam® (Can); Meval® (Can); Novo-Dipam® (Can); PMS-Diazepam (Can); Valium® Injection; Valium® Oral; Vivol® (Can)

Therapeutic Category Benzodiazepine

Controlled Substance C-IV

Use Management of general anxiety disorders, panic disorders; to provide preoperative sedation, light anesthesia, and amnesia; treatment of status epilepticus, alcohol withdrawal symptoms; used as a skeletal muscle relaxant

(Continued)

diazepam *(Continued)*

Usual Dosage

Children:

Sedation or muscle relaxation or anxiety:

Oral: 0.12-0.8 mg/kg/day in divided doses every 6-8 hours

I.M., I.V.: 0.04-0.3 mg/kg/dose every 2-4 hours to a maximum of 0.6 mg/kg within an 8-hour period if needed

Status epilepticus: I.V.:

Infants 30 days to 5 years: 0.05-0.3 mg/kg/dose administered over 2-3 minutes, every 15-30 minutes to a maximum total dose of 5 mg; repeat in 2-4 hours as needed or 0.2-0.5 mg/dose every 2-5 minutes to a maximum total dose of 5 mg

>5 years: 0.05-0.3 mg/kg/dose administered over 2-3 minutes, every 15-30 minutes to a maximum total dose of 10 mg; repeat in 2-4 hours as needed or 1 mg/dose every 2-5 minutes to a maximum of 10 mg;

Adults:

Anxiety:

Oral: 2-10 mg 2-4 times/day

I.M., I.V.: 2-10 mg, may repeat in 3-4 hours if needed

Skeletal muscle relaxation:

Oral: 2-10 mg 2-4 times/day

I.M., I.V.: 5-10 mg, may repeat in 2-4 hours

Status epilepticus: I.V.: 0.2-0.5 mg/kg/dose every 15-30 minutes for 2-3 doses; maximum dose: 30 mg

Dosage Forms

Gel, rectal:

Adult: 10 mg, 15 mg, 20 mg

Pediatric: 2.5 mg, 5 mg, 10 mg

Injection: 5 mg/mL (1 mL, 2 mL, 5 mL, 10 mL)

Injection, emulsified (Dizac®): 5 mg/mL (3 mL)

Solution, oral (wintergreen-spice flavor): 5 mg/5 mL (5 mL, 10 mL, 500 mL)

Solution, oral concentrate: 5 mg/mL (30 mL)

Tablet: 2 mg, 5 mg, 10 mg

Diazepam Intensol® *see* diazepam *on previous page*

diazoxide (dye az OKS ide)

U.S./Canadian Brand Names Hyperstat® I.V.; Proglycem® Oral

Therapeutic Category Antihypoglycemic Agent; Vasodilator

Use I.V.: Emergency lowering of blood pressure; Oral: Hypoglycemia related to hyperinsulinism secondary to islet cell adenoma, carcinoma, or hyperplasia; adenomatosis; nesidioblastosis (persistent hyperinsulinemic hypoglycemia of infancy); leucine sensitivity, or extrapancreatic malignancy

Usual Dosage

Hyperinsulinemic hypoglycemia: Oral:

Newborns and Infants: 8-15 mg/kg/day in divided doses every 8-12 hours

Children and Adults: 3-8 mg/kg/day in divided doses every 8-12 hours

Hypertension: Children and Adults: I.V.: 1-3 mg/kg (maximum: 150 mg in a single injection); repeat dose in 5-15 minutes until blood pressure adequately reduced; repeat administration every 4-24 hours; monitor blood pressure closely

Dosage Forms

Capsule (Proglycem®): 50 mg

Injection (Hyperstat®): 15 mg/mL (1 mL, 20 mL)

Suspension, oral (chocolate-mint flavor) (Proglycem®): 50 mg/mL (30 mL)

Dibent® Injection *see* dicyclomine *on page 177*

Dibenzyline® *see* phenoxybenzamine *on page 445*

dibucaine (DYE byoo kane)

U.S./Canadian Brand Names Nupercainal® [OTC]

Therapeutic Category Local Anesthetic

Use Fast, temporary relief of pain and itching due to hemorrhoids, minor burns, other minor skin conditions

Usual Dosage Children and Adults:

Rectal: Hemorrhoids: Insert ointment into rectum using a rectal applicator; administer each morning,evening, and after each bowel movement

Topical: Apply gently to the affected areas; no more than 30 g for adults or 7.5 g for children should be used in any 24-hour period

Dosage Forms

Cream: 0.5% (45 g)

Ointment, topical: 1% (30 g, 60 g)

dibucaine and hydrocortisone (DYE byoo kane & hye droe KOR ti sone)

Synonyms hydrocortisone and dibucaine

U.S./Canadian Brand Names Corticaine® Topical

Therapeutic Category Anesthetic/Corticosteroid

Use Relief of the inflammatory and pruritic manifestations of corticosteroid-responsive dermatoses and for external anal itching

Usual Dosage Topical: Apply to affected areas 2-4 times/day

Dosage Forms Cream: Dibucaine 5% and hydrocortisone 5%

DIC *see* dacarbazine *on page 157*

dicalcium phosphate *see* calcium phosphate, dibasic *on page 93*

Dicarbosil® [OTC] *see* calcium carbonate *on page 89*

Dicetel® (Can) *see* pinaverium *(Canada only) on page 452*

dichlorodifluoromethane and trichloromonofluoromethane

(dye klor oh dye flor oh METH ane & tri klor oh mon oh flor oh METH ane)

U.S./Canadian Brand Names Fluori-Methane® Topical Spray

Therapeutic Category Analgesic, Topical

Use Management of myofascial pain, restricted motion, muscle pain; control of pain associated with injections

Usual Dosage Topical: Apply to area from approximately 12" away

Dosage Forms Spray, topical: Dichlorodifluoromethane 15% and trichloromonofluoromethane 85%

dichlorotetrafluoroethane and ethyl chloride *see* ethyl chloride and dichlorotetrafluoroethane *on page 227*

dichlorphenamide (dye klor FEN a mide)

Synonyms diclofenamide

U.S./Canadian Brand Names Daranide®

Therapeutic Category Carbonic Anhydrase Inhibitor

Use Adjunct in treatment of open-angle glaucoma and perioperative treatment for angle-closure glaucoma

Usual Dosage Adults: Oral: 100-200 mg to start followed by 100 mg every 12 hours until desired response is obtained; maintenance dose: 25-50 mg 1-3 times/day

Dosage Forms Tablet: 50 mg

dichysterol *see* dihydrotachysterol *on page 181*

diclofenac (dye KLOE fen ak)

U.S./Canadian Brand Names Apo®-Diclo (Can); Cataflam® Oral; Novo-Difenac® (Can); Novo-Difenac-SR® (Can); Nu-Diclo® (Can); Voltaren® Ophthalmic; Voltaren® Oral; Voltaren®-XR Oral

(Continued)

diclofenac *(Continued)*

Therapeutic Category Analgesic, Non-narcotic; Nonsteroidal Anti-inflammatory Drug (NSAID)

Use Acute treatment of mild to moderate pain; acute and chronic treatment of rheumatoid arthritis, ankylosing spondylitis, and osteoarthritis; used for juvenile rheumatoid arthritis, gout, dysmenorrhea; ophthalmic solution for postoperative inflammation after cataract extraction; temporary relief of pain and photophobia in patients undergoing corneal refractive surgery

Usual Dosage Adults:

Oral:

Rheumatoid arthritis: 150-200 mg/day in 2-4 divided doses

Osteoarthritis: 100-150 mg/day in 2-3 divided doses

Ankylosing spondylitis: 100-125 mg/day in 4-5 divided doses

Ophthalmic: Instill 1 drop into affected eye 4 times/day beginning 24 hours after cataract surgery and continuing for 2 weeks

Dosage Forms

Diclofenac sodium:

Solution, ophthalmic (Voltaren®): 0.1% (2.5 mL, 5 mL)

Tablet, delayed release (Voltaren®): 25 mg, 50 mg, 75 mg

Tablet, extended release, as sodium (Voltaren-XR®): 100 mg

Diclofenac potassium:

Tablet (Cataflam®): 50 mg

diclofenac and misoprostol (dye KLOE fen ak & mye soe PROST ole)

Synonyms misoprostol and diclofenac

U.S./Canadian Brand Names Arthrotec®

Therapeutic Category Analgesic, Non-narcotic; Prostaglandin

Use The diclofenac component is indicated for the treatment of osteoarthritis and rheumatoid arthritis; the misoprostol component is indicated for the prophylaxis of NSAID-induced gastric and duodenal ulceration

Usual Dosage Adults: Oral: 1 tablet 2-3 times/day with food; tablets should be swallowed whole, not chewed

Dosage Forms Tablet: Diclofenac 50 mg and misoprostol 200 mcg; diclofenac 75 mg and misoprostol 200 mcg

diclofenamide *see* dichlorphenamide *on previous page*

dicloxacillin (dye kloks a SIL in)

U.S./Canadian Brand Names Dycill®; Dynapen®; Pathocil®

Therapeutic Category Penicillin

Use Treatment of skin and soft tissue infections, pneumonia and follow-up therapy of osteomyelitis caused by susceptible penicillinase-producing staphylococci

Usual Dosage Oral:

Children <40 kg: 12.5-50 mg/kg/day divided every 6 hours; doses of 50-100 mg/kg/day in divided doses every 6 hours have been used for follow-up therapy of osteomyelitis

Children >40 kg and Adults: 125-500 mg every 6 hours

Dosage Forms Dicloxacillin sodium:

Capsule: 125 mg, 250 mg, 500 mg

Powder for oral suspension: 62.5 mg/5 mL (80 mL, 100 mL, 200 mL)

dicumarol (dye KOO ma role)

Synonyms bishydroxycoumarin

Therapeutic Category Anticoagulant

Use Prophylaxis and treatment of thromboembolic disorders

Usual Dosage Adults: Oral: 25-200 mg/day based on prothrombin time (PT) determinations

Dosage Forms Tablet: 25 mg, 50 mg, 100 mg

dicyclomine (dye SYE kloe meen)

Synonyms dicycloverine

U.S./Canadian Brand Names Antispas® Injection; Bentyl® Hydrochloride Injection; Bentyl® Hydrochloride Oral; Bentylol® (Can); Byclomine® Injection; Dibent® Injection; Dilomine® Injection; Di-Spaz® Injection; Di-Spaz® Oral; Or-Tyl® Injection

Therapeutic Category Anticholinergic Agent

Use Treatment of functional disturbances of GI motility such as irritable bowel syndrome

Usual Dosage

Oral:

Infants >6 months: 5 mg/dose 3-4 times/day

Children: 10 mg/dose 3-4 times/day

Adults: Begin with 80 mg/day in 4 equally divided doses, then increase up to 160 mg/day

I.M. **(should not be used I.V.)**: 80 mg/day in 4 divided doses (20 mg/dose)

Dosage Forms Dicyclomine hydrochloride:

Capsule: 10 mg, 20 mg

Injection: 10 mg/mL (2 mL, 10 mL)

Syrup: 10 mg/5 mL (118 mL, 473 mL, 946 mL)

Tablet: 20 mg

dicycloverine *see* dicyclomine *on this page*

didanosine (dye DAN oh seen)

Synonyms ddI

U.S./Canadian Brand Names Videx®

Therapeutic Category Antiviral Agent

Use Treatment of patients with advanced HIV infection which is resistant to zidovudine therapy or in those patients with zidovudine intolerance; has been used in asymptomatic patients with very low $CD4^+$ lymphocyte counts (<200 cells/mm^3) with or without AIDS-related complex

Usual Dosage Administer on an empty stomach: Oral:

Children (dosing is based on body surface area (m^2)):

<0.4: 25 mg tablets twice daily or 31 mg powder twice daily

0.5-0.7: 50 mg tablets twice daily or 62 mg powder twice daily

0.8-1: 75 mg tablets twice daily or 94 mg powder twice daily

1.1-1.4: 100 mg tablets twice daily or 125 mg powder twice daily

Adults: Dosing is based on patient weight:

35-49 kg: 125 mg tablets twice daily or 167 mg buffered powder twice daily

50-74 kg: 200 mg tablets twice daily or 250 mg buffered powder twice daily

≥75 mg: 300 mg tablets twice daily or 375 mg buffered powder twice daily

Note: Children >1 year and Adults should receive 2 tablets per dose and children <1 year should receive 1 tablet per dose for adequate buffering and absorption; tablets should be chewed

Dosage Forms

Powder for oral solution:

Buffered (single dose packet): 100 mg, 167 mg, 250 mg, 375 mg

Pediatric: 2 g, 4 g

Tablet, buffered, chewable (mint flavor): 25 mg, 50 mg, 100 mg, 150 mg

dideoxycytidine *see* zalcitabine *on page 609*

Didrex® *see* benzphetamine *on page 69*

Didronel® *see* etidronate disodium *on page 227*

dienestrol (dye en ES trole)

U.S./Canadian Brand Names DV® Vaginal Cream; Ortho®-Dienestrol Vaginal

Therapeutic Category Estrogen Derivative

Use Symptomatic management of atrophic vaginitis in postmenopausal women

(Continued)

dienestrol *(Continued)*

Usual Dosage Adults: Vaginal: 1-2 applicatorfuls/day for 2 weeks and then 1/2 of that dose for 2 weeks; maintenance dose: 1 applicatorful 1-3 times/week for 3 weeks each month

Dosage Forms Cream, vaginal: 0.01% (30 g, 78 g)

dietary supplements *see* enteral nutritional products *on page 208*

diethylpropion (dye eth il PROE pee on)

Synonyms amfepramone

U.S./Canadian Brand Names Nobesine® (Can); Tenuate®; Tenuate® Dospan®

Therapeutic Category Anorexiant

Controlled Substance C-IV

Use Short-term adjunct in exogenous obesity

Usual Dosage Adults: Oral: 25 mg 3 times/day before meals or food or 75 mg controlled release tablet at midmorning

Dosage Forms Diethylpropion hydrochloride:

Tablet: 25 mg

Tablet, controlled release: 75 mg

diethylstilbestrol (dye eth il stil BES trole)

Synonyms DES; stilbestrol

U.S./Canadian Brand Names Honvol® (Can); Stilphostrol®

Therapeutic Category Estrogen Derivative

Use Management of severe vasomotor symptoms of menopause, for estrogen replacement, and for palliative treatment of inoperable metastatic prostatic carcinoma

Usual Dosage Adults:

Hypogonadism and ovarian failure: Oral: 0.2-0.5 mg/day

Menopausal symptoms: Oral: 0.1-2 mg/day for 3 weeks and then off 1 week

Postmenopausal breast carcinoma: Oral: 15 mg/day

Prostate carcinoma: Oral: 1-3 mg/day

Prostatic cancer: I.V.: 0.5 g to start, then 1 g every 2-5 days followed by 0.25-0.5 g 1-2 times/week as maintenance

Diphosphate:

Oral: 50 mg 3 times/day; increase up to 200 mg or more 3 times/day

I.V.: Administer 0.5 g, dissolved in 250 mL of saline or D_5W, administer slowly the first 10-15 minutes then adjust rate so that the entire amount is administered in 1 hour

Dosage Forms

Diethylstilbestrol base:

Tablet: 1 mg, 2.5 mg, 5 mg

Diethylstilbestrol diphosphate sodium:

Injection (Stilphostrol®): 0.25 g (5 mL)

Tablet (Stilphostrol®): 50 mg

difenoxin and atropine (dye fen OKS in & A troe peen)

Synonyms atropine and difenoxin

U.S./Canadian Brand Names Motofen®

Therapeutic Category Antidiarrheal

Controlled Substance C-IV

Use Treatment of diarrhea

Usual Dosage Adults: Oral: Initial: 2 tablets, then 1 tablet after each loose stool; 1 tablet every 3-4 hours, up to 8 tablets in a 24-hour period; if no improvement after 48 hours, continued administration is not indicated

Dosage Forms Tablet: Difenoxin hydrochloride 1 mg and atropine sulfate 0.025 mg

Differin® *see* adapalene *on page 11*

diflorasone (dye FLOR a sone)

U.S./Canadian Brand Names Florone®; Florone E®; Maxiflor®; Psorcon™

Therapeutic Category Corticosteroid, Topical

Use Relief of inflammation and pruritic symptoms of corticosteroid-responsive dermatosis

Usual Dosage Topical:

Cream: Apply 2-4 times/day

Ointment: Apply sparingly 1-3 times/day

Dosage Forms Diflorasone diacetate:

Cream: 0.05% (15 g, 30 g, 60 g)

Ointment, topical: 0.05% (15 g, 30 g, 60 g)

Diflucan® *see* fluconazole *on page 241*

diflunisal (dye FLOO ni sal)

U.S./Canadian Brand Names Apo-Diflunisal® (Can); Dolobid®; Novo-Diflunisal (Can); Nu-Diflunisal (Can)

Therapeutic Category Analgesic, Non-narcotic; Nonsteroidal Anti-inflammatory Drug (NSAID)

Use Management of inflammatory disorders usually including rheumatoid arthritis and osteoarthritis; can be used as an analgesic for treatment of mild to moderate pain

Usual Dosage Adults: Oral:

Pain: Initial: 500-1000 mg followed by 250-500 mg every 8-12 hours

Inflammatory condition: 500-1000 mg/day in 2 divided doses

Dosage Forms Tablet: 250 mg, 500 mg

Di-Gel® [OTC] *see* aluminum hydroxide, magnesium hydroxide, and simethicone *on page 23*

Digepepsin® *see* pancreatin *on page 426*

Digess®8000 (Can) *see* pancrelipase *on page 427*

Digibind® *see* digoxin immune Fab *on next page*

Digitaline® (Can) *see* digitoxin *on this page*

digitoxin (di ji TOKS in)

U.S./Canadian Brand Names Crystodigin®; Digitaline® (Can)

Therapeutic Category Antiarrhythmic Agent, Miscellaneous; Cardiac Glycoside

Use Congestive heart failure; atrial fibrillation; atrial flutter; paroxysmal atrial tachycardia; and cardiogenic shock

Usual Dosage Oral:

Children: Doses are very individualized; the maintenance range after neonatal period, the recommended digitalizing dose is as follows:

<1 year: 0.045 mg/kg

1-2 years: 0.04 mg/kg

2 years: 0.03 mg/kg which is equivalent to 0.75 mg/m^2

Maintenance: Approximately $^1/_{10}$ of the digitalizing dose

Adults:

Rapid loading dose: Initial: 0.6 mg followed by 0.4 mg and then 0.2 mg at intervals of 4-6 hours

Slow loading dose: 0.2 mg twice daily for a period of 4 days followed by a maintenance dose

Maintenance: 0.05-0.3 mg/day

Most common dose: 0.15 mg/day

Dosage Forms Tablet: 0.1 mg, 0.2 mg

digoxin (di JOKS in)

U.S./Canadian Brand Names Lanoxicaps®; Lanoxin®; Novo-Digoxin® (Can)

Therapeutic Category Antiarrhythmic Agent, Miscellaneous; Cardiac Glycoside

(Continued)

digoxin *(Continued)*

Use Treatment of congestive heart failure; slows the ventricular rate in tachyarrhythmias such as atrial fibrillation, atrial flutter, supraventricular tachycardia

Usual Dosage Adults (based on lean body weight and normal renal function for age. Decrease dose in patients with decreased renal function)

Total digitalizing dose: Administer ½ as initial dose, then administer ¼ of the total digitalizing dose (TDD) in each of 2 subsequent doses at 8- to 12-hour intervals; obtain EKG 6 hours after each dose to assess potential toxicity

Oral: 0.75-1.5 mg

I.M., I.V.: 0.5-1 mg

Daily maintenance dose:

Oral: 0.125-0.5 mg

I.M., I.V.: 0.1-0.4 mg

Dosage Forms

Capsule: 50 mcg, 100 mcg, 200 mcg

Elixir: 50 mcg/mL with alcohol 10% (60 mL)

Injection: 250 mcg/mL (1 mL, 2 mL)

Injection, pediatric: 100 mcg/mL (1 mL)

Tablet: 125 mcg, 250 mcg, 500 mcg

digoxin immune Fab (di JOKS in i MYUN fab)

Synonyms antidigoxin Fab fragments

U.S./Canadian Brand Names Digibind®

Therapeutic Category Antidote

Use Treatment of potentially life-threatening digoxin or digitoxin intoxication in carefully selected patients

Usual Dosage Each vial of Digibind® will bind approximately 0.5 mg of digoxin or digitoxin

I.V.: To determine the dose of digoxin immune Fab, first determine the total body load of digoxin (TBL using either an approximation of the amount ingested or a postdistribution serum digoxin concentration). If neither ingestion amount or serum level is known: Adult dosage is 20 vials (760 mg) I.V. infusion.

Dosage Forms Powder for injection, lyophilized: 38 mg

Dihistine® DH *see* chlorpheniramine, pseudoephedrine, and codeine *on page 126*

Dihistine® Expectorant *see* guaifenesin, pseudoephedrine, and codeine *on page 272*

dihydrocodeine compound (dye hye droe KOE deen KOM pound)

U.S./Canadian Brand Names DHC Plus®; Synalgos®-DC

Therapeutic Category Analgesic, Narcotic

Controlled Substance C-III

Use Management of mild to moderate pain that requires relaxation

Usual Dosage Adults: Oral: 1-2 capsules every 4-6 hours as needed for pain

Dosage Forms Capsule:

DHC Plus®: Dihydrocodeine bitartrate 16 mg, acetaminophen 356.4 mg, and caffeine 30 mg

Synalgos®-DC: Dihydrocodeine bitartrate 16 mg, aspirin 356.4 mg, and caffeine 30 mg

dihydroergotamine (dye hye droe er GOT a meen)

U.S./Canadian Brand Names D.H.E. 45® Injection; Migranal® Nasal Spray

Therapeutic Category Ergot Alkaloid and Derivative

Use Abort or prevent vascular headaches

Usual Dosage Adults:

I.M.: 1 mg at first sign of headache; repeat hourly to a maximum dose of 3 mg total

I.V.: Up to 2 mg maximum dose for faster effects; maximum dose: 6 mg/week

Intranasal: One spray (0.5 mg) of nasal spray should be administered into each nostril; if the condition has not sufficiently improved approximately fifteen minutes later, an additional spray should be administered to each nostril. The usual dosage required to obtain optimal efficacy is a total dosage of 4 sprays (2 mg); nasal spray is exclusively indicated for the symptomatic treatment of migraine attacks; no more than 4 sprays (2 mg) should be administered for any single migraine attack; an interval of at least 6-8 hours should be observed before treating another migraine attack with the nasal spray or any drug containing dihydroergotamine or ergotamine; no more than 8 sprays (4 mg) (corresponding to the use of 2 ampuls) should be administered during any 24-hour period; the maximum weekly dosage is 24 sprays (12 mg)

Dosage Forms Dihydroergotamine mesylate:

Injection: 1 mg/mL (1 mL)

Spray, nasal: 4 mg/mL [0.5 mg/spray] (1 mL)

dihydroergotoxine *see* ergoloid mesylates *on page 213*

dihydrohydroxycodeinone *see* oxycodone *on page 422*

dihydromorphinone *see* hydromorphone *on page 293*

dihydrotachysterol (dye hye droe tak IS ter ole)

Synonyms dichysterol

U.S./Canadian Brand Names DHT™; Hytakerol®

Therapeutic Category Vitamin D Analog

Use Treatment of hypocalcemia associated with hypoparathyroidism; prophylaxis of hypocalcemic tetany following thyroid surgery; suppress hyperparathyroidism and treat renal osteodystrophy in patients with chronic renal failure

Usual Dosage Oral:

Hypoparathyroidism:

Infants and young Children: 0.1-0.5 mg/day

Older Children and Adults: 0.5-1 mg/day

Nutritional rickets: 0.5 mg as a single dose or 13-50 mcg/day until healing occurs

Renal osteodystrophy: 0.6-6 mg/24 hours; maintenance: 0.25-0.6 mg/24 hours adjusted as necessary to achieve normal serum calcium levels and promote bone healing

Dosage Forms

Capsule (Hytakerol®): 0.125 mg

Solution:

Oral Concentrate (DHT™): 0.2 mg/mL (30 mL)

Oral, in oil (Hytakerol®): 0.25 mg/mL (15 mL)

Tablet (DHT™): 0.125 mg, 0.2 mg, 0.4 mg

dihydroxyaluminum sodium carbonate

(dye hye DROKS i a LOO mi num SOW dee um KAR bun ate)

U.S./Canadian Brand Names Rolaids® [OTC]

Therapeutic Category Antacid

Use Symptomatic relief of upset stomach associated with hyperacidity

Usual Dosage Oral: Chew 1-2 tablets as needed

Dosage Forms Tablet, chewable: 334 mg

1,25 dihydroxycholecalciferol *see* calcitriol *on page 89*

dihydroxypropyl theophylline *see* dyphylline *on page 201*

Dihyrex® Injection *see* diphenhydramine *on page 185*

diiodohydroxyquin *see* iodoquinol *on page 310*

diisopropyl fluorophosphate *see* isoflurophate *on page 314*

Dilacor XR® *see* diltiazem *on next page*

Dilantin® *see* phenytoin *on page 449*

Dilantin-30® Pediatric Suspension *(Discontinued)* *see page 700*

Dilantin® With Phenobarbital *(Discontinued)* *see page 700*

Dilatrate®-SR *see* isosorbide dinitrate *on page 315*

Dilaudid® 1 mg & 3 mg Tablet *(Discontinued)* *see page 700*

Dilaudid® Cough Syrup *see* hydromorphone *on page 293*

Dilaudid-HP® Injection *see* hydromorphone *on page 293*

Dilaudid® Injection *see* hydromorphone *on page 293*

Dilaudid® Oral *see* hydromorphone *on page 293*

Dilaudid® Suppository *see* hydromorphone *on page 293*

Dilocaine® Injection *see* lidocaine *on page 333*

Dilomine® Injection *see* dicyclomine *on page 177*

Dilor® *see* dyphylline *on page 201*

diltiazem (dil TYE a zem)

U.S./Canadian Brand Names Apo®-Diltiaz (Can); Cardizem® CD; Cardizem® Injectable; Cardizem® SR; Cardizem® Tablet; Dilacor XR®; Novo-Diltazem® (Can); Nu-Diltiaz® (Can); Syn-Diltiazem® (Can); Tiamate®; Tiazac®

Therapeutic Category Calcium Channel Blocker

Use

Oral: Hypertension; chronic stable angina or angina from coronary artery spasm

Injection: Atrial fibrillation or atrial flutter; paroxysmal supraventricular tachycardias (PSVT)

Usual Dosage Adults:

Oral: 30-120 mg 3-4 times/day; dosage should be increased gradually, at 1- to 2-day intervals until optimum response is obtained; usual maintenance dose: 240-360 mg/day

Sustained-release capsules (SR): Initial dose of 60-120 mg twice daily

Sustained-release capsules (CD, XR): 180-300 mg once daily

I.V.: Initial: 0.25 mg/kg as a bolus over 2 minutes, then continuous infusion of 5-15 mg/hour for up to 24 hours

Dosage Forms

Capsule, sustained release, as hydrochloride:

Cardizem® CD: 120 mg, 180 mg, 240 mg, 300 mg

Cardizem® SR: 60 mg, 90 mg, 120 mg

Dilacor™ XR: 180 mg, 240 mg

Tiazac™: 120 mg, 180 mg, 240 mg, 300 mg, 360 mg

Injection, as hydrochloride: 5 mg/mL (5 mL, 10 mL)

Cardizem®: 5 mg/mL (5 mL, 10 mL)

Tablet, as hydrochloride (Cardizem®): 30 mg, 60 mg, 90 mg, 120 mg

Tablet, extended release, as hydrochloride (Tiamate®): 120 mg, 180 mg, 240 mg

Dimacol® Caplets [OTC] *see* guaifenesin, pseudoephedrine, and dextromethorphan *on page 273*

Dimaphen® Elixir [OTC] *see* brompheniramine and phenylpropanolamine *on page 81*

Dimaphen® Tablets [OTC] *see* brompheniramine and phenylpropanolamine *on page 81*

dimenhydrinate (dye men HYE dri nate)

U.S./Canadian Brand Names Apo®-Dimenhydrinate (Can); Calm-X® Oral [OTC]; Dimetabs® Oral; Dinate® Injection; Dramamine® Oral [OTC]; Dramilin® Injection; Dymenate® Injection; Gravol® (Can); Hydrate® Injection; Marmine® Injection; Marmine® Oral [OTC]; PMS-Dimenhydrinate (Can); Tega-Vert® Oral; Travel Aid® (Can); Travel Tabs (Can); TripTone® Caplets® [OTC]

Therapeutic Category Antihistamine

Use Treatment and prevention of nausea, vertigo, and vomiting associated with motion sickness

Usual Dosage Oral:
Children:
2-5 years: 12.5-25 mg every 6-8 hours, maximum: 75 mg/day
6-12 years: 25-50 mg every 6-8 hours, maximum: 75 mg/day
or
Alternately: 5 mg/kg/day in 4 divided doses, not to exceed 300 mg/day
Adults: 50-100 mg every 4-6 hours, not to exceed 400 mg/day

Dosage Forms
Capsule: 50 mg
Injection: 50 mg/mL (1 mL, 5 mL, 10 mL)
Liquid: 12.5 mg/4 mL (90 mL, 473 mL); 16.62 mg/5 mL (480 mL)
Tablet: 50 mg
Chewable: 50 mg

dimercaprol (dye mer KAP role)

Synonyms BAL; British anti-lewisite; dithioglycerol
U.S./Canadian Brand Names BAL in Oil®
Therapeutic Category Chelating Agent
Use Antidote to gold, arsenic, and mercury poisoning; adjunct to edetate calcium disodium in lead poisoning
Usual Dosage Children and Adults: I.M.:
Mild arsenic and gold poisoning: 2.5 mg/kg/dose every 6 hours for 2 days, then every 12 hours on the third day, and once daily thereafter for 10 days
Severe arsenic and gold poisoning: 3 mg/kg/dose every 4 hours for 2 days then every 6 hours on the third day, then every 12 hours thereafter for 10 days
Mercury poisoning: Initial: 5 mg/kg followed by 2.5 mg/kg/dose 1-2 times/day for 10 days
Lead poisoning (use with edetate calcium disodium):
Mild: 3 mg/kg/dose every 4 hours for 5-7 days
Severe: 4 mg/kg/dose every 4 hours for 5-7 days
Acute encephalopathy: Initial: 4 mg/kg/dose, then every 4 hours
Dosage Forms Injection: 100 mg/mL (3 mL)

Dimetabs® Oral *see* dimenhydrinate *on previous page*

Dimetane®-DC *see* brompheniramine, phenylpropanolamine, and codeine *on page 82*

Dimetane® Decongestant Elixir [OTC] *see* brompheniramine and phenylephrine *on page 80*

Dimetane® *(Discontinued)* *see page 700*

Dimetane® Extentabs® [OTC] *see* brompheniramine *on page 80*

Dimetapp® 4-Hour Liqui-Gel Capsule [OTC] *see* brompheniramine and phenylpropanolamine *on page 81*

Dimetapp® Elixir [OTC] *see* brompheniramine and phenylpropanolamine *on page 81*

Dimetapp® Extentabs® [OTC] *see* brompheniramine and phenylpropanolamine *on page 81*

Dimetapp® Sinus Caplets [OTC] *see* pseudoephedrine and ibuprofen *on page 487*

Dimetapp® Tablet [OTC] *see* brompheniramine and phenylpropanolamine *on page 81*

β,β-dimethylcysteine *see* penicillamine *on page 433*

dimethyl sulfoxide (dye meth il sul FOKS ide)

Synonyms DMSO
U.S./Canadian Brand Names Rimso®-50
Therapeutic Category Urinary Tract Product
Use Symptomatic relief of interstitial cystitis
(Continued)

dimethyl sulfoxide *(Continued)*

Usual Dosage Instill 50 mL directly into bladder and allow to remain for 15 minutes; repeat every 2 weeks until maximum symptomatic relief is obtained

Dosage Forms Solution: 50% [500 mg/mL] (50 mL)

dimethyl tubocurarine iodide *see* metocurine iodide *on page 371*

Dinate® Injection *see* dimenhydrinate *on page 182*

dinoprostone (dye noe PROST one)

Synonyms PGE_2; prostaglandin E_2

U.S./Canadian Brand Names Cervidil® Vaginal Insert; Prepidil® Vaginal Gel; Prostin E_2® Vaginal Suppository

Therapeutic Category Prostaglandin

Use Terminate pregnancy from 12th through 28th week of gestation; evacuate uterus in cases of missed abortion or intrauterine fetal death; manage benign hydatidiform mole

Usual Dosage Vaginal: Insert 1 suppository high in vagina, repeat at 3- to 5-hour intervals until abortion occurs up to 240 mg (maximum dose)

Dosage Forms

Insert, vaginal (Cervidil®): 10 mg

Gel, vaginal: 0.5 mg in 3 g syringes [each package contains a 10-mm and 20-mm shielded catheter]

Suppository, vaginal: 20 mg

dinoprost tromethamine (DYE noe prost tro METH a meen)

Synonyms $PGF_{2\alpha}$; prostaglandin F_2 alpha

U.S./Canadian Brand Names Prostin F_2 Alpha®

Therapeutic Category Prostaglandin

Use Abort 2nd trimester pregnancy

Usual Dosage 40 mg (8 mL) via transabdominal tap; if abortion not completed in 24 hours, another 10-40 mg may be administered

Dosage Forms Injection: 5 mg/mL (4 mL, 8 mL)

Diocaine(Can) *see* proparacaine *on page 481*

Diocarpine (Can) *see* pilocarpine *on page 451*

Diochloram (Can) *see* chloramphenicol *on page 116*

Diocto® [OTC] *see* docusate *on page 191*

Diocto C® [OTC] *see* docusate and casanthranol *on page 191*

Diocto-K® [OTC] *see* docusate *on page 191*

Diocto-K Plus® [OTC] *see* docusate and casanthranol *on page 191*

Dioctolose Plus® [OTC] *see* docusate and casanthranol *on page 191*

dioctyl calcium sulfosuccinate *see* docusate *on page 191*

dioctyl potassium sulfosuccinate *see* docusate *on page 191*

dioctyl sodium sulfosuccinate *see* docusate *on page 191*

Diodoquin® (Can) *see* iodoquinol *on page 310*

Dioeze® [OTC] *see* docusate *on page 191*

Diomycin (Can) *see* erythromycin (systemic) *on page 215*

Dionephrine (Can) *see* phenylephrine *on page 445*

Dionosil Oily® *see* radiological/contrast media (ionic) *on page 495*

Diotrope (Can) *see* tropicamide *on page 587*

Dioval® Injection *see* estradiol *on page 217*

Diovan™ *see* valsartan *on page 594*

Diovan HCTZ™ *see* valsartan and hydrochlorothiazide *on page 595*

dipalmitoylphosphatidylcholine *see* colfosceril palmitate *on page 145*

Dipentum® *see* olsalazine *on page 415*

Diphenacen-50® Injection [OTC] *see* diphenhydramine *on this page*

Diphen® Cough [OTC] *see* diphenhydramine *on this page*

Diphenhist [OTC] *see* diphenhydramine *on this page*

diphenhydramine (dye fen HYE dra meen)

U.S./Canadian Brand Names Allerdryl® (Can); AllerMax® Oral [OTC]; Allernix® (Can); Banophen® Oral [OTC]; Belix® Oral [OTC]; Benadryl® Injection; Benadryl® Oral [OTC]; Benadryl® Topical; Ben-Allergin-50® Injection; Benylin® Cough Syrup [OTC]; Bydramine® Cough Syrup [OTC]; Compoz® Gel Caps [OTC]; Compoz® Nighttime Sleep Aid [OTC]; Dihyrex® Injection; Diphenacen-50® Injection [OTC]; Diphen® Cough [OTC]; Diphenhist [OTC]; Dormarex® 2 Oral [OTC]; Dormin® Oral [OTC]; Genahist® Oral; Hydramyn® Syrup [OTC]; Hyrexin-50® Injection; Maximum Strength Nytol® [OTC]; Miles Nervine® Caplets [OTC]; Nordryl® Injection; Nordryl® Oral; Nytol® Oral [OTC]; Phendry® Oral [OTC]; Siladryl® Oral [OTC]; Silphen® Cough [OTC]; Sleep-eze 3® Oral [OTC]; Sleepinal® [OTC]; Sleepwell 2-nite® [OTC]; Sominex® Oral [OTC]; Tusstat® Syrup; Twilite® Oral [OTC]; Uni-Bent® Cough Syrup; Winks® [OTC]

Therapeutic Category Antihistamine

Use Symptomatic relief of allergic symptoms caused by histamine release which include nasal allergies and allergic dermatosis; mild nighttime sedation, prevention of motion sickness, as an antitussive; treatment of phenothiazine-induced dystonic reactions

Usual Dosage

Children: Oral, I.M., I.V.: 5 mg/kg/day or 150 mg/m²/day in divided doses every 6-8 hours, not to exceed 300 mg/day

Adults:

- Oral: 25-50 mg every 4-6 hours
- I.M., I.V.: 10-50 mg in a single dose every 2-4 hours, not to exceed 400 mg/day
- Topical: For external application, not longer than 7 days

Dosage Forms Diphenhydramine hydrochloride:

Capsule: 25 mg, 50 mg
Cream: 1%, 2%
Elixir: 12.5 mg/5 mL (5 mL, 10 mL, 20 mL, 120 mL, 480 mL, 3780 mL)
Injection: 10 mg/mL (10 mL, 30 mL); 50 mg/mL (1 mL, 10 mL)
Lotion: 1% (75 mL)
Solution, topical spray: 1% (60 mL)
Syrup: 12.5 mg/5 mL (5 mL, 120 mL, 240 mL, 480 mL, 3780 mL)
Tablet: 25 mg, 50 mg

diphenhydramine and pseudoephedrine

(dye fen HYE dra meen & soo doe e FED rin)

U.S./Canadian Brand Names Actifed® Allergy Tablet (Night) [OTC]; Banophen® Decongestant Capsule [OTC]; Benadryl® Decongestant Allergy Tablet [OTC]

Therapeutic Category Antihistamine/Decongestant Combination

Use Relief of symptoms of upper respiratory mucosal congestion in seasonal and perennial nasal allergies, acute rhinitis, rhinosinusitis, and eustachian tube blockage

Usual Dosage Adults: Oral: 1 capsule or tablet every 4-6 hours, up to 4/day

Dosage Forms

Capsule: Diphenhydramine hydrochloride 25 mg and pseudoephedrine hydrochloride 60 mg

Tablet:

- Actifed® Allergy (Night): Diphenhydramine hydrochloride 25 mg and pseudoephedrine hydrochloride 30 mg
- Benadryl® Decongestant Allergy: Diphenhydramine hydrochloride 25 mg and pseudoephedrine hydrochloride 60 mg

diphenoxylate and atropine (dye fen OKS i late & A troe peen)

Synonyms atropine and diphenoxylate

U.S./Canadian Brand Names Logen®; Lomanate®; Lomotil®; Lonox®

Therapeutic Category Antidiarrheal

Controlled Substance C-V

Use Treatment of diarrhea

Usual Dosage Oral (as diphenoxylate): Initial dose:

Children: 0.3-0.4 mg/kg/day in 2-4 divided doses
- <2 years: Not recommended
- 2-5 years: 2 mg 3 times/day
- 5-8 years: 2 mg 4 times/day
- 8-12 years: 2 mg 5 times/day

Adults: 15-20 mg/day in 3-4 divided doses

Reduce dosage as soon as initial control of symptoms is achieved

Dosage Forms

Solution, oral: Diphenoxylate hydrochloride 2.5 mg and atropine sulfate 0.025 mg per 5 mL (4 mL, 10 mL, 60 mL)

Tablet: Diphenoxylate hydrochloride 2.5 mg and atropine sulfate 0.025 mg

Diphenylan Sodium® *see* phenytoin *on page 449*

diphenylhydantoin *see* phenytoin *on page 449*

diphtheria and tetanus toxoid (dif THEER ee a & TET a nus TOKS oyd)

Synonyms DT; Td; tetanus and diphtheria toxoid

Therapeutic Category Toxoid

Use Active immunity against diphtheria and tetanus

Usual Dosage I.M.:

Infants and Children:
- 6 weeks to 1 year: Three 0.5 mL doses at least 4 weeks apart; administer a reinforcing dose 6-12 months after the third injection
- 1-6 years: Administer two 0.5 mL doses at least 4 weeks apart; reinforcing dose 6-12 months after second injection; if final dose is administered after seventh birthday, use adult preparation
- 4-6 years (booster immunization): 0.5 mL; not necessary if all 4 doses were administered after fourth birthday - routinely administer booster doses at 10-year intervals with the adult preparation

Children >7 years and Adults: 2 primary doses of 0.5 mL each, administered at an interval of 4-6 weeks; third (reinforcing) dose of 0.5 mL 6-12 months later; boosters every 10 years

Dosage Forms Injection:

Pediatric use:
- Diphtheria 6.6 Lf units and tetanus 5 Lf units per 0.5 mL (5 mL)
- Diphtheria 10 Lf units and tetanus 5 Lf units per 0.5 mL (0.5 mL, 5 mL)
- Diphtheria 12.5 Lf units and tetanus 5 Lf units per 0.5 mL (5 mL)
- Diphtheria 15 Lf units and tetanus 10 Lf units per 0.5 mL (5 mL)

Adult use:
- Diphtheria 1.5 Lf units and tetanus 5 Lf units per 0.5 mL (0.5 mL, 5 mL)
- Diphtheria 2 Lf units and tetanus 5 Lf units per 0.5 mL (5 mL)
- Diphtheria 2 Lf units and tetanus 10 Lf units per 0.5 mL (5 mL)

diphtheria antitoxin (dif THEER ee a an tee TOKS in)

Therapeutic Category Antitoxin

Use Passive prevention and treatment of diphtheria

Usual Dosage I.M. or slow I.V. infusion: Dosage varies; range: 20,000-120,000 units

Dosage Forms Injection: 500 units/mL (20 mL, 40 mL)

diphtheria, tetanus toxoids, and acellular pertussis vaccine

(dif THEER ee a, TET a nus TOKS oyds & ay CEL yoo lar per TUS sis vak SEEN)

Synonyms DTAP

U.S./Canadian Brand Names Acel-Imune®; Certiva®; Infanrix™; Tripedia®

Therapeutic Category Toxoid

Use Fourth or fifth immunization of children 15 months to 7 years of age (prior to seventh birthday) who have been previously immunized with 3 or 4 doses of whole-cell pertussis DTP vaccine

Usual Dosage I.M.: After at least 3 doses of whole-cell DTP, administer 0.5 mL at ~18 months (at least 6 months after third DTWP dose), then another dose at 4-5 years of age

Dosage Forms Injection:

Acel-Imune®: Diphtheria 7.5 Lf units, tetanus 5 Lf units, and acellular pertussis vaccine 40 mcg per 0.5 mL (7.5 mL)

Certiva®: Diphtheria 15 Lf units, tetanus 6 Lf units, and acellular pertussis vaccine 40 mcg per 0.5 mL (7.5 mL)

Infanrix™: Diphtheria 25 Lf units, tetanus 10 Lf units, and acellular pertussis vaccine 25 mcg per 0.5 mL (7.5 mL)

Tripedia®: Diphtheria 6.7 Lf units, tetanus 5 Lf units, and acellular pertussis vaccine 46.8 mcg per 0.5 mL (7.5 mL)

diphtheria, tetanus toxoids, and whole-cell pertussis vaccine

(dif THEER ee a & TET a nus TOKS oyds & hole-sel per TUS sis vak SEEN)

Synonyms DPT

U.S./Canadian Brand Names Tri-Immunol®

Therapeutic Category Toxoid

Use Active immunization of infants and children through 6 years of age (between 2 months and the seventh birthday) against diphtheria, tetanus, and pertussis; recommended for both primary immunization and routine recall; start immunization at once if whooping cough or diphtheria is present in the community

Usual Dosage The primary immunization for children 2 months to 6 years of age, ideally beginning at the age of 2-3 months or at 6-week check-up. Administer 0.5 mL I.M. on 3 occasions at 4- to 8-week intervals with a re-enforcing dose administered 1 year after the third injection. The booster doses (0.5 mL I.M.) are administered when the child is 4-6 years of age.

Dosage Forms Injection:

Diphtheria 6.7 Lf units, tetanus 5 Lf units, and pertussis 4 protective units per 0.5 mL (7.5 mL)

Tri-Immunol®: Diphtheria 12.5 Lf units, tetanus 5 Lf units, and pertussis 4 protective units per 0.5 mL (7.5 mL)

diphtheria, tetanus toxoids, whole-cell pertussis, and *Haemophilus* B conjugate vaccine

(dif THEER ee a, TET a nus TOKS oyds, hole-sel per TUS sis, & hem OF fil us bee KON joo gate vak SEEN)

Synonyms DTwP-HIB

U.S./Canadian Brand Names Tetramune®

Therapeutic Category Toxoid

Use Active immunization of infants and children through 5 years of age (between 2 months and the sixth birthday) against diphtheria, tetanus, and pertussis and *Haemophilus* B disease when indications for immunization with DTP vaccine and HIB vaccine coincide

Usual Dosage The primary immunization for children 2 months to 5 years of age, ideally beginning at the age of 2-3 months or at 6-week check-up; administer 0.5 mL I.M. on 3 occasions at ~2 month intervals, followed by a fourth 0.5 mL dose at ~15 months of age

Dosage Forms Injection: Diphtheria toxoid 12.5 Lf units, tetanus toxoid 5 Lf units, and whole-cell pertussis vaccine 4 units, and *Haemophilus influenzae* type B oligosaccharide 10 mcg per 0.5 mL (5 mL)

dipivalyl epinephrine *see* dipivefrin *on next page*

dipivefrin (dye PI ve frin)

Synonyms dipivalyl epinephrine; DPE

U.S./Canadian Brand Names DPE™ (Can); Optho-Dipivefrin™ (Can); Propine®

Therapeutic Category Adrenergic Agonist Agent

Use Reduces elevated intraocular pressure in chronic open-angle glaucoma; treatment of ocular hypertension

Usual Dosage Adults: Ophthalmic: Initial: 1 drop every 12 hours

Dosage Forms Solution, ophthalmic, as hydrochloride: 0.1% (5 mL, 10 mL, 15 mL)

Diprivan® *see* propofol *on page 481*

Diprolene® AF Topical *see* betamethasone (topical) *on page 72*

Diprolene® Glycol (Can) *see* betamethasone (topical) *on page 72*

Diprolene® Topical *see* betamethasone (topical) *on page 72*

dipropylacetic acid *see* valproic acid and derivatives *on page 594*

Diprosone® Topical *see* betamethasone (topical) *on page 72*

dipyridamole (dye peer ID a mole)

U.S./Canadian Brand Names Apo®-Dipyridamole FC (Can); Apo®-Dipyridamole SC (Can); Asasantine® [with Aspirin also] (Can); Novo-Dipiradol® (Can); Persantine®

Therapeutic Category Antiplatelet Agent; Vasodilator

Use Maintain patency after surgical grafting procedures including coronary artery bypass; with warfarin to decrease thrombosis in patients after artificial heart valve replacement; for chronic management of angina pectoris; with aspirin to prevent coronary artery thrombosis; in combination with aspirin or warfarin to prevent other thromboembolic disorders; dipyridamole may also be administered 2 days prior to open heart surgery to prevent platelet activation by extracorporeal bypass pump; diagnostic agent I.V. (dipyridamole stress test) for coronary artery disease

Usual Dosage

Children: Oral: 3-6 mg/kg/day in 3 divided doses

Dipyridamole stress test (for evaluation of myocardial perfusion): I.V.: 0.14 mg/kg/minute for a total of 4 minutes

Adults: Oral: 75-400 mg/day in 3-4 divided doses

Dosage Forms

Injection: 10 mg/2 mL

Tablet: 25 mg, 50 mg, 75 mg

dipyridamole and aspirin *(Canada only)* (dye peer ID a mole & AS pir in)

U.S./Canadian Brand Names Asasantine® (Can)

Therapeutic Category Antiplatelet Agent

Use Combined therapy with dipyridamole and aspirin is indicated in patients who are recovering from a myocardial infarction; the rate of reinfarction is significantly reduced by such therapy; combined treatment is also indicated for the prevention of occlusion of saphenous vein coronary artery bypass grafts

Usual Dosage Adults: Oral:

Prevention of recurrent myocardial infarction: The recommended oral dose is one capsule 3 times/day, in patients who have suffered a previous myocardial infarction

Prevention of occlusion of saphenous vein coronary artery bypass grafts:

For 2 days preoperatively: Dipyridamole 100 mg four times/day;

Day of surgery: Morning of operation: Dipyridamole 100 mg; 1 hour post-op: Dipyridamole 100 mg (via nasogastric tube); 7 hours post-op: Asasantine® capsule; daily maintenance dosage: (for the next 12 months): One Asasantine® capsule three times/daily

Dosage Forms Capsule: Dipyridamole 75 mg and aspirin 330 mg

dirithromycin (dye RITH roe mye sin)

U.S./Canadian Brand Names Dynabac®

Therapeutic Category Macrolide (Antibiotic)

Use Treatment of mild to moderate upper and lower respiratory tract infections, infections of the skin and skin structure, and sexually transmitted diseases due to susceptible strains

Usual Dosage Adults: Oral: 500 mg once daily for 7-14 days

Dosage Forms Tablet, enteric coated: 250 mg

Disalcid® *see* salsalate *on page 515*

disalicylic acid *see* salsalate *on page 515*

Disanthrol® [OTC] *see* docusate and casanthranol *on page 191*

Disobrom® [OTC] *see* dexbrompheniramine and pseudoephedrine *on page 168*

disodium cromoglycate *see* cromolyn sodium *on page 150*

***d*-isoephedrine** *see* pseudoephedrine *on page 486*

Disonate® [OTC] *see* docusate *on page 191*

Disophrol® Chronotabs® [OTC] *see* dexbrompheniramine and pseudoephedrine *on page 168*

Disophrol® Tablet [OTC] *see* dexbrompheniramine and pseudoephedrine *on page 168*

disopyramide (dye soe PEER a mide)

U.S./Canadian Brand Names Norpace®; Norpace® CR; Rythmodan®, -LA (Can)

Therapeutic Category Antiarrhythmic Agent, Class I-A

Use Suppression and prevention of unifocal and multifocal ventricular premature complexes, coupled ventricular premature complexes, and/or paroxysmal ventricular tachycardia; also effective in the conversion and prevention of recurrence of atrial fibrillation, atrial flutter, and paroxysmal atrial tachycardia

Usual Dosage Oral:

Children:

<1 year: 10-30 mg/kg/24 hours in 4 divided doses
1-4 years: 10-20 mg/kg/24 hours in 4 divided doses
4-12 years: 10-15 mg/kg/24 hours in 4 divided doses
12-18 years: 6-15 mg/kg/24 hours in 4 divided doses

Adults:

<50 kg: 100 mg every 6 hours or 200 mg every 12 hours (controlled release)
>50 kg: 150 mg every 6 hours or 300 mg every 12 hours (controlled release); if no response, may increase to 200 mg every 6 hours; maximum dose required for patients with severe refractory ventricular tachycardia is 400 mg every 6 hours

Dosage Forms Disopyramide phosphate:

Capsule: 100 mg, 150 mg
Capsule, sustained action: 100 mg, 150 mg

Disotate® *see* edetate disodium *on page 203*

Di-Spaz® Injection *see* dicyclomine *on page 177*

Di-Spaz® Oral *see* dicyclomine *on page 177*

Dispos-a-Med® Isoproterenol *(Discontinued)* *see page 700*

Distaval® *see* thalidomide *on page 557*

disulfiram (dye SUL fi ram)

U.S./Canadian Brand Names Antabuse®

Therapeutic Category Aldehyde Dehydrogenase Inhibitor Agent

Use Management of chronic alcoholics

Usual Dosage Oral:

Maximum daily dose: 500 mg/day in a single dose for 1-2 weeks

(Continued)

disulfiram *(Continued)*

Average maintenance dose: 250 mg/day; range: 125-500 mg; duration of therapy is to continue until the patient is fully recovered socially and a basis for permanent self control has been established; maintenance therapy may be required for months or even years

Dosage Forms Tablet: 250 mg, 500 mg

Dital® *see* phendimetrazine *on page 442*

dithioglycerol *see* dimercaprol *on page 183*

dithranol *see* anthralin *on page 38*

Ditropan® *see* oxybutynin *on page 422*

Ditropan® XL *see* oxybutynin *on page 422*

Diucardin® *see* hydroflumethiazide *on page 293*

Diuchlor® (Can) *see* hydrochlorothiazide *on page 286*

Diupress® *(Discontinued)* *see page 700*

Diurigen® *see* chlorothiazide *on page 119*

Diuril® *see* chlorothiazide *on page 119*

Dixarit® (Can) *see* clonidine *on page 139*

Dizac® Injectable Emulsion *see* diazepam *on page 173*

Dizmiss® [OTC] *see* meclizine *on page 351*

Dizymes® Tablet *(Discontinued)* *see page 700*

***dl*-alpha tocopherol** *see* vitamin E *on page 604*

***dl*-norephedrine** *see* phenylpropanolamine *on page 447*

***d*-mannitol** *see* mannitol *on page 347*

4-dmdr *see* idarubicin *on page 301*

D-Med® Injection *see* methylprednisolone *on page 368*

DMSO *see* dimethyl sulfoxide *on page 183*

DNASE *see* dornase alfa *on page 194*

DNR *see* daunorubicin hydrochloride *on page 160*

Doan's®, Original [OTC] *see* magnesium salicylate *on page 346*

dobutamine (doe BYOO ta meen)

U.S./Canadian Brand Names Dobutrex®

Therapeutic Category Adrenergic Agonist Agent

Use Short-term management of patients with cardiac decompensation

Usual Dosage I.V. infusion:

Children: 2.5-15 mcg/kg/minute, titrate to desired response

Adults: 2.5-15 mcg/kg/minute; maximum: 40 mcg/kg/minute, titrate to desired response

Dosage Forms Infusion, as hydrochloride: 12.5 mg/mL (20 mL)

Dobutrex® *see* dobutamine *on this page*

docetaxel (doe se TAKS el)

U.S./Canadian Brand Names Taxotere®

Therapeutic Category Antineoplastic Agent

Use Treatment of breast cancer

Usual Dosage Adults: I.V.: 60-100 mg/m^2 administered over 1 hour every 3 weeks

Dosage Forms Injection: 40 mg/mL (0.5 mL, 2 mL)

docusate (DOK yoo sate)

Synonyms dioctyl calcium sulfosuccinate; dioctyl potassium sulfosuccinate; dioctyl sodium sulfosuccinate; DOSS; DSS

U.S./Canadian Brand Names Albert® Docusate (Can); Colace® [OTC]; Colax-C® (Can); DC 240® Softgel® [OTC]; Dialose® Tablet [OTC]; Diocto® [OTC]; Diocto-K® [OTC]; Dioeze® [OTC]; Disonate® [OTC]; DOK® [OTC]; DOS® Softgel® [OTC]; D-S-S® [OTC]; Kasof® [OTC]; Modane® Soft [OTC]; PMS-Docusate Calcium (Can); Pro-Cal-Sof® [OTC]; Regulax SS® [OTC]; Regulex® (Can); Selax® (Can); Soflax™ (Can); Sulfalax® [OTC]; Surfak® [OTC]

Therapeutic Category Stool Softener

Use Stool softener in patients who should avoid straining during defecation and constipation associated with hard, dry stools

Usual Dosage Docusate salts are interchangeable; the amount of sodium, calcium, or potassium per dosage unit is clinically insignificant

Infants and Children <3 years: Oral: 10-40 mg/day in 1-4 divided doses
Children: Oral:
- 3-6 years: 20-60 mg/day in 1-4 divided doses
- 6-12 years: 40-150 mg/day in 1-4 divided doses

Adolescents and Adults: Oral: 50-500 mg/day in 1-4 divided doses
Older Children and Adults: Rectal: Add 50-100 mg of docusate liquid to enema fluid (saline or water); administer as retention or flushing enema

Dosage Forms

Capsule:
- As calcium:
  - DC 240® Softgels®, Pro-Cal-Sof®, Sulfalax®: 240 mg
  - Surfak®: 50 mg, 240 mg
- As potassium:
  - Diocto-K®: 100 mg
  - Kasof®: 240 mg
- As sodium:
  - Colace®: 50 mg, 100 mg
  - Dioeze®: 250 mg
  - Disonate®: 100 mg, 240 mg
  - DOK®: 100 mg, 250 mg
  - DOS® Softgel®: 100 mg, 250 mg
  - D-S-S®: 100 mg
  - Modane® Soft: 100 mg
  - Regulax SS®: 100 mg, 250 mg

Liquid, as sodium (Diocto®, Colace®, Disonate®, DOK®): 150 mg/15 mL (30 mL, 60 mL, 480 mL)
Solution, oral, as sodium (Doxinate®): 50 mg/mL with alcohol 5% (60 mL, 3780 mL)
Syrup, as sodium:
- 50 mg/15 mL (15 mL, 30 mL)
- Colace®, Diocto®, Disonate®, DOK®: 60 mg/15 mL (240 mL, 480 mL, 3780 mL)

Tablet, as sodium: 100 mg

docusate and casanthranol (DOK yoo sate & ka SAN thra nole)

Synonyms casanthranol and docusate; DSS with casanthranol

U.S./Canadian Brand Names Dialose® Plus Capsule [OTC]; Diocto C® [OTC]; Diocto-K Plus® [OTC]; Dioctolose Plus® [OTC]; Disanthrol® [OTC]; DSMC Plus® [OTC]; Genasoft® Plus [OTC]; Peri-Colace® [OTC]; Pro-Sof® Plus [OTC]; Regulace® [OTC]; Silace-C® [OTC]

Therapeutic Category Laxative/Stool Softner

Use Treatment of constipation generally associated with dry, hard stools and decreased intestinal motility

Usual Dosage Oral:

Children: 5-15 mL of syrup at bedtime or 1 capsule at bedtime

(Continued)

docusate and casanthranol *(Continued)*

Adults: 1-2 capsules or 15-30 mL syrup at bedtime, may be increased to 2 capsules or 30 mL twice daily or 3 capsules at bedtime

Dosage Forms

Capsule:

Dialose® Plus, Diocto-K Plus®, Dioctolose Plus®, DSMC Plus®: Docusate potassium 100 mg and casanthranol 30 mg

Disanthrol®, Genasoft® Plus, Peri-Colace®, Pro-Sof® Plus, Regulace®: Docusate sodium 100 mg and casanthranol 30 mg

Syrup (Diocto C®, Peri-Colace®, Silace-C®): Docusate sodium 60 mg and casanthranol 30 mg per 15 mL with alcohol 10% (240 mL, 480 mL, 4000 mL)

DOK® [OTC] *see* docusate *on previous page*

Doktors® Nasal Solution [OTC] *see* phenylephrine *on page 445*

Dolacet® *see* hydrocodone and acetaminophen *on page 287*

dolasetron (dol A se tron)

U.S./Canadian Brand Names Anzemet®

Therapeutic Category Selective 5-HT_3 Receptor Antagonist

Use The prevention of nausea and vomiting associated with moderately emetogenic cancer chemotherapy, including initial and repeat courses; the prevention of postoperative nausea and vomiting.

Usual Dosage

Oral:

Prevention of cancer chemotherapy-induced nausea and vomiting:

Children 2-16 years: 1.8 mg/kg given within 1 hour before chemotherapy, up to a maximum of 100 mg; safety and effectiveness in pediatric patients <2 years of age have not been established

Adults: 100 mg given within 1 hour before chemotherapy

Use in the elderly, renal failure patients, or hepatically impaired patients: No dosage adjustment is recommended

Prevention of postoperative nausea and vomiting:

Children 2-16 years: 1.2 mg/kg given within 2 hours before surgery, up to a maximum of 100 mg; safety and effectiveness in pediatric patients <2 years of age have not been established

Adults: 100 mg within 2 hours before surgery

Use in the elderly, renal failure patients, or hepatically impaired patients: No dosage adjustment is recommended

Parenteral (injection):

Prevention of cancer chemotherapy-induced nausea and vomiting:

Children 2-16 years: 1.8 mg/kg given as a single dose approximately 30 minutes before chemotherapy, up to a maximum of 100 mg; safety and effectiveness in pediatric patients <2 years of age have not been established. Injection mixed in apple or apple-grape juice may be used for oral dosing of pediatric patients. When injection is administered orally, the recommended dosage in pediatric patients 2-16 years of age is 1.8 mg/kg up to a maximum 100 mg dose given within 1 hour before chemotherapy. The diluted product may be kept up to 2 hours at room temperature before use.

Adults: From clinical trials, the dose is 1.8 mg/kg given as a single dose approximately 30 minutes before chemotherapy; alternatively, for most patients, a fixed dose of 100 mg can be administered over 30 seconds

Use in the elderly, renal failure patients, or hepatically impaired patients: No dosage adjustment is recommended

Prevention of postoperative nausea and/or vomiting:

Children 2-16 years: 0.35 mg/kg, with a maximum dose of 12.5 mg, given as a single dose approximately 15 minutes before the cessation of anesthesia or as soon as nausea or vomiting presents. Safety and effectiveness in pediatric patients <2 years of age have not been established. Injection mixed in apple or apple-grape juice may be used for oral dosing of pediatric patients; dosage in pediatric patients 2-16 years is 1.2 mg/kg up to a maximum 100 mg dose given before surgery.

Adults: 12.5 mg given as a single dose approximately 15 minutes before the cessation of anesthesia (prevention) or as soon as nausea or vomiting presents (treatment)

Dosage Forms Dolasetron mesylate:

Injection: 20 mg/mL

Tablet: 50 mg, 100 mg

Dolene® *see* propoxyphene *on page 482*

Dolobid® *see* diflunisal *on page 179*

Dolophine® *see* methadone *on page 361*

Dolorac™ [OTC] *see* capsaicin *on page 96*

Domeboro® Topical [OTC] *see* aluminum acetate and calcium acetate *on page 22*

Dommanate® Injection *(Discontinued)* *see page 700*

domperidone *(Canada only)* (dom PE ri done)

U.S./Canadian Brand Names Motilium® (Can)

Therapeutic Category Dopamine Antagonist

Use Symptomatic management of upper gastrointestinal motility disorders associated with chronic and subacute gastritis and diabetic gastroparesis; may also be used to prevent gastrointestinal symptoms associated with the use of dopamine agonist anti-Parkinsonian's agents

Usual Dosage Adults: Oral:

Upper gastrointestinal motility disorders: Usual dosage in adults: 10 mg 3-4 times/day, 15-30 minutes before meals and at bedtime if required. In severe or resistant cases the dose may be increased to a maximum of 20 mg 3-4 times/day.

Nausea and vomiting associated with dopamine agonist anti-Parkinsonian's agents: Usual dosage in adults: 20 mg 3-4 times/day. Higher doses may be required to achieve symptom control while titration of the antiparkinsonian medication is occurring.

donepezil (don EH pa zil)

Synonyms E2020

U.S./Canadian Brand Names Aricept®

Therapeutic Category Acetylcholinesterase Inhibitor

Use Treatment of mild to moderate dementia of the Alzheimer's type

Usual Dosage Adults: Oral: Initial: 5 mg at bedtime; may be increased to 10 mg at bedtime after 4-6 weeks; a 10 mg dose may provide additional benefit for some patients

Dosage Forms Tablet: 5 mg, 10 mg

Donnagel®-MB (Can) *see* kaolin and pectin *on page 318*

Donnamar® *see* hyoscyamine *on page 297*

Donnapectolin-PG® *see* hyoscyamine, atropine, scopolamine, kaolin, pectin, and opium *on page 299*

Donnatal® *see* hyoscyamine, atropine, scopolamine, and phenobarbital *on page 298*

Donnazyme® *see* pancreatin *on page 426*

Donphen® Tablet *(Discontinued)* *see page 700*

Dopamet® (Can) *see* methyldopa *on page 367*

dopamine (DOE pa meen)

U.S./Canadian Brand Names Intropin®

Therapeutic Category Adrenergic Agonist Agent

Use Adjunct in the treatment of shock which persists after adequate fluid volume replacement

(Continued)

dopamine *(Continued)*

Usual Dosage I.V. infusion:

Children: 1-20 mcg/kg/minute, maximum: 50 mcg/kg/minute continuous infusion, titrate to desired response

Adults: 1 mcg/kg/minute up to 50 mcg/kg/minute, titrate to desired response

If dosages >20-30 mcg/kg/minute are needed, a more direct acting pressor may be more beneficial (ie, epinephrine, norepinephrine)

Hemodynamic effects of dopamine are dose-dependent:

- Low-dose: 1-5 mcg/kg/minute, increased renal blood flow and urine output
- Intermediate-dose: 5-15 mcg/kg/minute, increased renal blood flow, heart rate, cardiac contractility, and cardiac output
- High-dose: >15 mcg/kg/minute, alpha-adrenergic effects begin to predominate, vasoconstriction, increased blood pressure

Dosage Forms Dopamine hydrochloride:

Infusion in D_5W: 0.8 mg/mL (250 mL, 500 mL); 1.6 mg/mL (250 mL, 500 mL); 3.2 mg/mL (250 mL, 500 mL)

Injection: 40 mg/mL (5 mL, 10 mL, 20 mL); 80 mg/mL (5 mL, 20 mL); 160 mg/mL (5 mL)

Dopar® *see* levodopa *on page 331*

Dopastat® Injection *(Discontinued)* *see page 700*

Dopram® *see* doxapram *on next page*

Doral® *see* quazepam *on page 491*

Dorcol® [OTC] *see* acetaminophen *on page 3*

Doriden® Tablet *(Discontinued)* *see page 700*

Dormarex® 2 Oral [OTC] *see* diphenhydramine *on page 185*

Dormin® Oral [OTC] *see* diphenhydramine *on page 185*

dornase alfa (DOOR nase AL fa)

Synonyms DNASE; recombinant human deoxyribonuclease

U.S./Canadian Brand Names Pulmozyme®

Therapeutic Category Enzyme

Use Management of cystic fibrosis patients to reduce the frequency of respiratory infections and to improve pulmonary function

Usual Dosage Children >5 years and Adults: Inhalation: 2.5 mg once daily through selected nebulizers in conjunction with a Pulmo-Aide® or a Pari-Proneb® compressor

Dosage Forms Solution, inhalation: 1 mg/mL (2.5 mL)

Doryx® *see* doxycycline *on page 197*

dorzolamide (dor ZOLE a mide)

U.S./Canadian Brand Names Trusopt®

Therapeutic Category Carbonic Anhydrase Inhibitor

Use Lower intraocular pressure to treat glaucoma

Usual Dosage Adults: Ophthalmic: 1 drop in eye(s) 3 times/day

Dosage Forms Solution, ophthalmic, as hydrochloride: 2%

dorzolamide and timolol (dor ZOLE a mide & TYE moe lole)

U.S./Canadian Brand Names Cosopt™

Therapeutic Category Beta-Adrenergic Blocker; Carbonic Anhydrase Inhibitor

Use Lowers intraocular pressure to treat glaucoma in patients with ocular hypertension or open-angle glaucoma

Usual Dosage Adults: ophthalmic: One drop in eye(s) twice daily

Dosage Forms Solution, ophthalmic: Dorzolamide 2% and timolol 0.5% (5 mL, 10 mL)

DOSS *see* docusate *on page 191*

DOS® Softgel® [OTC] *see* docusate *on page 191*

Dostinex® *see* cabergoline *on page 87*

Dovonex® *see* calcipotriene *on page 88*

doxacurium (doks a KYOO ri um)

U.S./Canadian Brand Names Nuromax®

Therapeutic Category Skeletal Muscle Relaxant

Use Doxacurium is indicated for use as an adjunct to general anesthesia. It provides skeletal muscle relaxation during surgery or endotracheal intubation; increases pulmonary compliance during mechanical ventilation

Usual Dosage I.V. (in obese patients, use ideal body weight to calculate dosage):

Children >2 years: Initial: 0.03-0.05 mg/kg followed by maintenance doses of 0.005-0.01 mg/kg after 30-45 minutes

Adults: Surgery: 0.05 mg/kg with thiopental/narcotic or 0.025 mg/kg with succinylcholine; maintenance dose: 0.005-0.01 mg/kg after 60-100 minutes

Dosage Forms Injection, as chloride: 1 mg/mL (5 mL)

doxapram (DOKS a pram)

U.S./Canadian Brand Names Dopram®

Therapeutic Category Respiratory Stimulant

Use Respiratory and CNS stimulant; idiopathic apnea of prematurity refractory to xanthines

Usual Dosage I.V.:

Neonatal apnea (apnea of prematurity):

Initial: 0.5 mg/kg/hour

Maintenance: 0.5-2.5 mg/kg/hour, titrated to the lowest rate at which apnea is controlled

Adults: Respiratory depression following anesthesia:

Initial: 0.5-1 mg/kg; may repeat at 5-minute intervals; maximum total dose: 2 mg/kg; single doses should not exceed 1.5 mg/kg

I.V. infusion: Initial: 5 mg/minute until adequate response or adverse effects seen; decrease to 1-3 mg/minute; usual total dose: 0.5-4 mg/kg; maximum: 300 mg

Dosage Forms Injection, as hydrochloride: 20 mg/mL (20 mL)

doxazosin (doks AYE zoe sin)

U.S./Canadian Brand Names Cardura®

Therapeutic Category Alpha-Adrenergic Blocking Agent

Use Alpha-adrenergic blocking agent for treatment of hypertension

Usual Dosage Adults: Oral: 1 mg once daily, may be increased to 2 mg once daily thereafter up to 16 mg if needed

Dosage Forms Tablet: 1 mg, 2 mg, 4 mg, 8 mg

doxepin (DOKS e pin)

U.S./Canadian Brand Names Adapin® Oral; Apo®-Doxepin (Can); Novo-Doxepin® (Can); Sinequan® Oral; Triadapin® (Can); Zonalon® Topical Cream

Therapeutic Category Antidepressant, Tricyclic (Tertiary Amine); Topical Skin Product

Use

Oral: Treatment of various forms of depression, usually in conjunction with psychotherapy; treatment of anxiety disorders; analgesic for certain chronic and neuropathic pain

Topical: Adults: Short-term (<8 days) therapy of moderate pruritus due to atopic dermatitis or lichen simplex chronicus

Usual Dosage

Oral:

Adolescents: Initial: 25-50 mg/day in single or divided doses; gradually increase to 100 mg/day

(Continued)

doxepin *(Continued)*

Adults: Initial: 30-150 mg/day at bedtime or in 2-3 divided doses; may increase up to 300 mg/day; single dose should not exceed 150 mg; select patients may respond to 25-50 mg/day

Topical: Apply in a thin film 4 times/day

Dosage Forms Doxepin hydrochloride:

Capsule: 10 mg, 25 mg, 50 mg, 75 mg, 100 mg, 150 mg

Concentrate, oral: 10 mg/mL (120 mL)

Cream (Zonalon®): 5% (30 g)

doxercalciferol (dox er kal si fe FEER ole)

U.S./Canadian Brand Names Hectorol®

Therapeutic Category Vitamin D Analog

Use Reduction of elevated intact parathyroid hormone (iPTH) in the management of secondary hyperparathyroidism in patients on chronic hemodialysis.

Usual Dosage

Adults: Oral: If the iPTH >400 pg/mL, then the initial dose is 10 mcg 3 times/week at dialysis. The dose is adjusted at 8-week intervals based upon the iPTH levels. If the iPTH level is decreased by 50% and above 300 pg/mL, then the dose can be increased to 12.5 mcg 3 times/week for 8 more weeks. This titration process can continue at 8-week intervals up to a maximum dose of 20 mcg 3 times/week. Each increase should be by 2.5 mcg/dose. If the iPTH is between 150-300 pg/mL, maintain the current dose. If the iPTH is <100 pg/mL, then suspend the drug for 1 week. Resume doxercalciferol at a reduced dose. Decrease each dose (not weekly dose) by at least 2.5 mcg.

Dosage Forms Capsule: 2.5 mcg

Doxil® *see* doxorubicin (liposomal) *on this page*

Doxinate® Capsule *(Discontinued)* *see page 700*

doxorubicin (doks oh ROO bi sin)

Synonyms ADR; hydroxydaunomycin

U.S./Canadian Brand Names Adriamycin PFS™; Adriamycin RDF®; Rubex®

Therapeutic Category Antineoplastic Agent

Use Treatment of various solid tumors including ovarian, breast, and bladder tumors; various lymphomas and leukemias (ANL, ALL), soft tissue sarcomas, neuroblastoma, osteosarcoma

Usual Dosage I.V. (refer to individual protocols; patient's ideal weight should be used to calculate body surface area):

Children: 35-75 mg/m^2 as a single dose, repeat every 21 days; or 20 mg/m^2 once weekly

Adults: 60-75 mg/m^2 as a single dose, repeat every 21 days or other dosage regimens like 20-30 mg/m^2/day for 2-3 days, repeat in 4 weeks or 20 mg/m^2 once weekly

The lower dose regimen should be administered to patients with decreased bone marrow reserve, prior therapy or marrow infiltration with malignant cells

Dosage Forms Doxorubicin hydrochloride:

Aqueous injection with NS: 2 mg/mL (5 mL, 10 mL, 25 mL)

Preservative free injection: 2 mg/mL (5 mL, 10 mL, 25 mL, 100 mL)

Powder for injection, lyophilized: 10 mg, 20 mg, 50 mg, 100 mg

Powder for injection, lyophilized, rapid dissolution formula: 10 mg, 20 mg, 50 mg, 150 mg

doxorubicin (liposomal) (doks oh ROO bi sin lip pah SOW mal)

U.S./Canadian Brand Names Doxil®

Therapeutic Category Antineoplastic Agent

Use Treatment of AIDS-related Kaposi's sarcoma in patients with disease that has progressed on prior combination chemotherapy or in patients who are intolerant to such therapy

Usual Dosage I.V. (refer to individual protocols; patient's ideal weight should be used to calculate body surface area): I.V.: 20 mg/m^2 over 30 minutes, once every 3 weeks, for as long as patients respond satisfactorily and tolerate treatment

Dosage Forms Injection, as hydrochloride: 2 mg/mL (10 mL)

Doxy-200® *see* doxycycline *on this page*

Doxy-Caps® *see* doxycycline *on this page*

Doxychel® *see* doxycycline *on this page*

Doxycin (Can) *see* doxycycline *on this page*

doxycycline (doks i SYE kleen)

U.S./Canadian Brand Names Apo®-Doxy (Can); Apo®-Doxy Tabs (Can); Bio-Tab®; Doryx®; Doxy-200®; Doxy-Caps®; Doxychel®; Doxycin (Can); Doxy-Tabs®; Doxytec (Can); Dynacin®; Monodox®; Novo-Doxylin® (Can); Nu-Doxycycline® (Can); Vibramycin®; Vibra-Tabs®

Therapeutic Category Tetracycline Derivative

Use

Children, Adolescents, and Adults: Treatment of Rocky Mountain spotted fever caused by susceptible *Rickettsia* or brucellosis

Older Children, Adolescents, and Adults: Treatment of Lyme disease, mycoplasmal disease, or *Legionella*; management of malignant pleural effusions when intrapleural therapy is indicated

Adolescents and Adults: Treatment of nongonococcal pelvic inflammatory disease and urethritis due to *Chlamydia*; treatment for victims of sexual assault

Adults: Periostat™ (20 mg capsule) is used as an adjunct to scaling and root planing to promote attachment level gain and to reduce pocket depth in patients with adult periodontitis

Unapproved use: Treatment for syphilis in penicillin-allergic patients; sclerosing agent for pleural effusions

Usual Dosage Oral, I.V.:

Children ≥8 years (<45 kg): 2-5 mg/kg/day in 1-2 divided doses, not to exceed 200 mg/day

Children >8 years (>45 kg) and Adults: 100-200 mg/day in 1-2 divided doses

Sclerosing agent for pleural effusion injection: 500 mg as a single dose in 30-50 mL of NS or SWI

Adults: Periodontitis: 20 mg twice/day for up to 9 months; safety beyond 12 months and efficacy beyond 9 months have not been established

Dosage Forms

Doxycycline calcium:
- Syrup (raspberry-apple flavor) (Vibramycin®): 50 mg/5 mL (30 mL, 473 mL)

Doxycycline hyclate:
- Capsule:
  - Periostat™: 20 mg
  - Doxychel®, Vibramycin®: 50 mg
  - Doxy®, Doxychel®, Vibramycin®: 100 mg
- Capsule, coated pellets (Doryx®): 100 mg
- Powder for injection (Doxy®, Doxychel®, Vibramycin® IV): 100 mg, 200 mg

Tablet:
- Doxychel®: 50 mg
- Bio-Tab®, Doxychel®, Vibra-Tabs®: 100 mg

Doxycycline monohydrate:
- Capsule (Monodox®): 50 mg, 100 mg
- Powder for oral suspension (raspberry flavor) (Vibramycin®): 25 mg/5 mL (60 mL)

Doxy-Tabs® *see* doxycycline *on this page*

Doxytec (Can) *see* doxycycline *on this page*

DPA *see* valproic acid and derivatives *on page 594*

DPE *see* dipivefrin *on page 188*

DPE™ (Can) *see* dipivefrin *on page 188*

d-penicillamine *see* penicillamine *on page 433*

DPH *see* phenytoin *on page 449*

DPPC *see* colfosceril palmitate *on page 145*

DPT *see* diphtheria, tetanus toxoids, and whole-cell pertussis vaccine *on page 187*

Dramamine® II [OTC] *see* meclizine *on page 351*

Dramamine® Injection *(Discontinued)* *see page 700*

Dramamine® Oral [OTC] *see* dimenhydrinate *on page 182*

Dramilin® Injection *see* dimenhydrinate *on page 182*

Dramocen® *(Discontinued)* *see page 700*

Dramoject® *(Discontinued)* *see page 700*

Drenison® (Can) *see* flurandrenolide *on page 248*

Dri-Ear® Otic [OTC] *see* boric acid *on page 77*

Drisdol® *see* ergocalciferol *on page 212*

Dristan® Cold Caplets [OTC] *see* acetaminophen and pseudoephedrine *on page 5*

Dristan® Long Lasting Nasal Solution [OTC] *see* oxymetazoline *on page 423*

Dristan® Saline Spray [OTC] *see* sodium chloride *on page 526*

Dristan® Sinus Caplets [OTC] *see* pseudoephedrine and ibuprofen *on page 487*

Drithocreme® *see* anthralin *on page 38*

Drithocreme® HP 1% *see* anthralin *on page 38*

Dritho-Scalp® *see* anthralin *on page 38*

Drixomed® *see* dexbrompheniramine and pseudoephedrine *on page 168*

Drixoral® [OTC] *see* dexbrompheniramine and pseudoephedrine *on page 168*

Drixoral® Cough & Congestion Liquid Caps [OTC] *see* pseudoephedrine and dextromethorphan *on page 487*

Drixoral® Cough Liquid Caps [OTC] *see* dextromethorphan *on page 171*

Drixoral® Cough & Sore Throat Liquid Caps [OTC] *see* acetaminophen and dextromethorphan *on page 4*

Drixoral® Nasal (Can) *see* oxymetazoline *on page 423*

Drixoral® Non-Drowsy [OTC] *see* pseudoephedrine *on page 486*

Drixoral® Syrup [OTC] *see* brompheniramine and pseudoephedrine *on page 81*

dronabinol (droe NAB i nol)

Synonyms tetrahydrocannabinol; THC

U.S./Canadian Brand Names Marinol®

Therapeutic Category Antiemetic

Controlled Substance C-II

Use Treatment of nausea and vomiting secondary to cancer chemotherapy in patients who have not responded to conventional antiemetics; treatment of anorexia associated with weight loss in AIDS patients

Usual Dosage Oral:

Children: NCI protocol recommends 5 mg/m^2 starting 6-8 hours before chemotherapy and every 4-6 hours after to be continued for 12 hours after chemotherapy is discontinued

Adults: 5 mg/m^2 1-3 hours before chemotherapy, then administer 5 mg/m^2/dose every 2-4 hours after chemotherapy for a total of 4-6 doses/day; dose may be increased up to a maximum of 15 mg/m²/dose if needed (dosage may be increased by 2.5 mg/m² increments)

Dosage Forms Capsule: 2.5 mg, 5 mg, 10 mg

droperidol (droe PER i dole)

U.S./Canadian Brand Names Inapsine®

Therapeutic Category Antiemetic; Antipsychotic Agent, Butyrophenone

Use Tranquilizer and antiemetic in surgical and diagnostic procedures; antiemetic for cancer chemotherapy; preoperative medication

Usual Dosage Titrate carefully to desired effect

Children 2-12 years:

Premedication: I.M.: 0.088-0.165 mg/kg; smaller doses may be sufficient for control of nausea or vomiting

Adjunct to general anesthesia: I.V. induction: 0.088-0.165 mg/kg

Nausea and vomiting: I.M., I.V.: 0.05-0.06 mg/kg/dose every 4-6 hours as needed

Adults:

Premedication: I.M., I.V.: 2.5-10 mg 30 minutes to 1 hour preoperatively

Adjunct to general anesthesia: I.V. induction: 0.22-0.275 mg/kg; maintenance: 1.25-2.5 mg/dose

Alone in diagnostic procedures: I.M.: Initial: 2.5-10 mg 30 minutes to 1 hour before; then 1.25-2.5 mg if needed

Nausea and vomiting: I.M., I.V.: 2.5-5 mg/dose every 3-4 hours as needed

Dosage Forms Injection: 2.5 mg/mL (1 mL, 2 mL, 5 mL, 10 mL)

droperidol and fentanyl (droe PER i dole & FEN ta nil)

Synonyms fentanyl and droperidol

U.S./Canadian Brand Names Innovar®

Therapeutic Category Analgesic, Narcotic

Use Produce and maintain analgesia and sedation during diagnostic or surgical procedures (neuroleptanalgesia and neuroleptanesthesia); adjunct to general anesthesia

Usual Dosage

Children:

Premedication: I.M.: 0.03 mL/kg 30-60 minutes prior to surgery

Adjunct to general anesthesia: I.V.: Total dose: 0.05 mL/kg as slow infusion (1 mL/1-2 minutes) until sleep occurs

Adults:

Premedication: I.M.: 0.5-2 mL 30-60 minutes prior to surgery

Adjunct to general anesthesia: I.V.: 0.09-0.11 mL/kg as slow infusion (1 mL/1-2 minutes) until sleep occurs

Dosage Forms Injection: Droperidol 2.5 mg and fentanyl 50 mcg per mL (2 mL, 5 mL)

Droxia™ *see* hydroxyurea *on page 296*

Drug Products No Longer Available *see page 700*

Dry Eyes® Solution [OTC] *see* artificial tears *on page 47*

Dry Eye® Therapy Solution [OTC] *see* artificial tears *on page 47*

Dryox® Gel [OTC] *see* benzoyl peroxide *on page 68*

Dryox® Wash [OTC] *see* benzoyl peroxide *on page 68*

Drysol™ *see* aluminum chloride hexahydrate *on page 22*

DSCG *see* cromolyn sodium *on page 150*

DSMC Plus® [OTC] *see* docusate and casanthranol *on page 191*

DSS *see* docusate *on page 191*

D-S-S® [OTC] *see* docusate *on page 191*

D-S-S Plus® ***(Discontinued)*** *see page 700*

DSS with casanthranol *see* docusate and casanthranol *on page 191*

Dwelle® Ophthalmic Solution [OTC] *see* artificial tears *on page 47*

d-xylose (dee ZYE lose)

Synonyms wood sugar
U.S./Canadian Brand Names Xylo-Pfan® [OTC]
Therapeutic Category Diagnostic Agent
Use Evaluating intestinal absorption and diagnosing malabsorptive states
Usual Dosage Oral:
Infants and young Children: 500 mg/kg as a 5% to 10% aqueous solution
Children: 5 g is dissolved in 250 mL water; additional fluids are permitted and are encouraged for children
Adults: 25 g dissolved in 200-300 mL water followed with an additional 200-400 mL water **or** 5 g dissolved in 200-300 mL water followed by an additional 200-400 mL water
Dosage Forms Powder for oral solution: 25 g

Dyazide® *see* hydrochlorothiazide and triamterene *on page 287*

Dycill® *see* dicloxacillin *on page 176*

Dyclone® *see* dyclonine *on this page*

dyclonine (DYE kloe neen)

U.S./Canadian Brand Names Dyclone®; Sucrets® [OTC]
Therapeutic Category Local Anesthetic
Use Local anesthetic prior to laryngoscopy, bronchoscopy, or endotracheal intubation; used topically for temporary relief of pain associated with oral mucosa, skin, episiotomy, or anogenital lesions; the 0.5% topical solution may be used to block the gag reflex, and to relieve the pain of oral ulcers or stomatitis
Usual Dosage
Children and Adults: Topical solution:
Mouth sores: 5-10 mL of 0.5% or 1% to oral mucosa (swab or swish and then spit) 3-4 times/day as needed; maximum single dose: 200 mg (40 mL of 0.5% solution or 20 mL of 1% solution)
Bronchoscopy: Use 2 mL of the 1% solution or 4 mL of the 0.5% solution sprayed onto the larynx and trachea every 5 minutes until the reflex has been abolished
Children >3 years and Adults: Lozenge: Dissolve 1 in mouth slowly every 2 hours
Dosage Forms Dyclonine hydrochloride:
Lozenges: 1.2 mg, 3 mg
Solution, topical: 0.5% (30 mL); 1% (30 mL)

Dyflex-400® Tablet *(Discontinued)* *see page 700*

dyflos *see* isoflurophate *on page 314*

Dymelor® *see* acetohexamide *on page 8*

Dymenate® Injection *see* dimenhydrinate *on page 182*

Dynabac® *see* dirithromycin *on page 189*

Dynacin® *see* doxycycline *on page 197*

Dynacin® Oral *see* minocycline *on page 377*

DynaCirc® *see* isradipine *on page 317*

Dynafed®, Maximum Strength [OTC] *see* acetaminophen and pseudoephedrine *on page 5*

Dyna-Hex® [OTC] *see* chlorhexidine gluconate *on page 117*

Dynapen® *see* dicloxacillin *on page 176*

dyphylline (DYE fi lin)

Synonyms dihydroxypropyl theophylline
U.S./Canadian Brand Names Dilor®; Lufyllin®
Therapeutic Category Theophylline Derivative
(Continued)

dyphylline *(Continued)*

Use Bronchodilator in reversible airway obstruction due to asthma or COPD

Usual Dosage

Children: I.M.: 4.4-6.6 mg/kg/day in divided doses

Adults:

Oral: Up to 15 mg/kg 4 times/day, individualize dosage

I.M.: 250-500 mg, do not exceed total dosage of 15 mg/kg every 6 hours

Dosage Forms

Elixir:

Lufyllin®: 100 mg/15 mL with alcohol 20% (473 mL, 3780 mL)

Dilor®: 160 mg/15 mL with alcohol 18% (473 mL)

Injection (Dilor®, Lufyllin®): 250 mg/mL (2 mL)

Tablet: 200 mg, 400 mg

Dilor®, Lufyllin®: 200 mg, 400 mg

Dyrenium® *see* triamterene *on page 578*

Dyrexan-OD® *see* phendimetrazine *on page 442*

E2020 *see* donepezil *on page 193*

Easprin® *see* aspirin *on page 49*

echothiophate iodide (ek oh THYE oh fate EYE oh dide)

Synonyms ecostigmine iodide

U.S./Canadian Brand Names Phospholine Iodide® Ophthalmic

Therapeutic Category Cholinesterase Inhibitor

Use Reverse toxic CNS effects caused by anticholinergic drugs; used as miotic in treatment of glaucoma

Usual Dosage Adults: Ophthalmic: Glaucoma: Instill 1 drop twice daily into eyes with one dose just prior to bedtime; some patients have been treated with 1 dose/day or every other day. Use lowest concentration and frequency which gives satisfactory response, with a maximum dose of 0.125% once daily, although more intensive therapy may be used for short periods of time

Dosage Forms Powder for reconstitution, ophthalmic: 1.5 mg [0.03%] (5 mL); 3 mg [0.06%] (5 mL); 6.25 mg [0.125%] (5 mL); 12.5 mg [0.25%] (5 mL)

E-Complex-600® [OTC] *see* vitamin E *on page 604*

econazole (e KONE a zole)

U.S./Canadian Brand Names Ecostatin® (Can); Spectazole™

Therapeutic Category Antifungal Agent

Use Topical treatment of tinea pedis, tinea cruris, tinea corporis, tinea versicolor, and cutaneous candidiasis

Usual Dosage Children and Adults: Topical: Apply a sufficient amount to cover affected areas once daily; for cutaneous candidiasis: apply twice daily; candidal infections and tinea cruris, versicolor, and corporis should be treated for 2 weeks and tinea pedis for 1 month; occasionally, longer treatment periods may be required

Dosage Forms Cream, as nitrate: 1% (15 g, 30 g, 85 g)

Econopred® Ophthalmic *see* prednisolone (ophthalmic) *on page 471*

Econopred® Plus Ophthalmic *see* prednisolone (ophthalmic) *on page 471*

Ecostatin® (Can) *see* econazole *on this page*

ecostigmine iodide *see* echothiophate iodide *on this page*

Ecotrin® [OTC] *see* aspirin *on page 49*

Ectosone (Can) *see* betamethasone (topical) *on page 72*

Ed A-Hist® Liquid *see* chlorpheniramine and phenylephrine *on page 121*

edathamil disodium *see* edetate disodium *on next page*

Ecxtol

Edecrin® *see* ethacrynic acid *on page 221*

edetate calcium disodium (ED e tate KAL see um dye SOW dee um)

Synonyms calcium edta

U.S./Canadian Brand Names Calcium Disodium Versenate®

Therapeutic Category Chelating Agent

Use Treatment of acute and chronic lead poisoning; also used as an aid in the diagnosis of lead poisoning

Usual Dosage

Children:

Diagnosis of lead poisoning: Mobilization test: (Asymptomatic patients or lead levels <55 mcg/dL): (**Note:** Urine is collected for 24 hours after first EDTA dose and analyzed for lead content; if the ratio of mcg of lead in urine to mg calcium EDTA given is >1, then test is considered positive): Children: 500 mg/m^2 (maximum: 1 g/dose) I.M. or I.V. over 1 hour **or** 2 doses of 500 mg/m^2 at 12-hour intervals

Asymptomatic lead poisoning: (Blood lead concentration >55 mcg/dL or blood lead concentrations of 25-55 mcg/dL with blood erythrocyte protoporphyrin concentrations of ≥35 mcg/dL and positive mobilization test) or symptomatic lead poisoning without encephalopathy with lead level <100 mcg/dL: 1 g/m^2/day I.M./I.V. in divided doses every 8-12 hours for 3-5 days (usually 5 days); maximum: 1 g/24 hours or 50 mg/kg/day

Symptomatic lead poisoning with encephalopathy with lead level >100 mcg/dL (treatment with calcium EDTA and dimercaprol is preferred): 250 mg/m^2 I.M. or intermittent I.V. infusion 4 hours after dimercaprol, then at 4-hour intervals thereafter for 5 days (1.5 g/m^2/day); dose (1.5 g/m^2/day) can also be administered as a single I.V. continuous infusion over 12-24 hours/day for 5 days; maximum: 1 g/24 hours or 75 mg/kg/day

Note: Course of therapy may be repeated in 2-3 weeks until blood lead level is normal

Adults: I.M., I.V.:

Diagnosis of lead poisoning: 500 mg/m^2 (maximum: 1 g/dose) over 1 hour

Treatment: 2 g/day or 1.5 g/m^2/day in divided doses every 12-24 hours for 5 days; may repeat course one time after at least 2 days (usually after 2 weeks)

Dosage Forms Injection: 200 mg/mL (5 mL)

edetate disodium (ED e tate dye SOW dee um)

Synonyms edathamil disodium; EDTA; sodium edetate

U.S./Canadian Brand Names Chealamide®; Disotate®; Endrate®

Therapeutic Category Chelating Agent

Use Emergency treatment of hypercalcemia; control digitalis-induced cardiac dysrhythmias (ventricular arrhythmias)

Usual Dosage I.V.:

Hypercalcemia:

Children: 40-70 mg/kg slow infusion over 3-4 hours

Adults: 50 mg/kg/day over 3 or more hours

Dysrhythmias: Children and Adults: 15 mg/kg/hour up to 60 mg/kg/day

Dosage Forms Injection: 150 mg/mL (20 mL)

Edex® Injection *see* alprostadil *on page 20*

edrophonium (ed roe FOE nee um)

U.S./Canadian Brand Names Enlon®; Reversol®; Tensilon®

Therapeutic Category Cholinergic Agent

Use Diagnosis of myasthenia gravis; differentiation of cholinergic crises from myasthenia crises; reversal of nondepolarizing neuromuscular blockers; treatment of paroxysmal atrial tachycardia

Usual Dosage

Infants: I.V.: Initial: 0.1 mg, followed by 0.4 mg if no response; total dose: 0.5 mg

(Continued)

edrophonium *(Continued)*

Children:

Diagnosis: Initial: 0.04 mg/kg followed by 0.16 mg/kg if no response, to a maximum total dose of 5 mg for children ≤34 kg, or 10 mg for children >34 kg

Titration of oral anticholinesterase therapy: 0.04 mg/kg once; if strength improves, an increase in neostigmine or pyridostigmine dose is indicated

Adults:

Diagnosis: I.V.: 2 mg test dose administered over 15-30 seconds; 8 mg administered 45 seconds later if no response is seen. Test dose may be repeated after 30 minutes.

Titration of oral anticholinesterase therapy: 1-2 mg administered 1 hour after oral dose of anticholinesterase; if strength improves, an increase in neostigmine or pyridostigmine dose is indicated

Differentiation of cholinergic from myasthenic crisis: I.V.: 1 mg, may repeat after 1 minute (**Note:** Intubation and controlled ventilation may be required if patient has cholinergic crises.)

Reversal of nondepolarizing neuromuscular blocking agents (neostigmine with atropine usually preferred): I.V.: 10 mg, may repeat every 5-10 minutes up to 40 mg

Termination of paroxysmal atrial tachycardia: I.V.: 5-10 mg

Dosage Forms Injection, as chloride: 10 mg/mL (1 mL, 10 mL, 15 mL)

ED-SPAZ® *see* hyoscyamine *on page 297*

EDTA *see* edetate disodium *on previous page*

E.E.S.® *see* erythromycin (systemic) *on page 215*

E.E.S.® Chewable *see* erythromycin (systemic) *on page 215*

E.E.S.® Granules *see* erythromycin (systemic) *on page 215*

efavirenz (e FAV e renz)

U.S./Canadian Brand Names Sustiva™

Therapeutic Category Non-nucleoside Reverse Transciptase Inhibitor

Use Treatment of HIV-1 infections in combination with at least 2 other antiretroviral agents. Also has some activity against hepatitis B virus and herpes viruses.

Usual Dosage Dosing at bedtime is recommended to limit central nervous system effects; should not be used as single-agent therapy

Oral:

Adults: 600 mg once daily

Children: Dosage is based on body weight

10 to <15 kg: 200 mg

15 to <20 kg: 250 mg

20 to <25 kg: 300 mg

25 to <32.5 kg: 350 mg

32.5 to <40 kg: 400 mg

≥40 kg: 600 mg

Dosage Forms Capsule: 50 mg, 100 mg, 200 mg

Effer-K™ *see* potassium bicarbonate and potassium citrate, effervescent *on page 463*

Effer-Syllium® [OTC] *see* psyllium *on page 488*

Effexor® *see* venlafaxine *on page 598*

Effexor-XR® *see* venlafaxine *on page 598*

Efidac/24® [OTC] *see* pseudoephedrine *on page 486*

eflornithine (ee FLOR ni theen)

U.S./Canadian Brand Names Ornidyl®

Therapeutic Category Antiprotozoal

Use Treatment of meningoencephalitic stage of *Trypanosoma brucei gambiense* infection (sleeping sickness)

Usual Dosage I.V. infusion: 100 mg/kg/dose administered every 6 hours (over 45 minutes) for 14 days

Dosage Forms Injection, as hydrochloride: 200 mg/mL (100 mL)

Efodine® [OTC] *see* povidone-iodine *on page 467*

Efudex® Topical *see* fluorouracil *on page 246*

EHDP *see* etidronate disodium *on page 227*

Elase®-Chloromycetin® Ointment *(Discontinued)* *see page 700*

Elase® Ointment *(Discontinued)* *see page 700*

Elavil® *see* amitriptyline *on page 28*

Eldecort® Topical *see* hydrocortisone (topical) *on page 292*

Eldepryl® *see* selegiline *on page 518*

Eldepryl® Tablet (only) *(Discontinued)* *see page 700*

Eldercaps® [OTC] *see* vitamin, multiple (oral) *on page 604*

Eldopaque® [OTC] *see* hydroquinone *on page 294*

Eldopaque Forte® *see* hydroquinone *on page 294*

Eldoquin® [OTC] *see* hydroquinone *on page 294*

Eldoquin® Forte® *see* hydroquinone *on page 294*

Eldoquin® Lotion *(Discontinued)* *see page 700*

electrolyte lavage solution *see* polyethylene glycol-electrolyte solution *on page 459*

Elimite™ Cream *see* permethrin *on page 440*

Elixomin® *see* theophylline *on page 557*

Elixophyllin® *see* theophylline *on page 557*

Elixophyllin SR® *(Discontinued)* *see page 700*

Ellence™ *see* epirubicin *on page 211*

Elmiron® *see* pentosan polysulfate sodium *on page 438*

Elocom (Can) *see* mometasone furoate *on page 380*

Elocon® *see* mometasone furoate *on page 380*

E-Lor® Tablet *(Discontinued)* *see page 700*

Elspar® *see* asparaginase *on page 49*

Eltor® (Can) *see* pseudoephedrine *on page 486*

Eltroxin® *see* levothyroxine *on page 332*

Emcyt® *see* estramustine *on page 218*

Emecheck® [OTC] *see* phosphorated carbohydrate solution *on page 450*

Emete-Con Injection *(Discontinued)* *see page 700*

Emetine Hydrochloride *(Discontinued)* *see page 700*

Emetrol® [OTC] *see* phosphorated carbohydrate solution *on page 450*

Emgel™ Topical *see* erythromycin (ophthalmic/topical) *on page 214*

Eminase® *see* anistreplase *on page 38*

Emitrip® *see* amitriptyline *on page 28*

Emko® [OTC] *see* nonoxynol 9 *on page 406*

EMLA® *see* lidocaine and prilocaine *on page 334*

Emo-Cort™ (Can) *see* hydrocortisone (topical) *on page 292*

Empirin® [OTC] *see* aspirin *on page 49*

Empirin® With Codeine *see* aspirin and codeine *on page 50*

Empracet®-30, -60 (Can) *see* acetaminophen and codeine *on page 4*

Emtec-30® (Can) *see* acetaminophen and codeine *on page 4*

Emulsoil® [OTC] *see* castor oil *on page 103*

E-Mycin® *see* erythromycin (systemic) *on page 215*

E-Mycin-E® *see* erythromycin (systemic) *on page 215*

enalapril (e NAL a pril)

U.S./Canadian Brand Names Apo®-Enalapril (Can); Vasotec® I.V.; Vasotec® Oral

Therapeutic Category Angiotensin-Converting Enzyme (ACE) Inhibitor

Use Management of mild to severe hypertension, congestive heart failure, and asymptomatic left ventricular dysfunction

Usual Dosage Use lower listed initial dose in patients with hyponatremia, hypovolemia, severe congestive heart failure, decreased renal function, or in those receiving diuretics

Children:

Investigational initial oral doses of enalapril of 0.1 mg/kg/day increasing over 2 weeks to 0.12-0.43 mg/kg/day have been used to treat severe congestive heart failure in infants (n=8)

Investigational I.V. doses of enalaprilat of 5-10 mcg/kg/dose administered every 8-24 hours (as determined by blood pressure readings) have been used for the treatment of neonatal hypertension (n=10); monitor patients carefully; select patients may require higher doses

Adults:

Oral: **Enalapril**: 2.5-5 mg/day then increase as required, usually 10-40 mg/day in 1-2 divided doses

I.V.: **Enalaprilat**: 0.625-1.25 mg/dose, administered over 5 minutes every 6 hours

Dosage Forms

Enalaprilat: Injection: 1.25 mg/mL (1 mL, 2 mL)

Enalapril maleate: Tablet: 2.5 mg, 5 mg, 10 mg, 20 mg

enalapril and diltiazem (e NAL a pril & dil TYE a zem)

U.S./Canadian Brand Names Teczem®

Therapeutic Category Antihypertensive Agent, Combination

Use Combination drug for treatment of hypertension

Usual Dosage Adults: Oral: One tablet daily, if further blood pressure control is required, increase dosage to two tablets daily

Dosage Forms Tablet, extended release: Enalapril maleate 5 mg and diltiazem maleate 180 mg

enalapril and felodipine (e NAL a pril & fe LOE di peen)

U.S./Canadian Brand Names Lexxel™

Therapeutic Category Antihypertensive Agent, Combination

Use Treatment of hypertension

Usual Dosage Adults: Oral: The dose of this combination when given as a replacement to patients taking both components separately should be equal to the component doses previously used. Patients whose blood pressure is not sufficiently controlled on either component may be switched to one combination tablet (5 mg enalapril and 5 mg extended-release felodipine) daily. If control remains inadequate after 1 or 2 weeks, the dosage may be increased to two tablets daily, and if lack of control persists, a thiazide diuretic may be added

Dosage Forms Tablet, extended release: Enalapril maleate 5 mg and felodipine 5 mg

enalapril and hydrochlorothiazide

(e NAL a pril & hye droe klor oh THYE a zide)

Synonyms hydrochlorothiazide and enalapril

U.S./Canadian Brand Names Vaseretic® 10-25

Therapeutic Category Antihypertensive Agent, Combination

Use Treatment of hypertension
Usual Dosage Oral: Dose is individualized
Dosage Forms Tablet:
Enalapril maleate 5 mg and hydrochlorothiazide 12.5 mg
Enalapril maleate 10 mg and hydrochlorothiazide 25 mg

Enbrel® *see* etanercept *on page 221*

Encare® [OTC] *see* nonoxynol 9 *on page 406*

Endal® *see* guaifenesin and phenylephrine *on page 269*

Endantadine™ (Can) *see* amantadine *on page 24*

Endep® *see* amitriptyline *on page 28*

Endep® 25 mg, 50 mg, 100 mg *(Discontinued)* *see page 700*

End Lice® Liquid [OTC] *see* pyrethrins *on page 489*

Endocet® (Can) *see* oxycodone and acetaminophen *on page 422*

Endodan® (Can) *see* oxycodone and aspirin *on page 423*

Endolor® *see* butalbital compound and acetaminophen *on page 85*

Endrate® *see* edetate disodium *on page 203*

Enduron® *see* methyclothiazide *on page 366*

Enduron® 2.5 mg Tablet *(Discontinued)* *see page 700*

Enduronyl® *see* methyclothiazide and deserpidine *on page 366*

Enduronyl® Forte *see* methyclothiazide and deserpidine *on page 366*

Enecat® *see* radiological/contrast media (ionic) *on page 495*

Enemol™ (Can) *see* sodium phosphates *on page 529*

Ener-B® [OTC] *see* cyanocobalamin *on page 152*

enflurane (EN floo rane)

U.S./Canadian Brand Names Ethrane®
Therapeutic Category General Anesthetic
Use General induction and maintenance of anesthesia (inhalation)
Usual Dosage Inhalation: 0.5% to 3%
Dosage Forms Liquid: 125 mL, 250 mL

Engerix-B® *see* hepatitis B vaccine *on page 280*

Enisyl® [OTC] *see* **l**-lysine *on page 337*

Enkaid® *(Discontinued)* *see page 700*

Enlon® *see* edrophonium *on page 203*

Enomine® *see* guaifenesin, phenylpropanolamine, and phenylephrine *on page 272*

Enovid® *(Discontinued)* *see page 700*

Enovil® *see* amitriptyline *on page 28*

enoxacin (en OKS a sin)

U.S./Canadian Brand Names Penetrex™
Therapeutic Category Quinolone
Use Complicated and uncomplicated urinary tract infections caused by susceptible gram-negative and gram-positive bacteria
Usual Dosage Adults: Oral: 400 mg twice daily
Dosage Forms Tablet: 200 mg, 400 mg

enoxaparin (ee noks a PA rin)

U.S./Canadian Brand Names Lovenox®
Therapeutic Category Anticoagulant

(Continued)

enoxaparin *(Continued)*

Use Prophylaxis and treatment of thromboembolic disorders (deep vein thrombosis)
Usual Dosage Adults: S.C.: 30 mg twice daily
Dosage Forms Injection, as sodium, preservative free: 30 mg/0.3 mL

Ensure® [OTC] *see* enteral nutritional products *on this page*

Ensure Plus® [OTC] *see* enteral nutritional products *on this page*

E.N.T.® *(Discontinued)* *see page 700*

enteral nutritional products (noo TRISH un al FOR myoo la, EN ter al/OR al)

Synonyms dietary supplements
U.S./Canadian Brand Names Carnation Instant Breakfast® [OTC]; Citrisource® (Can); Citrotein® [OTC]; Criticare HN® [OTC]; Ensure® [OTC]; Ensure Plus® [OTC]; Glucerna™ (Can); Isocal® [OTC]; Isocal® with Fibre (Can): Isosource® (Can); Magnacal® [OTC]; Microlipid™ [OTC]; Nutrisource™ (Can); Optifast® 900 (Can); Osmolite® HN [OTC]; Palmocare® (Can); Pedialyte® [OTC]; Pediasure™ (Can); Portagen® [OTC]; Pregestimil® [OTC]; Propac™ [OTC]; Resource® (Can); Sandosource™ Peptide (Can), Sustacal® (Can); Soyalac® [OTC]; Tolerex® (Can); Travasol® (Can); Vital HN® [OTC]; Vitaneed™ [OTC]; Vivonex® [OTC]; Vivonex® Plus (Can); Vivonex® T.E.N. [OTC]
Therapeutic Category Nutritional Supplement
Dosage Forms
Liquid: Calcium and sodium caseinate, maltodextrin, sucrose, partially hydrogenated soy oil, soy lecithin
Powder: Amino acids, predigested carbohydrates, safflower oil

Entertainer's Secret® Spray [OTC] *see* saliva substitute *on page 514*

Entex® *see* guaifenesin, phenylpropanolamine, and phenylephrine *on page 272*

Entex® LA *see* guaifenesin and phenylpropanolamine *on page 270*

Entex® PSE *see* guaifenesin and pseudoephedrine *on page 270*

Entocort® (Can) *see* budesonide *on page 82*

Entozyme® *(Discontinued)* *see page 700*

Entrobar® *see* radiological/contrast media (ionic) *on page 495*

Entrophen® (Can) *see* aspirin *on page 49*

Entuss-D® LIquid *see* hydrocodone and pseudoephedrine *on page 289*

Enulose® *see* lactulose *on page 325*

Enzone® *see* pramoxine and hydrocortisone *on page 469*

E Pam® (Can) *see* diazepam *on page 173*

EPEG *see* etoposide *on page 228*

ephedrine (e FED rin)

U.S./Canadian Brand Names Kondon's Nasal® [OTC]; Pretz-D® [OTC]
Therapeutic Category Adrenergic Agonist Agent
Use Bronchial asthma; nasal congestion; acute bronchospasm; acute hypotensive states
Usual Dosage
Children:
Oral, S.C.: 3 mg/kg/day or 25-100 mg/m^2/day in 4-6 divided doses every 4-6 hours
I.M., slow I.V. push: 0.2-0.3 mg/kg/dose every 4-6 hours
Adults:
Oral: 25-50 mg every 3-4 hours as needed
I.M., S.C.: 25-50 mg, parenteral adult dose should not exceed 150 mg in 24 hours
I.V.: 5-25 mg/dose slow I.V. push repeated after 5-10 minutes as needed, then every 3-4 hours not to exceed 150 mg/24 hours
Dosage Forms Ephedrine sulfate:
Injection: 25 mg/mL (1 mL); 50 mg/mL (1 mL, 10 mL)

Jelly (Kondon's Nasal®): 1% (20 g)
Spray (Pretz-D®): 0.25% (15 mL)

ephedrine, theophylline, and hydroxyzine *see* theophylline, ephedrine, and hydroxyzine *on page 559*

ephedrine, theophylline, and phenobarbital *see* theophylline, ephedrine, and phenobarbital *on page 559*

Epi-C® *see* radiological/contrast media (ionic) *on page 495*

Epi E-Z Pen™, -Jr (Can) *see* epinephrine *on this page*

Epifrin® *see* epinephrine *on this page*

E-Pilo-x® Ophthalmic *see* pilocarpine and epinephrine *on page 452*

Epimorph® (Can) *see* morphine sulfate *on page 382*

Epinal® *see* epinephryl borate *on next page*

epinephrine (ep i NEF rin)

Synonyms adrenaline

U.S./Canadian Brand Names Adrenalin® Chloride; AsthmaHaler® Mist [OTC]; AsthmaNefrin® [OTC]; Bronitin® Mist [OTC]; Bronkaid® Mist [OTC]; Epi E-Z Pen™, -Jr (Can); Epifrin®; EpiPen®; EpiPen® Jr; Glaucon®; microNefrin® [OTC]; Primatene® Mist [OTC]; Sus-Phrine®; Vaponefrin® [OTC]

Therapeutic Category Adrenergic Agonist Agent

Use Treatment of bronchospasm, anaphylactic reactions, cardiac arrest, and management of open-angle (chronic simple) glaucoma

Usual Dosage

Bronchodilator:

Children: S.C.: 10 mcg/kg (0.01 mL/kg of 1:1000) (single doses not to exceed 0.5 mg); injection suspension (1:200): 0.005 mL/kg/dose (0.025 mg/kg/dose) to a maximum of 0.15 mL (0.75 mg for single dose) every 8-12 hours

Adults:

I.M., S.C. (1:1000): 0.1-0.5 mg every 10-15 minutes to 4 hours
Suspension (1:200) S.C.: 0.1-0.3 mL (0.5-1.5 mg)
I.V.: 0.1-0.25 mg (single dose maximum: 1 mg)

Cardiac arrest:

Neonates: I.V. or intratracheal: 0.01-0.03 mg/kg (0.1-0.3 mL/kg of 1:10,000 solution) every 3-5 minutes as needed; dilute intratracheal doses in 1-2 mL of normal saline

Infants and Children: Asystole or pulseless arrest:

I.V., intraosseous: First dose: 0.01 mg/kg (0.1 mL/kg of a 1:10,000 solution); subsequent doses: 0.1 mg/kg (0.1 mL/kg of a 1:1000 solution); doses as high as 0.2 mg/kg may be effective; repeat every 3-5 minutes

Intratracheal: 0.1 mg/kg (0.1 mL/kg of a 1:1000 solution); doses as high as 0.2 mg/kg may be effective

Adults: Asystole:

I.V.: 1 mg every 3-5 minutes; if this approach fails, alternative regimens include: Intermediate: 2-5 mg every 3-5 minutes; Escalating: 1 mg, 3 mg, 5 mg at 3-minute intervals; High: 0.1 mg/kg every 3-5 minutes

Intratracheal: Although optimal dose is unknown, doses of 2-2.5 times the I.V. dose may be needed

Bradycardia: Children:

I.V.: 0.01 mg/kg (0.1 mL/kg of 1:10,000 solution) every 3-5 minutes as needed (maximum: 1 mg/10 mL)

Intratracheal: 0.1 mg/kg (0.1 mL/kg of 1:1000 solution every 3-5 minutes); doses as high as 0.2 mg/kg may be effective

Refractory hypotension (refractory to dopamine/dobutamine): I.V. infusion administration requires the use of an infusion pump:

Children: Infusion rate 0.1-4 mcg/kg/minute

(Continued)

epinephrine *(Continued)*

Adults: I.V. infusion: 1 mg in 250 mL NS/D_5W at 0.1-1 mcg/kg/minute; titrate to desired effect

Hypersensitivity reaction:

Children: S.C.: 0.01 mg/kg every 15 minutes for 2 doses then every 4 hours as needed (single doses not to exceed 0.5 mg)

Adults: I.M., S.C.: 0.2-0.5 mg every 20 minutes to 4 hours (single dose maximum: 1 mg)

Nebulization:

Children <2 years: 0.25 mL of 1:1000 diluted in 3 mL NS with treatments ordered individually

Children >2 years and Adolescents: 0.5 mL of 1:1000 concentration diluted in 3 mL NS

Children >2 years and Adults (racemic epinephrine):

<10 kg: 2 mL of 1:8 dilution over 15 minutes every 1-4 hours

10-15 kg: 2 mL of 1:6 dilution over 15 minutes every 1-4 hours

15-20 kg: 2 mL of 1:4 dilution over 15 minutes every 1-4 hours

>20 kg: 2 mL of 1:3 dilution over 15 minutes every 1-4 hours

Adults: Instill 8-15 drops into nebulizer reservoirs; administer 1-3 inhalations 4-6 times/day

Ophthalmic: Instill 1-2 drops in eye(s) once or twice daily

Intranasal: Children ≥6 years and Adults: Apply locally as drops or spray or with sterile swab

Dosage Forms

Aerosol, oral:

Bitartrate (AsthmaHaler®, Bronitin®): 0.3 mg/spray [epinephrine base 0.16 mg/spray] (10 mL, 15 mL, 22.5 mL)

Bronkaid®: 0.5% (10 mL, 15 mL, 22.5 mL)

Primatene® Mist: 0.2 mg/spray (15 mL, 22.5 mL)

Auto-injector:

EpiPen®: Delivers 0.3 mg I.M. of epinephrine 1:1000 (2 mL)

EpiPen® Jr.: Delivers 0.15 mg I.M. of epinephrine 1:2000 (2 mL)

Solution:

Inhalation:

Adrenalin®: 1% [10 mg/mL, 1:100] (7.5 mL)

Injection:

Adrenalin®: 0.01 mg/mL [1:100,000] (5 mL); 0.1 mg/mL [1:10,000] (3 mL, 10 mL); 1 mg/mL [1:1000] (1 mL, 2 mL, 30 mL)

Suspension (Sus-Phrine®): 5 mg/mL [1:200] (0.3 mL, 5 mL)

Nasal (Adrenalin®): 0.1% [1 mg/mL, 1:1000] (30 mL)

Ophthalmic, as hydrochloride (Epifrin®, Glaucon®): 0.1% (1 mL, 30 mL); 0.5% (15 mL); 1% (1 mL, 10 mL, 15 mL); 2% (10 mL, 15 mL)

Topical (Adrenalin®): 0.1% [1 mg/mL, 1:1000] (10 mL, 30 mL)

epinephrine and lidocaine *see* lidocaine and epinephrine *on page 334*

epinephrine and pilocarpine *see* pilocarpine and epinephrine *on page 452*

epinephryl borate (ep i NEF ril BOR ate)

U.S./Canadian Brand Names Epinal®

Therapeutic Category Adrenergic Agonist Agent

Use Reduces elevated intraocular pressure in chronic open-angle glaucoma

Usual Dosage Adults: Ophthalmic: Instill 1 drop into the eyes once or twice daily

Dosage Forms Solution, ophthalmic: 0.5% (7.5 mL); 1% (7.5 mL)

EpiPen® *see* epinephrine *on previous page*

EpiPen® Jr *see* epinephrine *on previous page*

epirubicin (ep i ROO bi sin)

U.S./Canadian Brand Names Ellence™

Therapeutic Category Antineoplastic Agent, Anthracycline; Antineoplastic Agent, Antibiotic

Use As a component of adjuvant therapy following primary resection of primary breast cancer in patients with evidence of axillary node tumor involvement

Usual Dosage Adults: I.V. (refer to individual protocols): 100-120 mg/m^2, repeated in 3- to 4-week cycles. The total dose of epirubicin may be given on Day 1 of each cycle or the dose may be divided equally and given on Day 1 and Day 8 of each cycle.

Dosage Forms Injection: 2 mg/mL (25 mL, 100 mL)

Epitol® *see* carbamazepine *on page 97*

Epivir® *see* lamivudine *on page 325*

Epivir®-HBV™ *see* lamivudine *on page 325*

E.P. Mycin® Capsule *(Discontinued)* *see page 700*

EPO *see* epoetin alfa *on this page*

epoetin alfa (e POE e tin AL fa)

Synonyms EPO; erythropoietin; RHUEPO-α

U.S./Canadian Brand Names Epogen®; Eprex® (Can); Procrit®

Therapeutic Category Colony-Stimulating Factor

Use Anemia associated with end-stage renal disease; anemia related to therapy with AZT-treated HIV-infected patients; anemia in cancer patients receiving chemotherapy; anemia of prematurity

Usual Dosage

In patients on dialysis, epoetin alfa usually has been administered as an I.V. bolus 3 times/week; while the administration is independent of the dialysis procedure, it may be administered into the venous line at the end of the dialysis procedure to obviate the need for additional venous access. In patients with CRF not on dialysis, epoetin alfa may be administered either as an I.V. or S.C. injection.

AZT-treated HIV-infected patients: I.V., S.C.: Initial: 100 units/kg/dose 3 times/week for 8 weeks; after 8 weeks of therapy the dose can be adjusted by 50-100 units/kg increments 3 times/week to a maximum dose of 300 units/kg 3 times/week; if the hematocrit exceeds 40%, the dose should be discontinued until the hematocrit drops to 36%

Anemia of prematurity: S.C.: 25-100 units/kg/dose 3 times/week

Dosage Forms

1 mL single-dose vials: Preservative-free solution
- 2000 units/mL
- 3000 units/mL
- 4000 units/mL
- 10,000 units/mL

2 mL multidose vials: Preserved solution: 10,000 units/mL

Epogen® *see* epoetin alfa *on this page*

epoprostenol (e poe PROST en ole)

U.S./Canadian Brand Names Flolan®

Therapeutic Category Platelet Inhibitor

Use Long-term intravenous treatment of primary pulmonary hypertension (PPH)

Usual Dosage I.V. continuous infusion: 2 ng/kg/minute

Dosage Forms Injection, as sodium: 0.5 mg/vial and 1.5 mg/vial, each supplied with 50 mL of sterile diluent

Eprex® (Can) *see* epoetin alfa *on this page*

epsom salts *see* magnesium sulfate *on page 346*

EPT *see* teniposide *on page 549*

eptifibatide (ep TIF i ba tide)

U.S./Canadian Brand Names Integrilin®

Therapeutic Category Antiplatelet Agent

Use Treatment of patients with acute coronary syndrome (UA/NQMI), including patients who are to be managed medically and those undergoing percutaneous coronary intervention (PCI); it has been shown to decrease the rate of a combined endpoint of death or new myocardial infarction. For the treatment of patients undergoing PCI, it has been shown to decrease the rate of a combined endpoint of death, new myocardial infarction, or need for urgent intervention.

Usual Dosage Adults: I.V.:

Acute coronary syndrome: Bolus of 180 mcg/kg as soon as possible following diagnosis, followed by a continuous infusion of 2 mcg/kg/minute until hospital discharge or initiation of CABG surgery, up to 72 hours. If a patient is to undergo a percutaneous coronary intervention (PCI) while receiving eptifibatide, consideration can be given to decreasing the infusion rate to 0.5 mcg/kg/minute (the infusion rate in IMPACT II) at the time of the procedure. Infusion should be continued for an additional 20-24 hours after the procedure, allowing for up to 96 hours of therapy.

Percutaneous coronary intervention (PCI) in patients not presenting with an acute coronary syndrome: Bolus of 135 mcg/kg administered immediately before the initiation of PCI followed by a continuous infusion of 0.5 mcg/kg/minute for 20-24 hours. In the IMPACT II Study, there was little experience in patients weighing more than 143 kg.

Dosage Forms Injection: 0.75 mg/mL (100 mL); 2 mg/mL (10 mL)

Equagesic® *see* aspirin and meprobamate *on page 50*

Equalactin® Chewable Tablet [OTC] *see* calcium polycarbophil *on page 93*

Equanil® *see* meprobamate *on page 356*

Equilet® [OTC] *see* calcium carbonate *on page 89*

Ercaf® *see* ergotamine *on next page*

Ergamisol® *see* levamisole *on page 329*

ergocalciferol (er goe kal SIF e role)

Synonyms activated ergosterol; viosterol; vitamin D_2

U.S./Canadian Brand Names Calciferol™; Drisdol®; Ostoforte® (Can); Radiostol® (Can)

Therapeutic Category Vitamin D Analog

Use Refractory rickets; hypophosphatemia; hypoparathyroidism

Usual Dosage

Dietary supplementation: Oral:
- Premature infants: 10-20 mcg/day (400-800 units), up to 750 mcg/day (30,000 units)
- Infants and healthy Children: 10 mcg/day (400 units)

Renal failure: Oral:
- Children: 0.1-1 mg/day (4000-40,000 units)
- Adults: 0.5 mg/day (20,000 units)

Hypoparathyroidism: Oral:
- Children: 1.25-5 mg/day (50,000-200,000 units) and calcium supplements
- Adults: 625 mcg to 5 mg/day (25,000-200,000 units) and calcium supplements

Vitamin D-dependent rickets: Oral:
- Children: 75-125 mcg/day (3000-5000 units)
- Adults: 250 mcg to 1.5 mg/day (10,000-60,000 units)

Nutritional rickets and osteomalacia:
- Oral:
  - Children and Adults (with normal absorption): 25 mcg/day (1000 units)
  - Children with malabsorption: 250-625 mcg/day (10,000-25,000 units)
- I.M.: Adults: 250 mcg/day

Dosage Forms

Capsule (Drisdol®): 50,000 units [1.25 mg]

Injection (Calciferol™): 500,000 units/mL [12.5 mg/mL] (1 mL)

Liquid (Calciferol™, Drisdol®): 8000 units/mL [200 mcg/mL] (60 mL)

Tablet (Calciferol™): 50,000 units [1.25 mg]

ergoloid mesylates (ER goe loid MES i lates)

Synonyms dihydroergotoxine; hydrogenated ergot alkaloids

U.S./Canadian Brand Names Germinal®; Hydergine®; Hydergine® LC

Therapeutic Category Ergot Alkaloid and Derivative

Use Treatment of cerebrovascular insufficiency in primary progressive dementia, Alzheimer's dementia, and senile onset

Usual Dosage Adults: Oral: 1 mg 3 times/day up to 4.5-12 mg/day; up to 6 months of therapy may be necessary

Dosage Forms

Capsule, liquid (Hydergine® LC): 1 mg

Liquid (Hydergine®): 1 mg/mL (100 mL)

Tablet:

Oral: 0.5 mg

Gerimal®, Hydergine®: 1 mg

Sublingual: Gerimal®, Hydergine®: 0.5 mg, 1 mg

Ergomar® *see* ergotamine *on this page*

Ergostat *(Discontinued)* *see page 700*

ergotamine (er GOT a meen)

Synonyms ergotamine tartrate; ergotamine tartrate and caffeine; ergotamine tartrate with belladonna alkaloids, and phenobarbital

U.S./Canadian Brand Names Cafatine-PB®; Cafergot®; Cafetrate®; Ercaf®; Ergomar®; Ergotamine Tartrate and Caffeine Cafatine®; Gynergen® (Can); Phenerbel-S®; Wigraine®

Therapeutic Category Ergot Alkaloid and Derivative

Use Prevent or abort vascular headaches, such as migraine or cluster

Usual Dosage

Older Children and Adolescents: Oral: 1 tablet at onset of attack; then 1 tablet every 30 minutes as needed, up to a maximum of 3 tablets per attack

Adults:

Oral (Cafergot®): 2 tablets at onset of attack; then 1 tablet every 30 minutes as needed; maximum: 6 tablets per attack; do not exceed 10 tablets/week

Oral (Ergostat®): 1 tablet under tongue at first sign, then 1 tablet every 30 minutes, 3 tablets/24 hours, 5 tablets/week

Rectal (Cafergot® suppositories, Wigraine® suppositories, Cafatine-PB® suppositories): 1 at first sign of an attack; follow with second dose after 1 hour, if needed; maximum dose: 2 per attack; do not exceed 5/week

Dosage Forms

Suppository, rectal (Cafatine®, Cafergot®, Cafetrate®, Wigraine®): Ergotamine tartrate 2 mg and caffeine 100 mg (12s)

Tablet (Ercaf®, Wigraine®): Ergotamine tartrate 1 mg and caffeine 100 mg

Sublingual (Ergomar®): Ergotamine tartrate 2 mg

ergotamine tartrate *see* ergotamine *on this page*

ergotamine tartrate and caffeine *see* ergotamine *on this page*

Ergotamine Tartrate and Caffeine Cafatine® *see* ergotamine *on this page*

ergotamine tartrate, belladonna, and phenobarbital *see* belladonna, phenobarbital, and ergotamine tartrate *on page 63*

ergotamine tartrate with belladonna alkaloids, and phenobarbital *see* ergotamine *on this page*

Ergotrate® Maleate *(Discontinued)* *see page 700*

Eridium® *(Discontinued)* *see page 700*

E•R•O Ear [OTC] *see* carbamide peroxide *on page 98*

Erybid™ (Can) *see* erythromycin (systemic) *on page 215*

Eryc® *see* erythromycin (systemic) *on next page*

Eryderm® Topical *see* erythromycin (ophthalmic/topical) *on this page*

Erygel® Topical *see* erythromycin (ophthalmic/topical) *on this page*

Erymax® Topical *see* erythromycin (ophthalmic/topical) *on this page*

Ery-Sol® Topical Solution *(Discontinued)* *see page 700*

Ery-Tab® *see* erythromycin (systemic) *on next page*

erythrityl tetranitrate (e RI thri til te tra NYE trate)

U.S./Canadian Brand Names Cardilate®

Therapeutic Category Vasodilator

Use Prophylaxis and long-term treatment of frequent or recurrent anginal pain and reduced exercise tolerance associated with angina pectoris

Usual Dosage Adults: Oral: 5 mg under the tongue or in the buccal pouch 3 times/day or 10 mg before meals or food, chewed 3 times/day, increasing in 2-3 days if needed

Dosage Forms Tablet, oral or sublingual: 10 mg

Erythro-Base® (Can) *see* erythromycin (systemic) *on next page*

Erythrocin® *see* erythromycin (systemic) *on next page*

erythromycin and benzoyl peroxide

(er ith roe MYE sin & BEN zoe il per OKS ide)

Synonyms benzoyl peroxide and erythromycin

U.S./Canadian Brand Names Benzamycin®

Therapeutic Category Acne Products

Use Topical control of acne vulgaris

Usual Dosage Topical: Apply twice daily (morning and evening)

Dosage Forms Gel: Erythromycin 30 mg and benzoyl peroxide 50 mg per g

erythromycin and sulfisoxazole (er ith roe MYE sin & sul fi SOKS a zole)

Synonyms sulfisoxazole and erythromycin

U.S./Canadian Brand Names Eryzole®; Pediazole®

Therapeutic Category Macrolide (Antibiotic); Sulfonamide

Use Treatment of susceptible bacterial infections of the upper and lower respiratory tract; otitis media in children caused by susceptible strains of *Haemophilus influenzae*; other infections in patients allergic to penicillin

Usual Dosage Dosage recommendation is based on the product's erythromycin content; Oral:

Children ≥2 months: 40-50 mg/kg/day of erythromycin in divided doses every 6-8 hours; not to exceed 2 g erythromycin or 6 g sulfisoxazole/day or approximately 1.25 mL/kg/day divided every 6-8 hours

Adults: 400 mg erythromycin and 1200 mg sulfisoxazole every 6 hours

Dosage Forms Suspension, oral: Erythromycin ethylsuccinate 200 mg and sulfisoxazole acetyl 600 mg per 5 mL (100 mL, 150 mL, 200 mL, 250 mL)

erythromycin (ophthalmic/topical) (er ith roe MYE sin TOP i kal)

U.S./Canadian Brand Names Akne-Mycin® Topical; A/T/S® Topical; Del-Mycin® Topical; Emgel™ Topical; Eryderm® Topical; Erygel® Topical; Erymax® Topical; E-Solve-2® Topical; ETS-2%® Topical; Ilotycin® Ophthalmic; Staticin® Topical; T-Stat® Topical

Therapeutic Category Acne Products; Antibiotic, Ophthalmic; Antibiotic, Topical

Use Topical treatment of acne vulgaris

Usual Dosage Children and Adults:

Ophthalmic: Instill one or more times daily depending on the severity of the infection

Topical: Apply 2% solution over the affected area twice daily after the skin has been thoroughly washed and patted dry

Dosage Forms

Gel: 2% (30 g, 60 g)

Gel (A/T/S®, Emgel™, Erygel®): 2% (27 g, 30 g, 60 g)
Ointment:
Ophthalmic: 0.5% [5 mg/g] (3.5 g)
Ilotycin®: 0.5% [5 mg/g] (3.5 g)
Topical (Akne-Mycin®): 2% (25 g)
Solution, topical:
Staticin®: 1.5% (60 mL)
Akne-Mycin®, A/T/S®, Del-Mycin®, EryDerm®, ETS-2%®, Romycin®, Theramycin Z®, T-Stat®: 2% (60 mL, 66 mL, 120 mL)
Pad (T-Stat®): 2% (60s)
Pledgets: 2% (60s)
Swab: 2% (60s)

erythromycin (systemic) (er ith roe MYE sin)

U.S./Canadian Brand Names AK-Mycin®; Apo®-Erythro E-C (Can); Diomycin (Can); E.E.S.®; E.E.S.® Chewable; E.E.S.® Granules; E-Mycin®; E-Mycin-E®; Erybid™ (Can); Eryc®; Ery-Tab®; Erythro-Base® (Can); Erythrocin®; Ilosone®; Ilosone® Pulvules®; Ilotycin®; Ilotycin® (Can); Novo-Rythro Encap (Can); PCE®; PMS-Erythromycin (Can); Wyamycin® S

Therapeutic Category Macrolide (Antibiotic)

Use Treatment of mild to moderately severe infections of the upper and lower respiratory tract, pharyngitis and skin infections due to susceptible streptococci and staphylococci; other susceptible bacterial infections including *Mycoplasma* pneumonia, *Legionella* pneumonia, diphtheria, pertussis, chancroid, *Chlamydia*, and *Campylobacter* gastroenteritis; used in conjunction with neomycin for decontaminating the bowel for surgery; dental procedure prophylaxis in penicillin allergic patients

Usual Dosage
Infants and Children:
Oral: Do not exceed 2 g/day
Base and ethylsuccinate: 30-50 mg/kg/day divided every 6-8 hours
Estolate: 30-50 mg/kg/day divided every 8-12 hours
Stearate: 20-40 mg/kg/day divided every 6 hours
Pre-op bowel preparation: 20 mg/kg erythromycin base at 1, 2, and 11 PM on the day before surgery combined with mechanical cleansing of the large intestine and oral neomycin
I.V.: Lactobionate: 20-40 mg/kg/day divided every 6 hours, not to exceed 4 g/day
Adults:
Oral:
Base: 333 mg every 8 hours
Estolate, stearate or base: 250-500 mg every 6-12 hours
Ethylsuccinate: 400-800 mg every 6-12 hours
Pre-op bowel preparation: 1 g erythromycin base at 1, 2, and 11 PM on the day before surgery combined with mechanical cleansing of the large intestine and oral neomycin
I.V.: 15-20 mg/kg/day divided every 6 hours or administered as a continuous infusion over 24 hours

Dosage Forms
Erythromycin base:
Capsule:
Delayed release: 250 mg
Delayed release, enteric coated pellets (Eryc®): 250 mg
Tablet:
Delayed release: 333 mg
Enteric coated (E-Mycin®, Ery-Tab®, E-Base®): 250 mg, 333 mg, 500 mg
Film coated: 250 mg, 500 mg
Polymer coated particles (PCE®): 333 mg, 500 mg
Erythromycin estolate:
Capsule (Ilosone® Pulvules®): 250 mg
Suspension, oral (Ilosone®): 125 mg/5 mL (480 mL); 250 mg/5 mL (480 mL)
Tablet (Ilosone®): 500 mg
(Continued)

erythromycin (systemic) *(Continued)*

Erythromycin ethylsuccinate:
Granules for oral suspension (EryPed®): 400 mg/5 mL (60 mL, 100 mL, 200 mL)
Powder for oral suspension (E.E.S.®): 200 mg/5 mL (100 mL, 200 mL)
Suspension:
Oral (E.E.S.®, EryPed®): 200 mg/5 mL (5 mL, 100 mL, 200 mL, 480 mL); 400 mg/5 mL (5 mL, 60 mL, 100 mL, 200 mL, 480 mL)
Oral [drops] (EryPed®): 100 mg/2.5 mL (50 mL)
Tablet (E.E.S.®): 400 mg
Tablet, chewable (EryPed®): 200 mg
Erythromycin gluceptate: Injection: 1000 mg (30 mL)
Erythromycin lactobionate: Powder for injection: 500 mg, 1000 mg
Erythromycin stearate: Tablet, film coated (Eramycin®, Erythrocin®): 250 mg, 500 mg

erythropoietin *see* epoetin alfa *on page 211*

Eryzole® *see* erythromycin and sulfisoxazole *on page 214*

Esclim® Transdermal *see* estradiol *on next page*

Esgic® *see* butalbital compound and acetaminophen *on page 85*

Esgic-Plus® *see* butalbital compound and acetaminophen *on page 85*

Esidrix® *see* hydrochlorothiazide *on page 286*

Esidrix® 100 mg Tablet *(Discontinued)* *see page 700*

Eskalith® *see* lithium *on page 337*

esmolol (ES moe lol)

U.S./Canadian Brand Names Brevibloc®

Therapeutic Category Antiarrhythmic Agent, Class II; Beta-Adrenergic Blocker

Use Supraventricular tachycardia (primarily to control ventricular rate) and hypertension (especially perioperatively)

Usual Dosage Must be adjusted to individual response and tolerance

Children: An extremely limited amount of information regarding esmolol use in pediatric patients is currently available. Some centers have utilized doses of 100-500 mcg/kg administered over 1 minute for control of supraventricular tachycardias. Loading doses of 500 mcg/kg/minute over 1 minute with maximal doses of 50-250 mcg/kg/minute (mean 173) have been used in addition to nitroprusside in a small number of patients (7 patients; 7-19 years of age; median 13 years) to treat postoperative hypertension after coarctation of aorta repair.

Adults: I.V.: Loading dose: 500 mcg/kg over 1 minute; follow with a 50 mcg/kg/minute infusion for 4 minutes; if response is inadequate, rebolus with another 500 mcg/kg loading dose over 1 minute, and increase the maintenance infusion to 100 mcg/kg/minute. Repeat this process until a therapeutic effect has been achieved or to a maximum recommended maintenance dose of 200 mcg/kg/minute. Usual dosage range: 50-200 mcg/kg/minute with average dose = 100 mcg/kg/minute.

Dosage Forms Injection, as hydrochloride: 10 mg/mL (10 mL); 250 mg/mL (10 mL)

E-Solve-2® Topical *see* erythromycin (ophthalmic/topical) *on page 214*

Esoterica® Facial [OTC] *see* hydroquinone *on page 294*

Esoterica® Regular [OTC] *see* hydroquinone *on page 294*

Esoterica® Sensitive Skin Formula [OTC] *see* hydroquinone *on page 294*

Esoterica® Sunscreen [OTC] *see* hydroquinone *on page 294*

Estar® [OTC] *see* coal tar *on page 141*

estazolam (es TA zoe lam)

U.S./Canadian Brand Names ProSom™

Therapeutic Category Benzodiazepine

Controlled Substance C-IV

esomeprazole magnesium (Nexium)

Use Short-term management of insomnia

Usual Dosage Adults: Oral: 1 mg at bedtime, some patients may require 2 mg

Dosage Forms Tablet: 1 mg, 2 mg

esterified estrogen and methyltestosterone *see* estrogens and methyltestosterone *on page 219*

esterified estrogens *see* estrogens, esterified *on page 220*

Estinyl® *see* ethinyl estradiol *on page 222*

Estivin® II Ophthalmic [OTC] *see* naphazoline *on page 390*

Estrace® Oral *see* estradiol *on this page*

Estraderm® Transdermal *see* estradiol *on this page*

estradiol (es tra DYE ole)

U.S./Canadian Brand Names Alora® Transdermal; Climara® Transdermal; depGynogen® Injection; Depo®-Estradiol Injection; Depogen® Injection; Dioval® Injection; Esclim® Transdermal; Estrace® Oral; Estraderm® Transdermal; Estra-L® Injection; Estring®; Estro-Cyp® Injection; Gynogen L.A.® Injection; Vivelle™ Transdermal

Therapeutic Category Estrogen Derivative

Use Atrophic vaginitis, atrophic dystrophy of vulva, menopausal symptoms, female hypogonadism

Usual Dosage Adults (all dosage needs to be adjusted based upon the patient's response):

Male: Prostate cancer: Valerate:
- I.M.: ≥30 mg or more every 1-2 weeks
- Oral: 1-2 mg 3 times/day

Female:
- Hypogonadism:
  - Oral: 1-2 mg/day in a cyclic regimen for 3 weeks on drug, then 1 week off drug
  - I.M.: Cypionate: 1.5-2 mg/month; valerate: 10-20 mg/month
  - Transdermal: 0.05 mg patch initially (titrate dosage to response) applied twice weekly in a cyclic regimen, for 3 weeks on drug and 1 week off drug
- Atrophic vaginitis, kraurosis vulvae: Vaginal: Insert 2-4 g/day for 2 weeks then gradually reduce to 1/2 the initial dose for 2 weeks followed by a maintenance dose of 1 g 1-3 times/week
- Moderate to severe vasomotor symptoms: I.M.:
  - Cypionate: 1-5 mg every 3-4 weeks
  - Valerate: 10-20 mg every 4 weeks
- Postpartum breast engorgement: I.M.: Valerate: 10-25 mg at end of first stage of labor

Dosage Forms

Cream, vaginal (Estrace®): 0.1 mg/g (42.5 g)

Injection, as cypionate (depGynogen®, Depo®-Estradiol, Depogen®, Dura-Estrin®, Estra-D®, Estro-Cyp®, Estroject-L.A.®): 5 mg/mL (5 mL, 10 mL)

Injection, as valerate:
- Dioval®, Duragen®, Estra-L®, Gynogen L.A.®: 20 mg/mL (10 mL); 40 mg/mL (10 mL)

Tablet, micronized (Estrace®): 1 mg, 2 mg

Transdermal system
- Alora®:
  - 0.05 mg/24 hours [18 cm^2], total estradiol 1.5 mg
  - 0.075 mg/24 hours [27 cm^2], total estradiol 2.3 mg
  - 0.1 mg/24 hours [36 cm^2], total estradiol 3 mg
- Climara®:
  - 0.05 mg/24 hours [12.5 cm^2], total estradiol 3.9 mg
  - 0.1 mg/24 hours [25 cm^2], total estradiol 7.8 mg
- Esclim®:
  - 0.025 mg/day
  - 0.0375 mg/day
  - 0.05 mg/day

(Continued)

estradiol *(Continued)*

0.075 mg/day
0.1 mg/day
Estraderm®:
0.05 mg/24 hours [10 cm^2], total estradiol 4 mg
0.1 mg/24 hours [20 cm^2], total estradiol 8 mg
Vivelle®:
0.0375 mg/day
0.05 mg/day
0.075 mg/day
Vaginal ring (Estring®): 2 mg gradually released over 90 days

estradiol and norethindrone (es tra DYE ole & nor eth IN drone)

U.S./Canadian Brand Names Activelle™

Therapeutic Category Estrogen and Progestin Combination

Use Treatment of moderate to severe vasomotor symptoms associated with menopause; treatment of vulvar and vaginal atrophy

Usual Dosage Adults: Oral: Take one tablet daily

Dosage Forms Tablet: Estradiol 1 mg and norethindrone acetate 0.5 mg (28s)

estradiol and testosterone (es tra DYE ole & tes TOS ter one)

U.S./Canadian Brand Names Andro/Fem®; Deladumone®; depAndrogyn®; Depo-Testadiol®; Depotestogen®; Duo-Cyp®; Duratestrin®; Valertest No.1®

Therapeutic Category Estrogen and Androgen Combination

Use Vasomotor symptoms associated with menopause; postpartum breast engorgement

Usual Dosage Adults (all dosage needs to be adjusted based upon the patient's response)

Dosage Forms Injection:

Andro/Fem®, depAndrogyn®, Depo-Testadiol®, Depotestogen®, Duo-Cyp®, Duratestrin®: Estradiol cypionate 2 mg and testosterone cypionate 50 mg per mL in cottonseed oil (1 mL, 10 mL)

Androgyn L.A.®, Deladumone®, Estra-Testrin®, Valertest No.1®: Estradiol valerate 4 mg and testosterone enanthate 90 mg per mL in sesame oil (5 mL, 10 mL)

Estradurin® Injection *(Discontinued)* *see page 700*

Estra-L® Injection *see* estradiol *on previous page*

estramustine (es tra MUS teen)

U.S./Canadian Brand Names Emcyt®

Therapeutic Category Antineoplastic Agent

Use Palliative treatment of prostatic carcinoma

Usual Dosage Oral: 1 capsule for each 22 lb/day, in 3-4 divided doses

Dosage Forms Capsule, as phosphate sodium: 140 mg

Estratab® *see* estrogens, esterified *on page 220*

Estratest® *see* estrogens and methyltestosterone *on next page*

Estratest® H.S. *see* estrogens and methyltestosterone *on next page*

Estring® *see* estradiol *on previous page*

Estro-Cyp® Injection *see* estradiol *on previous page*

estrogenic substance aqueous *see* estrone *on page 220*

estrogens and medroxyprogesterone

(ES troe jenz & me DROKS ee proe JES te rone)

Synonyms medroxyprogesterone and estrogens

U.S./Canadian Brand Names Premphase™; Prempro™

Therapeutic Category Estrogen and Progestin Combination

Use Women with an intact uterus for the treatment of moderate to severe vasomotor symptoms associated with the menopause; treatment of atrophic vaginitis; primary ovarian failure; osteoporosis prophylactic

Usual Dosage Adults: Oral:

Premphase™: Conjugated estrogen 0.625 mg [Premarin®] and taken orally for 28 days and medroxyprogesterone acetate [Cycrin®] 5 mg (14s) which are taken orally with a Premarin® tablet on days 15 through 28

Prempro™: Conjugated estrogen 0.625 mg [Premarin®] and medroxyprogesterone acetate [Cycrin®] 2.5 mg are taken continuously one each day

Dosage Forms

Premphase™: Two separate tablets in therapy pack: Conjugated estrogens 0.625 mg [Premarin®] (28s) taken orally for 28 days and medroxyprogesterone acetate [Cycrin®] 5 mg (14s) which are taken orally with a Premarin® tablet on days 15 through 28

Prempro™: Conjugated estrogens 0.625 mg and medroxyprogesterone acetate 2.5 mg (14s)

estrogens and methyltestosterone (ES troe jenz & meth il tes TOS te rone)

Synonyms conjugated estrogen and methyltestosterone; esterified estrogen and methyltestosterone

U.S./Canadian Brand Names Estratest®; Estratest® H.S.; Premarin® With Methyltestosterone

Therapeutic Category Estrogen and Androgen Combination

Use Atrophic vaginitis; hypogonadism; primary ovarian failure; vasomotor symptoms of menopause; prostatic carcinoma; osteoporosis prophylactic

Usual Dosage Oral: Lowest dose that will control symptoms should be chosen, normally administered 3 weeks on and 1 week off

Dosage Forms Tablet:

Estratest®, Menogen®: Esterified estrogen 1.25 mg and methyltestosterone 2.5 mg

Estratest® H.S., Menogen H.S.®: Esterified estrogen 0.625 mg and methyltestosterone 1.25 mg

Premarin® With Methyltestosterone: Conjugated estrogen 0.625 mg and methyltestosterone 5 mg; conjugated estrogen 1.25 mg and methyltestosterone 10 mg

estrogens, conjugated, A (synthetic)

(ES troe jenz, KON joo gate ed, aye, sin THET ik)

U.S./Canadian Brand Names Cenestin™

Therapeutic Category Estrogen Derivative

Use Treatment of moderate to severe vasomotor symptoms of menopause

Usual Dosage Moderate to severe vasomotor symptoms: Oral: 0.625 mg/day; may be titrated up to 1.25 mg daily. Attempts to discontinue medication should be made at 3-6 month intervals.

Dosage Forms Tablet: 0.625 mg, 1.25 mg

estrogens, conjugated (equine) (ES troe jenz KON joo gate ed)

Synonyms CES; conjugated estrogens

U.S./Canadian Brand Names C.E.S.™ (Can); Congest (Can); Premarin®

Therapeutic Category Estrogen Derivative

Use Dysfunctional uterine bleeding, atrophic vaginitis, hypogonadism, vasomotor symptoms of menopause

Usual Dosage Adults:

Male: Prostate cancer: Oral: 1.25-2.5 mg 3 times/day

Female:

Hypogonadism: Oral: 2.5-7.5 mg/day for 20 days, off 10 days and repeat until menses occur

Abnormal uterine bleeding:

Oral: 2.5-5 mg/day for 7-10 days; then decrease to 1.25 mg/day for 2 weeks

I.V.: 25 mg every 6-12 hours until bleeding stops

Moderate to severe vasomotor symptoms: Oral: 0.625-1.25 mg/day

(Continued)

estrogens, conjugated (equine) *(Continued)*

Postpartum breast engorgement: Oral: 3.75 mg every 4 hours for 5 doses, then 1.25 mg every 4 hours for 5 days

Dosage Forms

Cream, vaginal: 0.625 mg/g (42.5 g)
Injection: 25 mg (5 mL)
Tablet: 0.3 mg, 0.625 mg, 0.9 mg, 1.25 mg, 2.5 mg

estrogens, esterified (ES troe jenz, es TER i fied)

Synonyms esterified estrogens

U.S./Canadian Brand Names Estratab®; Menest®

Therapeutic Category Estrogen Derivative

Use Atrophic vaginitis; hypogonadism; primary ovarian failure; vasomotor symptoms of menopause; prostatic carcinoma; osteoporosis prophylactic

Usual Dosage Adults: Oral:

Male: Prostate cancer: 1.25-2.5 mg 3 times/day
Female:
Hypogonadism: 2.5-7.5 mg/day for 20 days, off 10 days and repeat until menses occur
Moderate to severe vasomotor symptoms: 0.3-1.25 mg/day

Dosage Forms Tablet: 0.3 mg, 0.625 mg, 1.25 mg, 2.5 mg

Estroject-2® Injection *(Discontinued)* *see page 700*

Estroject-L.A.® Injection *(Discontinued)* *see page 700*

estrone (ES trone)

Synonyms estrogenic substance aqueous

U.S./Canadian Brand Names Aquest®; Femogen® (Can); Kestrone®; Neo-Estrone® (Can); Oestrillin® (Can)

Therapeutic Category Estrogen Derivative

Use Atrophic vaginitis; hypogonadism; primary ovarian failure; vasomotor symptoms of menopause; prostatic carcinoma; osteoporosis prophylactic

Usual Dosage Adults: I.M.:

Vasomotor symptoms, atrophic vaginitis: 0.1-0.5 mg 2-3 times/week
Primary ovarian failure, hypogonadism: 0.1-1 mg/week, up to 2 mg/week
Prostatic carcinoma: 2-4 mg 2-3 times/week

Dosage Forms Injection: 2 mg/mL (10 mL, 30 mL); 5 mg/mL (10 mL)

Estronol® Injection *(Discontinued)* *see page 700*

estropipate (ES troe pih pate)

Synonyms piperazine estrone sulfate

U.S./Canadian Brand Names Ogen® Oral; Ogen® Vaginal; Ortho-Est® Oral

Therapeutic Category Estrogen Derivative

Use Atrophic vaginitis; hypogonadism; primary ovarian failure; vasomotor symptoms of menopause; prostatic carcinoma; osteoporosis prophylactic

Usual Dosage Adults: Female:

Moderate to severe vasomotor symptoms: Oral: 0.625-5 mg/day
Hypogonadism: Oral: 1.25-7.5 mg/day for 3 weeks followed by an 8- to 10-day rest period
Atrophic vaginitis or kraurosis vulvae: Vaginal: Instill 2-4 g/day 3 weeks on and 1 week off

Dosage Forms Piperazine estrone sulfate:

Cream, vaginal: 0.15% [estropipate 1.5 mg/g] (42.5 g tube)
Tablet: 0.625 mg [estropipate 0.75 mg]; 1.25 mg [estropipate 1.5 mg]; 2.5 mg [estropipate 3 mg]; 5 mg [estropipate 6 mg]

Estrostep® 21 *see* ethinyl estradiol and norethindrone *on page 224*

Estrostep® Fe *see* ethinyl estradiol and norethindrone *on page 224*

Estrovis® ***(Discontinued)*** *see page 700*

etanercept (et a NER cept)

U.S./Canadian Brand Names Enbrel®

Therapeutic Category Antirheumatic, Disease Modifying

Use Reduction in signs and symptoms of moderately to severely active rheumatoid arthritis in patients who have had an inadequate response to one or more disease-modifying antirheumatic drugs (DMARDs).

Usual Dosage S.C.:

Children: 0.4 mg/kg (maximum: 25 mg dose)

Adult: 25 mg given twice weekly; if the physician determines that it is appropriate, patients may self-inject after proper training in injection technique

Dosage Forms Powder for injection: 25 mg

ethacrynic acid (eth a KRIN ik AS id)

Synonyms sodium ethacrynate

U.S./Canadian Brand Names Edecrin®

Therapeutic Category Diuretic, Loop

Use Management of edema secondary to congestive heart failure; hepatic or renal disease, hypertension

Usual Dosage

Children:

Oral: 25 mg/day to start, increase by 25 mg/day at intervals of 2-3 days as needed, to a maximum of 3 mg/kg/day

I.V.: 1 mg/kg/dose, (maximum: 50 mg/dose); repeat doses not recommended

Adults:

Oral: 50-100 mg/day increased in increments of 25-50 mg at intervals of several days to a maximum of 400 mg/24 hours

I.V.: 0.5-1 mg/kg/dose (maximum: 50 mg/dose); repeat doses not recommended

Dosage Forms

Powder for injection, as ethacrynate sodium: 50 mg (50 mL)

Tablet: 25 mg, 50 mg

ethambutol (e THAM byoo tole)

U.S./Canadian Brand Names Etibi® (Can); Myambutol®

Therapeutic Category Antimycobacterial Agent

Use Treatment of tuberculosis and other mycobacterial diseases in conjunction with other antimycobacterial agents

Usual Dosage Oral (not recommended in children <12 years of age):

Children >12 years: 15 mg/kg/day once daily

Adolescents and Adults: 15-25 mg/kg/day once daily, not to exceed 2.5 g/day

Dosage Forms Tablet, as hydrochloride: 100 mg, 400 mg

Ethamolin® *see* ethanolamine oleate *on this page*

ETH and C *see* terpin hydrate and codeine *on page 552*

ethanoic acid *see* acetic acid *on page 7*

ethanol *see* alcohol, ethyl *on page 16*

ethanolamine oleate (ETH a nol a meen OH lee ate)

U.S./Canadian Brand Names Ethamolin®

Therapeutic Category Sclerosing Agent

Use Mild sclerosing agent used for bleeding esophageal varices

Usual Dosage Adults: 1.5-5 mL per varix, up to 20 mL total or 0.4 mL/kg; patients with severe hepatic dysfunction should receive less than recommended maximum dose

Dosage Forms Injection: 5% [50 mg/mL] (2 mL)

Ethaquin® ***(Discontinued)*** *see page 700*

Ethatab® *(Discontinued)* *see page 700*

ethaverine (eth AV er een)

Therapeutic Category Vasodilator

Use Peripheral and cerebral vascular insufficiency associated with arterial spasm

Usual Dosage Adults: Oral: 100 mg 3 times/day

Dosage Forms Ethaverine hydrochloride:

Capsule: 100 mg

Tablet: 100 mg

Ethavex-100® *(Discontinued)* *see page 700*

ethchlorvynol (eth klor VI nole)

U.S./Canadian Brand Names Placidyl®

Therapeutic Category Hypnotic, Nonbarbiturate

Controlled Substance C-IV

Use Short-term management of insomnia

Usual Dosage Oral: 500-1000 mg at bedtime

Dosage Forms Capsule: 200 mg, 500 mg, 750 mg

ethinyl estradiol (ETH in il es tra DYE ole)

U.S./Canadian Brand Names Estinyl®

Therapeutic Category Estrogen Derivative

Use Atrophic vaginitis; hypogonadism; primary ovarian failure; vasomotor symptoms of menopause; prostatic carcinoma; osteoporosis prophylactic

Usual Dosage Adults: Oral:

Hypogonadism: 0.05 mg 1-3 times/day for 2 weeks

Prostatic carcinoma: 0.15-2 mg/day

Vasomotor symptoms: 0.02-0.05 mg for 21 days, off 7 days and repeat

Dosage Forms Tablet: 0.02 mg, 0.05 mg, 0.5 mg

ethinyl estradiol and desogestrel

(ETH in il es tra DYE ole & des oh JES trel)

Synonyms desogestrel and ethinyl estradiol

U.S./Canadian Brand Names Desogen®; Ortho-Cept®

Therapeutic Category Contraceptive, Oral

Use Prevention of pregnancy

Usual Dosage Contraception: Oral: 1 tablet daily, beginning on day 5 of menstrual cycle (first day of menstrual flow is day 1). With 21-tablet packages, new dosing cycle begins 7 days after last tablet taken. With 28-tablet packages, dosage is 1 tablet daily without interruption; extra tablets are placebos, If next menstrual period does not begin on schedule, rule out pregnancy before starting new dosing cycle. If menstrual period begins, start new dosing cycle 7 days after last tablet was taken. if all doses have been taken on schedule and 1 menstrual period is missed, continue dosing cycle. If 2 consecutive menstrual periods are missed, pregnancy test is required before new dosing cycle is started.

One dose missed: Take as soon as remembered or take 2 tablets next day

Two doses missed: Take 2 tablets as soon as remembered or 2 tablets next 2 days

Three doses missed: Begin new compact of tablets starting on day 1 of next cycle

Dosage Forms Tablet: Ethinyl estradiol 0.03 mg and desogestrel 0.15 mg (21s, 28s)

ethinyl estradiol and ethynodiol diacetate

(ETH in il es tra DYE ole & e thye noe DYE ole dye AS e tate)

Synonyms ethynodiol diacetate and ethinyl estradiol

U.S./Canadian Brand Names Demulen®; Zovia®

Therapeutic Category Contraceptive, Oral

Use Prevention of pregnancy; treatment of hypermenorrhea, endometriosis, female hypogonadism

Usual Dosage

For 21-tablet cycle packs, with 21 active tablets (28-day packs have 21 active tablets and 7 inert tablets): Administer 1 tablet daily starting on the fifth day of menstrual cycle, with day 1 being the first day of menstruation; begin taking a new cycle pack on the eighth day after taking the last tablet from the previous pack

With 28-tablet packages, dosage is 1 tablet daily without interruption; extra tablets are placebos or contain iron. If next menstrual period does not begin on schedule, rule out pregnancy before starting new dosing cycle. If menstrual period begins, start new dosing cycle 7 days after last tablet was administered. If all doses have been administered on schedule and 1 menstrual period is missed, continue dosing cycle. If 2 consecutive menstrual periods are missed, pregnancy test is required before new dosing cycle is started.

One dose missed: Administer as soon as remembered or administer 2 tablets next day

Two doses missed: Administer 2 tablets as soon as remembered or 2 tablets next 2 days

Three doses missed: Begin new compact of tablets starting on day 1 of next cycle

Dosage Forms Tablet:

1/35: Ethinyl estradiol 0.035 mg and ethynodiol diacetate 1 mg (21s, 28s)

1/50: Ethinyl estradiol 0.05 mg and ethynodiol diacetate 1 mg (21s, 28s)

ethinyl estradiol and levonorgestrel

(ETH in il es tra DYE ole & LEE voe nor jes trel)

Synonyms levonorgestrel and ethinyl estradiol

U.S./Canadian Brand Names Alesse™; Levlen®; Levlite®; Levora®; Nordette®; Preven™; Tri-Levlen®; Triphasil®

Therapeutic Category Contraceptive, Oral

Use Prevention of pregnancy; treatment of hypermenorrhea, endometriosis, female hypogonadism

Usual Dosage Adults: Female: Oral:

Contraception: 1 tablet daily, beginning on day 5 of menstrual cycle (first day of menstrual flow is day 1). With 20-tablet and 21-tablet packages, new dosing cycle begins 7 days after last tablet taken. With 28-tablet packages, dosage is 1 tablet daily without interruption; extra tablets are placebos or contain iron. If next menstrual period does not begin on schedule, rule out pregnancy before starting new dosing cycle. If menstrual period begins, start new dosing cycle 7 days after last tablet was taken. If all doses have been taken on schedule and one menstrual period is missed, continue dosing cycle. If two consecutive menstrual periods are missed, pregnancy test is required before new dosing cycle is started.

One dose missed: Take as soon as remembered or take 2 tablets next day

Two doses missed: Take 2 tablets as soon as remembered or 2 tablets next 2 days

Three doses missed: Begin new compact of tablets starting on day 1 of next cycle

Triphasic oral contraceptive (Tri-Levlen®, Triphasil®): 1 tablet/day in the sequence specified by the manufacturer

Post-intercourse pregnancy prevention: Take 2 tablets ≤72 hours after unprotected intercourse, take second dose of 2 tablets 12 hours later

Dosage Forms Tablet:

Alesse™, Levlite®: Ethinyl estradiol 0.02 mg and levonorgestrel 0.1 mg (21s, 28s)

Levlen®, Levora®, Nordette®: Ethinyl estradiol 0.03 mg and levonorgestrel 0.15 mg (21s, 28s)

Preven™: Ethinyl estradiol 0.05 mg and levonorgestrel 0.25 mg (4s)

Tri-Levlen®, Triphasil®: Phase 1 (6 brown tablets): Ethinyl estradiol 0.03 mg and levonorgestrel 0.05 mg; Phase 2 (5 white tablets): Ethinyl estradiol 0.04 mg and levonorgestrel 0.075 mg; Phase 3 (10 yellow tablets): Ethinyl estradiol 0.03 mg and levonorgestrel 0.125 mg (21s, 28s)

ethinyl estradiol and norethindrone

(ETH in il es tra DYE ole & nor eth IN drone)

Synonyms norethindrone acetate and ethinyl estradiol

U.S./Canadian Brand Names Brevicon®; Estrostep® 21; Estrostep® Fe; Genora® 0.5/35; Genora® 1/35; Jenest-28™; Loestrin®; Modicon™; N.E.E.® 1/35; Nelova™ 0.5/35E; Nelova™ 10/11; Norethin™ 1/35E; Norinyl® 1+35; Ortho® 0.5/35 (Can); Ortho-Novum® 1/35; Ortho-Novum® 7/7/7; Ortho-Novum® 10/11; Ovcon® 35; Ovcon® 50; Synphasic® (Can); Tri-Norinyl®

Therapeutic Category Contraceptive, Oral

Use Prevention of pregnancy; treatment of hypermenorrhea, endometriosis, female hypogonadism

Usual Dosage

For 21-tablet cycle packs, with 21 active tablets (28-day packs have 21 active tablets and 7 inert tablets): Administer 1 tablet daily starting on the fifth day of menstrual cycle, with day 1 being the first day of menstruation; begin taking a new cycle pack on the eighth day after taking the last tablet from the previous pack

With 28-tablet packages, dosage is 1 tablet daily without interruption; extra tablets are placebos or contain iron. If next menstrual period does not begin on schedule, rule out pregnancy before starting new dosing cycle. If menstrual period begins, start new dosing cycle 7 days after last tablet was administered. If all doses have been administered on schedule and 1 menstrual period is missed, continue dosing cycle. If 2 consecutive menstrual periods are missed, pregnancy test is required before new dosing cycle is started.

One dose missed: Administer as soon as remembered or administer 2 tablets next day

Two doses missed: Administer 2 tablets as soon as remembered or 2 tablets next 2 days

Three doses missed: Begin new compact of tablets starting on day 1 of next cycle

Biphasic oral contraceptive (Ortho-Novum™ 10/11): 1 color tablet/day for 10 days, then next color tablet for 11 days

Triphasic oral contraceptive (Ortho-Novum™ 7/7/7, Tri-Norinyl®, Triphasil®): 1 tablet/day in the sequence specified by the manufacturer

Dosage Forms Tablet:

Brevicon®, Genora® 0.5/35, Modicon™, Nelova™ 0.5/35E: Ethinyl estradiol 0.035 mg and norethindrone 0.5 mg (21s, 28s)

Estrostep®:

Triangular tablet (white): Ethinyl estradiol 0.02 mg and norethindrone acetate 1 mg
Square tablet (white): Ethinyl estradiol 0.03 mg and norethindrone acetate 1 mg
Round tablet (white): Ethinyl estradiol 0.035 mg and norethindrone acetate 1 mg

Estrostep® Fe:

Triangular tablet (white): Ethinyl estradiol 0.02 mg and norethindrone acetate 1 mg
Square tablet (white): Ethinyl estradiol 0.03 mg and norethindrone acetate 1 mg
Round tablet (white): Ethinyl estradiol 0.035 mg and norethindrone acetate 1 mg
Brown tablet: Ferrous fumarate 75 mg

Loestrin® 1.5/30: Ethinyl estradiol 0.03 mg and norethindrone acetate 1.5 mg (21s)

Loestrin® Fe 1.5/30: Ethinyl estradiol 0.03 mg and norethindrone acetate 1.5 mg with ferrous fumarate 75 mg in 7 inert tablets (28s)

Loestrin® 1/20: Ethinyl estradiol 0.02 mg and norethindrone acetate 1 mg (21s)

Loestrin® Fe 1/20: Ethinyl estradiol 0.02 mg and norethindrone acetate 1 mg with ferrous fumarate 75 mg in 7 inert tablets (28s)

Genora® 1/35, N.E.E.® 1/35, Nelova® 1/35E, Norethin™ 1/35E, Norinyl® 1+35, Ortho-Novum® 1/35: Ethinyl estradiol 0.035 mg and norethindrone 1 mg (21s, 28s)

Jenest-28™: Phase 1 (7 white tablets): Ethinyl estradiol 0.035 mg and norethindrone 0.5 mg; Phase 2 (14 peach tablets): Ethinyl estradiol 0.035 mg and norethindrone 1 mg and 7 green inert tablets (28s)

Ortho-Novum® 7/7/7: Phase 1 (7 white tablets): Ethinyl estradiol 0.035 mg and norethindrone 0.5 mg; Phase 2 (7 light peach tablets): Ethinyl estradiol 0.035 mg and norethindrone 0.75 mg; Phase 3 (7 peach tablets): Ethinyl estradiol 0.035 mg and norethindrone 1 mg (21s, 28s)

Ortho-Novum® 10/11: Phase 1 (10 white tablets): Ethinyl estradiol 0.035 mg and norethindrone 0.5 mg; Phase 2 (11 dark yellow tablets): Ethinyl estradiol 0.035 mg and norethindrone 1 mg (21s, 28s)

Ovcon® 35: Ethinyl estradiol 0.035 mg and norethindrone 0.4 mg (21s, 28s)

Ovcon® 50: Ethinyl estradiol 0.050 mg and norethindrone 1 mg (21s, 28s)

Tri-Norinyl®: Phase 1 (7 blue tablets): Ethinyl estradiol 0.035 mg and norethindrone 0.5 mg; Phase 2 (9 green tablets): Ethinyl estradiol 0.035 mg and norethindrone 1 mg; Phase 3 (5 blue tablets): Ethinyl estradiol 0.035 mg and norethindrone 0.5 mg (21s, 28s)

ethinyl estradiol and norgestimate

(ETH in il es tra DYE ole & nor JES ti mate)

Synonyms norgestimate and ethinyl estradiol

U.S./Canadian Brand Names Ortho-Cyclen®; Ortho Tri-Cyclen®

Therapeutic Category Contraceptive, Oral

Use Prevention of pregnancy

Usual Dosage

Contraception: Oral: 1 tablet daily, beginning on day 5 of menstrual cycle (first day of menstrual flow is day 1). With 21-tablet packages, new dosing cycle begins 7 days after last tablet administered. With 28-tablet packages, dosage is 1 tablet daily without interruption; extra tablets are placebos or contain iron. If next menstrual period does not begin on schedule, rule out pregnancy before starting new dosing cycle. If menstrual period begins, start new dosing cycle 7 days after last tablet was administered. If all doses have been administered on schedule and 1 menstrual period is missed, continue dosing cycle. If 2 consecutive menstrual periods are missed, pregnancy test is required before new dosing cycle is started.

One dose missed: Administer as soon as remembered or administer 2 tablets next day

Two doses missed: Administer 2 tablets as soon as remembered or 2 tablets next 2 days

Three doses missed: Begin new compact of tablets starting on day 1 of next cycle

Triphasic oral contraceptive: 1 tablet/day in the sequence specified by the manufacturer

Dosage Forms Tablet:

Ortho-Cyclen®: Ethinyl estradiol 0.035 mg and norgestimate 0.25 mg (21s, 28s)

Ortho Tri-Cyclen®: Phase 1 (7 white tablets): Ethinyl estradiol 0.035 mg and norgestimate 0.18 mg; Phase 2 (5 light blue tablets): Ethinyl estradiol 0.035 mg and norgestimate 0.215 mg; Phase 3 (10 blue tablets): Ethinyl estradiol 0.035 mg and norgestimate 0.25 mg (21s, 28s)

ethinyl estradiol and norgestrel (ETH in il es tra DYE ole & nor JES trel)

Synonyms norgestrel and ethinyl estradiol

U.S./Canadian Brand Names Lo/Ovral®; Ovral®

Therapeutic Category Contraceptive, Oral

Use Prevention of pregnancy; treatment of hypermenorrhea, endometriosis, female hypogonadism

Usual Dosage Contraception: Oral: 1 tablet daily, beginning on day 5 of menstrual cycle (first day of menstrual flow is day 1). With 20-tablet and 21-tablet packages, new dosing cycle begins 7 days after last tablet administered; with 28-tablet packages, dosage is 1 tablet daily without interruption; extra tablets are placebos or contain iron. If next menstrual period does not begin on schedule, rule out pregnancy before starting new dosing cycle; if menstrual period begins, start new dosing cycle 7 days after last tablet was administered; if all doses have been administered on schedule and 1 menstrual period is missed, continue dosing cycle; if two consecutive menstrual periods are missed, pregnancy test is required before new dosing cycle is started.

One dose missed: Administer as soon as remembered or administer 2 tablets next day

Two doses missed: Administer 2 tablets as soon as remembered or 2 tablets next 2 days

Three doses missed: Begin new compact of tablets starting on day 1 of next cycle

Dosage Forms Tablet:

Lo/Ovral®: Ethinyl estradiol 0.03 mg and norgestrel 0.3 mg (21s and 28s)

Ovral®: Ethinyl estradiol 0.05 mg and norgestrel 0.5 mg (21s and 28s)

Ethiodol® *see* radiological/contrast media (ionic) *on page 495*

ethiofos *see* amifostine *on page 25*

ethionamide (e thye on AM ide)

U.S./Canadian Brand Names Trecator®-SC

Therapeutic Category Antimycobacterial Agent

Use In conjunction with other antituberculosis agents in the treatment of tuberculosis and other mycobacterial diseases

Usual Dosage Oral:

Children: 15-20 mg/kg/day in 2 divided doses, not to exceed 1 g/day

Adults: 500-1000 mg/day in 1-3 divided doses

Dosage Forms Tablet, sugar coated: 250 mg

Ethmozine® *see* moricizine *on page 381*

ethosuximide (eth oh SUKS i mide)

U.S./Canadian Brand Names Zarontin®

Therapeutic Category Anticonvulsant

Use Management of absence (petit mal) seizures, myoclonic seizures, and akinetic epilepsy

Usual Dosage Oral:

Children 3-6 years:

Initial: 250 mg

Increment: 250 mg/day at 4- to 7-day intervals

Maintenance: 20-40 mg/kg/day

Maximum: 1500 mg/day in 2 divided doses

Children >6 years and Adults:

Initial: 500 mg/day

Increment: 250 mg/day at 4- to 7-day intervals

Maintenance: 20-40 mg/kg/day

Maximum: 1500 mg/day in 2 divided doses

Dosage Forms

Capsule: 250 mg

Syrup (raspberry flavor): 250 mg/5 mL (473 mL)

ethotoin (ETH oh toyn)

Synonyms ethylphenylhydantoin

U.S./Canadian Brand Names Peganone®

Therapeutic Category Hydantoin

Use Generalized tonic-clonic or complex-partial seizures

Usual Dosage Oral:

Children: 250 mg twice daily, up to 250 mg 4 times/day

Adults: 250 mg 4 times/day after meals, may be increased up to 3 g/day in divided doses 4 times/day

Dosage Forms Tablet: 250 mg, 500 mg

ethoxynaphthamido penicillin sodium *see* nafcillin *on page 388*

Ethrane® *see* enflurane *on page 207*

ethyl aminobenzoate *see* benzocaine *on page 66*

ethyl chloride (ETH il KLOR ide)

Synonyms chloroethane

Therapeutic Category Local Anesthetic

Use Local anesthetic in minor operative procedures and to relieve pain caused by insect stings and burns, and irritation caused by myofascial and visceral pain syndromes

Usual Dosage Topical: Dosage varies with use

Dosage Forms Spray: 100 mL, 120 mL

ethyl chloride and dichlorotetrafluoroethane
(ETH il KLOR ide & dye klor oh te tra floo or oh ETH ane)
Synonyms dichlorotetrafluoroethane and ethyl chloride
U.S./Canadian Brand Names Fluro-Ethyl® Aerosol
Therapeutic Category Local Anesthetic
Use Topical refrigerant anesthetic to control pain associated with minor surgical procedures, dermabrasion, injections, contusions, and minor strains
Usual Dosage Topical: Press gently on side of spray valve allowing the liquid to emerge as a fine mist approximately 2" to 4" from site of application
Dosage Forms Aerosol: Ethyl chloride 25% and dichlorotetrafluoroethane 75% (225 g)

ethylphenylhydantoin *see* ethotoin *on previous page*

ethynodiol diacetate and ethinyl estradiol *see* ethinyl estradiol and ethynodiol diacetate *on page 222*

Ethyol® *see* amifostine *on page 25*

Etibi® (Can) *see* ethambutol *on page 221*

etidocaine (e TI doe kane)
U.S./Canadian Brand Names Duranest®
Therapeutic Category Local Anesthetic
Use Infiltration anesthesia; peripheral nerve blocks; central neural blocks
Usual Dosage Varies with procedure; use 1% for peripheral nerve block, central nerve block, lumbar peridural caudal; use 1.5% for maxillary infiltration or inferior alveolar nerve block; use 1% or 1.5% for intra-abdominal or pelvic surgery, lower limb surgery, or caesarean section
Dosage Forms
Injection, as hydrochloride: 1% [10 mg/mL] (30 mL)
With epinephrine 1:200,000: 1% [10 mg/mL] (30 mL); 1.5% [15 mg/mL] (20 mL)

etidronate disodium (e ti DROE nate dye SOW dee um)
Synonyms EHDP; sodium etidronate
U.S./Canadian Brand Names Didronel®
Therapeutic Category Bisphosphonate Derivative
Use Symptomatic treatment of Paget's disease and heterotopic ossification due to spinal cord injury; hypercalcemia associated with malignancy
Usual Dosage Adults: Oral:
Paget's disease: 5 mg/kg/day administered every day for no more than 6 months; may administer 10 mg/kg/day for up to 3 months. Daily dose may be divided if adverse GI effects occur.
Heterotopic ossification with spinal cord injury: 20 mg/kg/day for 2 weeks, then 10 mg/kg/day for 10 weeks (this dosage has been used in children, however, treatment >1 year has been associated with a rachitic syndrome)
Hypercalcemia associated with malignancy: I.V.: 7.5 mg/kg/day for 3 days
Dosage Forms
Injection: 50 mg/mL (6 mL)
Tablet: 200 mg, 400 mg

etodolac (ee toe DOE lak)
Synonyms etodolic acid
U.S./Canadian Brand Names Lodine®; Lodine® XL
Therapeutic Category Analgesic, Non-narcotic; Nonsteroidal Anti-inflammatory Drug (NSAID)
Use Acute and long-term use in the management of signs and symptoms of osteoarthritis and management of pain
Usual Dosage Adults: Oral:
Acute pain: 200-400 mg every 6-8 hours, as needed, not to exceed total daily doses of 1200 mg
(Continued)

etodolac *(Continued)*

Osteoarthritis: Initial: 800-1200 mg/day administered in divided doses: 400 mg 2 or 3 times/day; 300 mg 2, 3 or 4 times/day; 200 mg 3 or 4 times/day; total daily dose should not exceed 1200 mg; for patients weighing <60 kg, total daily dose should not exceed 20 mg/kg; extended release dose: one tablet daily

Dosage Forms

Capsule (Lodine®): 200 mg, 300 mg

Tablet: 400 mg

Lodine®: 400 mg

Tablet, extended release (Lodine® XL): 400 mg, 600 mg

etodolic acid *see* etodolac *on previous page*

etomidate (e TOM i date)

U.S./Canadian Brand Names Amidate®

Therapeutic Category General Anesthetic

Use Induction of general anesthesia

Usual Dosage Children >10 years and Adults: I.V.: 0.2-0.6 mg/kg over period of 30-60 seconds

Dosage Forms Injection: 2 mg/mL (10 mL, 20 mL)

Etopophos® *see* etoposide phosphate *on this page*

etoposide (e toe POE side)

Synonyms EPEG; VP-16

U.S./Canadian Brand Names Toposar® Injection; VePesid®

Therapeutic Category Antineoplastic Agent

Use Treatment of testicular and lung carcinomas, malignant lymphoma, Hodgkin's disease, leukemias (ALL, AML), neuroblastoma; also used in the treatment of Ewing's sarcoma, rhabdomyosarcoma, Wilms' tumor, brain tumors, and as a conditioning regimen for bone marrow transplantation in patients with advanced hematologic malignancies

Usual Dosage Refer to individual protocols

Pediatric solid tumors: I.V.: 60-120 mg/m^2/day for 3-5 days every 3-6 weeks

Leukemia in children: I.V.: 100-200 mg/m^2/day for 5 days

Testicular cancer: I.V.: 50-100 mg/m^2/day on days 1-5 or 100 mg/m^2/day on days 1, 3 and 5 every 3-4 weeks for 3-4 courses

Small cell lung cancer:

Oral: Twice the I.V. dose rounded to the nearest 50 mg administered once daily if total dose ≤400 mg or in divided doses if >400 mg

I.V.: 35 mg/m^2/day for 4 days or 50 mg/m^2/day for 5 days every 3-4 weeks

Dosage Forms

Capsule: 50 mg

Injection: 20 mg/mL (5 mL, 10 mL, 25 mL)

etoposide phosphate (e toe POE side FOS fate)

U.S./Canadian Brand Names Etopophos®

Therapeutic Category Antineoplastic Agent

Use Treatment of refractory testicular tumors and small cell lung cancer

Usual Dosage Refer to individual protocols. Adults:

Small cell lung cancer:

I.V. (in combination with other approved chemotherapeutic drugs): **Equivalent doses of etoposide phosphate to an etoposide dosage** range of 35 mg/m^2/day for 4 days to 50 mg/m^2/day for 5 days. Courses are repeated at 3- to 4-week intervals after adequate recovery from any toxicity.

Testicular cancer:

I.V. (in combination with other approved chemotherapeutic agents): **Equivalent dose of etoposide phosphate to etoposide dosage** range of 50-100 mg/m^2/day on days 1-5 to 100 mg/m²/day on days 1, 3, and 5. Courses are repeated at 3- to 4-week intervals after adequate recovery from any toxicity.

Dosage Forms Powder for injection, lyophilized: 119.3 mg (100 mg base)

Etrafon® *see* amitriptyline and perphenazine *on page 29*

etretinate (e TRET i nate)

U.S./Canadian Brand Names Tegison®

Therapeutic Category Antipsoriatic Agent

Use Treatment of severe recalcitrant psoriasis in patients intolerant of or unresponsive to standard therapies

Usual Dosage Adults: Oral (individualized): Initial: 0.75-1 mg/kg/day in divided doses up to 1.5 mg/kg/day; maintenance dose established after 8-10 weeks of therapy 0.5-0.75 mg/kg/day

Dosage Forms Capsule: 10 mg, 25 mg

ETS-2%® Topical *see* erythromycin (ophthalmic/topical) *on page 214*

Eudal-SR® *see* guaifenesin and pseudoephedrine *on page 270*

Euflex® (Can) *see* flutamide *on page 249*

Euglucon® (Can) *see* glyburide *on page 263*

Eulexin® *see* flutamide *on page 249*

Eurax® Topical *see* crotamiton *on page 151*

Euthroid® Tablet *(Discontinued)* *see page 700*

Eutron® *see* methyclothiazide and pargyline *on page 366*

Evac-Q-Mag® [OTC] *see* magnesium citrate *on page 344*

Evalose® *see* lactulose *on page 325*

Everone® Injection *see* testosterone *on page 552*

Evista® *see* raloxifene *on page 497*

E-Vitamin® [OTC] *see* vitamin E *on page 604*

Exact® Cream [OTC] *see* benzoyl peroxide *on page 68*

Excedrin®, Extra Strength [OTC] *see* acetaminophen, aspirin, and caffeine *on page 6*

Excedrin® IB [OTC] *see* ibuprofen *on page 300*

Excedrin® P.M. [OTC] *see* acetaminophen and diphenhydramine *on page 5*

Exelderm® Topical *see* sulconazole *on page 539*

Exidine® Scrub [OTC] *see* chlorhexidine gluconate *on page 117*

Exna® *see* benzthiazide *on page 69*

Exosurf® Neonatal™ *see* colfosceril palmitate *on page 145*

Exsel® Shampoo *see* selenium sulfide *on page 518*

Extendryl® SR *see* chlorpheniramine, phenylephrine, and methscopolamine *on page 124*

Extra Action Cough Syrup [OTC] *see* guaifenesin and dextromethorphan *on page 268*

Extra Strength Doan's® [OTC] *see* magnesium salicylate *on page 346*

Eye-Lube-A® Solution [OTC] *see* artificial tears *on page 47*

Eye-Sed® Ophthalmic [OTC] *see* zinc sulfate *on page 612*

Eyesine® Ophthalmic [OTC] *see* tetrahydrozoline *on page 556*

Ezide® *see* hydrochlorothiazide *on page 286*

f_3t *see* trifluridine *on page 581*

factor IX complex (human) (FAK ter nyne KOM pleks HYU man)

U.S./Canadian Brand Names AlphaNine® SD; BeneFix™; Hemonyne®; Konȳne® 80; Profilnine® SD; Proplex® T

Therapeutic Category Antihemophilic Agent

Use

Control bleeding in patients with factor IX deficiency (hemophilia B or Christmas disease). **Note:** Factor IX concentrate containing ONLY factor IX is also available and preferable for this indication.

Prevention/control of bleeding in hemophilia A patients with inhibitors to factor VIII

Prevention/control of bleeding in patients with factor VII deficiency

Emergency correction of the coagulopathy of warfarin excess in critical situations

Usual Dosage Factor IX deficiency (1 unit/kg raises IX levels 1%)

Children and Adults: I.V.:

Hospitalized patients: 20-50 units/kg/dose; may be higher in special cases; may be administered every 24 hours or more often in special cases

Inhibitor patients: 75-100 units/kg/dose; may be administered every 6-12 hours

Dosage Forms Injection:

AlphaNine® SD: Single dose vial

BeneFix™: 250 units, 500 units, 1000 units

Konȳne® 80: 20 mL, 40 mL

Hemonyne®: 20 mL, 40 mL

Profilnine® SD: Single dose vial

Proplex® T: 30 mL vial

factor IX purified *see* factor IX, purified (human) *on this page*

factor IX, purified (human) (FAK ter nyne, PURE eh fide HYU man)

Synonyms factor IX purified; monoclonal antibody purified

U.S./Canadian Brand Names Mononine®

Therapeutic Category Antihemophilic Agent

Use

Control bleeding in patients with factor IX deficiency (hemophilia B or Christmas disease)

Mononine® contains **nondetectable levels of factors II, VII, and X** (<0.0025 units per factor IX unit using standard coagulation assays) and is, therefore, **NOT INDICATED** for replacement therapy of any of these clotting factors

Mononine® is also **NOT INDICATED** in the treatment or reversal of coumarin-induced anticoagulation or in a hemorrhagic state caused by hepatitis-induced lack of production of liver dependent coagulation factors.

Usual Dosage Children and Adults: Dosage is expressed in units of factor IX activity and must be individualized. I.V. only:

Formula for units required to raise blood level %:

Number of factor IX Units Required = body weight (in kg) x desired factor IX level increase (% normal) x 1 unit/kg

For example, for a 100% level a patient who has an actual level of 20%: Number of factor IX Units needed = 70 kg x 80% x 1 Unit/kg = 5,600 Units

Dosage Forms Factor IX units listed per vial and per lot to lot variation *$0.72*/unit of factor IX

Injection: 250 units, 500 units, 1000 units

factor VIIa, recombinant (factor seven ay ree KOM be nant)

Synonyms coagulation factor VIIa; rFVIIa

U.S./Canadian Brand Names Novo-Seven®

Therapeutic Category Antihemophilic Agent; Blood Product Derivative

Use Treatment of bleeding episodes in patients with hemophilia A or B when inhibitors to factor VIII or factor IX are present

Usual Dosage Children and Adults: I.V. administration only: 90 mcg/kg every 2 hours until hemostasis is achieved or until the treatment is judged ineffective. The dose and interval may be adjusted based upon the severity of bleeding and the degree of hemostasis achieved. The duration of therapy following hemostasis has not been fully established; for patients experiencing severe bleeds, dosing should be continued at 3- to 6-hour intervals after hemostasis has been achieved and the duration of dosing should be minimized.

In clinical trials, dosages have ranged from 35-120 mcg/kg and a decision on the final therapeutic dosages was reached within 8 hours in the majority of patients

Dosage Forms Powder for injection: 1.2 mg, 2.4 mg, 4.8 mg

factor VIII *see* antihemophilic factor (human) *on page 39*

factor VIII recombinant *see* antihemophilic factor (recombinant) *on page 40*

Factrel® *see* gonadorelin *on page 265*

famciclovir (fam SYE kloe veer)

U.S./Canadian Brand Names Famvir™

Therapeutic Category Antiviral Agent

Use Management of acute herpes zoster (shingles); treatment of recurrent herpes simplex in immunocompetent patients; treatment of recurrent mucocutaneous herpes simplex infections in HIV-infected patients

Usual Dosage Adults: Oral:

Acute herpes zoster: 500 mg every 8 hours for 7 days

Recurrent herpes simplex in immunocompetent patients: 125 mg twice daily for 5 days

Herpes simplex infections in HIV-infected patients: 500 mg twice daily

Dosage Forms Tablet: 125 mg, 250 mg, 500 mg

famotidine (fa MOE ti deen)

U.S./Canadian Brand Names Apo®-Famotidine (Can); Novo-Famotidine® (Can); Nu-Famotidine® (Can); Pepcid®; Pepcid® AC Acid Controller [OTC]; Pepcid RPD®

Therapeutic Category Histamine H_2 Antagonist

Use Therapy and treatment of duodenal ulcer, gastric ulcer, control gastric pH in critically ill patients, symptomatic relief in gastritis, gastroesophageal reflux, active benign ulcer, and pathological hypersecretory conditions

Usual Dosage

Children: Oral, I.V.: Doses of 1-2 mg/kg/day have been used; maximum dose: 40 mg

Adults:

Oral:

Duodenal ulcer, gastric ulcer: 40 mg/day at bedtime for 4-8 weeks

Hypersecretory conditions: Initial: 20 mg every 6 hours, may increase up to 160 mg every 6 hours

GERD: 20 mg twice daily for 6 weeks

I.V.: 20 mg every 12 hours

Dosage Forms

Infusion, premixed in NS: 20 mg (50 mL)

Injection: 10 mg/mL (2 mL, 4 mL)

Powder for oral suspension (cherry-banana-mint flavor): 40 mg/5 mL (50 mL)

Tablet, chewable (Pepcid® AC): 10 mg

Tablet, film coated: 20 mg, 40 mg

Tablet, orally disintegrating (Pepcid RPD™): 20 mg, 40 mg

Pepcid® AC Acid Controller: 10 mg

Famvir™ *see* famciclovir *on this page*

Fansidar® ***(Discontinued)*** *see page 700*

Fareston® *see* toremifene *on page 572*

Fastin® ***(Discontinued)*** *see page 700*

fat emulsion (fat e MUL shun)

Synonyms intravenous fat emulsion

U.S./Canadian Brand Names Intralipid®; Liposyn®; Nutrilipid®; Soyacal®

(Continued)

fat emulsion *(Continued)*

Therapeutic Category Intravenous Nutritional Therapy

Use Source of calories and essential fatty acids for patients requiring parenteral nutrition of extended duration

Usual Dosage Fat emulsion should not exceed 60% of the total daily calories

Initial dose:

Infants, premature: 0.25-0.5 g/kg/day, increase by 0.25-0.5 g/kg/day to a maximum of 3-4 g/kg/day; maximum rate of infusion: 0.15 g/kg/hour (0.75 mL/kg/hour of 20% solution)

Infants and Children: 0.5-1 g/kg/day, increase by 0.5 g/kg/day to a maximum of 3-4 g/kg/day; maximum rate of infusion: 0.25 g/kg/hour (1.25 mL/kg/hour of 20% solution)

Adolescents and Adults: 1 g/kg/day, increase by 0.5-1 g/kg/day to a maximum of 2.5 g/kg/day; maximum rate of infusion: 0.25 g/kg/hour (1.25 mL/kg/hour of 20% solution); do not exceed 50 mL/hour (20%) or 100 mL/hour (10%)

Fatty acid deficiency: Children and Adults: 8% to 10% of total caloric intake; infuse once or twice weekly

Note: At the onset of therapy, the patient should be observed for any immediate allergic reactions such as dyspnea, cyanosis, and fever. Slower initial rates of infusion may be used for the first 10-15 minutes of the infusion (eg, 0.1 mL/minute of 10% or 0.05 mL/minute of 20% solution).

Dosage Forms Injection: 10% [100 mg/mL] (100 mL, 250 mL, 500 mL); 20% [200 mg/mL] (100 mL, 250 mL, 500 mL)

5-FC *see* flucytosine *on page 242*

FC1157a *see* toremifene *on page 572*

Fedahist® Expectorant [OTC] *see* guaifenesin and pseudoephedrine *on page 270*

Fedahist® Expectorant Pediatric [OTC] *see* guaifenesin and pseudoephedrine *on page 270*

Fedahist® Tablet [OTC] *see* chlorpheniramine and pseudoephedrine *on page 122*

Feiba VH Immuno® *see* anti-inhibitor coagulant complex *on page 40*

felbamate (FEL ba mate)

U.S./Canadian Brand Names Felbatol®

Therapeutic Category Anticonvulsant

Use Not a first-line agent; reserved for patients who do not adequately respond to alternative agents and whose epilepsy is so severe that benefit outweighs risk of liver failure or aplastic anemia; used as monotherapy and adjunctive therapy in patients ≥14 years of age with partial seizures with and without secondary generalization; adjunctive therapy in children ≥2 years of age who have partial and generalized seizures associated with Lennox-Gastaut syndrome

Usual Dosage Oral:

Monotherapy: 1200 mg/day in divided doses 3 or 4 times/day; titrate previously untreated patients under close clinical supervision, increasing the dosage in 600 mg increments every 2 weeks to 2400 mg/day based on clinical response and thereafter to 3600 mg/day in clinically indicated

Conversion to monotherapy: Initiate at 1200 mg/day in divided doses 3 or 4 times/day, reduce the dosage of the concomitant anticonvulsant(s) by 33% at the initiation of felbamate therapy; at week 2, increase the felbamate dosage to 2400 mg/day while reducing the dosage of the other anticonvulsant(s) up to an additional 33% of their original dosage; at week 3, increase the felbamate dosage up to 3600 mg/day and continue to reduce the dosage of the other anticonvulsant(s) as clinically indicated

Adjunctive therapy:

Week 1:

Felbamate: 1200 mg/day initial dose

Concomitant anticonvulsant(s): Reduce original dosage by 20% to 33%

Week 2:
Felbamate: 2400 mg/day (Therapeutic range)
Concomitant anticonvulsant(s): Reduce original dosage by up to an additional 33%
Week 3:
Felbamate: 3600 mg/day (Therapeutic range)
Concomitant anticonvulsant(s): Reduce original dosage as clinically indicated

Dosage Forms
Suspension, oral: 600 mg/5 mL (240 mL, 960 mL)
Tablet: 400 mg, 600 mg

Felbatol® *see* felbamate *on previous page*

Feldene® *see* piroxicam *on page 454*

felodipine (fe LOE di peen)

U.S./Canadian Brand Names Plendil®

Therapeutic Category Calcium Channel Blocker

Use Management of angina pectoris due to coronary insufficiency, hypertension

Usual Dosage Oral:
Adults: Initial: 5 mg once daily; dosage range: 2.5-10 mg once daily; may increase dose up to a maximum of 10 mg
Elderly: Initial: 2.5 mg/day

Dosage Forms Tablet, extended release: 2.5 mg, 5 mg, 10 mg

Femara™ *see* letrozole *on page 328*

FemCare® ***(Discontinued)*** *see page 700*

Femcet® *see* butalbital compound and acetaminophen *on page 85*

Femguard® *see* sulfabenzamide, sulfacetamide, and sulfathiazole *on page 539*

Femiron® [OTC] *see* ferrous fumarate *on page 236*

Femizol-M® [OTC] *see* miconazole *on page 373*

Femogen® (Can) *see* estrone *on page 220*

Femstat® ***(Discontinued)*** *see page 700*

Fenesin™ *see* guaifenesin *on page 267*

Fenesin™ DM *see* guaifenesin and dextromethorphan *on page 268*

fenofibrate (fen oh FYE brate)

Synonyms procetofene; proctofene

U.S./Canadian Brand Names TriCor™

Therapeutic Category Antihyperlipidemic Agent, Miscellaneous

Use Adjunct to dietary therapy for the treatment of adults with very high elevations of serum triglyceride levels (types IV and V hyperlipidemia) who are at risk of pancreatitis and who do not respond adequately to a determined dietary effort; its efficacy can be enhanced by combination with other hypolipidemic agents that have a different mechanism of action; safety and efficacy may be greater than that of clofibrate

Usual Dosage Adults: Oral: Initial: 67 mg/day, up to 3 capsules (201 mg)

Dosage Forms Capsule: 67 mg

fenoldopam (fe NOL doe pam)

U.S./Canadian Brand Names Corlopam®

Therapeutic Category Antihypertensive Agent

Use Patients presenting with emergency hypertension and those requiring blood pressure control during hospitalization pose a challenge due to the associated risk of renal failure and end-organ compromise

Usual Dosage
Oral: 100 mg 2-4 times/day
(Continued)

fenoldopam *(Continued)*

I.V.: Severe hypertension: Initial: 0.1 mcg/kg/minute; may be increased in increments of 0.05-0.2 mcg/kg/minute; maximal infusion rate: 1.6 mcg/kg/minute

Dosage Forms Injection, as mesylate: 10 mg/mL

fenoprofen (fen oh PROE fen)

U.S./Canadian Brand Names Nalfon®

Therapeutic Category Analgesic, Non-narcotic; Nonsteroidal Anti-inflammatory Drug (NSAID)

Use Symptomatic treatment of acute and chronic rheumatoid arthritis and osteoarthritis; relief of mild to moderate pain

Usual Dosage Oral:

Children: Juvenile arthritis: 900 mg/m^2/day, then increase over 4 weeks to 1.8 g/m^2/day

Adults:

Arthritis: 300-600 mg 3-4 times/day up to 3.2 g/day

Pain: 200 mg every 4-6 hours as needed

Dosage Forms Fenoprofen calcium:

Capsule: 200 mg, 300 mg

Tablet: 600 mg

fenoterol *(Canada only)* (fen oh TER ole)

U.S./Canadian Brand Names Berotec® Forte Inhalation Aerosol (Can); Berotec® Inhalation Aerosol (Can); Berotec® Solution (Can)

Therapeutic Category Beta$_2$-Adrenergic Agonist Agent

Use For the symptomatic relief and acute prophylaxis of bronchial obstruction in asthma and other conditions in which reversible bronchospasm is a complicating factor, such as chronic bronchitis or emphysema.

Usual Dosage Adults:

MDI: Acute symptoms: One puff will usually be adequate to relieve bronchospasm in the majority of patients, however, if required, a second puff may be taken preferably after waiting 5 minutes for the effect of the first puff to be obtained. This delay allows better assessment of the effectiveness of 1 puff and deeper penetration of the second puff. If an attack has not been relieved by 2 puffs, further puffs may be required. In these cases, patients should immediately consult the physician or the nearest hospital. If, despite other adequate maintenance therapy, regular use of beta-agonists remains necessary for the control of bronchospasm, the recommended dose is 1-2 puffs of the 100 mcg inhaler 3-4 times/day. A maximum of 8 puffs/day should not be exceeded.

Solution: Dosage should be individualized, and patient response should be monitored by the prescribing physician on an ongoing basis. Should be used only under medical supervision.

Motorized, compressed air or ultrasonic nebulizers: These nebulizers generate low pressure, low velocity aerosols. The average single dose is 0.5 to 1 mg of fenoterol. In more refractory cases, up to 2.5 mg of fenoterol may be given. Fenoterol solution should be diluted to 5 mL with preservative-free sterile sodium chloride inhalation solution, USP 0.9% (normal saline) and the total volume should be nebulized over a period of 10 to 15 minutes. Optimal deposition in the lungs is achieved with the patient breathing quietly and slowly. Treatment may be repeated every 6 hours if necessary.

Intermittent positive pressure ventilation: Fenoterol solution may be used in conjunction with Intermittent Positive Pressure Ventilation (IPPV) when such therapy is indicated. The average single dose is 0.5 to 1 mg of fenoterol. In more refractory cases, up to 2.5 mg of fenoterol may be given. Fenoterol solution should be diluted to 5 mL with preservative-free sterile sodium chloride inhalation solution, USP 0.9% and the total volume should be nebulized over a period of 10-15 minutes. The inspiratory pressure is usually 10 to 20 cm H2O and optimal deposition of the drug in the lungs is achieved with the patient breathing quietly and slowly. Treatment may be repeated every 6 hours if necessary. If a previous effective dosage regimen fails to provide the usual relief, or the effects of a dose last for less than 3 hours, medical advice should be sought immediately; this is a sign of seriously worsening asthma that requires reassessment of therapy. In accordance with the present practice for asthma treatment, concomitant anti-inflammatory therapy should be part of the regimen if fenoterol inhalation solution needs to be used on a regular daily basis.

Dosage Forms

Metered dose inhalers: 100 mcg/actuation (200 doses; 200 mcg/actuation) (100 doses)

Solution, inhalation: 1 mg/mL (20 mL)

fentanyl (FEN ta nil)

U.S./Canadian Brand Names Actiq® Oral Transmucosal; Duragesic® Transdermal; Fentanyl Oralet®; Sublimaze® Injection

Therapeutic Category Analgesic, Narcotic; General Anesthetic

Controlled Substance C-II

Use Sedation; relief of pain; preoperative medication; adjunct to general or regional anesthesia; management of chronic pain (transdermal product)

Oral transmucosal: Hospital setting use only as preoperative anesthetic agent or to induce conscious sedation before procedures

Usual Dosage Doses should be titrated to appropriate effects; wide range of doses, dependent upon desired degree of analgesia/anesthesia

Children:

Sedation for minor procedures/analgesia: I.M., I.V.:

1-3 years: 2-3 mcg/kg/dose; may repeat after 30-60 minutes as required

3-12 years: 1-2 mcg/kg/dose; may repeat at 30- to 60-minute intervals as required. **Note:** Children 18-36 months of age may require 2-3 mcg/kg/dose

Continuous sedation/analgesia: Initial I.V. bolus: 1-2 mcg/kg then 1 mcg/kg/hour; titrate upward; usual: 1-3 mcg/kg/hour

Transdermal: Not recommended

Children <12 years and Adults:

Sedation for minor procedures/analgesia: 0.5-1 mcg/kg/dose; higher doses are used for major procedures

Preoperative sedation, adjunct to regional anesthesia, postoperative pain: I.M., I.V.: 50-100 mcg/dose

Adjunct to general anesthesia: I.M., I.V.: 2-50 mcg/kg

General anesthesia without additional anesthetic agents: I.V. 50-100 mcg/kg with O_2 and skeletal muscle relaxant

Transdermal: Initial: 25 mcg/hour system; if currently receiving opiates, convert to fentanyl equivalent and administer equianalgesic dosage (see package insert for further information)

Dosage Forms

Injection, as citrate: 0.05 mg/mL (2 mL, 5 mL, 10 mL, 20 mL, 50 mL)

Lozenge, oral transmucosal:

Fentanyl Oralet® (raspberry flavored): 200 mcg, 300 mcg, 400 mcg

Actiq® Oral Transmucosal: 200 mcg, 400 mcg, 600 mcg, 800 mcg, 1200 mcg, 1600 mcg

Transdermal system: 25 mcg/hour [10 cm^2]; 50 mcg/hour [20 cm^2]; 75 mcg/hour [30 cm^2]; 100 mcg/hour [40 cm^2] (all available in 5s)

fentanyl and droperidol *see* droperidol and fentanyl *on page 199*

Fentanyl Oralet® *see* fentanyl *on this page*

Feosol® [OTC] *see* ferrous sulfate *on page 237*

Feostat® [OTC] *see* ferrous fumarate *on next page*

Ferancee® [OTC] *see* ferrous salt and ascorbic acid *on page 237*

Feratab® [OTC] *see* ferrous sulfate *on page 237*

Fergon® [OTC] *see* ferrous gluconate *on next page*

Fergon Plus® ***(Discontinued)*** *see page 700*

Feridex I.V.® *see* ferumoxides *on page 238*

Fer-in-Sol® Capsule ***(Discontinued)*** *see page 700*

Fer-In-Sol® Drops [OTC] *see* ferrous sulfate *on next page*

Fer-Iron® [OTC] *see* ferrous sulfate *on next page*

Fermalac® (Can) *see* Lactobacillus *on page 324*

Fermalox® *(Discontinued)* *see page 700*

Ferndex® *(Discontinued)* *see page 700*

Fero-Grad 500® [OTC] *see* ferrous salt and ascorbic acid *on next page*

Fero-Gradumet® [OTC] *see* ferrous sulfate *on next page*

Ferospace® [OTC] *see* ferrous sulfate *on next page*

Ferralet® [OTC] *see* ferrous gluconate *on this page*

Ferralyn® Lanacaps® [OTC] *see* ferrous sulfate *on next page*

Ferra-TD® [OTC] *see* ferrous sulfate *on next page*

ferric gluconate (FER ik GLOO koe nate)

U.S./Canadian Brand Names Ferrlecit®

Therapeutic Category Iron Salt

Use Repletion of total body iron content in patients with iron deficiency anemia who are undergoing hemodialysis in conjunction with erythropoietin therapy

Usual Dosage Adults:

Test dose (recommended): 2 mL diluted in 50 mL 0.9% sodium chloride over 60 minutes

Repletion of iron in hemodialysis patients: I.V.: 125 mg (10 mL) in 100 mL 0.9% sodium chloride over 1 hour during hemodialysis. Most patients will require a cumulative dose of 1 g elemental iron over approximately 8 sequential dialysis treatments to achieve a favorable response.

Dosage Forms Injection: 12.5 mg/mL (5 mL)

Ferrlecit® *see* ferric gluconate *on this page*

Ferro-Sequels® [OTC] *see* ferrous fumarate *on this page*

ferrous fumarate (FER us FYOO ma rate)

U.S./Canadian Brand Names Femiron® [OTC]; Feostat® [OTC]; Ferro-Sequels® [OTC]; Fumasorb® [OTC]; Fumerin® [OTC]; Hemocyte® [OTC]; Ircon® [OTC]; Nephro-Fer™ [OTC]; Palafer® (Can); Span-FF® [OTC]

Therapeutic Category Electrolyte Supplement, Oral

Use Prevention and treatment of iron deficiency anemias

Usual Dosage Oral:

Children: 3 mg/kg 3 times/day

Adults: 200 mg 3-4 times/day

Dosage Forms Amount of elemental iron is listed in brackets

Capsule, controlled release (Span-FF®): 325 mg [106 mg]

Drops (Feostat®): 45 mg/0.6 mL [15 mg/0.6 mL] (60 mL)

Suspension, oral (Feostat®): 100 mg/5 mL [33 mg/5 mL] (240 mL)

Tablet: 325 mg [106 mg]

Chewable (chocolate flavor) (Feostat®): 100 mg [33 mg]

Femiron®: 63 mg [20 mg]

Fumerin®: 195 mg [64 mg]

Fumasorb®, Ircon®: 200 mg [66 mg]

Hemocyte®: 324 mg [106 mg]

Nephro-Fer™: 350 mg [115 mg]

Timed release (Ferro-Sequels®): Ferrous fumarate 150 mg [50 mg] and docusate sodium 100 mg

ferrous gluconate (FER us GLOO koe nate)

U.S./Canadian Brand Names Apo-Ferrous® Gluconate (Can); Fergon® [OTC]; Ferralet® [OTC]; Simron® [OTC]

Therapeutic Category Electrolyte Supplement, Oral

Use Prevention and treatment of iron deficiency anemias

Usual Dosage Oral (dose expressed in terms of elemental iron):

Iron deficiency anemia: 3-6 Fe mg/kg/day in 3 divided doses

Maintenance:

Preterm infants:

Birthweight <1000 g: 4 Fe mg/kg/day

Birthweight 1000-1500 g: 3 Fe mg/kg/day

Birthweight 1500-2500 g: 2 Fe mg/kg/day

Term Infants and Children: 1-2 Fe mg/kg/day in 3 divided doses, up to a maximum of 18 Fe mg/day

Adults: 60-100 Fe mg/day in 3 divided doses

Dosage Forms Amount of elemental iron is listed in brackets

Capsule, soft gelatin (Simron®): 86 mg [10 mg]

Elixir (Fergon®): 300 mg/5 mL [34 mg/5 mL] with alcohol 7% (480 mL)

Tablet: 300 mg [34 mg]; 325 mg [38 mg]

Fergon®, Ferralet®: 320 mg [37 mg]

Sustained release (Ferralet® Slow Release): 320 mg [37 mg]

ferrous salt and ascorbic acid (FER us SUL fate & a SKOR bik AS id)

Synonyms ascorbic acid and ferrous sulfate

U.S./Canadian Brand Names Ferancee® [OTC]; Fero-Grad 500® [OTC]

Therapeutic Category Vitamin

Use Treatment of iron deficiency in nonpregnant adults; treatment and prevention of iron deficiency in pregnant adults

Usual Dosage Adults: Oral: 1 tablet daily

Dosage Forms Amount of elemental iron is listed in brackets

Caplet, sustained release (Ferromar®): Ferrous fumarate 201.5 mg [65 mg] and ascorbic acid 200 mg

Tablet (Fero-Grad 500®): Ferrous sulfate 525 mg [105 mg] and ascorbic acid 500 mg

Chewable (Ferancee®): Ferrous fumarate 205 mg [67 mg] and ascorbic acid 150 mg

ferrous sulfate (FER us SUL fate)

Synonyms $FeSO_4$

U.S./Canadian Brand Names Apo-Ferrous® Sulfate (Can); Feosol® [OTC]; Feratab® [OTC]; Fer-In-Sol® Drops [OTC]; Fer-Iron® [OTC]; Fero-Gradumet® [OTC]; Ferospace® [OTC]; Ferralyn® Lanacaps® [OTC]; Ferra-TD® [OTC]; Mol-Iron® [OTC]; PMS-Ferrous Sulfate (Can); Slow FE® [OTC]

Therapeutic Category Electrolyte Supplement, Oral

Use Prevention and treatment of iron deficiency anemias

Usual Dosage Oral (dose expressed in terms of elemental iron):

Children:

Severe iron deficiency anemia: 4-6 mg Fe/kg/day in 3 divided doses

Mild to moderate iron deficiency anemia: 3 mg Fe/kg/day in 1-2 divided doses

Prophylaxis: 1-2 mg Fe/kg/day up to a maximum of 15 mg/day

Adults: Iron deficiency: 60-100 Fe/kg/day in divided doses

Dosage Forms Amount of elemental iron is listed in brackets

Capsule:

Exsiccated, timed release (Feosol®): 159 mg [50 mg]

Exsiccated, timed release (Ferralyn® Lanacaps®, Ferra-TD®): 250 mg [50 mg]

Ferospace®: 250 mg [50 mg]

Drops, oral:

Fer-In-Sol®: 75 mg/0.6 mL [15 mg/0.6 mL] (50 mL)

Fer-Iron®: 125 mg/mL [25 mg/mL] (50 mL)

Elixir (Feosol®): 220 mg/5 mL [44 mg/5 mL] with alcohol 5% (473 mL, 4000 mL)

Syrup (Fer-In-Sol®): 90 mg/5 mL [18 mg/5 mL] with alcohol 5% (480 mL)

Tablet: 324 mg [65 mg]

Exsiccated (Feosol®) 200 mg [65 mg]

Exsiccated, timed release (Slow FE®): 160 mg [50 mg]

(Continued)

ferrous sulfate *(Continued)*

Feratab®: 300 mg [60 mg]
Mol-Iron®: 195 mg [39 mg]
Timed release (Fero-Gradumet®): 525 mg [105 mg]

ferrous sulfate, ascorbic acid, and vitamin B-complex

(FER us SUL fate, a SKOR bik AS id, & VYE ta min bee KOM pleks)

U.S./Canadian Brand Names Iberet®-Liquid [OTC]

Therapeutic Category Vitamin

Use Treatment of conditions of iron deficiency with an increased need for B complex vitamins and vitamin C

Usual Dosage Oral:

Children 1-3 years: 5 mL twice daily after meals
Children >4 years and Adults: 10 mL 3 times/day after meals

Dosage Forms Liquid:

Ferrous sulfate: 78.75 mg
Ascorbic acid: 375 mg
B_1: 4.5 mg
B_2: 4.5 mg
B_3: 22.5 mg
B_5: 7.5 mg
B_6: 3.75 mg
B_{12}: 18.75 mg all per 15 mL

ferrous sulfate, ascorbic acid, vitamin B-complex, and folic acid

(FER us SUL fate, a SKOR bik AS id, VYE ta min bee KOM pleks, & FOE lik AS id)

U.S./Canadian Brand Names Iberet-Folic-500®

Therapeutic Category Vitamin

Use Treatment of iron deficiency and prevention of concomitant folic acid deficiency where there is an associated deficient intake or increased need for B complex vitamins

Usual Dosage Adults: Oral: 1 tablet daily

Dosage Forms Tablet, controlled release:

Ferrous sulfate: 105 mg
Ascorbic acid: 500 mg
B_1: 6 mg
B_2: 6 mg
B_3: 30 mg
B_5: 10 mg
B_6: 5 mg
B_{12}: 25 mcg
Folic acid: 800 mcg

Fertinex® *see* urofollitropin *on page 592*

ferumoxides (fer yoo MOX ides)

U.S./Canadian Brand Names Feridex I.V.®

Therapeutic Category Radiopaque Agents

Use For I.V. administration as an adjunct to MRI (in adult patients) to enhance the T2 weighted images used in the detection and evaluation of lesions of the liver

Usual Dosage Adults: 0.56 mg of iron (0.05 mL Feridex I.V.®)/kg body weight diluted in 100 mL of 5% dextrose and infused over 30 minutes; a 5-micron filter is recommended; do not administer undiluted

Dosage Forms Injection: Iron 11.2 mg and mannitol per mL (5 mL)

$FeSO_4$ *see* ferrous sulfate *on previous page*

Feverall™ [OTC] *see* acetaminophen *on page 3*

fexofenadine (feks oh FEN a deen)

U.S./Canadian Brand Names Allegra®

Therapeutic Category Antihistamine

Use Nonsedating antihistamine indicated for the relief of seasonal allergic rhinitis

Usual Dosage Children ≥12 years and Adults: Oral: 1 capsule (60 mg) twice daily

Dosage Forms Capsule, as hydrochloride: 60 mg

fexofenadine and pseudoephedrine
(feks oh FEN a deen & soo doe e FED rin)

U.S./Canadian Brand Names Allegra-D™

Therapeutic Category Antihistamine/Decongestant Combination

Use Relief of symptoms associated with seasonal allergic rhinitis in adults and children ≥12 years. Symptoms treated effectively include sneezing, rhinorrhea, itchy nose/palate/ and/or throat, itchy/watery/red eyes, and nasal congestion.

Usual Dosage Oral: Adults: 1 tablet twice daily for adults and children ≥12 years of age. It is recommended that the administration with food should be avoided. A dose of 1 tablet once daily is recommended as the starting dose in patients with decreased renal function.

Dosage Forms Tablet, extended release: Fexofenadine hydrochloride 60 mg and pseudoephedrine hydrochloride 120 mg

Fiberall® Chewable Tablet [OTC] *see* calcium polycarbophil *on page 93*

Fiberall® Powder [OTC] *see* psyllium *on page 488*

Fiberall® Wafer [OTC] *see* psyllium *on page 488*

FiberCon® Tablet [OTC] *see* calcium polycarbophil *on page 93*

Fiber-Lax® Tablet [OTC] *see* calcium polycarbophil *on page 93*

Fibrepur® (Can) *see* psyllium *on page 488*

filgrastim (fil GRA stim)

Synonyms G-CSF; granulocyte colony-stimulating factor

U.S./Canadian Brand Names Neupogen®

Therapeutic Category Colony-Stimulating Factor

Use To reduce the duration of neutropenia and the associated risk of infection in patients with nonmyeloid malignancies receiving myelosuppressive chemotherapeutic regimens associated with a significant incidence of severe neutropenia with fever; it has also been used in AIDS patients on zidovudine and in patients with noncancer chemotherapy-induced neutropenia

Usual Dosage Children and Adults (refer to individual protocols): I.V., S.C.: 5-10 mcg/kg/day (~150-300 mcg/m²/day) once daily for up to 14 days until ANC = 10,000/mm³; dose escalations at 5 mcg/kg/day may be required in some individuals when response at 5 mcg/kg/day is not adequate; dosages of 0.6-120 mcg/kg/day have been used in children ranging in age from 3 months to 18 years

Dosage Forms Injection, preservative free: 300 mcg/mL (1 mL, 1.6 mL)

finasteride (fi NAS teer ide)

U.S./Canadian Brand Names Proscar®

Therapeutic Category Antiandrogen

Use Early data indicate that finasteride is useful in the treatment of benign prostatic hyperplasia

Usual Dosage Benign prostatic hyperplasia: Adults: Oral: 5 mg/day as a single dose; clinical responses occur within 12 weeks to 6 months of initiation of therapy; long-term administration is recommended for maximal response

Dosage Forms

Tablet, film coated:

Propecia®: 1 mg

Proscar®: 5 mg

Fiorgen PF® *see* butalbital compound and aspirin *on page 85*

Fioricet® *see* butalbital compound and acetaminophen *on page 85*

Fiorinal® *see* butalbital compound and aspirin *on page 85*

Fiorinal® With Codeine *see* butalbital compound and codeine *on page 86*

fisalamine *see* mesalamine *on page 358*

FK506 *see* tacrolimus *on page 546*

Flagyl® Oral *see* metronidazole *on page 372*

Flamazine® (Can) *see* silver sulfadiazine *on page 522*

Flarex® *see* fluorometholone *on page 245*

Flatulex® [OTC] *see* simethicone *on page 522*

Flavorcee® [OTC] *see* ascorbic acid *on page 48*

flavoxate (fla VOKS ate)

U.S./Canadian Brand Names Urispas®

Therapeutic Category Antispasmodic Agent, Urinary

Use Antispasmodic to provide symptomatic relief of dysuria, nocturia, suprapubic pain, urgency, and incontinence

Usual Dosage Children >12 years and Adults: Oral: 100-200 mg 3-4 times/day

Dosage Forms Tablet, film coated, as hydrochloride: 100 mg

Flaxedil® *see* gallamine triethiodide *on page 256*

flecainide (fle KAY nide)

U.S./Canadian Brand Names Tambocor™

Therapeutic Category Antiarrhythmic Agent, Class I-C

Use Prevention and suppression of documented life-threatening ventricular arrhythmias (ie, sustained ventricular tachycardia); prevention of symptomatic, disabling supraventricular tachycardias in patients without structural heart disease

Usual Dosage Oral:

Children: Initial: 3 mg/kg/day in 3 divided doses; usual 3-6 mg/kg/day in 3 divided doses; up to 11 mg/kg/day for uncontrolled patients with subtherapeutic levels

Adults: Initial: 100 mg every 12 hours, increase by 100 mg/day (administer in 2 doses/day) every 4 days to maximum of 400 mg/day; for patients receiving 400 mg/day who are not controlled and have trough concentrations <0.6 mcg/mL, dosage may be increased to 600 mg/day

Dosage Forms Tablet, as acetate: 50 mg, 100 mg, 150 mg

Fleet® Babylax® Rectal [OTC] *see* glycerin *on page 263*

Fleet® Enema [OTC] *see* sodium phosphates *on page 529*

Fleet® Flavored Castor Oil [OTC] *see* castor oil *on page 103*

Fleet® Laxative [OTC] *see* bisacodyl *on page 74*

Fleet® Pain Relief [OTC] *see* pramoxine *on page 469*

Fleet® Phospho®-Soda [OTC] *see* sodium phosphates *on page 529*

Flexaphen® *see* chlorzoxazone *on page 128*

Flexeril® *see* cyclobenzaprine *on page 153*

Flo-Coat® *see* radiological/contrast media (ionic) *on page 495*

floctafenine *(Canada only)* (flok ta FEN een)

U.S./Canadian Brand Names Idarac® (Can)

Therapeutic Category Nonsteroidal Anti-inflammatory Drug (NSAID), Oral

Use Short-term use in acute pain of mild and moderate severity

Usual Dosage Adults: Oral: 200-400 mg every 6-8 hours as required; maximum recommended daily dose: 1200 mg

Dosage Forms Tablet: 200 mg, 400 mg

Flodine® (Can) *see* folic acid *on page 251*

Flolan® *see* epoprostenol *on page 211*

Flomax® *see* tamsulosin *on page 547*

Flonase® *see* fluticasone (nasal) *on page 249*

Flonase® 9 g *(Discontinued)* *see page 700*

Florical® [OTC] *see* calcium carbonate *on page 89*

Florinef® Acetate *see* fludrocortisone *on next page*

Florone® *see* diflorasone *on page 179*

Florone E® *see* diflorasone *on page 179*

Floropryl® Ophthalmic *see* isoflurophate *on page 314*

Flovent® *see* fluticasone (oral inhalation) *on page 249*

Flovent® Rotadisk® *see* fluticasone (oral inhalation) *on page 249*

Floxin® *see* ofloxacin *on page 414*

floxuridine (floks YOOR i deen)

Synonyms fluorodeoxyuridine

U.S./Canadian Brand Names Fludara® (Can); FUDR®

Therapeutic Category Antineoplastic Agent

Use Palliative management of carcinomas of head, neck, and brain as well as liver, gallbladder, and bile ducts

Usual Dosage Adults:

Intra-arterial infusion: 0.1-0.6 mg/kg/day for 14 days followed by heparinized saline for 14 days

Investigational: I.V.: 0.5-1 mg/kg/day for 6-15 days

Dosage Forms

Injection, preservative free: 100 mg/mL (5 mL)

Powder for injection: 500 mg (5 mL, 10 mL)

Fluanxol® Depot (Can) *see* flupenthixol *(Canada only) on page 247*

Fluanxol® Tablet (Can) *see* flupenthixol *(Canada only) on page 247*

flubenisolone *see* betamethasone (topical) *on page 72*

fluconazole (floo KOE na zole)

U.S./Canadian Brand Names Diflucan®

Therapeutic Category Antifungal Agent

Use Treatment of susceptible fungal infections including oropharyngeal, esophageal, and vaginal candidiasis; treatment of systemic candidal infections including urinary tract infection, peritonitis, cystitis, and pneumonia; treatment and suppression of cryptococcal meningitis; prophylaxis of candidiasis in patients undergoing bone marrow transplantation; alternative to amphotericin B in patients with pre-existing renal impairment or when requiring concomitant therapy with other potentially nephrotoxic drugs

Usual Dosage Daily dose of fluconazole is the same for oral and I.V. administration

Infants and Children: Oral, I.V.: Safety profile of fluconazole has been studied in 577 children, ages 1 day to 17 years; doses as high as 12 mg/kg/day once daily (equivalent to adult doses of 400 mg/day) have been used to treat candidiasis in immunocompromised children; 10-12 mg/kg/day doses once daily have been used prophylactically against fungal infections in pediatric bone marrow transplantation patients. Do not exceed 600 mg/day.

Adults:

Vaginal candidiasis: Oral: 150 mg single dose

(Continued)

fluconazole *(Continued)*

Prophylaxis against fungal infections in bone marrow transplantation patients: Oral, I.V.: 400 mg/day once daily

Dosage Forms

Injection: 2 mg/mL (100 mL, 200 mL)
Powder for oral suspension: 10 mg/mL (35 mL); 40 mg/mL (35 mL)
Tablet: 50 mg, 100 mg, 150 mg, 200 mg

flucytosine (floo SYE toe seen)

Synonyms 5-FC; 5-flurocytosine

U.S./Canadian Brand Names Ancobon®; Ancotil® (Can)

Therapeutic Category Antifungal Agent

Use In combination with amphotericin B in the treatment of serious *Candida, Aspergillus, Cryptococcus*, and *Torulopsis* infections

Usual Dosage Children and Adults: Oral: 50-150 mg/kg/day in divided doses every 6 hours

Dosage Forms Capsule: 250 mg, 500 mg

Fludara® *see* fludarabine *on this page*

fludarabine (floo DARE a been)

U.S./Canadian Brand Names Fludara®

Therapeutic Category Antineoplastic Agent

Use Treatment of B-cell chronic lymphocytic leukemia unresponsive to previous therapy with an alkylating agent containing regimen. Fludarabine has been tested in patients with refractory acute lymphocytic leukemia and acute nonlymphocytic leukemia, but required a highly toxic dose to achieve response.

Usual Dosage Adults: I.V.:

Chronic lymphocytic leukemia: 25 mg/m^2/day over a 30-minute period for 5 days
Non-Hodgkin's lymphoma: Loading dose: 20 mg/m^2 followed by 30 mg/m^2/day for 48 hours

Dosage Forms Powder for injection, as phosphate, lyophilized: 50 mg (6 mL)

Fludara® (Can) *see* floxuridine *on previous page*

fludrocortisone (floo droe KOR ti sone AS e tate)

Synonyms fluohydrocortisone; 9α-fluorohydrocortisone

U.S./Canadian Brand Names Florinef® Acetate

Therapeutic Category Adrenal Corticosteroid (Mineralocorticoid)

Use Addison's disease; partial replacement therapy for adrenal insufficiency; treatment of salt-losing forms of congenital adrenogenital syndrome; has been used with increased sodium intake for the treatment of idiopathic orthostatic hypotension

Usual Dosage Oral:

Infants and Children: 0.05-0.1 mg/day
Adults: 0.05-0.2 mg/day

Dosage Forms Tablet, as acetate: 0.1 mg

Flumadine® *see* rimantadine *on page 506*

flumazenil (FLO may ze nil)

U.S./Canadian Brand Names Anexate® (Can); Romazicon®

Therapeutic Category Antidote

Use Benzodiazepine antagonist; reverses sedative effects of benzodiazepines used in general anesthesia or conscious sedation; management of benzodiazepine overdose; not indicated for ethanol, barbiturate, general anesthetic or narcotic overdose

Usual Dosage Reversal of conscious sedation or general anesthesia: 0.2 mg (2 mL) administered I.V. over 15 seconds; if desired effect is not achieved after 60 seconds, repeat in 0.2 mg (2 mL) increments every 60 seconds up to a total of 1 mg (10 mL); in event of resedation, repeat doses may be administered at 20-minute intervals with no more than 1 mg (10 mL) administered at any one time, with a maximum of 3 mg in any 1 hour

Dosage Forms Injection: 0.1 mg/mL (5 mL, 10 mL)

flunisolide (floo NIS oh lide)

U.S./Canadian Brand Names AeroBid®-M Oral Aerosol Inhaler; AeroBid® Oral Aerosol Inhaler; Bronalide® (Can); Nasalide® Nasal Aerosol; Nasarel™ Nasal Spray; Rhinalar® (Can); Rhinaris-F® (Can); Syn-Flunisolide® (Can)

Therapeutic Category Adrenal Corticosteroid

Use Steroid-dependent asthma; nasal solution is used for seasonal or perennial rhinitis

Usual Dosage

Children:

Oral inhalation: >6 years: 2 inhalations twice daily up to 4 inhalations/day

Nasal: 6-14 years: 1 spray each nostril 2-3 times/day, not to exceed 4 sprays/day each nostril

Adults:

Oral inhalation: 2 inhalations twice daily up to 8 inhalations/day

Nasal: 2 sprays each nostril twice daily; maximum dose: 8 sprays/day in each nostril

Dosage Forms

Inhalant:

Nasal (Nasalide®): 25 mcg/actuation [200 sprays] (25 mL)

Nasal (Nasarel™): 25 mcg/actuation [200 sprays] (25 mL)

Oral:

AeroBid®: 250 mcg/actuation [100 metered doses] (7 g)

AeroBid-M® (menthol flavor): 250 mcg/actuation [100 metered doses] (7 g)

Solution, spray: 0.025% [200 actuations] (25 mL)

fluocinolone (floo oh SIN oh lone)

U.S./Canadian Brand Names Derma-Smoothe/FS® Topical; Fluonid® Topical; Flurosyn® Topical; FS Shampoo® Topical; Lidemol® (Can); Synalar-HP® Topical; Synalar® Topical; Synemol® Topical

Therapeutic Category Corticosteroid, Topical

Use Relief of susceptible inflammatory dermatosis

Usual Dosage Children and Adults: Topical: Apply 2-4 times/day

Dosage Forms Fluocinolone acetonide:

Cream, topical: 0.01% (15 g, 60 g); 0.025% (15 g, 60 g)

Flurosyn®, Synalar®: 0.01% (15 g, 30 g, 60 g, 425 g)

Flurosyn®, Synalar®, Synemol®: 0.025% (15 g, 60 g, 425 g)

Synalar-HP®: 0.2% (12 g)

Ointment, topical: 0.025% (15 g, 60 g)

Flurosyn®, Synalar®: 0.025% (15 g, 30 g, 60 g, 425 g)

Oil (Derma-Smoothe/FS®): 0.01% (120 mL)

Shampoo (FS Shampoo®): 0.01% (180 mL)

Solution, topical: 0.01% (20 mL, 60 mL)

Fluonid®, Synalar®: 0.01% (20 mL, 60 mL)

fluocinonide (floo oh SIN oh nide)

U.S./Canadian Brand Names Fluoderm (Can); Lidex®; Lidex-E®; Lyderm® (Can); Tiamol® (Can); Topactin® (Can); Topsyn® (Can)

Therapeutic Category Corticosteroid, Topical

Use Inflammation of corticosteroid-responsive dermatoses

Usual Dosage Children and Adults: Topical: Apply thin layer to affected area 2-4 times/day depending on the severity of the condition

Dosage Forms

Cream: 0.05% (15 g, 30 g, 60 g, 120 g)

Anhydrous, emollient (Lidex®): 0.05% (15 g, 30 g, 60 g, 120 g)

Aqueous, emollient (Lidex-E®): 0.05% (15 g, 30 g, 60 g, 120 g)

(Continued)

fluocinonide *(Continued)*

Gel, topical: 0.05% (15 g, 60 g)
Lidex®: 0.05% (15 g, 30 g, 60 g, 120 g)
Ointment, topical: 0.05% (15 g, 30 g, 60 g)
Lidex®: 0.05% (15 g, 30 g, 60 g, 120 g)
Solution, topical: 0.05% (20 mL, 60 mL)
Lidex®: 0.05% (20 mL, 60 mL)

Fluoderm (Can) *see* fluocinonide *on previous page*

Fluogen® *see* influenza virus vaccine *on page 306*

fluohydrocortisone *see* fludrocortisone *on page 242*

Fluonid® Topical *see* fluocinolone *on previous page*

Fluoracaine® Ophthalmic *see* proparacaine and fluorescein *on page 481*

Fluor-A-Day® (Can) *see* fluoride *on this page*

FluorCare® Neutral *see* fluoride *on this page*

fluorescein sodium (FLURE e seen SOW dee um)

Synonyms soluble fluorescein

U.S./Canadian Brand Names AK-Fluor Injection; Fluorescite® Injection; Fluorets® Ophthalmic Strips; Fluor-I-Strip®; Fluor-I-Strip-AT®; Flurate® Ophthalmic Solution; Fluress® Ophthalmic Solution; Ful-Glo® Ophthalmic Strips; Funduscein® Injection

Therapeutic Category Diagnostic Agent

Use Demonstrates defects of corneal epithelium; diagnostic aid in ophthalmic angiography

Usual Dosage

Injection: Perform intradermal skin test before use to avoid possible allergic reaction
Children: 3.5 mg/lb (7.5 mg/kg) injected rapidly into antecubital vein
Adults: 500-750 mg injected rapidly into antecubital vein
Strips: Moisten with sterile water or irrigating solution, touch conjunctiva with moistened tip, blink several times after application
Topical solution: Instill 1-2 drops, allow a few seconds for staining, then wash out excess with sterile irrigation solution

Dosage Forms

Injection (AK-Fluor, Fluorescite®, Funduscein®, Ophthifluor®): 10% [100 mg/mL] (5 mL); 25% [250 mg/mL] (2 mL, 3 mL)
Ophthalmic:
Solution: 2% [20 mg/mL] (1 mL, 2 mL, 15 mL)
Flurate®, Fluress®: 0.25% [2.5 mg/mL] with benoxinate 0.4% (5 mL)
Strip:
Ful-Glo®: 0.6 mg
Fluorets®, Fluor-I-Strip-AT®: 1 mg
Fluor-I-Strip®: 9 mg

Fluorescite® Injection *see* fluorescein sodium *on this page*

Fluorets® Ophthalmic Strips *see* fluorescein sodium *on this page*

fluoride (FLOR ide)

U.S./Canadian Brand Names ACT® [OTC]; Fluor-A-Day® (Can); FluorCare® Neutral; Fluorigard® [OTC]; Fluorinse®; Fluoritab®; Fluotic® (Can); Flura®; Flura-Drops®; Flura-Loz®; Gel-Kam®; Gel-Tin® [OTC]; Karidium®; Karigel®; Karigel®-N; Listermint® with Fluoride [OTC]; Lozi-Tab®; Luride®; Luride®-SF; Minute-Gel®; Pediaflor®; Pedi-Dent™ (Can); Pharmaflur®; Phos-Flur®; Point-Two®; Prevident®; Stop® [OTC]; Thera-Flur®; Thera-Flur-N®

Therapeutic Category Mineral, Oral

Use Prevention of dental caries

Usual Dosage Oral: Dental rinse or gel:

Children 6-12 years: 5-10 mL rinse or apply to teeth and spit daily after brushing

Adults: 10 mL rinse or apply to teeth and spit daily after brushing

Dosage Forms Fluoride ion content listed in brackets

Acidulated phosphate fluoride: Rinse, topical:

Minute-Gel®: 1.23% (480 mL)

Sodium fluoride:

Drops, oral:

Fluoritab®, Flura-Drops®: 0.55 mg/drop [0.25 mg/drop] (22.8 mL, 24 mL)

Karidium®, Luride®: 0.275 mg/drop [0.125 mg/drop] (30 mL, 60 mL)

Pediaflor®: 1.1 mg/mL [0.5 mg/mL] (50 mL)

Gel, topical:

Karigel®, Karigel®-N, PreviDent®: 1.1% [0.5%] (24 g, 30 g, 60 g, 120 g, 130 g, 250 g)

Rinse, topical:

ACT®, Fluorigard®: 0.05% [0.02%] (90 mL, 180 mL, 300 mL, 360 mL, 480 mL)

Fluorinse®, Point-Two®: 0.2% [0.09%] (240 mL, 480 mL, 3780 mL)

Listermint® with Fluoride: 0.02% [0.01%] (180 mL, 300 mL, 360 mL, 480 mL, 540 mL, 720 mL, 960 mL, 1740 mL)

Solution, oral, as sodium (Phos-Flur®): 0.44 mg/mL [0.2 mg/mL] (250 mL, 500 mL, 3780 mL)

Tablet:

Chewable:

Fluoritab®, Luride® Lozi-Tab®, Pharmaflur®: 1.1 mg [0.5 mg]

Fluoritab®, Karidium®, Luride® Lozi-Tab®, Luride®-SF Lozi-Tab®, Pharmaflur®: 2.2 mg [1 mg]

Oral: Flura®, Karidium®: 2.2 mg [1 mg]

Stannous fluoride: Rinse, topical:

Gel-Kam®, Gel-Tin®, Stop®: 0.4% [0.1%] (60 g, 15 g, 105 g, 120 g)

Fluorigard® [OTC] *see* fluoride *on previous page*

Fluori-Methane® Topical Spray *see* dichlorodifluoromethane and trichloromonofluoromethane *on page 175*

Fluorinse® *see* fluoride *on previous page*

Fluor-I-Strip® *see* fluorescein sodium *on previous page*

Fluor-I-Strip-AT® *see* fluorescein sodium *on previous page*

Fluoritab® *see* fluoride *on previous page*

fluorodeoxyuridine *see* floxuridine *on page 241*

9α-fluorohydrocortisone *see* fludrocortisone *on page 242*

fluorometholone (flure oh METH oh lone)

U.S./Canadian Brand Names Flarex®; Fluor-Op®; FML®; FML® Forte

Therapeutic Category Adrenal Corticosteroid

Use Inflammatory conditions of the eye, including keratitis, iritis, cyclitis, and conjunctivitis

Usual Dosage Children >2 years and Adults: Ophthalmic: 1-2 drops into conjunctival sac every hour during day, every 2 hours at night until favorable response is obtained, then use 1 drop every 4 hours; in mild or moderate inflammation: 1-2 drops into conjunctival sac 2-4 times/day. Ointment may be applied every 4 hours in severe cases or 1-3 times/day in mild to moderate cases.

Dosage Forms Ophthalmic:

Ointment (FML®): 0.1% (3.5 g)

Suspension:

Flarex®, Fluor-Op®, FML®: 0.1% (2.5 mL, 5 mL, 10 mL)

FML® Forte: 0.25% (2 mL, 5 mL, 10 mL, 15 mL)

fluorometholone and sulfacetamide *see* sulfacetamide sodium and fluorometholone *on page 541*

Fluor-Op® *see* fluorometholone *on this page*

Fluoroplex® Topical *see* fluorouracil *on next page*

fluorouracil (flure oh YOOR a sil)

Synonyms 5-fluorouracil; 5-FU

U.S./Canadian Brand Names Adrucil® Injection; Efudex® Topical; Fluoroplex® Topical

Therapeutic Category Antineoplastic Agent

Use Treatment of carcinoma of stomach, colon, rectum, breast, and pancreas; also used topically for management of multiple actinic keratoses and superficial basal cell carcinomas

Usual Dosage Children and Adults (refer to individual protocol):

I.V.: Initial: 12 mg/kg/day (maximum: 800 mg/day) for 4-5 days; maintenance: 6 mg/kg every other day for 4 doses

Single weekly bolus dose of 15 mg/kg can be administered depending on the patient's reaction to the previous course of treatment; maintenance dose of 5-15 mg/kg/week as a single dose not to exceed 1 g/week

I.V. infusion: 15 mg/kg/day (maximum daily dose: 1 g) has been administered by I.V. infusion over 4 hours for 5 days

Oral: 20 mg/kg/day for 5 days every 5 weeks for colorectal carcinoma; 15 mg/kg/week for hepatoma

Topical: 5% cream twice daily

Dosage Forms

Cream, topical:

Efudex®: 5% (25 g)

Fluoroplex®: 1% (30 g)

Injection (Adrucil®): 50 mg/mL (10 mL, 20 mL, 50 mL, 100 mL)

Solution, topical:

Efudex®: 2% (10 mL); 5% (10 mL)

Fluoroplex®: 1% (30 mL)

5-fluorouracil *see* fluorouracil *on this page*

fluostigmin *see* isoflurophate *on page 314*

Fluothane® *see* halothane *on page 277*

Fluotic® (Can) *see* fluoride *on page 244*

fluoxetine (floo OKS e teen)

U.S./Canadian Brand Names Prozac®

Therapeutic Category Antidepressant, Selective Serotonin Reuptake Inhibitor

Use Treatment of major depression; preliminary studies report use for obsessive-compulsive disorders in children and adolescents

Usual Dosage Oral:

Children <18 years: Dose not established

Adults: 20 mg/day in the morning; may increase after several weeks by 20 mg/day increments; maximum: 80 mg/day; doses >20 mg should be divided into 2 daily doses

Note: Lower doses of 5 mg/day have been used for initial treatment

Dosage Forms Fluoxetine hydrochloride:

Capsule: 10 mg, 20 mg

Liquid (mint flavor): 20 mg/5 mL (120 mL)

Tablet: 10 mg

fluoxymesterone (floo oks i MES te rone)

U.S./Canadian Brand Names Halotestin®

Therapeutic Category Androgen

Use Replacement of endogenous testicular hormone; in female used as palliative treatment of breast cancer, postpartum breast engorgement

Usual Dosage Adults: Oral:

Male:

Hypogonadism: 5-20 mg/day

Delayed puberty: 2.5-20 mg/day for 4-6 months

Female:

Breast carcinoma: 10-40 mg/day in divided doses for 1-3 months

Breast engorgement: 2.5 mg after delivery, 5-10 mg/day in divided doses for 4-5 days

Dosage Forms Tablet: 2 mg, 5 mg, 10 mg

flupenthixol *(Canada only)* (floo pen THIKS ol)

U.S./Canadian Brand Names Fluanxol® Depot (Can); Fluanxol® Tablet (Can)

Therapeutic Category Antipsychotic Agent; Thioxanthene Derivative

Use Maintenance therapy of chronic schizophrenic patients whose main manifestations do not include excitement, agitation, or hyperactivity

Usual Dosage

Injection: Flupenthixol is administered by deep I.M. injection, preferably in the gluteus maximus, NOT for I.V. use

Patients not previously treated with long acting depot neuroleptics should be given an initial test dose of 5 mg (0.25 mL) to 20 mg (1 mL). An initial dose of 20 mg (1 mL) is usually well tolerated; however, a 5 mg (0.25 mL) test dose is recommended in elderly, frail and cachectic patients, and in patients whose individual or family history suggests a predisposition to extrapyramidal reactions. In the subsequent 5-10 days, the therapeutic response and the appearance of extrapyramidal symptoms should be carefully monitored. Oral neuroleptic drugs may be continued, but in diminishing dosage, during this period.

Tablets: The dosage should be individualized and adjusted according to the severity of symptoms and tolerance to the drug. Initial recommended dose: 1 mg, 3 times/day. This may be increased, if necessary by 1 mg every 2-3 days until there is effective control of psychotic symptoms. The usual maintenance dosage: 3-6 mg/day in divided doses, although doses of up to 12 mg/day or more have been used in some patients.

Dosage Forms

Injection, depot: 20 mg/mL (10 mL); 100 mg/mL (2 mL)

Tablet: 0.5 mg, 3 mg

fluphenazine (floo FEN a zeen)

U.S./Canadian Brand Names Apo®-Fluphenazine (Can); Modecate® (Can); Modecate® Enanthate (Can); Moditen® Hydrochloride (Can); Permitil® Oral; PMS-Fluphenazine (Can); Prolixin Decanoate® Injection; Prolixin Enanthate® Injection; Prolixin® Injection; Prolixin® Oral

Therapeutic Category Phenothiazine Derivative

Use Management of manifestations of psychotic disorders

Usual Dosage Adults:

Oral: 0.5-10 mg/day in divided doses every 6-8 hours; usual maximum dose 20 mg/day

I.M.: 2.5-10 mg/day in divided doses every 6-8 hours; usual maximum dose 10 mg/day

I.M., S.C. (Decanoate®): Oral to I.M., S.C. conversion ratio = 12.5 mg, I.M., S.C. every 3 weeks for every 10 mg of oral fluphenazine

Dosage Forms

Fluphenazine decanoate: Injection:

Prolixin Decanoate®: 25 mg/mL (1 mL, 5 mL)

Fluphenazine enanthate: Injection:

Prolixin Enanthate®: 25 mg/mL (5 mL)

Fluphenazine hydrochloride:

Concentrate, oral:

Permitil®: 5 mg/mL with alcohol 1% (118 mL)

Prolixin®: 5 mg/mL with alcohol 14% (120 mL)

Elixir (Prolixin®): 2.5 mg/5 mL with alcohol 14% (60 mL, 473 mL)

Injection: Prolixin®: 2.5 mg/mL (10 mL)

Tablet:

Permitil®: 2.5 mg, 5 mg, 10 mg

Prolixin®: 1 mg, 2.5 mg, 5 mg, 10 mg

Flura® *see* fluoride *on page 244*

Flura-Drops® *see* fluoride *on page 244*

Flura-Loz® *see* fluoride *on page 244*

flurandrenolide (flure an DREN oh lide)

Synonyms flurandrenolone

U.S./Canadian Brand Names Cordran®; Cordran® SP; Drenison® (Can)

Therapeutic Category Corticosteroid, Topical

Use Inflammation of corticosteroid-responsive dermatoses

Usual Dosage Topical:

Children:

Ointment or cream: Apply 1-2 times/day

Tape: Apply once daily

Adults: Cream, lotion, ointment: Apply 2-3 times/day

Dosage Forms

Cream, emulsified base (Cordran® SP): 0.025% (30 g, 60 g); 0.05% (15 g, 30 g, 60 g)

Lotion (Cordran®): 0.05% (15 mL, 60 mL)

Ointment, topical (Cordran®): 0.025% (30 g, 60 g); 0.05% (15 g, 30 g, 60 g)

Tape, topical (Cordran®): 4 mcg/cm^2 (7.5 cm x 60 cm, 7.5 cm x 200 cm rolls)

flurandrenolone *see* flurandrenolide *on this page*

Flurate® Ophthalmic Solution *see* fluorescein sodium *on page 244*

flurazepam (flure AZ e pam)

U.S./Canadian Brand Names Apo®-Flurazepam (Can); Dalmane®; Novo-Flupam® (Can); PMS-Flupam (Can); Somnol® (Can); Som Pam® (Can)

Therapeutic Category Benzodiazepine

Controlled Substance C-IV

Use Short-term treatment of insomnia

Usual Dosage Oral:

Children:

<15 years: Dose not established

>15 years: 15 mg at bedtime

Adults: 15-30 mg at bedtime

Dosage Forms Capsule, as hydrochloride: 15 mg, 30 mg

flurbiprofen (flure BI proe fen)

U.S./Canadian Brand Names Ansaid® Oral; Apro-Flurbiprofen® (Can); Froben® (Can); Froben-SR® (Can); Novo-Flurprofen® (Can); Nu-Flurprofen® (Can); Ocufen® Ophthalmic

Therapeutic Category Analgesic, Non-narcotic; Nonsteroidal Anti-inflammatory Drug (NSAID)

Use

Ophthalmic: For inhibition of intraoperative trauma-induced miosis; the value of flurbiprofen for the prevention and management of postoperative ocular inflammation and postoperative cystoid macular edema remains to be determined

Systemic: Management of inflammatory disease and rheumatoid disorders; dysmenorrhea; pain

Usual Dosage

Oral: Rheumatoid arthritis and osteoarthritis: 200-300 mg/day in 2, 3, or 4 divided doses

Ophthalmic: Instill 1 drop every 30 minutes, 2 hours prior to surgery (total of 4 drops to each affected eye)

Dosage Forms Flurbiprofen sodium:

Solution, ophthalmic (Ocufen®): 0.03% (2.5 mL, 5 mL, 10 mL)

Tablet (Ansaid®): 50 mg, 100 mg

Fluress® Ophthalmic Solution *see* fluorescein sodium *on page 244*

5-flurocytosine *see* flucytosine *on page 242*

Fluro-Ethyl® Aerosol *see* ethyl chloride and dichlorotetrafluoroethane *on page 227*

Flurosyn® Topical *see* fluocinolone *on page 243*

flutamide (FLOO ta mide)

U.S./Canadian Brand Names Euflex® (Can); Eulexin®

Therapeutic Category Antiandrogen

Use In combination with LHRH agonistic analogs for the treatment of metastatic prostatic carcinoma

Usual Dosage Oral: 2 capsules every 8 hours

Dosage Forms Capsule: 125 mg

Flutex® Topical *see* triamcinolone (topical) *on page 578*

fluticasone (nasal) (floo TIK a sone)

U.S./Canadian Brand Names Flonase®

Therapeutic Category Adrenal Corticosteroid

Use Management of seasonal and perennial allergic rhinitis in patients ≥12 years of age

Usual Dosage

Adolescents:

Intranasal: Initial: 1 spray (50 mcg/spray) per nostril once daily. Patients not adequately responding or patients with more severe symptoms may use 2 sprays (200 mcg) per nostril. Depending on response, dosage may be reduced to 100 mcg daily. Total daily dosage should not exceed 4 sprays (200 mcg)/day.

Adults:

Intranasal: Initial: 2 sprays (50 mcg/spray) per nostril once daily. After the first few days, dosage may be reduced to 1 spray per nostril once daily for maintenance therapy. Maximum total daily dose should not exceed 4 sprays (200 mcg)/day.

Dosage Forms Fluticasone propionate:

Spray, aerosol, oral inhalation (Flovent®): 44 mcg/actuation (7.9 g = 60 actuations or 13 g = 120 actuations), 110 mcg/actuation (13 g = 120 actuations); 220 mcg/actuation (13 g = 120 actuations)

Spray, intranasal (Flonase®): 50 mcg/actuation (16 g = 120 actuations)

Topical (Cutivate™):

Cream: 0.05% (15 g, 30 g, 60 g)

Ointment: 0.005% (15 g, 60 g)

fluticasone (oral inhalation) (floo TIK a sone)

U.S./Canadian Brand Names Flovent®; Flovent® Rotadisk®

Therapeutic Category Adrenal Corticosteroid

Use Inhalation: Maintenance treatment of asthma as prophylactic therapy. It is also indicated for patients requiring oral corticosteroid therapy for asthma to assist in total discontinuation or reduction of total oral dose. NOT indicated for the relief of acute bronchospasm.

Usual Dosage Oral inhalation: If adequate response is not seen after 2 weeks of initial dosage, increase dosage; doses should be titrated to the lowest effective dose once asthma is controlled; Manufacturer recommendations:

Inhalation aerosol (Flovent®): Children ≥12 years and Adults:

Patients previously treated with bronchodilators only: Initial: 88 mcg twice daily; maximum dose: 440 mcg twice daily

Patients treated with an inhaled corticosteroid: Initial: 88-220 mcg twice daily; maximum dose: 440 mcg twice daily; may start doses above 88 mcg twice daily in poorly controlled patients or in those who previously required higher doses of inhaled corticosteroids

Patients previously treated with oral corticosteroids: Initial: 880 mcg twice daily; maximum dose: 880 mcg twice daily

(Continued)

fluticasone (oral inhalation) *(Continued)*

Inhalation powder (Flovent® Rotadisk®):

Children 4-11 years: Patients previously treated with bronchodilators alone or inhaled corticosteroids: Initial: 50 mcg twice daily; maximum dose: 100 mcg twice daily; may start higher initial dose in poorly controlled patients or in those who previously required higher doses of inhaled corticosteroids

Adolescents and Adults:

Patients previously treated with bronchodilators alone: Initial: 100 mcg twice daily; maximum dose: 500 mcg twice daily

Patients previously treated with inhaled corticosteroids: Initial: 100-250 mcg twice daily; maximum dose: 500 mcg twice daily; may start doses above 100 mcg twice daily in poorly controlled patients or in those who previously required higher doses of inhaled corticosteroids

Patients previously treated with oral corticosteroids: Initial: 1000 mcg twice daily; maximum dose: 1000 mcg twice daily

Dosage Forms Fluticasone propionate:

Powder (in 4 blisters containing 15 Rotodisks® with inhalation device): 50 mcg, 100 mcg, 250 mcg

Spray, aerosol, oral inhalation (Flovent®): 44 mcg/actuation (7.9 g = 60 actuations or 13 g = 120 actuations), 110 mcg/actuation (13 g = 120 actuations); 220 mcg/actuation (13 g = 120 actuations)

fluticasone (topical) (floo TIK a sone)

U.S./Canadian Brand Names Cutivate™

Therapeutic Category Adrenal Corticosteroid; Corticosteroid, Topical

Use Relief of inflammation and pruritus associated with corticosteroid-responsive dermatoses [medium potency topical corticosteroid]

Usual Dosage

Adolescents:

Topical: Apply sparingly in a thin film twice daily

Adults:

Topical: Apply sparingly in a thin film twice daily

Dosage Forms Fluticasone propionate:

Cream: 0.05% (15 g, 30 g, 60 g)

Ointment: 0.005% (15 g, 60 g)

fluvastatin (FLOO va sta tin)

U.S./Canadian Brand Names Lescol®

Therapeutic Category HMG-CoA Reductase Inhibitor

Use Adjunct to dietary therapy to decrease elevated serum total and LDL cholesterol concentrations in primary hypercholesterolemia; slowing of progression of coronary atherosclerosis in patients with coronary heart disease as part of a treatment strategy to lower serum total and LDL cholesterol to target levels

Usual Dosage Adults: Oral: 20 mg at bedtime

Dosage Forms Capsule: 20 mg, 40 mg

Fluviral® (Can) *see* influenza virus vaccine *on page 306*

fluvoxamine (floo VOKS ah meen)

U.S./Canadian Brand Names Luvox®

Therapeutic Category Antidepressant, Selective Serotonin Reuptake Inhibitor

Use Treatment of major depression and obsessive-compulsive disorder (OCD)

Usual Dosage Adults: Initial: 50 mg at bedtime; adjust in 50 mg increments at 4- to 7-day intervals; usual dose range: 100-300 mg/day; divide total daily dose into 2 doses; administer larger portion at bedtime

Dosage Forms Tablet: 50 mg, 100 mg

Fluzone® *see* influenza virus vaccine *on page 306*

FML® *see* fluorometholone *on page 245*

FML® Forte *see* fluorometholone *on page 245*

FML-S® Ophthalmic Suspension *see* sulfacetamide sodium and fluorometholone *on page 541*

Foille® [OTC] *see* benzocaine *on page 66*

Foille® Medicated First Aid [OTC] *see* benzocaine *on page 66*

folacin *see* folic acid *on this page*

folate *see* folic acid *on this page*

Folex® Injection *(Discontinued)* *see page 700*

Folex® PFS *see* methotrexate *on page 364*

folic acid (FOE lik AS id)

Synonyms folacin; folate; pteroylglutamic acid

U.S./Canadian Brand Names Apo®-Folic (Can); Flodine® (Can); Folvite®; Novo-Folacid® (Can)

Therapeutic Category Vitamin, Water Soluble

Use Treatment of megaloblastic and macrocytic anemias due to folate deficiency

Usual Dosage Folic acid deficiency:

Infants: 15 mcg/kg/dose daily or 50 mcg/day

Children: Oral, I.M., I.V., S.C.: 1 mg/day initial dosage; maintenance dose: 1-10 years: 0.1-0.3 mg/day

Children >11 years and Adults: Oral, I.M., I.V., S.C.: 1 mg/day initial dosage; maintenance dose: 0.5 mg/day

Dosage Forms

Injection, as sodium folate: 5 mg/mL (10 mL); 10 mg/mL (10 mL)

Folvite®: 5 mg/mL (10 mL)

Tablet: 0.1 mg, 0.4 mg, 0.8 mg, 1 mg

Folvite®: 1 mg

folinic acid *see* leucovorin *on page 328*

Follistim® *see* follitropin beta *on this page*

follitropin alpha (foe li TRO pin AL fa)

U.S./Canadian Brand Names Gonal-F®

Therapeutic Category Ovulation Stimulator

Use Induction of ovulation in the anovulatory infertile patient in whom the cause of infertility is functional and not caused by primary ovarian failure

Usual Dosage Adults (women): S.C.: Initial: 75 units/day for the first cycle; an incremental dose adjustment of up to 37.5 units may be considered after 14 days; treatment duration should not exceed 35 days unless an E2 rise indicates follicular development

Dosage Forms Injection: 75 FSH units, 150 FSH units

follitropin beta (foe li TRO pin BAY ta)

U.S./Canadian Brand Names Follistim®

Therapeutic Category Ovulation Stimulator

Use The development of multiple follicles in infertility patients treated in Assisted Reproductive Technology (ART) program and for the induction of ovulation

Usual Dosage Adults (female): I.M./S.C.:

Ovulation: In general, a sequential treatment scheme is recommended. This usually starts with daily administration of 75 int. units (International Units) FSH activity. The starting dose is maintained for at least seven days. If there is no ovarian response, the daily dose is then gradually increased until follicle growth and/or plasma estradiol levels indicate an adequate pharmacodynamic response. A daily increase in estradiol levels of 40% to 100% is considered to be optimal. The daily dose is then maintained until preovulatory conditions are reached. Preovulatory conditions are reached when there

(Continued)

follitropin beta *(Continued)*

ultrasonographic evidence of a dominant follicle of at least 18 mm in diameter and/or when plasma estradiol levels of 300-900 picograms/mL (1000-3000 pmol/L) are attained; usually, 7-14 days of treatment are sufficient to reach this state. The administration is then discontinued and ovulation can be induced by administering human chorionic gonadotropin (hCG). If the number of responding follicles is too high or estradiol levels increase too rapidly (ie, more than a daily doubling of estradiol for 2-3 consecutive days), the daily dose should be decreased. Since follicles of >14 mm may lead to pregnancies, multiple preovulatory follicles exceeding 14 mm carry the risk of multiple gestations. In that case, hCG should be withheld and pregnancy should be avoided in order to prevent multiple gestations.

ART: Various stimulation protocols are applied; starting dose of 150-225 units is recommended for at least the first four days; thereafter, the dose may be adjusted individually, based upon ovarian response. In clinical studies, it was shown that maintenance dosages ranging from 75-375 units for 6-12 days are sufficient, although longer treatment may be necessary. May be given either alone, or in combination with a GnRH agonist to prevent premature luteinization; in the latter case, a higher total treatment dose of Follistim® may be required. Ovarian response is monitored by ultrasonography and measurement of plasma estradiol levels; when ultrasonographic evaluation indicates the presence of at least three follicles of 16-20 mm, and there is evidence of a good estradiol (plasma levels of about 300-400 picogram/mL (1000-1300 pmol/L) for each follicle with a diameter >18 mm), the final phase of maturation of the follicles is induced by administration of hCG. Oocyte retrieval is performed 34-35 hours later.

Dosage Forms Injection: 75 FSH units

Follutein® *see* chorionic gonadotropin *on page 130*

Folvite® *see* folic acid *on previous page*

fomepizole (foe ME pi zole)

Synonyms 4-methylpyrazole; 4-MP

U.S./Canadian Brand Names Antizol™

Therapeutic Category Antidote

Use Ethylene glycol and methanol toxicity (antifreeze); may be useful in propylene glycol; unclear whether it is useful in disulfiram-ethanol reactions

Usual Dosage Oral: 15 mg/kg followed by 5 mg/kg in 12 hours and then 10 mg/kg every 12 hours until levels of toxin are not present

One other protocol (from France) suggests an infusion of 10-20 mg/kg before dialysis and intravenous infusion of 1-1.5 mg/kg/hour during hemodialysis

META (methylpyrazole for toxic alcohol) study in U.S. (investigational): Loading I.V. dose of 15 mg/kg followed by 10 mg/kg I.V. every 12 hours for 48 hours; continue treatment until methanol or ethylene glycol levels are <20 mg/dL; supplemental doses required during dialysis; contact your local poison center regarding this study

Dosage Forms Injection: 1 g/mL (1.5 mL)

fomivirsen (foe MI vir sen)

U.S./Canadian Brand Names Vitravene™

Therapeutic Category Antiviral Agent, Ophthalmic

Use Treatment of cytomegalovirus (CMV); CMV can affect one or both eyes in patients with acquired immunodeficiency syndrome (AIDS) who cannot take other treatment(s) for CMV retinitis or who did not respond to other treatments for CMV retinitis; the diagnosis should be made after a comprehensive eye exam, including indirect ophthalmoscopy

Usual Dosage Treatment with Vitravene™ consists of two phases:

Phase I (induction phase): One injection (6.6 mg) every other week for 2 doses

Phase II (maintenance phase): One injection (6.6 mg) once every 4 weeks

Dosage Forms Injection, intravitreal: 6.6 mg

Foradil® (Can) *see* formoterol *(Canada only)* *on next page*

Forane® *see* isoflurane *on page 313*

formoterol *(Canada only)* (for MOT ter ol)

U.S./Canadian Brand Names Foradil® (Can)

Therapeutic Category Adrenergic Agonist Agent; $Beta_2$-Adrenergic Agonist Agent; Bronchodilator

Use Long-term treatment in maintenance of asthma and in prevention of bronchospasm in patients >12 years of age with reversible obstructive airway disease

Usual Dosage Inhalation: One capsule (12 mcg) inhaled using the Aerolizer inhaler twice daily, morning and evening

Dosage Forms Capsule, for inhalation use, as fumarate: 12 mcg

Formula Q® *see* quinine *on page 493*

5-formyl tetrahydrofolate *see* leucovorin *on page 328*

Fortaz® *see* ceftazidime *on page 108*

Fortovase® *see* saquinavir *on page 515*

Fosamax® *see* alendronate *on page 17*

foscarnet (fos KAR net)

Synonyms PFA; phosphonoformic acid

U.S./Canadian Brand Names Foscavir®

Therapeutic Category Antiviral Agent

Use Alternative to ganciclovir for treatment of CMV infections and is possibly the preferred initial agent for the treatment of CMV retinitis except for those patients with decreased renal function; treatment of acyclovir-resistant mucocutaneous herpes simplex virus infections in immunocompromised patients; and acyclovir-resistant herpes zoster infections

Usual Dosage

Induction treatment: 60 mg/kg 3 times/day for 14-21 days

Maintenance therapy: 90-120 mg/kg/day

Dosage Forms Injection: 24 mg/mL (250 mL, 500 mL)

Foscavir® *see* foscarnet *on this page*

fosfomycin (fos foe MYE sin)

U.S./Canadian Brand Names Monurol™

Therapeutic Category Antibiotic, Miscellaneous

Use Treatment of uncomplicated urinary tract infections

Usual Dosage Adults: Oral: Single dose of 3 g in 4 oz of water

Dosage Forms Powder, as tromethamine: 3 g, to be mixed in 4 oz of water

fosinopril (foe SIN oh pril)

U.S./Canadian Brand Names Monopril®

Therapeutic Category Angiotensin-Converting Enzyme (ACE) Inhibitor

Use Treatment of hypertension, either alone or in combination with other antihypertensive agents

Usual Dosage Adults: Oral: 20-40 mg/day

Dosage Forms Tablet: 10 mg, 20 mg

fosphenytoin (FOS fen i toyn)

U.S./Canadian Brand Names Cerebyx®

Therapeutic Category Hydantoin

Use Indicated for short-term parenteral administration when other means of phenytoin administration are unavailable, inappropriate or deemed less advantageous; the safety and effectiveness of fosphenytoin in this use has not been systematically evaluated for more than 5 days; may be used for the control of generalized convulsive status epilepticus and prevention and treatment of seizures occurring during neurosurgery

(Continued)

fosphenytoin *(Continued)*

Usual Dosage **The dose, concentration in solutions, and infusion rates for fosphenytoin are expressed as phenytoin sodium equivalents; fosphenytoin should always be prescribed and dispensed in phenytoin sodium equivalents**

Status epilepticus: I.V.: Adults: Loading dose: Phenytoin equivalent 15-20 mg/kg I.V. administered at 100-150 mg/minute

Nonemergent loading and maintenance dosing: I.V. or I.M.: Adults:

Loading dose: Phenytoin equivalent 10-20 mg/kg I.V. or I.M. (max I.V. rate 150 mg/minute)

Initial daily maintenance dose: Phenytoin equivalent 4-6 mg/kg/day I.V. or I.M.

I.M. or I.V. substitution for oral phenytoin therapy: May be substituted for oral phenytoin sodium at the same total daily dose, however, Dilantin® capsules are ~90% bioavailable by the oral route; phenytoin, supplied as fosphenytoin, is 100% bioavailable by both the I.M. and I.V. routes; for this reason, plasma phenytoin concentrations may increase when I.M. or I.V. fosphenytoin is substituted for oral phenytoin sodium therapy; in clinical trials I.M. fosphenytoin was administered as a single daily dose utilizing either 1 or 2 injection sites; some patients may require more frequent dosing

Dosage Forms Injection, as sodium: 150 mg [equivalent to phenytoin sodium 100 mg]; 750 mg, [equivalent to phenytoin sodium 500 mg]

Fostex® [OTC] *see* sulfur and salicylic acid *on page 543*

Fostex® 10% BPO Gel [OTC] *see* benzoyl peroxide *on page 68*

Fostex® 10% Wash [OTC] *see* benzoyl peroxide *on page 68*

Fostex® Bar [OTC] *see* benzoyl peroxide *on page 68*

Fototar® [OTC] *see* coal tar *on page 141*

Fragmin® *see* dalteparin *on page 158*

Fraxiparine® (Can) *see* nadroparin *(Canada only) on page 387*

Freezone® Solution [OTC] *see* salicylic acid *on page 513*

Froben® (Can) *see* flurbiprofen *on page 248*

Froben-SR® (Can) *see* flurbiprofen *on page 248*

frusemide *see* furosemide *on next page*

FS Shampoo® Topical *see* fluocinolone *on page 243*

5-FU *see* fluorouracil *on page 246*

Fucidin® I.V. (Can) *see* fusidic acid *(Canada only) on next page*

Fucidin® Oral Suspension (Can) *see* fusidic acid *(Canada only) on next page*

Fucidin® Tablet (Can) *see* fusidic acid *(Canada only) on next page*

FUDR® *see* floxuridine *on page 241*

Ful-Glo® Ophthalmic Strips *see* fluorescein sodium *on page 244*

Fulvicin® P/G *see* griseofulvin *on page 267*

Fulvicin-U/F® *see* griseofulvin *on page 267*

Fumasorb® [OTC] *see* ferrous fumarate *on page 236*

Fumerin® [OTC] *see* ferrous fumarate *on page 236*

Funduscein® Injection *see* fluorescein sodium *on page 244*

Fungizone® *see* amphotericin B (conventional) *on page 33*

Fungoid® AF Topical Solution [OTC] *see* undecylenic acid and derivatives *on page 590*

Fungoid® Creme *see* miconazole *on page 373*

Fungoid® Tincture *see* miconazole *on page 373*

Furacin® Topical *see* nitrofurazone *on page 403*

Furadantin® *see* nitrofurantoin *on page 403*

Furalan® *see* nitrofurantoin *on page 403*

Furan® *see* nitrofurantoin *on page 403*

Furanite® *see* nitrofurantoin *on page 403*

furazolidone (fyoor a ZOE li done)

U.S./Canadian Brand Names Furoxone®

Therapeutic Category Antiprotozoal

Use Treatment of bacterial or protozoal diarrhea and enteritis caused by susceptible organisms: *Giardia lamblia* and *Vibrio cholerae*

Usual Dosage Oral:

Children >1 month: 5-8.8 mg/kg/day in 3-4 divided doses for 7-10 days, not to exceed 400 mg/day

Adults: 100 mg 4 times/day for 7-10 days

Dosage Forms

Liquid: 50 mg/15 mL (60 mL, 473 mL)

Tablet: 100 mg

furazosin *see* prazosin *on page 470*

furosemide (fyoor OH se mide)

Synonyms frusemide

U.S./Canadian Brand Names Apo®-Furosemide (Can); Furoside® (Can); Lasix®; Lasix® Special (Can); Novo-Semide® (Can); Uritol® (Can)

Therapeutic Category Diuretic, Loop

Use Management of edema associated with congestive heart failure and hepatic or renal disease; used alone or in combination with antihypertensives in treatment of hypertension

Usual Dosage

Infants and Children:

Oral: 2 mg/kg/dose increased in increments of 1 mg/kg/dose with each succeeding dose until a satisfactory effect is achieved to a maximum of 6 mg/kg/dose no more frequently than 6 hours

I.M., I.V.: 1 mg/kg/dose, increasing by each succeeding dose at 1 mg/kg/dose at intervals of 6-12 hours until a satisfactory response up to 6 mg/kg/dose

Adults:

Oral: Initial: 20-80 mg/dose, increase in increments of 20-40 mg/dose at intervals of 6-8 hours; usual maintenance dose interval is twice daily or every day

I.M., I.V.: 20-40 mg/dose, may be repeated in 1-2 hours as needed and increased by 20 mg/dose with each succeeding dose up to 600 mg/day; usual dosing interval: 6-12 hours

Dosage Forms

Injection: 10 mg/mL (2 mL, 4 mL, 5 mL, 6 mL, 8 mL, 10 mL, 12 mL)

Solution, oral: 10 mg/mL (60 mL, 120 mL); 40 mg/5 mL (5 mL, 10 mL, 500 mL)

Tablet: 20 mg, 40 mg, 80 mg

Furoside® (Can) *see* furosemide *on this page*

Furoxone® *see* furazolidone *on this page*

fusidic acid *(Canada only)* (fyoo SI dik AS id)

Synonyms Sodium Fusidate

U.S./Canadian Brand Names Fucidin® I.V. (Can); Fucidin® Oral Suspension (Can); Fucidin® Tablet (Can)

Therapeutic Category Antifungal Agent, Systemic

Use The treatment of the following infections when due to susceptible strains of *S. aureus*, both penicillinase producing and nonpenicillinase producing: skin and soft tissue infections, osteomyelitis. For patients with staphylococcal infections where other antibiotics have failed (ie, patients with staphylococcal septicemia, burns, endocarditis, pneumonia, (Continued)

fusidic acid *(Canada only)* *(Continued)*

cystic fibrosis). Appropriate culture and susceptibility studies should be performed. Fucidin® may be administered to those patients in whom a staphylococcal infection is suspected. This antibiotic treatment may subsequently require modification once these results become available.

Usual Dosage Adults:

I.V.: 500 mg 3 times/day

Oral: 500 mg 3 times/day

Dosage Forms

Powder for injection: 500 mg

Suspension, oral (banana flavor): 246 mg/5 mL (50 mL)

Tablet, sodium fusidate: 250 mg (equivalent to 240 mg fusidic acid)

G-1® *see* butalbital compound and acetaminophen *on page 85*

gabapentin (GA ba pen tin)

U.S./Canadian Brand Names Neurontin®

Therapeutic Category Anticonvulsant

Use Adjunct for treatment of drug-refractory partial and secondarily generalized seizures

Usual Dosage Adults: Oral: 900-1800 mg/day administered in 3 divided doses; therapy is initiated with a rapid titration, beginning with 300 mg on day 1, 300 mg twice daily on day 2, and 300 mg 3 times/day on day 3

Discontinuing therapy or replacing with an alternative agent should be done gradually over a minimum of 7 days

Dosage Forms Capsule: 100 mg, 300 mg, 400 mg

Gabitril® *see* tiagabine *on page 565*

gallamine triethiodide (GAL a meen trye eth EYE oh dide)

U.S./Canadian Brand Names Flaxedil®

Therapeutic Category Skeletal Muscle Relaxant

Use Produce skeletal muscle relaxation during surgery after general anesthesia has been induced

Usual Dosage I.V.: 1 mg/kg then repeat dose of 0.5-1 mg/kg in 30-40 minutes for prolonged procedures

Dosage Forms Injection: 20 mg/mL (10 mL)

gallium nitrate (GAL ee um NYE trate)

U.S./Canadian Brand Names Ganite™

Therapeutic Category Antidote

Use Treatment of clearly symptomatic cancer-related hypercalcemia that has not responded to adequate hydration

Usual Dosage Adults: I.V. infusion: 200 mg/m^2 for 5 consecutive days

Dosage Forms Injection: 25 mg/mL (20 mL)

Gamastan® ***(Discontinued)*** *see page 700*

Gamimune® N *see* immune globulin, intravenous *on page 303*

gamma benzene hexachloride *see* lindane *on page 335*

Gammabulin Immuno (Can) *see* immune globulin, intramuscular *on page 303*

Gammagard® Injection ***(Discontinued)*** *see page 700*

Gammagard® S/D *see* immune globulin, intravenous *on page 303*

gamma globulin *see* immune globulin, intramuscular *on page 303*

gammaphos *see* amifostine *on page 25*

Gammar® ***(Discontinued)*** *see page 700*

Gammar®-P I.V. *see* immune globulin, intravenous *on page 303*

Gamulin® Rh *see* Rh_0(D) immune globulin (intramuscular) *on page 502*

ganciclovir (gan SYE kloe veer)

Synonyms DHPG sodium; GCV sodium; nordeoxyguanosine

U.S./Canadian Brand Names Cytovene®; Vitrasert®

Therapeutic Category Antiviral Agent

Use

Parenteral: Treatment of CMV retinitis in immunocompromised individuals, including patients with acquired immunodeficiency syndrome; prophylaxis of CMV infection in transplant patients

Oral: Alternative to the I.V. formulation for maintenance treatment of CMV retinitis in immunocompromised patients, including patients with AIDS, in whom retinitis is stable following appropriate induction therapy and for whom the risk of more rapid progression is balanced by the benefit associated with avoiding daily I.V. infusions.

Usual Dosage Slow I.V. infusion:

Retinitis: Children >3 months and Adults: Induction therapy: 5 mg/kg/dose every 12 hours for 14-21 days followed by maintenance therapy; maintenance therapy: 5 mg/kg/day as a single daily dose for 7 days/week or 6 mg/kg/day for 5 days/week

Other CMV infections: 5 mg/kg/dose every 12 hours for 14-21 days or 2.5 mg/kg/dose every 8 hours; maintenance therapy: 5 mg/kg/day as a single daily dose for 7 days/week or 6 mg/kg/day for 5 days/week

Dosage Forms

Capsule: 250 mg, 500 mg

Implant, intravitreal: 4.5 mg released gradually over 5-8 months

Powder for injection, lyophilized: 500 mg (10 mL)

ganirelix (ga ni REL ix)

U.S./Canadian Brand Names Antagon™

Therapeutic Category Antigonadotropic Agent

Use Inhibits premature luteinizing hormone (LH) surges in women undergoing controlled ovarian hyperstimulation in fertility clinics.

Usual Dosage Adult: S.C.: 250 mcg/day during the early to midfollicular phase after initiating follicle-stimulating hormone. Treatment should be continued daily until the day of chorionic gonadotropin administration.

Dosage Forms Injection: Prefilled glass syringe: 250 mcg/0.5 mL with 27-gauge x $^1/_2$ inch needle

Ganite™ *see* gallium nitrate *on previous page*

Gantanol® *see* sulfamethoxazole *on page 542*

Gantrisin® *see* sulfisoxazole *on page 543*

Gantrisin® Ophthalmic *(Discontinued)* *see page 700*

Gantrisin® Tablet *(Discontinued)* *see page 700*

Garamycin® *see* gentamicin *on page 260*

Garatec (Can) *see* gentamicin *on page 260*

Gas-Ban DS® [OTC] *see* aluminum hydroxide, magnesium hydroxide, and simethicone *on page 23*

Gastrocrom® *see* cromolyn sodium *on page 150*

Gastrografin® *see* radiological/contrast media (ionic) *on page 495*

Gastrosed™ *see* hyoscyamine *on page 297*

Gas-X® [OTC] *see* simethicone *on page 522*

Gaviscon®-2 Tablet [OTC] *see* aluminum hydroxide and magnesium trisilicate *on page 23*

Gaviscon® Liquid [OTC] *see* aluminum hydroxide and magnesium carbonate *on page 23*

Gaviscon® Tablet [OTC] *see* aluminum hydroxide and magnesium trisilicate *on page 23*

G-CSF *see* filgrastim *on page 239*

GCV sodium *see* ganciclovir *on previous page*

Gee Gee® [OTC] *see* guaifenesin *on page 267*

gelatin, absorbable (JEL a tin, ab SORB a ble)

Synonyms absorbable gelatin sponge

U.S./Canadian Brand Names Gelfilm® Ophthalmic; Gelfoam® Topical

Therapeutic Category Hemostatic Agent

Use Adjunct to provide hemostasis in surgery; also used in oral and dental surgery; in open prostatic surgery

Usual Dosage Topical: Hemostasis: Apply packs or sponges dry or saturated with sodium chloride. When applied dry, hold in place with moderate pressure. When applied wet, squeeze to remove air bubbles. Prostatectomy cones are designed for use with the Foley bag catheter. The powder is applied as a paste prepared by adding approximately 4 mL of sterile saline solution to the powder.

Dosage Forms

Gelfilm® (sterile)
- Film: 100 mm x 125 mm (1s)
- Ophthalmic: 25 mm x 50 mm (6s)

Gelfoam®
- Cones, prostatectomy:
  - Size 13 cm (13 cm in diameter) (6s)
  - Size 18 cm (18 cm in diameter) (6s)
- Packs:
  - Size 2 cm (40 cm x 2 cm) (1s)
  - Size 6 cm (40 cm x 6 cm) (6s)
- Packs, dental:
  - Size 2 (10 mm x 20 mm x 7 mm) (15s)
  - Size 4 (20 mm x 20 mm x 7 mm) (15s)
- Sponges:
  - Size 12-3 mm (20 mm x 60 mm x 3 mm) (4s)
  - Size 12-7 mm (20 mm x 60 mm x 7 mm) (4s)
  - Size 50 (80 mm x 62.5 mm x 10 mm) (4s)
  - Size 100 (80 mm x 125 mm x 10 mm) (6s)
  - Size 100, compressed (80 mm x 125 mm) (6s)
  - Size 200 (80 mm x 250 mm x 10 mm) (6s)

gelatin, pectin, and methylcellulose

(JEL a tin, PEK tin, & meth il SEL yoo lose)

U.S./Canadian Brand Names Orabase® Plain [OTC]

Therapeutic Category Protectant, Topical

Use Temporary relief from minor oral irritations

Usual Dosage Oral: Press small dabs into place until the involved area is coated with a thin film; do not try to spread onto area; may be used as often as needed

Dosage Forms Paste, oral: 5 g, 15 g

Gelfilm® Ophthalmic *see* gelatin, absorbable *on this page*

Gelfoam® Topical *see* gelatin, absorbable *on this page*

Gel-Kam® *see* fluoride *on page 244*

Gelpirin® [OTC] *see* acetaminophen, aspirin, and caffeine *on page 6*

Gel-Tin® [OTC] *see* fluoride *on page 244*

Gelucast® *see* zinc gelatin *on page 612*

Gelusil® Liquid *(Discontinued)* *see* *page 700*

gemcitabine (jem SIT a been)

U.S./Canadian Brand Names Gemzar®

Therapeutic Category Antineoplastic Agent

Use Treatment of patients with inoperable pancreatic cancer

Usual Dosage Adults: I.V.: 1000 mg/^{2} over 30 minutes once weekly for up to 7 weeks

Dosage Forms Powder for injection, as hydrochloride, lyophilized: 20 mg/mL (10 mL, 50 mL)

gemfibrozil (jem FI broe zil)

Synonyms CI-719

U.S./Canadian Brand Names Apo-Gemfibrozil® (Can); Lopid®; Nu-Gemfibrozil (Can)

Therapeutic Category Antihyperlipidemic Agent, Miscellaneous

Use Hypertriglyceridemia in types IV and V hyperlipidemia; increases HDL cholesterol

Usual Dosage Oral: 1200 mg/day in 2 divided doses, 30 minutes before breakfast and supper

Dosage Forms

Capsule: 300 mg

Tablet, film coated: 600 mg

Gemzar® *see* gemcitabine *on this page*

Genabid® *see* papaverine *on page 428*

Genac® Tablet [OTC] *see* triprolidine and pseudoephedrine *on page 584*

Genagesic® *see* guaifenesin and phenylpropanolamine *on page 270*

Genahist® Oral *see* diphenhydramine *on page 185*

Genamin® Cold Syrup [OTC] *see* chlorpheniramine and phenylpropanolamine *on page 122*

Genamin® Expectorant [OTC] *see* guaifenesin and phenylpropanolamine *on page 270*

Genapap® [OTC] *see* acetaminophen *on page 3*

Genasoft® Plus [OTC] *see* docusate and casanthranol *on page 191*

Genaspor® [OTC] *see* tolnaftate *on page 571*

Genatap® Elixir [OTC] *see* brompheniramine and phenylpropanolamine *on page 81*

Genatuss® [OTC] *see* guaifenesin *on page 267*

Genatuss DM® [OTC] *see* guaifenesin and dextromethorphan *on page 268*

Gencalc® 600 [OTC] *see* calcium carbonate *on page 89*

Gen-Clobetasol (Can) *see* clobetasol *on page 137*

Gen-D-phen® *(Discontinued)* *see page 700*

Genebs® [OTC] *see* acetaminophen *on page 3*

Geneye® Ophthalmic [OTC] *see* tetrahydrozoline *on page 556*

Gen-Glybe (Can) *see* glyburide *on page 263*

Gen-K® *see* potassium chloride *on page 464*

Gen-Lac (Can) *see* lactulose *on page 325*

Gen-Minoxidil (Can) *see* minoxidil *on page 377*

Gen-Nifedipine (Can) *see* nifedipine *on page 402*

Genoptic® *see* gentamicin *on next page*

Genora® 0.5/35 *see* ethinyl estradiol and norethindrone *on page 224*

Genora® 1/35 *see* ethinyl estradiol and norethindrone *on page 224*

Genora® 1/50 *see* mestranol and norethindrone *on page 359*

Genotropin® *see* human growth hormone *on page 283*

Gen-Pindolol (Can) *see* pindolol *on page 452*

Genpril® [OTC] *see* ibuprofen *on page 300*

Gentacidin® *see* gentamicin *on this page*

Gent-AK® *see* gentamicin *on this page*

gentamicin (jen ta MYE sin)

U.S./Canadian Brand Names Cidomycin® (Can); Garamycin®; Garatec (Can); Genoptic®; Gentacidin®; Gent-AK®; Gentrasul®; G-myticin®; Jenamicin®; Lomicin® Ophthalmic (Can); Ocugram® (Can)

Therapeutic Category Aminoglycoside (Antibiotic); Antibiotic, Ophthalmic; Antibiotic, Topical

Use Treatment of susceptible bacterial infections, normally due to gram-negative organisms including *Pseudomonas*, *Proteus*, *Serratia*, and gram-positive *Staphylococcus*; treatment of bone infections, CNS infections, respiratory tract infections, skin and soft tissue infections, as well as abdominal and urinary tract infections, endocarditis, and septicemia; used in combination with ampicillin as empiric therapy for sepsis in newborns; used topically to treat superficial infections of the skin or ophthalmic infections caused by susceptible bacteria

Usual Dosage Dosage should be based on an estimate of ideal body weight

Infants and Children >3 months: Intrathecal: 1-2 mg/day

Infants and Children <5 years: 2.5 mg/kg/dose every 8 hours

Children >5 years: 1.5-2.5 mg/kg/dose every 8 hours

Ophthalmic: Solution: 1-2 drops every 2-4 hours, up to 2 drops every hour for severe infections; ointment: 2-3 times/day

Topical: Apply 3-4 times/day

Adults:

I.M., I.V.: 3-5 mg/kg/day in divided doses every 8 hours

Topical: Apply 3-4 times/day

Ophthalmic: Solution: 1-2 drops every 2-4 hours; ointment: 2-3 times/day

Dosage Forms Gentamicin sulfate:

Cream, topical, (Garamycin®, G-myticin®): 0.1% (15 g)

Infusion, in D_5W: 60 mg, 80 mg, 100 mg

Infusion, in NS: 40 mg, 60 mg, 80 mg, 90 mg, 100 mg, 120 mg

Injection: 40 mg/mL (1 mL, 1.5 mL, 2 mL)

Pediatric: 10 mg/mL (2 mL)

Intrathecal, preservative free (Garamycin®): 2 mg/mL (2 mL)

Ointment:

Ophthalmic: 0.3% [3 mg/g] (3.5 g)

Garamycin®, Genoptic® S.O.P., Gentacidin®, Gentak®: 0.3% [3 mg/g] (3.5 g)

Topical (Garamycin®, G-myticin®): 0.1% (15 g)

Solution, ophthalmic: 0.3% (5 mL, 15 mL)

Garamycin®, Genoptic®, Gentacidin®, Gentak®: 0.3% (1 mL, 5 mL, 15 mL)

gentamicin and prednisolone *see* prednisolone and gentamicin *on page 471*

Gen-Timolol® (Can) *see* timolol *on page 567*

Gentran® *see* dextran *on page 170*

Gentrasul® *see* gentamicin *on this page*

Gen-Triazolam® (Can) *see* triazolam *on page 579*

Gen-XENE® *see* clorazepate *on page 140*

Geocillin® *see* carbenicillin *on page 98*

Geopen® (Can) *see* carbenicillin *on page 98*

Geref® *see* sermorelin acetate *on page 519*

Geridium® *see* phenazopyridine *on page 442*

german measles vaccine *see* rubella virus vaccine, live *on page 511*

Germinal® *see* ergoloid mesylates *on page 213*

Gevrabon® [OTC] *see* vitamin B complex *on page 603*

GG *see* guaifenesin *on page 267*

GG-Cen® [OTC] *see* guaifenesin *on page 267*

glatiramer acetate (gla TIR a mer AS e tate)

Synonyms copolymer-1

U.S./Canadian Brand Names Copaxone®

Therapeutic Category Biological, Miscellaneous

Use Reduce the frequency of relapses in relapsing-remitting multiple sclerosis (MS)

Usual Dosage Adults: S.C.: 20 mg/day

Dosage Forms Injection: 20 mg (2 mL)

Glaucon® *see* epinephrine *on page 209*

GlaucTabs® *see* methazolamide *on page 362*

glibenclamide *see* glyburide *on page 263*

gliclazide *(Canada only)* (GLYE kla zide)

U.S./Canadian Brand Names Diamicron® (Can)

Therapeutic Category Antidiabetic Agent; Hypoglycemic Agent, Oral; Sulfonylurea Agent

Use Control of hyperglycemia in gliclazide responsive diabetes mellitus of stable, mild, nonketosis prone, maturity onset or adult type which cannot be controlled by proper dietary management and exercise, or when insulin therapy is not appropriate.

Usual Dosage Adults: Oral: There is no fixed dosage regimen for the management of diabetes mellitus with gliclazide or any other hypoglycemic agent. Determination of the proper dosage for gliclazide for each patient should be made on the basis of frequent determinations of blood glucose during dose titration and throughout maintenance. Recommended daily dosage: 80-320 mg. Dosage of ≥160 mg should be divided into 2 equal parts for twice daily administration. Gliclazide should be taken preferentially with meals. Recommended starting dose: 160 mg/day taken as 1 tablet twice daily with meals. Total daily dose should not exceed 320 mg.

Dosage Forms Tablet: 80 mg

glimepiride (GLYE me pye ride)

U.S./Canadian Brand Names Amaryl®

Therapeutic Category Antidiabetic Agent, Oral

Use

Management of noninsulin-dependent diabetes mellitus (type II) as an adjunct to diet and exercise to lower blood glucose

In combination with insulin to lower blood glucose in patients whose hyperglycemia cannot be controlled by diet and exercise in conjunction with an oral hypoglycemic agent

Usual Dosage Oral (allow several days between dose titrations):

Adults: Initial: 1-2 mg once daily, administered with breakfast or the first main meal; usual maintenance dose: 1-4 mg once daily; after a dose of 2 mg once daily, increase in increments of 2 mg at 1- to 2-week intervals based upon the patient's blood glucose response to a maximum of 8 mg once daily

Elderly: Initial: 1 mg/day

Combination with insulin therapy (fasting glucose level for instituting combination therapy is in the range of >150 mg/dL in plasma or serum depending on the patient): 8 mg once daily with the first main meal

After starting with low-dose insulin, upward adjustments of insulin can be done approximately weekly as guided by frequent measurements of fasting blood glucose. Once stable, combination-therapy patients should monitor their capillary blood glucose on an ongoing basis, preferably daily.

Dosage Forms Tablet: 1 mg, 2 mg, 4 mg

glipizide (GLIP i zide)

Synonyms glydiazinamide

U.S./Canadian Brand Names Glucotrol®; Glucotrol® XL

Therapeutic Category Antidiabetic Agent, Oral

Use Management of noninsulin-dependent diabetes mellitus (type II)

Usual Dosage Adults: Oral: 2.5-40 mg/day; doses larger than 15-20 mg/day should be divided and administered twice daily

Dosage Forms

Tablet: 5 mg, 10 mg

Tablet, extended release: 5 mg, 10 mg

glucagon (GLOO ka gon)

Therapeutic Category Antihypoglycemic Agent

Use Hypoglycemia; diagnostic aid in the radiologic examination of GI tract when a hypotonic state is needed; used with some success as a cardiac stimulant in management of severe cases of beta-adrenergic blocking agent overdosage

Usual Dosage

Hypoglycemia or insulin shock therapy: I.M., I.V., S.C.:

Children: 0.025-0.1 mg/kg/dose, not to exceed 1 mg/dose, repeated in 20 minutes as needed

Adults: 0.5-1 mg, may repeat in 20 minutes as needed

Diagnostic aid: Adults: I.M., I.V.: 0.25-2 mg 10 minutes prior to procedure

Dosage Forms Powder for injection, lyophilized: 1 mg [1 unit]; 10 mg [10 units]

Glucerna™ (Can) *see* enteral nutritional products *on page 208*

glucocerebrosidase *see* alglucerase *on page 18*

Glucophage® *see* metformin *on page 360*

glucose, instant (GLOO kose, IN stant)

U.S./Canadian Brand Names B-D Glucose® [OTC]; Glutose® [OTC]; Insta-Glucose® [OTC]

Therapeutic Category Antihypoglycemic Agent

Use Management of hypoglycemia

Usual Dosage Oral: 10-20 g

Dosage Forms

Gel, oral (Glutose®, Insta-Glucose®): Dextrose 40% (25 g, 30.8 g, 80 g)

Tablet, chewable (B-D Glucose®): 5 g

glucose polymers (GLOO kose POL i merz)

U.S./Canadian Brand Names Moducal® [OTC]; Polycose® [OTC]; Sumacal® [OTC]

Therapeutic Category Nutritional Supplement

Use Supplies calories for those persons not able to meet the caloric requirement with usual food intake

Usual Dosage Adults: Oral: Add to foods or beverages or mix in water

Dosage Forms

Liquid (Polycose®): 126 mL

Powder (Moducal®, Polycose®, Sumacal®): 350 g, 368 g, 400 g

Glucotrol® *see* glipizide *on this page*

Glucotrol® XL *see* glipizide *on this page*

Glukor® *see* chorionic gonadotropin *on page 130*

glutamic acid (gloo TAM ik AS id)

Therapeutic Category Gastrointestinal Agent, Miscellaneous

Use Treatment of hypochlorhydria and achlorhydria

Usual Dosage Adults: Oral: 340 mg to 1.02 g 3 times/day before meals or food

Dosage Forms
Capsule, as hydrochloride: 340 mg
Powder: 100 g
Tablet: 500 mg

glutethimide (gloo TETH i mide)

Therapeutic Category Hypnotic, Nonbarbiturate
Controlled Substance C-II
Use Short-term treatment of insomnia
Usual Dosage Oral:
Adults: 250-500 mg at bedtime, dose may be repeated but not less than 4 hours before intended awakening; maximum: 1 g/day
Elderly/debilitated patients: Total daily dose should not exceed 500 mg
Dosage Forms Tablet: 250 mg

Glutose® [OTC] *see* glucose, instant *on previous page*

Glyate® [OTC] *see* guaifenesin *on page 267*

glyburide (GLYE byoor ide)

Synonyms glibenclamide
U.S./Canadian Brand Names Albert® Glyburide (Can); Apo-Glyburide® (Can); Diaβeta®; Euglucon® (Can); Gen-Glybe (Can); Glynase™ PresTab™; Micronase®; Novo-Glyburide (Can); Nu-Glyburide (Can)
Therapeutic Category Antidiabetic Agent, Oral
Use Management of noninsulin-dependent diabetes mellitus (type II)
Usual Dosage Oral:
Diaβeta®, Micronase®:
Adults: Initial: 1.25-5 mg, then increase at weekly intervals to 1.25-20 mg maintenance dose/day divided in 1-2 doses
Elderly: Initial: 1.25-2.5 mg/day, increase by 1.25-2.5 mg/day every 1-3 weeks
Glynase™ PresTab™: Adults: Initial: 0.75-3 mg/day, increase by 1.5 mg/day in weekly intervals, maximum: 12 mg/day
Dosage Forms
Tablet (Diaβeta®, Micronase®): 1.25 mg, 2.5 mg, 5 mg
Tablet, micronized (Glynase™ PresTab™): 1.5 mg, 3 mg, 6 mg

glycerin (GLIS er in)

Synonyms glycerol
U.S./Canadian Brand Names Fleet® Babylax® Rectal [OTC]; Ophthalgan® Ophthalmic; Osmoglyn®; Sani-Supp® Suppository [OTC]
Therapeutic Category Laxative; Ophthalmic Agent, Miscellaneous
Use Constipation; reduction of intraocular pressure; reduction of corneal edema; glycerin has been administered orally to reduce intracranial pressure
Usual Dosage
Constipation: Rectal:
Children <6 years: 1 infant suppository 1-2 times/day as needed or 2-5 mL as an enema
Children >6 years and Adults: 1 adult suppository 1-2 times/day as needed or 5-15 mL as an enema

Children and Adults:
Reduction of intraocular pressure: Oral: 1-1.8 g/kg 1-1½ hours preoperatively; additional doses may be administered at 5-hour intervals
Reduction of corneal edema: Instill 1-2 drops in eye(s) every 3-4 hours
Reduction of intracranial pressure: Oral: 1.5 g/kg/day divided every 4 hours; dose of 1 g/kg/dose every 6 hours has also been used
Dosage Forms
Solution:
Ophthalmic, sterile (Ophthalgan®): Glycerin with chlorobutanol 0.55% (7.5 mL)
Oral (lime flavor)(Osmoglyn®): 50% (220 mL)
(Continued)

glycerin *(Continued)*

Rectal (Fleet® Babylax®): 4 mL/applicator (6s)
Suppository, rectal (Sani-Supp®): Glycerin with sodium stearate (infant and adult sizes)

glycerin, lanolin, and peanut oil (GLIS er in, LAN oh lin, & PEE nut oyl)

U.S./Canadian Brand Names Massé® Breast Cream [OTC]
Therapeutic Category Topical Skin Product
Use Nipple care of pregnant and nursing women
Usual Dosage Topical: Apply as often as needed
Dosage Forms Cream: 2 oz

glycerol *see* glycerin *on previous page*

glycerol guaiacolate *see* guaifenesin *on page 267*

Glycerol-T® *see* theophylline and guaifenesin *on page 559*

glycerol triacetate *see* triacetin *on page 576*

glyceryl trinitrate *see* nitroglycerin *on page 404*

Glycofed® *see* guaifenesin and pseudoephedrine *on page 270*

glycopyrrolate (glye koe PYE roe late)

U.S./Canadian Brand Names Robinul®; Robinul® Forte
Therapeutic Category Anticholinergic Agent
Use Adjunct in treatment of peptic ulcer disease; inhibit salivation and excessive secretions of the respiratory tract; reversal of cholinergic agents such as neostigmine and pyridostigmine; control of upper airway secretions
Usual Dosage
Children: Control of secretions:
Oral: 40-100 mcg/kg/dose 3-4 times/day
I.M., I.V.: 4-10 mcg/kg/dose every 3-4 hours; maximum: 0.2 mg/dose or 0.8 mg/24 hours
Children:
Intraoperative: I.V.: 4 mcg/kg not to exceed 0.1 mg; repeat at 2- to 3-minute intervals as needed
Preoperative: I.M.:
<2 years: 4.4-8.8 mcg/kg 30-60 minutes before procedure
>2 years: 4.4 mcg/kg 30-60 minutes before procedure
Children and Adults: Reverse neuromuscular blockade: I.V.: 0.2 mg for each 1 mg of neostigmine or 5 mg of pyridostigmine administered
Adults:
Intraoperative: I.V.: 0.1 mg repeated as needed at 2- to 3-minute intervals
Peptic ulcer:
Oral: 1-2 mg 2-3 times/day
I.M., I.V.: 0.1-0.2 mg 3-4 times/day
Preoperative: I.M.: 4.4 mcg/kg 30-60 minutes before procedure
Dosage Forms
Glycopyrrolate bromide:
Injection: 0.2 mg/mL (1 mL, 2 mL, 5 mL, 20 mL)
Robinul®: 0.2 mg/mL (1 mL, 2 mL, 5 mL, 20 mL)
Tablet:
Robinul®: 1 mg
Robinul® Forte: 2 mg

Glycotuss® [OTC] *see* guaifenesin *on page 267*

Glycotuss-dM® [OTC] *see* guaifenesin and dextromethorphan *on page 268*

glydiazinamide *see* glipizide *on page 262*

Glynase™ PresTab™ *see* glyburide *on previous page*

Gly-Oxide® Oral [OTC] *see* carbamide peroxide *on page 98*

Glysennid® (Can) *see* senna *on page 518*

Glyset® *see* miglitol *on page 376*

Glytuss® [OTC] *see* guaifenesin *on page 267*

GM-CSF *see* sargramostim *on page 515*

G-myticin® *see* gentamicin *on page 260*

GnRH *see* gonadorelin *on this page*

Go-Evac® *see* polyethylene glycol-electrolyte solution *on page 459*

gold sodium thiomalate (gold SOW dee um thye oh MAL ate)

U.S./Canadian Brand Names Aurolate®

Therapeutic Category Gold Compound

Use Treatment of progressive rheumatoid arthritis

Usual Dosage I.M.:

Children: Initial: Test dose of 10 mg I.M. is recommended, followed by 1 mg/kg I.M. weekly for 20 weeks; not to exceed 50 mg in a single injection; maintenance: 1 mg/kg/dose at 2- to 4-week intervals thereafter for as long as therapy is clinically beneficial and toxicity does not develop. Administration for 2-4 months is usually required before clinical improvement is observed.

Adults: 10 mg first week; 25 mg second week; then 25-50 mg/week until 1 g cumulative dose has been administered. If improvement occurs without adverse reactions, administer 25-50 mg every 2-3 weeks, then every 3-4 weeks.

Dosage Forms Injection: 25 mg/mL (1 mL); 50 mg/mL (1 mL, 2 mL, 10 mL)

GoLYTELY® *see* polyethylene glycol-electrolyte solution *on page 459*

gonadorelin (goe nad oh REL in)

Synonyms GnRH; gonadotropin-releasing hormone; LHRH; LRH; luteinizing hormone-releasing hormone

U.S./Canadian Brand Names Factrel®; Lutrepulse®

Therapeutic Category Diagnostic Agent; Gonadotropin

Use Evaluation of hypothalamic-pituitary gonadotropic function; used to evaluate abnormal gonadotropin regulation as in precocious puberty and delayed puberty; treatment of primary hypothalamic amenorrhea

Usual Dosage Female:

Diagnostic test: Children >12 years and Adults: I.V., S.C. hydrochloride salt: 100 mcg administered in women during early phase of menstrual cycle (day 1-7)

Primary hypothalamic amenorrhea: Adults: Acetate: I.V.: 5 mcg every 90 minutes via Lutrepulse® pump kit at treatment intervals of 21 days (pump will pulsate every 90 minutes for 7 days)

Dosage Forms

Injection, as acetate (Lutrepulse®): 0.8 mg, 3.2 mg

Injection, as hydrochloride (Factrel®): 100 mcg, 500 mcg

gonadotropin-releasing hormone *see* gonadorelin *on this page*

Gonak™ [OTC] *see* hydroxypropyl methylcellulose *on page 296*

Gonal-F® *see* follitropin alpha *on page 251*

Gonic® *see* chorionic gonadotropin *on page 130*

gonioscopic ophthalmic solution *see* hydroxypropyl methylcellulose *on page 296*

Goniosol® [OTC] *see* hydroxypropyl methylcellulose *on page 296*

Goody's® Headache Powders *see* acetaminophen, aspirin, and caffeine *on page 6*

Gordofilm® Liquid *see* salicylic acid *on page 513*

Gormel® Creme [OTC] *see* urea *on page 591*

goserelin (GOE se rel in)

U.S./Canadian Brand Names Zoladex® Implant

Therapeutic Category Gonadotropin Releasing Hormone Analog

Use Palliative treatment of advanced prostate cancer and breast cancer

Usual Dosage Adults: S.C.:

Breast/prostatic cancer: 3.6 mg as a depot injection every 28 days into upper abdominal wall using sterile technique under the supervision of a physician. At the physician's option, local anesthesia may be used prior to injection. The injection should be repeated every 28 days as long as the patient can tolerate the side effects and there is satisfactory disease regression. While a delay of a few days is permissible, every effort should be made to adhere to the 28-day schedule.

Prostatic cancer: 10.8 mg as a depot injection every 12 weeks into upper abdominal wall using sterile technique under the supervision of a physician. At the physician's option, local anesthesia may be used prior to injection. The injection should be repeated every 12 weeks as long as the patient can tolerate the side effects and there is satisfactory disease regression. While a delay of a few days is permissible, every effort should be made to adhere to the 12-week schedule.

Dosage Forms Injection, implant, as acetate: 3.6 mg, 10.8 mg

gramicidin, neomycin, and polymyxin B *see* neomycin, polymyxin B, and gramicidin *on page 396*

granisetron (gra NI se tron)

U.S./Canadian Brand Names Kytril™

Therapeutic Category Selective 5-HT_3 Receptor Antagonist

Use Prophylaxis and treatment of chemotherapy-related emesis

Usual Dosage

Oral: 1 tablet (1 mg) twice daily

I.V.:

10-40 mcg/kg for 1-3 doses; doses should be administered as a single IVPB over 5 minutes to 1 hour, administer just prior to chemotherapy (15-60 minutes before)

As intervention therapy for breakthrough nausea and vomiting, during the first 24 hours following chemotherapy, 2 or 3 repeat infusions (same dose) have been administered, separated by at least 10 minutes

Dosage Forms

Injection: 1 mg/mL

Tablet: 1 mg (2s), (20s)

Granulex *see* trypsin, balsam Peru, and castor oil *on page 587*

granulocyte colony-stimulating factor *see* filgrastim *on page 239*

granulocyte-macrophage colony-stimulating factor *see* sargramostim *on page 515*

Gravol® (Can) *see* dimenhydrinate *on page 182*

grepafloxacin ***Withdrawn from U.S. market 10/27/99***

(grep a FLOX a sin)

Synonyms OPC-17116

U.S./Canadian Brand Names Raxar®

Therapeutic Category Antibiotic, Quinolone

Use Treatment of acute bacterial exacerbations of chronic bronchitis caused by *Haemophilus influenzae*, *Streptococcus pneumoniae*, or *Moraxella catarrhalis*; community-acquired pneumonia caused by *Mycoplasma pneumoniae* or the organisms previously mentioned; uncomplicated gonorrhea caused by *Neisseria gonorrhoeae*, and nongonococcal cervicitis and urethritis caused by *Chlamydia trachomatis*

Usual Dosage Adults: Oral: 400-600 mg every 24 hours (given in a single dose)

Dosage Forms Tablet, as hydrochloride: 200 mg, 400 mg, 600 mg

Grifulvin® V *see* griseofulvin *on next page*

Grisactin® *see* griseofulvin *on this page*

Grisactin® *(Discontinued)* *see page 700*

Grisactin® Ultra *see* griseofulvin *on this page*

griseofulvin (gri see oh FUL vin)

Synonyms griseofulvin microsize; griseofulvin ultramicrosize

U.S./Canadian Brand Names Fulvicin® P/G; Fulvicin-U/F®; Grifulvin® V; Grisactin®; Grisactin® Ultra; Grisovin®-FP (Can); Gris-PEG®

Therapeutic Category Antifungal Agent

Use Treatment of tinea infections of the skin, hair, and nails caused by susceptible species of *Microsporum*, *Epidermophyton*, or *Trichophyton*

Usual Dosage Oral:

Children:

Microsize: 10-15 mg/kg/day in single or divided doses;

Ultramicrosize: >2 years: 5.5-7.3 mg/kg/day in single or divided doses

Adults:

Microsize: 500-1000 mg/day in single or divided doses

Ultramicrosize: 330-375 mg/day in single or divided doses; doses up to 750 mg/day have been used for infections more difficult to eradicate such as tinea unguium

Duration of therapy depends on the site of infection:

Tinea corporis: 2-4 weeks

Tinea capitis: 4-6 weeks or longer

Tinea pedis: 4-8 weeks

Tinea unguium: 3-6 months

Dosage Forms

Microsize:

Capsule (Grisactin®): 125 mg, 250 mg

Suspension, oral (Grifulvin® V): 125 mg/5 mL with alcohol 0.2% (120 mL)

Tablet:

Fulvicin-U/F®, Grifulvin® V: 250 mg

Fulvicin-U/F®, Grifulvin® V, Grisactin-500®: 500 mg

Ultramicrosize:

Tablet:

Fulvicin® P/G: 165 mg, 330 mg

Fulvicin® P/G, Grisactin® Ultra, Gris-PEG®: 125 mg, 250 mg

Grisactin® Ultra: 330 mg

griseofulvin microsize *see* griseofulvin *on this page*

griseofulvin ultramicrosize *see* griseofulvin *on this page*

Grisovin®-FP (Can) *see* griseofulvin *on this page*

Gris-PEG® *see* griseofulvin *on this page*

Guaifed® [OTC] *see* guaifenesin and pseudoephedrine *on page 270*

Guaifed-PD® *see* guaifenesin and pseudoephedrine *on page 270*

guaifenesin (gwye FEN e sin)

Synonyms GG; glycerol guaiacolate

U.S./Canadian Brand Names Anti-Tuss® Expectorant [OTC]; Balminil® Expectorant (Can); Breonesin® [OTC]; Calmylin Expectorant (Can); Diabetic Tussin® EX [OTC]; Duratuss-G®; Fenesin™; Gee Gee® [OTC]; Genatuss® [OTC]; GG-Cen® [OTC]; Glyate® [OTC]; Glycotuss® [OTC]; Glytuss® [OTC]; Guaifenex® LA; GuiaCough® Expectorant [OTC]; Guiatuss® [OTC]; Halotussin® [OTC]; Humibid® L.A.; Humibid® Sprinkle; Hytuss® [OTC]; Hytuss-2X® [OTC]; Liquibid®; Medi-Tuss® [OTC]; Monafed®; Muco-Fen-LA®; Mytussin® [OTC]; Naldecon® Senior EX [OTC]; Organidin® NR; Pneumomist®; Respa-GF®; Robitussin® [OTC]; Scot-Tussin® [OTC]; Siltussin® [OTC]; Sinumist®-SR Capsulets®; Touro Ex®; Tusibron® [OTC]; Uni-tussin® [OTC]

Therapeutic Category Expectorant

(Continued)

guaifenesin *(Continued)*

Use Temporary control of cough due to minor throat and bronchial irritation

Usual Dosage Oral:

Children:

<2 years: 12 mg/kg/day in 6 divided doses

2-5 years: 50-100 mg (2.5-5 mL) every 4 hours, not to exceed 600 mg/day

6-11 years: 100-200 mg (5-10 mL) every 4 hours, not to exceed 1.2 g/day

Children >12 years and Adults: 200-400 mg (10-20 mL) every 4 hours to a maximum of 2.4 g/day (60 mL/day)

Dosage Forms

Caplet, sustained release (Touro Ex®): 600 mg

Capsule (Breonesin®, GG-Cen®, Hytuss-2X®): 200 mg

Sustained release (Humibid® Sprinkle): 300 mg

Liquid:

Diabetic Tussin® EX, Organidin® NR, Tusibron®: 100 mg/5 mL (118 mL)

Naldecon® Senior EX: 200 mg/5 mL (118 mL, 480 mL)

Syrup (Anti-Tuss® Expectorant, Genatuss®, Glyate®, GuiaCough® Expectorant, Guiatuss®, Halotussin®, Malotuss®, Medi-Tuss®, Mytussin®, Robitussin®, Scot-Tussin®, Siltussin®, Tusibron®, Uni-Tussin®): 100 mg/5 mL with alcohol 3.5% (30 mL, 120 mL, 240 mL, 473 mL, 946 mL)

Tablet:

Duratuss-G®: 1200 mg

Gee Gee®, Glytuss®, Organidin® NR: 200 mg

Glycotuss®, Hytuss®: 100 mg

Sustained release:

Fenesin™, Guaifenex® LA, Humibid® L.A., Liquibid®, Monafed®, Muco-Fen-LA®, Pneumomist®, Respa-GF®, Sinumist®-SR Capsulets®: 600 mg

guaifenesin and codeine (gwye FEN e sin & KOE deen)

Synonyms codeine and guaifenesin

U.S./Canadian Brand Names Brontex® Liquid; Brontex® Tablet; Cheracol®; Guaituss AC®; Guiatussin® With Codeine; Mytussin® AC; Robafen® AC; Robitussin® A-C; Tussi-Organidin® NR

Therapeutic Category Antitussive/Expectorant

Controlled Substance C-V

Use Temporary control of cough due to minor throat and bronchial irritation

Usual Dosage Oral:

Children:

2-6 years: 1-1.5 mg/kg codeine/day divided into 4 doses administered every 4-6 hours

6-12 years: 5 mL every 4 hours, not to exceed 30 mL/24 hours

>12 years: 10 mL every 4 hours, up to 60 mL/24 hours

Adults: 10 mL or 1 tablet every 6-8 hours

Dosage Forms

Liquid [C-V] (Brontex®): Guaifenesin 75 mg and codeine phosphate 2.5 mg per 5 mL

Syrup [C-V] (Cheracol®, Guaituss AC®, Guiatussin® with Codeine, Mytussin® AC, Robafen® AC, Robitussin® A-C, Tussi-Organidin® NR): Guaifenesin 100 mg and codeine phosphate 10 mg per 5 mL (60 mL, 120 mL, 480 mL)

Tablet [C-III] (Brontex®): Guaifenesin 300 mg and codeine phosphate 10 mg

guaifenesin and dextromethorphan

(gwye FEN e sin & deks troe meth OR fan)

Synonyms dextromethorphan and guaifenesin

U.S./Canadian Brand Names Benylin® Expectorant [OTC]; Cheracol® D [OTC]; Clear Tussin® 30; Contac® Cough Formula Liquid [OTC]; Diabetic Tussin DM® [OTC]; Extra Action Cough Syrup [OTC]; Fenesin™ DM; Genatuss DM® [OTC]; Glycotuss-dM® [OTC]; Guaifenex® DM; GuiaCough® [OTC]; Guiatuss-DM® [OTC]; Halotussin® DM [OTC]; Humibid® DM [OTC]; Iobid DM®; Kolephrin® GG/DM [OTC]; Monafed® DM; Muco-Fen-DM®; Mytussin® DM [OTC]; Naldecon® Senior DX [OTC]; Phanatuss® Cough Syrup

[OTC]; Phenadex® Senior [OTC]; Respa-DM®; Rhinosyn-DMX® [OTC]; Robafen DM® [OTC]; Robitussin®-DM [OTC]; Safe Tussin® 30 [OTC]; Scot-Tussin® Senior Clear [OTC]; Siltussin DM® [OTC]; Synacol® CF [OTC]; Syracol-CF® [OTC]; Tolu-Sed® DM [OTC]; Tusibron-DM® [OTC]; Tuss-DM® [OTC]; Tussi-Organidin® DM NR; Uni-tussin® DM [OTC]; Vicks® 44E [OTC]; Vicks® Pediatric Formula 44E [OTC]

Therapeutic Category Antitussive/Expectorant

Use Temporary control of cough due to minor throat and bronchial irritation

Usual Dosage Oral:

Children:

2-5 years: 2.5 mL every 6-8 hours; maximum: 10 mL/day

6-12 years: 5 mL every 6-8 hours; maximum: 20 mL/24 hours

>12 years: 10 mL every 6-8 hours; maximum: 40 mL/24 hours

Alternatively: 0.1-0.15 mL/kg/dose every 6-8 hours as needed

Adults: 10 mL every 6-8 hours

Dosage Forms

Syrup:

Benylin® Expectorant: Guaifenesin 100 mg and dextromethorphan hydrobromide 5 mg per 5 mL (118 mL, 236 mL)

Cheracol® D, Clear Tussin® 30, Genatuss DM®, Mytussin® DM, Robitussin®-DM, Siltussin DM®, Tolu-Sed® DM, Tussi-Organidin® DM NR: Guaifenesin 100 mg and dextromethorphan hydrobromide 10 mg per 5 mL (5 mL, 10 mL, 120 mL, 240 mL, 360 mL, 480 mL, 3780 mL)

Contac® Cough Formula Liquid: Guaifenesin 67 mg and dextromethorphan hydrobromide 10 mg per 5 mL (120 mL)

Extra Action Cough Syrup, GuiaCough®, Guiatuss DM®, Halotussin® DM, Rhinosyn-DMX®, Tusibron-DM®, Uni-tussin® DM: Guaifenesin 100 mg and dextromethorphan hydrobromide 15 mg per 5 mL (120 mL, 240 mL, 480 mL)

Kolephrin® GG/DM: Guaifenesin 150 mg and dextromethorphan hydrobromide 10 mg per 5 mL (120 mL)

Naldecon® Senior DX: Guaifenesin 200 mg and dextromethorphan hydrobromide 15 mg per 5 mL (118 mL, 480 mL)

Phanatuss®: Guaifenesin 85 mg and dextromethorphan hydrobromide 10 mg per 5 mL

Vicks® 44E: Guaifenesin 66.7 mg and dextromethorphan hydrobromide 6.7 mg per 5 mL

Tablet:

Extended release

Guaifenex DM®, Iobid DM®, Fenesin™ DM, Humibid® DM, Monafed® DM, Respa-DM®: Guaifenesin 600 mg and dextromethorphan hydrobromide 30 mg

Glycotuss-dM®: Guaifenesin 100 mg and dextromethorphan hydrobromide 10 mg

Queltuss®: Guaifenesin 100 mg and dextromethorphan hydrobromide 15 mg

Syracol-CF®: Guaifenesin 200 mg and dextromethorphan hydrobromide 15 mg

Tuss-DM®: Guaifenesin 200 mg and dextromethorphan hydrobromide 10 mg

guaifenesin and hydrocodone *see* hydrocodone and guaifenesin *on page 288*

guaifenesin and phenylephrine (gwye FEN e sin & fen il EF rin)

Synonyms phenylephrine and guaifenesin

U.S./Canadian Brand Names Deconsal® Sprinkle®; Endal®; Sinupan®

Therapeutic Category Cold Preparation

Use Symptomatic relief of those respiratory conditions where tenacious mucous plugs and congestion complicate the problem such as sinusitis, pharyngitis, bronchitis, asthma, and as an adjunctive therapy in serous otitis media

Usual Dosage Adults: Oral: 1-2 tablets/capsules every 12 hours

Dosage Forms

Capsule, sustained release:

Deconsal® Sprinkle®: Guaifenesin 300 mg and phenylephrine hydrochloride 10 mg

Sinupan®: Guaifenesin 200 mg and phenylephrine hydrochloride 40 mg

Tablet, timed release (Endal®): Guaifenesin 300 mg and phenylephrine hydrochloride 20 mg

guaifenesin and phenylpropanolamine

(gwye FEN e sin & fen il proe pa NOLE a meen)

Synonyms phenylpropanolamine and guaifenesin

U.S./Canadian Brand Names Ami-Tex LA®; Coldlac-LA®; Conex® [OTC]; Contuss® XT; Dura-Vent®; Entex® LA; Genagesic®; Genamin® Expectorant [OTC]; Guaifenex® PPA 75; Guaipax®; Myminic® Expectorant [OTC]; Naldecon-EX® Children's Syrup [OTC]; Nolex® LA; Partuss® LA; Phenylfenesin® L.A.; Profen II®; Profen LA®; Rymed-TR®; Silaminic® Expectorant [OTC]; Sildicon-E® [OTC]; Snaplets-EX® [OTC]; Triaminic® Expectorant [OTC]; Tri-Clear® Expectorant [OTC]; Triphenyl® Expectorant [OTC]; ULR-LA®; Vicks® DayQuil® Sinus Pressure & Congestion Relief [OTC]

Therapeutic Category Expectorant/Decongestant

Use Symptomatic relief of those respiratory conditions where tenacious mucous plugs and congestion complicate the problem such as sinusitis, pharyngitis, bronchitis, asthma, and as an adjunctive therapy in serous otitis media

Usual Dosage Oral:

Children:

2-6 years: 2.5 mL every 4 hours

6-12 years: $^1/_2$ tablet every 12 hours or 5 mL every 4 hours

Children >12 years and Adults: 1 tablet every 12 hours or 10 mL every 4 hours

Dosage Forms

Caplet:

Vicks® DayQuil® Sinus Pressure & Congestion Relief: Guaifenesin 200 mg and phenylpropanolamine hydrochloride 25 mg

Rymed-TR®: Guaifenesin 400 mg and phenylpropanolamine hydrochloride 75 mg

Drops:

Sildicon-E®: Guaifenesin 30 mg and phenylpropanolamine hydrochloride 6.25 mg per mL (30 mL)

Granules (Snaplets-EX®): Guaifenesin 50 mg and phenylpropanolamine hydrochloride 6.25 mg (pack)

Liquid:

Conex®, Genamin® Expectorant, Myminic® Expectorant, Silaminic® Expectorant, Triaminic® Expectorant, Tri-Clear® Expectorant, Triphenyl® Expectorant: Guaifenesin 100 mg and phenylpropanolamine hydrochloride 12.5 mg per 5 mL (120 mL, 240 mL, 480 mL, 3780 mL)

Naldecon-EX® Children's Syrup: Guaifenesin 100 mg and phenylpropanolamine hydrochloride 6.25 mg per 5 mL (120 mL)

Tablet, extended release:

Ami-Tex LA®, Contuss® XT, Entex® LA, Guaipax®, Nolex® LA, Partuss® LA, Phenylfenesin® L.A., ULR-LA®: Guaifenesin 400 mg and phenylpropanolamine hydrochloride 75 mg

Dura-Vent®, Profen LA®: Guaifenesin 600 mg and phenylpropanolamine hydrochloride 75 mg

Coldlac-LA®, Guaifenex® PPA 75, Profen II®: Guaifenesin 600 mg and phenylpropanolamine hydrochloride 37.5 mg

guaifenesin and pseudoephedrine (gwye FEN e sin & soo doe e FED rin)

Synonyms pseudoephedrine and guaifenesin

U.S./Canadian Brand Names Congess® Jr; Congess® Sr; Congestac®; Deconsal® II; Defen-LA®; Entex® PSE; Eudal-SR®; Fedahist® Expectorant [OTC]; Fedahist® Expectorant Pediatric [OTC]; Glycofed®; Guaifed® [OTC]; Guaifed-PD®; Guaifenex® PSE; GuaiMAX-D®; Guaitab®; Guaivent®; Guai-Vent/PSE®; Guiatuss PE® [OTC]; Halotussin® PE [OTC]; Histalet® X; Nasabid™; Respa-1st®; Respaire®-60 SR; Respaire®-120 SR; Robitussin-PE® [OTC]; Robitussin® Severe Congestion Liqui-Gels® [OTC]; Ru-Tuss® DE; Rymed®; Sinufed® Timecelles®; Touro LA®; Tuss-LA®; V-Dec-M®; Versacaps®; Zephrex®; Zephrex LA®

Therapeutic Category Expectorant/Decongestant

Use Enhance the output of respiratory tract fluid and reduce mucosal congestion and edema in the nasal passage

Usual Dosage Oral:

Children:

2-6 years: 2.5 mL every 4 hours not to exceed 15 mL/24 hours

6-12 years: 5 mL every 4 hours not to exceed 30 mL/24 hours

Children >12 years and Adults: 10 mL every 4 hours not to exceed 60 mL/24 hours

Dosage Forms

Capsule:

Guaivent®: Guaifenesin 250 mg and pseudoephedrine hydrochloride 120 mg

Robitussin® Severe Congestion Liqui-Gels®: Guaifenesin 200 mg and pseudoephedrine hydrochloride 30 mg

Rymed®: Guaifenesin 250 mg and pseudoephedrine hydrochloride 30 mg

Capsule, extended release:

Congess® Jr: Guaifenesin 125 mg and pseudoephedrine hydrochloride 60 mg

Nasabid®: Guaifenesin 250 mg and pseudoephedrine hydrochloride 90 mg

Congess® SR, Guaifed®, Respaire®-120 SR,: Guaifenesin 250 mg and pseudoephedrine hydrochloride 120 mg

Guaifed-PD®, Sinufed® Timecelles®, Versacaps®: Guaifenesin 300 mg and pseudoephedrine hydrochloride 60 mg

Respaire®-60 SR: Guaifenesin 200 mg and pseudoephedrine hydrochloride 60 mg

Tuss-LA® Capsule: Guaifenesin 500 mg and pseudoephedrine hydrochloride 120 mg

Drops, oral (Fedahist® Expectorant Pediatric): Guaifenesin 40 mg and pseudoephedrine hydrochloride 7.5 mg per mL (30 mL)

Syrup:

Fedahist® Expectorant, Guaifed®: Guaifenesin 200 mg and pseudoephedrine hydrochloride 30 mg per 5 mL (120 mL, 240 mL)

Guiatuss® PE, Halotussin® PE, Robitussin-PE®, Rymed®: Guaifenesin 100 mg and pseudoephedrine hydrochloride 30 mg per 5 mL (120 mL, 240 mL, 480 mL)

Histalet® X: Guaifenesin 200 mg and pseudoephedrine hydrochloride 45 mg per 5 mL (473 mL)

Tablet:

Congestac®, Guaitab®, Zephrex®: Guaifenesin 400 mg and pseudoephedrine hydrochloride 60 mg

Glycofed®: Guaifenesin 100 mg and pseudoephedrine hydrochloride 30 mg

Tablet, extended release:

Deconsal® II, Defen-LA®, Respa-1st®: Guaifenesin 600 mg and pseudoephedrine hydrochloride 60 mg

Entex® PSE, Guaifenex® PSE, GuaiMax-D®, Guai-Vent/PSE®, Ru-Tuss® DE, Sudex®, Zephrex LA®: Guaifenesin 600 mg and pseudoephedrine hydrochloride 120 mg

Eudal-SR®, Histalet® X, Touro LA®: Guaifenesin 400 mg and pseudoephedrine hydrochloride 120 mg

Tuss-LA® Tablet, V-Dec-M®: Guaifenesin 5mg and pseudoephedrine hydrochloride 120 mg

guaifenesin and theophylline *see* theophylline and guaifenesin *on page 559*

guaifenesin, hydrocodone, and pseudoephedrine *see* hydrocodone, pseudoephedrine, and guaifenesin *on page 290*

guaifenesin, phenylpropanolamine, and dextromethorphan

(gwye FEN e sin, fen il proe pa NOLE a meen, & deks troe meth OR fan)

Synonyms dextromethorphan, guaifenesin, and phenylpropanolamine; phenylpropanolamine, guaifenesin, and dextromethorphan

U.S./Canadian Brand Names Anatuss® [OTC]; Guiatuss CF® [OTC]; Naldecon® DX Adult Liquid [OTC]; Profen II DM®; Robafen® CF [OTC]; Robitussin-CF® [OTC]; Siltussin-CF® [OTC]

Therapeutic Category Antitussive/Decongestant/Expectorant

Use Temporarily relieves nasal congestion and controls cough due to minor throat and bronchial irritation; helps loosen phlegm and thin bronchial secretions to make coughs more productive

(Continued)

guaifenesin, phenylpropanolamine, and dextromethorphan *(Continued)*

Usual Dosage Oral:

Children:

2-6 years: 2.5 mL every 4 hours not to exceed 15 mL/24 hours

6-12 years: 5 mL every 4 hours not to exceed 30 mL/24 hours

Children >12 years and Adults: 10 mL every 4 hours not to exceed 60 mL/24 hours

Dosage Forms

Syrup:

Anatuss®: Guaifenesin 100 mg, phenylpropanolamine hydrochloride 25 mg, and dextromethorphan hydrobromide 15 mg per 5 mL (120 mL, 473 mL)

Guiatuss® CF, Robafen® CF, Robitussin-CF®: Guaifenesin 100 mg, phenylpropanolamine hydrochloride 12.5 mg, and dextromethorphan hydrobromide 10 mg per 5 mL (120 mL, 240 mL, 360 mL, 480 mL)

Naldecon® DX Adult: Guaifenesin 200 mg, phenylpropanolamine hydrochloride 12.5 mg, and dextromethorphan hydrobromide 10 mg per 5 mL (120 mL, 473 mL)

Siltussin-CF®: Guaifenesin 100 mg, phenylpropanolamine hydrochloride 12.5 mg, and dextromethorphan hydrobromide 10 mg per 5 mL

Tablet: Anatuss®: Guaifenesin 100 mg, phenylpropanolamine hydrochloride 25 mg, and dextromethorphan hydrobromide 15 mg

Timed release (Profen II DM®): Guaifenesin 600 mg, phenylpropanolamine hydrochloride 37.5 mg, and dextromethorphan hydrobromide 30 mg

guaifenesin, phenylpropanolamine, and phenylephrine

(gwye FEN e sin, fen il proe pa NOLE a meen, & fen il EF rin)

Synonyms phenylephrine, guaifenesin, and phenylpropanolamine; phenylpropanolamine, guaifenesin, and phenylephrine

U.S./Canadian Brand Names Coldloc®; Contuss®; Dura-Gest®; Enomine®; Entex®; Guaifenex®; Guiatex®

Therapeutic Category Expectorant/Decongestant

Use Temporary relief of nasal congestion, running nose, sneezing, itching of nose and throat, and itchy, watery eyes due to common cold, hay fever, or other upper respiratory allergies

Usual Dosage Children >12 years and Adults: Oral: 1 capsule 4 times/day (every 6 hours) with food or fluid

Dosage Forms

Capsule (Contuss®, Dura-Gest®, Enomine®, Entex®, Guiatex®): Guaifenesin 200 mg, phenylpropanolamine hydrochloride 45 mg, and phenylephrine hydrochloride 5 mg

Liquid (Coldloc®, Contuss®, Entex®, Guaifenex®): Guaifenesin 100 mg, phenylpropanolamine hydrochloride 20 mg, and phenylephrine hydrochloride 5 mg per 5 mL (118 mL, 480 mL)

Tablet (Respinol-G®): Guaifenesin 200 mg, phenylpropanolamine hydrochloride 45 mg, and phenylephrine hydrochloride 5 mg

guaifenesin, pseudoephedrine, and codeine

(gwye FEN e sin, soo doe e FED rin, & KOE deen)

Synonyms codeine, guaifenesin, and pseudoephedrine; pseudoephedrine, guaifenesin, and codeine

U.S./Canadian Brand Names Codafed® Expectorant; Cycofed® Pediatric; Decohistine® Expectorant; Deproist® Expectorant With Codeine; Dihistine® Expectorant; Guiatuss DAC®; Guiatussin® DAC; Halotussin® DAC; Isoclor® Expectorant; Mytussin® DAC; Nucofed®; Nucofed® Pediatric Expectorant; Nucotuss®; Phenhist® Expectorant; Robitussin®-DAC; Ryna-CX®; Tussar® SF Syrup

Therapeutic Category Antitussive/Decongestant/Expectorant

Controlled Substance C-III; C-V

Use Temporarily relieves nasal congestion and controls cough due to minor throat and bronchial irritation; helps loosen phlegm and thin bronchial secretions to make coughs more productive

Usual Dosage Oral:

Children 6-12 years: 5 mL every 4 hours, not to exceed 40 mL/24 hours

Children >12 years and Adults: 10 mL every 4 hours, not to exceed 40 mL/24 hours

Dosage Forms Liquid:

C-III: Nucoted®, Nucotuss®: Guaifenesin 200 mg, pseudoephedrine hydrochloride 60 mg, and codeine phosphate 20 mg per 5 mL (480 mL)

C-V: Codafed® Expectorant, Decohistine® Expectorant, Deproist® Expectorant with Codeine, Dihistine® Expectorant, Guiatuss DAC®, Guiatussin® DAC, Halotussin® DAC, Isoclor® Expectorant, Mytussin® DAC, Nucofed® Pediatric Expectorant, Phenhist® Expectorant, Robitussin®-DAC, Ryna-CX®, Tussar® SF: Guaifenesin 100 mg, pseudoephedrine hydrochloride 30 mg, and codeine phosphate 10 mg per 5 mL (120 mL, 480 mL, 4000 mL)

guaifenesin, pseudoephedrine, and dextromethorphan

(gwye FEN e sin, soo doe e FED rin, & deks troe meth OR fan)

Synonyms dextromethorphan, guaifenesin, and pseudoephedrine; pseudoephedrine, dextromethorphan, and guaifenesin

U.S./Canadian Brand Names Anatuss® DM [OTC]; Dimacol® Caplets [OTC]; Rhinosyn-X® Liquid [OTC]; Ru-Tuss® Expectorant [OTC]; Sudafed® Cold & Cough Liquid Caps [OTC]

Therapeutic Category Cold Preparation

Use Temporarily relieves nasal congestion and controls cough due to minor throat and bronchial irritation; helps loosen phlegm and thin bronchial secretions to make coughs more productive

Usual Dosage Adults: Oral: 2 capsules (caplets) or 10 mL every 4 hours

Dosage Forms

Caplets (Dimacol®): Guaifenesin 100 mg, pseudoephedrine hydrochloride 30 mg, and dextromethorphan hydrobromide 10 mg

Capsule (Sudafed® Cold & Cough Liquid Caps): Guaifenesin 100 mg, pseudoephedrine hydrochloride 30 mg, and dextromethorphan hydrobromide 10 mg

Liquid (Anatuss® DM, Rhinosyn-X® Liquid, Ru-Tuss® Expectorant): Guaifenesin 100 mg, pseudoephedrine hydrochloride 30 mg, and dextromethorphan hydrobromide 10 mg per 5 mL

Guaifenex® *see* guaifenesin, phenylpropanolamine, and phenylephrine *on previous page*

Guaifenex® DM *see* guaifenesin and dextromethorphan *on page 268*

Guaifenex® LA *see* guaifenesin *on page 267*

Guaifenex® PPA 75 *see* guaifenesin and phenylpropanolamine *on page 270*

Guaifenex® PSE *see* guaifenesin and pseudoephedrine *on page 270*

GuaiMAX-D® *see* guaifenesin and pseudoephedrine *on page 270*

Guaipax® *see* guaifenesin and phenylpropanolamine *on page 270*

Guaitab® *see* guaifenesin and pseudoephedrine *on page 270*

Guaituss AC® *see* guaifenesin and codeine *on page 268*

Guaivent® *see* guaifenesin and pseudoephedrine *on page 270*

Guai-Vent/PSE® *see* guaifenesin and pseudoephedrine *on page 270*

guanabenz (GWAHN a benz)

U.S./Canadian Brand Names Wytensin®

Therapeutic Category Alpha-Adrenergic Agonist

Use Management of hypertension

Usual Dosage Adults: Oral: Initial: 4 mg twice daily, increase in increments of 4-8 mg/day every 1-2 weeks to a maximum of 32 mg twice daily

Dosage Forms Tablet, as acetate: 4 mg, 8 mg

guanadrel (GWAHN a drel)

U.S./Canadian Brand Names Hylorel®

Therapeutic Category Alpha-Adrenergic Agonist

Use Step 2 agent in stepped-care treatment of hypertension, usually with a diuretic

Usual Dosage Oral: Initial: 10 mg/day (5 mg twice daily); adjust dosage until blood pressure is controlled, usual dosage: 20-75 mg/day, administered twice daily

Dosage Forms Tablet, as sulfate: 10 mg, 25 mg

guanethidine (gwahn ETH i deen)

U.S./Canadian Brand Names Apo-Guanethidine® (Can); Ismelin®

Therapeutic Category Alpha-Adrenergic Agonist

Use Treatment of moderate to severe hypertension

Usual Dosage Oral:

Children:

Initial: 0.2 mg/kg/day administered daily

Maximum dose: Up to 3 mg/kg/24 hours

Adults: Initial: 10-12.5 mg/day, then 25-50 mg/day in 3 divided doses

Dosage Forms Tablet, as monosulfate: 10 mg, 25 mg

guanfacine (GWAHN fa seen)

U.S./Canadian Brand Names Tenex®

Therapeutic Category Alpha-Adrenergic Agonist

Use Management of hypertension

Usual Dosage Adults: Oral: 1 mg (usually at bedtime), may increase if needed at 3- to 4-week intervals to a maximum of 3 mg/day; 1 mg/day is most common dose

Dosage Forms Tablet, as hydrochloride: 1 mg, 2 mg

guanidine (GWAHN i deen)

Therapeutic Category Cholinergic Agent

Use Reduction of the symptoms of muscle weakness associated with the myasthenic syndrome of Eaton-Lambert, not for myasthenia gravis

Usual Dosage Adults: Oral: Initial: 10-15 mg/kg/day in 3-4 divided doses, gradually increase to 35 mg/kg/day

Dosage Forms Tablet, as hydrochloride: 125 mg

GuiaCough® [OTC] *see* guaifenesin and dextromethorphan *on page 268*

GuiaCough® Expectorant [OTC] *see* guaifenesin *on page 267*

Guiatex® *see* guaifenesin, phenylpropanolamine, and phenylephrine *on page 272*

Guiatuss® [OTC] *see* guaifenesin *on page 267*

Guiatuss CF® [OTC] *see* guaifenesin, phenylpropanolamine, and dextromethorphan *on page 271*

Guiatuss DAC® *see* guaifenesin, pseudoephedrine, and codeine *on page 272*

Guiatuss-DM® [OTC] *see* guaifenesin and dextromethorphan *on page 268*

Guiatussin® DAC *see* guaifenesin, pseudoephedrine, and codeine *on page 272*

Guiatussin® With Codeine *see* guaifenesin and codeine *on page 268*

Guiatuss PE® [OTC] *see* guaifenesin and pseudoephedrine *on page 270*

gum benjamin *see* benzoin *on page 68*

G-well® *see* lindane *on page 335*

Gynecort® Topical [OTC] *see* hydrocortisone (topical) *on page 292*

Gyne-Lotrimin® Vaginal [OTC] *see* clotrimazole *on page 140*

Gynergen® (Can) *see* ergotamine *on page 213*

Gyne-Sulf® *see* sulfabenzamide, sulfacetamide, and sulfathiazole *on page 539*

Gynogen® Injection *(Discontinued)* *see page 700*

Gynogen L.A.® Injection *see* estradiol *on page 217*

Gynol II® [OTC] *see* nonoxynol 9 *on page 406*

H_2Oxyl® (Can) *see* benzoyl peroxide *on page 68*

Habitrol™ Patch *see* nicotine *on page 401*

Haemophilus B conjugate and hepatitis B vaccine

(hem OF fi lus bee KON joo gate & hep a TYE tis bee vak SEEN)

U.S./Canadian Brand Names Comvax®

Therapeutic Category Vaccine, Inactivated Virus

Use For vaccination against *Haemophilus influenzae* type B and hepatitis B virus in infants 6 weeks to 15 months old of HGsAG-negative mothers

Usual Dosage Children: I.M.: 0.5 mL as a single dose should be administered

Dosage Forms Injection: *Haemophilus* B conjugate purified capsular polysaccharide 7.5 mcg and hepatitis B vaccine surface antigen 5 mcg per 0.5 mL (0.5 mL)

Haemophilus B conjugate vaccine

(hem OF fi lus bee KON joo gate vak SEEN)

Synonyms HIB polysaccharide conjugate; PRP-D

U.S./Canadian Brand Names HibTITER®; OmniHIB™; PedvaxHIB™; ProHIBiT®

Therapeutic Category Vaccine, Inactivated Bacteria

Use Immunization of children 24 months to 6 years of age against diseases caused by *H. influenzae* type B

Usual Dosage Children: I.M.: 0.5 mL as a single dose should be administered

Dosage Forms Injection:

HibTITER®, OmniHIB™: Capsular oligosaccharide 10 mcg and diphtheria CRM_{197} protein ~25 mcg per 0.5 mL (0.5 mL, 2.5 mL, 5 mL)

PedvaxHIB™: Purified capsular polysaccharide 15 mcg and *Neisseria meningitidis* OMPC 250 mcg per dose (0.5 mL)

ProHIBiT®: Purified capsular polysaccharide 25 mcg and conjugated diphtheria toxoid protein 18 mcg per dose (0.5 mL, 2.5 mL, 5 mL)

halazepam (hal AZ e pam)

U.S./Canadian Brand Names Paxipam®

Therapeutic Category Benzodiazepine

Controlled Substance C-IV

Use Management of anxiety disorders; short-term relief of the symptoms of anxiety

Usual Dosage Adults: Oral: 20-40 mg 3 or 4 times/day

Dosage Forms Tablet: 20 mg, 40 mg

Halazone Tablet *(Discontinued)* *see page 700*

halcinonide (hal SIN oh nide)

U.S./Canadian Brand Names Halog®; Halog®-E

Therapeutic Category Corticosteroid, Topical

Use Inflammation of corticosteroid-responsive dermatoses

Usual Dosage Children and Adults: Topical: Apply sparingly 1-3 times/day; occlusive dressing may be used for severe or resistant dermatoses

Dosage Forms

Cream (Halog®): 0.025% (15 g, 60 g, 240 g); 0.1% (15 g, 30 g, 60 g, 240 g)

Cream, emollient base (Halog®-E) : 0.1% (15 g, 30 g, 60 g)

Ointment, topical (Halog®): 0.1% (15 g, 30 g, 60 g, 240 g)

Solution (Halog®): 0.1% (20 mL, 60 mL)

Halcion® *see* triazolam *on page 579*

Haldol® *see* haloperidol *on next page*

Haldol® Decanoate *see* haloperidol *on this page*

Haldrone® *see* paramethasone acetate *on page 429*

Halenol® Tablet *(Discontinued)* *see page 700*

Haley's M-O® [OTC] *see* magnesium hydroxide and mineral oil emulsion *on page 345*

Halfan® *see* halofantrine *on this page*

Halfprin® [OTC] *see* aspirin *on page 49*

halobetasol (hal oh BAY ta sol)

U.S./Canadian Brand Names Ultravate™

Therapeutic Category Corticosteroid, Topical

Use Relief of inflammatory and pruritic manifestations of corticosteroid-response dermatoses

Usual Dosage Children and Adults: Topical: Apply sparingly to skin twice daily; rub in gently and completely

Dosage Forms Halobetasol propionate:

Cream: 0.05% (15 g, 45 g)

Ointment, topical: 0.05% (15 g, 45 g)

halofantrine (ha loe FAN trin)

U.S./Canadian Brand Names Halfan®

Therapeutic Category Antimalarial Agent

Use Treatment of mild to moderate acute malaria caused by susceptible strains of *Plasmodium falciparum* and *Plasmodium vivax*

Usual Dosage Oral:

Children <40 kg: 8 mg/kg every 6 hours for 3 doses

Adults: 500 mg every 6 hours for 3 doses

Dosage Forms Halofantrine hydrochloride:

Suspension: 100 mg/5 mL

Tablet: 250 mg

Halog® *see* halcinonide *on previous page*

Halog®-E *see* halcinonide *on previous page*

haloperidol (ha loe PER i dole)

U.S./Canadian Brand Names Haldol®; Haldol® Decanoate; Peridol (Can)

Therapeutic Category Antipsychotic Agent, Butyrophenone

Use Treatment of psychoses, Tourette's disorder, and severe behavioral problems in children

Usual Dosage

Children:

<3 years: Not recommended

3-6 years: Dose and indications are not well established

Control of agitation or hyperkinesia in disturbed children: Oral: 0.01-0.03 mg/kg/day once daily

Infantile autism: Oral: Daily doses of 0.5-4 mg have been reported to be helpful in this disorder

6-12 years: Dose not well established

I.M.: 1-3 mg/dose every 4-8 hours, up to a maximum of 0.1 mg/kg/day

Acute psychoses: Oral: Begin with 0.5-1.5 mg/day and increase gradually in increments of 0.5 mg/day, to a maintenance dose of 2-4 mg/day (0.05-0.1 mg/kg/day).

Tourette's syndrome and mental retardation with hyperkinesia: Oral: Begin with 0.5 mg/day and increase by 0.5 mg/day each day until symptoms are controlled or a maximum dose of 15 mg is reached

Children >12 years and Adults:

I.M.:

Acute psychoses: 2-5 mg/dose every 1-8 hours PRN up to a total of 10-30 mg, until control of symptoms is achieved

Mental retardation with hyperkinesia: Begin with 20 mg/day in divided doses, then increase slowly, up to a maximum of 60 mg/day; change to oral administration as soon as symptoms are controlled

Oral:

Acute psychoses: Begin with 1-15 mg/day in divided doses, then gradually increase until symptoms are controlled, up to a maximum of 100 mg/day; after control of symptoms is achieved, reduce dose to the minimal effective dose

Tourette's syndrome: Begin with 6-15 mg/day in divided doses, increase in increments of 2-10 mg/day until symptoms are controlled or adverse reactions become disabling; when symptoms are controlled, reduce to approximately 9 mg/day for maintenance

Dosage Forms

Haloperidol lactate:

Concentrate, oral: 2 mg/mL (5 mL, 10 mL, 15 mL, 120 mL, 240 mL)

Injection: 5 mg/mL (1 mL, 2 mL, 2.5 mL, 10 mL)

Haloperidol decanoate:

Injection: 50 mg/mL (1 mL, 5 mL); 100 mg/mL (1 mL, 5 mL)

Tablet: 0.5 mg, 1 mg, 2 mg, 5 mg, 10 mg, 20 mg

haloprogin (ha loe PROE jin)

U.S./Canadian Brand Names Halotex®

Therapeutic Category Antifungal Agent

Use Topical treatment of tinea pedis, tinea cruris, tinea corporis, tinea manuum caused by *Trichophyton rubrum*, *Trichophyton tonsurans*, *Trichophyton mentagrophytes*, *Microsporum canis*, or *Epidermophyton floccosum*

Usual Dosage Children and Adults: Topical: Twice daily for 2-3 weeks; intertriginous areas may require up to 4 weeks of treatment

Dosage Forms

Cream: 1% (15 g, 30 g)

Solution, topical: 1% with alcohol 75% (10 mL, 30 mL)

Halotestin® *see* fluoxymesterone *on page 246*

Halotex® *see* haloprogin *on this page*

halothane (HA loe thane)

U.S./Canadian Brand Names Fluothane®

Therapeutic Category General Anesthetic

Use General induction and maintenance of anesthesia (inhalation)

Usual Dosage Maintenance concentration varies from 0.5% to 1.5%

Dosage Forms Liquid: 125 mL, 250 mL

Halotussin® [OTC] *see* guaifenesin *on page 267*

Halotussin® DAC *see* guaifenesin, pseudoephedrine, and codeine *on page 272*

Halotussin® DM [OTC] *see* guaifenesin and dextromethorphan *on page 268*

Halotussin® PE [OTC] *see* guaifenesin and pseudoephedrine *on page 270*

Haltran® [OTC] *see* ibuprofen *on page 300*

hamamelis water *see* witch hazel *on page 607*

Harmonyl® *(Discontinued)* *see page 700*

Havrix® *see* hepatitis A vaccine *on page 279*

Hayfebrol® Liquid [OTC] *see* chlorpheniramine and pseudoephedrine *on page 122*

HBIG *see* hepatitis B immune globulin *on page 280*

H-BIG® *see* hepatitis B immune globulin *on page 280*

HCG *see* chorionic gonadotropin *on page 130*

HCTZ *see* hydrochlorothiazide *on page 286*

HD 85® *see* radiological/contrast media (ionic) *on page 495*

HD 200 Plus® *see* radiological/contrast media (ionic) *on page 495*

HDCV *see* rabies virus vaccine *on page 494*

HDRS *see* rabies virus vaccine *on page 494*

Head & Shoulders® [OTC] *see* pyrithione zinc *on page 491*

Healon® *see* sodium hyaluronate *on page 527*

Healon® GV *see* sodium hyaluronate *on page 527*

Hectorol® *see* doxercalciferol *on page 196*

Helidac™ *see* bismuth subsalicylate, metronidazole, and tetracycline *on page 75*

Helistat® *see* microfibrillar collagen hemostat *on page 374*

Helixate® *see* antihemophilic factor (recombinant) *on page 40*

Hemabate™ *see* carboprost tromethamine *on page 100*

HemFe® ***(Discontinued)*** *see page 700*

hemiacidrin *see* citric acid bladder mixture *on page 134*

hemin (HEE min)

U.S./Canadian Brand Names Panhematin®

Therapeutic Category Blood Modifiers

Use Treatment of recurrent attacks of acute intermittent porphyria (AIP) only after an appropriate period of alternate therapy has been tried

Usual Dosage I.V.: 1-4 mg/kg/day administered over 10-15 minutes for 3-14 days; may be repeated no earlier than every 12 hours; not to exceed 6 mg/kg in any 24-hour period

Dosage Forms Powder for injection, preservative free: 313 mg/vial [hematin 7 mg/mL] (43 mL)

Hemocyte® [OTC] *see* ferrous fumarate *on page 236*

Hemofil® M *see* antihemophilic factor (human) *on page 39*

Hemonyne® *see* factor IX complex (human) *on page 230*

Hemotene® *see* microfibrillar collagen hemostat *on page 374*

Hepalean®, -LOK, -LCO (Can) *see* heparin *on this page*

heparin (HEP a rin)

Synonyms heparin lock flush

U.S./Canadian Brand Names Calcilean® [HepCalium] (Can); Hepalean®, -LOK, -LCO (Can); Hep-Lock®; Liquaemin®

Therapeutic Category Anticoagulant

Use Prophylaxis and treatment of thromboembolic disorders

Usual Dosage Note: For full-dose heparin (ie, nonlow-dose), the dose should be titrated according to PTT results. For anticoagulation, an APTT 1.5-2.5 times normal is usually desired. APTT is usually measured prior to heparin therapy, 6-8 hours after initiation of a continuous infusion (following a loading dose), and 6-8 hours after changes in the infusion rate; increase or decrease infusion by 2-4 units/kg/hour dependent on PTT. Continuous I.V. infusion is preferred vs I.V. intermittent injections. For intermittent I.V. injections, PTT is measured 3.5-4 hours after I.V. injection.

Children:

Intermittent I.V.: Initial: 50-100 units/kg, then 50-100 units/kg every 4 hours

I.V. infusion: Initial: 50 units/kg, then 15-25 units/kg/hour; increase dose by 2-4 units/kg/hour every 6-8 hours as required

Adults:

Prophylaxis (low-dose heparin): S.C.: 5000 units every 8-12 hours

Intermittent I.V.: Initial: 10,000 units, then 50-70 units/kg (5000-10,000 units) every 4-6 hours

I.V. infusion: Initial: 75-100 units/kg, then 15 units/kg/hour with dose adjusted according to PTT results; usual range: 10-30 units/kg/hour

Dosage Forms

Heparin sodium:

Lock flush injection:

Beef lung source: 10 units/mL (1 mL, 2 mL, 2.5 mL, 3 mL, 5 mL, 10 mL, 30 mL); 100 units/mL (1 mL, 2 mL, 2.5 mL, 3 mL, 5 mL, 10 mL, 30 mL)

Porcine intestinal mucosa source: 10 units/mL (1 mL, 2 mL, 10 mL, 30 mL); 100 units/mL (1 mL, 2 mL, 10 mL, 30 mL)

Porcine intestinal mucosa source, preservative free: 10 units/mL (1 mL); 100 units/mL (1 mL)

Multiple-dose vial injection:

Beef lung source, with preservative: 1000 units/mL (5 mL, 10 mL, 30 mL); 5000 units/mL (10 mL); 10,000 units/mL (4 mL, 5 mL, 10 mL); 20,000 units/mL (2 mL, 5 mL, 10 mL); 40,000 units/mL (5 mL)

Porcine intestinal mucosa source, with preservative: 1000 units/mL (10 mL, 30 mL); 5000 units/mL (10 mL); 10,000 units/mL (4 mL); 20,000 units/mL (2 mL, 5 mL)

Single-dose vial injection:

Beef lung source: 1000 units/mL (1 mL); 5000 units/mL (1 mL); 10,000 units/mL (1 mL); 20,000 units/mL (1 mL); 40,000 units/mL (1 mL)

Porcine intestinal mucosa: 1000 units/mL (1 mL); 5000 units/mL (1 mL); 10,000 units/mL (1 mL); 20,000 units/mL (1 mL); 40,000 units/mL (1 mL)

Unit dose injection:

Porcine intestinal mucosa source, with preservative: 1000 units/dose (1 mL, 2 mL); 2500 units/dose (1 mL); 5000 units/dose (0.5 mL, 1 mL); 7500 units/dose (1 mL); 10,000 units/dose (1 mL); 15,000 units/dose (1 mL); 20,000 units/dose (1 mL)

Heparin sodium infusion, porcine intestinal mucosa source:

D_5W: 40 units/mL (500 mL); 50 units/mL (250 mL, 500 mL); 100 units/mL (100 mL, 250 mL)

NaCl 0.45%: 2 units/mL (500 mL, 1000 mL); 50 units/mL (250 mL); 100 units/mL (250 mL)

NaCl 0.9%: 2 units/mL (500 mL, 1000 mL); 5 units/mL (1000 mL); 50 units/mL (250 mL, 500 mL, 1000 mL)

Heparin calcium:

Unit dose injection, porcine intestinal mucosa, preservative free: 5000 units/dose (0.2 mL); 12,500 units/dose (0.5 mL); 20,000 units/dose (0.8 mL)

heparin cofactor I *see* antithrombin III *on page 41*

heparin lock flush *see* heparin *on previous page*

hepatitis A vaccine (hep a TYE tis aye vak SEEN)

U.S./Canadian Brand Names Havrix®

Therapeutic Category Vaccine, Inactivated Virus

Use For populations desiring protection against hepatitis A or for populations at high risk of exposure to hepatitis A virus (travelers to developing countries, household and sexual contacts of persons infected with hepatitis A), child day care employees, illicit drug users, male homosexuals, institutional workers (eg, institutions for the mentally and physically handicapped persons, prisons, etc), and healthcare workers who may be exposed to hepatitis A virus (eg, laboratory employees)

Usual Dosage I.M.:

Children: 0.5 mL (360 units) on days 1 and 30, with a booster dose 6-12 months late; completion of the first 2 doses (ie, the primary series) should be accomplished at least 2 weeks before anticipated exposure to hepatitis A

Adults: 1 mL (1440 units), with a booster dose at 6-12 months

(Continued)

hepatitis A vaccine *(Continued)*

Dosage Forms

Injection: 360 ELISA units/0.5 mL (0.5 mL); 1440 ELISA units/mL (1 mL)

Injection, pediatric: 720 ELISA units/0.5 mL (0.5 mL)

hepatitis B immune globulin (hep a TYE tis bee i MYUN GLOB yoo lin)

Synonyms HBIG

U.S./Canadian Brand Names H-BIG®; HyperHep®; Nabi-HB™

Therapeutic Category Immune Globulin

Use Provide prophylactic passive immunity to hepatitis B infection to those individuals exposed. Hepatitis B immune globulin is not indicated for treatment of active hepatitis B infections and is ineffective in the treatment of chronic active hepatitis B infection.

Usual Dosage I.M.:

Newborns: Hepatitis B: 0.5 mL as soon after birth as possible (within 12 hours)

Adults: Postexposure prophylaxis: 0.06 mL/kg; usual dose: 3-5 mL; repeat at 28-30 days after exposure

Dosage Forms Injection:

H-BIG®: 4 mL, 5 mL

HyperHep®: 0.5 mL, 1 mL, 5 mL

Nabi-HB™: 1 mL, 5 mL

hepatitis B inactivated virus vaccine (plasma derived) *see* hepatitis B vaccine *on this page*

hepatitis B inactivated virus vaccine (recombinant DNA) *see* hepatitis B vaccine *on this page*

hepatitis B vaccine (hep a TYE tis bee vak SEEN)

Synonyms hepatitis B inactivated virus vaccine (plasma derived); hepatitis B inactivated virus vaccine (recombinant DNA)

U.S./Canadian Brand Names Engerix-B®; Recombivax HB®

Therapeutic Category Vaccine, Inactivated Virus

Use Immunization against infection caused by all known subtypes of hepatitis B virus in individuals considered at high risk of potential exposure to hepatitis B virus or HB_sAg-positive materials

Usual Dosage I.M.:

Children:

≤11 years: 2.5 mcg doses

11-19 years: 5 mcg doses

Adults >20 years: 10 mcg doses

Dosage Forms Injection:

Recombinant DNA (Engerix-B®): Hepatitis B surface antigen 20 mcg/mL (1 mL)

Pediatric, recombinant DNA (Engerix-B®): Hepatitis B surface antigen 10 mcg/0.5 mL (0.5 mL)

Recombinant DNA (Recombivax HB®): Hepatitis B surface antigen 10 mcg/mL (1 mL, 3 mL)

Dialysis formulation, recombinant DNA (Recombivax HB®): Hepatitis B surface antigen 40 mcg/mL (1 mL)

Hep-B-Gammagee® ***(Discontinued)*** *see page 700*

Hep-Lock® *see* heparin *on page 278*

Heptalac® *see* lactulose *on page 325*

Herceptin® *see* trastuzumab *on page 575*

Herplex® ***(Discontinued)*** *see page 700*

HES *see* hetastarch *on next page*

Hespan® *see* hetastarch *on next page*

hetastarch (HET a starch)

Synonyms HES; hydroxyethyl starch

U.S./Canadian Brand Names Hespan®

Therapeutic Category Plasma Volume Expander

Use Blood volume expander used in treatment of shock or impending shock when blood or blood products are not available; does not have oxygen-carrying capacity and is not a substitute for blood or plasma; an adjunct in leukapheresis to enhance the yield of granulocytes by centrifugal means

Usual Dosage I.V.: Up to 1500 mL/day

Dosage Forms Infusion, in sodium chloride 0.9%: 6% (500 mL)

Hetrazan® ***(Discontinued)*** *see page 700*

Hexabrix™ *see* radiological/contrast media (ionic) *on page 495*

hexachlorocyclohexane *see* lindane *on page 335*

hexachlorophene (heks a KLOR oh feen)

U.S./Canadian Brand Names pHisoHex®; Septisol®

Therapeutic Category Antibacterial, Topical

Use Surgical scrub and as a bacteriostatic skin cleanser; to control an outbreak of gram-positive staphylococcal infection when other infection control procedures have been unsuccessful

Usual Dosage Children and Adults: Topical: Apply 5 mL cleanser and water to area to be cleansed; lather and rinse thoroughly under running water

Dosage Forms

Foam (Septisol®): 0.23% with alcohol 56% (180 mL, 600 mL)

Liquid, topical (pHisoHex®): 3% (8 mL, 150 mL, 500 mL, 3840 mL)

Hexadrol® *see* dexamethasone (systemic) *on page 167*

Hexalen® *see* altretamine *on page 21*

hexamethylenetetramine *see* methenamine *on page 362*

hexamethylmelamine *see* altretamine *on page 21*

Hexit® (Can) *see* lindane *on page 335*

hexylresorcinol (heks il re ZOR si nole)

U.S./Canadian Brand Names Sucrets® Sore Throat [OTC]

Therapeutic Category Local Anesthetic

Use Minor antiseptic and local anesthetic for sore throat

Usual Dosage May be used as needed, allow to dissolve slowly in mouth

Dosage Forms Lozenge: 2.4 mg

Hibiclens® [OTC] *see* chlorhexidine gluconate *on page 117*

Hibidil® 1:2000 (Can) *see* chlorhexidine gluconate *on page 117*

Hibistat® [OTC] *see* chlorhexidine gluconate *on page 117*

Hibitane® Skin Cleanser (Can) *see* chlorhexidine gluconate *on page 117*

HIB polysaccharide conjugate *see* *Haemophilus* B conjugate vaccine *on page 275*

HibTITER® *see* *Haemophilus* B conjugate vaccine *on page 275*

Hi-Cor-1.0® Topical *see* hydrocortisone (topical) *on page 292*

Hi-Cor-2.5® Topical *see* hydrocortisone (topical) *on page 292*

Hiprex® *see* methenamine *on page 362*

Hismanal® ***(Discontinued)*** *see page 700*

Histaject® ***(Discontinued)*** *see page 700*

Histalet Forte® Tablet *see* chlorpheniramine, pyrilamine, phenylephrine, and phenylpropanolamine *on page 126*

Histalet® Syrup [OTC] *see* chlorpheniramine and pseudoephedrine *on page 122*

Histalet® X *see* guaifenesin and pseudoephedrine *on page 270*

Histamine Phosphate Injection *(Discontinued)* *see page 700*

Histantil (Can) *see* promethazine *on page 478*

Histatab® Plus Tablet [OTC] *see* chlorpheniramine and phenylephrine *on page 121*

Hista-Vadrin® Tablet *see* chlorpheniramine, phenylephrine, and phenylpropanolamine *on page 124*

Histerone® Injection *see* testosterone *on page 552*

Histolyn-CYL® *see* histoplasmin *on this page*

histoplasmin (his toe PLAZ min)

Synonyms histoplasmosis skin test antigen

U.S./Canadian Brand Names Histolyn-CYL®

Therapeutic Category Diagnostic Agent

Use Diagnosing histoplasmosis; to assess cell-mediated immunity

Usual Dosage Adults: Intradermally: 0.1 mL of 1:100 dilution 5-10 cm apart into volar surface of forearm; induration of ≥5 mm in diameter indicates a positive reaction

Dosage Forms Injection: 1:100 (0.1 mL, 1.3 mL)

histoplasmosis skin test antigen *see* histoplasmin *on this page*

Histor-D® Syrup *see* chlorpheniramine and phenylephrine *on page 121*

Histor-D® Timecelles® *see* chlorpheniramine, phenylephrine, and methscopolamine *on page 124*

histrelin (his TREL in)

U.S./Canadian Brand Names Supprelin™

Therapeutic Category Gonadotropin Releasing Hormone Analog

Use Central idiopathic precocious puberty; also used to treat estrogen-associated gynecological disorders (ie, endometriosis, intermittent porphyria, possibly premenstrual syndrome, leiomyomata uteri [uterine fibroids])

Usual Dosage

Central idiopathic precocious puberty: S.C.: Usual dose is 10 mcg/kg/day administered as a single daily dose at the same time each day

Acute intermittent porphyria in women:

- S.C.: 5 mcg/day
- Intranasal: 400-800 mcg/day

Endometriosis: S.C.: 100 mcg/day

Leiomyomata uteri: S.C.: 20-50 mcg/day or 4 mcg/kg/day

Dosage Forms Injection: 7-day kits of single use: 120 mcg/0.6 mL; 300 mcg/0.6 mL; 600 mcg/0.6 mL

Histussin D® Liquid *see* hydrocodone and pseudoephedrine *on page 289*

Hi-Vegi-Lip® *see* pancreatin *on page 426*

Hivid® *see* zalcitabine *on page 609*

HMS Liquifilm® *see* medrysone *on page 353*

HN_2 *see* mechlorethamine *on page 351*

Hold® DM [OTC] *see* dextromethorphan *on page 171*

homatropine (hoe MA troe peen)

U.S./Canadian Brand Names AK-Homatropine® Ophthalmic; Isopto® Homatropine Ophthalmic

Therapeutic Category Anticholinergic Agent

Use Producing cycloplegia and mydriasis for refraction; treatment of acute inflammatory conditions of the uveal tract

Usual Dosage Ophthalmic:

Children:

Mydriasis and cycloplegia for refraction: 1 drop of 2% solution immediately before the procedure; repeat at 10-minute intervals as needed

Uveitis: 1 drop of 2% solution 2-3 times/day

Adults:

Mydriasis and cycloplegia for refraction: 1-2 drops of 2% solution or 1 drop of 5% solution before the procedure; repeat at 5- to 10-minute intervals as needed

Uveitis: 1-2 drops 2-3 times/day up to every 3-4 hours as needed

Dosage Forms Solution, ophthalmic, as hydrobromide:

2% (1 mL, 5 mL); 5% (1 mL, 2 mL, 5 mL)

AK-Homatropine®: 5% (15 mL)

Isopto® Homatropine 2% (5 mL, 15 mL); 5% (5 mL, 15 mL)

homatropine and hydrocodone *see* hydrocodone and homatropine *on page 289*

Honvol® (Can) *see* diethylstilbestrol *on page 178*

horse antihuman thymocyte gamma globulin *see* lymphocyte immune globulin *on page 343*

H.P. Acthar® Gel *see* corticotropin *on page 148*

Humalog® *see* insulin preparations *on page 307*

human growth hormone (HYU man grothe HOR mone)

Synonyms somatrem; somatropin

U.S./Canadian Brand Names Genotropin®; Humatrope®; Norditropin®; Nutropin®; Nutropin® AQ; Protropin®; Saizen®; Serostim®

Therapeutic Category Growth Hormone

Use Long-term treatment of growth failure from lack of adequate endogenous growth hormone secretion

Usual Dosage Children: I.M., S.C.:

Somatrem: Up to 0.1 mg (0.26 units)/kg/dose 3 times/week

Somatropin: Up to 0.06 mg (0.16 units)/kg/dose 3 times/week

Therapy should be discontinued when patient has reached satisfactory adult height, when epiphyses have fused, or when the patient ceases to respond

Dosage Forms Powder for injection (lyophilized):

Somatropin:

Genotropin®: 1.5 mg ~4.5 units (5 mL); 5.8 mg ~17.4 units (5 mL)

Humatrope®: 5 mg ~15 units

Norditropin®: 4 mg ~12 units; 8 mg ~24 units

Nutropin®: 5 mg ~15 units (10 mL); 10 mg ~30 units (10 mL)

Nutropin® AQ: 10 mg ~30 units (2 mL)

Saizen® (rDNA origin): 5 mg ~15 units

Serostim®: 5 mg ~15 units (5 mL); 6 mg ~18 units (5 mL)

Somatrem, Protropin®: 5 mg ~15 units (10 mL); 10 mg ~26 units (10 mL)

human thyroid-stimulating hormone *see* thyrotropin alpha *on page 564*

Humate-P® *see* antihemophilic factor (human) *on page 39*

Humatin® *see* paromomycin *on page 430*

Humatrope® *see* human growth hormone *on this page*

Humegon™ *see* menotropins *on page 354*

Humibid® DM [OTC] *see* guaifenesin and dextromethorphan *on page 268*

Humibid® L.A. *see* guaifenesin *on page 267*

Humibid® Sprinkle *see* guaifenesin *on page 267*

HuMist® Nasal Mist [OTC] *see* sodium chloride *on page 526*

Humorsol® Ophthalmic *see* demecarium *on page 163*

Humulin® 50/50 *see* insulin preparations *on page 307*

Humulin® 70/30 *see* insulin preparations *on page 307*

Humulin® L *see* insulin preparations *on page 307*

Humulin® N *see* insulin preparations *on page 307*

Humulin® R *see* insulin preparations *on page 307*

Humulin® U *see* insulin preparations *on page 307*

Hurricaine® *see* benzocaine *on page 66*

hyaluronic acid *see* sodium hyaluronate *on page 527*

hyaluronidase (hye al yoor ON i dase)

U.S./Canadian Brand Names Wydase®

Therapeutic Category Antidote

Use Increase the dispersion and absorption of other drugs; increase rate of absorption of parenteral fluids administered by hypodermoclysis; management of I.V. extravasations

Usual Dosage

Infants and Children:

Management of I.V. extravasation: Reconstitute the 150 unit vial of lyophilized powder with 1 mL normal saline; administer 0.1 mL of this solution and dilute with 0.9 mL normal saline to yield 15 units/mL; using a 25- or 26-gauge needle, five 0.2 mL injections are made subcutaneously or intradermally into the extravasation site at the leading edge, changing the needle after each injection

Hypodermoclysis: S.C.: 15 units is added to each 100 mL of I.V. fluid to be administered

Adults: Absorption and dispersion of drugs: 150 units is added to the vehicle containing the drug

Dosage Forms

Injection, stabilized solution: 150 units/mL (1 mL, 10 mL)

Powder for injection, lyophilized: 150 units, 1500 units

Hyate®:C *see* antihemophilic factor (porcine) *on page 39*

Hybolin™ Decanoate *see* nandrolone *on page 390*

Hybolin™ Improved Injection *see* nandrolone *on page 390*

hycamptamine *see* topotecan *on page 572*

Hycamtin™ *see* topotecan *on page 572*

HycoClear Tuss® *see* hydrocodone and guaifenesin *on page 288*

Hycodan® *see* hydrocodone and homatropine *on page 289*

Hycomine® *see* hydrocodone and phenylpropanolamine *on page 289*

Hycomine® Compound *see* hydrocodone, chlorpheniramine, phenylephrine, acetaminophen, and caffeine *on page 290*

Hycomine® Pediatric *see* hydrocodone and phenylpropanolamine *on page 289*

Hycort® Topical *see* hydrocortisone (topical) *on page 292*

Hycotuss® Expectorant Liquid *see* hydrocodone and guaifenesin *on page 288*

Hydeltra-T.B.A.® *(Discontinued)* *see page 700*

Hydergine® *see* ergoloid mesylates *on page 213*

Hydergine® LC *see* ergoloid mesylates *on page 213*

Hyderm (Can) *see* hydrocortisone (topical) *on page 292*

hydralazine (hye DRAL a zeen)

U.S./Canadian Brand Names Apo®-Hydralazine (Can); Apresoline®; Novo-Hylazin® (Can); Nu-Hydral® (Can)

Therapeutic Category Vasodilator

Use Management of moderate to severe hypertension, congestive heart failure, hypertension secondary to pre-eclampsia/eclampsia, primary pulmonary hypertension

Usual Dosage

Children:

Oral: Initial: 0.75-1 mg/kg/day in 2-4 divided doses, not to exceed 25 mg/dose; increase over 3-4 weeks to maximum of 7.5 mg/kg/day in 2-4 divided doses; maximum daily dose: 200 mg/day

I.M., I.V.: 0.1-0.5 mg/kg/dose (initial dose not to exceed 20 mg) every 4-6 hours as needed

Adults:

Oral: Initial: 10 mg 4 times/day, increase by 10-25 mg/dose every 2-5 days to maximum of 300 mg/day

I.M., I.V.:

Hypertensive initial: 10-20 mg/dose every 4-6 hours as needed, may increase to 40 mg/dose

Pre-eclampsia/eclampsia: 5 mg/dose then 5-10 mg every 20-30 minutes as needed

Dosage Forms Hydralazine hydrochloride:

Injection: 20 mg/mL (1 mL)

Tablet: 10 mg, 25 mg, 50 mg, 100 mg

hydralazine and hydrochlorothiazide

(hye DRAL a zeen & hye droe klor oh THYE a zide)

Synonyms hydrochlorothiazide and hydralazine

U.S./Canadian Brand Names Apresazide®

Therapeutic Category Antihypertensive Agent, Combination

Use Management of moderate to severe hypertension and treatment of congestive heart failure

Usual Dosage Adults: Oral: 1 capsule twice daily

Dosage Forms Capsule:

25/25: Hydralazine hydrochloride 25 mg and hydrochlorothiazide 25 mg

50/50: Hydralazine hydrochloride 50 mg and hydrochlorothiazide 50 mg

100/50: Hydralazine hydrochloride 100 mg and hydrochlorothiazide 50 mg

hydralazine, hydrochlorothiazide, and reserpine

(hye DRAL a zeen, hye droe klor oh THYE a zide, & re SER peen)

Synonyms hydrochlorothiazide, hydralazine, and reserpine; reserpine, hydralazine, and hydrochlorothiazide

U.S./Canadian Brand Names Hydrap-ES®; Marpres®; Ser-Ap-Es®

Therapeutic Category Antihypertensive Agent, Combination

Use Hypertensive disorders

Usual Dosage Adults: Oral: 1-2 tablets 3 times/day

Dosage Forms Tablet: Hydralazine 25 mg, hydrochlorothiazide 15 mg, and reserpine 0.1 mg

Hydramine® *(Discontinued)* *see page 700*

Hydramyn® Syrup [OTC] *see* diphenhydramine *on page 185*

Hydrap-ES® *see* hydralazine, hydrochlorothiazide, and reserpine *on this page*

Hydrate® Injection *see* dimenhydrinate *on page 182*

Hydrea® *see* hydroxyurea *on page 296*

Hydrobexan® Injection *(Discontinued)* *see page 700*

Hydrocet® *see* hydrocodone and acetaminophen *on page 287*

hydrochlorothiazide (hye droe klor oh THYE a zide)

Synonyms HCTZ

U.S./Canadian Brand Names Apo®-Hydro (Can); Diuchlor® (Can); Esidrix®; Ezide®; HydroDIURIL®; Hydro-Par®; Microzide®; Neo-Codema® (Can); Novo-Hydrazide® (Can); Oretic®; Urozide® (Can)

Therapeutic Category Diuretic, Thiazide

Use Management of mild to moderate hypertension; treatment of edema in congestive heart failure and nephrotic syndrome

Usual Dosage Oral:

Children (daily dosages should be decreased if used with other antihypertensives):
- <6 months: 2-3 mg/kg/day in 2 divided doses
- >6 months: 2 mg/kg/day in 2 divided doses

Adults: 25-50 mg/day in 1-2 doses; maximum: 200 mg/day

Dosage Forms

Capsule: 12.5 mg
Solution, oral (mint flavor): 50 mg/5 mL (50 mL)
Tablet: 25 mg, 50 mg, 100 mg

hydrochlorothiazide and amiloride *see* amiloride and hydrochlorothiazide *on page 26*

hydrochlorothiazide and benazepril *see* benazepril and hydrochlorothiazide *on page 64*

hydrochlorothiazide and bisoprolol *see* bisoprolol and hydrochlorothiazide *on page 76*

hydrochlorothiazide and captopril *see* captopril and hydrochlorothiazide *on page 96*

hydrochlorothiazide and enalapril *see* enalapril and hydrochlorothiazide *on page 206*

hydrochlorothiazide and hydralazine *see* hydralazine and hydrochlorothiazide *on previous page*

hydrochlorothiazide and lisinopril *see* lisinopril and hydrochlorothiazide *on page 337*

hydrochlorothiazide and losartan *see* losartan and hydrochlorothiazide *on page 341*

hydrochlorothiazide and methyldopa *see* methyldopa and hydrochlorothiazide *on page 367*

hydrochlorothiazide and propranolol *see* propranolol and hydrochlorothiazide *on page 484*

hydrochlorothiazide and reserpine

(hye droe klor oh THYE a zide & re SER peen)

Synonyms reserpine and hydrochlorothiazide

U.S./Canadian Brand Names Hydropres®; Hydro-Serp®; Hydroserpine®

Therapeutic Category Antihypertensive Agent, Combination

Use Management of mild to moderate hypertension; treatment of edema in congestive heart failure and nephrotic syndrome

Usual Dosage Adults: Oral: 1-2 tablets once or twice daily

Dosage Forms Tablet:

25: Hydrochlorothiazide 25 mg and reserpine 0.125 mg
50: Hydrochlorothiazide 50 mg and reserpine 0.125 mg

hydrochlorothiazide and spironolactone

(hye droe klor oh THYE a zide & speer on oh LAK tone)

Synonyms spironolactone and hydrochlorothiazide

U.S./Canadian Brand Names Alazide®; Aldactazide®; Spironazide®; Spirozide®

Therapeutic Category Antihypertensive Agent, Combination

Use Management of mild to moderate hypertension; treatment of edema in congestive heart failure and nephrotic syndrome

Usual Dosage Oral:

Children: 1.66-3.3 mg/kg/day (of spironolactone) in 2-4 divided doses

Adults: 1-8 tablets in 1-2 divided doses

Dosage Forms Tablet:

25/25: Hydrochlorothiazide 25 mg and spironolactone 25 mg

50/50: Hydrochlorothiazide 50 mg and spironolactone 50 mg

hydrochlorothiazide and triamterene

(hye droe klor oh THYE a zide & trye AM ter een)

Synonyms triamterene and hydrochlorothiazide

U.S./Canadian Brand Names Apo-Triazide® (Can); Dyazide®; Maxzide®; Novo-Triamzide (Can); Nu-Triazide (Can)

Therapeutic Category Antihypertensive Agent, Combination

Use Management of mild to moderate hypertension; treatment of edema in congestive heart failure and nephrotic syndrome

Usual Dosage Adults: Oral: 1-2 capsules twice daily after meals

Dosage Forms

Capsule (Dyazide®): Hydrochlorothiazide 25 mg and triamterene 37.5 mg

Tablet:

Maxzide®-25: Hydrochlorothiazide 25 mg and triamterene 37.5 mg

Maxzide®: Hydrochlorothiazide 50 mg and triamterene 75 mg

hydrochlorothiazide, hydralazine, and reserpine *see* hydralazine, hydrochlorothiazide, and reserpine *on page 285*

Hydrocil® [OTC] *see* psyllium *on page 488*

Hydro Cobex® *see* hydroxocobalamin *on page 294*

hydrocodone and acetaminophen

(hye droe KOE done & a seet a MIN oh fen)

Synonyms acetaminophen and hydrocodone

U.S./Canadian Brand Names Anexsia®; Anodynos-DHC®; Bancap HC®; Co-Gesic®; Dolacet®; DuoCet™; Duradyne DHC®; Hydrocet®; Hydrogesic®; Hy-Phen®; Lorcet® 10/650; Lorcet®-HD; Lorcet® Plus; Lortab®; Margesic® H; Norcet®; Stagesic®; T-Gesic®; Vapocet® (Can); Vicodin®; Vicodin® ES; Zydone®

Therapeutic Category Analgesic, Narcotic

Controlled Substance C-III

Use Relief of moderate to severe pain; antitussive (hydrocodone)

Usual Dosage Doses should be titrated to appropriate analgesic effect

Adults: Oral: 1-2 tablets or capsules every 4-6 hours

Dosage Forms

Capsule:

Bancap HC®, Dolacet®, Hydrocet®, Hydrogesic®, Lorcet®-HD, Margesic® H, Medipain 5®, Norcet®, Stagesic®, T-Gesic®, Zydone®: Hydrocodone bitartrate 5 mg and acetaminophen 500 mg

Elixir (tropical fruit punch flavor) (Lortab®): Hydrocodone bitartrate 2.5 mg and acetaminophen 167 mg per 5 mL with alcohol 7% (480 mL)

Solution, oral (tropical fruit punch flavor) (Lortab®): Hydrocodone bitartrate 2.5 mg and acetaminophen 167 mg per 5 mL with alcohol 7% (480 mL)

Tablet: Hydrocodone bitartrate 5 mg and acetaminophen 400 mg; hydrocodone bitartrate 7.5 mg and acetaminophen 400 mg; hydrocodone bitartrate 10 mg and acetaminophen 400 mg; hydrocodone bitartrate 5 mg and acetaminophen 500 mg; hydrocodone bitartrate 7.5 mg and acetaminophen 750 mg; hydrocodone bitartrate 7.5 mg and acetaminophen 500 mg; hydrocodone bitartrate 7.5 mg and acetaminophen 650 mg; hydrocodone bitartrate 10 mg and acetaminophen 650 mg

Lortab® 2.5/500: Hydrocodone bitartrate 2.5 mg and acetaminophen 500 mg

(Continued)

hydrocodone and acetaminophen *(Continued)*

Anexsia® 5/500, Anodynos-DHC®, Co-Gesic®, DuoCet™, DHC®; Hy-Phen®, Lorcet®, Lortab®® 5/500, Vicodin®: Hydrocodone bitartrate 5 mg and acetaminophen 500 mg

Lortab® 7.5/500: Hydrocodone bitartrate 7.5 mg and acetaminophen 500 mg

Anexsia® 7.5/650, Lorcet® Plus: Hydrocodone bitartrate 7.5 mg and acetaminophen 650 mg

Vicodin® ES: Hydrocodone bitartrate 7.5 mg and acetaminophen 750 mg

Norco®: Hydrocodone bitartrate 10 mg and acetaminophen 325 mg

Lortab® 10/500: Hydrocodone bitartrate 10 mg and acetaminophen 500 mg

Lorcet® 10/650: Hydrocodone bitartrate 10 mg and acetaminophen 650 mg

Vicodin® HP: Hydrocodone bitartrate 10 mg and acetaminophen 660 mg

Zydone®: Hydrocodone bitartrate 5 mg and acetaminophen 400 mg; hydrocodone bitartrate 7.5 mg and acetaminophen 400 mg; hydrocodone bitartrate 10 mg and acetaminophen 400 mg

hydrocodone and aspirin (hye droe KOE done & AS pir in)

Synonyms aspirin and hydrocodone

U.S./Canadian Brand Names Alor® 5/500; Azdone®; Damason-P®; Lortab® ASA; Panasal® 5/500

Therapeutic Category Analgesic, Narcotic

Controlled Substance C-III

Use Relief of moderate to moderately severe pain

Usual Dosage Adults: Oral: 1-2 tablets every 4-6 hours as needed for pain

Dosage Forms Tablet: Hydrocodone bitartrate 5 mg and aspirin 500 mg

hydrocodone and chlorpheniramine

(hye droe KOE done & klor fen IR a meen)

Synonyms chlorpheniramine and hydrocodone

U.S./Canadian Brand Names Tussionex®

Therapeutic Category Antihistamine/Antitussive

Controlled Substance C-III

Use Symptomatic relief of cough

Usual Dosage Oral:

Children 6-12 years: 2.5 mL every 12 hours; do not exceed 5 mL/24 hours

Adults: 5 mL every 12 hours; do not exceed 10 mL/24 hours

Dosage Forms Syrup, alcohol free: Hydrocodone polistirex 10 mg and chlorpheniramine polistirex 8 mg per 5 mL (480 mL, 900 mL)

hydrocodone and guaifenesin (hye droe KOE done & gwye FEN e sin)

Synonyms guaifenesin and hydrocodone

U.S./Canadian Brand Names Codiclear® DH; HycoClear Tuss®; Hycotuss® Expectorant Liquid; Kwelcof®

Therapeutic Category Antitussive/Expectorant

Controlled Substance C-III

Use Symptomatic relief of nonproductive coughs associated with upper and lower respiratory tract congestion

Usual Dosage Oral:

Children:

<2 years: 0.3 mg/kg/day (hydrocodone) in 4 divided doses

2-12 years: 2.5 mL every 4 hours, after meals and at bedtime

>12 years: 5 mL every 4 hours, after meals and at bedtime

Adults: 5 mL every 4 hours, after meals and at bedtime, up to 30 mL/24 hours

Dosage Forms Liquid: Hydrocodone bitartrate 5 mg and guaifenesin 100 mg per 5 mL (120 mL, 480 mL)

hydrocodone and homatropine (hye droe KOE done & hoe MA troe peen)

Synonyms homatropine and hydrocodone

U.S./Canadian Brand Names Hycodan®; Hydromet®; Oncet®; Tussigon®

Therapeutic Category Antitussive

Controlled Substance C-III

Use Symptomatic relief of cough

Usual Dosage Oral (based on hydrocodone component):

Children: 0.6 mg/kg/day in 3-4 divided doses; do not administer more frequently than every 4 hours

A single dose should not exceed 10 mg in children >12 years, 5 mg in children 2-12 years, and 1.25 mg in children <2 years of age

Adults: 5-10 mg every 4-6 hours, a single dose should not exceed 15 mg; do not administer more frequently than every 4 hours

Dosage Forms

Syrup (Hycodan®, Hydromet®, Hydropane®, Hydrotropine®): Hydrocodone bitartrate 5 mg and homatropine methylbromide 1.5 mg per 5 mL (120 mL, 480 mL, 4000 mL)

Tablet (Hycodan®, Tussigon®): Hydrocodone bitartrate 5 mg and homatropine methylbromide 1.5 mg

hydrocodone and ibuprofen (hye droe KOE done & eye byoo PROE fen)

Synonyms ibuprofen and hydrocodone

U.S./Canadian Brand Names Vicoprofen®

Therapeutic Category Analgesic, Narcotic

Controlled Substance C-III

Use Relief of moderate to moderately severe pain (short-term, less than 10 days)

Usual Dosage Adults: Oral: 1-2 tablets every 4-6 hours as needed for pain

Dosage Forms Tablet: Hydrocodone bitartrate 7.5 mg and ibuprofen 200 mg

hydrocodone and phenylpropanolamine

(hye droe KOE done & fen il proe pa NOLE a meen)

Synonyms phenylpropanolamine and hydrocodone

U.S./Canadian Brand Names Codamine®; Codamine® Pediatric; Hycomine®; Hycomine® Pediatric; Hydrocodone PA® Syrup

Therapeutic Category Antitussive/Decongestant

Controlled Substance C-III

Use Symptomatic relief of cough and nasal congestion

Usual Dosage Oral:

Children 6-12 years: 2.5 mL every 4 hours, up to 6 doses/24 hours

Adults: 5 mL every 4 hours, up to 6 doses/24 hours

Dosage Forms Syrup:

Codamine®, Hycomine®: Hydrocodone bitartrate 5 mg and phenylpropanolamine hydrochloride 25 mg per 5 mL (480 mL)

Codamine® Pediatric, Hycomine® Pediatric: Hydrocodone bitartrate 2.5 mg and phenylpropanolamine hydrochloride 12.5 mg per 5 mL (480 mL)

hydrocodone and pseudoephedrine

(hye droe KOE done & soo doe e FED rin)

U.S./Canadian Brand Names Detussin® Liquid; Entuss-D® LIquid; Histussin D® Liquid; Tyrodone® Liquid

Therapeutic Category Cough and Cold Combination

Use Symptomatic relief of cough due to colds, etc

Usual Dosage Oral: Adults: 5 mL four times/day

Dosage Forms Liquid:

Entuss-D®: Hydrocodone bitartrate 5 mg and pseudoephedrine hydrochloride 30 mg per 5 mL

Detussin®, Histussin D®, Tyrodone®: Hydrocodone bitartrate 5 mg and pseudoephedrine hydrochloride 60 mg per 5 mL

hydrocodone, chlorpheniramine, phenylephrine, acetaminophen, and caffeine

(hye droe KOE done, klor fen IR a meen, fen il EF rin, a seet a MIN oh fen, & KAF een)

Synonyms acetaminophen, caffeine, hydrocodone, chlorpheniramine, and phenylephrine; caffeine, hydrocodone, chlorpheniramine, phenylephrine, and acetaminophen; chlorpheniramine, hydrocodone, phenylephrine, acetaminophen, and caffeine; phenylephrine, hydrocodone, chlorpheniramine, acetaminophen, and caffeine

U.S./Canadian Brand Names Hycomine® Compound

Therapeutic Category Antitussive

Use Symptomatic relief of cough and symptoms of upper respiratory infections

Usual Dosage Adults: Oral: 1 tablet every 4 hours, up to 4 times/day

Dosage Forms Tablet: Hydrocodone bitartrate 5 mg, chlorpheniramine maleate 2 mg, phenylephrine hydrochloride 10 mg, acetaminophen 250 mg, and caffeine 30 mg

Hydrocodone PA® Syrup *see* hydrocodone and phenylpropanolamine *on previous page*

hydrocodone, phenylephrine, pyrilamine, phenindamine, chlorpheniramine, and ammonium chloride

(hye droe KOE done, fen il EF rin, peer IL a meen, fen IN da meen, klor fen IR a meen, & a MOE nee um KLOR ide)

U.S./Canadian Brand Names P-V-Tussin®

Therapeutic Category Antihistamine/Decongestant/Antitussive

Use Symptomatic relief of cough and nasal congestion

Usual Dosage Adults: Oral: 10 mL every 4-6 hours, up to 40 mL/day

Dosage Forms Syrup: Hydrocodone bitartrate 2.5 mg, phenylephrine hydrochloride 5 mg, pyrilamine maleate 6 mg, phenindamine tartrate 5 mg, chlorpheniramine maleate 2 mg, and ammonium chloride 50 mg per 5 mL with alcohol 5% (480 mL, 3780 mL)

hydrocodone, pseudoephedrine, and guaifenesin

(hye droe KOE done, soo doe e FED rin & gwye FEN e sin)

Synonyms guaifenesin, hydrocodone, and pseudoephedrine; pseudoephedrine, hydrocodone, and guaifenesin

U.S./Canadian Brand Names Cophene XP®; Detussin® Expectorant; SRC® Expectorant; Tussafin® Expectorant

Therapeutic Category Antitussive/Decongestant/Expectorant

Controlled Substance C-III

Use Symptomatic relief of irritating, nonproductive cough associated with respiratory conditions such as bronchitis, bronchial asthma, tracheobronchitis, and the common cold

Usual Dosage Adults: Oral: 5 mL every 4-6 hours

Dosage Forms Liquid: Hydrocodone bitartrate 5 mg, pseudoephedrine hydrochloride 60 mg, and guaifenesin 200 mg per 5 mL with alcohol 12.5% (480 mL)

hydrocortisone and benzoyl peroxide *see* benzoyl peroxide and hydrocortisone *on page 69*

hydrocortisone and clioquinol *see* clioquinol and hydrocortisone *on page 137*

hydrocortisone and dibucaine *see* dibucaine and hydrocortisone *on page 175*

hydrocortisone and iodoquinol *see* iodoquinol and hydrocortisone *on page 311*

hydrocortisone and lidocaine *see* lidocaine and hydrocortisone *on page 334*

hydrocortisone and neomycin *see* neomycin and hydrocortisone *on page 395*

hydrocortisone and oxytetracycline *see* oxytetracycline and hydrocortisone *on page 425*

hydrocortisone and polymyxin B *see* polymyxin B and hydrocortisone *on page 460*

hydrocortisone and pramoxine *see* pramoxine and hydrocortisone *on page 469*

hydrocortisone and urea *see* urea and hydrocortisone *on page 591*

hydrocortisone, bacitracin, neomycin, and polymyxin B *see* bacitracin, neomycin, polymyxin B, and hydrocortisone *on page 59*

hydrocortisone, colistin, and neomycin *see* colistin, neomycin, and hydrocortisone *on page 145*

hydrocortisone, neomycin, and polymyxin B *see* neomycin, polymyxin B, and hydrocortisone *on page 396*

hydrocortisone (rectal) (hye droe KOR ti sone)

U.S./Canadian Brand Names Anusol-HC® Suppository; Cortenema® Rectal; Cortifoam® Rectal; Proctocort™ Rectal; Rectocort (Can)

Therapeutic Category Adrenal Corticosteroid

Use Management of adrenocortical insufficiency; adjunctive treatment of ulcerative colitis

Usual Dosage Ulcerative colitis: Adults: Rectal: 10-100 mg 1-2 times/day for 2-3 weeks

Dosage Forms

Acetate:

Aerosol, rectal: 10% [90 mg/applicatorful] 20 g

Suppository, rectal: 25 mg

Base:

Rectal: 1% (30 g)

Suspension, rectal: 100 mg/60 mL (7s)

hydrocortisone (systemic) (hye droe KOR ti sone)

Synonyms compound F

U.S./Canadian Brand Names A-hydroCort® Injection; Cortef® Oral; Hydrocortone® Acetate Injection; Hydrocortone® Oral; Hydrocortone® Phosphate Injection; Solu-Cortef® Injection

Therapeutic Category Adrenal Corticosteroid

Use Management of adrenocortical insufficiency; relief of inflammation of corticosteroid-responsive dermatoses

Usual Dosage Dose should be based on severity of disease and patient response

Acute adrenal insufficiency: I.M., I.V.:

Infants and young Children: Succinate: 1-2 mg/kg/dose bolus, then 25-150 mg/day in divided doses every 6-8 hours

Older Children: Succinate: 1-2 mg/kg bolus then 150-250 mg/day in divided doses every 6-8 hours

Adults: Succinate: 100 mg I.V. bolus, then 300 mg/day in divided doses every 8 hours or as a continuous infusion for 48 hours; once patient is stable change to oral, 50 mg every 8 hours for 6 doses, then taper to 30-50 mg/day in divided doses

Chronic adrenal corticoid insufficiency: Adults: Oral: 20-30 mg/day

Anti-inflammatory or immunosuppressive:

Infants and Children:

Oral: 2.5-10 mg/kg/day **or** 75-300 mg/m^2/day every 6-8 hours

I.M., I.V.: Succinate: 1-5 mg/kg/day **or** 30-150 mg/m^2/day divided every 12-24 hours

Adolescents and Adults: Oral, I.M., I.V.: Succinate: 15-240 mg every 12 hours

Congenital adrenal hyperplasia: Oral: Initial: 30-36 mg/m^2/day with $^1/_3$ of dose every morning and $^2/_3$ every evening or $^1/_4$ every morning and mid-day and $^1/_2$ every evening; maintenance: 20-25 mg/m^2/day in divided doses

Physiologic replacement: Children:

Oral: 0.5-0.75 mg/kg/day **or** 20-25 mg/m^2/day every 8 hours

I.M.: Succinate: 0.25-0.35 mg/kg/day **or** 12-15 mg/m^2/day once daily

Shock: I.M., I.V.: Succinate:

Children: Initial: 50 mg/kg, then repeated in 4 hours and/or every 24 hours as needed

Adolescents and Adults: 500 mg to 2 g every 2-6 hours

Status asthmaticus: Children and Adults: I.V.: Succinate: 1-2 mg/kg/dose every 6 hours for 24 hours, then maintenance of 0.5-1 mg/kg every 6 hours

(Continued)

hydrocortisone (systemic) *(Continued)*

Rheumatic diseases:

Adults: Intralesional, intra-articular, soft tissue injection: Acetate:

Large joints: 25 mg (up to 37.5 mg)

Small joints: 10-25 mg

Tendon sheaths: 5-12.5 mg

Soft tissue infiltration: 25-50 mg (up to 75 mg)

Bursae: 25-37.5 mg

Ganglia: 12.5-25 mg

Dermatosis: Children >2 years and Adults: Topical: Apply to affected area 3-4 times/day (Buteprate: Apply once or twice daily)

Ulcerative colitis: Adults: Rectal: 10-100 mg 1-2 times/day for 2-3 weeks

Dosage Forms

Injection, suspension: 25 mg/mL (5 mL, 10 mL); 50 mg/mL (5 mL, 10 mL)

Tablet: 5 mg, 10 mg, 20 mg

Suspension, oral: 10 mg/5 mL (120 mL)

hydrocortisone (topical) (hye droe KOR ti sone)

U.S./Canadian Brand Names Acticort® Topical; Aeroseb-HC® Topical; Ala-Cort® Topical; Ala-Scalp® Topical; Anusol® HC-1 Topical [OTC]; Anusol® HC-2.5% Topical [OTC]; Aquacort® (Can); Bactine® Hydrocortisone [OTC]; CaldeCort® Anti-Itch Topical Spray; CaldeCort® Topical [OTC]; Cetacort® Topical; Clocort® Maximum Strength [OTC]; CortaGel® Topical [OTC]; Cortaid® Maximum Strength Topical [OTC]; Cortaid® with Aloe Topical [OTC]; Cortamed® (Can); Cortate® (Can); Cort-Dome® Topical; Cortef® Feminine Itch Topical; Corticreme® (Can); Cortiment® (Can); Cortizone®-5 Topical [OTC]; Cortizone®-10 Topical [OTC]; Cortoderm (Can); Delcort® Topical; Dermacort® Topical; Dermarest Dricort® Topical; Dermolate® Topical [OTC]; Dermtex® HC with Aloe Topical [OTC]; Eldecort® Topical; Emo-Cort™ (Can); Gynecort® Topical [OTC]; Hi-Cor-1.0® Topical; Hi-Cor-2.5® Topical; Hycort® Topical; Hyderm (Can); Hydrocort® Topical; Hydro-Tex® Topical [OTC]; Hytone® Topical; LactiCare-HC® Topical; Lanacort® Topical [OTC]; Locoid® Topical; Nutracort® Topical; Orabase® HCA Topical; Penecort® Topical; Prevex™ HC (Can); Scalpicin® Topical; S-T Cort® Topical; Synacort® Topical; Tegrin®-HC Topical [OTC]; Texacort® Topical; U-Cort™ Topical; Westcort® Topical

Therapeutic Category Corticosteroid, Topical

Use Management of adrenocortical insufficiency; relief of inflammation of corticosteroid-responsive dermatoses; adjunctive treatment of ulcerative colitis

Usual Dosage Children >2 years and Adults: Topical: Apply to affected area 3-4 times/day (Buteprate: Apply once or twice daily)

Dosage Forms

Aerosol, topical:

Cream: 0.5%, 1%, 2.5%

Gel: 0.5%

Ointment, topical: 0.5%, 1%, 2.5%

Lotion: 0.5%, 1%, 2.5%

Paste: 0.5% (5 g)

Solution, topical; 1%

Butyrate:

Cream: 0.1%

Ointment, topical: 0.1%

Solution, topical: 0.1%

Valerate:

Cream: 0.2%

Ointment, topical: 0.2%

Hydrocortone® Acetate Injection *see* hydrocortisone (systemic) *on previous page*

Hydrocortone® Oral *see* hydrocortisone (systemic) *on previous page*

Hydrocortone® Phosphate Injection *see* hydrocortisone (systemic) *on previous page*

Hydrocort® Topical *see* hydrocortisone (topical) *on previous page*

Hydro-Crysti-12® *see* hydroxocobalamin *on next page*

HydroDIURIL® *see* hydrochlorothiazide *on page 286*

hydroflumethiazide (hye droe floo meth EYE a zide)

U.S./Canadian Brand Names Diucardin®; Saluron®

Therapeutic Category Diuretic, Thiazide

Use Management of mild to moderate hypertension; treatment of edema in congestive heart failure and nephrotic syndrome

Usual Dosage Oral: 1 tablet 1-2 times/day

Dosage Forms Tablet: 50 mg

hydroflumethiazide and reserpine

(hye droe floo meth EYE a zide & re SER peen)

Synonyms reserpine and hydroflumethiazide

U.S./Canadian Brand Names Salutensin®

Therapeutic Category Antihypertensive Agent, Combination

Use Management of hypertension

Usual Dosage Oral (determined by individual titration): Usually 1 tablet once or twice daily

Dosage Forms

Tablet (Salutensin®): Hydroflumethiazide 50 mg and reserpine 0.125 mg

Tablet (Hydro-Fluserpine®, Salutensin-Demi®): Hydroflumethiazide 25 mg and reserpine 0.125 mg

hydrogenated ergot alkaloids *see* ergoloid mesylates *on page 213*

Hydrogesic® *see* hydrocodone and acetaminophen *on page 287*

hydromagnesium aluminate *see* magaldrate *on page 344*

Hydromet® *see* hydrocodone and homatropine *on page 289*

hydromorphone (hye droe MOR fone)

Synonyms dihydromorphinone

U.S./Canadian Brand Names Dilaudid® Cough Syrup; Dilaudid-HP® Injection; Dilaudid® Injection; Dilaudid® Oral; Dilaudid® Suppository; PMS-Hydromorphone (Can)

Therapeutic Category Analgesic, Narcotic

Controlled Substance C-II

Use Management of moderate to severe pain; antitussive at lower doses

Usual Dosage Doses should be titrated to appropriate analgesic effects; when changing routes of administration, note that oral doses are less than half as effective as parenteral doses (may be only $^1/_5$ as effective)

Pain: Older Children and Adults: Oral, I.M., I.V., S.C.: 1-4 mg/dose every 4-6 hours as needed; usual adult dose: 2 mg/dose

Antitussive: Oral:

- Children 6-12 years: 0.5 mg every 3-4 hours as needed
- Children >12 years and Adults: 1 mg every 3-4 hours as needed

Dosage Forms Hydromorphone hydrochloride:

Injection:

- Dilaudid®: 1 mg/mL (1 mL); 2 mg/mL (1 mL, 20 mL); 3 mg/mL (1 mL); 4 mg/mL (1 mL)
- Dilaudid-HP®: 10 mg/mL (1 mL, 2 mL, 5 mL)

Liquid: 5 mg/5 mL (480 mL)

Powder for injection: (Dilaudid-HP®): 250 mg

Suppository, rectal: 3 mg (6s)

Tablet: 1 mg, 2 mg, 3 mg, 4 mg, 8 mg

Hydromox® *see* quinethazone *on page 492*

Hydro-Par® *see* hydrochlorothiazide *on page 286*

Hydrophed® *see* theophylline, ephedrine, and hydroxyzine *on page 559*

Hydropres® *see* hydrochlorothiazide and reserpine *on page 286*

Hydropres® 25 mg Tablet *(Discontinued)* *see page 700*

hydroquinol *see* hydroquinone *on this page*

hydroquinone (HYE droe kwin one)

Synonyms hydroquinol; quinol

U.S./Canadian Brand Names Ambi® Skin Tone [OTC]; Eldopaque® [OTC]; Eldopaque Forte®; Eldoquin® [OTC]; Eldoquin® Forte®; Esoterica® Facial [OTC]; Esoterica® Regular [OTC]; Esoterica® Sensitive Skin Formula [OTC]; Esoterica® Sunscreen [OTC]; Melanex®; Neostrata® HQ (Can); Porcelana® [OTC]; Porcelana® Sunscreen [OTC]; Solaquin® [OTC]; Solaquin Forte®; Ultraquin™ (Can)

Therapeutic Category Topical Skin Product

Use Gradual bleaching of hyperpigmented skin conditions

Usual Dosage Topical: Apply thin layer and rub in twice daily

Dosage Forms

Cream, topical:

Esoterica® Sensitive Skin Formula: 1.5% [OTC] (85 g)

Eldopaque®, Eldoquin®, Esoterica® Facial, Esoterica® Regular, Porcelana®: 2% [OTC] (14.2 g, 28.4 g, 60 g, 85 g, 120 g)

Eldopaque Forte®, Eldoquin® Forte®, Melquin HP®: 4% (14.2 g, 28.4 g)

Cream, topical, with sunblock:

Esoterica® Sunscreen, Porcelana®, Solaquin®: 2% [OTC] (28.4 g, 120 g)

Melpaque HP®, Nuquin HP®, Solaquin Forte®: 4% (14.2 g, 28.4 g)

Gel, topical, with sunscreen (Solaquin Forte®): 4% (14.2 g, 28.4 g)

Solution, topical (Melanex®): 3% (30 mL)

Hydro-Serp® *see* hydrochlorothiazide and reserpine *on page 286*

Hydroserpine® *see* hydrochlorothiazide and reserpine *on page 286*

Hydro-Tex® Topical [OTC] *see* hydrocortisone (topical) *on page 292*

Hydroxacen® *(Discontinued)* *see page 700*

hydroxocobalamin (hye droks oh koe BAL a min)

Synonyms vitamin B_{12a}

U.S./Canadian Brand Names Acti-B_{12}® (Can); Hydro Cobex®; Hydro-Crysti-12®; LA-12®

Therapeutic Category Vitamin, Water Soluble

Use Pernicious anemia, vitamin B_{12} deficiency, increased B_{12} requirements due to pregnancy, thyrotoxicosis, hemorrhage, malignancy, liver or kidney disease

Usual Dosage

Children:

Congenital pernicious anemia (if evidence of neurologic involvement): I.M.: 1000 mcg/day for at least 2 weeks; maintenance: 50 mcg/month

Vitamin B_{12} deficiency: I.M., S.C.: 1-5 mg administered in single or S.C. doses of 100 mcg over 2 or more weeks

Adults:

Pernicious anemia: I.M., S.C.: 100 mcg/day for 6-7 days

Vitamin B_{12} deficiency:

Oral: Usually not recommended, maximum absorbed from a single oral dose is 2-3 mcg

I.M., S.C.: 30 mcg/day for 5-10 days, followed by 100-200 mcg/month

Dosage Forms Injection: 1000 mcg/mL (10 mL, 30 mL)

hydroxyamphetamine (hye droks ee am FET a meen)

U.S./Canadian Brand Names Paredrine®

Therapeutic Category Adrenergic Agonist Agent

Use Produce mydriasis in diagnostic eye examination

Usual Dosage Instill 1-2 drops into conjunctival sac

Dosage Forms Solution, as hydrobromide: 1%

hydroxyamphetamine and tropicamide

(hye droks ee am FET a meen & troe PIK a mide)

U.S./Canadian Brand Names Paremyd® Ophthalmic

Therapeutic Category Adrenergic Agonist Agent

Use Mydriasis with cycloplegia

Usual Dosage Adults: Ophthalmic: Instill 1-2 drops into conjunctival sac(s)

Dosage Forms Solution, ophthalmic: Hydroxyamphetamine hydrobromide 1% and tropicamide 0.25% (5 mL, 15 mL)

hydroxycarbamide *see* hydroxyurea *on next page*

hydroxychloroquine (hye droks ee KLOR oh kwin)

U.S./Canadian Brand Names Plaquenil®

Therapeutic Category Aminoquinoline (Antimalarial)

Use Suppression or chemoprophylaxis of malaria caused by susceptible *P. vivax*, *P. ovale*, *P. malariae*, and some strains of *P. falciparum* (not active against pre-erythrocytic or exoerythrocytic tissue stages of *Plasmodium*); treatment of systemic lupus erythematosus (SLE) and rheumatoid arthritis

Usual Dosage Oral:

Children:

Chemoprophylaxis of malaria: 5 mg/kg (base) once weekly; should not exceed the recommended adult dose; begin 2 weeks before exposure; continue for 8 weeks after leaving endemic area

Acute attack: 10 mg/kg (base) initial dose; followed by 5 mg/kg in 6 hours on day 1; 5 mg/kg in 1 dose on day 2 and on day 3

Juvenile rheumatoid arthritis or SLE: 3-5 mg/kg/day divided 1-2 times/day to a maximum of 400 mg/day; not to exceed 7 mg/kg/day

Adults:

Chemoprophylaxis of malaria: 2 tablets weekly on same day each week; begin 2 weeks before exposure; continue for 6-8 weeks after leaving epidemic area

Acute attack: 4 tablets first dose day 1; 2 tablets in 6 hours day 1; 2 tablets in 1 dose day 2; and 2 tablets in 1 dose on day 3

Rheumatoid arthritis: 2-3 tablets/day to start with food or milk; increase dose until optimum response level is reached; usually after 4-12 weeks dose should be reduced by $1/2$ and a maintenance dose of 1-2 tablets/day

Lupus erythematosus: 2 tablets every day or twice daily for several weeks depending on response; 1-2 tablets/day for prolonged maintenance therapy

Dosage Forms Tablet, as sulfate: 200 mg [base 155 mg]

25-hydroxycholecalciferol *see* calcifediol *on page 88*

hydroxydaunomycin *see* doxorubicin *on page 196*

hydroxyethyl starch *see* hetastarch *on page 281*

hydroxyprogesterone caproate (hye droks ee proe JES te rone KAP roe ate)

U.S./Canadian Brand Names Hylutin®; Hyprogest® 250

Therapeutic Category Progestin

Use Treatment of amenorrhea, abnormal uterine bleeding, submucous fibroids, endometriosis, uterine carcinoma, and testing of estrogen production

Usual Dosage Adults: I.M.:

Amenorrhea: 375 mg; if no bleeding, begin cyclic treatment with estradiol valerate

Endometriosis: Start cyclic therapy with estradiol valerate

Uterine carcinoma: 1 g one or more times/day (1-7 g/week) for up to 12 weeks

Test for endogenous estrogen production: 250 mg anytime; bleeding 7-14 days after injection indicate positive test

Dosage Forms Hydroxyprogesterone caproate:

Injection: 125 mg/mL (10 mL)

(Continued)

hydroxyprogesterone caproate *(Continued)*

Hylutin®, Hyprogest®: 250 mg/mL (5 mL)

hydroxypropyl cellulose (hye droks ee PROE pil SEL yoo lose)

U.S./Canadian Brand Names Lacrisert®

Therapeutic Category Ophthalmic Agent, Miscellaneous

Use Dry eyes

Usual Dosage Adults: Ophthalmic: Apply once daily into the inferior cul-de-sac beneath the base of tarsus, not in apposition to the cornea nor beneath the eyelid at the level of the tarsal plate

Dosage Forms Insert, ophthalmic: 5 mg

hydroxypropyl methylcellulose (hye droks ee PROE pil meth il SEL yoo lose)

Synonyms gonioscopic ophthalmic solution

U.S./Canadian Brand Names Gonak™ [OTC]; Goniosol® [OTC]

Therapeutic Category Ophthalmic Agent, Miscellaneous

Use Ophthalmic surgical aid in cataract extraction and intraocular implantation; gonioscopic examinations

Usual Dosage Introduced into anterior chamber of eye with 20-gauge or larger cannula

Dosage Forms Solution: 2.5% (15 mL)

hydroxyurea (hye droks ee yoor EE a)

Synonyms hydroxycarbamide

U.S./Canadian Brand Names Droxia™; Hydrea®

Therapeutic Category Antineoplastic Agent

Use CML in chronic phase; radiosensitizing agent in the treatment of primary brain tumors; head and neck tumors; uterine cervix and nonsmall cell lung cancer; psoriasis; sickle cell anemia and other hemoglobinopathies; resistant chronic myelocytic leukemia; hematologic conditions such as essential thrombocythemia, polycythemia vera, hypereosinophilia, and hyperleukocytosis due to acute leukemia. Has shown activity against renal cell cancer; malignant melanoma; metastatic or inoperable carcinoma of the ovary; head, neck, and lip cancer; and prostate cancer.

Droxia™: Approved - specifically for patients >18 years of age who have had at least three "painful crises" in the previous year - to reduce frequency of these crises and the need for blood transfusions; Droxia™ is not a cure for sickle cell disease, but it may help control the symptoms of the disease.

Unlabeled use: Thrombocythemia

Usual Dosage Adults: Oral (refer to individual protocols): Dosage based on patient's actual or ideal weight, whichever is less

Solid tumors: Intermittent therapy: 80 mg/kg as a single dose every third day; continuous therapy: 20-30 mg/kg/day given as a single dose/day

Concomitant therapy with irradiation: 80 mg/kg as a single dose every third day starting at least 7 days before initiation of irradiation

Resistant chronic myelocytic leukemia: 20-30 mg/kg/day divided daily

Sickle cell anemia: Droxia™: Initial: 15 mg/kg as a single daily dose (dose based on IBW or actual body weight whichever is less); dose may be increased by 5 mg/kg every 12 weeks to highest dose which does not produce toxic blood counts over 24 weeks, or a maximum of 35 mg/kg

Do not increase dose if counts are between acceptable and toxic; if counts are considered toxic, discontinue hydroxyurea until hematologic recovery; resume dosing at a dose which is 2.5 mg/kg/day less than the dose which resulted in toxicity; further titration should proceed at 2.5 mg/kg/day increments, adjusted every 12 weeks as above; do not attempt any dosage which results in toxicity on two occasions

Acceptable: Neutrophils ≥2500 cells/mm^3, platelets ≥95,000/mm^3, hemoglobin >5.3 g/dL and reticulocytes ≥95,000/mm^3 if the hemoglobin concentration is <9 g/dL

Toxic: Neutrophils <2000 cells/mm^3, platelets <80,000/mm^3, hemoglobin <4.5 g/dL and reticulocytes ≥80,000/mm^3 if the hemoglobin concentration is <9 g/dL

Dosage Forms

Capsule: 500 mg

Capsule (Droxia™): 200 mg, 300 mg, 400 mg

25-hydroxyvitamin D_3 *see* calcifediol *on page 88*

hydroxyzine (hye DROKS i zeen)

U.S./Canadian Brand Names Anxanil® Oral; Apo®-Hydroxyzine (Can); Atarax® Oral; Atozine® Oral; Durrax® Oral; Hy-Pam® Oral; Hyzine-50® Injection; Multipax® (Can); Neucalm-50® Injection; Novo-Hydroxyzine® (Can); PMS-Hydroxyzine (Can); Quiess® Injection; Vamate® Oral; Vistacon-50® Injection; Vistaquel® Injection; Vistaril® Injection; Vistaril® Oral; Vistazine® Injection

Therapeutic Category Antiemetic; Antihistamine

Use Treatment of anxiety; preoperative sedative; antipruritic; antiemetic

Usual Dosage

Children:

Oral: 2 mg/kg/day divided every 6-8 hours

I.M.: 0.5-1 mg/kg/dose every 4-6 hours as needed

Adults:

Antiemetic: I.M.: 25-100 mg/dose every 4-6 hours as needed

Anxiety: Oral: 25-100 mg 4 times/day; maximum dose: 600 mg/day

Preoperative sedation:

Oral: 50-100 mg

I.M.: 25-100 mg

Management of pruritus: Oral: 25 mg 3-4 times/day

Dosage Forms

Hydroxyzine hydrochloride:

Injection:

Vistaril®: 25 mg/mL (1 mL, 2 mL, 10 mL)

Hyzine-50®, Neucalm®, Quiess®, Vistacon-50®, Vistaquel®, Vistaril®, Vistazine®: 50 mg/mL (1 mL, 2 mL, 10 mL)

Syrup (Atarax®): 10 mg/5 mL (120 mL, 480 mL, 4000 mL)

Tablet:

Anxanil®: 25 mg

Atarax®: 10 mg, 25 mg, 50 mg, 100 mg

Atozine®: 10 mg, 25 mg, 50 mg

Durrax®: 10 mg, 25 mg

Hydroxyzine pamoate:

Capsule:

Hy-Pam®: 25 mg, 50 mg

Vamate®: 25 mg, 50 mg, 100 mg

Vistaril®: 25 mg, 50 mg, 100 mg

Suspension, oral (Vistaril®:) 25 mg/5 mL (120 mL, 480 mL)

hydroxyzine, theophylline, and ephedrine *see* theophylline, ephedrine, and hydroxyzine *on page 559*

Hygroton® *see* chlorthalidone *on page 128*

Hylorel® *see* guanadrel *on page 274*

Hylutin® *see* hydroxyprogesterone caproate *on page 295*

hyoscine *see* scopolamine *on page 516*

hyoscyamine (hye oh SYE a meen)

Synonyms *l*-hyoscyamine sulfate

U.S./Canadian Brand Names Anaspaz®; A-Spas® S/L; Cystospaz®; Cystospaz-M®; Donnamar®; ED-SPAZ®; Gastrosed™; Levbid®; Levsin®; Levsinex®; Levsin/SL®

Therapeutic Category Anticholinergic Agent

Use GI tract disorders caused by spasm, adjunctive therapy for peptic ulcers

(Continued)

hyoscyamine *(Continued)*

Usual Dosage

Children:

<2 years: 1/4 adult dosage

2-10 years: 1/2 adult dosage

Adults:

Oral, S.L.: 0.125-0.25 mg 3-4 times/day before meals or food and at bedtime; 0.375-0.75 mg (timed release) every 12 hours

I.M., I.V., S.C.: 0.25-0.5 mg every 6 hours

Dosage Forms

Capsule, as sulfate, timed release (Cystospaz-M®, Levsinex®): 0.375 mg

Elixir, as sulfate (Levsin®): 0.125 mg/5 mL with alcohol 20% (480 mL)

Injection, as sulfate (Levsin®): 0.5 mg/mL (1 mL, 10 mL)

Solution, oral (Gastrosed™, Levsin®): 0.125 mg/mL (15 mL)

Tablet, as sulfate:

Anaspaz®, Gastrosed™, Levsin®: 0.125 mg

Cystospaz®: 0.15 mg

hyoscyamine, atropine, scopolamine, and phenobarbital

(hye oh SYE a meen, A troe peen, skoe POL a meen & fee noe BAR bi tal)

Synonyms atropine, hyoscyamine, scopolamine, and phenobarbital; phenobarbital, hyoscyamine, atropine, and scopolamine; scopolamine, hyoscyamine, atropine, and phenobarbital

U.S./Canadian Brand Names Barbidonna®; Bellatal®; Donnatal®; Hyosophen®; Spasmolin®

Therapeutic Category Anticholinergic Agent

Use Adjunct in treatment of peptic ulcer disease, irritable bowel, spastic colitis, spastic bladder, and renal colic

Usual Dosage Oral:

Children 2-12 years:

Kinesed® dose: 1/2 to 1 tablet 3-4 times/day

Donnatal®: 0.1 mL/kg/dose every 4 hours; maximum dose: 5 mL

Adults: 0.125-0.25 mg (1-2 capsules or tablets) 3-4 times/day; or 0.375-0.75 mg (1 Donnatal® Extentab®) in sustained release form every 12 hours; or 5-10 mL elixir 3-4 times/day or every 8 hours

Dosage Forms

Capsule (Donnatal®, Spasmolin®): Hyoscyamine sulfate 0.1037 mg, atropine sulfate 0.0194 mg, scopolamine hydrobromide 0.0065 mg, and phenobarbital 16.2 mg

Elixir (Donnatal®, Hyosophen®, Spasmophen®): Hyoscyamine sulfate 0.1037 mg, atropine sulfate 0.0194 mg, scopolamine hydrobromide 0.0065 mg, and phenobarbital 16.2 mg per 5 mL (120 mL, 480 mL, 4000 mL)

Tablet:

Barbidonna®: Hyoscyamine hydrobromide 0.1286 mg, atropine sulfate 0.025 mg, scopolamine hydrobromide 0.0074 mg, and phenobarbital 16 mg

Barbidonna® No. 2: Hyoscyamine hydrobromide 0.1286 mg, atropine sulfate 0.025 mg, scopolamine hydrobromide 0.0074 mg, and phenobarbital 32 mg

Bellatal®, Donnatal®, Hyosophen®: Hyoscyamine sulfate 0.1037 mg, atropine sulfate 0.0194 mg, scopolamine hydrobromide 0.0065 mg, and phenobarbital 16.2 mg

Long-acting (Donnatal®): Hyoscyamine sulfate 0.3111 mg, atropine sulfate 0.0582 mg, scopolamine hydrobromide 0.0195 mg, and phenobarbital 48.6 mg

Spasmophen®: Hyoscyamine sulfate 0.1037 mg, atropine sulfate 0.0194 mg, scopolamine hydrobromide 0.0065 mg, and phenobarbital 15 mg

hyoscyamine, atropine, scopolamine, kaolin, and pectin

(hye oh SYE a meen, A troe peen, skoe POL a meen, KAY oh lin & PEK tin)

Therapeutic Category Anticholinergic Agent

Use Antidiarrheal; also used in gastritis, enteritis, colitis, and acute gastrointestinal upsets, and nausea which may accompany any of these conditions

Usual Dosage Oral:
Children:
10-20 lb: 2.5 mL
20-30 lb: 5 mL
>30 lb: 5-10 mL
Adults:
Diarrhea: 30 mL at once and 15-30 mL with each loose stool
Other conditions: 15 mL every 3 hours as needed

Dosage Forms Suspension, oral: Hyoscyamine sulfate 0.1037 mg, atropine sulfate 0.0194 mg, scopolamine hydrobromide 0.0065 mg, kaolin 6 g, and pectin 142.8 mg per 30 mL

hyoscyamine, atropine, scopolamine, kaolin, pectin, and opium

(hye oh SYE a meen, A troe peen, skoe POL a meen, KAY oh lin, PEK tin, & OH pee um)

U.S./Canadian Brand Names Donnapectolin-PG®; Kapectolin PG®

Therapeutic Category Anticholinergic Agent

Controlled Substance C-V

Use Treatment of diarrhea

Usual Dosage Oral:
Children 6-12 years: Initial: 10 mL, then 5-10 mL every 3 hours thereafter
Dosage recommendations (body weight/dosage): 10 lb/2.5 mL; 20 lb/5 mL; 30 lb and over/5-10 mL; do not administer more than 4 doses in any 24-hour period
Children >12 years and Adults: Initial: 30 mL (1 fluid oz) followed by 15 mL every 3 hours

Dosage Forms Suspension, oral: Hyoscyamine sulfate 0.1037 mg, atropine sulfate 0.0194 mg, scopolamine hydrobromide 0.0065 mg, kaolin 6 g, pectin 142.8 mg, and powdered opium 24 mg per 30 mL with alcohol 5%

Hyosophen® *see* hyoscyamine, atropine, scopolamine, and phenobarbital *on previous page*

Hy-Pam® Oral *see* hydroxyzine *on page 297*

Hypaque-Cysto® *see* radiological/contrast media (ionic) *on page 495*

Hypaque® Meglumine *see* radiological/contrast media (ionic) *on page 495*

Hypaque® Sodium *see* radiological/contrast media (ionic) *on page 495*

Hyperab® *see* rabies immune globulin (human) *on page 494*

HyperHep® *see* hepatitis B immune globulin *on page 280*

Hyperstat® I.V. *see* diazoxide *on page 174*

Hyper-Tet® *see* tetanus immune globulin (human) *on page 553*

Hy-Phen® *see* hydrocodone and acetaminophen *on page 287*

HypoTears PF Solution [OTC] *see* artificial tears *on page 47*

HypoTears Solution [OTC] *see* artificial tears *on page 47*

HypRho®-D *see* Rh_o(D) immune globulin (intramuscular) *on page 502*

HypRho®-D Mini-Dose *see* Rh_o(D) immune globulin (intramuscular) *on page 502*

Hyprogest® 250 *see* hydroxyprogesterone caproate *on page 295*

Hyrexin-50® Injection *see* diphenhydramine *on page 185*

Hytakerol® *see* dihydrotachysterol *on page 181*

Hytinic® [OTC] *see* polysaccharide-iron complex *on page 460*

Hytone® Topical *see* hydrocortisone (topical) *on page 292*

Hytrin® *see* terazosin *on page 550*

Hytuss® [OTC] *see* guaifenesin *on page 267*

Hytuss-2X® [OTC] *see* guaifenesin *on page 267*

Hyzaar® *see* losartan and hydrochlorothiazide *on page 341*

Hyzine-50® Injection *see* hydroxyzine *on page 297*

ibenzmethyzin *see* procarbazine *on page 476*

Iberet-Folic-500® *see* ferrous sulfate, ascorbic acid, vitamin B-complex, and folic acid *on page 238*

Iberet®-Liquid [OTC] *see* ferrous sulfate, ascorbic acid, and vitamin B-complex *on page 238*

ibidomide *see* labetalol *on page 323*

Ibuprin® [OTC] *see* ibuprofen *on this page*

ibuprofen (eye byoo PROE fen)

Synonyms *p*-isobutylhydratropic acid

U.S./Canadian Brand Names Aches-N-Pain® [OTC]; Actiprofen® (Can); Advil® [OTC]; Apo®-Ibuprofen (Can); Children's Advil® Suspension; Children's Motrin® Suspension [OTC]; Excedrin® IB [OTC]; Genpril® [OTC]; Haltran® [OTC]; Ibuprin® [OTC]; Ibuprohm® [OTC]; Ibu-Tab®; Junior Strength Motrin® [OTC]; Medipren® [OTC]; Menadol® [OTC]; Midol® IB [OTC]; Motrin®; Motrin® IB [OTC]; Novo-Profen® (Can); Nu-Ibuprofen® (Can); Nuprin® [OTC]; Pamprin IB® [OTC]; Pedia-Profen™; Saleto-200® [OTC]; Saleto-400®; Trendar® [OTC]; Uni-Pro® [OTC]

Therapeutic Category Analgesic, Non-narcotic; Antipyretic; Nonsteroidal Anti-inflammatory Drug (NSAID)

Use Inflammatory diseases and rheumatoid disorders including juvenile rheumatoid arthritis (JRA); mild to moderate pain; fever; dysmenorrhea; gout

Usual Dosage Oral:

Children:

Antipyretic: 6 months to 12 years: Temperature <102.5°F (39°C): 5 mg/kg/dose; temperature >102.5°F: 10 mg/kg/dose administered every 6-8 hours; maximum daily dose: 40 mg/kg/day

Juvenile rheumatoid arthritis: 30-50 mg/kg/day in 4 divided doses; start at lower end of dosing range and titrate upward; maximum: 2.4 g/day

Analgesic: 4-10 mg/kg/dose every 6-8 hours

Adults:

Inflammatory disease: 400-800 mg/dose 3-4 times/day; maximum dose: 3.2 g/day

Pain/fever/dysmenorrhea: 200-400 mg/dose every 4-6 hours; maximum daily dose: 1.2 g

Dosage Forms

Caplet: 100 mg

Drops, oral (berry flavor): 40 mg/mL (15 mL)

Suspension, oral: 100 mg/5 mL [OTC] (60 mL, 120 mL, 480 mL)

Drops: 40 mg/mL [OTC]

Tablet: 100 mg [OTC], 200 mg [OTC], 300 mg, 400 mg, 600 mg, 800 mg

Chewable: 50 mg, 100 mg

ibuprofen and hydrocodone *see* hydrocodone and ibuprofen *on page 289*

Ibuprohm® [OTC] *see* ibuprofen *on this page*

Ibu-Tab® *see* ibuprofen *on this page*

ibutilide (i BYOO ti lide)

U.S./Canadian Brand Names Corvert®

Therapeutic Category Antiarrhythmic Agent, Class III

Use Acute termination of atrial fibrillation or flutter of recent onset; the effectiveness of ibutilide has not been determined in patients with arrhythmias of >90 days in duration

Usual Dosage I.V.: Initial:

<60 kg: 0.01 mg/kg over 10 minutes

≥60 kg: 1 mg over 10 minutes

If the arrhythmia does not terminate within 10 minutes after the end of the initial infusion, a second infusion of equal strength may be infused over a 10-minute period

Dosage Forms Injection, as fumarate: 0.1 mg/mL (10 mL)

Icaps® (Can) *see* vitamin, multiple (oral) *on page 604*

ICI 204, 219 *see* zafirlukast *on page 609*

ICRF-187 *see* dexrazoxane *on page 169*

Idamycin® *see* idarubicin *on this page*

Idamycin® PFS *see* idarubicin *on this page*

Idarac® (Can) *see* floctafenine *(Canada only)* *on page 240*

idarubicin (eye da ROO bi sin)

Synonyms 4-demethoxydaunorubicin; 4-dmdr

U.S./Canadian Brand Names Idamycin®; Idamycin® PFS

Therapeutic Category Antineoplastic Agent

Use In combination with other antineoplastic agents for treatment of acute myelogenous leukemia (AML) in adults and acute lymphocytic leukemia (ALL) in children

Usual Dosage I.V.:

Children:

Leukemia: 10-12 mg/m^2 once daily for 3 days and repeat every 3 weeks

Solid tumors: 5 mg/m^2 once daily for 3 days and repeat every 3 weeks

Adults: 12 mg/m^2/day for 3 days by slow I.V. injection (10-15 minutes) in combination with Ara-C. The Ara-C may be given as 100 mg/m^2/day by continuous infusion for 7 days or 25 mg/m^2 bolus followed by Ara-C 200 mg/m^2/day for 5 days continuous infusion.

Dosage Forms

Injection: 1 mg/mL (5 mL, 10 mL, 20 mL)

Powder for injection, lyophilized, as hydrochloride: 5 mg, 10 mg

Ifex® *see* ifosfamide *on this page*

IFLrA *see* interferon alfa-2a *on page 308*

ifosfamide (eye FOSS fa mide)

U.S./Canadian Brand Names Ifex®

Therapeutic Category Antineoplastic Agent

Use In combination with other antineoplastics in treatment of lung cancer, Hodgkin's and non-Hodgkin's lymphoma, breast cancer, acute and chronic lymphocytic leukemia, ovarian cancer, testicular cancer, and sarcomas

Usual Dosage I.V. (refer to individual protocols):

Children: 1800 mg/m^2/day for 3-5 days every 21-28 days or 5000 mg/m^2 as a single 24-hour infusion or 3 g/m^2/day for 2 days

Adults: 700-2000 mg/m^2/day for 5 days or 2400 mg/m^2/day for 3 days every 21-28 days; 5000 mg/m^2 as a single dose over 24 hours

Dosage Forms Powder for injection: 1 g, 3 g

IG *see* immune globulin, intramuscular *on page 303*

IGIM *see* immune globulin, intramuscular *on page 303*

IGIV *see* immune globulin, intravenous *on page 303*

IL-11 *see* oprelvekin *on page 416*

Iletin® (Can) *see* insulin preparations *on page 307*

Iletin® II Pork (Can) *see* insulin preparations *on page 307*

Ilopan-Choline® Oral *see* dexpanthenol *on page 169*

Ilopan® Injection *see* dexpanthenol *on page 169*

Ilosone® *see* erythromycin (systemic) *on page 215*

Ilosone® Pulvules® *see* erythromycin (systemic) *on page 215*

Ilotycin® *see* erythromycin (systemic) *on page 215*

Ilotycin® (Can) *see* erythromycin (systemic) *on page 215*

Ilotycin® Ophthalmic *see* erythromycin (ophthalmic/topical) *on page 214*

Ilozyme® *see* pancrelipase *on page 427*

Imdur™ *see* isosorbide mononitrate *on page 316*

imidazole carboxamide *see* dacarbazine *on page 157*

imiglucerase (i mi GLOO ser ace)

U.S./Canadian Brand Names Cerezyme®

Therapeutic Category Enzyme

Use Long-term enzyme replacement therapy for patients with Type 1 Gaucher's disease

Usual Dosage I.V.: 2.5 units/kg 3 times/week up to as much as 60 units/kg administered as frequently as once weekly or as infrequently as every 4 weeks; 60 units/kg administered every 2 weeks is the most common dose

Dosage Forms Powder for injection, preservative free (lyophilized): 212 units [equivalent to a withdrawal dose of 200 units]

imipemide *see* imipenem and cilastatin *on this page*

imipenem and cilastatin (i mi PEN em & sye la STAT in)

Synonyms cilastatin and imipenem; imipemide

U.S./Canadian Brand Names Primaxin®

Therapeutic Category Carbapenem (Antibiotic)

Use Treatment of documented multidrug resistant gram-negative infection due to organisms proven or suspected to be susceptible to imipenem/cilastatin; treatment of multiple organism infection in which other agents have an insufficient spectrum of activity or are contraindicated due to toxic potential; therapeutic alternative for treatment of gram negative sepsis in immunocompromised patients

Usual Dosage I.V. infusion (dosage recommendation based on imipenem component):

Children: 60-100 mg/kg/day in 4 divided doses

Adults:

- Serious infection: 2-4 g/day in 3-4 divided doses
- Mild to moderate infection: 1-2 g/day in 3-4 divided doses

Dosage Forms Powder for injection:

I.M.:

- Imipenem 500 mg and cilastatin 500 mg
- Imipenem 750 mg and cilastatin 750 mg

I.V.:

- Imipenem 250 mg and cilastatin 250 mg
- Imipenem 500 mg and cilastatin 500 mg

imipramine (im IP ra meen)

U.S./Canadian Brand Names Apo®-Imipramine (Can); Janimine®; Novo-Pramine® (Can); PMS-Imipramine (Can); Tofranil®; Tofranil-PM®

Therapeutic Category Antidepressant, Tricyclic (Tertiary Amine)

Use Treatment of various forms of depression, often in conjunction with psychotherapy; enuresis in children; analgesic for certain chronic and neuropathic pain

Usual Dosage

Children: Oral (safety and efficacy of imipramine therapy for treatment of depression in children <12 years have not been established):

- Enuresis: ≥6 years: Initial: 10-25 mg at bedtime, if inadequate response still seen after 1 week of therapy, increase by 25 mg/day; dose should not exceed 2.5 mg/kg/day or 50 mg at bedtime if 6-12 years of age or 75 mg at bedtime if ≥12 years of age
- Adjunct in the treatment of cancer pain: Initial: 0.2-0.4 mg/kg at bedtime; dose may be increased by 50% every 2-3 days up to 1-3 mg/kg/dose at bedtime

Adolescents: Oral: Initial: 25-50 mg/day; increase gradually; maximum: 100 mg/day in single or divided doses

Adults:
Oral: Initial: 25 mg 3-4 times/day, increase dose gradually, total dose may be administered at bedtime; maximum: 300 mg/day
I.M.: Initial: Up to 100 mg/day in divided doses; change to oral as soon as possible

Dosage Forms
Imipramine hydrochloride:
Injection (Tofranil®): 12.5 mg/mL (2 mL)
Tablet (Janimine®, Tofranil®): 10 mg, 25 mg, 50 mg
Imipramine pamoate: Capsule (Tofranil-PM®): 75 mg, 100 mg, 125 mg, 150 mg

imiquimod (i mi KWI mod)

U.S./Canadian Brand Names Aldara™

Therapeutic Category Immune Response Modifier

Use Genital and perianal warts (condyloma acuminata)

Usual Dosage Adults: Topical: Apply 3 times/week, prior to bedtime, leave on for 6-10 hours; remove cream by washing area with mild soap and water

Dosage Forms Cream: 5% (250 mg single dose packets)

Imitrex® *see* sumatriptan succinate *on page 544*

ImmuCyst® (Can) *see* BCG vaccine *on page 61*

immune globulin, intramuscular

(i MYUN GLOB yoo lin, IN tra MUS kyoo ler)

Synonyms gamma globulin; IG; IGIM; immune serum globulin; ISG

U.S./Canadian Brand Names Gammabulin Immuno (Can)

Therapeutic Category Immune Globulin

Use Prophylaxis against hepatitis A, measles, varicella, and possibly rubella and immunoglobulin deficiency, idiopathic thrombocytopenia purpura, Kawasaki syndrome, lymphocytic leukemia

Usual Dosage I.M.:
Hepatitis A: 0.02 mL/kg
IgG: 1.3 mL/kg then 0.66 mL/kg in 3-4 weeks
Measles: 0.25 mL/kg
Rubella: 0.55 mL/kg
Varicella: 0.6-1.2 mL/kg

Dosage Forms Injection: I.M.: 165±15 mg (of protein)/mL (2 mL, 10 mL)

immune globulin, intravenous (i MYUN GLOB yoo lin, IN tra VEE nus)

Synonyms IGIV; IVIG

U.S./Canadian Brand Names Gamimune® N; Gammagard® S/D; Gammar®-P I.V.; Polygam® S/D; Sandoglobulin®; Venoglobulin®-I; Venoglobulin®-S

Therapeutic Category Immune Globulin

Use Immunodeficiency syndrome, idiopathic thrombocytopenic purpura (ITP) and B-cell chronic lymphocytic leukemia (CLL); used in conjunction with appropriate anti-infective therapy to prevent or modify acute bacterial or viral infections in patients with iatrogenically-induced or disease-associated immunodepression; autoimmune neutropenia, bone marrow transplantation patients, Kawasaki disease, Guillain-Barré syndrome, demyelinating polyneuropathies

Usual Dosage Children and Adults: I.V. infusion:
Immunodeficiency syndrome: 100-200 mg/kg/dose every month; may increase to 400 mg/kg/dose as needed
Idiopathic thrombocytopenic purpura: 400-1000 mg/kg/dose for 2-5 consecutive days; maintenance dose: 400-1000 mg/kg/dose every 3-6 weeks based on clinical response and platelet count
Kawasaki disease: 400 mg/kg/day for 4 days or 2 g/kg as a single dose
Congenital and acquired antibody deficiency syndrome: 100-400 mg/kg/dose every 3-4 weeks
Bone marrow transplant: 500 mg/kg/week
(Continued)

immune globulin, intravenous *(Continued)*

Severe systemic viral and bacterial infections: Children: 500-1000 mg/kg/week

Dosage Forms

Injection: Gamimune® N: 5% [50 mg/mL] (10 mL, 50 mL, 100 mL); 10% [100 mg/mL] (50 mL, 100 mL, 200 mL)

Powder for injection, lyophilized:

Gammar-P®-IV: 1 g, 2.5 g, 5 g

Sandoglobulin®: 1 g, 3 g, 6 g

Venoglobulin®-I: 2.5 g, 5 g

Detergent treated:

Gammagard® S/D: 2.5 g, 5 g, 10 g

Polygam® S/D: 2.5 g, 5 g, 10 g

Venoglobulin®-S: 2.5 g, 5 g, 10 g

immune serum globulin *see* immune globulin, intramuscular *on previous page*

Imodium® *see* loperamide *on page 339*

Imodium® A-D [OTC] *see* loperamide *on page 339*

Imodium® Advanced *see* loperamide *on page 339*

Imogam® *see* rabies immune globulin (human) *on page 494*

Imovax® Rabies I.D. Vaccine *see* rabies virus vaccine *on page 494*

Imovax® Rabies Vaccine *see* rabies virus vaccine *on page 494*

Imuran® *see* azathioprine *on page 55*

I-Naphline® Ophthalmic *see* naphazoline *on page 390*

Inapsine® *see* droperidol *on page 199*

indapamide (in DAP a mide)

U.S./Canadian Brand Names Lozide® (Can); Lozol®

Therapeutic Category Diuretic, Miscellaneous

Use Management of mild to moderate hypertension; treatment of edema in congestive heart failure and nephrotic syndrome

Usual Dosage Adults: Oral: 2.5-5 mg/day

Dosage Forms Tablet: 1.25 mg, 2.5 mg

Inderal® *see* propranolol *on page 483*

Inderal® LA *see* propranolol *on page 483*

Inderide® *see* propranolol and hydrochlorothiazide *on page 484*

indinavir (in DIN a veer)

U.S./Canadian Brand Names Crixivan®

Therapeutic Category Antiviral Agent

Use Treatment of HIV infection, especially advanced disease; usually administered as part of a three-drug regimen (two nucleosides plus a protease inhibitor) or double therapy (one nucleoside plus a protease inhibitor)

Usual Dosage Adults: Oral: 800 mg every 8 hours

Dosage Forms Capsule: 200 mg, 400 mg

Indocin® I.V. Injection *see* indomethacin *on next page*

Indocin® Oral *see* indomethacin *on next page*

Indocin® SR Oral *see* indomethacin *on next page*

Indocollyre® (Can) *see* indomethacin *on next page*

indocyanine green (in doe SYE a neen green)

U.S./Canadian Brand Names Cardio-Green®

Therapeutic Category Diagnostic Agent

Use Determining hepatic function, cardiac output and liver blood flow and for ophthalmic angiography

Usual Dosage Dilute dose in sterile water for injection or 0.9% NaCl to final volume of 1 mL if necessary doses may be repeated periodically; total dose should not exceed 2 mg/kg

Infants: 1.25 mg
Children: 2.5 mg
Adults: 5 mg

Dosage Forms Injection: 25 mg, 50 mg

indometacin *see* indomethacin *on this page*

indomethacin (in doe METH a sin)

Synonyms indometacin

U.S./Canadian Brand Names Apo®-Indomethacin (Can); Indocin® I.V. Injection; Indocin® Oral; Indocin® SR Oral; Indocollyre® (Can); Indotec (Can); Novo-Methacin® (Can); Nu-Indo® (Can); Pro-Indo® (Can)

Therapeutic Category Analgesic, Non-narcotic; Nonsteroidal Anti-inflammatory Drug (NSAID)

Use Management of inflammatory diseases and rheumatoid disorders; moderate pain; acute gouty arthritis; I.V. form used as alternative to surgery for closure of patent ductus arteriosus (PDA) in neonates

Usual Dosage

Patent ductus arteriosus: Neonates: I.V.: Initial: 0.2 mg/kg; followed with: 2 doses of 0.1 mg/kg at 12- to 24-hour intervals if age <48 hours at time of first dose; 0.2 mg/kg 2 times if 2-7 days old at time of first dose; or 0.25 mg/kg 2 times if over 7 days at time of first dose; discontinue if significant adverse effects occur. Dose should be withheld if patient has anuria or oliguria.

Analgesia:

Children: Oral: Initial: 1-2 mg/kg/day in 2-4 divided doses; maximum: 4 mg/kg/day; not to exceed 150-200 mg/day

Adults: Oral, rectal: 25-50 mg/dose 2-3 times/day; maximum dose: 200 mg/day; extended release capsule should be administered on a 1-2 times/day schedule

Dosage Forms

Capsule: 25 mg, 50 mg
Indocin®: 25 mg, 50 mg
Capsule, sustained release (Indocin® SR): 75 mg
Powder for injection, as sodium trihydrate (Indocin® I.V.): 1 mg
Suppository, rectal (Indocin®): 50 mg
Suspension, oral (Indocin®): 25 mg/5 mL (5 mL, 10 mL, 237 mL, 500 mL)

Indotec (Can) *see* indomethacin *on this page*

INF-alpha 2 *see* interferon alfa-2b *on page 308*

Infanrix™ *see* diphtheria, tetanus toxoids, and acellular pertussis vaccine *on page 187*

Infantol® (Can) *see* vitamin, multiple (oral) *on page 604*

Infasurf® *see* calfactant *on page 94*

InFeD™ *see* iron dextran complex *on page 312*

Inflamase® Forte Ophthalmic *see* prednisolone (ophthalmic) *on page 471*

Inflamase® Mild Ophthalmic *see* prednisolone (ophthalmic) *on page 471*

infliximab (in FLIKS e mab)

U.S./Canadian Brand Names Remicade®

Therapeutic Category Gastrointestinal Agent, Miscellaneous

Use Treatment of moderately to severely active Crohn's disease for the reduction of the signs and symptoms in patients who have an inadequate response to conventional

(Continued)

infliximab *(Continued)*

therapy or for the treatment of patients with fistulizing Crohn's disease for the reduction in the number of draining enterocutaneous fistula(s)

Usual Dosage

Moderately to severely active Crohn's disease: Adults: I.V.: 5 mg/kg as a single infusion over a minimum of 2 hours

Fistulizing Crohn's disease: 5 mg/kg as an infusion over a minimum of 2 hours, dose repeated at 2 and 6 weeks after the initial infusion

Dosage Forms Powder for injection: 100 mg

influenza virus vaccine (in floo EN za VYE rus vak SEEN)

Synonyms influenza virus vaccine (inactivated whole-virus); influenza virus vaccine (purified surface antigen); influenza virus vaccine (split-virus)

U.S./Canadian Brand Names Fluogen®; Fluviral® (Can); Fluzone®

Therapeutic Category Vaccine, Inactivated Virus

Use Provide active immunity to influenza virus strains contained in the vaccine

Usual Dosage Annual vaccination with current vaccine; either whole- or split-virus vaccine may be used

Dosage Forms Injection:

Purified surface antigen (Flu-Imune®): 5 mL
Split-virus (Fluogen®, Fluzone®): 0.5 mL, 5 mL
Whole-virus (Fluzone®): 5 mL

influenza virus vaccine (inactivated whole-virus) *see* influenza virus vaccine *on this page*

influenza virus vaccine (purified surface antigen) *see* influenza virus vaccine *on this page*

influenza virus vaccine (split-virus) *see* influenza virus vaccine *on this page*

INH *see* isoniazid *on page 314*

Inhibace® (Can) *see* cilazapril *(Canada only)* *on page 131*

Innohep® (Can) *see* tinzaparin *(Canada only)* *on page 567*

Innovar® *see* droperidol and fentanyl *on page 199*

Inocor® *see* amrinone *on page 35*

insect sting kit (IN sekt sting kit)

U.S./Canadian Brand Names Ana-Kit®

Therapeutic Category Antidote

Use Anaphylaxis emergency treatment of insect bites or stings by the sensitive patient that may occur within minutes of insect sting or exposure to an allergic substance

Usual Dosage Children and Adults:

Epinephrine:
- <2 years: 0.05-0.1 mL
- 2-6 years: 0.15 mL
- 6-12 years: 0.2 mL
- >12 years : 0.3 mL

Chlorpheniramine:
- <6 years: 1 tablet
- 6-12 years: 2 tablets
- >12 years: 4 tablets

Dosage Forms Kit: Epinephrine hydrochloride 1:1000 (1 mL syringe), chlorpheniramine maleate chewable tablet 2 mg (4), sterile alcohol pads (2), tourniquet

Insta-Glucose® [OTC] *see* glucose, instant *on page 262*

Insulin Lente® L *see* insulin preparations *on next page*

insulin preparations (IN su lin prep a RAY shuns)

U.S./Canadian Brand Names Humalog®; Humulin® 50/50; Humulin® 70/30; Humulin® L; Humulin® N; Humulin® R; Humulin® U; Iletin® (Can); Iletin® II Pork (Can); Insulin Lente® L; Lente®; Lente® Iletin® I; Lente® Iletin® II; Novolin® 70/30; Novolin® ge (Can); Novolin® L; Novolin® N; Novolin-Pen® II, -3 (Can); Novolin® R; NPH Iletin® I; NPH Insulin; NPH-N; Pork NPH; Pork Regular Iletin® II; Regular Iletin® I; Regular [Concentrated] Iletin® II U-500; Regular Insulin; Regular Purified Pork Insulin; Velosulin®

Therapeutic Category Antidiabetic Agent, Parenteral

Use Treatment of insulin-dependent diabetes mellitus, also noninsulin-dependent diabetes mellitus unresponsive to treatment with diet and/or oral hypoglycemics; to assure proper utilization of glucose and reduce glucosuria in nondiabetic patients receiving parenteral nutrition whose glucosuria cannot be adequately controlled with infusion rate adjustments or those who require assistance in achieving optimal caloric intakes

Usual Dosage Dose requires continuous medical supervision; only regular insulin may be administered I.V. The daily dose should be divided up depending upon the product used and the patient's response, eg, regular insulin every 4-6 hours; NPH insulin every 8-12 hours.

Children and Adults: S.C.: 0.5-1 unit/kg/day
Adolescents (during growth spurt): S.C.: 0.8-1.2 units/kg/day

Diabetic ketoacidosis: Children: I.V. loading dose: 0.1 unit/kg, then maintenance continuous infusion: 0.1 unit/kg/hour (range: 0.05-0.2 units/kg/hour depending upon the rate of decrease of serum glucose - too rapid decrease of serum glucose may lead to cerebral edema).
Optimum rate of decrease (serum glucose): 80-100 mg/dL/hour

Note: Newly diagnosed patients with JODM presenting in DKA and patients with blood sugars <800 mg/dL may be relatively "sensitive" to insulin and should receive loading and initial maintenance doses approximately ½ of those indicated above.

Note: The term "purified" refers to insulin preparations containing no more than 10 ppm proinsulin (purified and human insulins are less immunogenic)

Dosage Forms All insulins are 100 units/mL (10 mL) except where indicated:

RAPID ACTING:
Insulin lispro rDNA origin: Humalog® [*Lilly*] (1.5 mL, 10 mL)
Insulin Injection (Regular Insulin)
Beef and pork: Regular Iletin® I [*Lilly*]
Human:
rDNA: Humulin® R [*Lilly*], Novolin® R [*Novo Nordisk*]
Semisynthetic: Velosulin® Human [*Novo Nordisk*]
Pork: Regular Insulin [*Novo Nordisk*]
Purified pork:
Pork Regular Iletin® II [*Lilly*], Regular Purified Pork Insulin [*Novo Nordisk*]
Regular (Concentrated) Iletin® II U-500 (*Lilly*): 500 units/mL

INTERMEDIATE-ACTING:
Insulin Zinc Suspension (Lente®)
Beef and pork: Lente® Iletin® I [*Lilly*]
Human, rDNA: Humulin® L [*Lilly*], Novolin® L [*Novo Nordisk*]
Purified pork: Lente® Iletin® II [*Lilly*], Lente® L [*Novo Nordisk*]

Isophane Insulin Suspension (NPH)
Beef and pork: NPH Iletin® I [*Lilly*]
Human, rDNA: Humulin® N [*Lilly*], Novolin® N [*Novo Nordisk*]
Purified pork: Pork NPH Iletin® II [*Lilly*], NPH-N [*Novo Nordisk*]

LONG-ACTING:
Insulin zinc suspension, extended (Ultralente®)
Human, rDNA: Humulin® U [Lilly]

COMBINATIONS:
Isophane Insulin Suspension and Insulin Injection
Isophane insulin suspension (50%) and insulin injection (50%) human (rDNA): Humulin® 50/50 [*Lilly*]

(Continued)

insulin preparations *(Continued)*

Isophane insulin suspension (70%) and insulin injection (30%) human (rDNA): Humulin® 70/30 [*Lilly*], Novolin® 70/30 [*Novo Nordisk*]

Intal® *see* cromolyn sodium *on page 150*

Intal® Inahalation Capsule *(Discontinued)* *see page 700*

Integrilin® *see* eptifibatide *on page 212*

Intercept® *(Discontinued)* *see page 700*

α-2-interferon *see* interferon alfa-2b *on this page*

interferon alfa-2a (in ter FEER on AL fa too aye)

Synonyms IFLrA; rIFN-A

U.S./Canadian Brand Names Roferon-A®

Therapeutic Category Biological Response Modulator

Use Hairy cell leukemia, AIDS-related Kaposi's sarcoma in patients >18 years of age, multiple unlabeled uses

Usual Dosage

Children: S.C.: Pulmonary hemangiomatosis: 1-3 million units/m²/day once daily

Adults >18 years:

Hairy cell leukemia: I.M., S.C.: Induction dose is 3 million units/day for 16-24 weeks; maintenance: 3 million units 3 times/week

AIDS-related Kaposi's sarcoma: I.M., S.C.: Induction dose is 36 million units for 10-12 weeks; maintenance: 36 million units 3 times/week (may begin with dose escalation from 3-9-18 million units each day over 3 consecutive days followed by 36 million units daily for the remainder of the 10-12 weeks of induction)

Dosage Forms

Injection: 3 million units/mL (1 mL); 6 million units/mL (3 mL); 9 million units/mL (0.9 mL, 3 mL); 36 million units/mL (1 mL)

Powder for injection: 6 million units/mL when reconstituted

interferon alfa-2b (in ter FEER on AL fa too bee)

Synonyms INF-alpha 2; α-2-interferon; rLFN-α2

U.S./Canadian Brand Names Intron® A

Therapeutic Category Biological Response Modulator

Use Induce hairy cell leukemia remission; treatment of AIDS-related Kaposi's sarcoma; condylomata acuminata; chronic hepatitis C

Usual Dosage Adults (refer to individual protocols):

Hairy cell leukemia: I.M., S.C.: 2 million units/m² 3 times/week

AIDS-related Kaposi's sarcoma: I.M., S.C.: 30 million units/m² 3 times/week or 50 million units/m² I.V. 5 days/week every other week

Condylomata acuminata: Intralesionally: 1 million units/lesion 3 times/week for 3 weeks; not to exceed 5 million units per treatment (maximum: 5 lesions at one time)

Chronic hepatitis C: I.M., S.C.: 3 million units 3 times/week for approximately a 6-month course

Dosage Forms

Injection, albumin free: 3 million units (0.5 mL); 5 million units (0.5 mL); 10 million units (1 mL); 25 million units

Powder for injection, lyophilized: 18 million units, 50 million units

interferon alfa-2b and ribavirin combination pack

(in ter FEER on AL fa too bee)

U.S./Canadian Brand Names Rebetron™

Therapeutic Category Antiviral Agent; Biological Response Modulator

Use The combination therapy is indicated for the treatment of chronic hepatitis C in patients with compensated liver disease who have relapsed following alpha interferon therapy

Usual Dosage The recommended dosage of combination therapy is 3 million int. units of Intron® A injected subcutaneously three times per week and 1000-1200 mg of Rebtrol® capsules administered orally in a divided daily (morning and evening) dose for 24 weeks; patients weighing 75 kg (165 pounds) or less should receive 1000 mg of Rebetrol® daily, while patients weighing more than 75 kg should receive 1200 mg of Rebetrol® daily

Dosage Forms Combination package:

For patients ≤75 kg:

Each Rebetron™ combination package consists of:

A box containing 6 vials of Intron® A (3 million int. units in 0.5 mL per vial) and 6 syringes and alcohol swabs; two boxes containing 35 Rebetrol® capsules each for a total of 70 capsules (5 capsules per blister card)

One 18 million int. units multidose vial of Intron® A injection (22.8 million int. units per 3.8 mL; 3 million int. units/0.5 mL) and 6 syringes and alcohol swabs; two boxes containing 35 Rebetrol® capsules each for a total of 70 capsules (5 capsules per blister card)

One 18 million int. units Intron® A injection multidose pen (22.5 million int. units per 1.5 mL; 3 million int. units/0.2 mL) and 6 disposable needles and alcohol swabs; two boxes containing 35 Rebetrol® capsules each for a total of 70 capsules (5 capsules per blister card)

For patients >75 kg:

A box containing 6 vials of Intron® A injection (3 million int. units in 0.5 mL per vial) and 6 syringes and alcohol swabs; two boxes containing 42 Rebetrol® capsules each for a total of 84 capsules (6 capsules per blister card)

One 18 million int. units multidose vial of Intron® A injection (22.5 million int. units per 3.8 mL; 3 million int. units/0.5 mL) and 6 syringes and alcohol swabs; two boxes containing 42 Rebetrol® capsules each for a total of 84 capsules (6 capsules per blister card)

One 18 million int. units Intron® A injection multidose pen (22.5 million int. units per 1.5 mL; 3 million int. units/0.2 mL) and 6 disposable needles and alcohol swabs; two boxes containing 42 Rebetrol® capsules each for a total of 84 capsules (6 capsules per blister card)

For Rebetrol® dose reduction:

A box containing 6 vials of Intron® A injection (3 million int. units in 0.5 mL per vial) and 6 syringes and alcohol swabs; one box containing 42 Rebetrol® capsules (6 capsules per blister card)

One 18 million int. units multidose vial of Intron® A injection (22.8 million int. units per 3.8 mL; 3 million int. units/0.5 mL) and 6 syringes and alcohol swabs; one box containing 42 Rebetrol® capsules (6 capsules per blister card)

One 18 million int. units Introl® A injection multidose pen (22.5 million int. units per 1.5 mL; 3 million int. units/0.2 mL) and 6 disposable needles and alcohol swabs; one box containing 42 Rebetrol® capsules (6 capsules per blister card)

interferon alfa-n3 (in ter FEER on AL fa en three)

U.S./Canadian Brand Names Alferon® N

Therapeutic Category Biological Response Modulator

Use Intralesional treatment of refractory or recurring genital or venereal warts; useful in patients who do not respond or are not candidates for usual treatments; indications and dosage regimens are specific for a particular brand of interferon

Usual Dosage Adults: Inject 250,000 units (0.05 mL) in each wart twice weekly for a maximum of 8 weeks; therapy should not be repeated for at least 3 months after the initial 8-week course of therapy

Dosage Forms Injection: 5 million units (1 mL)

interferon beta-1a (in ter FEER on BAY ta won aye)

U.S./Canadian Brand Names Avonex™

Therapeutic Category Biological Response Modulator

Use Treatment of relapsing forms of multiple sclerosis (MS); to slow the accumulation of physical disability and decrease the frequency of clinical exacerbations

Usual Dosage Adults >18 years: I.M.: 30 mcg once weekly

Dosage Forms Powder for injection, lyophilized: 33 mcg [6.6 million units]

interferon beta-1b (in ter FEER on BAY ta won bee)
U.S./Canadian Brand Names Betaseron®
Therapeutic Category Biological Response Modulator
Use Reduce the frequency of clinical exacerbations in ambulatory patients with relapsing-remitting multiple sclerosis
Usual Dosage Adults: S.C.: 0.25 mg every other day
Dosage Forms Powder for injection, lyophilized: 0.3 mg [9.6 million units]

interferon gamma-1b (in ter FEER on GAM ah won bee)
U.S./Canadian Brand Names Actimmune®
Therapeutic Category Biological Response Modulator
Use Reduce the frequency and severity of serious infections associated with chronic granulomatous disease
Usual Dosage Adults: S.C. (dosing is based on body surface (m^2)):
≤0.5: 1.5 mcg/kg/dose
>0.5: 50 mcg/m^2 (1.5 million units/m^2) 3 times/week
Dosage Forms Injection: 100 mcg [3 million units]

interleukin-2 *see* aldesleukin *on page 16*

Interleukin-11 *see* oprelvekin *on page 416*

Intralipid® *see* fat emulsion *on page 231*

intravenous fat emulsion *see* fat emulsion *on page 231*

Intron® A *see* interferon alfa-2b *on page 308*

Intropin® *see* dopamine *on page 193*

Inversine® *see* mecamylamine *on page 351*

Invirase® *see* saquinavir *on page 515*

Iobid DM® *see* guaifenesin and dextromethorphan *on page 268*

Iodex® [OTC] *see* povidone-iodine *on page 467*

Iodex-p® [OTC] *see* povidone-iodine *on page 467*

iodine (EYE oh dyne)
Therapeutic Category Topical Skin Product
Use Topically as an antiseptic in the management of minor, superficial skin wounds and has been used to disinfect the skin preoperatively
Usual Dosage Topical: Apply as necessary to affected areas of skin
Dosage Forms
Solution: 2%
Tincture: 2%

iodochlorhydroxyquin and hydrocortisone *see* clioquinol and hydrocortisone *on page 137*

Iodo-Niacin® Tablet *(Discontinued)* *see page 700*

Iodopen® *see* trace metals *on page 573*

iodoquinol (eye oh doe KWIN ole)
Synonyms diiodohydroxyquin
U.S./Canadian Brand Names Diodoquin® (Can); Yodoxin®
Therapeutic Category Amebicide
Use Treatment of acute and chronic intestinal amebiasis due to *Entamoeba histolytica*; asymptomatic cyst passers; *Blastocystis hominis* infections; iodoquinol alone is ineffective for amebic hepatitis or hepatic abscess
Usual Dosage Oral:
Children: 30-40 mg/kg/day in 3 divided doses for 20 days; not to exceed 1.95 g/day
Adults: 650 mg 3 times/day after meals for 20 days; not to exceed 2 g/day

Dosage Forms
Powder: 25 g
Tablet: 210 mg, 650 mg

iodoquinol and hydrocortisone

(eye oh doe KWIN ole & hye droe KOR ti sone)

Synonyms hydrocortisone and iodoquinol

U.S./Canadian Brand Names Vytone® Topical

Therapeutic Category Antifungal/Corticosteroid

Use Treatment of eczema; infectious dermatitis; chronic eczematoid otitis externa; mycotic dermatoses

Usual Dosage Topical: Apply 3-4 times/day

Dosage Forms Cream: Iodoquinol 1% and hydrocortisone 1% (30 g)

Iofed® *see* brompheniramine and pseudoephedrine *on page 81*

Iofed® PD *see* brompheniramine and pseudoephedrine *on page 81*

Ionamin® ***(Discontinued)*** *see page 700*

Ionil-T® Plus (Can) *see* coal tar *on page 141*

Iophen-C® ***(Discontinued)*** *see page 700*

Iophen® ***(Discontinued)*** *see page 700*

Iophen-DM® ***(Discontinued)*** *see page 700*

Iophylline® ***(Discontinued)*** *see page 700*

Iopidine® *see* apraclonidine *on page 45*

Iotuss® ***(Discontinued)*** *see page 700*

Iotuss-DM® ***(Discontinued)*** *see page 700*

I-Paracaine® *see* proparacaine *on page 481*

ipecac syrup (IP e kak SIR up)

Therapeutic Category Antidote

Use Treatment of acute oral drug overdosage and certain poisonings

Usual Dosage Oral:

Children:

6-12 months: 5-10 mL followed by 10-20 mL/kg of water; repeat dose one time if vomiting does not occur within 20 minutes

1-12 years: 15 mL followed by 10-20 mL/kg of water; repeat dose one time if vomiting does not occur within 20 minutes

Adults: 30 mL followed by 200-300 mL of water; repeat dose one time if vomiting does not occur within 20 minutes

Dosage Forms Syrup: 70 mg/mL (15 mL, 30 mL, 473 mL, 4000 mL)

I-Pentolate® *see* cyclopentolate *on page 153*

I-Phrine® Ophthalmic Solution *see* phenylephrine *on page 445*

I-Picamide® *see* tropicamide *on page 587*

IPOL™ *see* poliovirus vaccine, inactivated *on page 458*

ipratropium (i pra TROE pee um)

U.S./Canadian Brand Names Atrovent®

Therapeutic Category Anticholinergic Agent

Use Bronchodilator used in bronchospasm associated with asthma, COPD, bronchitis, and emphysema; nasal spray used for symptomatic relief of rhinorrhea

Usual Dosage Children >12 years and Adults: 2 inhalations 4 times/day up to 12 inhalations/24 hours

Dosage Forms Solution, as bromide:

Inhalation: 18 mcg/actuation (14 g)

(Continued)

ipratropium *(Continued)*

Nasal spray: 0.03% (30 mL); 0.06% (15 mL)
Nebulizing: 0.02% (2.5 mL)

ipratropium and albuterol (i pra TROE pee um & al BYOO ter ole)

U.S./Canadian Brand Names Combivent®

Therapeutic Category Bronchodilator

Use Treatment of chronic obstructive pulmonary disease (COPD) in those patients that are currently on a regular bronchodilator who continue to have bronchospasms and require a second bronchodilator

Usual Dosage Adults: 2 inhalations 4 times/day, maximum of 12 inhalations/24 hours

Dosage Forms Aerosol: Ipratropium bromide 18 mcg and albuterol sulfate 103 mcg per actuation [200 doses] (14.7 g)

iproveratril *see* verapamil *on page 598*

IPV *see* poliovirus vaccine, inactivated *on page 458*

irbesartan (ir be SAR tan)

U.S./Canadian Brand Names Avapro®

Therapeutic Category Angiotensin II Antagonist

Use Treatment of hypertension alone or in combination with other antihypertensives

Usual Dosage Adults: Oral: 150 mg once daily with or without food; patients may be titrated to 300 mg once daily

Dosage Forms Tablet: 75 mg, 150 mg, 300 mg

irbesartan and hydrochlorothiazide

(ir be SAR tan & hye droe klor oh THYE a zide)

U.S./Canadian Brand Names Avapro® HCT

Therapeutic Category Antihypertensive Agent, Combination

Use Combination therapy for the management of hypertension

Dosage Forms Tablet: Irbesartan 150 mg and hydrochlorothiazide 12.5 mg; irbesartan 300 mg and hydrochlorothiazide 12.5 mg

Ircon® [OTC] *see* ferrous fumarate *on page 236*

irinotecan (eye rye no TEE kan)

U.S./Canadian Brand Names Camptosar®

Therapeutic Category Antineoplastic Agent

Use Treatment of patients with metastatic carcinoma of the colon or rectum whose disease has progressed following 5-FU based therapy

Usual Dosage Adults: I.V.: The recommended starting dose is 125 mg/m^2 (I.V. infusion over 90 minutes) once a week for 4 weeks, followed by a 2-week rest period; additional 6-week cycles of treatment may be repeated indefinitely in patients who remain stable or do not develop intolerable toxicities

Dosage Forms Injection: 20 mg/mL (5 mL)

iron dextran complex (EYE ern DEKS tran KOM pleks)

U.S./Canadian Brand Names Dexferrum®; InFeD™

Therapeutic Category Electrolyte Supplement, Oral

Use Treatment of microcytic, hypochromic anemia resulting from iron deficiency when oral iron administration is infeasible or ineffective

Usual Dosage I.M., I.V.:

A 0.5 mL test dose (0.25 mL in infants) should be administered prior to starting iron dextran therapy

Total replacement dosage of iron dextran (mL) = 0.0476 x weight (kg) x (Hb_n-Hb_o) + 1 mL/per 5 kg body weight (up to maximum of 14 mL)

Hb_n = desired hemoglobin (g/dL)

Hb_o = measured hemoglobin (g/dL)
Maximum daily dose:
Infants <5 kg: 25 mg iron
Children:
5-10 kg: 50 mg iron
10-50 kg: 100 mg iron
Adults >50 kg: 100 mg iron

Dosage Forms Injection: 50 mg/mL (2 mL, 10 mL)

ISD *see* isosorbide dinitrate *on page 315*

ISDN *see* isosorbide dinitrate *on page 315*

ISG *see* immune globulin, intramuscular *on page 303*

Ismelin® *see* guanethidine *on page 274*

ISMN *see* isosorbide mononitrate *on page 316*

Ismo® *see* isosorbide mononitrate *on page 316*

Ismotic® *see* isosorbide *on page 315*

isoamyl nitrite *see* amyl nitrite *on page 36*

isobamate *see* carisoprodol *on page 101*

Iso-Bid® ***(Discontinued)*** *see page 700*

Isocaine® HCl *see* mepivacaine *on page 356*

Isocal® [OTC] *see* enteral nutritional products *on page 208*

Isocal® with Fibre (Can): Isosource® (Can) *see* enteral nutritional products *on page 208*

Isoclor® Expectorant *see* guaifenesin, pseudoephedrine, and codeine *on page 272*

Isocom® *see* acetaminophen, isometheptene, and dichloralphenazone *on page 6*

isoetharine (eye soe ETH a reen)

U.S./Canadian Brand Names Arm-a-Med® Isoetharine; Beta-2®; Bronkometer®; Bronkosol®; Dey-Lute® Isoetharine

Therapeutic Category Adrenergic Agonist Agent

Use Bronchodilator used in asthma and for the reversible bronchospasm occurring with bronchitis and emphysema

Usual Dosage Treatments are usually not repeated more often than every 4 hours, except in severe cases, and may be repeated up to 5 times/day if necessary

Nebulizer: Children: 0.1-0.2 mg/kg/dose every 2-6 hours as needed; adult: 0.5 mL diluted in 2-3 mL normal saline or 4 inhalations of undiluted 1% solution

Dosage Forms
Isoetharine hydrochloride:
Solution, inhalation: 0.062% (4 mL); 0.08% (3.5 mL); 0.1% (2.5 mL, 5 mL); 0.125% (4 mL); 0.167% (3 mL); 0.17% (3 mL); 0.2% (2.5 mL); 0.25% (2 mL, 3.5 mL); 0.5% (0.5 mL); 1% (0.5 mL, 0.25 mL, 10 mL, 14 mL, 30 mL)
Isoetharine mesylate: Aerosol, oral: 340 mcg/metered spray

isoflurane (eye soe FLURE ane)

U.S./Canadian Brand Names Forane®

Therapeutic Category General Anesthetic

Use General induction and maintenance of anesthesia (inhalation)

Usual Dosage 1.5% to 3%

Dosage Forms Solution: 100 mL, 125 mL, 250 mL

isoflurophate (eye soe FLURE oh fate)

Synonyms DFP; diisopropyl fluorophosphate; dyflos; fluostigmin

U.S./Canadian Brand Names Floropryl® Ophthalmic

Therapeutic Category Cholinergic Agent

Use Treat primary open-angle glaucoma and conditions that obstruct aqueous outflow and to treat accommodative convergent strabismus

Usual Dosage Adults: Ophthalmic:

Glaucoma: Instill 1/4" strip in eye every 8-72 hours

Strabismus: Instill 1/4" strip to each eye every night for 2 weeks then reduce to 1/4" every other night to once weekly for 2 months

Dosage Forms Ointment, ophthalmic: 0.025% in polyethylene mineral oil gel (3.5 g)

Isollyl® Improved *see* butalbital compound and aspirin *on page 85*

isoniazid (eye soe NYE a zid)

Synonyms INH; isonicotinic acid hydrazide

U.S./Canadian Brand Names Laniazid® Syrup; PMS-Isoniazid (Can)

Therapeutic Category Antitubercular Agent

Use Treatment of susceptible mycobacterial infection due to *M. tuberculosis* and prophylactically to those individuals exposed to tuberculosis

Usual Dosage Oral, I.M.:

Children: 10-20 mg/kg/day in 1-2 divided doses (maximum: 300 mg total dose)

Prophylaxis: 10 mg/kg/day administered daily (up to 300 mg total dose) for 12 months

Adults: 5 mg/kg/day administered daily (usual dose: 300 mg)

Disseminated disease: 10 mg/kg/day in 1-2 divided doses

Treatment should be continued for 9 months with rifampin or for 6 months with rifampin and pyrazinamide

Prophylaxis: 300 mg/day administered daily for 12 months

American Thoracic Society and CDC currently recommend twice weekly therapy as part of a short-course regimen which follows 1-2 months of daily treatment for uncomplicated pulmonary tuberculosis in compliant patients

Children: 20-40 mg/kg/dose (up to 900 mg) twice weekly

Adults: 15 mg/kg/dose (up to 900 mg) twice weekly

Dosage Forms

Injection: 100 mg/mL (10 mL)

Syrup (orange flavor): 50 mg/5 mL (473 mL)

Tablet: 50 mg, 100 mg, 300 mg

isoniazid and rifampin *see* rifampin and isoniazid *on page 505*

isoniazid, rifampin, and pyrazinamide *see* rifampin, isoniazid, and pyrazinamide *on page 505*

isonicotinic acid hydrazide *see* isoniazid *on this page*

isonipecaine *see* meperidine *on page 355*

Isopap® *see* acetaminophen, isometheptene, and dichloralphenazone *on page 6*

isoproterenol (eye soe proe TER e nole)

U.S./Canadian Brand Names Arm-a-Med® Isoproterenol; Dey-Dose® Isoproterenol; Isuprel®; Medihaler-Iso®

Therapeutic Category Adrenergic Agonist Agent

Use Asthma or COPD (reversible airway obstruction); ventricular arrhythmias due to A-V nodal block; hemodynamically compromised bradyarrhythmias or atropine-resistant bradyarrhythmias, temporary use in third degree A-V block until pacemaker insertion; low cardiac output or vasoconstrictive shock states

Usual Dosage

Children:

Bronchodilation: Inhalation 1-2 metered doses up to 5 times/day

Nebulization: 0.01 mL/kg; minimum dose: 0.1 mL; maximum dose: 0.5 mL diluted in 2-3 mL normal saline

I.V. infusion: 0.05-2 mcg/kg/minute; rate (mL/hour) = dose (mcg/kg/minute) x weight (kg) x 60 minutes/hour divided by concentration (mcg/mL)

Adults:

Bronchodilation: 1-2 inhalations 4-6 times/day

A-V nodal block: I.V. infusion: 2-20 mcg/minute

Dosage Forms Isoprenaline hydrochloride:

Inhalation:

Aerosol: 0.2% (1:500) (15 mL, 22.5 mL); 0.25% (1:400) (15 mL)

Solution for nebulization: 0.031% (4 mL); 0.062% (4 mL); 0.25% (0.5 mL, 30 mL); 0.5% (0.5 mL, 10 mL, 60 mL); 1% (10 mL)

Injection: 0.2 mg/mL (1:5000) (1 mL, 5 mL, 10 mL)

Tablet, sublingual: 10 mg, 15 mg

isoproterenol and phenylephrine (eye soe proe TER e nole & fen il EF rin)

Synonyms phenylephrine and isoproterenol

Therapeutic Category Adrenergic Agonist Agent

Use Treatment of bronchospasm associated with acute and chronic bronchial asthma, bronchitis, pulmonary emphysema, and bronchiectasis

Usual Dosage Daily maintenance: 1-2 inhalations 4-6 times/day, no more than 2 inhalations at any one time or more than 6 in any 1 hour within 24 hours

Dosage Forms Aerosol: Each actuation releases isoproterenol hydrochloride 0.16 mg and phenylephrine bitartrate 0.24 mg (15 mL, 22.5 mL)

Isoptin® *see* verapamil *on page 598*

Isoptin® SR *see* verapamil *on page 598*

Isopto® Atropine *see* atropine *on page 52*

Isopto® Carbachol Ophthalmic *see* carbachol *on page 97*

Isopto® Carpine Ophthalmic *see* pilocarpine *on page 451*

Isopto® Cetapred® Ophthalmic *see* sulfacetamide and prednisolone *on page 540*

Isopto® Frin Ophthalmic Solution *see* phenylephrine *on page 445*

Isopto® Homatropine Ophthalmic *see* homatropine *on page 282*

Isopto® Hyoscine *see* scopolamine *on page 516*

Isopto® P-ES *(Discontinued)* *see page 700*

Isopto® Plain Solution [OTC] *see* artificial tears *on page 47*

Isopto® Tears Solution [OTC] *see* artificial tears *on page 47*

Isordil® *see* isosorbide dinitrate *on this page*

isosorbide (eye soe SOR bide)

U.S./Canadian Brand Names Ismotic®

Therapeutic Category Diuretic, Osmotic

Use Short-term emergency treatment of acute angle-closure glaucoma

Usual Dosage Adults: Oral: Initial: 1.5 g/kg; usual range: 1-3 g/kg 2-4 times/day

Dosage Forms Solution: 45% [450 mg/mL] (220 mL)

isosorbide dinitrate (eye soe SOR bide dye NYE trate)

Synonyms ISD; ISDN

U.S./Canadian Brand Names Apo-ISDN® (Can); Cedocard-SR® (Can); Coradur® (Can); Dilatrate®-SR; Isordil®; Sorbitrate®

Therapeutic Category Vasodilator

Use Prevention and treatment of angina pectoris; for congestive heart failure; to relieve pain, dysphagia, and spasm in esophageal spasm with GE reflux

(Continued)

isosorbide dinitrate *(Continued)*

Usual Dosage Adults:

Oral: 5-30 mg 4 times/day or 40 mg every 6-12 hours in sustained-released dosage form
Chewable: 5-10 mg every 2-3 hours
Sublingual: 2.5-10 mg every 4-6 hours

Dosage Forms

Capsule, sustained release: 40 mg
Tablet:
Chewable: 5 mg, 10 mg
Oral: 5 mg, 10 mg, 20 mg, 30 mg
Sublingual: 2.5 mg, 5 mg, 10 mg
Sustained release: 40 mg

isosorbide mononitrate (eye soe SOR bide mon oh NYE trate)

Synonyms ISMN

U.S./Canadian Brand Names Imdur™; Ismo®; Monoket®

Therapeutic Category Vasodilator

Use Long-acting metabolite of the vasodilator isosorbide dinitrate used for the prophylactic treatment of angina pectoris

Usual Dosage Adults: Oral:

Regular tablet: 20 mg twice daily separated by 7 hours
Extended-release tablet: 30 mg (1/2 of 60 mg tablet) or 60 mg (administered as a single tablet) once daily; after several days the dosage may be increased to 120 mg (administered as two 60 mg tablets) once daily; the daily dose should be administered in the morning upon arising

Dosage Forms

Tablet: 10 mg, 20 mg
Ismo®, Monoket®: 10 mg, 20 mg
Tablet, extended release: 60 mg
Imdur™: 30 mg, 60 mg, 120 mg

isotretinoin (eye soe TRET i noyn)

Synonyms 13-*cis*-retinoic acid

U.S./Canadian Brand Names Accutane®; Isotrex® (Can)

Therapeutic Category Retinoic Acid Derivative

Use Treatment of severe recalcitrant cystic and/or conglobate acne unresponsive to conventional therapy

Investigational use: Treatment of children with metastatic neuroblastoma or leukemia that does not respond to conventional therapy

Usual Dosage Oral:

Children: Maintenance therapy for neuroblastoma: 100-250 mg/m^2/day in 2 divided doses has been used investigationally
Children and Adults: 0.5-2 mg/kg/day in 2 divided doses for 15-20 weeks

Dosage Forms Capsule: 10 mg, 20 mg, 40 mg

Isotrex® (Can) *see* isotretinoin *on this page*

Isovex® *(Discontinued)* *see page 700*

Isovue® *see* radiological/contrast media (non-ionic) *on page 496*

isoxsuprine (eye SOKS syoo preen)

U.S./Canadian Brand Names Vasodilan®

Therapeutic Category Vasodilator

Use Treatment of peripheral vascular diseases, such as arteriosclerosis obliterans and Raynaud's disease

Usual Dosage Adults: Oral: 10-20 mg 3-4 times/day

Dosage Forms Tablet, as hydrochloride: 10 mg, 20 mg

isradipine (iz RA di peen)

U.S./Canadian Brand Names DynaCirc®

Therapeutic Category Calcium Channel Blocker

Use Management of hypertension, alone or concurrently with thiazide-type diuretics

Usual Dosage Adults: Oral: Initial: 2.5 mg twice daily, if satisfactory response does not occur after 2-4 weeks the dose may be adjusted in increments of 5 mg/day at 2- to 4-week intervals up to a maximum of 20 mg/day

Dosage Forms Capsule: 2.5 mg, 5 mg

I-Sulfacet® *see* sulfacetamide *on page 540*

Isuprel® *see* isoproterenol *on page 314*

Isuprel® Glossets® ***(Discontinued)*** *see page 700*

Itch-X® [OTC] *see* pramoxine *on page 469*

itraconazole (i tra KOE na zole)

U.S./Canadian Brand Names Sporanox®

Therapeutic Category Antifungal Agent

Use Treatment of systemic fungal infections in immunocompromised and nonimmunocompromised patients including the treatment of susceptible blastomycosis, histoplasmosis, and aspergillosis in patients who do not respond to or cannot tolerate amphotericin B; it also has activity against *Cryptococcus*, *Coccidioides*, and sporotrichosis species; has also been used for prophylaxis against aspergillosis infection

Usual Dosage Adults: Oral: 200 mg once daily, if no obvious improvement or there is evidence of progressive fungal disease, increase the dose in 100 mg increments to a maximum of 400 mg/day; doses >200 mg/day are administered in 2 divided doses

Life-threatening: Loading dose: 200 mg administered 3 times/day (600 mg/day) should be administered for the first 3 days

Dosage Forms

Capsule: 100 mg

Solution, oral: 100 mg/10 mL (150 mL)

I-Tropine® *see* atropine *on page 52*

ivermectin (eye ver MEK tin)

U.S./Canadian Brand Names Stromectol®

Therapeutic Category Antibiotic, Miscellaneous

Use Treatment of the following infections: Strongyloidiasis of the intestinal tract due the nematode parasite *Strongyloides stercoralis*. Onchocerciasis due to the nematode parasite *Onchocerca volvulus*. Note: Ivermectin is ineffective against adult *Onchocerca volvulus* parasites because they reside in subcutaneous nodules which are infrequently palpable. Surgical excision of these nodules may be considered in the management of patients with onchocerciasis.

Usual Dosage Oral:

Children >5 years: 150 mcg/kg as a single dose once every 12 months

Adults: 150 mcg/kg as a single dose; may be repeated every 6-12 **months**

Dosage Forms Tablet: 6 mg

IVIG *see* immune globulin, intravenous *on page 303*

IvyBlock® *see* bentoquatam *on page 65*

Jaa Amp® (Can) *see* ampicillin *on page 34*

Jaa-Prednisone® (Can) *see* prednisone *on page 472*

Janimine® *see* imipramine *on page 302*

Japanese encephalitis virus vaccine, inactivated

(jap a NEESE en sef a LYE tis VYE rus vak SEEN, in ak ti VAY ted)

U.S./Canadian Brand Names JE-VAX®

Therapeutic Category Vaccine, Inactivated Virus

Use Active immunization against Japanese encephalitis for persons spending a month or longer in endemic areas, especially if travel will include rural areas

Usual Dosage S.C. (administered on days 0, 7, and 30):

Children 1-3 years: 3 doses of 0.5 mL; booster doses of 0.5 mL may administer 2 years after primary immunization series

Children >3 years and Adults: 3 doses of 1 mL; booster doses of 1 mL may be administered 2 years after primary immunization series

Dosage Forms Powder for injection, lyophilized: 1 mL, 10 mL

Jenamicin® *see* gentamicin *on page 260*

Jenest-28™ *see* ethinyl estradiol and norethindrone *on page 224*

JE-VAX® *see* Japanese encephalitis virus vaccine, inactivated *on this page*

Junior Strength Motrin® [OTC] *see* ibuprofen *on page 300*

Just Tears® Solution [OTC] *see* artificial tears *on page 47*

K+ 10® *see* potassium chloride *on page 464*

Kabikinase® *see* streptokinase *on page 535*

Kalcinate® *see* calcium gluconate *on page 92*

kanamycin (kan a MYE sin)

U.S./Canadian Brand Names Kantrex®

Therapeutic Category Aminoglycoside (Antibiotic)

Use

Oral: Preoperative bowel preparation in the prophylaxis of infections and adjunctive treatment of hepatic coma (oral kanamycin is not indicated in the treatment of systemic infections)

Parenteral: Initial therapy of severe infections where the strain is thought to be susceptible in patients allergic to other antibiotics, or in mixed staphylococcal or gram-negative infections

Usual Dosage

Children: Infections: I.M., I.V.: 15 mg/kg/day in divided doses every 8-12 hours

Adults:

Infections: I.M., I.V.: 15 mg/kg/day in divided doses every 8-12 hours

Preoperative intestinal antisepsis: Oral: 1 g every 4-6 hours for 36-72 hours

Dosage Forms Kanamycin sulfate:

Capsule: 500 mg

Injection:

Pediatrics: 75 mg (2 mL)

Adults: 500 mg (2 mL); 1 g (3 mL)

Kantrex® *see* kanamycin *on this page*

Kaochlor® *see* potassium chloride *on page 464*

Kaochlor-Eff® *see* potassium bicarbonate, potassium chloride, and potassium citrate *on page 463*

Kaochlor® SF *see* potassium chloride *on page 464*

Kaodene® [OTC] *see* kaolin and pectin *on this page*

kaolin and pectin (KAY oh lin & PEK tin)

Synonyms pectin and kaolin

U.S./Canadian Brand Names Donnagel®-MB (Can); Kaodene® [OTC]; Kao-Spen® [OTC]; Kapectolin® [OTC]

Therapeutic Category Antidiarrheal

Use Treatment of uncomplicated diarrhea

Usual Dosage Oral:

Children:

<6 years: Do not use

6-12 years: 30-60 mL after each loose stool

Adults: 60-120 mL after each loose stool

Dosage Forms Suspension, oral: Kaolin 975 mg and pectin 22 mg per 5 mL

kaolin and pectin with opium (KAY oh lin & PEK tin with OH pee um)

Synonyms pectin with opium and kaolin

U.S./Canadian Brand Names Parepectolin®

Therapeutic Category Antidiarrheal

Controlled Substance C-V

Use Symptomatic relief of diarrhea

Usual Dosage Oral:

Children:

3-6 years: 7.5 mL with each loose bowel movement, not to exceed 30 mL in 12 hours

6-12 years: 5-10 mL with each loose bowel movement, not to exceed 40 mL in 12 hours

Children >12 years and Adults: 15-30 mL with each loose bowel movement, not to exceed 120 mL in 12 hours

Dosage Forms Suspension, oral: Kaolin 5.5 g, pectin 162 mg, and opium 15 mg per 30 mL [3.7 mL paregoric] (240 mL)

Kaon® *see* potassium gluconate *on page 465*

Kaon-Cl® *see* potassium chloride *on page 464*

Kaon-Cl-10® *see* potassium chloride *on page 464*

Kaopectate® Advanced Formula [OTC] *see* attapulgite *on page 53*

Kaopectate® Children's Tablet *(Discontinued)* *see page 700*

Kaopectate® II [OTC] *see* loperamide *on page 339*

Kaopectate® Maximum Strength Caplets *see* attapulgite *on page 53*

Kao-Spen® [OTC] *see* kaolin and pectin *on previous page*

Kapectolin® [OTC] *see* kaolin and pectin *on previous page*

Kapectolin PG® *see* hyoscyamine, atropine, scopolamine, kaolin, pectin, and opium *on page 299*

Karidium® *see* fluoride *on page 244*

Karigel® *see* fluoride *on page 244*

Karigel®-N *see* fluoride *on page 244*

Kasof® [OTC] *see* docusate *on page 191*

Kato® Powder *(Discontinued)* *see page 700*

Kaybovite-1000® *see* cyanocobalamin *on page 152*

Kay Ciel® *see* potassium chloride *on page 464*

Kayexalate® *see* sodium polystyrene sulfonate *on page 530*

K+ Care® *see* potassium chloride *on page 464*

K+ Care® Effervescent *see* potassium bicarbonate *on page 462*

KCl *see* potassium chloride *on page 464*

K-Dur® 10 *see* potassium chloride *on page 464*

K-Dur® 20 *see* potassium chloride *on page 464*

Keflex® *see* cephalexin *on page 111*

Keflin® *(Discontinued)* *see page 700*

Keftab® *see* cephalexin *on page 111*

Kefurox® Injection *see* cefuroxime *on page 109*

Kefzol® *see* cefazolin *on page 105*

K-Electrolyte® Effervescent *see* potassium bicarbonate *on page 462*

Kemadrin® *see* procyclidine *on page 477*

Kenacort® Oral *see* triamcinolone (systemic) *on page 577*

Kenaject® Injection *see* triamcinolone (systemic) *on page 577*

Kenalog® Injection *see* triamcinolone (systemic) *on page 577*

Kenalog® in Orabase® *see* triamcinolone (topical) *on page 578*

Kenalog® Topical *see* triamcinolone (topical) *on page 578*

Kenonel® Topical *see* triamcinolone (topical) *on page 578*

Keralyt® Gel *see* salicylic acid and propylene glycol *on page 514*

Kerlone® Oral *see* betaxolol *on page 73*

Kestrin® Injection *(Discontinued)* *see page 700*

Kestrone® *see* estrone *on page 220*

Ketalar® *see* ketamine *on this page*

ketamine (KEET a meen)

U.S./Canadian Brand Names Ketalar®

Therapeutic Category General Anesthetic

Controlled Substance C-III

Use Anesthesia, short surgical procedures, dressing changes

Usual Dosage

Children:

I.M.: 3-7 mg/kg

I.V.: Range: 0.5-2 mg/kg, use smaller doses (0.5-1 mg/kg) for sedation for minor procedures; usual induction dosage: 1-2 mg/kg

Adults:

I.M.: 3-8 mg/kg

I.V.: Range: 1-4.5 mg/kg; usual induction dosage: 1-2 mg/kg

Children and Adults: Maintenance: Supplemental doses of 1/3 to 1/2 of initial dose

Dosage Forms Injection, as hydrochloride: 10 mg/mL (20 mL, 25 mL, 50 mL); 50 mg/mL (10 mL); 100 mg/mL (5 mL)

ketoconazole (kee toe KOE na zole)

U.S./Canadian Brand Names Nizoral®

Therapeutic Category Antifungal Agent

Use Treatment of susceptible fungal infections, including candidiasis, oral thrush, blastomycosis, histoplasmosis, coccidioidomycosis, paracoccidioidomycosis, chronic mucocutaneous candidiasis, as well as certain recalcitrant cutaneous dermatophytoses; used topically for treatment of tinea corporis, tinea cruris, tinea versicolor, and cutaneous candidiasis; shampoo is used for dandruff

Usual Dosage

Children: Oral: 5-10 mg/kg/day divided every 12-24 hours until lesions clear

Adults:

Oral: 200-400 mg/day as a single daily dose

Topical: Rub gently into the affected area once daily to twice daily for two weeks

Dosage Forms

Cream: 2% (15 g, 30 g, 60 g)

Shampoo: 2% (120 mL)

Tablet: 200 mg

ketoprofen (kee toe PROE fen)

U.S./Canadian Brand Names Actron® [OTC]; Apo-Keto-E® (Can); Novo-Keto-EC (Can); Nu-Ketoprofen (Can); Nu-Ketoprofen-E (Can); Orudis®; Orudis® KT [OTC]; Oruvail®; PMS-Ketoprofen (Can); Rhodis® (Can); Rhodis-EC® (Can)

Therapeutic Category Analgesic, Non-narcotic; Nonsteroidal Anti-inflammatory Drug (NSAID)

Use Acute or long-term treatment of rheumatoid arthritis and osteoarthritis; primary dysmenorrhea; mild to moderate pain

Usual Dosage Oral:

Children 3 months to 14 years: Fever: 0.5-1 mg/kg

Children >12 years and Adults:

Rheumatoid arthritis or osteoarthritis: 50-75 mg 3-4 times/day up to a maximum of 300 mg/day

Mild to moderate pain: 25-50 mg every 6-8 hours up to a maximum of 300 mg/day

Dosage Forms

Capsule (Orudis®): 25 mg, 50 mg, 75 mg

Actron®, Orudis® KT [OTC]: 12.5 mg

Capsule, extended release: 100 mg, 150 mg, 200 mg

Oruvail®: 100 mg, 200 mg

ketorolac tromethamine (KEE toe role ak troe METH a meen)

U.S./Canadian Brand Names Acular® Ophthalmic; Toradol®

Therapeutic Category Analgesic, Non-narcotic; Nonsteroidal Anti-inflammatory Drug (NSAID)

Use

Oral, I.M., I.V.,: Short-term (≤5 days) management of moderate to severe pain, including postoperative pain, visceral pain associated with cancer, pain associated with trauma, acute renal colic

Ophthalmic: Ocular itch associated with seasonal allergic conjunctivitis

Usual Dosage Adults (pain relief usually begins within 10 minutes with parenteral forms):

Oral: 10 mg every 4-6 hours as needed for a maximum of 40 mg/day; on day of transition from I.M. to oral: maximum oral dose: 40 mg (or 120 mg combined oral and I.M.); maximum 5 days administration

I.M.: Initial: 30-60 mg, then 15-30 mg every 6 hours as needed for up to 5 days maximum; maximum dose in the first 24 hours: 150 mg with 120 mg/24 hours for up to 5 days total

I.V.: Initial: 30 mg, then 15-30 mg every 6 hours as needed for up to 5 days **maximum**; maximum daily dose: 120 mg for up to 5 days total

Ophthalmic: Instill 1 drop in eye(s) 4 times/day

Dosage Forms

Injection: 15 mg/mL (1 mL); 30 mg/mL (1 mL, 2 mL)

Solution, ophthalmic: 0.5% (5 mL)

Tablet: 10 mg

ketotifen (kee toe TYE fen)

U.S./Canadian Brand Names Zaditor™

Therapeutic Category Antihistamine, H_1 Blocker, Ophthalmic

Use Temporary prevention of eye itching due to allergic conjunctivitis

Usual Dosage Adults: Ophthalmic: Instill 1 drop in the affected eye(s) every 8-12 hours

Dosage Forms Solution, ophthalmic: 0.025% (5 mL)

Kevadon® *see* thalidomide *on page 557*

Key-Pred® Injection *see* prednisolone (systemic) *on page 471*

Key-Pred-SP® Injection *see* prednisolone (systemic) *on page 471*

K-G® *see* potassium gluconate *on page 465*

K-Gen® Effervescent *see* potassium bicarbonate *on page 462*

KI *see* potassium iodide *on page 466*

K-Ide® *see* potassium bicarbonate and potassium citrate, effervescent *on page 463*

Kidrolase® (Can) *see* asparaginase *on page 49*

Kinevac® *see* sincalide *on page 523*

Kionex® *see* sodium polystyrene sulfonate *on page 530*

Klean-Prep® (Can) *see* polyethylene glycol-electrolyte solution *on page 459*

K-Lease® *see* potassium chloride *on page 464*

Klerist-D® Tablet [OTC] *see* chlorpheniramine and pseudoephedrine *on page 122*

Klonopin™ *see* clonazepam *on page 138*

K-Lor™ *see* potassium chloride *on page 464*

Klor-Con® *see* potassium chloride *on page 464*

Klor-Con® 8 *see* potassium chloride *on page 464*

Klor-Con® 10 *see* potassium chloride *on page 464*

Klor-Con®/25 *see* potassium chloride *on page 464*

Klor-con®/EF *see* potassium bicarbonate and potassium citrate, effervescent *on page 463*

Klorominr® Oral [OTC] *see* chlorpheniramine *on page 120*

Klorvess® *see* potassium chloride *on page 464*

Klorvess® Effervescent *see* potassium bicarbonate and potassium chloride, effervescent *on page 463*

Klotrix® *see* potassium chloride *on page 464*

K-Lyte® *see* potassium bicarbonate and potassium citrate, effervescent *on page 463*

K/Lyte/CL® *see* potassium bicarbonate and potassium chloride, effervescent *on page 463*

K-Lyte®/Cl *see* potassium chloride *on page 464*

K-Lyte® Effervescent *see* potassium bicarbonate *on page 462*

K-Norm® *see* potassium chloride *on page 464*

Koāte®-HP *see* antihemophilic factor (human) *on page 39*

Koate®-HS Injection *(Discontinued)* *see page 700*

Koate®-HT Injection *(Discontinued)* *see page 700*

Koffex® DM, -DM Children (Can) *see* dextromethorphan *on page 171*

Kogenate® *see* antihemophilic factor (recombinant) *on page 40*

Kolephrin® GG/DM [OTC] *see* guaifenesin and dextromethorphan *on page 268*

Kolyum® Powder *(Discontinued)* *see page 700*

Konakion® Injection *see* phytonadione *on page 451*

Kondon's Nasal® [OTC] *see* ephedrine *on page 208*

Konsyl® [OTC] *see* psyllium *on page 488*

Konsyl-D® [OTC] *see* psyllium *on page 488*

Konȳne® 80 *see* factor IX complex (human) *on page 230*

Konyne-HT® Injection *(Discontinued)* *see page 700*

Koromex® [OTC] *see* nonoxynol 9 *on page 406*

K-Phos® Neutral *see* potassium phosphate and sodium phosphate *on page 467*

K-Phos® Original *see* potassium acid phosphate *on page 462*

Kristalose® *see* lactulose *on page 325*

K-Tab® *see* potassium chloride *on page 464*

Ku-Zyme® HP *see* pancrelipase *on page 427*

K-Vescent® *see* potassium bicarbonate and potassium citrate, effervescent *on page 463*

Kwelcof® *see* hydrocodone and guaifenesin *on page 288*

Kwellada™ (Can) *see* lindane *on page 335*

Kwell® ***(Discontinued)*** *see page 700*

Kytril™ *see* granisetron *on page 266*

***L*-3-hydroxytyrosine** *see* levodopa *on page 331*

LA-12® *see* hydroxocobalamin *on page 294*

labetalol (la BET a lole)

Synonyms ibidomide

U.S./Canadian Brand Names Normodyne®; Trandate®

Therapeutic Category Alpha-/Beta- Adrenergic Blocker

Use Treatment of mild to severe hypertension; I.V. for hypertensive emergencies

Usual Dosage

Children: Limited information regarding labetalol use in pediatric patients is currently available in literature. Some centers recommend initial oral doses of 4 mg/kg/day in 2 divided doses. Reported oral doses have started at 3 mg/kg/day and 20 mg/kg/day and have increased up to 40 mg/kg/day.

I.V., intermittent bolus doses of 0.3-1 mg/kg/dose have been reported

For treatment of pediatric hypertensive emergencies, initial continuous infusions of 0.4-1 mg/kg/hour with a maximum of 3 mg/kg/hour have been used.

Due to limited documentation of its use, labetalol should be initiated cautiously in pediatric patients with careful dosage adjustment and blood pressure monitoring

Adults:

Oral: Initial: 100 mg twice daily, may increase as needed every 2-3 days by 100 mg until desired response is obtained; usual dose: 200-400 mg twice daily; not to exceed 2.4 g/day

I.V.: 20 mg or 1-2 mg/kg whichever is lower, IVP over 2 minutes, may administer 40-80 mg at 10-minute intervals, up to 300 mg total dose

I.V. infusion: Initial: 2 mg/minute; titrate to response

Dosage Forms Labetalol hydrochloride:

Injection: 5 mg/mL (20 mL, 40 mL, 60 mL)

Tablet: 100 mg, 200 mg, 300 mg

Lac-Hydrin® *see* lactic acid with ammonium hydroxide *on next page*

Lacril® Ophthalmic Solution [OTC] *see* artificial tears *on page 47*

Lacrisert® *see* hydroxypropyl cellulose *on page 296*

LactAid® [OTC] *see* lactase *on this page*

lactase (LAK tase)

U.S./Canadian Brand Names Dairy Ease® [OTC]; LactAid® [OTC]; Lactrase® [OTC]

Therapeutic Category Nutritional Supplement

Use Help digest lactose in milk for patients with lactose intolerance

Usual Dosage Oral:

Capsule: 1-2 capsules administered with milk or meal; pretreat milk with 1-2 capsules per quart of milk

Liquid: 5-15 drops per quart of milk

Tablet: 1-3 tablets with meals

Dosage Forms

Caplet: 3000 FCC lactase units

Capsule: 250 mg

Liquid: 1250 neutral lactase units/5 drops

(Continued)

lactase *(Continued)*

Tablet, chewable: 3300 FCC lactase units

lactic acid and salicylic acid *see* salicylic acid and lactic acid *on page 513*

lactic acid and sodium-PCA (LAK tik AS id & SOW dee um-pee see aye)

Synonyms sodium-pca and lactic acid

U.S./Canadian Brand Names LactiCare® [OTC]

Therapeutic Category Topical Skin Product

Use Lubricate and moisturize the skin counteracting dryness and itching

Usual Dosage Topical: Apply as needed

Dosage Forms Lotion, topical: Lactic acid 5% and sodium-PCA 2.5% (240 mL)

lactic acid with ammonium hydroxide

(LAK tik AS id with a MOE nee um hye DROKS ide)

Synonyms ammonium lactate

U.S./Canadian Brand Names Lac-Hydrin®

Therapeutic Category Topical Skin Product

Use Treatment of moderate to severe xerosis and ichthyosis vulgaris

Usual Dosage Topical: Shake well; apply to affected areas, use twice daily, rub in well

Dosage Forms Lotion: Lactic acid 12% with ammonium hydroxide (150 mL)

LactiCare® [OTC] *see* lactic acid and sodium-PCA *on this page*

LactiCare-HC® Topical *see* hydrocortisone (topical) *on page 292*

Lactinex® [OTC] *see* Lactobacillus *on this page*

Lactobacillus (lak toe ba SIL us)

Synonyms *Lactobacillus acidophilus*; *Lactobacillus acidophilus* and *Lactobacillus bulgaricus*

U.S./Canadian Brand Names Bacid® [OTC]; Fermalac® (Can); Lactinex® [OTC]; MoreDophilus® [OTC]

Therapeutic Category Gastrointestinal Agent, Miscellaneous

Use Uncomplicated diarrhea particularly that caused by antibiotic therapy; re-establish normal physiologic and bacterial flora of the intestinal tract

Usual Dosage Children >3 years and Adults: Oral:

Capsules: 2 capsules 2-4 times/day

Granules: 1 packet added to or taken with cereal, food, milk, fruit juice, or water, 3-4 times/day

Powder: $^1/_4$-1 teaspoonful 1-3 times/daily with liquid

Tablet, chewable: 4 tablets 3-4 times/day; may follow each dose with a small amount of milk, fruit juice, or water

Dosage Forms

Capsule:

Bacid®: *Lactobacillus acidophilus* cultured strain ≥500 million viable (50s, 100s)

Pro-Bionate®: *Lactobacillus acidophilus* strain NAS 2 billion units/g

Granules (Lactinex®): *Lactobacillus acidophilus* and *Lactobacillus bulgaricus* mixed culture (1 g/packet-12s)

Powder:

MoreDophilus®: Acidophilus-carrot derivative 4 billion units/g

Pro-Bionate®: *Lactobacillus acidophilus* strain NAS 2 billion units/g

Tablet, chewable (Lactinex®): *Lactobacillus acidophilus* and *Lactobacillus bulgaricus* mixed culture (50s)

Lactobacillus acidophilus *see* Lactobacillus *on this page*

Lactobacillus acidophilus* and *Lactobacillus bulgaricus *see* Lactobacillus *on this page*

lactoflavin *see* riboflavin *on page 504*

Lactrase® [OTC] *see* lactase *on page 323*

Lactulax (Can) *see* lactulose *on this page*

lactulose (LAK tyoo lose)

U.S./Canadian Brand Names Acilac (Can); Cephulac®; Cholac®; Chronulac®; Comalose-R (Can); Constilac®; Constulose®; Duphalac®; Enulose®; Evalose®; Gen-Lac (Can); Heptalac®; Kristalose®; Lactulax (Can); Lactulose PSE®; Laxilose (Can); PMS-Lactulose (Can)

Therapeutic Category Ammonium Detoxicant; Laxative

Use Adjunct in the prevention and treatment of portal-systemic encephalopathy (PSE); treatment of chronic constipation

Usual Dosage Oral:

Infants: 2.5-10 mL/day divided 3-4 times/day

Children: 40-90 mL/day divided 3-4 times/day

Adults:

Acute episodes of portal systemic encephalopathy: 30-45 mL at 1- to 2-hour intervals until laxative effect observed

Chronic therapy: 30-45 mL/dose 3-4 times/day; titrate dose to produce 2-3 soft stools per day

Rectal: 300 mL diluted with 700 mL of water or normal saline, and administered via a rectal balloon catheter and retained for 30-60 minutes; may administer every 4-6 hours

Dosage Forms Syrup: 10 g/15 mL (15 mL, 30 mL, 237 mL, 473 mL, 946 mL, 1890 mL)

Lactulose PSE® *see* lactulose *on this page*

ladakamycin *see* azacitidine *on page 55*

L-AmB *see* amphotericin B (liposomal) *on page 34*

Lamictal® *see* lamotrigine *on this page*

Lamisil® Cream *see* terbinafine, topical *on page 550*

Lamisil® Oral *see* terbinafine, oral *on page 550*

lamivudine (la MI vyoo deen)

Synonyms 3TC

U.S./Canadian Brand Names Epivir®; Epivir®-HBV™; 3TC® (Can)

Therapeutic Category Antiviral Agent

Use

Epivir®: In combination with zidovudine for treatment of HIV infection when therapy is warranted based on clinical and/or immunological evidence of disease progression

Epivir®-HBV™: Treatment of chronic hepatitis B associated with evidence of hepatitis B viral replication and active liver inflammation

Usual Dosage Oral:

Hepatitis B virus (HBV): 100 mg once daily

HIV:

Adolescents 12-16 years and Adults: 150 mg twice daily with zidovudine

Adults <50 kg: 2 mg/kg twice daily with zidovudine

Dosage Forms

Solution, oral: 10 mg/mL (240 mL)

Tablet: 150 mg

lamotrigine (la MOE tri jeen)

Synonyms LTG

U.S./Canadian Brand Names Lamictal®

Therapeutic Category Anticonvulsant

Use Adjunctive treatment of partial seizures, with or without secondary generalized seizures; investigations for absence, generalized tonic-clonic, atypical absence, myoclonic seizures, and Lennox-Gastaut syndrome are in progress

(Continued)

lamotrigine *(Continued)*

Usual Dosage Oral:

Initial dose: 50-100 mg/day then titrate to daily maintenance dose of 100-400 mg/day in 1-2 divided daily doses

With concomitant valproic acid therapy: Start initial dose at 25 mg/day then titrate to maintenance dose of 50-200 mg/day in 1-2 divided daily doses

Dosage Forms Tablet: 25 mg, 100 mg, 150 mg, 200 mg

Lamprene® *see* clofazimine *on page 137*

Lamprene® 100 mg *(Discontinued)* *see page 700*

Lanacane® [OTC] *see* benzocaine *on page 66*

Lanacort® Topical [OTC] *see* hydrocortisone (topical) *on page 292*

Lanaphilic® Topical [OTC] *see* urea *on page 591*

Laniazid® Syrup *see* isoniazid *on page 314*

Laniazid® Tablet *(Discontinued)* *see page 700*

lanolin, cetyl alcohol, glycerin, and petrolatum

(LAN oh lin, SEE til AL koe hol, GLIS er in, & pe troe LAY tum)

U.S./Canadian Brand Names Lubriderm® [OTC]

Therapeutic Category Topical Skin Product

Use Treatment of dry skin

Usual Dosage Topical: Apply to skin as necessary

Dosage Forms Lotion: 480 mL

Lanorinal® *see* butalbital compound and aspirin *on page 85*

Lanoxicaps® *see* digoxin *on page 179*

Lanoxin® *see* digoxin *on page 179*

lansoprazole (lan SOE pra zole)

U.S./Canadian Brand Names Prevacid®

Therapeutic Category Gastric Acid Secretion Inhibitor

Use Short-term treatment (up to 4 weeks) for healing and symptom relief of active duodenal ulcers (should not be used for maintenance therapy of duodenal ulcers); up to 8 weeks of treatment for all grades of erosive esophagitis (8 additional weeks can be given for incompletely healed esophageal erosions or for recurrence); and long-term treatment of pathological hypersecretory conditions, including Zollinger-Ellison syndrome

Usual Dosage

Duodenal or gastric ulcer:

Treatment: 15 mg once daily for 4 weeks

Maintenance (healed): 15 mg once daily

Erosive esophagitis:

Treatment: 30 mg once daily for up to 8 weeks; may give for additional 8 weeks for patients who do not heal with the first 8 weeks; if recurrence or erosive esophagitis, consider an additional 8-week course

Maintenance (healing): 15 mg once daily

Hypersecretory conditions: 30-180 mg once daily, titrated to reduce acid secretion to <10 mEq/hour (5 mEq/hour in patients with prior gastric surgery)

Dosage Forms Capsule, delayed release: 15 mg, 30 mg

Lanvis® (Can) *see* thioguanine *on page 561*

Largactil® (Can) *see* chlorpromazine *on page 127*

Lariam® *see* mefloquine *on page 353*

Larodopa® *see* levodopa *on page 331*

Lasan® HP-1 Topical *(Discontinued)* *see page 700*

Lasan® Topical *(Discontinued)* *see page 700*

Lasix® *see* furosemide *on page 255*

Lasix® Special (Can) *see* furosemide *on page 255*

Lassar's zinc paste *see* zinc oxide *on page 612*

latanoprost (la TAN oh prost)

U.S./Canadian Brand Names Xalatan®

Therapeutic Category Prostaglandin

Use Prostaglandin analog to reduce intraocular pressure that occurs in patients with glaucoma who cannot tolerate or have not responded to any other available treatments

Usual Dosage Ophthalmic:

Children: Not recommended

Adults: 1 drop in affected eye(s) once daily in the evening

Dosage Forms Solution, ophthalmic: 0.005% (2.5 mL)

***Latrodectus mactans* antivenin** *see* antivenin (*Latrodectus mactans*) *on page 42*

Lavacol® [OTC] *see* alcohol, ethyl *on page 16*

Laxilose (Can) *see* lactulose *on page 325*

***l*-bunolol** *see* levobunolol *on page 330*

***l*-carnitine** *see* levocarnitine *on page 330*

LCD *see* coal tar *on page 141*

LCR *see* vincristine *on page 600*

***l*-deprenyl** *see* selegiline *on page 518*

***l*-dopa** *see* levodopa *on page 331*

Lectopam® (Can) *see* bromazepam *(Canada only) on page 79*

Ledercillin VK® *(Discontinued)* *see page 700*

Lederplex® [OTC] *see* vitamin B complex *on page 603*

leflunomide (le FLU no mide)

U.S./Canadian Brand Names Arava™

Therapeutic Category Anti-inflammatory Agent

Use Treatment of active rheumatoid arthritis to reduce signs and symptoms and to retard structural damage as evidenced by X-ray erosions and joint space narrowing

Usual Dosage Oral:

Adults: Initial: 100 mg/day for 3 days, followed by 20 mg/day; dosage may be decreased to 10 mg/day in patients who have difficulty tolerating the 20 mg dose. Due to the long half-life of the active metabolite, plasma levels may require a prolonged period to decline after dosage reduction.

Guidelines for dosage adjustment or discontinuation based on the severity and persistence of ALT elevation have been developed. For ALT elevations >2 times the upper limit of normal, dosage reduction to 10 mg/day may allow continued administration. Cholestyramine 8 g 3 times/day for 1-3 days may be administered to decrease plasma levels. If elevations >2 times but less than or equal to 3 times the upper limit of normal persist, liver biopsy is recommended. If elevations >3 times the upper limit of normal persist despite cholestyramine administration and dosage reduction, leflunomide should be discontinued and drug elimination should be enhanced with additional cholestyramine as indicated.

Elderly: Although hepatic function may decline with age, no specific dosage adjustment is recommended; patients should be monitored closely for adverse effects which may require dosage adjustment

Dosage Forms Tablet: 10 mg, 20 mg, 100 mg

Lenoltec® No.1, 2, 3, 4 (Can) *see* acetaminophen and codeine *on page 4*

Lente® *see* insulin preparations *on page 307*

Lente® Iletin® I *see* insulin preparations *on page 307*

Lente® Iletin® II *see* insulin preparations *on page 307*

lepirudin (leh puh ROO din)

U.S./Canadian Brand Names Refludan®

Therapeutic Category Anticoagulant

Use Indicated for anticoagulation in patient with heparin-induced thrombocytopenia (HIT) and associated thromboembolic disease in order to prevent further thromboembolic complications

Usual Dosage Maximum dose: Do not exceed 0.21 mg/kg/hour unless an evaluation of coagulation abnormalities limiting response has been completed; dosing is weight-based, however patients weighing >110 kg should not receive doses greater than the recommended dose for a patient weighing 110 kg (44 mg bolus and initial maximal infusion rate of 16.5 mg/hour)

Use in patients with heparin-induced thrombocytopenia: Bolus dose: 0.4 mg/kg IVP (over 15-20 seconds), followed by continuous infusion at 0.15 mg/kg/hour; bolus and infusion must be reduced in renal insufficiency

Concomitant use with thrombolytic therapy: Bolus dose: 0.2 mg/kg IVP (over 15-20 seconds), followed by continuous infusion at 0.1 mg/kg/hour

Dosing adjustments during infusions: Monitor first APTT 4 hours after the start of the infusion; subsequent determinations of APTT should be obtained at least once daily during treatment; more frequent monitoring is recommended in renally impaired patients; any APTT out of range should be confirmed prior to adjusting dose, unless a clinical need for immediate reaction exists; if the APTT is below target range, increase infusion by 20%; if the APTT is in excess of the target range, decrease infusion rate by 50%; a repeat APTT should be obtained 4 hours after any dosing change

Dosage Forms Injection: 50 mg

Lescol® *see* fluvastatin *on page 250*

letrozole (LET roe zole)

U.S./Canadian Brand Names Femara™

Therapeutic Category Antineoplastic Agent, Hormone (Antiestrogen)

Use Treatment of advanced breast cancer in postmenopausal women with disease progression following tamoxifen therapy. Patients with ER-negative disease and patients who did not respond to tamoxifen therapy rarely responded to anastrozole.

Usual Dosage Adults: Oral: 2.5 mg once/day, without regard to meals

Dosage Forms Tablet: 2.5 mg

leucovorin (loo koe VOR in)

Synonyms citrovorum factor; folinic acid; 5-formyl tetrahydrofolate

U.S./Canadian Brand Names Wellcovorin®

Therapeutic Category Folic Acid Derivative

Use Antidote for folic acid antagonists; treatment of folate deficient megaloblastic anemias of infancy, sprue, pregnancy; nutritional deficiency when oral folate therapy is not possible

Usual Dosage Children and Adults:

Adjunctive therapy with antimicrobial agents (pyrimethamine): Oral: 2-15 mg/day for 3 days or until blood counts are normal or 5 mg every 3 days; doses of 6 mg/day are needed for patients with platelet counts <100,000/mm^3

Folate-deficient megaloblastic anemia: I.M.: 1 mg/day

Megaloblastic anemia secondary to congenital deficiency of dihydrofolate reductase: I.M.: 3-6 mg/day

Rescue dose: I.V.: 10 mg/m^2 to start, then 10 mg/m^2 every 6 hours orally for 72 hours; if serum creatinine 24 hours after methotrexate is elevated 50% or more **or** the serum

MTX concentration is >5 x 10^{-6}M, increase dose to 100 mg/m^2/dose every 3 hours until serum methotrexate level is less than 1 x 10^{-8}M

Dosage Forms Leucovorin calcium:
- Injection: 3 mg/mL (1 mL)
- Powder for injection: 25 mg, 50 mg, 100 mg, 350 mg
- Powder for oral solution: 1 mg/mL (60 mL)
- Tablet: 5 mg, 10 mg, 15 mg, 25 mg

Leukeran® *see* chlorambucil *on page 115*

Leukine™ *see* sargramostim *on page 515*

leuprolide acetate (loo PROE lide AS e tate)

U.S./Canadian Brand Names Lupron®; Lupron Depot®; Lupron Depot-3® Month; Lupron Depot-4® Month; Lupron Depot-Ped®

Therapeutic Category Antineoplastic Agent; Luteinizing Hormone-Releasing Hormone Analog

Use Treatment of precocious puberty; palliative treatment of advanced prostate carcinoma

Usual Dosage
- Children: S.C.: Precocious puberty: 20-45 mcg/kg/day
- Adults:
  - Advanced prostatic carcinoma:
    - S.C.: 1 mg/day **or**
    - I.M. (suspension): 7.5 mg/dose administered monthly
  - Endometriosis: ≥18 years: I.M.: 3.75 mg/month for 6 months

Dosage Forms Leuprolide acetate:
- Injection: 5 mg/mL (2.8 mL)
- Powder for injection (depot):
  - Depot®: 3.75 mg, 7.5 mg
  - Depot-3® Month: 11.25 mg, 22.5 mg
  - Depot-Ped™: 7.5 mg, 11.25 mg, 15 mg

leurocristine *see* vincristine *on page 600*

Leustatin™ *see* cladribine *on page 134*

levalbuterol (leve al BYOO ter ole)

Synonyms R-albuterol

U.S./Canadian Brand Names Xopenex™

Therapeutic Category Adrenergic Agonist Agent; Beta$_2$-Adrenergic Agonist Agent; Bronchodilator

Use Treatment or prevention of bronchospasm in adults and adolescents 12 years of age and older with reversible obstructive airway disease.

Usual Dosage
- Pediatric: Safety and efficacy in patients <12 years of age not established.
- Children >12 years and Adults: Inhalation: 0.63 mg 3 times/day at intervals of 6-8 hours, via nebulization. Dosage may be increased to 1.25 mg 3 times/day with close monitoring for adverse effects. Most patients gain optimal benefit from regular use
- Elderly: Only a small number of patients have been studied. Although greater sensitivity of some elderly patients cannot be ruled out, no overall differences in safety or effectiveness were observed. An initial dose of 0.63 mg should be used in all patients >65 years of age.

Dosage Forms Solution, inhalation: 0.63 mg/3 mL, 1.25 mg/3 mL

levamisole (lee VAM i sole)

U.S./Canadian Brand Names Ergamisol®

Therapeutic Category Immune Modulator

Use Adjuvant treatment with fluorouracil in Dukes stage C colon cancer

Usual Dosage Oral: Initial: 50 mg every 8 hours for 3 days, then 50 mg every 8 hours for 3 days every 2 weeks (fluorouracil is always administered concomitantly)

(Continued)

levamisole *(Continued)*

Dosage Forms Tablet, as base: 50 mg

Levaquin™ *see* levofloxacin *on next page*

Levate® (Can) *see* amitriptyline *on page 28*

Levatol® *see* penbutolol *on page 432*

Levbid® *see* hyoscyamine *on page 297*

Levlen® *see* ethinyl estradiol and levonorgestrel *on page 223*

Levlite® *see* ethinyl estradiol and levonorgestrel *on page 223*

levobunolol (lee voe BYOO noe lole)

Synonyms *l*-bunolol

U.S./Canadian Brand Names AKBeta® Ophthalmic; Betagan® Liquifilm® Ophthalmic; Optho-Bunolol® (Can)

Therapeutic Category Beta-Adrenergic Blocker

Use To lower intraocular pressure in chronic open-angle glaucoma or ocular hypertension

Usual Dosage Adults: Ophthalmic: 1-2 drops of 0.5% solution in eye(s) once daily or 1-2 drops of 0.25% solution twice daily

Dosage Forms Solution, ophthalmic, as hydrochloride: 0.25% (5 mL, 10 mL, 15 mL); 0.5% (2 mL, 5 mL, 10 mL, 15 mL)

levobupivacaine (LEE voe byoo PIV a kane)

U.S./Canadian Brand Names Chirocaine®

Therapeutic Category Local Anesthetic, Injectable

Use Production of local or regional anesthesia for surgery and obstetrics, and for postoperative pain management

Usual Dosage Adults: **Note:** Rapid injection of a large volume of local anesthetic solution should be avoided. Fractional (incremental) doses are recommended.

Maximum dosage: Epidural doses up to 375 mg have been administered incrementally to patients during a surgical procedure

Intraoperative block and postoperative pain: 695 mg in 24 hours

Postoperative epidural infusion over 24 hours: 570 mg

Single-fractionated injection for brachial plexus block: 300 mg

Dosage Forms Injection: 2.5 mg/mL (10 mL, 30 mL); 5 mg/mL (10 mL, 30 mL); 7.5 mg/mL (10 mL, 30 mL)

levocabastine (LEE voe kab as teen)

U.S./Canadian Brand Names Livostin®

Therapeutic Category Antihistamine

Use Temporary relief of the signs and symptoms of seasonal allergic conjunctivitis

Usual Dosage Adults: Ophthalmic: Instill 1 drop in affected eye 4 times/day for up to 2 weeks

Dosage Forms Suspension, ophthalmic, as hydrochloride: 0.05% (2.5 mL, 5 mL, 10 mL)

levocarnitine (lee voe KAR ni teen)

Synonyms *l*-carnitine

U.S./Canadian Brand Names Carnitor® Injection; Carnitor® Oral; VitaCarn® Oral

Therapeutic Category Dietary Supplement

Use Treatment of primary or secondary carnitine deficiency

Usual Dosage Oral:

Children: 50-100 mg/kg/day divided 2-3 times/day, maximum: 3 g/day; dosage must be individualized based upon patient response; higher dosages have been used

Adults: 1-3 g/day for 50 kg subject; start at 1 g/day, increase slowly assessing tolerance and response

Dosage Forms

Capsule: 250 mg

Injection: 1 g/5 mL (5 mL)
Liquid (cherry flavor): 100 mg/mL (10 mL)
Tablet: 330 mg

levodopa (lee voe DOE pa)

Synonyms *L*-3-hydroxytyrosine; *l*-dopa
U.S./Canadian Brand Names Dopar®; Larodopa®
Therapeutic Category Diagnostic Agent; Dopaminergic Agent (Anti-Parkinson's)
Use Diagnostic agent for growth hormone deficiency
Usual Dosage Children: Oral (administered as a single dose to evaluate growth hormone deficiency): 0.5 g/m^2

or

<30 lbs: 125 mg
30-70 lbs: 250 mg
>70 lbs: 500 mg

Dosage Forms
Capsule: 100 mg, 250 mg, 500 mg
Tablet: 100 mg, 250 mg, 500 mg

levodopa and carbidopa (lee voe DOE pa & kar bi DOE pa)

Synonyms carbidopa and levodopa
U.S./Canadian Brand Names Sinemet®
Therapeutic Category Anti-Parkinson's Agent; Dopaminergic Agent (Anti-Parkinson's)
Use Treatment of Parkinsonian syndrome
Usual Dosage Adults: Oral (carbidopa/levodopa): 75/300 to 150/1500 mg/day in 3-4 divided doses; can increase up to 200/2000 mg/day
Dosage Forms Tablet:
10/100: Carbidopa 10 mg and levodopa 100 mg
25/100: Carbidopa 25 mg and levodopa 100 mg
25/250: Carbidopa 25 mg and levodopa 250 mg
Sustained release: Carbidopa 25 mg and levodopa 100 mg; carbidopa 50 mg and levodopa 200 mg

Levo-Dromoran® *see* levorphanol *on next page*

levofloxacin (lee voe FLOKS a sin)

U.S./Canadian Brand Names Levaquin™
Therapeutic Category Quinolone
Use Treatment of bacterial respiratory tract infections
Usual Dosage Adults: Oral, I.V.: 500 mg every 24 hours for at least 7 days (dose and duration varies with indication); at least 2 hours before or 2 hours after antacids containing magnesium or aluminum
Dosage Forms
Infusion, in D_5W: 5 mg/mL (50 mL, 100 mL)
Injection: 25 mg/mL (20 mL)
Tablet: 250 mg, 500 mg

levomepromazine *see* methotrimeprazine *on page 364*

levomethadyl acetate hydrochloride

(lee voe METH a dil AS e tate hye droe KLOR ide)

U.S./Canadian Brand Names ORLAAM®
Therapeutic Category Analgesic, Narcotic
Controlled Substance C-II
Use Management of opiate dependence
Usual Dosage Adults: Oral: 20-40 mg 3 times/week; range: 10 mg to as high as 140 mg 3 times/week
Dosage Forms Solution, oral: 10 mg/mL (474 mL)

levonorgestrel (LEE voe nor jes trel)

U.S./Canadian Brand Names Norplant® Implant

Therapeutic Category Contraceptive, Implant (Progestin); Contraceptive, Progestin Only

Use Prevention of pregnancy

Usual Dosage Each Norplant® silastic capsule releases 80 mcg of drug/day for 6-18 months, following which a rate of release of 25-30 mcg/day is maintained for ≤5 years

Dosage Forms Capsule, subdermal implantation: 36 mg (6s)

levonorgestrel and ethinyl estradiol *see* ethinyl estradiol and levonorgestrel *on page 223*

Levophed® *see* norepinephrine *on page 406*

Levoprome® *see* methotrimeprazine *on page 364*

Levora® *see* ethinyl estradiol and levonorgestrel *on page 223*

levorphanol (lee VOR fa nole)

U.S./Canadian Brand Names Levo-Dromoran®

Therapeutic Category Analgesic, Narcotic

Controlled Substance C-II

Use Relief of moderate to severe pain; also used parenterally for preoperative sedation and an adjunct to nitrous oxide/oxygen anesthesia

Usual Dosage Adults: Oral, S.C.: 2 mg, up to 3 mg if necessary

Dosage Forms Levorphanol tartrate:

Injection: 2 mg/mL (1 mL, 10 mL)

Tablet: 2 mg

Levo-T™ *see* levothyroxine *on this page*

Levothroid® *see* levothyroxine *on this page*

levothyroxine (lee voe thye ROKS een)

Synonyms *l*-thyroxine; t_4 thyroxine

U.S./Canadian Brand Names Eltroxin®; Levo-T™; Levothroid®; Levoxyl®; PMS-Levothyroxine Sodium (Can); Synthroid®

Therapeutic Category Thyroid Product

Use Replacement or supplemental therapy in hypothyroidism; management of nontoxic goiter, chronic lymphocytic thyroiditis, as an adjunct to thyrotoxicosis

Usual Dosage

Children:

- Oral:
  - 0-6 months: 8-10 mcg/kg/day
  - 6-12 months: 6-8 mcg/kg/day
  - 1-5 years: 5-6 mcg/kg/day
  - 6-12 years: 4-5 mcg/kg/day
  - >12 years: 2-3 mcg/kg/day
- I.M., I.V.: 75% of the oral dose

Adults:

- Oral: 12.5-50 mcg/day to start, then increase by 25-50 mcg/day at intervals of 2-4 weeks; average adult dose: 100-200 mcg/day
- I.M., I.V.: 50% of the oral dose

Myxedema coma or stupor: I.V.: 200-500 mcg one time, then 100-300 mcg the next day if necessary

Dosage Forms

Powder for injection, as sodium, lyophilized: 200 mcg/vial (6 mL, 10 mL); 500 mcg/vial (6 mL, 10 mL)

Tablet, as sodium: 25 mcg, 50 mcg, 75 mcg, 88 mcg, 100 mcg, 112 mcg, 125 mcg, 137 mcg, 150 mcg, 175 mcg, 200 mcg, 300 mcg

Levoxyl® *see* levothyroxine *on previous page*

Levsin® *see* hyoscyamine *on page 297*

Levsinex® *see* hyoscyamine *on page 297*

Levsin/SL® *see* hyoscyamine *on page 297*

levulose, dextrose and phosphoric acid *see* phosphorated carbohydrate solution *on page 450*

Lexxel™ *see* enalapril and felodipine *on page 206*

LHRH *see* gonadorelin *on page 265*

***l*-hyoscyamine sulfate** *see* hyoscyamine *on page 297*

Librax® *see* clidinium and chlordiazepoxide *on page 136*

Libritabs® *see* chlordiazepoxide *on page 116*

Libritabs® 5 mg *(Discontinued)* *see page 700*

Librium® *see* chlordiazepoxide *on page 116*

Lice-Enz® Shampoo [OTC] *see* pyrethrins *on page 489*

Lida-Mantle HC® Topical *see* lidocaine and hydrocortisone *on next page*

Lidemol® (Can) *see* fluocinolone *on page 243*

Lidex® *see* fluocinonide *on page 243*

Lidex-E® *see* fluocinonide *on page 243*

lidocaine (LYE doe kane)

Synonyms lignocaine

U.S./Canadian Brand Names Anestacon® Topical Solution; Dilocaine® Injection; Duo-Trach® Injection; Lidodan® (Can); LidoPen® I.M. Injection Auto-Injector; Nervocaine® Injection; PMS-Lidocaine Viscous (Can); Solarcaine® Topical; Xylocaine® HCl I.V. Injection for Cardiac Arrhythmias; Xylocaine® Oral; Xylocaine® Topical Ointment; Xylocaine® Topical Solution; Xylocaine® Topical Spray; Xylocard® (Can)

Therapeutic Category Analgesic, Topical; Antiarrhythmic Agent, Class I-B; Local Anesthetic

Use Drug of choice for ventricular ectopy, ventricular tachycardia (VT), ventricular fibrillation (VF); for pulseless VT or VF preferably administer **after** defibrillation and epinephrine; control of premature ventricular contractions, wide-complex PSVT; local anesthetic

Usual Dosage

Topical: Apply to affected area as needed; maximum: 3 mg/kg/dose; do not repeat within 2 hours

Injectable local anesthetic: Varies with procedure, degree of anesthesia needed, vascularity of tissue, duration of anesthesia required, and physical condition of patient; maximum: 4.5 mg/kg/dose; do not repeat within 2 hours

Children: Endotracheal, I.O., I.V.: Loading dose: 1 mg/kg; may repeat in 10-15 minutes to a maximum total dose of 5 mg/kg; after loading dose, start I.V. continuous infusion 20-50 mcg/kg/minute. Use 20 mcg/kg/minute in patients with shock, hepatic disease, mild congestive heart failure (CHF); moderate to severe CHF may require 1/2 loading dose and lower infusion rates to avoid toxicity. Endotracheal doses should be diluted to 1-2 mL with normal saline prior to endotracheal administration and may need 2-3 times the I.V. dose.

Adults: Antiarrhythmic:

Endotracheal: Total dose: 5 mg/kg; follow with 0.5 mg/kg in 10 minutes if effective

I.M.: 300 mg may be repeated in 1-1 1/2 hours

I.V.: Loading dose: 1 mg/kg/dose, then 50-100 mg bolus over 2-3 minutes; may repeat in 5-10 minutes up to 200-300 mg in a 1-hour period; continuous infusion of 20-50 mcg/kg/minute or 1-4 mg/minute; decrease the dose in patients with CHF, shock, or hepatic disease

Dosage Forms Lidocaine hydrochloride:

Cream: 2% (56 g)

(Continued)

lidocaine *(Continued)*

Injection: 0.5% [5 mg/mL] (50 mL); 1% [10 mg/mL] (2 mL, 5 mL, 10 mL, 20 mL, 30 mL, 50 mL); 1.5% [15 mg/mL] (20 mL); 2% [20 mg/mL] (2 mL, 5 mL, 10 mL, 20 mL, 30 mL, 50 mL); 4% [40 mg/mL] (5 mL); 10% [100 mg/mL] (10 mL); 20% [200 mg/mL] (10 mL, 20 mL)

Injection:

I.M. use: 10% [100 mg/mL] (3 mL, 5 mL)

Direct I.V.: 1% [10 mg/mL] (5 mL, 10 mL); 20 mg/mL (5 mL)

I.V. admixture, preservative free: 4% [40 mg/mL] (25 mL, 30 mL); 10% [100 mg/mL] (10 mL); 20% [200 mg/mL] (5 mL, 10 mL)

I.V. infusion, in D_5W: 0.2% [2 mg/mL] (500 mL); 0.4% [4 mg/mL] (250 mL, 500 mL, 1000 mL); 0.8% [8 mg/mL] (250 mL, 500 mL)

Gel, topical: 2% (30 mL); 2.5% (15 mL)

Liquid:

Topical: 2.5% (7.5 mL)

Viscous: 2% (20 mL, 100 mL)

Ointment, topical: 2.5% [OTC], 5% (35 g)

Solution, topical: 2% (15 mL, 240 mL); 4% (50 mL)

lidocaine and epinephrine (LYE doe kane & ep i NEF rin)

Synonyms epinephrine and lidocaine

U.S./Canadian Brand Names Octocaine®; Xylocaine® With Epinephrine

Therapeutic Category Local Anesthetic

Use Local infiltration anesthesia

Usual Dosage Children (dosage varies with the anesthetic procedure): Use lidocaine concentrations of 0.5% or 1% (or even more dilute) to decrease possibility of toxicity; lidocaine dose should not exceed 4.5 mg/kg/dose; do not repeat within 2 hours

Dosage Forms Injection with epinephrine:

Epinephrine 1:200,000: Lidocaine hydrochloride 0.5% [5 mg/mL] (50 mL); 1% [10 mg/mL] (30 mL); 1.5% [15 mg/mL] (5 mL, 10 mL, 30 mL); 2% [20 mg/mL] (20 mL)

Epinephrine 1:100,000: Lidocaine hydrochloride 1% [10 mg/mL] (20 mL, 50 mL); 2% [20 mg/mL] (1.8 mL, 20 mL, 50 mL)

Epinephrine 1:50,000: Lidocaine hydrochloride 2% [20 mg/mL] (1.8 mL)

lidocaine and hydrocortisone (LYE doe kane & hye droe KOR ti sone)

Synonyms hydrocortisone and lidocaine

U.S./Canadian Brand Names Lida-Mantle HC® Topical

Therapeutic Category Anesthetic/Corticosteroid

Use Topical anti-inflammatory and anesthetic for skin disorders

Usual Dosage Topical: Apply 2-4 times/day

Dosage Forms Cream: Lidocaine 3% and hydrocortisone 0.5% (15 g, 30 g)

lidocaine and prilocaine (LYE doe kane & PRIL oh kane)

Synonyms prilocaine and lidocaine

U.S./Canadian Brand Names EMLA®

Therapeutic Category Analgesic, Topical

Use Topical anesthetic for use on normal intact skin to provide local analgesia for minor procedures such as I.V. cannulation or venipuncture; has also been used for painful procedures such as lumbar puncture and skin graft harvesting

Usual Dosage Children and Adults: Topical: Apply a thick layer of cream to intact skin and cover with an occlusive dressing; for minor procedures, apply 2.5 g/site for at least 60 minutes; for painful procedures, apply 2 g/10 cm^2 of skin and leave on for at least 2 hours

Dosage Forms Cream: Lidocaine 2.5% and prilocaine 2.5% [2 Tegaderm® dressings] (5 g, 30 g)

Lidodan® (Can) *see* lidocaine *on previous page*

LidoPen® I.M. Injection Auto-Injector *see* lidocaine *on page 333*

lignocaine *see* lidocaine *on page 333*

Limbitrol® DS 10-25 *see* amitriptyline and chlordiazepoxide *on page 29*

Lincocin® *see* lincomycin *on this page*

lincomycin (lin koe MYE sin)

U.S./Canadian Brand Names Lincocin®; Lincorex® Injection

Therapeutic Category Macrolide (Antibiotic)

Use Treatment of susceptible bacterial infections, mainly those caused by streptococci and staphylococci

Usual Dosage

Children >1 month:
- Oral: 30-60 mg/kg/day in 3-4 divided doses
- I.M.: 10 mg/kg every 12-24 hours
- I.V.: 10-20 mg/kg/day in divided doses 2-3 times/day

Adults:
- Oral: 500 mg every 6-8 hours
- I.M.: 600 mg every 12-24 hours
- I.V.: 600-1 g every 8-12 hours up to 8 g/day

Dosage Forms Lincomycin hydrochloride:

Capsule: 250 mg, 500 mg
Injection: 300 mg/mL (2 mL, 10 mL)

Lincorex® Injection *see* lincomycin *on this page*

Linctus Codeine Blac (Can) *see* codeine *on page 143*

Linctus With Codeine Phosphate (Can) *see* codeine *on page 143*

lindane (LIN dane)

Synonyms benzene hexachloride; gamma benzene hexachloride; hexachlorocyclohexane

U.S./Canadian Brand Names G-well®; Hexit® (Can); Kwellada™ (Can); PMS-Lindane (Can)

Therapeutic Category Scabicides/Pediculicides

Use Treatment of scabies (*Sarcoptes scabiei*), *Pediculus capitis* (head lice), and *Pediculus pubis* (crab lice)

Usual Dosage Children and Adults: Topical:

Scabies: Apply a thin layer of lotion and massage it on skin from the neck to the toes. For adults, bathe and remove the drug after 8-12 hours; for children, wash off 6 hours after application.

Pediculosis: 15-30 mL of shampoo is applied and lathered for 4-5 minutes; rinse hair thoroughly and comb with a fine tooth comb to remove nits; repeat treatment in 7 days if lice or nits are still present

Dosage Forms

Cream: 1% (60 g, 454 g)
Lotion: 1% (60 mL, 473 mL, 4000 mL)
Shampoo: 1% (60 mL, 473 mL, 4000 mL)

Lioresal® *see* baclofen *on page 59*

liothyronine (lye oh THYE roe neen)

Synonyms *l*-triiodothyronine; t_3 thyronine

U.S./Canadian Brand Names Cytomel® Oral; Triostat™ Injection

Therapeutic Category Thyroid Product

Use Replacement or supplemental therapy in hypothyroidism, management of nontoxic goiter, chronic lymphocytic thyroiditis, as an adjunct in thyrotoxicosis and as a diagnostic aid; levothyroxine is recommended for chronic therapy; (if rapid correction of thyroid is needed, T_3 is preferred, but use cautiously and with lower recommended doses)

(Continued)

liothyronine *(Continued)*

Usual Dosage

Mild hypothyroidism: 25 mcg/day; daily dosage may then be increased by 12.5 or 25 mcg/day every 1 or 2 weeks; maintenance: 25-75 mcg/day

Myxedema: 5mcg/day; may be increased by 5-10 mcg/day every 1-2 weeks; when 25 mcg is reached, dosage may often be increased by 12.5 or 25 mcg every 1 or 2 weeks; maintenance: 50-100 mcg/day

Cretinism: 5 mcg/day with a 5 mcg increment every 3-4 days until the desired response is achieved

Simple (nontoxic) goiter: 5 mcg/day; may be increased every week or two by 5 or 10 mcg; when 25 mcg/day is reached, dosage may be increased every week or two by 12.5 or 25 mcg; maintenance: 75 mcg/day

T_3 suppression test: I^{131} thyroid uptake is in the borderline-high range, administer 75-100 mcg/day for 7 days then repeat I^{131} thyroid uptake test

Children and Elderly: Start therapy with 5 mcg/day; increase only by 5 mcg increments at the recommended intervals

Dosage Forms Liothyronine sodium:

Injection: 10 mcg/mL (1 mL)

Tablet: 5 mcg, 25 mcg, 50 mcg

liotrix (LYE oh triks)

Synonyms t_3/t_4 liotrix

U.S./Canadian Brand Names Thyrolar®

Therapeutic Category Thyroid Product

Use Replacement or supplemental therapy in hypothyroidism

Usual Dosage Congenital hypothyroidism: Oral:

Children (dose/day):
- 0-6 months: 8-10 mcg/kg
- 6-12 months: 6-8 mcg/kg
- 1-5 years: 5-6 mcg/kg
- 6-12 years: 4-5 mcg/kg
- >12 years: 2-3 mcg/kg

Adults: 30 mg/day, increasing by 15 mg/day at 2- to 3-week intervals to a maximum of 180 mg/day

Dosage Forms Tablet: 30 mg, 60 mg, 120 mg, 180 mg [thyroid equivalent]

lipancreatin *see* pancrelipase *on page 427*

lipase, protease, and amylase *see* pancrelipase *on page 427*

Lipitor® *see* atorvastatin *on page 51*

Liposyn® *see* fat emulsion *on page 231*

Lipovite® [OTC] *see* vitamin B complex *on page 603*

Liquaemin® *see* heparin *on page 278*

Liquibid® *see* guaifenesin *on page 267*

Liqui-Char® [OTC] *see* charcoal *on page 114*

liquid antidote *see* charcoal *on page 114*

Liquid Barosperse® *see* radiological/contrast media (ionic) *on page 495*

Liquid Pred® *see* prednisone *on page 472*

Liqui-E® *see* tocophersolan *on page 570*

Liquifilm® Forte Solution [OTC] *see* artificial tears *on page 47*

Liquifilm® Tears Solution [OTC] *see* artificial tears *on page 47*

Liquipake® *see* radiological/contrast media (ionic) *on page 495*

Liquiprin® [OTC] *see* acetaminophen *on page 3*

lisinopril (lyse IN oh pril)

U.S./Canadian Brand Names Prinivil®; Zestril®

Therapeutic Category Angiotensin-Converting Enzyme (ACE) Inhibitor

Use Treatment of hypertension, either alone or in combination with other antihypertensive agents

Usual Dosage Adults: Oral: 10-40 mg/day in a single dose

Dosage Forms Tablet: 2.5 mg, 5 mg, 10 mg, 20 mg, 40 mg

lisinopril and hydrochlorothiazide

(lyse IN oh pril & hye droe klor oh THYE a zide)

Synonyms hydrochlorothiazide and lisinopril

U.S./Canadian Brand Names Prinzide®; Zestoretic®

Therapeutic Category Antihypertensive Agent, Combination

Use Treatment of hypertension

Usual Dosage Adults: Oral: Dosage is individualized; see each component for appropriate dosing suggestions

Dosage Forms Tablet:

Lisinopril 10 mg and hydrochlorothiazide 12.5 mg
[12.5]-Lisinopril 20 mg and hydrochlorothiazide 12.5 mg
[25]-Lisinopril 20 mg and hydrochlorothiazide 25 mg

Listerex® Scrub *(Discontinued)* *see page 700*

Listermint® with Fluoride [OTC] *see* fluoride *on page 244*

Lithane® *see* lithium *on this page*

lithium (LITH ee um)

U.S./Canadian Brand Names Carbolith™ (Can); Duralith® (Can); Eskalith®; Lithane®; Lithobid®; Lithonate®; Lithotabs®

Therapeutic Category Antimanic Agent

Use Management of acute manic episodes, bipolar disorders, and depression

Usual Dosage Oral: Monitor serum concentrations and clinical response (efficacy and toxicity) to determine proper dose

Children: 15-60 mg/kg/day in 3-4 divided doses; dose not to exceed usual adult dosage
Adults: 300 mg 3-4 times/day; usual maximum maintenance dose: 2.4 g/day

Dosage Forms

Lithium carbonate:
- Capsule: 150 mg, 300 mg, 600 mg
- Tablet: 300 mg
- Tablet, controlled release: 450 mg (Eskalith CR®)
- Tablet, slow release: 300 mg (Lithobid®)

Lithium citrate:
- Syrup: 300 mg/5 mL (5 mL, 10 mL, 480 mL)

Lithobid® *see* lithium *on this page*

Lithonate® *see* lithium *on this page*

Lithostat® *see* acetohydroxamic acid *on page 8*

Lithotabs® *see* lithium *on this page*

Livostin® *see* levocabastine *on page 330*

LKV-Drops® [OTC] *see* vitamin, multiple (pediatric) *on page 606*

l-lysine (el LYE seen)

U.S./Canadian Brand Names Enisyl® [OTC]; Lycolan® Elixir [OTC]

Therapeutic Category Dietary Supplement

Use Improves utilization of vegetable proteins

Usual Dosage Adults: Oral: 334-1500 mg/day

(Continued)

l-lysine *(Continued)*

Dosage Forms *l*-lysine hydrochloride:
Capsule: 500 mg
Elixir: 100 mg/15 mL with glycine 1800 mg/15 mL and alcohol 12%
Tablet: 312 mg, 334 mg, 500 mg, 1000 mg

8-*l*-lysine vasopressin *see* lypressin *on page 343*

LMD® *see* dextran *on page 170*

LoCHOLEST® *see* cholestyramine resin *on page 129*

LoCHOLEST® Light *see* cholestyramine resin *on page 129*

Locoid® Topical *see* hydrocortisone (topical) *on page 292*

Lodine® *see* etodolac *on page 227*

Lodine® XL *see* etodolac *on page 227*

Lodosyn® *see* carbidopa *on page 99*

lodoxamide tromethamine (loe DOKS a mide troe METH a meen)

U.S./Canadian Brand Names Alomide® Ophthalmic
Therapeutic Category Mast Cell Stabilizer
Use Symptomatic treatment of vernal keratoconjunctivitis, vernal conjunctivitis, and vernal keratitis
Usual Dosage Children >2 years and Adults: Ophthalmic: Instill 1-2 drops in eye(s) 4 times/day for up to 3 months
Dosage Forms Solution, ophthalmic: 0.1% (10 mL)

Loestrin® *see* ethinyl estradiol and norethindrone *on page 224*

Logen® *see* diphenoxylate and atropine *on page 186*

Lomanate® *see* diphenoxylate and atropine *on page 186*

lomefloxacin (loe me FLOKS a sin)

U.S./Canadian Brand Names Maxaquin®
Therapeutic Category Quinolone
Use Quinolone antibiotic for skin and skin structure, lower respiratory and urinary tract infections, and sexually transmitted diseases
Usual Dosage Adults: Oral: 400 mg once daily for 10-14 days
Dosage Forms Tablet, as hydrochloride: 400 mg

Lomicin® Ophthalmic (Can) *see* gentamicin *on page 260*

Lomotil® *see* diphenoxylate and atropine *on page 186*

lomustine (loe MUS teen)

Synonyms CCNU
U.S./Canadian Brand Names CeeNU®
Therapeutic Category Antineoplastic Agent
Use Treatment of brain tumors, Hodgkin's and non-Hodgkin's lymphomas, melanoma, renal carcinoma, lung cancer, colon cancer
Usual Dosage Oral (refer to individual protocol):
Children: 75-150 mg/m^2 as a single dose every 6 weeks. Subsequent doses are readjusted after initial treatment according to platelet and leukocyte counts
Adults: 100-130 mg/m^2 as a single dose every 6 weeks; readjust after initial treatment according to platelet and leukocyte counts
Dosage Forms
Capsule: 10 mg, 40 mg, 100 mg
Dose Pack: 10 mg (2s); 100 mg (2s); 40 mg (2s)

Loniten® Oral *see* minoxidil *on page 377*

Lonox® *see* diphenoxylate and atropine *on page 186*

Lo/Ovral® *see* ethinyl estradiol and norgestrel *on page 225*

loperamide (loe PER a mide)

U.S./Canadian Brand Names Diar-aid® [OTC]; Imodium®; Imodium® A-D [OTC]; Imodium® Advanced; Kaopectate® II [OTC]; Pepto® Diarrhea Control [OTC]; PMS-Loperamine (Can)

Therapeutic Category Antidiarrheal

Use Treatment of acute diarrhea and chronic diarrhea associated with inflammatory bowel disease; chronic functional diarrhea (idiopathic), chronic diarrhea caused by bowel resection or organic lesions; to decrease the volume of ileostomy discharge

Usual Dosage Oral:

Children:

Acute diarrhea: 0.4-0.8 mg/kg/day divided every 6-12 hours, maximum: 2 mg/dose

Chronic diarrhea: 0.08-0.24 mg/kg/day divided 2-3 times/day, maximum: 2 mg/dose

Adults: Initial: 4 mg (2 capsules), followed by 2 mg after each loose stool, up to 16 mg/day (8 capsules)

Dosage Forms Loperamide hydrochloride:

Caplet: 2 mg

Capsule: 2 mg

Liquid, oral: 1 mg/5 mL (60 mL, 90 mL, 120 mL)

Tablet: 2 mg

Lopid® *see* gemfibrozil *on page 259*

lopremone *see* protirelin *on page 485*

Lopressor® *see* metoprolol *on page 371*

Loprox® *see* ciclopirox *on page 130*

Lorabid™ *see* loracarbef *on this page*

loracarbef (lor a KAR bef)

U.S./Canadian Brand Names Lorabid™

Therapeutic Category Antibiotic, Carbacephem

Use Treatment of mild to moderate community-acquired infections of the respiratory tract, skin and skin structure, and urinary tract that are caused by susceptible *S. pneumoniae*, *H. influenzae*, *B. catarrhalis*, *S. aureus*, and *E. coli*

Usual Dosage Oral:

Acute otitis media: Children: 15 mg/kg twice a day for 10 days

Urinary tract infections: Women: 200 mg once a day for 7 days

Dosage Forms

Capsule: 200 mg, 400 mg

Suspension, oral: 100 mg/5 mL (50 mL, 100 mL); 200 mg/5 mL (50 mL, 100 mL)

loratadine (lor AT a deen)

U.S./Canadian Brand Names Claritin®; Claritin® RediTab®

Therapeutic Category Antihistamine

Use Perennial and seasonal allergic rhinitis and other allergic symptoms including urticaria

Usual Dosage Adults: Oral: 10 mg/day on an empty stomach

Dosage Forms

Solution, oral: 1 mg/mL

Tablet: 10 mg

Rapid-disintegrating tablets: 10 mg (RediTabs®)

loratadine and pseudoephedrine (lor AT a deen & soo doe e FED rin)

Synonyms pseudoephedrine and loratadine

U.S./Canadian Brand Names Claritin-D®; Claritin-D® 24-Hour

Therapeutic Category Antihistamine/Decongestant Combination

(Continued)

loratadine and pseudoephedrine *(Continued)*

Use Temporary relief of symptoms of seasonal and perennial allergic rhinitis, and vasomotor rhinitis, including nasal obstruction

Usual Dosage Adults: Oral: 1 tablet every 12 hours

Dosage Forms

Tablet: Loratadine 5 mg and pseudoephedrine sulfate 120 mg

Tablet, extended release: Loratadine 10 mg and pseudoephedrine sulfate 240 mg

lorazepam (lor A ze pam)

U.S./Canadian Brand Names Apo®-Lorazepam (Can); Ativan®; Novo-Lorazepam® (Can); Nu-Loraz® (Can); PMS-Lorazepam (Can); Pro-Lorazepam® (Can)

Therapeutic Category Benzodiazepine

Controlled Substance C-IV

Use Management of anxiety; status epilepticus; preoperative sedation and amnesia

Usual Dosage

Anxiety and sedation:

Infants and Children: Oral, I.V.: Usual: 0.05 mg/kg/dose (range: 0.02-0.09 mg/kg) every 4-8 hours

Adults: Oral: 1-10 mg/day in 2-3 divided doses; usual dose: 2-6 mg/day in divided doses

Insomnia: Adults: Oral: 2-4 mg at bedtime

Preoperative: Adults:

I.M.: 0.05 mg/kg administered 2 hours before surgery; maximum: 4 mg/dose

I.V.: 0.044 mg/kg 15-20 minutes before surgery; usual maximum: 2 mg/dose

Operative amnesia: Adults: I.V.: up to 0.05 mg/kg; maximum: 4 mg/dose

Status epilepticus: I.V.:

Infants and Children: 0.1 mg/kg slow I.V. over 2-5 minutes, do not exceed 4 mg/single dose; may repeat second dose of 0.05 mg/kg slow I.V. in 10-15 minutes if needed

Adolescents: 0.07 mg/kg slow I.V. over 2-5 minutes; maximum: 4 mg/dose; may repeat in 10-15 minutes

Adults: 4 mg/dose administered slowly over 2-5 minutes; may repeat in 10-15 minutes; usual maximum dose: 8 mg

Dosage Forms

Injection: 2 mg/mL (1 mL, 10 mL); 4 mg/mL (1 mL, 10 mL)

Solution, oral concentrated, alcohol and dye free: 2 mg/mL (30 mL)

Tablet: 0.5 mg, 1 mg, 2 mg

Lorcet® 10/650 *see* hydrocodone and acetaminophen *on page 287*

Lorcet® *(Discontinued)* *see page 700*

Lorcet®-HD *see* hydrocodone and acetaminophen *on page 287*

Lorcet® Plus *see* hydrocodone and acetaminophen *on page 287*

Lorelco® *(Discontinued)* *see page 700*

Loroxide® [OTC] *see* benzoyl peroxide *on page 68*

Lortab® *see* hydrocodone and acetaminophen *on page 287*

Lortab® ASA *see* hydrocodone and aspirin *on page 288*

losartan (loe SAR tan)

Synonyms DuP 753; MK594

U.S./Canadian Brand Names Cozaar®

Therapeutic Category Angiotensin II Antagonist

Use Treatment of hypertension alone or in combination with other antihypertensives; in considering the use of monotherapy with Cozaar®, it should be noted that in controlled trials Cozaar® had an effect on blood pressure that was notably less in black patients than in nonblacks, a finding similar to the small effect of ACE inhibitors in blacks

Usual Dosage Adults: Oral: Initial: 50 mg once daily, with 25 mg used in patients with possible depletion of intravascular volume (eg, patients treated with diuretics) and patients with a history of hepatic impairment; can be administered once or twice daily with total daily doses ranging from 25-100 mg; if the antihypertensive effect measured at trough using once daily dosing is inadequate, a twice daily regimen at the same total daily dose or an increase in dose may give a more satisfactory response; if blood pressure is not controlled by Cozaar® alone, a low dose of a diuretic may be added; hydrochlorothiazide has been shown to have an additive effect

Dosage Forms Tablet, film coated, as potassium: 25 mg, 50 mg

losartan and hydrochlorothiazide

(loe SAR tan & hye droe klor oh THYE a zide)

Synonyms hydrochlorothiazide and losartan

U.S./Canadian Brand Names Hyzaar®

Therapeutic Category Antihypertensive Agent, Combination

Use Treatment of hypertension

Usual Dosage Adults: Oral: 1 tablet daily

Dosage Forms Tablet: Losartan potassium 50 mg and hydrochlorothiazide 12.5 mg

Losec® (Can) *see* omeprazole *on page 415*

Lotemax® *see* loteprednol *on this page*

Lotensin® *see* benazepril *on page 64*

Lotensin® HCT *see* benazepril and hydrochlorothiazide *on page 64*

loteprednol (loe te PRED nol)

U.S./Canadian Brand Names Alrex™; Lotemax®

Therapeutic Category Corticosteroid, Ophthalmic

Use Temporary relief of signs and symptoms of seasonal allergic conjunctivitis

Usual Dosage Adults: Ophthalmic: Instill 1 drop in eye(s) 4 times/day

Dosage Forms Suspension, ophthalmic, as etabonate: 0.2% (2.5 mL, 5 mL, 10 mL)

Lotrel® *see* amlodipine and benazepril *on page 29*

Lotrimin® AF Powder [OTC] *see* miconazole *on page 373*

Lotrimin® AF Spray Liquid [OTC] *see* miconazole *on page 373*

Lotrimin® AF Spray Powder [OTC] *see* miconazole *on page 373*

Lotrimin AF® Topical [OTC] *see* clotrimazole *on page 140*

Lotrimin® Topical *see* clotrimazole *on page 140*

Lotrisone® *see* betamethasone and clotrimazole *on page 71*

lovastatin (LOE va sta tin)

Synonyms mevinolin; monacolin k

U.S./Canadian Brand Names Mevacor®

Therapeutic Category HMG-CoA Reductase Inhibitor

Use Adjunct to dietary therapy to decrease elevated serum total and LDL cholesterol concentrations in primary hypercholesterolemia

Usual Dosage Adults: Oral: Initial: 20 mg with evening meal, then adjust at 4-week intervals; maximum dose: 80 mg/day

Dosage Forms Tablet: 10 mg, 20 mg, 40 mg

Lovenox® *see* enoxaparin *on page 207*

Loxapac® (Can) *see* loxapine *on this page*

loxapine (LOKS a peen)

Synonyms oxilapine

U.S./Canadian Brand Names Loxapac® (Can); Loxitane®

Therapeutic Category Antipsychotic Agent, Dibenzoxazepine

Use Management of psychotic disorders

(Continued)

loxapine *(Continued)*

Usual Dosage Adults:

Oral: 10 mg twice daily, increase dose until psychotic symptoms are controlled; usual dose range: 60-100 mg/day in divided doses 2-4 times/day; dosages >250 mg/day are not recommended

I.M.: 12.5-50 mg every 4-6 hours or longer as needed and change to oral therapy as soon as possible

Dosage Forms

Loxapine hydrochloride:

Concentrate, oral: 25 mg/mL (120 mL dropper bottle)

Injection: 50 mg/mL (1 mL)

Loxapine succinate:

Capsule: 5 mg, 10 mg, 25 mg, 50 mg

Loxitane® *see* loxapine *on previous page*

Lozide® (Can) *see* indapamide *on page 304*

Lozi-Tab® *see* fluoride *on page 244*

Lozol® *see* indapamide *on page 304*

l-PAM *see* melphalan *on page 354*

LRH *see* gonadorelin *on page 265*

l-sarcolysin *see* melphalan *on page 354*

LTG *see* lamotrigine *on page 325*

l-thyroxine *see* levothyroxine *on page 332*

l-triiodothyronine *see* liothyronine *on page 335*

Lubriderm® [OTC] *see* lanolin, cetyl alcohol, glycerin, and petrolatum *on page 326*

LubriTears® Solution [OTC] *see* artificial tears *on page 47*

Ludiomil® *see* maprotiline *on page 348*

Lufyllin® *see* dyphylline *on page 201*

Lugol's solution *see* potassium iodide *on page 466*

Luminal® *see* phenobarbital *on page 443*

Lupron® *see* leuprolide acetate *on page 329*

Lupron Depot® *see* leuprolide acetate *on page 329*

Lupron Depot-3® Month *see* leuprolide acetate *on page 329*

Lupron Depot-4® Month *see* leuprolide acetate *on page 329*

Lupron Depot-Ped® *see* leuprolide acetate *on page 329*

Luride® *see* fluoride *on page 244*

Luride®-SF *see* fluoride *on page 244*

luteinizing hormone-releasing hormone *see* gonadorelin *on page 265*

Lutrepulse® *see* gonadorelin *on page 265*

Luvox® *see* fluvoxamine *on page 250*

LY170053 *see* olanzapine *on page 414*

Lycolan® Elixir [OTC] *see* l-lysine *on page 337*

Lyderm® (Can) *see* fluocinonide *on page 243*

Lyme disease vaccine (LIME dee seas vak SEEN)

U.S./Canadian Brand Names LYMErix®

Therapeutic Category Vaccine

Use Active immunization against Lyme disease in individuals between 15-70 years of age

Usual Dosage Adults: I.M.: Vaccination with three doses of 30 mcg (0.5 mL), administered at 0, 1 and 12 months, is recommended for optimal protection

Dosage Forms Injection:

Vial: 30 mcg/0.5 mL

Prefilled syringe (Tip-Lok™): 30 mcg/0.5 mL

LYMErix® *see* Lyme disease vaccine *on previous page*

Lymphazurin® *see* radiological/contrast media (ionic) *on page 495*

lymphocyte immune globulin (LIM foe site i MYUN GLOB yoo lin)

Synonyms antithymocyte globulin (equine); ATG; horse antihuman thymocyte gamma globulin

U.S./Canadian Brand Names Atgam®

Therapeutic Category Immunosuppressant Agent

Use Prevention and treatment of acute allograft rejection; treatment of moderate to severe aplastic anemia in patients not considered suitable candidates for bone marrow transplantation; prevention of graft-vs-host disease following bone marrow transplantation

Usual Dosage An intradermal skin test is recommended prior to administration of the initial dose of ATG. Use 0.1 mL of a 1:1000 dilution of ATG in normal saline

Aplastic anemia protocol: I.V.: 10-20 mg/kg/day for 8-14 days, then administer every other day for 7 more doses

Rejection prevention: Children and Adults: I.V.: 15 mg/kg/day for 14 days, then administer every other day for 7 more doses; initial dose should be administered within 24 hours before or after transplantation

Rejection treatment: Children and Adults: I.V. 10-15 mg/kg/day for 14 days, then administer every other day for 7 more doses

Dosage Forms Injection: 50 mg/mL (5 mL)

Lyphocin® Injection *see* vancomycin *on page 595*

lypressin (lye PRES in)

Synonyms 8-*l*-lysine vasopressin

U.S./Canadian Brand Names Diapid® Nasal Spray

Therapeutic Category Antidiuretic Hormone Analog

Use Control or prevent signs and complications of neurogenic diabetes insipidus

Usual Dosage Children and Adults: Nasal: 1-2 sprays into one or both nostrils 4 times/day; approximately 2 USP posterior pituitary pressor units per spray

Dosage Forms Spray: 0.185 mg/mL (equivalent to 50 USP posterior pituitary units/mL) (8 mL)

Lysatec-rt-PA® (Can) *see* alteplase *on page 21*

Lysodren® *see* mitotane *on page 378*

Maalox® [OTC] *see* aluminum hydroxide and magnesium hydroxide *on page 23*

Maalox Anti-Gas® [OTC] *see* simethicone *on page 522*

Maalox® Plus [OTC] *see* aluminum hydroxide, magnesium hydroxide, and simethicone *on page 23*

Maalox® Therapeutic Concentrate [OTC] *see* aluminum hydroxide and magnesium hydroxide *on page 23*

Macrobid® *see* nitrofurantoin *on page 403*

Macrodantin® *see* nitrofurantoin *on page 403*

Macrodex® *see* dextran *on page 170*

mafenide (MA fe nide)

Synonyms succinate mafenide acetate

U.S./Canadian Brand Names Sulfamylon® Topical

(Continued)

mafenide *(Continued)*

Therapeutic Category Antibacterial, Topical

Use Adjunct in the treatment of second and third degree burns to prevent septicemia caused by susceptible organisms such as *Pseudomonas aeruginosa*

Usual Dosage Children and Adults: Topical: Apply once or twice daily with a sterile gloved hand; apply to a thickness of approximately 16 mm; the burned area should be covered with cream at all times

Dosage Forms Cream, topical, as acetate: 85 mg/g (56.7 g, 113.4 g, 411 g)

magaldrate (MAG al drate)

Synonyms hydromagnesium aluminate

U.S./Canadian Brand Names Riopan® [OTC]

Therapeutic Category Antacid

Use Symptomatic relief of hyperacidity associated with peptic ulcer, gastritis, peptic esophagitis and hiatal hernia

Usual Dosage Adults: Oral: 540-1080 mg between meals and at bedtime

Dosage Forms Suspension, oral: 540 mg/5 mL (360 mL)

magaldrate and simethicone (MAG al drate & sye METH i kone)

Synonyms simethicone and magaldrate

U.S./Canadian Brand Names Riopan Plus® [OTC]

Therapeutic Category Antacid; Antiflatulent

Use Relief of hyperacidity associated with peptic ulcer, gastritis, peptic esophagitis and hiatal hernia which are accompanied by symptoms of gas

Usual Dosage Adults: Oral: 5-10 mL between meals and at bedtime

Dosage Forms Suspension, oral: Magaldrate 540 mg and simethicone 40 mg per 5 mL (360 mL)

Magalox Plus® [OTC] *see* aluminum hydroxide, magnesium hydroxide, and simethicone *on page 23*

Magan® *see* magnesium salicylate *on page 346*

Maglucate™ (Can) *see* magnesium gluconate *on next page*

Magnacal® [OTC] *see* enteral nutritional products *on page 208*

magnesia magma *see* magnesium hydroxide *on next page*

magnesium chloride (mag NEE zhum KLOR ide)

U.S./Canadian Brand Names Slow-Mag® [OTC]

Therapeutic Category Electrolyte Supplement, Oral

Use Correct or prevent hypomagnesemia

Usual Dosage I.V. in TPN:

Children: 2-10 mEq/day; the usual recommended pediatric maintenance intake of magnesium ranges from 0.2-0.6 mEq/kg/day. The dose of magnesium may also be based on the caloric intake; on that basis, 3-10 mEq/day of magnesium are needed; maximum maintenance dose: 8-16 mEq/day

Adults: 8-24 mEq/day

Dosage Forms

Injection: 200 mg/mL [1.97 mEq/mL] (30 mL, 50 mL)

Tablet: Elemental magnesium 64 mg

magnesium citrate (mag NEE zhum SIT rate)

Synonyms citrate of magnesia

U.S./Canadian Brand Names Evac-Q-Mag® [OTC]

Therapeutic Category Laxative

Use Evacuation of bowel prior to certain surgical and diagnostic procedures

Usual Dosage Cathartic: Oral:

Children:
<6 years: 2-4 mL/kg administered as a single daily dose or in divided doses
6-12 years: 1/3 to 1/2 bottle
Children ≥12 years and Adults: 1/2 to 1 full bottle

Dosage Forms Solution, oral: 300 mL

magnesium gluconate (mag NEE zhum GLOO koe nate)

U.S./Canadian Brand Names Maglucate™ (Can); Magonate® [OTC]

Therapeutic Category Electrolyte Supplement, Oral

Use Dietary supplement for treatment of magnesium deficiencies

Usual Dosage The recommended dietary allowance (RDA) of magnesium is 4.5 mg/kg which is a total daily allowance of 350-400 mg for adult men and 280-300 mg for adult women. During pregnancy the RDA is 300 mg and during lactation the RDA is 355 mg. Average daily intakes of dietary magnesium have declined in recent years due to processing of food. The latest estimate of the average American dietary intake was 349 mg/day.

Dietary supplement: Oral:
Children: 3-6 mg/kg/day in divided doses 3-4 times/day; maximum: 400 mg/day
Adults: 27-54 mg 2-3 times/day or 100 mg 4 times/day

Dosage Forms Tablet: 500 mg [elemental magnesium 27 mg]

magnesium hydroxide (mag NEE zhum hye DROKS ide)

Synonyms magnesia magma; milk of magnesia; MOM

U.S./Canadian Brand Names Phillips'® Milk of Magnesia [OTC]

Therapeutic Category Antacid; Electrolyte Supplement, Oral; Laxative

Use Short-term treatment of occasional constipation and symptoms of hyperacidity

Usual Dosage Oral:
Laxative:
<2 years: 0.5 mL/kg/dose
2-5 years: 5-15 mL/day or in divided doses
6-12 years: 15-30 mL/day or in divided doses
≥12 years: 30-60 mL/day or in divided doses
Antacid:
Children: 2.5-5 mL as needed
Adults: 5-15 mL as needed

Dosage Forms
Liquid: 390 mg/5 mL (10 mL, 15 mL, 20 mL, 30 mL, 100 mL, 120 mL, 180 mL, 360 mL, 720 mL)
Liquid, concentrate: 10 mL equivalent to 30 mL milk of magnesia USP (3 times as potent as regular strength product)
Suspension, oral: 2.5 g/30 mL (10 mL, 15 mL, 30 mL)
Tablet: 300 mg, 600 mg

magnesium hydroxide and aluminum hydroxide *see* aluminum hydroxide and magnesium hydroxide *on page 23*

magnesium hydroxide and mineral oil emulsion

(mag NEE zhum hye DROKS ide & MIN er al oyl e MUL shun)

Synonyms mom/mineral oil emulsion

U.S./Canadian Brand Names Haley's M-O® [OTC]

Therapeutic Category Laxative

Use Short-term treatment of occasional constipation

Usual Dosage Adults: Oral: 5-45 mL at bedtime

Dosage Forms Suspension, oral: Equivalent to magnesium hydroxide 24 mL/mineral oil emulsion 6 mL (30 mL unit dose)

magnesium oxide (mag NEE zhum OKS ide)

U.S./Canadian Brand Names Maox®

Therapeutic Category Antacid; Electrolyte Supplement, Oral; Laxative

Use Treatment of magnesium deficiencies, short-term treatment of occasional constipation, and symptoms of hyperacidity

Usual Dosage Oral:

Antacid: 250 mg to 1.5 g with water or milk 4 times/day after meals and at bedtime
Laxative: 2-4 g at bedtime with full glass of water

Dosage Forms

Capsule: 140 mg
Tablet: 400 mg, 425 mg

magnesium salicylate (mag NEE zhum sa LIS i late)

U.S./Canadian Brand Names Doan's®, Original [OTC]; Extra Strength Doan's® [OTC]; Magan®; Magsal®; Mobidin®

Therapeutic Category Nonsteroidal Anti-inflammatory Drug (NSAID)

Use Mild to moderate pain, fever, various inflammatory conditions

Usual Dosage Adults: Oral: 650 mg 4 times/day or 1090 mg 3 times/day; may increase to 3.6-4.8 mg/day in 3-4 divided doses

Dosage Forms

Caplet:
Doan's®, Original: 325 mg
Extra Strength Doan's®: 500 mg
Tablet:
Magan®: 545 mg
Magsal®: 600 mg
Mobidin®: 600 mg

magnesium sulfate (mag NEE zhum SUL fate)

Synonyms epsom salts

Therapeutic Category Anticonvulsant; Electrolyte Supplement, Oral; Laxative

Use Treatment and prevention of hypomagnesemia; hypertension; encephalopathy and seizures associated with acute nephritis in children; also used as a cathartic

Usual Dosage Dose represented as $MgSO_4$ unless stated otherwise

Hypomagnesemia:
Children:
I.M., I.V.: 25-50 mg/kg/dose (0.2-0.4 mEq/kg/dose) every 4-6 hours for 3-4 doses, maximum single dose: 2000 mg (16 mEq), may repeat if hypomagnesemia persists (higher dosage up to 100 mg/kg/dose $MgSO_4$ I.V. has been used)
Oral: 100-200 mg/kg/dose 4 times/day
Maintenance: I.V.: 30-60 mg/kg/day (0.25-0.5 mEq/kg/day)
Adults: I.M., I.V.: 1 g every 6 hours for 4 doses or 250 mg/kg over a 4-hour period; for severe hypomagnesemia: 8-12 g $MgSO_4$/day in divided doses has been used; Oral: 3 g every 6 hours for 4 doses as needed
Management of seizures and hypertension: Children: I.M., I.V.: 20-100 mg/kg/dose every 4-6 hours as needed; in severe cases doses as high as 200 mg/kg/dose have been used

Cathartic: Oral:
Children: 0.25 g/kg/dose
Adults: 10-30 g

Dosage Forms

Granules: ~40 mEq magnesium/5 g (240 g)
Injection: 100 mg/mL (20 mL); 125 mg/mL (8 mL); 250 mg/mL (150 mL); 500 mg/mL (2 mL, 5 mL, 10 mL, 30 mL, 50 mL)
Solution, oral: 50% [500 mg/mL] (30 mL)

Magnevist® *see* radiological/contrast media (ionic) *on page 495*

Magonate® [OTC] *see* magnesium gluconate *on previous page*

Magsal® *see* magnesium salicylate *on previous page*

Malatal® ***(Discontinued)*** *see page 700*

malathion (mal a THYE on)

U.S./Canadian Brand Names Ovide™ Topical

Therapeutic Category Scabicides/Pediculicides

Use Treatment of head lice and their ova

Usual Dosage Topical: Sprinkle Ovide™ lotion on dry hair and rub gently until the scalp is thoroughly moistened; pay special attention to the back of the head and neck. Allow to dry naturally, use no heat and leave uncovered. After 8-12 hours, the hair should be washed with a nonmedicated shampoo; rinse and use a fine-toothed comb to remove dead lice and eggs. If required, repeat with second application in 7-9 days. Further treatment is generally not necessary. Other family members should be evaluated to determine if infested and if so, receive treatment.

Dosage Forms Lotion: 0.5% (59 mL)

Mallamint® [OTC] *see* calcium carbonate *on page 89*

Mallazine® Eye Drops [OTC] *see* tetrahydrozoline *on page 556*

Mallisol® [OTC] *see* povidone-iodine *on page 467*

Malotuss® Syrup ***(Discontinued)*** *see page 700*

Maltlevol® (Can) *see* vitamin, multiple (oral) *on page 604*

malt soup extract (malt soop EKS trakt)

U.S./Canadian Brand Names Maltsupex® [OTC]

Therapeutic Category Laxative

Use Short-term treatment of constipation

Usual Dosage Oral:

Infants >1 month:

Breast fed: 1-2 teaspoonfuls in 2-4 oz of water or fruit juice 1-2 times/day

Bottle fed: ½ to 2 tablespoonfuls/day in formula for 3-4 days, then 1-2 teaspoonfuls/day

Children 2-11 years: 1-2 tablespoonfuls 1-2 times/day

Adults ≥12 years: 2 tablespoonfuls twice daily for 3-4 days, then 1-2 tablespoonfuls every evening

Dosage Forms

Liquid: Nondiastatic barley malt extract 16 g/15 mL

Powder: Nondiastatic barley malt extract 16 g/heaping tablespoonful

Tablet: Nondiastatic barley malt extract 750 mg

Maltsupex® [OTC] *see* malt soup extract *on this page*

Mandelamine® *see* methenamine *on page 362*

Mandelamine® Tablet ***(Discontinued)*** *see page 700*

Mandol® *see* cefamandole *on page 104*

mandrake *see* podophyllum resin *on page 458*

manganese injection *see* trace metals *on page 573*

mannitol (MAN i tole)

Synonyms *d*-mannitol

U.S./Canadian Brand Names Osmitrol® Injection; Resectisol® Irrigation Solution

Therapeutic Category Diuretic, Osmotic

Use Reduction of increased intracranial pressure (ICP) associated with cerebral edema; promotion of diuresis in the prevention and/or treatment of oliguria or anuria due to acute renal failure; reduction of increased intraocular pressure; promotion of urinary excretion of toxic substances

(Continued)

mannitol *(Continued)*

Usual Dosage

Children:

Test dose (to assess adequate renal function): 200 mg/kg over 3-5 minutes to produce a urine flow of at least 1 mL/kg/hour for 1-3 hours

Initial: 0.5-1 g/kg

Maintenance: 0.25-0.5 g/kg/hour administered every 4-6 hours

Adults:

Test dose: 12.5 g (200 mg/kg) over 3-5 minutes to produce a urine flow of at least 30-50 mL of urine per hour over the next 2-3 hours

Initial: 0.5-1 g/kg

Maintenance: 0.25-0.5 g/kg every 4-6 hours

Dosage Forms

Injection: 5% [50 mg/mL] (1000 mL); 10% [100 mg/mL] (500 mL, 1000 mL); 15% [150 mg/mL] (150 mL, 500 mL); 20% [200 mg/mL] (150 mL, 250 mL, 500 mL); 25% [250 mg/mL] (50 mL)

Solution, urogenital: 0.54% [5.4 mg/mL] (2000 mL)

Mantadil® Cream *(Discontinued)* *see page 700*

Mantoux *see* tuberculin tests *on page 588*

Maolate® *see* chlorphenesin *on page 120*

Maox® *see* magnesium oxide *on page 346*

Mapap® [OTC] *see* acetaminophen *on page 3*

maprotiline (ma PROE ti leen)

U.S./Canadian Brand Names Ludiomil®

Therapeutic Category Antidepressant, Tetracyclic

Use Treatment of depression and anxiety associated with depression

Usual Dosage Oral:

Children 6-14 years: 10 mg/day, increase to a maximum daily dose of 75 mg

Adults: 75 mg/day to start, increase by 25 mg every 2 weeks up to 150-225 mg/day; administered in 3 divided doses or in a single daily dose

Dosage Forms Tablet, as hydrochloride: 25 mg, 50 mg, 75 mg

Maranox® [OTC] *see* acetaminophen *on page 3*

Marax® *see* theophylline, ephedrine, and hydroxyzine *on page 559*

Marcaine® *see* bupivacaine *on page 83*

Marcillin® *see* ampicillin *on page 34*

Marezine® Injection *(Discontinued)* *see page 700*

Marezine® Oral [OTC] *see* cyclizine *on page 152*

Margesic® H *see* hydrocodone and acetaminophen *on page 287*

Marinol® *see* dronabinol *on page 198*

Marmine® Injection *see* dimenhydrinate *on page 182*

Marmine® Oral [OTC] *see* dimenhydrinate *on page 182*

Marplan® *(Discontinued)* *see page 700*

Marpres® *see* hydralazine, hydrochlorothiazide, and reserpine *on page 285*

Marthritic® *see* salsalate *on page 515*

masoprocol (ma SOE pro kole)

U.S./Canadian Brand Names Actinex® Topical

Therapeutic Category Topical Skin Product

Use Treatment of actinic keratosis

Usual Dosage Adults: Topical: Wash and dry area; gently massage into affected area every morning and evening for 28 days

Dosage Forms Cream: 10% (30 g)

Massé® Breast Cream [OTC] *see* glycerin, lanolin, and peanut oil *on page 264*

Massengill® Medicated Douche w/Cepticin [OTC] *see* povidone-iodine *on page 467*

Materna® (Can) *see* vitamin, multiple (oral) *on page 604*

Materna® *(Discontinued)* *see page 700*

Matulane® *see* procarbazine *on page 476*

Mavik® *see* trandolapril *on page 574*

Maxair™ Inhalation Aerosol *see* pirbuterol *on page 454*

Maxalt® *see* rizatriptan *on page 508*

Maxalt-MLT™ *see* rizatriptan *on page 508*

Maxaquin® *see* lomefloxacin *on page 338*

Max-Caro® *(Discontinued)* *see page 700*

Maxeran® (Can) *see* metoclopramide *on page 370*

Maxidex® *see* dexamethasone (ophthalmic) *on page 167*

Maxiflor® *see* diflorasone *on page 179*

Maximum Strength Anbesol® [OTC] *see* benzocaine *on page 66*

Maximum Strength Desenex® Antifungal Cream [OTC] *see* miconazole *on page 373*

Maximum Strength Dex-A-Diet® [OTC] *see* phenylpropanolamine *on page 447*

Maximum Strength Dexatrim® [OTC] *see* phenylpropanolamine *on page 447*

Maximum Strength Nytol® [OTC] *see* diphenhydramine *on page 185*

Maximum Strength Orajel® [OTC] *see* benzocaine *on page 66*

Maxipime® *see* cefepime *on page 105*

Maxitrol® *see* neomycin, polymyxin B, and dexamethasone *on page 396*

Maxivate® Topical *see* betamethasone (topical) *on page 72*

Maxolon® *see* metoclopramide *on page 370*

Maxzide® *see* hydrochlorothiazide and triamterene *on page 287*

may apple *see* podophyllum resin *on page 458*

Mazanor® *see* mazindol *on this page*

Mazepine® (Can) *see* carbamazepine *on page 97*

mazindol (MAY zin dole)

U.S./Canadian Brand Names Mazanor®; Sanorex®

Therapeutic Category Anorexiant

Controlled Substance C-IV

Use Short-term adjunct in exogenous obesity

Usual Dosage Adults: Oral:

Initial: 1 mg once daily; adjust to patient response

Usual dose: 1 mg 3 times/day one hour before meals, or 2 mg once daily one hour before lunch; administer with meals to avoid GI discomfort

Dosage Forms Tablet:

Mazanor®: 1 mg

Sanorex®: 1 mg, 2 mg

MCH *see* microfibrillar collagen hemostat *on page 374*

m-cresyl acetate (em-KREE sil AS e tate)

U.S./Canadian Brand Names Cresylate®

Therapeutic Category Otic Agent, Anti-infective

Use Provides an acid medium; for external otitis infections caused by susceptible bacteria or fungus

Usual Dosage Otic: Instill 2-4 drops as required

Dosage Forms Solution: 25% with isopropanol 25%, chlorobutanol 1%, benzyl alcohol 1%, and castor oil 5% in propylene glycol (15 mL dropper bottle)

MCT Oil® [OTC] *see* medium chain triglycerides *on page 352*

MD-Gastroview® *see* radiological/contrast media (ionic) *on page 495*

measles and rubella vaccines, combined

(MEE zels & roo BEL a vak SEENS, kom BINED)

Synonyms rubella and measles vaccines, combined

U.S./Canadian Brand Names M-R-VAX® II

Therapeutic Category Vaccine, Live Virus

Use Simultaneous immunization against measles and rubella

Usual Dosage S.C.: Inject into outer aspect of upper arm

Dosage Forms Injection: 1000 $TCID_{50}$ each of live attenuated measles virus vaccine and live rubella virus vaccine

measles, mumps and rubella vaccines, combined

(MEE zels, mumpz & roo BEL a vak SEENS, kom BINED)

Synonyms MMR

U.S./Canadian Brand Names M-M-R® II

Therapeutic Category Vaccine, Live Virus

Use Measles, mumps, and rubella prophylaxis

Usual Dosage S.C.: Inject in outer aspect of the upper arm to children ≥15 months of age; each dose contains 1000 $TCID_{50}$ (tissue culture infectious doses) of live attenuated measle virus vaccine, 5000 $TCID_{50}$ of live mumps virus vaccine and 1000 $TCID_{50}$ of live rubella virus vaccine

Dosage Forms Injection: 1000 $TCID_{50}$ each of measles virus vaccine and rubella virus vaccine, 5000 $TCID_{50}$ mumps virus vaccine

measles virus vaccine, live (MEE zels VYE rus vak SEEN, live)

Synonyms more attenuated enders strain; rubeola vaccine

U.S./Canadian Brand Names Attenuvax®

Therapeutic Category Vaccine, Live Virus

Use Immunization against measles (rubeola) in persons ≥15 months of age

Usual Dosage Children >15 months and Adults: S.C.: 0.5 mL in outer aspect of the upper arm

Dosage Forms Injection: 1000 $TCID_{50}$ per dose

Measurin® [OTC] *see* aspirin *on page 49*

Mebaral® *see* mephobarbital *on page 356*

mebendazole (me BEN da zole)

U.S./Canadian Brand Names Vermox®

Therapeutic Category Anthelmintic

Use Treatment of enterobiasis (pinworm infection), trichuriasis (whipworm infections), ascariasis (roundworm infection), and hookworm infections caused by *Necator americanus* or *Ancylostoma duodenale*; drug of choice in the treatment of capillariasis

Usual Dosage Children and Adults: Oral:

Pinworms: Single chewable tablet; may need to repeat after 2 weeks

Whipworms, roundworms, hookworms: 1 tablet twice daily, morning and evening on 3 consecutive days; if patient is not cured within 3-4 weeks, a second course of treatment may be administered

Dosage Forms Tablet, chewable: 100 mg

mecamylamine (mek a MIL a meen)

U.S./Canadian Brand Names Inversine®

Therapeutic Category Ganglionic Blocking Agent

Use Treatment of moderately severe to severe hypertension and in uncomplicated malignant hypertension

Usual Dosage Adults: Oral: 2.5 mg twice daily after meals for 2 days; increased by increments of 2.5 mg at intervals of ≥2 days until desired blood pressure response is achieved

Dosage Forms Tablet, as hydrochloride: 2.5 mg

mechlorethamine (me klor ETH a meen)

Synonyms HN_2; mustine; nitrogen mustard

U.S./Canadian Brand Names Mustargen® Hydrochloride

Therapeutic Category Antineoplastic Agent

Use Combination therapy of Hodgkin's disease, brain tumors, non-Hodgkin's lymphoma, and malignant lymphomas; palliative treatment of bronchogenic, breast, and ovarian carcinoma; sclerosing agent in intracavitary therapy of pleural, pericardial, and other malignant effusions

Usual Dosage Refer to individual protocols

Children: MOPP: I.V.: 6 mg/m^2 on days 1 and 8 of a 28-day cycle

Adults:

I.V.: 0.4 mg/kg or 12-16 mg/m^2 for one dose or divided into 0.1 mg/kg/day for 4 days

Intracavitary: 10-20 mg or 0.2-0.4 mg/kg

Dosage Forms Powder for injection, as hydrochloride: 10 mg

Meclan® Topical *see* meclocycline *on this page*

meclizine (MEK li zeen)

Synonyms meclozine

U.S./Canadian Brand Names Antivert®; Antrizine®; Bonamine® (Can); Bonine® [OTC]; Dizmiss® [OTC]; Dramamine® II [OTC]; Meni-D®; Nico-Vert® [OTC]; Ru-Vert-M®; Vergon® [OTC]

Therapeutic Category Antihistamine

Use Prevention and treatment of motion sickness; management of vertigo

Usual Dosage Children >12 years and Adults: Oral:

Motion sickness: 25-50 mg 1 hour before travel, repeat dose every 24 hours if needed

Vertigo: 25-100 mg/day in divided doses

Dosage Forms Meclizine hydrochloride:

Capsule: 15 mg, 25 mg, 30 mg

Tablet: 12.5 mg, 25 mg, 50 mg

Tablet:

Chewable: 25 mg

Film coated: 25 mg

meclocycline (me kloe SYE kleen)

U.S./Canadian Brand Names Meclan® Topical

Therapeutic Category Antibiotic, Topical

Use Topical treatment of inflammatory acne vulgaris

Usual Dosage Topical: Apply to affected areas twice daily

Dosage Forms Cream, topical, as sulfosalicylate: 1% (20 g, 45 g)

meclofenamate (me kloe fen AM ate)

Therapeutic Category Analgesic, Non-narcotic; Nonsteroidal Anti-inflammatory Drug (NSAID)

Use Treatment of inflammatory disorders

Usual Dosage Adults: Oral: 200-300 mg 3-4 times/day

Dosage Forms Capsule, as sodium: 50 mg, 100 mg

Meclomen® *(Discontinued)* *see page 700*

meclozine *see* meclizine *on previous page*

Meda-Cap® [OTC] *see* acetaminophen *on page 3*

Meda® Tab [OTC] *see* acetaminophen *on page 3*

medicinal carbon *see* charcoal *on page 114*

Medigesic® *see* butalbital compound and acetaminophen *on page 85*

Medihaler-Epi® *(Discontinued)* *see page 700*

Medihaler Ergotamine® *(Discontinued)* *see page 700*

Medihaler-Iso® *see* isoproterenol *on page 314*

Medilium® (Can) *see* chlordiazepoxide *on page 116*

Medimet® (Can) *see* methyldopa *on page 367*

Mediplast® Plaster [OTC] *see* salicylic acid *on page 513*

Medipren® [OTC] *see* ibuprofen *on page 300*

Medi-Quick® Topical Ointment [OTC] *see* bacitracin, neomycin, and polymyxin B *on page 59*

Meditran® (Can) *see* meprobamate *on page 356*

Medi-Tuss® [OTC] *see* guaifenesin *on page 267*

medium chain triglycerides (mee DEE um chane trye GLIS er ides)

Synonyms triglycerides, medium chain

U.S./Canadian Brand Names MCT Oil® [OTC]

Therapeutic Category Nutritional Supplement

Use Dietary supplement for those who cannot digest long chain fats; malabsorption associated with disorders such as pancreatic insufficiency, bile salt deficiency, and bacterial overgrowth of the small bowel; induce ketosis as a prevention for seizures (akinetic, clonic, and petit mal)

Usual Dosage Oral: 15 mL 3-4 times/day

Dosage Forms Oil: 14 g/15 mL (960 mL)

Medralone® Injection *see* methylprednisolone *on page 368*

Medrapred® *(Discontinued)* *see page 700*

Medrol® Acetate Topical *(Discontinued)* *see page 700*

Medrol® Oral *see* methylprednisolone *on page 368*

Medrol® Veriderm® Cream (Can) *see* methylprednisolone *on page 368*

medroxyprogesterone acetate (me DROKS ee proe JES te rone AS e tate)

Synonyms acetoxymethylprogesterone; methylacetoxyprogesterone

U.S./Canadian Brand Names Amen® Oral; Curretab® Oral; Cycrin® Oral; Depo-Provera® Injection; Provera® Oral

Therapeutic Category Contraceptive, Progestin Only; Progestin

Use Secondary amenorrhea or abnormal uterine bleeding due to hormonal imbalance

Usual Dosage

Adolescents and Adults: Oral:

Amenorrhea: 5-10 mg/day for 5-10 days or 2.5 mg/day

Abnormal uterine bleeding: 5-10 mg for 5-10 days starting on day 16 or 21 of cycle

Accompanying cyclic estrogen therapy, postmenopausal: 2.5-10 mg the last 10-13 days of estrogen dosing each month

Adults:

Contraception: Deep I.M.: 150 mg every 3 months or 450 mg every 6 months

Endometrial or renal carcinoma: I.M.: 400-1000 mg/week

Dosage Forms Medroxyprogesterone acetate:

Injection, suspension: 100 mg/mL (5 mL); 150 mg/mL (1 mL); 400 mg/mL (1 mL, 2.5 mL, 10 mL)

Tablet: 2.5 mg, 5 mg, 10 mg

medroxyprogesterone and estrogens *see* estrogens and medroxyprogesterone *on page 218*

medrysone (ME dri sone)

U.S./Canadian Brand Names HMS Liquifilm®

Therapeutic Category Adrenal Corticosteroid

Use Treatment of allergic conjunctivitis, vernal conjunctivitis, episcleritis, ophthalmic epinephrine sensitivity reaction

Usual Dosage Children and Adults: Ophthalmic: 1 drop in conjunctival sac 2-4 times/day up to every 4 hours; may use every 1-2 hours during first 1-2 days

Dosage Forms Solution, ophthalmic: 1% (5 mL, 10 mL)

mefenamic acid (me fe NAM ik AS id)

U.S./Canadian Brand Names Ponstan® (Can); Ponstel®

Therapeutic Category Analgesic, Non-narcotic; Nonsteroidal Anti-inflammatory Drug (NSAID)

Use Short-term relief of mild to moderate pain including primary dysmenorrhea

Usual Dosage Children >14 years and Adults: Oral: 500 mg to start then 250 mg every 4 hours as needed; maximum therapy: 1 week

Dosage Forms Capsule: 250 mg

mefloquine (ME floe kwin)

U.S./Canadian Brand Names Lariam®

Therapeutic Category Antimalarial Agent

Use Treatment of acute malarial infections and prevention of malaria

Usual Dosage Adults: Oral:

Mild to moderate malaria infection: 5 tablets (1250 mg) as a single dose with at least 8 oz of water

Malaria prophylaxis: 1 tablet (250 mg) weekly starting 1 week before travel, continuing weekly during travel and for 4 weeks after leaving endemic area

Dosage Forms Tablet, as hydrochloride: 250 mg

Mefoxin® *see* cefoxitin *on page 107*

Mega B® [OTC] *see* vitamin B complex *on page 603*

Megace® *see* megestrol acetate *on this page*

Megacillin® Susp (Can) *see* penicillin G benzathine *on page 433*

Megaton™ [OTC] *see* vitamin B complex *on page 603*

megestrol acetate (me JES trole AS e tate)

U.S./Canadian Brand Names Megace®

Therapeutic Category Antineoplastic Agent; Progestin

Use Palliative treatment of breast and endometrial carcinomas, appetite stimulation and promotion of weight gain in cachexia

Usual Dosage Adults: Oral:

Breast carcinoma: 40 mg 4 times/day

Endometrial: 40-320 mg/day in divided doses

(Continued)

megestrol acetate *(Continued)*

Dosage Forms Megestrol acetate:

Suspension, oral: 40 mg/mL with alcohol 0.06% (240 mL)
Tablet: 20 mg, 40 mg

Melanex® *see* hydroquinone *on page 294*

Melfiat-105® Unicelles® *see* phendimetrazine *on page 442*

Melfiat® Tablet *(Discontinued)* *see page 700*

Mellaril® *see* thioridazine *on page 563*

Mellaril-S® *see* thioridazine *on page 563*

melphalan (MEL fa lan)

Synonyms l-PAM; l-sarcolysin; phenylalanine mustard

U.S./Canadian Brand Names Alkeran®

Therapeutic Category Antineoplastic Agent

Use Palliative treatment of multiple myeloma and nonresectable epithelial ovarian carcinoma; neuroblastoma, rhabdomyosarcoma, breast cancer, sarcoma; I.V. formulation: Use in patients in whom oral therapy is not appropriate

Usual Dosage Refer to individual protocols

Children: I.V. (investigational, distributed under the auspices of the NCI for authorized studies):

Pediatric rhabdomyosarcoma: 10-35 mg/m^2 bolus every 21-28 days
Chemoradiotherapy supported by marrow infusions for neuroblastoma: 70-140 mg/m^2 on day 7 and 6 before BMT

Adults: Oral:

Multiple myeloma: 6 mg/day or 10 mg/day for 7-10 days, or 0.15 mg/kg/day for 7 days
Ovarian carcinoma: 0.2 mg/kg/day for 5 days, repeat in 4-5 weeks

Dosage Forms

Powder for injection: 50 mg
Tablet: 2 mg

Menadol® [OTC] *see* ibuprofen *on page 300*

Menest® *see* estrogens, esterified *on page 220*

Meni-D® *see* meclizine *on page 351*

meningococcal polysaccharide vaccine, groups A, C, Y and W-135

(me NIN joe kok al pol i SAK a ride vak SEEN groops aye, see, why & dubl yoo won thur tee fyve)

U.S./Canadian Brand Names Menomune®-A/C/Y/W-135

Therapeutic Category Vaccine, Live Bacteria

Use Immunization against infection caused by *Neisseria meningitidis* groups A,C,Y, and W-135 in persons ≥2 years

Usual Dosage S.C.: 0.5 mL; do not inject intradermally or I.V.

Dosage Forms Injection: 10 dose, 50 dose

Menomune®-A/C/Y/W-135 *see* meningococcal polysaccharide vaccine, groups A, C, Y and W-135 *on this page*

menotropins (men oh TROE pins)

U.S./Canadian Brand Names Humegon™; Pergonal®; Repronex™

Therapeutic Category Gonadotropin

Use Sequentially with hCG to induce ovulation and pregnancy in the infertile woman with functional anovulation; used with hCG in men to stimulate spermatogenesis in those with primary hypogonadotropic hypogonadism

Usual Dosage I.M.:

Male: Following pretreatment with hCG, 1 ampul 3 times/week and hCG 2000 units twice weekly until sperm is detected in the ejaculate (4-6 months) then may be increased to 2 ampuls of menotropins 3 times/week

Female: 1 ampul/day (75 units of FSH and LH) for 9-12 days followed by 10,000 units hCG 1 day after the last dose; repeated at least twice at same level before increasing dosage to 2 ampuls

Dosage Forms Injection: Follicle-stimulating hormone activity 75 units and luteinizing hormone activity 75 units per 2 mL ampul; follicle stimulating hormone activity 150 units and luteinizing hormone activity 150 units per 2 mL ampul

Mentax® *see* butenafine *on page 86*

mepenzolate (me PEN zoe late)

U.S./Canadian Brand Names Cantil®

Therapeutic Category Anticholinergic Agent

Use Management of peptic ulcer disease; inhibit salivation and excessive secretions in respiratory tract preoperatively

Usual Dosage Adults: Oral: 25-50 mg 4 times/day with meals and at bedtime

Dosage Forms Tablet, as bromide: 25 mg

Mepergan® *see* meperidine and promethazine *on this page*

meperidine (me PER i deen)

Synonyms isonipecaine; pethidine

U.S./Canadian Brand Names Demerol®

Therapeutic Category Analgesic, Narcotic

Controlled Substance C-II

Use Management of moderate to severe pain; adjunct to anesthesia and preoperative sedation

Usual Dosage Doses should be titrated to appropriate analgesic effect; when changing route of administration, note that oral doses are about half as effective as parenteral dose

Oral, I.M., I.V., S.C.:

Children: 1-1.5 mg/kg/dose every 3-4 hours as needed; 1-2 mg/kg as a single dose preoperative medication may be used; maximum 100 mg/dose

Adults: 50-150 mg/dose every 3-4 hours as needed

Dosage Forms Meperidine hydrochloride:

Injection:

Multiple-dose vials: 50 mg/mL (30 mL); 100 mg/mL (20 mL)

Single dose: 10 mg/mL (5 mL, 10 mL, 30 mL); 25 mg/dose (0.5 mL, 1 mL); 50 mg/dose (1 mL); 75 mg/dose (1 mL, 1.5 mL); 100 mg/dose (1 mL)

Syrup: 50 mg/5 mL (500 mL)

Tablet: 50 mg, 100 mg

meperidine and promethazine (me PER i deen & proe METH a zeen)

Synonyms promethazine and meperidine

U.S./Canadian Brand Names Mepergan®

Therapeutic Category Analgesic, Narcotic

Use Management of moderate to severe pain

Usual Dosage Adults:

Oral: 1 capsule every 4-6 hours

I.M.: 1-2 mL every 3-4 hours

Dosage Forms

Capsule: Meperidine hydrochloride 50 mg and promethazine hydrochloride 25 mg

Injection: Meperidine hydrochloride 25 mg and promethazine hydrochloride 25 per mL (2 mL, 10 mL)

mephentermine (me FEN ter meen)

U.S./Canadian Brand Names Wyamine® Sulfate

Therapeutic Category Adrenergic Agonist Agent

Use Treatment of hypotension secondary to ganglionic blockade or spinal anesthesia; may be used as an emergency measure to maintain blood pressure until whole blood replacement becomes available

Usual Dosage

Hypotension: I.M., I.V.:

Children: 0.4 mg/kg

Adults: 0.5 mg/kg

Hypotensive emergency: I.V. infusion: 20-60 mg

Dosage Forms Injection, as sulfate: 15 mg/mL (2 mL, 10 mL); 30 mg/mL (10 mL)

mephenytoin (me FEN i toyn)

Synonyms methoin; methylphenylethylhydantoin; phenantoin

U.S./Canadian Brand Names Mesantoin®

Therapeutic Category Anticonvulsant

Use Treatment of tonic-clonic and partial seizures in patients who are uncontrolled with less toxic anticonvulsants

Usual Dosage Oral:

Children: 3-15 mg/kg/day in 3 divided doses; usual maintenance dose: 100-400 mg/day in 3 divided doses

Adults: Initial dose: 50-100 mg/day administered daily; increase by 50-100 mg at weekly intervals; usual maintenance dose: 200-600 mg/day in 3 divided doses; maximum: 800 mg/day

Dosage Forms Tablet: 100 mg

mephobarbital (me foe BAR bi tal)

Synonyms methylphenobarbital

U.S./Canadian Brand Names Mebaral®

Therapeutic Category Barbiturate

Controlled Substance C-IV

Use Treatment of generalized tonic-clonic and simple partial seizures

Usual Dosage Epilepsy: Oral:

Children: 4-10 mg/kg/day in 2-4 divided doses

Adults: 200-600 mg/day in 2-4 divided doses

Dosage Forms Tablet: 32 mg, 50 mg, 100 mg

Mephyton® Oral *see* phytonadione *on page 451*

mepivacaine (me PIV a kane)

U.S./Canadian Brand Names Carbocaine®; Isocaine® HCl; Polocaine®

Therapeutic Category Local Anesthetic

Use Local anesthesia by nerve block; infiltration in dental procedures

Usual Dosage

Injectable local anesthetic: Varies with procedure, degree of anesthesia needed, vascularity of tissue, duration of anesthesia required, and physical condition of patient

Topical: Apply to affected area as needed

Dosage Forms Injection, as hydrochloride: 1% [10 mg/mL] (30 mL, 50 mL); 1.5% [15 mg/mL] (30 mL); 2% [20 mg/mL] (20 mL, 50 mL); 3% [30 mg/mL] (1.8 mL)

meprobamate (me proe BA mate)

U.S./Canadian Brand Names Apo-Meprobamate® (Can); Equanil®; Meditran® (Can); Miltown®; Neuramate®; Novo-Mepro® (Can)

Therapeutic Category Antianxiety Agent, Miscellaneous

Controlled Substance C-IV

Use Management of anxiety disorders

Usual Dosage Oral:
Children 6-12 years: 100-200 mg 2-3 times/day
Sustained release: 200 mg twice daily
Adults: 400 mg 3-4 times/day, up to 2400 mg/day
Sustained release: 400-800 mg twice daily
Dosage Forms
Capsule, sustained release: 200 mg, 400 mg
Tablet: 200 mg, 400 mg, 600 mg

meprobamate and aspirin *see* aspirin and meprobamate *on page 50*

Mepron™ *see* atovaquone *on page 52*

Meprospan® ***(Discontinued)*** *see page 700*

merbromin (mer BROE min)

U.S./Canadian Brand Names Mercurochrome®
Therapeutic Category Topical Skin Product
Use Topical antiseptic
Usual Dosage Topical: Apply freely, until injury has healed
Dosage Forms Solution, topical: 2%

mercaptopurine (mer kap toe PYOOR een)

Synonyms 6-mercaptopurine; 6-MP
U.S./Canadian Brand Names Purinethol®
Therapeutic Category Antineoplastic Agent
Use Treatment of acute leukemias (ALL, CML)
Usual Dosage Oral (refer to individual protocols):
Induction: 2.5 mg/kg/day for several weeks or more; if, after 4 weeks there is no improvement and no myelosuppression, increase dosage up to 5 mg/kg/day
Maintenance: 1.5-2.5 mg/kg/day
Dosage Forms Tablet: 50 mg

6-mercaptopurine *see* mercaptopurine *on this page*

mercapturic acid *see* acetylcysteine *on page 8*

mercuric oxide (mer KYOOR ik OKS ide)

Synonyms yellow mercuric oxide
Therapeutic Category Antibiotic, Ophthalmic
Use Treatment of irritation and minor infections of the eyelids
Usual Dosage Ophthalmic: Apply small amount to inner surface of lower eyelid once or twice daily
Dosage Forms Ointment, ophthalmic: 1%, 2% [OTC]

Mercurochrome® *see* merbromin *on this page*

Meridia™ *see* sibutramine *on page 520*

meropenem (mer oh PEN em)

U.S./Canadian Brand Names Merrem® I.V.
Therapeutic Category Carbapenem (Antibiotic)
Use Meropenem is indicated as single agent therapy for the treatment of intra-abdominal infections including complicated appendicitis and peritonitis in adults and bacterial meningitis in pediatric patients >3 months of age caused by *S. pneumoniae*, *H. influenzae*, and *N. meningitidis* (penicillin-resistant pneumococci have not been studied in clinical trials); it is better tolerated than imipenem and highly effective against a broad range of bacteria
Usual Dosage
Children:
Intra-abdominal infections: 20 mg/kg every 8 hours (maximum dose: 1 g every 8 hours)
(Continued)

meropenem *(Continued)*

Meningitis: 40 mg/kg every 8 hours (maximum dose: 2 g every 8 hours)
Adults: 1 g every 8 hours

Dosage Forms
Infusion: 500 mg (100 mL); 1 g (100 mL)
Infusion, ADD-vantage®: 500 mg (15 mL); 1 g (15 mL)
Injection: 25 mg/mL (20 mL); 33.3 mg/mL (30 mL)

Merrem® I.V. *see* meropenem *on previous page*

Mersol® [OTC] *see* thimerosal *on page 561*

Merthiolate® [OTC] *see* thimerosal *on page 561*

Meruvax® II *see* rubella virus vaccine, live *on page 511*

mesalamine (me SAL a meen)

Synonyms 5-aminosalicylic acid; 5-ASA; fisalamine; mesalazine
U.S./Canadian Brand Names Asacol® Oral; Pentasa® Oral; Rowasa® Rectal
Therapeutic Category 5-Aminosalicylic Acid Derivative
Use Treatment of ulcerative colitis, proctosigmoiditis, and proctitis
Usual Dosage Adults (usual course of therapy is 3-6 weeks): Oral: 800 mg 3 times/day
Retention enema: 60 mL (4 g) at bedtime, retained overnight, approximately 8 hours
Rectal suppository: Insert 1 suppository in rectum twice daily

Dosage Forms
Capsule, controlled release (Pentasa®): 250 mg
Suppository, rectal (Rowasa®): 500 mg
Suspension, rectal (Rowasa®): 4 g/60 mL (7s)
Tablet, enteric coated (Asacol®): 400 mg

mesalazine *see* mesalamine *on this page*

Mesantoin® *see* mephenytoin *on page 356*

M-Eslon® (Can) *see* morphine sulfate *on page 382*

mesna (MES na)

Synonyms sodium 2-mercaptoethane sulfonate
U.S./Canadian Brand Names Mesnex™
Therapeutic Category Antidote
Use Detoxifying agent used as a protectant against hemorrhagic cystitis induced by ifosfamide and cyclophosphamide
Usual Dosage Children and Adults (refer to individual protocols):
Ifosfamide: I.V.: 20% W/W of ifosfamide dose at time of administration and 4 and 8 hours after each dose of ifosfamide
Cyclophosphamide: I.V.: 20% W/W of cyclophosphamide dose prior to administration and 3, 6, 9, 12 hours after cyclophosphamide dose (total daily dose: 120% to 180% of cyclophosphamide dose)
Oral dose: 40% W/W of the antineoplastic agent dose in 3 doses at 4-hour intervals
Dosage Forms Injection: 100 mg/mL (2 mL, 4 mL, 10 mL)

Mesnex™ *see* mesna *on this page*

mesoridazine (mez oh RID a zeen)

U.S./Canadian Brand Names Serentil®
Therapeutic Category Phenothiazine Derivative
Use Symptomatic management of psychotic disorders, including schizophrenia, behavioral problems, alcoholism as well as reducing anxiety and tension occurring in neurosis
Usual Dosage Initial: 25 mg for most patients; may repeat dose in 30-60 minutes, if necessary; usual optimum dosage range: 25-200 mg/day. Concentrate may be diluted

just prior to administration with distilled water, acidified tap water, orange or grape juice; do not prepare and store bulk dilutions.

Dosage Forms Mesoridazine besylate:
Injection: 25 mg/mL (1 mL)
Liquid, oral: 25 mg/mL (118 mL)
Tablet: 10 mg, 25 mg, 50 mg, 100 mg

Mestatin® (Can) *see* nystatin *on page 412*

Mestinon® Injection *see* pyridostigmine *on page 489*

Mestinon® Oral *see* pyridostigmine *on page 489*

mestranol and norethindrone (MES tra nole & nor eth IN drone)

Synonyms norethindrone and mestranol

U.S./Canadian Brand Names Genora® 1/50; Nelova® 1/50M; Norethin 1/50M; Norinyl® 1+50; Ortho-Novum® 1/50

Therapeutic Category Contraceptive, Oral

Use Prevention of pregnancy; treatment of hypermenorrhea, endometriosis, female hypogonadism

Usual Dosage Contraception: Oral: 1 tablet daily, beginning on day 5 of menstrual cycle (first day of menstrual flow is day 1). With 20-tablet and 21-tablet packages, new dosing cycle begins 7 days after last tablet taken; with 28-tablet packages, dosage is 1 tablet daily without interruption; extra tablets are placebos or contain iron. If next menstrual period does not begin on schedule, rule out pregnancy before starting new dosing cycle; if menstrual period begins, start new dosing cycle 7 days after last tablet was taken. If all doses have been taken on schedule and 1 menstrual period is missed, continue dosing cycle; if 2 consecutive menstrual periods are missed, pregnancy test is required before new dosing cycle is started.

Dosage Forms Tablet: Mestranol 0.05 mg and norethindrone 1 mg (21s and 28s)

metacortandralone *see* prednisolone (ophthalmic) *on page 471*

metacortandralone *see* prednisolone (systemic) *on page 471*

Metahydrin® *see* trichlormethiazide *on page 579*

Metamucil® [OTC] *see* psyllium *on page 488*

Metamucil® Instant Mix [OTC] *see* psyllium *on page 488*

Metaprel® Aerosol *(Discontinued)* *see page 700*

Metaprel® Inhalation Solution *(Discontinued)* *see page 700*

Metaprel® Syrup *see* metaproterenol *on this page*

Metaprel® Tablet *(Discontinued)* *see page 700*

metaproterenol (met a proe TER e nol)

Synonyms orciprenaline

U.S./Canadian Brand Names Alupent®; Arm-a-Med® Metaproterenol; Dey-Dose® Metaproterenol; Metaprel® Syrup; Prometa®

Therapeutic Category Adrenergic Agonist Agent

Use Bronchodilator in reversible airway obstruction due to asthma or COPD

Usual Dosage
- Oral:
  - Children:
    - <2 years: 0.4 mg/kg/dose administered 3-4 times/day; in infants, the dose can be administered every 8-12 hours
    - 2-6 years: 1-2.6 mg/kg/day divided every 6-8 hours
    - 6-9 years: 10 mg/dose administered 3-4 times/day
  - Children >9 years and Adults: 20 mg/dose administered 3-4 times/day
- Inhalation: Children >12 years and Adults: 2-3 inhalations every 3-4 hours, up to 12 inhalations in 24 hours

(Continued)

metaproterenol *(Continued)*

Nebulizer:

Infants: 6 mg/dose administered over 5 minutes

Children <12 years: 0.01-0.02 mL/kg of 5% solution; diluted in 2-3 mL normal saline every 4-6 hours (may be administered more frequently according to need), maximum dose: 15 mg/dose every 4-6 hours

Adolescents and Adults: 5-20 breaths of full strength 5% metaproterenol **or** 0.2-0.3 mL of 5% metaproterenol in 2.5-3 mL normal saline nebulized every 4-6 hours (can be administered more frequently according to need)

Dosage Forms Metaproterenol sulfate:

Aerosol, oral: 0.65 mg/dose (5 mL, 10 mL)

Solution for inhalation, preservative free: 0.4% [4 mg/mL] (2.5 mL); 0.6% [6 mg/mL] (2.5 mL); 5% [50 mg/mL] (10 mL, 30 mL)

Syrup: 10 mg/5 mL (480 mL)

Tablet: 10 mg, 20 mg

metaraminol (met a RAM i nole)

U.S./Canadian Brand Names Aramine®

Therapeutic Category Adrenergic Agonist Agent

Use Acute hypotensive crisis in the treatment of shock

Usual Dosage Adults:

Prevention of hypotension: I.M., S.C.: 2-10 mg

Adjunctive treatment of hypotension: I.V.: 15-100 mg in 250-500 mL NS or 5% dextrose in water

Severe shock: I.V.: 0.5-5 mg direct I.V. injection then use I.M. dose

Dosage Forms Injection, as bitartrate: 10 mg/mL (10 mL)

Metasep® [OTC] *see* parachlorometaxylenol *on page 429*

Metastron® *see* strontium-89 *on page 537*

metaxalone (me TAKS a lone)

U.S./Canadian Brand Names Skelaxin®

Therapeutic Category Skeletal Muscle Relaxant

Use Relief of discomfort associated with acute, painful musculoskeletal conditions

Usual Dosage Children >12 years and Adults: Oral: 800 mg 3-4 times/day

Dosage Forms Tablet: 400 mg

metformin (met FOR min)

U.S./Canadian Brand Names Glucophage®; Novo-Metformin (Can)

Therapeutic Category Antidiabetic Agent, Oral

Use Management of noninsulin-dependent diabetes mellitus (type II) as monotherapy when hyperglycemia cannot be managed on diet alone. May be used concomitantly with a sulfonylurea when diet and metformin or sulfonylurea alone do not result in adequate glycemic control.

Usual Dosage Oral (allow 1-2 weeks between dose titrations):

Adults:

500 mg tablets: Initial: 500 mg twice daily (administered with the morning and evening meals). Dosage increases should be made in increments of one tablet every week, administered in divided doses, up to a maximum of 2,500 mg/day. Doses of up to 2000 mg/day may be administered twice daily. If a dose of 2,500 mg/day is required, it may be better tolerated 3 times/day (with meals).

850 mg tablets: Initial: 850 mg once daily (administered with the morning meal). Dosage increases should be made in increments of one tablet every OTHER week, administered in divided doses, up to a maximum of 2550 mg/day. The usual maintenance dose is 850 mg twice daily (with the morning and evening meals). Some patients may be administered 850 mg 3 times/day (with meals).

Elderly patients: The initial and maintenance dosing should be conservative, due to the potential for decreased renal function. Generally, elderly patients should not be titrated to the maximum dose of metformin.

Transfer from other antidiabetic agents: No transition period is generally necessary except when transferring from chlorpropamide. When transferring from chlorpropamide, care should be exercised during the first 2 weeks because of the prolonged retention of chlorpropamide in the body, leading to overlapping drug effects and possible hypoglycemia.

Concomitant metformin and oral sulfonylurea therapy: If patients have not responded to 4 weeks of the maximum dose of metformin monotherapy, consideration to a gradually addition of an oral sulfonylurea while continuing metformin at the maximum dose, even if prior primary or secondary failure to a sulfonylurea has occurred.

Dosage Forms Tablet, as hydrochloride: 500 mg, 850 mg

methacholine (meth a KOLE leen)

U.S./Canadian Brand Names Provocholine®

Therapeutic Category Diagnostic Agent

Use Diagnosis of bronchial airway hyperactivity in subjects who do not have clinically apparent asthma

Usual Dosage The table is a suggested schedule for administration of methacholine challenge. Calculate cumulative units by multiplying number of breaths by concentration given. Total cumulative units is the sum of cumulative units for each concentration given.

Vial	Serial Concentration (mg/mL)	No. of Breaths	Cumulative Units per Concentration	Total Cumulative Units
E	0.025	5	0.125	0.125
D	0.25	5	1.25	1.375
C	2.5	5	12.5	13.88
B	10	5	50	63.88
A	25	5	125	188.88

Dosage Forms Powder for reconstitution, inhalation, as chloride: 100 mg/5 mL

methadone (METH a done)

U.S./Canadian Brand Names Dolophine®; Methadose® (Can)

Therapeutic Category Analgesic, Narcotic

Controlled Substance C-II

Use Management of severe pain, used in narcotic detoxification maintenance programs and for the treatment of iatrogenic narcotic dependency

Usual Dosage Doses should be titrated to appropriate effects:

Children: Analgesia:

Oral, I.M., S.C.: 0.7 mg/kg/24 hours divided every 4-6 hours as needed or 0.1-0.2 mg/kg every 4-12 hours as needed; maximum: 10 mg/dose

I.V.: Initial: 0.1 mg/kg every 4 hours for 2-3 doses, then every 6-12 hours as needed; maximum: 10 mg/dose

Adults:

Analgesia: Oral, I.M., S.C.: 2.5-10 mg every 3-8 hours as needed, up to 5-20 mg every 6-8 hours

Detoxification: Oral: 15-40 mg/day

Maintenance of opiate dependence: Oral: 20-120 mg/day

Dosage Forms Methadone hydrochloride:

Injection: 10 mg/mL (1 mL, 10 mL, 20 mL)

Solution:

Oral: 5 mg/5 mL (5 mL, 500 mL); 10 mg/5 mL (500 mL)

Oral, concentrate: 10 mg/mL (30 mL)

Tablet: 5 mg, 10 mg

(Continued)

methadone *(Continued)*

Tablet, dispersible: 40 mg

Methadose® (Can) *see* methadone *on previous page*

methaminodiazepoxide *see* chlordiazepoxide *on page 116*

methamphetamine (meth am FET a meen)

Synonyms desoxyephedrine

U.S./Canadian Brand Names Desoxyn®

Therapeutic Category Amphetamine

Controlled Substance C-II

Use Narcolepsy; exogenous obesity; abnormal behavioral syndrome in children (minimal brain dysfunction)

Usual Dosage Oral:

Attention deficit disorder: Children >6 years: 2.5-5 mg 1-2 times/day, may increase by 5 mg increments weekly until optimum response is achieved, usually 20-25 mg/day

Exogenous obesity: Children >12 years and Adults: 5 mg, 30 minutes before each meal, 10-15 mg in morning; treatment duration should not exceed a few weeks

Dosage Forms Methamphetamine hydrochloride:

Tablet: 5 mg

Tablet, extended release (Gradumet®): 5 mg, 10 mg, 15 mg

methantheline (meth AN tha leen)

Synonyms methanthelinium

U.S./Canadian Brand Names Banthine®

Therapeutic Category Anticholinergic Agent

Use Adjunctive treatment of peptic ulcer, irritable bowel syndrome, pancreatitis, ureteral and urinary bladder spasm; to reduce duodenal motility during diagnostic radiologic procedures and treatment of an uninhibited neurogenic bladder

Usual Dosage Oral:

Children:

<1 year: 12.5-25 mg 4 times/day

>1 year: 12.5-50 mg 4 times/day

Adults: 50-100 mg every 6 hours

Dosage Forms Tablet, as bromide: 50 mg

methanthelinium *see* methantheline *on this page*

methazolamide (meth a ZOE la mide)

U.S./Canadian Brand Names GlaucTabs®; Neptazane®

Therapeutic Category Carbonic Anhydrase Inhibitor

Use Adjunctive treatment of open-angle or secondary glaucoma; short-term therapy of narrow-angle glaucoma when delay of surgery is desired

Usual Dosage Adults: Oral: 50-100 mg 2-3 times/day

Dosage Forms Tablet: 25 mg, 50 mg

methenamine (meth EN a meen)

Synonyms hexamethylenetetramine

U.S./Canadian Brand Names Dehydral™ (Can); Hiprex®; Mandelamine®; Urasal® (Can); Urex®

Therapeutic Category Antibiotic, Miscellaneous

Use Prophylaxis or suppression of recurrent urinary tract infections

Usual Dosage Oral:

Children:

Hippurate: 6-12 years: 25-50 mg/kg/day divided every 12 hours

Mandelate: 50-75 mg/kg/day divided every 6 hours

Adults:
Hippurate: 1 g twice daily
Mandelate: 1 g 4 times/day after meals and at bedtime

Dosage Forms
Methenamine hippurate:
Tablet, (Hiprex®, Urex®): 1 g (Hiprex® contains tartrazine dye)
Methenamine mandelate:
Tablet, enteric coated: 500 mg, 1 g

Methergine® *see* methylergonovine *on page 368*

methimazole (meth IM a zole)

Synonyms thiamazole
U.S./Canadian Brand Names Tapazole®
Therapeutic Category Antithyroid Agent
Use Palliative treatment of hyperthyroidism, to return the hyperthyroid patient to a normal metabolic state prior to thyroidectomy, and to control thyrotoxic crisis that may accompany thyroidectomy
Usual Dosage Oral:
Children: Initial: 0.4 mg/kg/day in 3 divided doses; maintenance: 0.2 mg/kg/day in 3 divided doses
Adults: Initial: 10 mg every 8 hours; maintenance dose ranges from 5-30 mg/day
Dosage Forms Tablet: 5 mg, 10 mg

methionine (me THYE oh neen)

U.S./Canadian Brand Names Pedameth®
Therapeutic Category Dietary Supplement
Use Treatment of diaper rash and control of odor, dermatitis and ulceration caused by ammoniacal urine
Usual Dosage Oral:
Children: Control of diaper rash: 75 mg in formula or other liquid 3-4 times/day for 3-5 days
Adults:
Control of odor in incontinent adults: 200-400 mg 3-4 times/day
Dietary supplement: 500 mg/day
Dosage Forms
Capsule: 200 mg, 300 mg, 500 mg
Liquid: 75 mg/5 mL (473 mL)
Tablet: 500 mg

methocarbamol (meth oh KAR ba mole)

U.S./Canadian Brand Names Robaxin®
Therapeutic Category Skeletal Muscle Relaxant
Use Treatment of muscle spasm associated with acute painful musculoskeletal conditions; supportive therapy in tetanus
Usual Dosage
Children: Recommended **only** for use in tetanus I.V.: 15 mg/kg/dose or 500 mg/m^2/dose, may repeat every 6 hours if needed; maximum dose: 1.8 g/m^2/day for 3 days only
Adults: Muscle spasm:
Oral: 1.5 g 4 times/day for 2-3 days, then decrease to 4-4.5 g/day in 3-6 divided doses
I.M., I.V.: 1 g every 8 hours if oral not possible
Dosage Forms
Injection: 100 mg/mL in polyethylene glycol 50% (10 mL)
Tablet: 500 mg, 750 mg

methocarbamol and aspirin (meth oh KAR ba mole & AS pir in)

Synonyms aspirin and methocarbamol
U.S./Canadian Brand Names Robaxisal®
(Continued)

methocarbamol and aspirin *(Continued)*

Therapeutic Category Skeletal Muscle Relaxant

Use Adjunct to rest, physical therapy, and other measures for the relief of discomfort associated with acute, painful musculoskeletal disorders

Usual Dosage Children >12 years and Adults: Oral: 2 tablets 4 times/day

Dosage Forms Tablet: Methocarbamol 400 mg and aspirin 325 mg

methohexital (meth oh HEKS i tal)

U.S./Canadian Brand Names Brevital® Sodium; Brietal Sodium® (Can)

Therapeutic Category Barbiturate

Controlled Substance C-IV

Use Induction and maintenance of general anesthesia for short procedures

Usual Dosage Doses must be titrated to effect

Children:

- I.M.: Preop: 5-10 mg/kg/dose
- I.V.: Induction: 1-2 mg/kg/dose
- Rectal: Preop/induction: 20-35 mg/kg/dose; usual: 25 mg/kg/dose; administer as 10% aqueous solution

Adults: I.V.: Induction: 50-120 mg to start; 20-40 mg every 4-7 minutes

Dosage Forms Injection, as sodium: 500 mg, 2.5 g, 5 g

methoin *see* mephenytoin *on page 356*

methotrexate (meth oh TREKS ate)

Synonyms amethopterin; MTX

U.S./Canadian Brand Names Folex® PFS; Rheumatrex®

Therapeutic Category Antineoplastic Agent

Use Treatment of trophoblastic neoplasms, leukemias, osteosarcoma, non-Hodgkin's lymphoma; psoriasis, rheumatoid arthritis

Usual Dosage Refer to individual protocols

Children:

- High-dose MTX for acute lymphocytic leukemia: I.V.: Loading dose of 200 mg/m² and a 24-hour infusion of 1200 mg/m²/day
- Induction of remission in acute lymphoblastic leukemias: Oral, I.M., I.V.: 3.3 mg/m²/day for 4-6 weeks
- Leukemia: Remission maintenance: Oral, I.M.: 20-30 mg/m² 2 times/week
- Juvenile rheumatoid arthritis: Oral: 5-15 mg/m²/week as a single dose or as 3 divided doses administered 12 hours apart
- Osteosarcoma:
  - I.T.: 10-15 mg/m² (maximum dose: 15 mg) by protocol
  - I.V.: <12 years: 12 g/m² (12-18 g); >12 years: 8 g/m² (maximum dose: 18 g)
- Non-Hodgkin's lymphoma: I.V.: 200-300 mg/m²

Adults:

- Trophoblastic neoplasms: Oral, I.M.: 15-30 mg/day for 5 days, repeat in 7 days for 3-5 courses
- Rheumatoid arthritis: Oral: 7.5 mg once weekly or 2.5 mg every 12 hours for 3 doses/week; not to exceed 20 mg/week

Dosage Forms Methotrexate sodium:

- Injection: 2.5 mg/mL (2 mL); 25 mg/mL (2 mL, 4 mL, 8 mL, 10 mL)
- Injection, preservative free: 25 mg (2 mL, 4 mL, 8 mL, 10 mL)
- Powder, for injection: 20 mg, 25 mg, 50 mg, 100 mg, 250 mg, 1 g
- Tablet: 2.5 mg
- Tablet, dose pack: 2.5 mg (4 cards with 2, 3, 4, 5, or 6 tablets each)

methotrimeprazine (meth oh trye MEP ra zeen)

Synonyms levomepromazine

U.S./Canadian Brand Names Levoprome®

Therapeutic Category Analgesic, Non-narcotic

Use Relief of moderate to severe pain in nonambulatory patients; for analgesia and sedation when respiratory depression is to be avoided, as in obstetrics; preanesthetic for producing sedation, somnolence and relief of apprehension and anxiety

Usual Dosage Adults: I.M.:

Sedation analgesia: 10-20 mg every 4-6 hours as needed

Preoperative medication: 2-20 mg, 45 minutes to 3 hours before surgery

Postoperative analgesia: 2.5-7.5 mg every 4-6 hours is suggested as necessary since residual effects of anesthetic may be present

Pre- and postoperative hypotension: I.M.: 5-10 mg

Dosage Forms Injection, as hydrochloride: 20 mg/mL (10 mL)

methoxamine (meth OKS a meen)

U.S./Canadian Brand Names Vasoxyl®

Therapeutic Category Adrenergic Agonist Agent

Use Treatment of hypotension occurring during general anesthesia; to terminate episodes of supraventricular tachycardia; treatment of shock

Usual Dosage Adults:

Emergencies: I.V.: 3-5 mg

Supraventricular tachycardia: I.V.: 10 mg

During spinal anesthesia: I.M.: 10-20 mg

Dosage Forms Injection, as hydrochloride: 20 mg/mL (1 mL)

methoxsalen (meth OKS a len)

Synonyms methoxypsoralen

U.S./Canadian Brand Names Oxsoralen-Ultra®; Ultramop™ (Can)

Therapeutic Category Psoralen

Use Symptomatic control of severe, recalcitrant, disabling psoriasis in conjunction with long wave ultraviolet radiation; induce repigmentation in vitiligo topical repigmenting agent in conjunction with controlled doses of ultraviolet A (UVA) or sunlight

Usual Dosage

Psoriasis: Adults: Oral: 10-70 mg 1½-2 hours before exposure to ultraviolet light, 2-3 times at least 48 hours apart; dosage is based upon patient's body weight and skin type

Vitiligo: Children >12 years and Adults:

Oral: 20 mg 2-4 hours before exposure to UVA light or sunlight

Topical: Apply lotion 1-2 hours before exposure to UVA light, no more than once weekly

Dosage Forms

Capsule: 10 mg

Lotion: 1% (30 mL)

methoxycinnamate and oxybenzone

(meth OKS ee SIN a mate & oks i BEN zone)

Synonyms sunscreen (paba-free)

U.S./Canadian Brand Names PreSun® 29 [OTC]; Ti-Screen® [OTC]

Therapeutic Category Sunscreen

Use Reduce the chance of premature aging of the skin and skin cancer from overexposure to the sun

Usual Dosage Adults: Topical: Apply liberally to all exposed areas at least 30 minutes prior to sun exposure

Dosage Forms Lotion:

SPF 15: 120 mL

SPF 29: 120 mL

methoxyflurane (meth oks ee FLOO rane)

U.S./Canadian Brand Names Penthrane®

Therapeutic Category General Anesthetic

Use Adjunct to provide anesthesia procedures <4 hours in duration

Usual Dosage 0.3% to 0.8% for analgesia and anesthesia, with 0.1% to 2% for maintenance when used with nitrous oxide

(Continued)

methoxyflurane *(Continued)*

Dosage Forms Liquid: 15 mL, 125 mL

methoxypsoralen *see* methoxsalen *on previous page*

methscopolamine (meth skoe POL a meen)

U.S./Canadian Brand Names Pamine®

Therapeutic Category Anticholinergic Agent

Use Adjunctive therapy in the treatment of peptic ulcer

Usual Dosage Oral: 2.5 mg 30 minutes before meals or food and 2.5-5 mg at bedtime

Dosage Forms Tablet, as bromide: 2.5 mg

methsuximide (meth SUKS i mide)

U.S./Canadian Brand Names Celontin®

Therapeutic Category Anticonvulsant

Use Control of absence (petit mal) seizures; useful adjunct in refractory, partial complex (psychomotor) seizures

Usual Dosage Oral:

Children: Initial: 10-15 mg/kg/day in 3-4 divided doses; increase weekly up to maximum of 30 mg/kg/day

Adults: 300 mg/day for the first week; may increase by 300 mg/day at weekly intervals up to 1.2 g in 2-4 divided doses/day

Dosage Forms Capsule: 150 mg, 300 mg

methyclothiazide (meth i kloe THYE a zide)

U.S./Canadian Brand Names Aquatensen®; Enduron®

Therapeutic Category Diuretic, Thiazide

Use Management of mild to moderate hypertension; treatment of edema in congestive heart failure and nephrotic syndrome

Usual Dosage Adults: Oral:

Edema: 2.5-10 mg/day

Hypertension: 2.5-5 mg/day

Dosage Forms Tablet: 2.5 mg, 5 mg

methyclothiazide and deserpidine

(meth i kloe THYE a zide & de SER pi deen)

Synonyms deserpidine and methyclothiazide

U.S./Canadian Brand Names Enduronyl®; Enduronyl® Forte

Therapeutic Category Antihypertensive Agent, Combination

Use Management of mild to moderately severe hypertension

Usual Dosage Oral: Individualized, normally 1-4 tablets/day

Dosage Forms Tablet: Methyclothiazide 5 mg and deserpidine 0.25 mg; methyclothiazide 5 mg and deserpidine 0.5 mg

methyclothiazide and pargyline (meth i kloe THYE a zide & PAR gi leen)

Synonyms pargyline and methyclothiazide

U.S./Canadian Brand Names Eutron®

Therapeutic Category Antihypertensive Agent, Combination

Use Management of hypertension

Usual Dosage Oral: Individualized, normally 1-4 tablets/day

Dosage Forms Tablet: Methyclothiazide 5 mg and pargyline hydrochloride 25 mg

methylacetoxyprogesterone *see* medroxyprogesterone acetate *on page 352*

methylbenzethonium chloride (meth il ben ze THOE nee um KLOR ide)

U.S./Canadian Brand Names Diaparene® [OTC]; Puri-Clens™ [OTC]; Sween Cream® [OTC]

Therapeutic Category Topical Skin Product
Use Treatment of diaper rash and ammonia dermatitis
Usual Dosage Topical: Apply to area as needed
Dosage Forms
Cream: 0.1% (30 g, 60 g, 120 g)
Ointment, topical: 0.1% (30 g, 60 g, 120 g)
Powder: 0.055% (120 g, 270 g, 420 g)

methylcellulose (meth il SEL yoo lose)

U.S./Canadian Brand Names Citrucel® [OTC]
Therapeutic Category Laxative
Use Adjunct in treatment of constipation
Usual Dosage Oral:
Children: 5-10 mL 1-2 times/day
Adults: 5-20 mL 3 times/day
Dosage Forms Powder: 105 mg/g

methyldopa (meth il DOE pa)

U.S./Canadian Brand Names Aldomet®; Apo®-Methyldopa (Can); Dopamet® (Can); Medimet® (Can); Novo-Medopa® (Can); Nu-Medopa® (Can)
Therapeutic Category Alpha-Adrenergic Blocking Agent
Use Management of moderate to severe hypertension
Usual Dosage
Children:
Oral: Initial: 10 mg/kg/day in 2-4 divided doses; increase every 2 days as needed to maximum dose of 65 mg/kg/day; do not exceed 3 g/day
I.V.: 5-10 mg/kg/dose every 6-8 hours
Adults:
Oral: Initial: 250 mg 2-3 times/day; increase every 2 days as needed; usual dose 1-1.5 g/day in 2-4 divided doses; maximum dose: 3 g/day
I.V.: 250-1000 mg every 6-8 hours
Dosage Forms
Suspension, oral: 250 mg/5 mL (5 mL, 473 mL)
Tablet: 125 mg, 250 mg, 500 mg
Methyldopate hydrochloride: Injection: 50 mg/mL (5 mL, 10 mL)

methyldopa and chlorothiazide *see* chlorothiazide and methyldopa *on page 119*

methyldopa and hydrochlorothiazide

(meth il DOE pa & hye droe klor oh THYE a zide)
Synonyms hydrochlorothiazide and methyldopa
U.S./Canadian Brand Names Aldoril®
Therapeutic Category Antihypertensive Agent, Combination
Use Management of moderate to severe hypertension
Usual Dosage Oral: 1 tablet 2-3 times/day for first 48 hours, then decrease or increase at intervals of not less than 2 days until an adequate response is achieved
Dosage Forms Tablet:
15: Methyldopa 250 mg and hydrochlorothiazide 15 mg
25: Methyldopa 250 mg and hydrochlorothiazide 25 mg
D30: Methyldopa 500 mg and hydrochlorothiazide 30 mg
D50: Methyldopa 500 mg and hydrochlorothiazide 50 mg

methylene blue (METH i leen bloo)

U.S./Canadian Brand Names Urolene Blue®
Therapeutic Category Antidote
Use Antidote for cyanide poisoning and drug-induced methemoglobinemia, indicator dye, bacteriostatic genitourinary antiseptic
(Continued)

methylene blue *(Continued)*

Usual Dosage

Children:

NADH-methemoglobin reductase deficiency: Oral: 1.5-5 mg/kg/day (maximum: 300 mg/day) administered with 5-8 mg/kg/day of ascorbic acid

Methemoglobinemia: I.V.: 1-2 mg/kg over several minutes

Adults:

Genitourinary antiseptic: Oral: 55-130 mg 3 times/day (maximum: 390 mg/day)

Methemoglobinemia: I.V.: 1-2 mg/kg over several minutes; may be repeated in 1 hour if necessary

Dosage Forms

Injection: 10 mg/mL (1 mL, 10 mL)

Tablet: 65 mg

methylergonovine (meth il er goe NOE veen)

U.S./Canadian Brand Names Methergine®

Therapeutic Category Ergot Alkaloid and Derivative

Use Prevention and treatment of postpartum and postabortion hemorrhage caused by uterine atony or subinvolution

Usual Dosage Adults:

Oral: 0.2-0.4 mg every 6-12 hours for 2-7 days

I.M., I.V.: 0.2 mg every 2-4 hours for 5 doses then change to oral dosage

Dosage Forms Methylergonovine maleate:

Injection: 0.2 mg/mL (1 mL)

Tablet: 0.2 mg

methylmorphine *see* codeine *on page 143*

methylphenidate (meth il FEN i date)

U.S./Canadian Brand Names PMS-Methylphenidate (Can); Ritalin®; Ritalin-SR®

Therapeutic Category Central Nervous System Stimulant, Nonamphetamine

Controlled Substance C-II

Use Attention-deficit/hyperactivity disorder (ADHD); narcolepsy

Usual Dosage Oral:

Children ≥6 years: Attention deficit disorder: Initial: 0.3 mg/kg/dose or 2.5-5 mg/dose administered before breakfast and lunch; increase by 0.1 mg/kg/dose or by 5-10 mg/day at weekly intervals; usual dose: 0.5-1 mg/kg/day; maximum dose: 2 mg/kg/day or 60 mg/day

Adults: Narcolepsy: 10 mg 2-3 times/day, up to 60 mg/day

Dosage Forms Methylphenidate hydrochloride:

Tablet: 5 mg, 10 mg, 20 mg

Tablet, sustained release: 20 mg

methylphenobarbital *see* mephobarbital *on page 356*

methylphenylethylhydantoin *see* mephenytoin *on page 356*

methylphenyl isoxazolyl penicillin *see* oxacillin *on page 420*

methylphytyl napthoquinone *see* phytonadione *on page 451*

methylprednisolone (meth il pred NIS oh lone)

Synonyms 6-α-methylprednisolone

U.S./Canadian Brand Names Adlone® Injection; A-methaPred® Injection; depMedalone® Injection; Depoject® Injection; Depo-Medrol® Injection; Depopred® Injection; D-Med® Injection; Duralone® Injection; Medralone® Injection; Medrol® Oral; Medrol® Veriderm® Cream (Can); M-Prednisol® Injection; Solu-Medrol® Injection

Therapeutic Category Adrenal Corticosteroid

Use Anti-inflammatory or immunosuppressant agent in the treatment of a variety of diseases including those of hematologic, allergic, inflammatory, neoplastic, and autoimmune origin

Usual Dosage Methylprednisolone sodium succinate is highly soluble and has a rapid effect by I.M. and I.V. routes. Methylprednisolone acetate has a low solubility and has a sustained I.M. effect.

Children:
- Anti-inflammatory or immunosuppressive: Oral, I.M., I.V. (sodium succinate): 0.16-0.8 mg/kg/day or 5-25 mg/m²/day in divided doses every 6-12 hours
- Status asthmaticus: I.V. (sodium succinate): Loading dose: 2 mg/kg/dose, then 0.5-1 mg/kg/dose every 6 hours for up to 5 days
- Lupus nephritis: I.V. (sodium succinate): 30 mg/kg every other day for 6 doses

Adults:
- Anti-inflammatory or immunosuppressive: Oral: 4-48 mg/day to start, followed by gradual reduction in dosage to the lowest possible level consistent with maintaining an adequate clinical response
- I.M. (sodium succinate): 10-80 mg/day once daily
- I.M. (acetate): 40-120 mg every 1-2 weeks
- I.V. (sodium succinate): 10-40 mg over a period of several minutes and repeated I.V. or I.M. at intervals depending on clinical response; when high dosages are needed, administer 30 mg/kg over a period of 10-20 minutes and may be repeated every 4-6 hours for 48 hours
- Status asthmaticus: I.V. (sodium succinate): Loading dose: 2 mg/kg/dose, then 0.5-1 mg/kg/dose every hours for up to 5 days
- Lupus nephritis:
  - I.V. (sodium succinate): 1 g/day for 3 days
- Intra-articular (acetate):
  - Large joints: 20-80 mg
  - Small joints: 4-10 mg
- Intralesional (acetate): 20-60 mg

Dosage Forms

Injection:
- As acetate: 20 mg/mL (5 mL, 10 mL); 40 mg/mL (1 mL, 5 mL, 10 mL); 80 mg/mL (1 mL, 5 mL)
- As sodium succinate: 40 mg (1 mL, 3 mL); 125 mg (2 mL, 5 mL); 500 mg (1 mL, 4 mL, 8 mL, 20 mL); 1000 mg (1 mL, 8 mL, 50 mL); 2000 mg (30.6 mL)

Tablet: 2 mg, 4 mg, 8 mg, 16 mg, 24 mg, 32 mg
- Dose pack: 4 mg (21s)

6-α-methylprednisolone *see* methylprednisolone *on previous page*

4-methylpyrazole *see* fomepizole *on page 252*

methyltestosterone (meth il tes TOS te rone)

U.S./Canadian Brand Names Android®; Oreton® Methyl; Testred®; Virilon®

Therapeutic Category Androgen

Use
- Male: Hypogonadism; delayed puberty; impotence and climacteric symptoms
- Female: Palliative treatment of metastatic breast cancer; postpartum breast pain and/or engorgement

Usual Dosage Adults:
- Male:
  - Oral: 10-40 mg/day
  - Buccal: 5-20 mg/day
- Female:
  - Breast pain/engorgement:
    - Oral: 80 mg/day for 3-5 days
    - Buccal: 40 mg/day for 3-5 days
  - Breast cancer:
    - Oral: 200 mg/day

(Continued)

methyltestosterone *(Continued)*

Buccal: 100 mg/day

Dosage Forms

Capsule: 10 mg

Tablet: 10 mg, 25 mg

Buccal: 5 mg, 10 mg

methysergide (meth i SER jide)

U.S./Canadian Brand Names Sansert®

Therapeutic Category Ergot Alkaloid and Derivative

Use Prophylaxis of vascular headache

Usual Dosage Oral: 4-8 mg/day with meals; if no improvement is noted after 3 weeks, drug is unlikely to be beneficial; must not be administered continuously for longer than 6 months, and a drug-free interval of 3-4 weeks must follow each 6-month course; dosage should be tapered over the 2- to 3-week period before drug discontinuation to avoid rebound headaches

Dosage Forms Tablet, as maleate: 2 mg

Meticorten® *see* prednisone *on page 472*

Metimyd® Ophthalmic *see* sulfacetamide and prednisolone *on page 540*

metipranolol (met i PRAN oh lol)

U.S./Canadian Brand Names OptiPranolol® Ophthalmic

Therapeutic Category Beta-Adrenergic Blocker

Use Agent for lowering intraocular pressure

Usual Dosage Adults: Ophthalmic: 1 drop in the affected eye(s) twice daily

Dosage Forms Solution, ophthalmic, as hydrochloride: 0.3% (5 mL, 10 mL)

Metizol® Tablet *(Discontinued)* *see page 700*

metoclopramide (met oh kloe PRA mide)

U.S./Canadian Brand Names Apo®-Metoclop (Can); Clopra®; Maxeran® (Can); Maxolon®; Octamide®; Reglan®

Therapeutic Category Gastrointestinal Agent, Prokinetic

Use Gastroesophageal reflux; prevention of nausea associated with chemotherapy; facilitates intubation of the small intestine and symptomatic treatment of diabetic gastric stasis

Usual Dosage

Children:

- Gastroesophageal reflux: Oral: 0.1 mg/kg/dose up to 4 times/day; efficacy of continuing metoclopramide beyond 12 weeks in reflux has not been determined; total daily dose should not exceed 0.5 mg/kg/day
- Gastrointestinal hypomotility: Oral, I.M., I.V.: 0.1 mg/kg/dose up to 4 times/day, not to exceed 0.5 mg/kg/day
- Antiemetic: I.V.: 1-2 mg/kg 30 minutes before chemotherapy and every 2-4 hours
- Facilitate intubation: I.V.: <6 years: 0.1 mg/kg; 6-14 years: 2.5-5 mg

Adults:

- Stasis/reflux: Oral: 10-15 mg/dose up to 4 times/day 30 minutes before meals or food and at bedtime; efficacy of continuing metoclopramide beyond 12 weeks in reflux has not been determined
- Gastrointestinal hypomotility: Oral, I.M., I.V.: 10 mg 30 minutes before each meal and at bedtime
- Antiemetic: I.V.: 1-2 mg/kg 30 minutes before chemotherapy and every 2-4 hours
- Facilitate intubation: I.V.: 10 mg

Dosage Forms

Injection: 5 mg/mL (2 mL, 10 mL, 30 mL, 50 mL, 100 mL)

Solution, oral, concentrated: 10 mg/mL (10 mL, 30 mL)

Syrup, sugar free: 5 mg/5 mL (10 mL, 480 mL)

Tablet: 5 mg, 10 mg

metocurine iodide (met oh KYOOR een EYE oh dide)

Synonyms dimethyl tubocurarine iodide

U.S./Canadian Brand Names Metubine® Iodide

Therapeutic Category Skeletal Muscle Relaxant

Use Adjunct to anesthesia to induce skeletal muscle relaxation

Usual Dosage I.V.:

Children:

Chronic respiratory paralysis in neonates: Start 0.25-0.5 mg/kg/dose (repeat once if paralysis is not achieved in 3 minutes); maintenance: repeat previous dose as soon as movement is observed. The dose should be titrated to achieve a dosage interval of 3-4 hours, then plateau at 10-20 mg/kg/24 hours

Neuromuscular blockade for surgery: Initial: 0.2-0.4 mg/kg/dose; maintenance: 0.1-0.25 mg/kg/dose every 25-90 minutes

Adults:

Surgery: Initial: 0.2-0.4 mg/kg; supplement dose: 0.5-1 mg; use of anesthetics that potentiate effect of neuromuscular blocking drug requires less metocurine

Electric shock therapy: 1.75-5.5 mg

Dosage Forms Injection: 2 mg/mL (20 mL)

metolazone (me TOLE a zone)

U.S./Canadian Brand Names Mykrox®; Zaroxolyn®

Therapeutic Category Diuretic, Miscellaneous

Use Management of mild to moderate hypertension; treatment of edema in congestive heart failure, nephrotic syndrome, and impaired renal function

Usual Dosage Oral:

Children: 0.2-0.4 mg/kg/day divided every 12-24 hours

Adults:

Edema: 5-20 mg/dose every 24 hours

Hypertension: 2.5-5 mg/dose every 24 hours

Dosage Forms Tablet:

Zaroxolyn® (slow acting): 2.5 mg, 5 mg, 10 mg

Mykrox® (rapidly acting): 0.5 mg

Metopirone® Tablet *(Discontinued)* *see page 700*

metoprolol (me toe PROE lole)

U.S./Canadian Brand Names Apo-Metoprolol® (Can); Betaloc® (Can); Betaloc Durules® (Can); Lopressor®; Novo-Metoprolol® (Can); Nu-Metop (Can); Toprol XL®

Therapeutic Category Beta-Adrenergic Blocker

Use Treatment of hypertension and angina pectoris; prevention of myocardial infarction; selective inhibitor of $beta_1$-adrenergic receptors

Usual Dosage Safety and efficacy in children have not been established.

Children: Oral: 1-5 mg/kg/24 hours divided twice daily; allow 3 days between dose adjustments

Adults:

Oral: 100-450 mg/day in 2-3 divided doses, begin with 50 mg twice daily and increase doses at weekly intervals to desired effect

I.V.: 5 mg every 2 minutes for 3 doses in early treatment of myocardial infarction; thereafter administer 50 mg orally every 6 hours 15 minutes after last I.V. dose and continue for 48 hours; then administer a maintenance dose of 100 mg twice daily

Dosage Forms

Metoprolol succinate:

Tablet, sustained release: 50 mg, 100 mg, 200 mg

Metoprolol tartrate:

Injection: 1 mg/mL (5 mL)

Tablet: 50 mg, 100 mg

Metra® *(Discontinued)* *see page 700*

Metreton® Ophthalmic *see* prednisolone (ophthalmic) *on page 471*

Metrocream™ (Can) *see* metronidazole *on this page*

Metrodin® *see* urofollitropin *on page 592*

MetroGel® Topical *see* metronidazole *on this page*

MetroGel®-Vaginal *see* metronidazole *on this page*

Metro I.V.® Injection *see* metronidazole *on this page*

metronidazole (me troe NI da zole)

U.S./Canadian Brand Names Apo®-Metronidazole (Can); Flagyl® Oral; Metrocream™ (Can); MetroGel® Topical; MetroGel®-Vaginal; Metro I.V.® Injection; Nidagel™ (Can); Noritate® (Can); Novo-Nidazol® (Can); Protostat® Oral; TriKacide® (Can)

Therapeutic Category Amebicide; Antibiotic, Topical; Antibiotic, Miscellaneous; Antiprotozoal

Use Treatment of susceptible anaerobic bacterial and protozoal infections in the following conditions: amebiasis (liver abscess, dysentery), giardiasis, symptomatic and asymptomatic trichomoniasis; skin and skin structure infections, CNS infections, intra-abdominal infections, and systemic anaerobic bacterial infections; topically for the treatment of acne rosacea; treatment of antibiotic-associated pseudomembranous colitis (AAPC) caused by *C. difficile*; bacterial vaginosis

Usual Dosage

Infants and Children:

- Amebiasis: Oral: 35-50 mg/kg/day in divided doses every 8 hours
- Other parasitic infections: Oral: 15-30 mg/kg/day in divided doses every 8 hours
- Anaerobic infections: Oral, I.V.: 30 mg/kg/day in divided doses every 6 hours
- *Clostridium difficile* (antibiotic-associated colitis): Oral: 20 mg/kg/day divided every 6 hours
- Maximum dose: 2 g/day

Adults:

- Amebiasis: Oral: 500-750 mg every 8 hours
- Other parasitic infections: Oral: 250 mg every 8 hours or 2 g as a single dose
- Anaerobic infections: Oral, I.V.: 30 mg/kg/day in divided doses every 6 hours; not to exceed 4 g/day
- AAPC: Oral: 250-500 mg 3-4 times/day for 10-14 days
- Topical: Apply a thin film twice daily to affected areas
- Vaginal: One applicatorful in vagina each morning and evening or given once daily at bedtime

Dosage Forms

Capsule: 375 mg
Cream: 0.75% (45 g); 1% (30 g)
Gel, topical: 0.75% [7.5 mg/mL] (30 g)
Gel, vaginal: 0.75% (5 g applicator delivering 37.5 mg in 70 g tube)
Injection, ready to use: 5 mg/mL (100 mL)
Lotion: 0.75%
Powder for injection, as hydrochloride: 500 mg
Tablet: 250 mg, 500 mg
Tablet, extended release: 750 mg

Metubine® Iodide *see* metocurine iodide *on previous page*

metyrapone (me TEER a pone)

Therapeutic Category Diagnostic Agent

Use Diagnostic test for hypothalamic-pituitary ACTH function

Usual Dosage Oral:

Children: 15 mg/kg every 4 hours for 6 doses; minimum dose: 250 mg
Adults: 750 mg every 4 hours for 6 doses

Dosage Forms Capsule, as tartrate: 250 mg

metyrosine (me TYE roe seen)

Synonyms AMPT; OGMT

U.S./Canadian Brand Names Demser®

Therapeutic Category Tyrosine Hydroxylase Inhibitor

Use Short-term management of pheochromocytoma before surgery, long-term management when surgery is contraindicated or when malignant

Usual Dosage Children >12 years and Adults: Oral: Initial: 250 mg 4 times/day, increased by 250-500 mg/day up to 4 g/day; maintenance: 2-3 g/day in 4 divided doses; for preoperative preparation, administer optimum effective dosage for 5-7 days

Dosage Forms Capsule: 250 mg

Mevacor® *see* lovastatin *on page 341*

Meval® (Can) *see* diazepam *on page 173*

mevinolin *see* lovastatin *on page 341*

mexiletine (MEKS i le teen)

U.S./Canadian Brand Names Mexitil®

Therapeutic Category Antiarrhythmic Agent, Class I-B

Use Management of serious ventricular arrhythmias; suppression of PVCs

Unlabeled use: Diabetic neuropathy

Usual Dosage Oral:

Children: Range: 1.4-5 mg/kg/dose (mean: 3.3 mg/kg/dose) administered every 8 hours; start with lower initial dose and increase according to effects and serum concentrations

Adults: Initial: 200 mg every 8 hours (may load with 400 mg if necessary); adjust dose every 2-3 days; usual dose: 200-300 mg every 8 hours; maximum dose: 1.2 g/day (some patients respond to every 12-hour dosing)

Dosage Forms Capsule: 150 mg, 200 mg, 250 mg

Mexitil® *see* mexiletine *on this page*

Mezlin® *see* mezlocillin *on this page*

mezlocillin (mez loe SIL in)

U.S./Canadian Brand Names Mezlin®

Therapeutic Category Penicillin

Use Treatment of infections caused by susceptible gram-negative aerobic bacilli (*Klebsiella*, *Proteus*, *Escherichia coli*, *Enterobacter*, *Pseudomonas aeruginosa*, *Serratia*) involving the skin and skin structure, bone and joint, respiratory tract, urinary tract, gastrointestinal tract, as well as septicemia

Usual Dosage I.M., I.V.:

Children: 200-300 mg/kg/day divided every 4-6 hours; maximum: 24 g/day

Adults:

Uncomplicated urinary tract infection: 1.5-2 g every 6 hours

Serious infections: 3-4 g every 4-6 hours

Dosage Forms Powder for injection, as sodium: 1 g, 2 g, 3 g, 4 g, 20 g

Miacalcin® *see* calcitonin *on page 88*

Miacalcin® Nasal Spray *see* calcitonin *on page 88*

Micanol® Cream *see* anthralin *on page 38*

Micardis® *see* telmisartan *on page 549*

Micatin® Topical [OTC] *see* miconazole *on this page*

miconazole (mi KON a zole)

U.S./Canadian Brand Names Absorbine® Antifungal Foot Powder [OTC]; Breezee® Mist Antifungal [OTC]; Femizol-M® [OTC]; Fungoid® Creme; Fungoid® Tincture; Lotrimin® AF Powder [OTC]; Lotrimin® AF Spray Liquid [OTC]; Lotrimin® AF Spray Powder [OTC]; Maximum Strength Desenex® Antifungal Cream [OTC]; Micatin® Topical [OTC];

(Continued)

miconazole *(Continued)*

Monistat-Derm™ Topical; Monistat i.v.™ Injection; Monistat™ Vaginal; M-Zole® 7 Dual Pack [OTC]; Ony-Clear® Spray; Prescription Strength Desenex® [OTC]; Zeasorb-AF® Powder [OTC]

Therapeutic Category Antifungal Agent

Use

I.V.: Treatment of severe systemic fungal infections and fungal meningitis due to susceptible *Cryptococcus* neoformans, *Candida albicans*, *Candida tropicalis*, *Candida parapsilosis*, *Coccidioides immitis*, and *Histoplasma capsulatum* that are refractory to standard treatment

Topical: Treatment of vulvovaginal candidiasis; topical treatment of superficial fungal infections

Usual Dosage

Children:

I.V.: 20-40 mg/kg/day divided every 8 hours

Topical: Apply twice daily for 2-4 weeks

Vaginal: Insert contents of one applicator of vaginal cream or 100 mg suppository at bedtime for 7 days, or 200 mg suppository at bedtime for 3 days

Adults:

I.T.: 20 mg every 3-7 days

I.V.: Candidiasis: 600-1800 mg/day divided every 8 hours

Topical: Apply twice daily for 2-4 weeks

Vaginal: Insert contents of one applicator of vaginal cream or 100 mg suppository at bedtime for 7 days, or 200 mg suppository at bedtime for 3 days

Coccidioidomycosis: 1800-3600 mg/day divided every 8 hours

Cryptococcosis: 1200-2400 mg/day divided every 8 hours

Paracoccidioidomycosis: 200-1200 mg/day divided every 8 hours

Dosage Forms Miconazole nitrate:

Cream:

Topical: 2% (15 g, 30 g, 56.7 g, 85 g)

Vaginal: 2% (45 g is equivalent to 7 doses)

Injection: 1% [10 mg/mL] (20 mL)

Lotion: 2% (30 mL, 60 mL)

Powder, topical: 2% (45 g, 90 g, 113 g)

Spray, topical: 2% (105 mL)

Suppository, vaginal: 100 mg (7s); 200 mg (3s)

Tincture: 2% with alcohol (7.39 mL, 29.57 mL)

MICRhoGAM™ *see* Rh_o(D) immune globulin (intramuscular) *on page 502*

microfibrillar collagen hemostat

(mye kro FI bri lar KOL la jen HEE moe stat)

Synonyms MCH

U.S./Canadian Brand Names Avitene®; Helistat®; Hemotene®

Therapeutic Category Hemostatic Agent

Use Adjunct to hemostasis when control of bleeding by ligature is ineffective or impractical

Usual Dosage Apply dry directly to source of bleeding

Dosage Forms

Fibrous: 1 g, 5 g

Nonwoven web: 70 mm x 70 mm x 1 mm; 70 mm x 35 mm x 1 mm

Sponge: 1" x 2" (10s); 3" x 4" (10s); 9" x 10" (5s)

Micro-K® 10 *see* potassium chloride *on page 464*

Micro-K® 10 Extencaps® *see* potassium chloride *on page 464*

Micro-K® LS *see* potassium chloride *on page 464*

Microlipid™ [OTC] *see* enteral nutritional products *on page 208*

Micronase® *see* glyburide *on page 263*

microNefrin® [OTC] *see* epinephrine *on page 209*

Micronor® *see* norethindrone *on page 406*

Microzide® *see* hydrochlorothiazide *on page 286*

Midamor® *see* amiloride *on page 26*

midazolam (MID aye zoe lam)

Synonyms midazolam hydrochloride

U.S./Canadian Brand Names Versed®

Therapeutic Category Benzodiazepine

Controlled Substance C-IV

Use Preoperative sedation; conscious sedation prior to diagnostic or radiographic procedures

Usual Dosage

Preoperative sedation: Children:

Oral:

<5 years: 0.5 mg/kg;

>5 years: 0.4-0.5 mg/kg; doses as high as 0.5-0.75 mg/kg have provided effective preanesthetic sedation

I.M.: 0.07-0.08 mg/kg 30 minutes to 1 hour before surgery; range: 0.05-0.1 mg/kg

I.V.: 0.035 mg/kg/dose, repeat over several minutes as required to achieve the desired sedative effect up to a total dose of 0.1-0.2 mg/kg or 5 mg total

Conscious sedation during mechanical ventilation:

Neonates: I.V. continuous infusion: 0.15-1 mcg/kg/minute

Children:

I.V.: 0.1-0.2 mg/kg; follow loading dose with a 1-2 mcg/kg/minute continuous infusion; titrate to the desired effect; range: 0.4-6 mcg/kg/minute

I.V. intermittent infusion: 0.05-0.2 mg/kg every 1-2 hours as needed

Conscious sedation for procedures:

Children:

Oral: 0.2-0.4 mg/kg; dose as high as 1 mg/kg have been used in younger (6 months to <6 years of age) and less cooperative patients; (maximum: 20 mg) 30-45 minutes before the procedure

Intranasal: 0.2-0.4 mg/kg (use undiluted 5 mg/mL injectable drug for intranasal administration)

I.V.: 0.05-0.1 mg/kg 3 minutes before procedure

Adolescents >12 years:

Sedation for procedure: I.V.: 0.5 mg every 3-4 minutes until effect achieved

Preoperative sedation: I.M.: 0.07-0.08 mg/kg 30-60 minutes before surgery; usual dose: 5 mg

Conscious sedation: I.V.: Initial: 0.5-2 mg; slowly titrate to effect by repeating doses every 2-3 minutes; usual total dose: 2.5-5 mg

Adults, healthy <60 years: Some patients respond to doses as low as 1 mg; no more than 2.5 mg should be administered over a period of 2 minutes. Additional doses of midazolam may be administered after a 2-minute waiting period and evaluation of sedation after each dose increment. A total dose >5 mg is generally not needed. If narcotics or other CNS depressants are administered concomitantly, the midazolam dose should be reduced by 30%.

Dosage Forms

Injection, as hydrochloride: 1 mg/mL (2 mL, 5 mL, 10 mL); 5 mg/mL (1 mL, 2 mL, 5 mL, 10 mL)

Syrup, as hydrochloride: 2 mg/mL (118 mL)

midazolam hydrochloride *see* midazolam *on this page*

Midchlor® *see* acetaminophen, isometheptene, and dichloralphenazone *on page 6*

midodrine (MI doe dreen)

U.S./Canadian Brand Names ProAmatine

Therapeutic Category Alpha-Adrenergic Agonist

Use Treatment of symptomatic orthostatic hypotension in patients whose lives are considerably impaired despite standard clinical care.

Usual Dosage Adults: Oral: 10 mg 3 times/day (every 3-4 hours); dosing should take place during daytime hours when the patient needs to be upright, pursuing activities of daily living; a suggested dosing schedule is as follows:

Dose 1: Shortly before or upon rising in the morning

Dose 2: At midday

Dose 3: In the late afternoon (not later than 6 PM)

Dosage Forms Tablet, as hydrochloride: 2.5 mg, 5 mg

Midol® IB [OTC] *see* ibuprofen *on page 300*

Midol® PM [OTC] *see* acetaminophen and diphenhydramine *on page 5*

Midrin® *see* acetaminophen, isometheptene, and dichloralphenazone *on page 6*

Miflex® Tablet *(Discontinued)* *see page 700*

miglitol (MIG li tol)

U.S./Canadian Brand Names Glyset®

Therapeutic Category Antidiabetic Agent, Oral

Use As an adjunct to diet to lower blood glucose in patients with noninsulin-dependent diabetes mellitus (NIDDM)

Usual Dosage Adults: Oral: 25 mg 3 times/day with the first bite of food at each meal; dose may be increased to 50 mg 3 times/day after 4-8 weeks; maximum recommended dose: 100 mg 3 times/day

Dosage Forms Tablet: 25 mg, 50 mg, 100 mg

Migranal® Nasal Spray *see* dihydroergotamine *on page 180*

Migratine® *see* acetaminophen, isometheptene, and dichloralphenazone *on page 6*

MIH *see* procarbazine *on page 476*

Miles Nervine® Caplets [OTC] *see* diphenhydramine *on page 185*

milk of magnesia *see* magnesium hydroxide *on page 345*

Milontin® *see* phensuximide *on page 445*

Milophene® *see* clomiphene *on page 138*

Milprem® *(Discontinued)* *see page 700*

milrinone (MIL ri none)

U.S./Canadian Brand Names Primacor®

Therapeutic Category Cardiovascular Agent, Other

Use Short-term I.V. therapy of congestive heart failure

Usual Dosage Adults: I.V.: Loading dose: 50 mcg/kg administered over 10 minutes, then 0.375-0.75 mcg/kg/min as a continuous infusion for a total daily dose of 0.59-1.13 mg/kg

Dosage Forms Injection, as lactate: 1 mg/mL (5 mL, 10 mL, 20 mL)

Miltown® *see* meprobamate *on page 356*

Minidyne® [OTC] *see* povidone-iodine *on page 467*

Mini-Gamulin® Rh *see* Rh_o(D) immune globulin (intramuscular) *on page 502*

Minims® Pilocarpine (Can) *see* pilocarpine *on page 451*

Minipress® *see* prazosin *on page 470*

Minitran® Patch *see* nitroglycerin *on page 404*

Minizide® *see* prazosin and polythiazide *on page 470*

Minocin® *see* minocycline *on this page*

Minocin® IV Injection *see* minocycline *on this page*

Minocin® Tablet *(Discontinued)* *see page 700*

minocycline (mi noc SYE kleen)

U.S./Canadian Brand Names Apo-Minocycline® (Can); Dynacin® Oral; Minocin®; Minocin® IV Injection; Syn-Minocycline® (Can); Vectrin®

Therapeutic Category Tetracycline Derivative

Use Treatment of susceptible bacterial infections of both gram-negative and gram-positive organisms; acne

Usual Dosage

Children 8-12 years: 4 mg/kg stat, then 4 mg/kg/day (maximum: 200 mg/day) in divided doses every 12 hours

Adults:

Infection: Oral, I.V.: 200 mg stat, 100 mg every 12 hours

Acne: Oral: 50 mg 1-3 times/day

Dosage Forms Minocycline hydrochloride:

Capsule: 50 mg, 100 mg

Capsule (Dynacin®): 50 mg, 100 mg

Capsule, pellet-filled (Minocin®): 50 mg, 100 mg

Injection (Minocin® IV): 100 mg

Suspension, oral (Minocin®): 50 mg/5 mL (60 mL)

minoxidil (mi NOKS i dil)

U.S./Canadian Brand Names Apo®-Gain (Can); Gen-Minoxidil (Can); Loniten® Oral; Minoxigaine™ (Can); Rogaine® Topical

Therapeutic Category Topical Skin Product; Vasodilator

Use Management of severe hypertension; topically for management of alopecia or male pattern alopecia

Usual Dosage

Children <12 years: Hypertension: Oral: Initial: 0.1-0.2 mg/kg once daily; maximum: 5 mg/day; increase gradually every 3 days; usual dosage: 0.25-1 mg/kg/day in 1-2 divided doses; maximum: 50 mg/day

Adults:

Hypertension: Oral: Initial: 5 mg once daily, increase gradually every 3 days; usual dose: 10-40 mg/day in 1-2 divided doses; maximum: 100 mg/day

Alopecia: Topical: Apply twice daily

Dosage Forms

Solution, topical: 2% = 20 mg/metered dose (60 mL); 5% = 50 mg/metered dose (60 mL)

Tablet: 2.5 mg, 10 mg

Minoxigaine™ (Can) *see* minoxidil *on this page*

Mintezol® *see* thiabendazole *on page 560*

Minute-Gel® *see* fluoride *on page 244*

Miocarpine® (Can) *see* pilocarpine *on page 451*

Miochol® *(Discontinued)* *see page 700*

Miochol-E® *see* acetylcholine *on page 8*

Miostat® Intraocular *see* carbachol *on page 97*

Miradon® (Can) *see* anisotropine *on page 38*

Mirapex® *see* pramipexole *on page 468*

mirtazapine (mir TAZ a peen)

U.S./Canadian Brand Names Remeron®

Therapeutic Category Antidepressant, Selective Serotonin Reuptake Inhibitor

(Continued)

mirtazapine *(Continued)*

Use Treatment of depression, works through noradrenergic and serotonergic pharmacologic action

Usual Dosage Adults: Oral: Initial: 15 mg/day, then 15-45 mg/day

Dosage Forms Tablet: 15 mg, 30 mg

misoprostol (mye soe PROST ole)

U.S./Canadian Brand Names Cytotec®

Therapeutic Category Prostaglandin

Use Prevention of NSAID-induced gastric ulcers

Usual Dosage Oral: 200 mcg 4 times/day with food

Dosage Forms Tablet: 100 mcg, 200 mcg

misoprostol and diclofenac *see* diclofenac and misoprostol *on page 176*

Mithracin® *see* plicamycin *on page 456*

mithramycin *see* plicamycin *on page 456*

mitomycin (mye toe MYE sin)

Synonyms mitomycin-c; MTC

U.S./Canadian Brand Names Mutamycin®

Therapeutic Category Antineoplastic Agent

Use Therapy of disseminated adenocarcinoma of stomach, colon, or pancreas in combination with other approved chemotherapeutic agents; bladder cancer, breast cancer

Usual Dosage Children and Adults (refer to individual protocols): I.V.: 10-20 mg/m^2/dose every 6-8 weeks, or 2 mg/m^2/day for 5 days, stop for 2 days then repeat; subsequent doses should be adjusted to platelet and leukocyte response

Dosage Forms Powder for injection: 5 mg, 20 mg, 40 mg

mitomycin-c *see* mitomycin *on this page*

mitotane (MYE toe tane)

Synonyms o,p′-DDD

U.S./Canadian Brand Names Lysodren®

Therapeutic Category Antineoplastic Agent

Use Treatment of inoperable adrenal cortical carcinoma

Usual Dosage Adults: Oral: 8-10 g/day in 3-4 divided doses; dose is changed based on side effects with aim of administering as high a dose as tolerated

Dosage Forms Tablet: 500 mg

mitoxantrone (mye toe ZAN trone)

Synonyms DHAD

U.S./Canadian Brand Names Novantrone®

Therapeutic Category Antineoplastic Agent

Use FDA approved for remission-induction therapy of acute nonlymphocytic leukemia (ANLL); mitoxantrone is also active against other various leukemias, lymphoma, and breast cancer, and moderately active against pediatric sarcoma

Usual Dosage I.V. (refer to individual protocols):

Leukemias:

- Children ≤2 years: 0.4 mg/kg/day once daily for 3-5 days
- Children >2 years and Adults: 8-12 mg/m^2/day once daily for 5 days or 12 mg/m^2/day once daily for 3 days

Solid tumors:

- Children: 18-20 mg/m^2 every 3-4 weeks
- Adults: 12-14 mg/m^2 every 3-4 weeks

Dosage Forms Injection, as base: 2 mg/mL (10 mL, 12.5 mL, 15 mL)

Mitran® Oral *see* chlordiazepoxide *on page 116*

Mitrolan® Chewable Tablet [OTC] *see* calcium polycarbophil *on page 93*

Mivacron® *see* mivacurium *on this page*

mivacurium (mye va KYOO ree um)

U.S./Canadian Brand Names Mivacron®

Therapeutic Category Skeletal Muscle Relaxant

Use Short-acting nondepolarizing neuromuscular blocking agent; an adjunct to general anesthesia; facilitates endotracheal intubation; provides skeletal muscle relaxation during surgery or mechanical ventilation

Usual Dosage I.V.:

Children 2-12 years: 0.2 mg/kg over 5-15 seconds; continuous infusion: 14 mcg/kg

Adults: Initial: 0.15 mg/kg administered over 5-15 seconds

Dosage Forms Mivacurium chloride:

Infusion, in D_5W: 0.5 mg/mL (50 mL)

Injection: 2 mg/mL (5 mL, 10 mL)

MK594 *see* losartan *on page 340*

MMR *see* measles, mumps and rubella vaccines, combined *on page 350*

M-M-R® II *see* measles, mumps and rubella vaccines, combined *on page 350*

Moban® *see* molindone *on next page*

Mobenol® (Can) *see* tolbutamide *on page 570*

Mobidin® *see* magnesium salicylate *on page 346*

Moctanin® *see* monoctanoin *on page 381*

modafinil (moe DAF i nil)

U.S./Canadian Brand Names Provigil®

Therapeutic Category Central Nervous System Stimulant, Nonamphetamine

Controlled Substance C-IV

Use Indicated to improve wakefulness in patients with excessive daytime sleepiness associated with narcolepsy

Usual Dosage Adults: Oral: Initial: 200 mg as a single daily dose

Dosage Forms Tablet: 100 mg, 200 mg

Modane® Bulk [OTC] *see* psyllium *on page 488*

Modane® Soft [OTC] *see* docusate *on page 191*

Modecate® (Can) *see* fluphenazine *on page 247*

Modecate® Enanthate (Can) *see* fluphenazine *on page 247*

Modicon™ *see* ethinyl estradiol and norethindrone *on page 224*

modified Dakin's solution *see* sodium hypochlorite solution *on page 528*

Moditen® Hydrochloride (Can) *see* fluphenazine *on page 247*

Moducal® [OTC] *see* glucose polymers *on page 262*

Modulon® (Can) *see* trimebutine *(Canada only) on page 582*

Moduretic® *see* amiloride and hydrochlorothiazide *on page 26*

moexipril (mo EKS i pril)

U.S./Canadian Brand Names Univasc®

Therapeutic Category Angiotensin-Converting Enzyme (ACE) Inhibitor

Use Treatment of hypertension, alone or in combination with thiazide diuretics

Usual Dosage Oral:

Patients not receiving diuretics: Initial: 7.5 mg 1 hour prior to meals once daily; if antihypertensive effect diminishes toward end of dosing interval, increase or divide dose; maintenance dose of 7.5-30 mg/day in 1 or 2 divided doses

(Continued)

moexipril *(Continued)*

Patients receiving diuretics: Discontinue diuretic 2-3 days before starting moexipril to avoid symptomatic hypotension; if blood pressure is not controlled, resume diuretic therapy; if diuretic cannot be held, initiate moexipril at 3.75 mg/day

Dosage Forms Tablet, as hydrochloride: 7.5 mg, 15 mg

moexipril and hydrochlorothiazide

(mo EKS i pril & hye droe klor oh THYE a zide)

U.S./Canadian Brand Names Uniretic™

Therapeutic Category Angiotensin-Converting Enzyme (ACE) Inhibitor; Diuretic, Thiazide

Use Treatment of hypertension

Usual Dosage Adults: Oral: 7.5-30 mg of moexipril, taken either in a single or divided dose one hour before meals

Dosage Forms Tablet: Moexipril hydrochloride 7.5 mg and hydrochlorothiazide 12.5 mg; moexipril hydrochloride 15 mg and hydrochlorothiazide 25 mg

Moi-Stir® Solution [OTC] *see* saliva substitute *on page 514*

Moi-Stir® Swabsticks [OTC] *see* saliva substitute *on page 514*

Moisturel® Lotion *(Discontinued)* *see page 700*

Moisture® Ophthalmic Drops [OTC] *see* artificial tears *on page 47*

molindone (moe LIN done)

U.S./Canadian Brand Names Moban®

Therapeutic Category Antipsychotic Agent, Dihydroindoline

Use Management of psychotic disorder

Usual Dosage Oral: 50-75 mg/day; up to 225 mg/day

Dosage Forms Molindone hydrochloride:

Concentrate, oral: 20 mg/mL (120 mL)

Tablet: 5 mg, 10 mg, 25 mg, 50 mg, 100 mg

Mol-Iron® [OTC] *see* ferrous sulfate *on page 237*

Mollifene® Ear Wax Removing Formula [OTC] *see* carbamide peroxide *on page 98*

molybdenum injection *see* trace metals *on page 573*

Molypen® *see* trace metals *on page 573*

MOM *see* magnesium hydroxide *on page 345*

mometasone furoate (moe MET a sone FYOOR oh ate)

U.S./Canadian Brand Names Elocom (Can); Elocon®; Nasonex®

Therapeutic Category Corticosteroid, Topical

Use Relief of inflammatory and pruritic manifestations of corticosteroid-responsive dermatoses

Usual Dosage Topical: Apply to area once daily, do not use occlusive dressings

Dosage Forms Mometasone furoate:

Cream: 0.1% (15 g, 45 g)

Lotion: 0.1% (30 mL, 60 mL)

Ointment, topical: 0.1% (15 g, 45 g)

mom/mineral oil emulsion *see* magnesium hydroxide and mineral oil emulsion *on page 345*

monacolin k *see* lovastatin *on page 341*

Monafed® *see* guaifenesin *on page 267*

Monafed® DM *see* guaifenesin and dextromethorphan *on page 268*

***Monilia* skin test** *see Candida albicans* (*Monilia*) *on page 95*

Monistat-Derm™ Topical *see* miconazole *on page 373*

Monistat i.v.™ Injection *see* miconazole *on page 373*

Monistat™ Vaginal *see* miconazole *on page 373*

Monitan® (Can) *see* acebutolol *on page 3*

monobenzone (mon oh BEN zone)

U.S./Canadian Brand Names Benoquin®

Therapeutic Category Topical Skin Product

Use Final depigmentation in extensive vitiligo

Usual Dosage Adults: Topical: Apply 2-3 times/day

Dosage Forms Cream: 20% (35.4 g)

Monocete® Topical Liquid *(Discontinued)* *see page 700*

Monocid® *see* cefonicid *on page 106*

Monoclate-P® *see* antihemophilic factor (human) *on page 39*

monoclonal antibody *see* muromonab-CD3 *on page 385*

monoclonal antibody purified *see* factor IX, purified (human) *on page 230*

monoctanoin (mon OK ta noyn)

Synonyms monooctanoin

U.S./Canadian Brand Names Moctanin®

Therapeutic Category Gallstone Dissolution Agent

Use Solubilize cholesterol gallstones that are retained in the biliary tract after cholecystectomy

Usual Dosage Administer via T-tube into common bile duct at rate of 3-5 mL/hour at pressure of 10 mL water for 7-21 days

Dosage Forms Solution: 120 mL

Monodox® *see* doxycycline *on page 197*

Mono-Gesic® *see* salsalate *on page 515*

Monoket® *see* isosorbide mononitrate *on page 316*

Mononine® *see* factor IX, purified (human) *on page 230*

monooctanoin *see* monoctanoin *on this page*

Monopril® *see* fosinopril *on page 253*

montelukast (mon te LOO kast)

U.S./Canadian Brand Names Singulair®

Therapeutic Category Leukotriene Receptor Antagonist

Use Prophylaxis and chronic treatment of asthma in adults and children ≥6 years

Usual Dosage Oral:
- Children 6-14 years: 5 mg once daily
- Children >14 years and Adults: 10 mg once daily

Dosage Forms Montelukast sodium:
- Tablet: 10 mg
- Tablet, chewable: 5 mg

Monurol™ *see* fosfomycin *on page 253*

more attenuated enders strain *see* measles virus vaccine, live *on page 350*

More-Dophilus® [OTC] *see* Lactobacillus *on page 324*

moricizine (mor EYE siz een)

U.S./Canadian Brand Names Ethmozine®

Therapeutic Category Antiarrhythmic Agent, Class I

(Continued)

moricizine *(Continued)*

Use Treatment of ventricular tachycardia and life-threatening ventricular arrhythmias; a Class I antiarrhythmic agent

Usual Dosage Adults: Oral: 200-300 mg every 8 hours, adjust dosage at 150 mg/day at 3-day intervals

Dosage Forms Tablet, as hydrochloride: 200 mg, 250 mg, 300 mg

Morphine-HP® (Can) *see* morphine sulfate *on this page*

morphine sulfate (MOR feen SUL fate)

Synonyms MS

U.S./Canadian Brand Names Astramorph™ PF Injection; Duramorph® Injection; Epimorph® (Can); M-Eslon® (Can); Morphine-HP® (Can); MS Contin® Oral; MS-IR® (Can); MSIR® Oral; OMS® Oral; Oramorph SR™ Oral; RMS® Rectal; Roxanol™ Oral; Roxanol SR™ Oral; Statex® (Can)

Therapeutic Category Analgesic, Narcotic

Controlled Substance C-II

Use Relief of moderate to severe acute and chronic pain; pain of myocardial infarction; relieves dyspnea of acute left ventricular failure and pulmonary edema; preanesthetic medication

Usual Dosage Doses should be titrated to appropriate effect; when changing routes of administration in chronically treated patients, please note that oral doses are approximately $^1/_6$ as effective as parenteral dose

Infants and Children:

Oral: Tablet and solution (prompt-release): 0.2-0.5 mg/kg/dose every 4-6 hours as needed; tablet (controlled-release): 0.3-0.6 mg/kg/dose every 12 hours

I.M., I.V., S.C.: 0.1-0.2 mg/kg/dose every 2-4 hours as needed; usual maximum: 15 mg/dose; may initiate at 0.05 mg/kg/dose

I.V., S.C. continuous infusion: Sickle cell or cancer pain: 0.025-2 mg/kg/hour; postoperative pain: 0.01-0.04 mg/kg/hour

Sedation/analgesia for procedures: I.V.: 0.05-0.1 mg/kg 5 minutes before the procedure

Adolescents >12 years: Sedation/analgesia for procedures: I.V.: 3-4 mg and repeat in 5 minutes if necessary

Adults:

Oral: Prompt-release: 10-30 mg every 4 hours as needed; controlled release: 15-30 mg every 8-12 hours

I.M., I.V., S.C.: 2.5-20 mg/dose every 2-6 hours as needed; usual: 10 mg/dose every 4 hours as needed

I.V., S.C. continuous infusion: 0.8-10 mg/hour; may increase depending on pain relief/adverse effects; usual range up to 80 mg/hour

Epidural: Initial: 5 mg in lumbar region; if inadequate pain relief within 1 hour, administer 1-2 mg, maximum dose: 10 mg/24 hours

Intrathecal ($^1/_{10}$ of epidural dose): 0.2-1 mg/dose; repeat doses **not** recommended

Dosage Forms

Capsule (MSIR®): 15 mg, 30 mg

Capsule, sustained release (Kadian™): 20 mg, 50 mg, 100 mg

Injection: 0.5 mg/mL (10 mL); 1 mg/mL (10 mL, 30 mL, 60 mL); 2 mg/mL (1 mL, 2 mL, 60 mL); 3 mg/mL (50 mL); 4 mg/mL (1 mL, 2 mL); 5 mg/mL (1 mL, 30 mL); 8 mg/mL (1 mL, 2 mL); 10 mg/mL (1 mL, 2 mL, 10 mL); 15 mg/mL (1 mL, 2 mL, 20 mL); 25 mg/mL (4 mL, 10 mL, 20 mL, 40 mL); 50 mg/mL (10 mL, 20 mL, 40 mL)

Injection:

Preservative free (Astramorph™ PF, Duramorph®): 0.5 mg/mL (2 mL, 10 mL); 1 mg/mL (2 mL, 10 mL); 10 mg/mL (20 mL); 25 mg/mL (20 mL)

I.V. via PCA pump: 1 mg/mL (10 mL, 30 mL, 60 mL); 5 mg/mL (30 mL)

I.V. infusion preparation: 25 mg/mL (4 mL, 10 mL, 20 mL)

Solution, oral: 10 mg/5 mL (5 mL, 10 mL, 100 mL, 120 mL, 500 mL); 20 mg/5 mL (5 mL, 100 mL, 120 mL, 500 mL)

MSIR®: 10 mg/5 mL (5 mL, 120 mL, 500 mL); 20 mg/5 mL (5 mL 120 mL, 500 mL); 20 mg/mL (30 mL, 120 mL)
MS/L®: 100 mg/5 mL (120 mL) 20 mg/5 mL
OMS®: 20 mg/mL (30 mL, 120 mL)
Roxanol™: 10 mg/2.5 mL (2.5 mL); 20 mg/mL (1 mL, 1.5 mL, 30 mL, 120 mL, 240 mL)
Suppository, rectal: 5 mg, 10 mg, 20 mg, 30 mg
MS/S®, RMS®, Roxanol™: 5 mg, 10 mg, 20 mg, 30 mg
Tablet: 15 mg, 30 mg
MSIR®: 15 mg, 30 mg
Controlled release:
MS Contin®: 15 mg, 30 mg, 60 mg, 100 mg, 200 mg
Roxanol™ SR: 30 mg
Soluble: 10 mg, 15 mg, 30 mg
Sustained release (Oramorph SR™): 30 mg, 60 mg, 100 mg

morrhuate sodium (MOR yoo ate SOW dee um)

U.S./Canadian Brand Names Scleromate™

Therapeutic Category Sclerosing Agent

Use Treatment of small, uncomplicated varicose veins of the lower extremities

Usual Dosage I.V.:

Children 1-18 years: Esophageal hemorrhage: 2, 3, or 4 mL of 5% solution repeated every 3-4 days until bleeding is controlled, then every 6 weeks until varices obliterated

Adults: 50-250 mg, repeat at 5- to 7-day intervals (50-100 mg for small veins, 150-250 mg for large veins)

Dosage Forms Injection: 50 mg/mL (5 mL)

Motilium® (Can) *see* domperidone *(Canada only)* *on page 193*

Motofen® *see* difenoxin and atropine *on page 178*

Motrin® *see* ibuprofen *on page 300*

Motrin® IB [OTC] *see* ibuprofen *on page 300*

Motrin® IB Sinus [OTC] *see* pseudoephedrine and ibuprofen *on page 487*

Mouthkote® Solution [OTC] *see* saliva substitute *on page 514*

Moxam® Injection *(Discontinued)* *see page 700*

4-MP *see* fomepizole *on page 252*

6-MP *see* mercaptopurine *on page 357*

M-Prednisol® Injection *see* methylprednisolone *on page 368*

M-R-VAX® II *see* measles and rubella vaccines, combined *on page 350*

MS *see* morphine sulfate *on previous page*

MS Contin® Oral *see* morphine sulfate *on previous page*

MSD® Enteric Coated ASA (Can) *see* aspirin *on page 49*

MS-IR® (Can) *see* morphine sulfate *on previous page*

MSIR® Oral *see* morphine sulfate *on previous page*

MSTA *see* mumps skin test antigen *on next page*

MTC *see* mitomycin *on page 378*

M.T.E.-4® *see* trace metals *on page 573*

M.T.E.-5® *see* trace metals *on page 573*

M.T.E.-6® *see* trace metals *on page 573*

MTX *see* methotrexate *on page 364*

Muco-Fen-DM® *see* guaifenesin and dextromethorphan *on page 268*

Muco-Fen-LA® *see* guaifenesin *on page 267*

Mucomyst® *see* acetylcysteine *on page 8*

Mucoplex® [OTC] *see* vitamin B complex *on page 603*

Mucosil™ *see* acetylcysteine *on page 8*

MulTE-PAK-4® *see* trace metals *on page 573*

MulTE-PAK-5® *see* trace metals *on page 573*

Multipax® (Can) *see* hydroxyzine *on page 297*

multiple sulfonamides *see* sulfadiazine, sulfamethazine, and sulfamerazine *on page 541*

Multitest CMI® *see* skin test antigens, multiple *on page 524*

multivitamins/fluoride *see* vitamin, multiple (pediatric) *on page 606*

Multi Vit® Drops [OTC] *see* vitamin, multiple (pediatric) *on page 606*

mumps skin test antigen (mumpz skin test AN ti jen)

Synonyms MSTA

Therapeutic Category Diagnostic Agent

Use Assess the status of cell-mediated immunity

Usual Dosage Children and Adults: 0.1 mL intradermally into flexor surface of the forearm; examine reaction site in 24-48 hours; a positive reaction is ≥1.5 mm diameter induration

Dosage Forms Injection: 1 mL (10 tests)

Mumpsvax® *see* mumps virus vaccine, live, attenuated *on this page*

mumps virus vaccine, live, attenuated

(mumpz VYE rus vak SEEN, live, a ten YOO ate ed)

U.S./Canadian Brand Names Mumpsvax®

Therapeutic Category Vaccine, Live Virus

Use Immunization against mumps in children ≥12 months and adults

Usual Dosage S.C.: 1 vial (5000 units) in outer aspect of the upper arm

Dosage Forms Injection: Single dose

mupirocin (myoo PEER oh sin)

Synonyms pseudomonic acid A

U.S./Canadian Brand Names Bactroban®; Bactroban® Nasal

Therapeutic Category Antibiotic, Topical

Use Topical treatment of impetigo caused by *Staphylococcus aureus* and *Streptococcus pyogenes*; also effective for the topical treatment of folliculitis, furunculosis, minor wounds, burns, and ulcers caused by susceptible organisms; used as a prophylactic agent applied to intravenous catheter exit sites; used for eradication of *S. aureus* from nasal and perineal carriage sites

Usual Dosage

Children and Adults: Topical: Apply small amount to affected area 2-5 times/day for 5-14 days

Children ≥12 years and Adults: Intranasal: ~½ of a single use tube (0.5 g) to each nostril twice daily for 5 days

Dosage Forms Mupirocin calcium: Ointment:

Intranasal: 2% (1 g single use tube)

Topical: 2% (15 g)

Murine® Ear Drops [OTC] *see* carbamide peroxide *on page 98*

Murine® Plus Ophthalmic [OTC] *see* tetrahydrozoline *on page 556*

Murine® Solution [OTC] *see* artificial tears *on page 47*

Muro 128® Ophthalmic [OTC] *see* sodium chloride *on page 526*

Murocel® Ophthalmic Solution [OTC] *see* artificial tears *on page 47*

Murocoll-2® Ophthalmic *see* phenylephrine and scopolamine *on page 447*

muromonab-CD3 (myoo roe MOE nab see dee three)

Synonyms monoclonal antibody; OKT3

U.S./Canadian Brand Names Orthoclone® OKT3

Therapeutic Category Immunosuppressant Agent

Use Treatment of acute allograft rejection in renal transplant patients; effective in reversing acute hepatic, cardiac, and bone marrow transplant rejection episodes resistant to conventional treatment

Usual Dosage I.V. (refer to individual protocols):

Children <30 kg: 2.5 mg/day once daily for 10-14 days

Adults: 5 mg/day once daily for 10-14 days

Children and Adults: Methylprednisolone sodium succinate 1 mg/kg I.V. administered prior to first muromonab-CD3 administration and I.V. hydrocortisone sodium succinate 50-100 mg administered 30 minutes after administration are strongly recommended to decrease the incidence of reactions to the first dose; patient temperature should not exceed 37.8°C (100°F) at time of administration

Dosage Forms Injection: 5 mg/5 mL

Muroptic-5® [OTC] *see* sodium chloride *on page 526*

Muse® Pellet *see* alprostadil *on page 20*

Mus-Lax® ***(Discontinued)*** *see page 700*

Mustargen® Hydrochloride *see* mechlorethamine *on page 351*

mustine *see* mechlorethamine *on page 351*

Mutamycin® *see* mitomycin *on page 378*

M.V.C.® 9 + 3 *see* vitamin, multiple (injectable) *on page 604*

M.V.I.®-12 *see* vitamin, multiple (injectable) *on page 604*

M.V.I.® Concentrate *see* vitamin, multiple (injectable) *on page 604*

M.V.I.® Pediatric *see* vitamin, multiple (injectable) *on page 604*

Myambutol® *see* ethambutol *on page 221*

Myapap® [OTC] *see* acetaminophen *on page 3*

Mycelex®-G Topical *see* clotrimazole *on page 140*

Mycelex®-G Vaginal [OTC] *see* clotrimazole *on page 140*

Mycelex® Troche *see* clotrimazole *on page 140*

Mycifradin® Sulfate *see* neomycin *on page 394*

Myciguent® (Can) *see* neomycin *on page 394*

Mycinettes® [OTC] *see* benzocaine *on page 66*

Mycitracin® Topical [OTC] *see* bacitracin, neomycin, and polymyxin B *on page 59*

Myclo-Derm® (Can) *see* clotrimazole *on page 140*

Myclo-Gyne® (Can) *see* clotrimazole *on page 140*

Mycobutin® *see* rifabutin *on page 504*

Mycogen II Topical *see* nystatin and triamcinolone *on page 412*

Mycolog®-II Topical *see* nystatin and triamcinolone *on page 412*

Myconel® Topical *see* nystatin and triamcinolone *on page 412*

mycophenolate (mye koe FEN oh late)

U.S./Canadian Brand Names CellCept®

Therapeutic Category Immunosuppressant Agent

Use Immunosuppressant used with corticosteroids and cyclosporine to prevent organ rejection in patients receiving allogenic renal transplants

(Continued)

mycophenolate *(Continued)*

Usual Dosage Adults: I.V./Oral: 1 g twice daily (2 g daily dose), administered within 72 hours of transplantation, when administered in combination with corticosteroids and cyclosporine

Dosage Forms

Capsule, as mofetil: 250 mg

Powder for injection, as hydrochloride: 500 mg

Tablet, as mofetil: 500 mg

Mycostatin® *see* nystatin *on page 412*

Myco-Triacet® II *see* nystatin and triamcinolone *on page 412*

Mydfrin® Ophthalmic Solution *see* phenylephrine *on page 445*

Mydriacyl® *see* tropicamide *on page 587*

Mykrox® *see* metolazone *on page 371*

Mylanta® [OTC] *see* aluminum hydroxide, magnesium hydroxide, and simethicone *on page 23*

Mylanta Gas® [OTC] *see* simethicone *on page 522*

Mylanta® Gelcaps® *see* calcium carbonate and magnesium carbonate *on page 90*

Mylanta®-II [OTC] *see* aluminum hydroxide, magnesium hydroxide, and simethicone *on page 23*

Mylaxen® Injection *(Discontinued)* *see page 700*

Myleran® *see* busulfan *on page 84*

Mylicon® [OTC] *see* simethicone *on page 522*

Mylosar® *see* azacitidine *on page 55*

Myminic® Expectorant [OTC] *see* guaifenesin and phenylpropanolamine *on page 270*

Myochrysine® *(Discontinued)* *see page 700*

Myoflex® [OTC] *see* triethanolamine salicylate *on page 580*

Myotonachol™ *see* bethanechol *on page 73*

Myphetane DC® *see* brompheniramine, phenylpropanolamine, and codeine *on page 82*

Mysoline® *see* primidone *on page 474*

Mytelase® Caplets® *see* ambenonium *on page 24*

Mytrex® F Topical *see* nystatin and triamcinolone *on page 412*

Mytussin® [OTC] *see* guaifenesin *on page 267*

Mytussin® AC *see* guaifenesin and codeine *on page 268*

Mytussin® DAC *see* guaifenesin, pseudoephedrine, and codeine *on page 272*

Mytussin® DM [OTC] *see* guaifenesin and dextromethorphan *on page 268*

M-Zole® 7 Dual Pack [OTC] *see* miconazole *on page 373*

Nabi-HB™ *see* hepatitis B immune globulin *on page 280*

nabilone (NA bi lone)

U.S./Canadian Brand Names Cesamet®

Therapeutic Category Antiemetic

Use Treatment of nausea and vomiting associated with cancer chemotherapy

Usual Dosage Oral:

Children >4 years:

- <18 kg: 0.5 mg twice daily
- 18-30 kg: 1 mg twice daily
- >30 kg: 1 mg 3 times/day

Adults: 1-2 mg twice daily beginning 1-3 hours before chemotherapy is administered and continuing around-the-clock until 1 dose after chemotherapy is completed; maximum daily dose: 6 mg divided in 3 doses

Dosage Forms Capsule: 1 mg

nabumetone (na BYOO me tone)

U.S./Canadian Brand Names Relafen®

Therapeutic Category Analgesic, Non-narcotic; Nonsteroidal Anti-inflammatory Drug (NSAID)

Use Management of osteoarthritis and rheumatoid arthritis

Usual Dosage Adults: Oral: 1000 mg/day; an additional 500-1000 mg may be needed in some patients to obtain more symptomatic relief; may be administered once or twice daily

Dosage Forms Tablet: 500 mg, 750 mg

NAC *see* acetylcysteine *on page 8*

***N*-acetylcysteine** *see* acetylcysteine *on page 8*

***N*-acetyl-L-cysteine** *see* acetylcysteine *on page 8*

n-acetyl-p-aminophenol *see* acetaminophen *on page 3*

NaCl *see* sodium chloride *on page 526*

nadolol (nay DOE lole)

U.S./Canadian Brand Names Apo®-Nadol (Can); Corgard®; Syn-Nadolol® (Can)

Therapeutic Category Beta-Adrenergic Blocker

Use Treatment of hypertension and angina pectoris; prevention of myocardial infarction; prophylaxis of migraine headaches

Usual Dosage Adults: Oral: Initial: 40 mg once daily; increase gradually; usual dosage: 40-80 mg/day; may need up to 240-320 mg/day; doses as high as 640 mg/day have been used

Dosage Forms Tablet: 20 mg, 40 mg, 80 mg, 120 mg, 160 mg

Nadopen-V® (Can) *see* penicillin V potassium *on page 435*

Nadostine® (Can) *see* nystatin *on page 412*

nadroparin *(Canada only)* (nad roe PA rin)

U.S./Canadian Brand Names Fraxiparine® (Can)

Therapeutic Category Low Molecular Weight Heparin

Use Prevention of clotting during hemodialysis; Prophylaxis of thromboembolic disorders (particularly deep vein thrombosis and pulmonary embolism) in general surgery and in orthopedic surgery; treatment of deep vein thrombosis

Usual Dosage Adult: S.C.:

Thromboembolism prophylaxis: 0.3 mL daily S.C for 7 days.

Orthopaedic surgery: 0.2-0.4 mL daily for 3 days then 0.3-0.6 mL daily; doses should be adjusted for bodyweight.

Thromboembolism treatment: 0.4-0.9 mL twice daily for 10 days. Doses should be adjusted for bodyweight.

Hemodialysis: 0.3-0.6 mL into the arterial line at start of 4 hour session. Dose should be adjusted for bodyweight.

Child: Hemodialysis: 60-120 int. units/kg at the start of 4 hour session. Duration of therapy should be determined by the clinical need. Dosage should be individualized.

Dosage Forms Injection, as calcium: in pre-filled syringes or graduated syringes: 9500 int. units anti-Xa/mL (0.2mL, 0.3 mL, 0.4 mL, 0.6 mL, 0.8 mL, 1 mL)

nafarelin (NAF a re lin)

U.S./Canadian Brand Names Synarel®

Therapeutic Category Hormone, Posterior Pituitary

(Continued)

nafarelin *(Continued)*

Use Treatment of endometriosis, including pain and reduction of lesions; treatment of central precocious puberty (gonadotropin-dependent precocious puberty) in children of both sexes

Usual Dosage Adults: 1 spray in one nostril each morning and evening for 6 months

Dosage Forms Solution, nasal, as acetate: 2 mg/mL (10 mL)

Nafazair® Ophthalmic *see* naphazoline *on page 390*

Nafcil® *(Discontinued)* *see page 700*

nafcillin (naf SIL in)

Synonyms ethoxynaphthamido penicillin sodium

U.S./Canadian Brand Names Nallpen®

Therapeutic Category Penicillin

Use Treatment of bacterial infections such as osteomyelitis, septicemia, endocarditis, and CNS infections due to susceptible penicillinase-producing strains of *Staphylococcus*

Usual Dosage

Children: I.M., I.V.:

- Mild to moderate infections: 50-100 mg/kg/day in divided doses every 6 hours
- Severe infections: 100-200 mg/kg/day in divided doses every 4-6 hours
- Maximum dose: 12 g/day
- Oral: 50-100 mg/kg/day divided every 6 hours

Adults:

- Oral: 250-500 mg every 4-6 hours, up to 1 g every 4-6 hours for more severe infections
- I.M.: 500 mg every 4-6 hours
- I.V.: 500-2000 mg every 4-6 hours

Dosage Forms Nafcillin sodium:

- Capsule: 250 mg
- Powder for injection: 500 mg, 1 g, 2 g, 4 g, 10 g
- Solution: 250 mg/5 mL (100 mL)
- Tablet: 500 mg

naftifine (NAF ti feen)

U.S./Canadian Brand Names Naftin®

Therapeutic Category Antifungal Agent

Use Topical treatment of tinea cruris and tinea corporis

Usual Dosage Adults: Topical: Apply twice daily

Dosage Forms Naftifine hydrochloride:

- Cream: 1% (15 g, 30 g, 60 g)
- Gel, topical: 1% (20 g, 40 g, 60 g)

Naftin® *see* naftifine *on this page*

$NaHCO_3$ *see* sodium bicarbonate *on page 525*

nalbuphine (NAL byoo feen)

U.S./Canadian Brand Names Nubain®

Therapeutic Category Analgesic, Narcotic

Use Relief of moderate to severe pain

Usual Dosage I.M., I.V., S.C.: 10 mg/70 kg every 3-6 hours

Dosage Forms Injection, as hydrochloride: 10 mg/mL (1 mL, 10 mL); 20 mg/mL (1 mL, 10 mL)

Naldecon® *see* chlorpheniramine, phenyltoloxamine, phenylpropanolamine, and phenylephrine *on page 125*

Naldecon® DX Adult Liquid [OTC] *see* guaifenesin, phenylpropanolamine, and dextromethorphan *on page 271*

Naldecon-EX® Children's Syrup [OTC] *see* guaifenesin and phenylpropanolamine *on page 270*

Naldecon® Senior DX [OTC] *see* guaifenesin and dextromethorphan *on page 268*

Naldecon® Senior EX [OTC] *see* guaifenesin *on page 267*

Naldelate® *see* chlorpheniramine, phenyltoloxamine, phenylpropanolamine, and phenylephrine *on page 125*

Nalfon® *see* fenoprofen *on page 234*

Nalfon® Tablet *(Discontinued)* *see page 700*

Nalgest® *see* chlorpheniramine, phenyltoloxamine, phenylpropanolamine, and phenylephrine *on page 125*

nalidixic acid (nal i DIKS ik AS id)

Synonyms nalidixinic acid

U.S./Canadian Brand Names NegGram®

Therapeutic Category Quinolone

Use Lower urinary tract infections due to susceptible gram-negative organisms including *E. coli*, *Enterobacter*, *Klebsiella*, and *Proteus* (inactive against *Pseudomonas*)

Usual Dosage Oral:

Children: 55 mg/kg/day divided every 6 hours; suppressive therapy is 33 mg/kg/day divided every 6 hours

Adults: 1 g 4 times/day for 2 weeks; then suppressive therapy of 500 mg 4 times/day

Dosage Forms

Suspension, oral (raspberry flavor): 250 mg/5 mL (473 mL)

Tablet: 250 mg, 500 mg, 1 g

nalidixinic acid *see* nalidixic acid *on this page*

Nallpen® *see* nafcillin *on previous page*

***n*-allylnoroxymorphone** *see* naloxone *on this page*

nalmefene (NAL me feen)

U.S./Canadian Brand Names Revex®

Therapeutic Category Antidote

Use Complete or partial of opioid drug effects; management of known or suspected opioid overdose

Usual Dosage Titrate to reverse the undesired effects of opioids; once adequate reversal has been established, additional administration is not required and may actually be harmful due to unwanted reversal of analgesia or precipitated withdrawal; the recommended initial dose for nonopioid dependent patient is 0.5 mg/70 kg, a second dose of 1 mg/70 kg 2-5 minutes later may be administered, after a total dose of 1.5 mg/70 kg has been administered with no clinical response, additional nalmefene is not likely to have an effect

Dosage Forms Injection, as hydrochloride: 100 mcg/mL [blue label] (1 mL); 1000 mcg/mL [green label] (2 mL)

naloxone (nal OKS one)

Synonyms *n*-allylnoroxymorphone

U.S./Canadian Brand Names Narcan®

Therapeutic Category Antidote

Use Reverses CNS and respiratory depression in suspected narcotic overdose; neonatal opiate depression; coma of unknown etiology

Investigational use: Shock, phencyclidine, and alcohol ingestion

(Continued)

naloxone *(Continued)*

Usual Dosage I.M., I.V. (preferred), intratracheal, S.C. (administer undiluted injection):
Infants and Children:
Postanesthesia narcotic reversal: 0.01 mg/kg; may repeat every 2-3 minutes as needed based on response
Opiate intoxication:
Birth (including premature infants) to 5 years or <20 kg: 0.1 mg/kg; repeat every 2-3 minutes if needed; may need to repeat doses every 20-60 minutes
>5 years or ≥20 kg: 2 mg/dose; if no response, repeat every 2-3 minutes; may need to repeat doses every 20-60 minutes
Children and Adults: Continuous infusion: I.V.: If continuous infusion is required, calculate dosage/hour based on effective intermittent dose used and duration of adequate response seen, titrate dose
Adults: 0.4-2 mg every 2-3 minutes as needed; may need to repeat doses every 20-60 minutes; if no response is observed for a total of 10 mg, re-evaluate patient for possibility of a drug or disease process unresponsive to naloxone. **Note:** Use 0.1-0.2 mg increments in patients who are opioid dependent and in postoperative patients to avoid large cardiovascular changes

Dosage Forms Injection, as hydrochloride: 0.4 mg/mL (1 mL, 2 mL, 10 mL)

Nalspan® *see* chlorpheniramine, phenyltoloxamine, phenylpropanolamine, and phenylephrine *on page 125*

naltrexone (nal TREKS one)

U.S./Canadian Brand Names Depade®; ReVia®
Therapeutic Category Antidote
Use Adjunct to the maintenance of an opioid-free state in detoxified individual
Usual Dosage Do not administer until patient is opioid-free for 7-10 days as required by urine analysis

Adults: Oral: 25 mg; if no withdrawal signs within 1 hour administer another 25 mg; maintenance regimen is flexible, variable and individualized (50 mg/day to 100-150 mg 3 times/week)

Dosage Forms Tablet, as hydrochloride: 50 mg

Nandrobolic® Injection *(Discontinued)* *see page 700*

nandrolone (NAN droe lone)

U.S./Canadian Brand Names Anabolin®; Androlone®; Androlone®-D; Deca-Durabolin®; Hybolin™ Decanoate; Hybolin™ Improved Injection; Neo-Durabolic
Therapeutic Category Androgen
Controlled Substance C-III
Use Control of metastatic breast cancer; management of anemia of renal insufficiency
Usual Dosage
Children 2-13 years: 25-50 mg every 3-4 weeks
Adults:
Male: 100-200 mg/week
Female: 50-100 mg/week

Dosage Forms
Nandrolone phenpropionate: Injection in oil: 25 mg/mL (5 mL); 50 mg/mL (2 mL)
Nandrolone decanoate:
Injection in oil: 50 mg/mL (1 mL, 2 mL); 100 mg/mL (1 mL, 2 mL); 200 mg/mL (1 mL)
Injection, repository: 50 mg/mL (2 mL); 100 mg/mL (2 mL); 200 mg/mL (2 mL)

naphazoline (naf AZ oh leen)

U.S./Canadian Brand Names AK-Con® Ophthalmic; Albalon® Liquifilm® Ophthalmic; Allerest® Eye Drops [OTC]; Clear Eyes® [OTC]; Comfort® Ophthalmic [OTC]; Degest® 2 Ophthalmic [OTC]; Estivin® II Ophthalmic [OTC]; I-Naphline® Ophthalmic; Nafazair® Ophthalmic; Naphcon Forte® Ophthalmic; Naphcon® Ophthalmic [OTC]; Opcon®

Ophthalmic; Privine® Nasal [OTC]; Red Away® (Can); VasoClear® Ophthalmic [OTC]; Vasocon Regular® Ophthalmic

Therapeutic Category Adrenergic Agonist Agent

Use Topical ocular vasoconstrictor (to soothe, refresh, moisturize, and relieve redness due to minor eye irritation); temporarily relieves nasal congestion associated with rhinitis, sinusitis, hay fever, or the common cold

Usual Dosage

Nasal:

Children:

<6 years: Not recommended (especially infants) due to CNS depression

6-12 years: 1 spray of 0.05% into each nostril, repeat in 3 hours if necessary

Children >12 years and Adults: 0.05%, instill 2 drops or sprays every 3-6 hours if needed; therapy should not exceed 3-5 days or more frequently than every 3 hours

Ophthalmic:

Children <6 years: Not recommended for use due to CNS depression (especially in infants)

Children >6 years and Adults: Instill 1-2 drops into conjunctival sac of affected eye(s) every 3-4 hours; therapy generally should not exceed 3-4 days

Dosage Forms Solution, as hydrochloride:

Nasal:

Drops: 0.05% (20 mL)

Spray: 0.05% (15 mL)

Ophthalmic: 0.012% (7.5 mL, 30 mL); 0.02% (15 mL); 0.03% (15 mL); 0.1% (15 mL)

naphazoline and antazoline (naf AZ oh leen & an TAZ oh leen)

U.S./Canadian Brand Names Albalon-A® Ophthalmic; Antazoline-V® Ophthalmic; Vasocon-A® [OTC] Ophthalmic

Therapeutic Category Antihistamine/Decongestant Combination

Use Topical ocular congestion, irritation, and itching

Usual Dosage Ophthalmic: 1-2 drops every 3-4 hours

Dosage Forms Solution: Naphazoline hydrochloride 0.05% and antazoline phosphate 0.5% (15 mL)

naphazoline and pheniramine (naf AZ oh leen & fen NIR a meen)

Synonyms pheniramine and naphazoline

U.S./Canadian Brand Names Naphcon-A® Ophthalmic [OTC]

Therapeutic Category Antihistamine/Decongestant Combination

Use Topical ocular vasoconstrictor

Usual Dosage Ophthalmic: 1-2 drops every 3-4 hours

Dosage Forms Solution, ophthalmic: Naphazoline hydrochloride 0.025% and pheniramine 0.3% (15 mL)

Naphcon-A® Ophthalmic [OTC] *see* naphazoline and pheniramine *on this page*

Naphcon Forte® Ophthalmic *see* naphazoline *on previous page*

Naphcon® Ophthalmic [OTC] *see* naphazoline *on previous page*

Naprosyn® *see* naproxen *on this page*

naproxen (na PROKS en)

U.S./Canadian Brand Names Aleve® [OTC]; Anaprox®; Apo®-Naproxen (Can); Naprosyn®; Naxen® (Can); Novo-Naprox® (Can); Nu-Naprox® (Can); Synflex® (Can)

Therapeutic Category Analgesic, Non-narcotic; Antipyretic; Nonsteroidal Anti-inflammatory Drug (NSAID)

Use Management of inflammatory disease and rheumatoid disorders (including juvenile rheumatoid arthritis); acute gout; mild to moderate pain; dysmenorrhea; fever

Usual Dosage Oral (as naproxen):

Children >2 years:

Antipyretic or analgesic: 5-7 mg/kg/dose every 8-12 hours

(Continued)

naproxen *(Continued)*

Juvenile rheumatoid arthritis: 10 mg/kg/day, up to a maximum of 1000 mg/day divided twice daily

Adults:

Rheumatoid arthritis, osteoarthritis, and ankylosing spondylitis: 500-1000 mg/day in 2 divided doses

Mild to moderate pain or dysmenorrhea: Initial: 500 mg, then 250 mg every 6-8 hours; maximum: 1250 mg/day

Dosage Forms

Suspension, oral: 125 mg/5 mL (15 mL, 30 mL, 480 mL)

Tablet:

Aleve®: 200 mg

Naprosyn®: 250 mg, 375 mg, 500 mg

Tablet, controlled release (Naprelan®): 375 mg, 500 mg

Naproxen sodium:

Tablet, as sodium: 220 mg (200 mg base)

Anaprox®: 220 mg (200 mg base); 275 mg (250 mg base); 550 mg (500 mg base)

Naqua® *see* trichlormethiazide *on page 579*

naratriptan (NAR a trip tan)

U.S./Canadian Brand Names Amerge®

Therapeutic Category Antimigraine Agent; Serotonin Agonist

Use Acute treatment of migraine with or without aura

Usual Dosage Oral: Adults: 1 mg or 2.5 mg (maximum dose: 5 mg); if no response, dose may be repeated in 4 hours

Dosage Forms Tablet, as hydrochloride: 1 mg, 2.5 mg

Narcan® *see* naloxone *on page 389*

Narcan® 1 mg/mL Injection *(Discontinued)* *see page 700*

Nardil® *see* phenelzine *on page 442*

Naropin™ *see* ropivacaine *on page 510*

Nasabid™ *see* guaifenesin and pseudoephedrine *on page 270*

Nasacort® *see* triamcinolone (inhalation, nasal) *on page 577*

Nasacort® AQ *see* triamcinolone (inhalation, nasal) *on page 577*

Nasahist B® *see* brompheniramine *on page 80*

NaSal™ [OTC] *see* sodium chloride *on page 526*

Nasalcrom® [OTC] *see* cromolyn sodium *on page 150*

Nasalide® Nasal Aerosol *see* flunisolide *on page 243*

Nasal Moist® [OTC] *see* sodium chloride *on page 526*

Nasarel™ Nasal Spray *see* flunisolide *on page 243*

Nasonex® *see* mometasone furoate *on page 380*

Natabec® [OTC] *see* vitamin, multiple (prenatal) *on page 606*

Natabec® FA [OTC] *see* vitamin, multiple (prenatal) *on page 606*

Natabec® Rx *see* vitamin, multiple (prenatal) *on page 606*

Natacyn® *see* natamycin *on this page*

Natalins® [OTC] *see* vitamin, multiple (prenatal) *on page 606*

Natalins® Rx *see* vitamin, multiple (prenatal) *on page 606*

natamycin (na ta MYE sin)

Synonyms pimaricin

U.S./Canadian Brand Names Natacyn®

Therapeutic Category Antifungal Agent

Use Treatment of blepharitis, conjunctivitis, and keratitis caused by susceptible fungi (*Aspergillus*, *Candida*), *Cephalosporium*, *Curvularia*, *Fusarium*, *Penicillium*, *Microsporum*, *Epidermophyton*, *Blastomyces dermatitidis*, *Coccidioides immitis*, *Cryptococcus neoformans*, *Histoplasma capsulatum*, *Sporothrix schenckii*, *Trichomonas vaginalis*

Usual Dosage Adults: Ophthalmic: 1 drop in conjunctival sac every 1-2 hours, after 3-4 days dose may be reduced to one drop 6-8 times/day; usual course of therapy: 2-3 weeks

Dosage Forms Suspension, ophthalmic: 5% (15 mL)

Natulan® (Can) *see* procarbazine *on page 476*

natural lung surfactant *see* beractant *on page 70*

Nature's Tears® Solution [OTC] *see* artificial tears *on page 47*

Naturetin® *see* bendroflumethiazide *on page 64*

Naus-A-Way® [OTC] *see* phosphorated carbohydrate solution *on page 450*

Nausetrol® [OTC] *see* phosphorated carbohydrate solution *on page 450*

Navane® Capsule *see* thiothixene *on page 563*

Navane® Concentrate & Injection *(Discontinued)* *see page 700*

Navelbine® *see* vinorelbine *on page 601*

Naxen® (Can) *see* naproxen *on page 391*

N-B-P® Ointment *(Discontinued)* *see page 700*

ND-Stat® *see* brompheniramine *on page 80*

Nebcin® Injection *see* tobramycin *on page 569*

NebuPent™ Inhalation *see* pentamidine *on page 436*

nedocromil (ne doe KROE mil)

U.S./Canadian Brand Names Tilade® Inhalation Aerosol

Therapeutic Category Mast Cell Stabilizer

Use Maintenance therapy in patients with mild to moderate bronchial asthma

Usual Dosage Adults: Inhalation: 2 inhalations 4 times/day

Dosage Forms Aerosol, as sodium: 1.75 mg/activation (16.2 g)

N.E.E.® 1/35 *see* ethinyl estradiol and norethindrone *on page 224*

nefazodone (nef AY zoe done)

U.S./Canadian Brand Names Serzone®

Therapeutic Category Antidepressant, Miscellaneous

Use Treatment of depression

Usual Dosage Adults: Oral: Initial: 200 mg/day administered in two divided doses with a range of 300-600 mg/day in two divided doses thereafter

Dosage Forms Tablet, as hydrochloride: 100 mg, 150 mg, 200 mg, 250 mg

NegGram® *see* nalidixic acid *on page 389*

nelfinavir (nel FIN a veer)

U.S./Canadian Brand Names Viracept®

Therapeutic Category Antiviral Agent

Use As monotherapy or preferably in combination with nucleoside analogs in the treatment of HIV infection, in adults and children, when antiretroviral therapy is warranted

Usual Dosage Oral:

Children 2-13 years: 20-30 mg/kg 3 times/day with a meal or light snack; if tablets are unable to be taken, use oral powder in small amount of water, milk, formula, or dietary supplements; do not use acidic food/juice or store for >6 hours

Adults: 750 mg 3 times/day with meals

(Continued)

nelfinavir *(Continued)*

Dosage Forms Nelfinavir mesylate:
Powder, oral: 50 mg/g [144 g] (contains 11.2 mg phenylalanine)
Tablet: 250 mg

Nelova™ 0.5/35E *see* ethinyl estradiol and norethindrone *on page 224*

Nelova® 1/50M *see* mestranol and norethindrone *on page 359*

Nelova™ 10/11 *see* ethinyl estradiol and norethindrone *on page 224*

Nembutal® *see* pentobarbital *on page 437*

Neo-Calglucon® [OTC] *see* calcium glubionate *on page 91*

Neo-Castaderm *(Discontinued)* *see page 700*

Neo-Codema® (Can) *see* hydrochlorothiazide *on page 286*

Neo-Cortef® Ophthalmic *see* neomycin and hydrocortisone *on next page*

Neo-Cortef® Topical *(Discontinued)* *see page 700*

NeoDecadron® Ophthalmic *see* neomycin and dexamethasone *on next page*

NeoDecadron® Topical *(Discontinued)* *see page 700*

Neo-Dexameth® Ophthalmic *see* neomycin and dexamethasone *on next page*

Neo-Durabolic *see* nandrolone *on page 390*

Neo-Estrone® (Can) *see* estrone *on page 220*

Neofed® [OTC] *see* pseudoephedrine *on page 486*

Neo-fradin® *see* neomycin *on this page*

Neoloid® [OTC] *see* castor oil *on page 103*

Neo-Medrol® Acetate Topical *(Discontinued)* *see page 700*

Neomixin® Topical *see* bacitracin, neomycin, and polymyxin B *on page 59*

neomycin (nee oh MYE sin)

U.S./Canadian Brand Names Mycifradin® Sulfate; Myciguent® (Can); Neo-fradin®; Neo-Tabs®

Therapeutic Category Aminoglycoside (Antibiotic); Antibiotic, Topical

Use Administered orally to prepare GI tract for surgery; treat minor skin infections; treat diarrhea caused by *E. coli*; adjunct in the treatment of hepatic encephalopathy

Usual Dosage
Children: Oral:
Preoperative intestinal antisepsis: 90 mg/kg/day divided every 4 hours for 2 days; or 25 mg/kg at 1 PM, 2 PM, and 11 PM on the day preceding surgery as an adjunct to mechanical cleansing of the intestine and in combination with erythromycin base
Hepatic coma: 50-100 mg/kg/day in divided doses every 6-8 hours or 2.5-7 g/m^2/day divided every 4-6 hours for 5-6 days not to exceed 12 g/day
Children and Adults: Topical: Apply ointment 1-4 times/day; topical solutions containing 0.1% to 1% neomycin have been used for irrigation
Adults: Oral:
Preoperative intestinal antisepsis: 1 g each hour for 4 doses then 1 g every 4 hours for 5 doses; or 1 g at 1 PM, 2 PM, and 11 PM on day preceding surgery as an adjunct to mechanical cleansing of the bowel and oral erythromycin; or 6 g/day divided every 4 hours for 2-3 days
Hepatic coma: 500-2000 mg every 6-8 hours or 4-12 g/day divided every 4-6 hours for 5-6 days
Chronic hepatic insufficiency: Oral: 4 g/day for an indefinite period

Dosage Forms Neomycin sulfate:
Cream: 0.5% (15 g)
Ointment, topical: 0.5% (15 g, 30 g, 120 g)
Solution, oral: 125 mg/5 mL (480 mL)
Tablet: 500 mg [base 300 mg]

neomycin and dexamethasone (nee oh MYE sin & deks a METH a sone)

Synonyms dexamethasone and neomycin

U.S./Canadian Brand Names AK-Neo-Dex® Ophthalmic; NeoDecadron® Ophthalmic; Neo-Dexameth® Ophthalmic

Therapeutic Category Antibiotic/Corticosteroid, Ophthalmic; Antibiotic/Corticosteroid, Topical

Use Treatment of steroid responsive inflammatory conditions of the palpebral and bulbar conjunctiva, lid, cornea, and anterior segment of the globe

Usual Dosage

Ophthalmic: Instill 1-2 drops in eye(s) every 3-4 hours

Topical: Apply thin coat 3-4 times/day until favorable response is observed, then reduce dose to one application/day

Dosage Forms

Cream: Neomycin sulfate 0.5% [5 mg/g] and dexamethasone 0.1% [1 mg/g] (15 g, 30 g)

Ointment, ophthalmic: Neomycin sulfate 0.35% [3.5 mg/g] and dexamethasone 0.05% [0.5 mg/g] (3.5 g)

Solution, ophthalmic: Neomycin sulfate 0.35% [3.5 mg/mL] and dexamethasone 0.1% [1 mg/mL] (5 mL)

neomycin and hydrocortisone (nee oh MYE sin & hye droe KOR ti sone)

Synonyms hydrocortisone and neomycin

U.S./Canadian Brand Names Neo-Cortef® Ophthalmic

Therapeutic Category Antibiotic/Corticosteroid, Ophthalmic; Antibiotic/Corticosteroid, Topical

Use Treatment of susceptible topical bacterial infections with associated inflammation

Usual Dosage Topical: Apply to area in a thin film 2-4 times/day

Dosage Forms

Cream: Neomycin sulfate 0.5% and hydrocortisone 1% (20 g)

Ointment, topical: Neomycin sulfate 0.5% and hydrocortisone 0.5% (20 g); neomycin sulfate 0.5% and hydrocortisone 1% (20 g)

Solution, ophthalmic: Neomycin sulfate 0.5% and hydrocortisone 0.5% (5 mL)

neomycin and polymyxin B (nee oh MYE sin & pol i MIKS in bee)

Synonyms polymyxin B and neomycin

U.S./Canadian Brand Names Neosporin® Cream [OTC]; Neosporin® G.U. Irrigant

Therapeutic Category Antibiotic, Topical; Genitourinary Irrigant

Use Short-term use as a continuous irrigant or rinse in the urinary bladder to prevent bacteriuria and gram-negative rod septicemia associated with the use of indwelling catheters; to help prevent infection in minor cuts, scrapes, and burns

Usual Dosage Children and Adults:

Topical: Apply cream 2-4 times/day

Bladder irrigation: Continuous irrigant or rinse in the urinary bladder for up to 10 days where 1 mL is added to 1 L of normal saline with administration rate adjusted to patient's urine output; usually no more than 1 L of irrigant is used per day

Dosage Forms

Cream: Neomycin sulfate 3.5 mg and polymyxin B sulfate 10,000 units per g (0.94 g, 15 g)

Solution, irrigant: Neomycin sulfate 40 mg and polymyxin B sulfate 200,000 units per mL (1 mL, 20 mL)

neomycin, bacitracin, and polymyxin B *see* bacitracin, neomycin, and polymyxin B *on page 59*

neomycin, bacitracin, polymyxin B, and hydrocortisone *see* bacitracin, neomycin, polymyxin B, and hydrocortisone *on page 59*

neomycin, colistin, and hydrocortisone *see* colistin, neomycin, and hydrocortisone *on page 145*

neomycin, colistin, hydrocortisone, and thonzonium

(nee oh MYE sin, koe LIS tin, hye droe KOR ti sone, & thon ZOE nee um)

U.S./Canadian Brand Names Cortisporin®-TC Otic Suspension

Therapeutic Category Antibiotic/Corticosteroid, Otic

Use Treatment of superficial and susceptible bacterial infections of the external auditory canal; for treatment of susceptible bacterial infections of mastoidectomy and fenestration cavities

Usual Dosage

Children: 4 drops in affected ear 3-4 times/day

Adults: 5 drops in affected ear 3-4 times/day

Dosage Forms Suspension, otic: Neomycin sulfate 3.3 mg, colistin sulfate 3 mg, hydrocortisone acetate 1%, and thonzonium bromide 0.5 mg per mL (10 mL)

neomycin, polymyxin B, and dexamethasone

(nee oh MYE sin, pol i MIKS in bee, & deks a METH a sone)

Synonyms dexamethasone, neomycin, and polymyxin B; polymyxin B, neomycin, and dexamethasone

U.S./Canadian Brand Names AK-Trol®; Dexacidin®; Dexasporin®; Maxitrol®

Therapeutic Category Antibiotic/Corticosteroid, Ophthalmic

Use Steroid-responsive inflammatory ocular conditions in which a corticosteroid is indicated and where bacterial infection or a risk of bacterial infection exists

Usual Dosage Children and Adults: Ophthalmic:

Ointment: Place a small amount (~½") in the affected eye 3-4 times/day or apply at bedtime as an adjunct with drops

Solution: Instill 1-2 drops into affected eye(s) every 4-6 hours; in severe disease, drops may be used hourly and tapered to discontinuation

Dosage Forms

Ointment, ophthalmic: Neomycin sulfate 3.5 mg, polymyxin B sulfate 10,000 units, and dexamethasone 0.1% per g (3.5 g)

Suspension, ophthalmic: Neomycin sulfate 3.5 mg, polymyxin B sulfate 10,000 units, and dexamethasone 0.1% per mL (5 mL)

neomycin, polymyxin B, and gramicidin

(nee oh MYE sin, pol i MIKS in bee, & gram i SYE din)

Synonyms gramicidin, neomycin, and polymyxin B; polymyxin B, neomycin, and gramicidin

U.S./Canadian Brand Names AK-Spore® Ophthalmic Solution; Neosporin® Ophthalmic Solution

Therapeutic Category Antibiotic, Ophthalmic

Use Treatment of superficial ocular infection, infection prophylaxis in minor skin abrasions

Usual Dosage Ophthalmic: Drops: 1-2 drops 4-6 times/day or more frequently as required for severe infections

Dosage Forms Solution, ophthalmic: Neomycin sulfate 1.75 mg, polymyxin B sulfate 10,000 units, and gramicidin 0.025 mg per mL (2 mL, 10 mL)

neomycin, polymyxin B, and hydrocortisone

(nee oh MYE sin, pol i MIKS in bee, & hye droe KOR ti sone)

Synonyms hydrocortisone, neomycin, and polymyxin B; polymyxin B, neomycin, and hydrocortisone

U.S./Canadian Brand Names AK-Spore® H.C. Ophthalmic Suspension; AK-Spore® H.C. Otic; AntibiOtic® Otic; Cortatrigen® Otic; Cortisporin® Ophthalmic Suspension; Cortisporin® Otic; Cortisporin® Topical Cream; Octicair® Otic; Otic-Care® Otic; Otocort® Otic; Otosporin® Otic; Pediotic® Otic; UAD Otic®

Therapeutic Category Antibiotic/Corticosteroid, Ophthalmic; Antibiotic/Corticosteroid, Otic; Antibiotic/Corticosteroid, Topical

Use Steroid-responsive inflammatory condition for which a corticosteroid is indicated and where bacterial infection or a risk of bacterial infection exists

Usual Dosage Duration of use should be limited to 10 days unless otherwise directed by the physician

Ophthalmic: Adults and Children:

Ointment: Apply to the affected eye every 3-4 hours

Suspension: 1 drop every 3-4 hours

Otic: Solution/suspension:

Children: 3 drops into affected ear 3-4 times/day

Adults: 4 drops into affected ear 3-4 times/day

Dosage Forms

Cream, topical: Neomycin sulfate 5 mg, polymyxin B sulfate 10,000 units, and hydrocortisone 10 mg per mL (7.5 g)

Solution, otic: Neomycin sulfate 5 mg, polymyxin B sulfate 10,000 units, and hydrocortisone 10 mg per mL (10 mL)

Suspension:

Ophthalmic: Neomycin sulfate 5 mg, polymyxin B sulfate 10,000 units, and hydrocortisone 10 mg per mL (7.5 mL)

Otic: Neomycin sulfate 5 mg, polymyxin B sulfate 10,000 units, and hydrocortisone 10 mg per mL (10 mL)

neomycin, polymyxin B, and prednisolone

(nee oh MYE sin, pol i MIKS in bee, & pred NIS oh lone)

Synonyms polymyxin B, neomycin, and prednisolone; prednisolone, neomycin, and polymyxin B

U.S./Canadian Brand Names Poly-Pred® Ophthalmic Suspension

Therapeutic Category Antibiotic/Corticosteroid, Ophthalmic

Use Steroid-responsive inflammatory ocular condition in which bacterial infection or a risk of bacterial ocular infection exists

Usual Dosage Children and Adults: Ophthalmic: Instill 1-2 drops every 3-4 hours; acute infections may require every 30-minute instillation initially with frequency of administration reduced as the infection is brought under control. To treat the lids: Instill 1-2 drops every 3-4 hours, close the eye and rub the excess on the lids and lid margins.

Dosage Forms Suspension, ophthalmic: Neomycin sulfate 0.35%, polymyxin B sulfate 10,000 units, and prednisolone acetate 0.5% per mL (5 mL, 10 mL)

neonatal trace metals *see* trace metals *on page 573*

Neopap® [OTC] *see* acetaminophen *on page 3*

Neoquess® Injection *(Discontinued)* *see page 700*

Neoquess® Tablet *(Discontinued)* *see page 700*

Neoral® *see* cyclosporine *on page 154*

Neosar® *see* cyclophosphamide *on page 153*

Neosporin® Cream [OTC] *see* neomycin and polymyxin B *on page 395*

Neosporin® G.U. Irrigant *see* neomycin and polymyxin B *on page 395*

Neosporin® Ophthalmic Ointment *see* bacitracin, neomycin, and polymyxin B *on page 59*

Neosporin® Ophthalmic Solution *see* neomycin, polymyxin B, and gramicidin *on previous page*

Neosporin® Topical Ointment [OTC] *see* bacitracin, neomycin, and polymyxin B *on page 59*

neostigmine (nee oh STIG meen)

U.S./Canadian Brand Names Prostigmin®

Therapeutic Category Cholinergic Agent

Use Treatment of myasthenia gravis; prevention and treatment of postoperative bladder distention and urinary retention; reversal of the effects of nondepolarizing neuromuscular blocking agents after surgery

(Continued)

neostigmine *(Continued)*

Usual Dosage

Myasthenia gravis: Diagnosis: I.M.:
Children: 0.04 mg/kg as a single dose
Adults: 0.02 mg/kg as a single dose

Myasthenia gravis: Treatment:
Children:
Oral: 2 mg/kg/day divided every 3-4 hours
I.M., I.V., S.C.: 0.01-0.04 mg/kg every 2-4 hours
Adults:
Oral: 15 mg/dose every 3-4 hours
I.M., I.V., S.C.: 0.5-2.5 mg every 1-3 hours

Reversal of nondepolarizing neuromuscular blockade after surgery in conjunction with atropine or glycopyrrolate: I.V.:
Infants: 0.025-0.1 mg/kg/dose
Children: 0.025-0.08 mg/kg/dose
Adults: 0.5-2.5 mg; total dose not to exceed 5 mg

Bladder atony: Adults: I.M., S.C.:
Prevention: 0.25 mg every 4-6 hours for 2-3 days
Treatment: 0.5-1 mg every 3 hours for 5 doses after bladder has emptied

Dosage Forms

Injection, as methylsulfate: 0.25 mg/mL (1 mL); 0.5 mg/mL (1 mL, 10 mL); 1 mg/mL (10 mL)

Tablet, as bromide: 15 mg

Neostrata® HQ (Can) *see* hydroquinone *on page 294*

Neo-Synalar® Topical *(Discontinued)* *see page 700*

Neo-Synephrine® 12 Hour Nasal Solution [OTC] *see* oxymetazoline *on page 423*

Neo-Synephrine® 12 Hour Nasal Solution *(Discontinued)* *see page 700*

Neo-Synephrine® Nasal Solution [OTC] *see* phenylephrine *on page 445*

Neo-Synephrine® Ophthalmic Solution *see* phenylephrine *on page 445*

Neo-Tabs® *see* neomycin *on page 394*

Neotopic® (Can) *see* bacitracin, neomycin, and polymyxin B *on page 59*

Neotrace-4® *see* trace metals *on page 573*

Neotricin HC® Ophthalmic Ointment *see* bacitracin, neomycin, polymyxin B, and hydrocortisone *on page 59*

NeoVadrin® [OTC] *see* vitamin, multiple (oral) *on page 604*

NeoVadrin® B Complex [OTC] *see* vitamin B complex *on page 603*

Nephro-Calci® [OTC] *see* calcium carbonate *on page 89*

Nephrocaps® *see* vitamin B complex with vitamin C and folic acid *on page 603*

Nephro-Fer™ [OTC] *see* ferrous fumarate *on page 236*

Nephronex® (Can) *see* nitrofurantoin *on page 403*

Nephrox Suspension [OTC] *see* aluminum hydroxide *on page 22*

Neptazane® *see* methazolamide *on page 362*

Nervocaine® Injection *see* lidocaine *on page 333*

Nesacaine® *see* chloroprocaine *on page 118*

Nesacaine®-MPF *see* chloroprocaine *on page 118*

Nestrex® *see* pyridoxine *on page 490*

1-*n*-ethyl sisomicin *see* netilmicin *on next page*

netilmicin (ne til MYE sin)

Synonyms 1-*n*-ethyl sisomicin

U.S./Canadian Brand Names Netromycin®

Therapeutic Category Aminoglycoside (Antibiotic)

Use Short-term treatment of serious or life-threatening infections including septicemia, peritonitis, intra-abdominal abscess, lower respiratory tract infections, urinary tract infections, skin, bone and joint infections caused by sensitive *Pseudomonas aeruginosa*, *Escherichia coli*, *Proteus*, *Klebsiella*, *Serratia*, *Enterobacter*, *Citrobacter*, and *Staphylococcus*

Usual Dosage I.M., I.V.:

Children 6 weeks to 12 years: 1-2.5 mg/kg/dose every 8 hours

Children >12 years and Adults: 1.5-2 mg/kg/dose every 8-12 hours

Dosage Forms Injection, as sulfate: 100 mg/mL (1.5 mL)

Netromycin® *see* netilmicin *on this page*

Neucalm-50® Injection *see* hydroxyzine *on page 297*

Neuleptil® (Can) *see* pericyazine *(Canada only) on page 439*

Neumega® *see* oprelvekin *on page 416*

Neupogen® *see* filgrastim *on page 239*

Neuramate® *see* meprobamate *on page 356*

Neurontin® *see* gabapentin *on page 256*

Neut® *see* sodium bicarbonate *on page 525*

Neutra-Phos® Capsule *(Discontinued)* *see page 700*

Neutra-Phos®-K *see* potassium phosphate *on page 466*

Neutrexin® *see* trimetrexate glucuronate *on page 583*

Neutrogena® Acne Mask [OTC] *see* benzoyl peroxide *on page 68*

Neutrogena® T/Derm *see* coal tar *on page 141*

nevirapine (ne VYE ra peen)

U.S./Canadian Brand Names Viramune®

Therapeutic Category Antiviral Agent

Use In combination therapy with nucleoside antiretroviral agents in HIV-1 infected adults previously treated for whom current therapy is deemed inadequate

Usual Dosage Adults: Oral: 200 mg once daily for 2 weeks followed by 200 mg twice daily

Dosage Forms

Suspension, oral: 50 mg/5 mL (240 mL)

Tablet: 200 mg

New Decongestant® *see* chlorpheniramine, phenyltoloxamine, phenylpropanolamine, and phenylephrine *on page 125*

N.G.T.® Topical *see* nystatin and triamcinolone *on page 412*

Niac® *(Discontinued)* *see page 700*

Niacels® *(Discontinued)* *see page 700*

niacin (NYE a sin)

Synonyms nicotinic acid; vitamin B_3

U.S./Canadian Brand Names Niaspan®; Nicobid® [OTC]; Nicolar® [OTC]; Nicotinex [OTC]; Slo-Niacin® [OTC]

Therapeutic Category Vitamin, Water Soluble

Use Adjunctive treatment of hyperlipidemias; peripheral vascular disease and circulatory disorders; treatment of pellagra; dietary supplement

Usual Dosage

Children: Pellagra: Oral, I.M., I.V.: 50-100 mg/dose 3 times/day

(Continued)

niacin *(Continued)*

Oral: Recommended daily allowances:
0-1 year: 6-8 mg/day
2-6 years: 9-11 mg/day
7-10 years: 16 mg/day
>10 years: 15-18 mg/day
Adults: Oral:
Hyperlipidemia: 1.5-6 g/day in 3 divided doses with or after meals
Pellagra: 50 mg 3-10 times/day, maximum: 500 mg/day
Niacin deficiency: 10-20 mg/day, maximum: 100 mg/day

Dosage Forms
Capsule, timed release: 125 mg, 250 mg, 300 mg, 400 mg, 500 mg
Elixir: 50 mg/5 mL (473 mL, 4000 mL)
Injection: 100 mg/mL (30 mL)
Tablet: 25 mg, 50 mg, 100 mg, 250 mg, 500 mg
Extended release: 500 mg, 750 mg, 1000 mg
Timed release: 150 mg, 250 mg, 500 mg, 750 mg

niacinamide (nye a SIN a mide)

Synonyms nicotinamide
Therapeutic Category Vitamin, Water Soluble
Use Prophylaxis and treatment of pellagra
Usual Dosage Oral:
Children: Pellagra: 100-300 mg/day
Adults: 50 mg 3-10 times/day
Pellagra: 300-500 mg/day
Hyperlipidemias: 1-2 g 3 times/day
Dosage Forms Tablet: 50 mg, 100 mg, 125 mg, 250 mg, 500 mg

Niaspan® *see* niacin *on previous page*

nicardipine (nye KAR de peen)

U.S./Canadian Brand Names Cardene®; Cardene® SR
Therapeutic Category Calcium Channel Blocker
Use Chronic stable angina; management of essential hypertension
Usual Dosage Adults:
Oral: 40 mg 3 times/day (allow 3 days between dose increases)
Oral, sustained release: Initial: 30 mg twice daily, titrate up to 60 mg twice daily
I.V.: (Dilute to 0.1 mg/mL) Initial: 5 mg/hour increased by 2.5 mg/hour every 15 minutes to a maximum of 15 mg/hour
Oral to I.V. dose:
20 mg every 8 hours = I.V. 0.5 mg/hour
30 mg every 8 hours = I.V. 1.2 mg/hour
40 mg every 8 hours = I.V. 2.2 mg/hour
Dosage Forms Nicardipine hydrochloride:
Capsule: 20 mg, 30 mg
Capsule, sustained release: 30 mg, 45 mg, 60 mg
Injection: 2.5 mg/mL (10 mL)

N'ice® *see* ascorbic acid *on page 48*

Niclocide® ***(Discontinued)*** *see page 700*

Nicobid® [OTC] *see* niacin *on previous page*

Nicoderm® Patch *see* nicotine *on next page*

Nicolar® [OTC] *see* niacin *on previous page*

Nicorette® DS Gum *see* nicotine *on next page*

Nicorette® Gum *see* nicotine *on next page*

Nicorette® Plus (Can) *see* nicotine *on this page*

nicotinamide *see* niacinamide *on previous page*

nicotine (nik oh TEEN)

U.S./Canadian Brand Names Habitrol™ Patch; Nicoderm® Patch; Nicorette® DS Gum; Nicorette® Gum; Nicorette® Plus (Can); Nicotrol® Inhaler; Nicotrol® NS Nasal Spray; Nicotrol® Patch [OTC]; ProStep® Patch

Therapeutic Category Smoking Deterrent

Use Treatment aid to giving up smoking while participating in a behavioral modification program, under medical supervision

Usual Dosage

Gum: Chew 1 piece of gum when urge to smoke, up to 30 pieces/day; most patients require 10-12 pieces of gum/day

Inhaler: Usually 6 to 16 cartridges per day; best effect was achieved by frequent continuous puffing (20 minutes); recommended duration of treatment is 3 months, after which patients may be weaned from the inhaler by gradual reduction of the daily dose over 6-12 weeks

Transdermal patch (patients should be advised to completely stop smoking upon initiation of therapy): Apply new patch every 24 hours to nonhairy, clean, dry skin on the upper body or upper outer arm; each patch should be applied to a different site

Initial starting dose: 21 mg/day for 4-8 weeks for most patients

First weaning dose: 14 mg/day for 2-4 weeks

Second weaning dose: 7 mg/day for 2-4 weeks

Initial starting dose for patients <100 pounds, smoke <10 cigarettes/day, have a history of cardiovascular disease: 14 mg/day for 4-8 weeks followed by 7 mg/day for 2-4 weeks

In patients who are receiving >600 mg/day of cimetidine: Decrease to the next lower patch size

Benefits of use of nicotine transdermal patches beyond 3 months have not been demonstrated

Spray: 1-2 sprays/hour; do not exceed more than 5 doses (10 sprays) per hour; each dose (2 sprays) contains 1 mg of nicotine. **Warning:** A dose of 40 mg can cause fatalities

Dosage Forms

Inhaler, oral (cartridge): 10 mg [delivering 4 mg] (42s); each unit consists of one mouthpiece, 7 storage trays each containing 6 cartridges and one storage case

Patch, transdermal:

Habitrol™: 21 mg/day; 14 mg/day; 7 mg/day (30 systems/box)

Nicoderm®: 21 mg/day; 14 mg/day; 7 mg/day (14 systems/box)

Nicotrol® [OTC]: 15 mg/day (gradually released over 16 hours)

ProStep®: 22 mg/day; 11 mg/day (7 systems/box)

Pieces, chewing gum, as polacrilex: 2 mg/square [OTC] (96 pieces/box); 4 mg/square (96 pieces/box)

Spray, nasal: 0.5 mg/actuation [10 mg/mL - 200 actuations] (10 mL)

Nicotinex [OTC] *see* niacin *on page 399*

nicotinic acid *see* niacin *on page 399*

Nicotrol® Inhaler *see* nicotine *on this page*

Nicotrol® NS Nasal Spray *see* nicotine *on this page*

Nicotrol® Patch [OTC] *see* nicotine *on this page*

nicoumalone *(Canada only)* (nye KYOO ma lone)

U.S./Canadian Brand Names Sintrom® (Can)

Therapeutic Category Anticoagulant

Use Prophylaxis and treatment of venous thrombosis and its extension, the treatment of atrial fibrillation with embolization, the prophylaxis and treatment of pulmonary embolism and as an adjunct in the treatment of coronary occlusion and transient cerebral ischemic attacks

(Continued)

nicoumalone *(Canada only)* *(Continued)*

Usual Dosage Adults: Oral:
- First day: 8-12 mg
- Second day: 4-8 mg; if the thromboplastin time is initially abnormal, treatment must be commenced with great caution
- Maintenance therapy and coagulation tests: In view of the marked individual differences encountered, the maintenance dose should be established and adjusted by reference to the results of periodically performed laboratory tests to determine the patient's blood coagulation time.

Dosage Forms Tablet: 1 mg, 4 mg

Nico-Vert® [OTC] *see* meclizine *on page 351*

Nidagel™ (Can) *see* metronidazole *on page 372*

Nidryl® *(Discontinued)* *see page 700*

nifedipine (nye FED i peen)

U.S./Canadian Brand Names Adalat®; Adalat® CC; Adalat PA® (Can); Apo®-Nifed (Can); Gen-Nifedipine (Can); Novo-Nifedin® (Can); Nu-Nifedin® (Can); Procardia®; Procardia XL®

Therapeutic Category Calcium Channel Blocker

Use Angina, hypertrophic cardiomyopathy, hypertension

Usual Dosage
- Children: Oral:
  - Hypertensive emergencies: 0.25-0.5 mg/kg/dose
  - Hypertrophic cardiomyopathy: 0.6-0.9 mg/kg/24 hours in 3-4 divided doses
- Adults: Initial: 10 mg 3 times/day as capsules or 30-60 mg once daily as sustained release tablet; maintenance: 10-30 mg 3-4 times/day (capsules); maximum: 180 mg/24 hours (capsules) or 120 mg/day (sustained release)

Dosage Forms
- Capsule, liquid-filled (Adalat®, Procardia®): 10 mg, 20 mg
- Tablet, extended release (Adalat® CC): 30 mg, 60 mg, 90 mg
- Tablet, sustained release (Procardia XL®): 30 mg, 60 mg, 90 mg

Niferex® [OTC] *see* polysaccharide-iron complex *on page 460*

Niferex Forte® *(Discontinued)* *see page 700*

Niferex®-PN *see* vitamin, multiple (oral) *on page 604*

Nilandron™ *see* nilutamide *on this page*

Niloric® *(Discontinued)* *see page 700*

Nilstat® *see* nystatin *on page 412*

nilutamide (ni LU ta mide)

U.S./Canadian Brand Names Anandron® (Can); Nilandron™

Therapeutic Category Antineoplastic Agent

Use With orchiectomy (surgical castration) for the treatment of metastatic prostate cancer

Usual Dosage Adults: Oral: 300 mg (6-50 mg tablets) once daily for 30 days, then 150 mg (3-50 mg tablets) once daily; starting on the same day or day after surgical castration

Dosage Forms Tablet: 50 mg

Nimbex® *see* cisatracurium *on page 133*

nimodipine (nye MOE di peen)

U.S./Canadian Brand Names Nimotop®

Therapeutic Category Calcium Channel Blocker

Use Improvement of neurological deficits due to spasm following subarachnoid hemorrhage from ruptured congenital intracranial aneurysms who are in good neurological condition postictus

Usual Dosage Adults: Oral: 60 mg every 4 hours for 21 days, start therapy within 96 hours after subarachnoid hemorrhage

Dosage Forms Capsule, liquid-filled: 30 mg

Nimotop® *see* nimodipine *on previous page*

Nipent™ *see* pentostatin *on page 438*

Nipride® Injection *(Discontinued)* *see page 700*

Nisaval® *(Discontinued)* *see page 700*

nisoldipine (NYE sole di peen)

U.S./Canadian Brand Names Sular®

Therapeutic Category Calcium Channel Blocker

Use Management of hypertension, may be used alone or in combination with other antihypertensive agents

Usual Dosage Adults: Oral: Initial: 20 mg once daily, then increase by 10 mg per week (or longer intervals) to attain adequate control of blood pressure; doses >60 mg once daily are not recommended

Dosage Forms Tablet, extended release: 10 mg, 20 mg, 30 mg, 40 mg

Nitalapram *see* citalopram *on page 134*

Nitoman® (Can) *see* tetrabenazine *(Canada only) on page 554*

Nitro-Bid® I.V. Injection *see* nitroglycerin *on next page*

Nitro-Bid® Ointment *see* nitroglycerin *on next page*

Nitro-Bid® Oral *(Discontinued)* *see page 700*

Nitrocine® Oral *(Discontinued)* *see page 700*

Nitrodisc® Patch *see* nitroglycerin *on next page*

Nitro-Dur® Patch *see* nitroglycerin *on next page*

nitrofural *see* nitrofurazone *on this page*

nitrofurantoin (nye troe fyoor AN toyn)

U.S./Canadian Brand Names Apo®-Nitrofurantoin (Can); Furadantin®; Furalan®; Furan®; Furanite®; Macrobid®; Macrodantin®; Nephronex® (Can); Novo-Furan® (Can)

Therapeutic Category Antibiotic, Miscellaneous

Use Prevention and treatment of urinary tract infections caused by susceptible gram-negative and some gram-positive organisms including *E. coli*, *Klebsiella*, *Enterobacter*, *Enterococa*, and *S. aureus*; *Pseudomonas*, *Serratia*, and most species of *Proteus* are generally resistant to nitrofurantoin

Usual Dosage Oral:

Children >1 month: 5-7 mg/kg/day divided every 6 hours; maximum: 400 mg/day

Chronic therapy: 1-2 mg/kg/day in divided doses every 12-24 hours; maximum dose: 400 mg/day

Adults: 50-100 mg/dose every 6 hours (not to exceed 400 mg/24 hours)

Prophylaxis: 50-100 mg/dose at bedtime

Dosage Forms

Capsule: 50 mg, 100 mg

Capsule:

Macrocrystal: 25 mg, 50 mg, 100 mg

Macrocrystal/monohydrate: 100 mg

Suspension, oral: 25 mg/5 mL (470 mL)

nitrofurazone (nye troe FYOOR a zone)

Synonyms nitrofural

U.S./Canadian Brand Names Furacin® Topical

Therapeutic Category Antibacterial, Topical

Use Antibacterial agent used in second- and third-degree burns and skin grafting

(Continued)

nitrofurazone *(Continued)*

Usual Dosage Children and Adults: Topical: Apply once daily or every few days to lesion or place on gauze

Dosage Forms

Cream: 0.2% (4 g, 28 g)
Ointment, soluble dressing: 0.2% (28 g, 56 g, 454 g, 480 g)
Solution, topical: 0.2% (480 mL, 3780 mL)

Nitrogard® Buccal *see* nitroglycerin *on this page*

nitrogen mustard *see* mechlorethamine *on page 351*

nitroglycerin (nye troe GLI ser in)

Synonyms glyceryl trinitrate; nitroglycerol; NTG

U.S./Canadian Brand Names Deponit® Patch; Minitran® Patch; Nitro-Bid® I.V. Injection; Nitro-Bid® Ointment; Nitrodisc® Patch; Nitro-Dur® Patch; Nitrogard® Buccal; Nitroglyn® Oral; Nitrolingual® Translingual Spray; Nitrol® Ointment; Nitrong® Oral Tablet; Nitrong® SR (Can); Nitrostat® Sublingual; Transdermal-NTG® Patch; Transderm-Nitro® Patch; Tridil® Injection

Therapeutic Category Vasodilator

Use Angina pectoris; I.V. for congestive heart failure (especially when associated with acute myocardial infarction); pulmonary hypertension; hypertensive emergencies occurring perioperatively (especially during cardiovascular surgery)

Usual Dosage Note: Hemodynamic and antianginal tolerance often develops within 24-48 hours of continuous nitrate administration

Children: Pulmonary hypertension: Continuous infusion: Start 0.25-0.5 mcg/kg/minute and titrate by 1 mcg/kg/minute at 20- to 60-minute intervals to desired effect; usual dose: 1-3 mcg/kg/minute; maximum: 5 mcg/kg/minute

Adults:

Oral: 2.5-9 mg 2-4 times/day (up to 26 mg 4 times/day)

I.V.: 5 mcg/minute, increase by 5 mcg/minute every 3-5 minutes to 20 mcg/minute; if no response at 20 mcg/minute increase by 10 mcg/minute every 3-5 minutes, up to 200 mcg/minute

Sublingual: 0.2-0.6 mg every 5 minutes for maximum of 3 doses in 15 minutes; may also use prophylactically 5-10 minutes prior to activities which may provoke an attack

Ointment: 1" to 2" every 8 hours up to 4" to 5" every 4 hours

Patch, transdermal: 0.2-0.4 mg/hour initially and titrate to doses of 0.4-0.8 mg/hour; tolerance is minimized by using a patch on period of 12-14 hours and patch off period of 10-12 hours

Translingual: 1-2 sprays into mouth under tongue every 3-5 minutes for maximum of 3 doses in 15 minutes, may also be used 5-10 minutes prior to activities which may provoke an attack prophylactically

Buccal: Initial: 1 mg every 3-5 hours while awake (3 times/day); titrate dosage upward if angina occurs with tablet in place

May need to use nitrate-free interval (10-12 hours/day) to avoid tolerance development; tolerance may possibly be reversed with acetylcysteine; gradually decrease dose in patients receiving NTG for prolonged period to avoid withdrawal reaction

Dosage Forms

Capsule, sustained release: 2.5 mg, 6.5 mg, 9 mg
Injection: 0.5 mg/mL (10 mL); 0.8 mg/mL (10 mL); 5 mg/mL (1 mL, 5 mL, 10 mL, 20 mL); 10 mg/mL (5 mL, 10 mL)
Ointment, topical (Nitrol®): 2% [20 mg/g] (30 g, 60 g)
Patch, transdermal, topical: Systems designed to deliver 2.5, 5, 7.5, 10, or 15 mg NTG over 24 hours
Spray, translingual: 0.4 mg/metered spray (13.8 g)
Tablet:
Buccal, controlled release: 1 mg, 2 mg, 3 mg
Sublingual (Nitrostat®): 0.3 mg, 0.4 mg, 0.6 mg
Sustained release: 2.6 mg, 6.5 mg, 9 mg

nitroglycerol *see* nitroglycerin *on previous page*

Nitroglyn® Oral *see* nitroglycerin *on previous page*

Nitrolingual® Translingual Spray *see* nitroglycerin *on previous page*

Nitrol® Ointment *see* nitroglycerin *on previous page*

Nitrong® Oral Tablet *see* nitroglycerin *on previous page*

Nitrong® SR (Can) *see* nitroglycerin *on previous page*

Nitropress® *see* nitroprusside *on this page*

nitroprusside (nye troe PRUS ide)

Synonyms sodium nitroferricyanide

U.S./Canadian Brand Names Nitropress®

Therapeutic Category Vasodilator

Use Management of hypertensive crises; congestive heart failure; used for controlled hypotension during anesthesia

Usual Dosage I.V.:

Children: Continuous infusion:

Initial: 1 mcg/kg/minute by continuous I.V. infusion; increase in increments of 1 mcg/kg/minute at intervals of 20-60 minutes; titrating to the desired response

Usual dose: 3 mcg/kg/minute; rarely need >4 mcg/kg/minute

Maximum: 10 mcg/kg/minute. Dilute 15 mg x weight (kg) to 250 mL D_5W, then dose in mcg/kg/minute = infusion rate in mL/hour

Adults: Begin at 5 mcg/kg/minute; increase in increments of 5 mcg/kg/minute (up to 20 mcg/kg/minute), then in increments of 10-20 mcg/kg/minute; titrating to the desired hemodynamic effect or the appearance of headache or nausea. When >500 mcg/kg is administered by prolonged infusion of faster than 2 mcg/kg/minute, cyanide is generated faster than an unaided patient can handle.

Dosage Forms Injection, as sodium: 10 mg/mL (5 mL); 25 mg/mL (2 mL)

Nitrostat® 0.15 mg Tablet *(Discontinued)* *see* *page 700*

Nitrostat® Sublingual *see* nitroglycerin *on previous page*

Nix™ Creme Rinse *see* permethrin *on page 440*

nizatidine (ni ZA ti deen)

U.S./Canadian Brand Names Axid®; Axid® AR [OTC]

Therapeutic Category Histamine H_2 Antagonist

Use Treatment and maintenance of duodenal ulcer; treatment of gastroesophageal reflux disease (GERD)

Usual Dosage Adults: Active duodenal ulcer: Oral:

Treatment: 300 mg at bedtime or 150 mg twice daily

Maintenance: 150 mg/day

Dosage Forms

Capsule: 150 mg, 300 mg

Tablet: 75 mg

Nizoral® *see* ketoconazole *on page 320*

n-methylhydrazine *see* procarbazine *on page 476*

Nobesine® (Can) *see* diethylpropion *on page 178*

Noctec® *(Discontinued)* *see* *page 700*

Nolahist® [OTC] *see* phenindamine *on page 443*

Nolamine® *see* chlorpheniramine, phenindamine, and phenylpropanolamine *on page 123*

Nolex® LA *see* guaifenesin and phenylpropanolamine *on page 270*

Noludar® *(Discontinued)* *see* *page 700*

Nolvadex® *see* tamoxifen *on page 547*

nonoxynol 9 (non OKS i nole nine)

U.S./Canadian Brand Names Because® [OTC]; Delfen® [OTC]; Emko® [OTC]; Encare® [OTC]; Gynol II® [OTC]; Koromex® [OTC]; Ramses® [OTC]; Semicid® [OTC]; Shur-Seal® [OTC]

Therapeutic Category Spermicide

Use Spermatocide in contraception

Usual Dosage Insert into vagina at least 15 minutes before intercourse

Dosage Forms Vaginal:

Cream: 2% (103.5 g)
Foam: 12.5% (60 g)
Jelly: 2% (81 g, 126 g)

No Pain-HP® [OTC] *see* capsaicin *on page 96*

noradrenaline acid tartrate *see* norepinephrine *on this page*

Norcet® *see* hydrocodone and acetaminophen *on page 287*

Norcuron® *see* vecuronium *on page 597*

nordeoxyguanosine *see* ganciclovir *on page 257*

Nordette® *see* ethinyl estradiol and levonorgestrel *on page 223*

Norditropin® *see* human growth hormone *on page 283*

Nordryl® Injection *see* diphenhydramine *on page 185*

Nordryl® Oral *see* diphenhydramine *on page 185*

norepinephrine (nor ep i NEF rin)

Synonyms noradrenaline acid tartrate

U.S./Canadian Brand Names Levophed®

Therapeutic Category Adrenergic Agonist Agent

Use Treatment of shock which persists after adequate fluid volume replacement; severe hypotension; cardiogenic shock

Usual Dosage **Note:** Dose stated in terms of norepinephrine base. I.V.:

Children: Initial: 0.05-0.1 mcg/kg/minute, titrate to desired effect; rate (mL/hour) = dose (mcg/kg/minute) x weight (kg) x 60 minutes/hour divided by concentration (mcg/mL)

Adults: 8-12 mcg/minute as an infusion; initiate at 4 mcg/minute and titrate to desired response

Dosage Forms Injection, as bitartrate: 1 mg/mL (4 mL)

Norethin™ 1/35E *see* ethinyl estradiol and norethindrone *on page 224*

Norethin 1/50M *see* mestranol and norethindrone *on page 359*

norethindrone (nor eth IN drone)

Synonyms norethisterone

U.S./Canadian Brand Names Aygestin®; Micronor®; NOR-QD®

Therapeutic Category Contraceptive, Progestin Only; Progestin

Use Treatment of amenorrhea; abnormal uterine bleeding; endometriosis

Usual Dosage Adolescents and Adults: Oral:

Amenorrhea and abnormal uterine bleeding: 2.5-10 mg on days 5-25 of menstrual cycle

Endometriosis: 5 mg/day for 14 days; increase at increments of 2.5 mg/day every 2 weeks up to 15 mg/day

Dosage Forms

Tablet: 0.35 mg, 5 mg
Tablet, as acetate: 5 mg

norethindrone acetate and ethinyl estradiol *see* ethinyl estradiol and norethindrone *on page 224*

norethindrone and mestranol *see* mestranol and norethindrone *on page 359*

norethisterone *see* norethindrone *on this page*

Norflex™ *see* orphenadrine *on page 418*

norfloxacin (nor FLOKS a sin)

U.S./Canadian Brand Names Chibroxin™ Ophthalmic; Noroxin® Oral

Therapeutic Category Quinolone

Use Complicated and uncomplicated urinary tract infections caused by susceptible gram-negative and gram-positive bacteria

Usual Dosage

Children >1 year and Adults: Ophthalmic: Instill 1-2 drops in affected eye(s) 4 times/day for up to 7 days

Adults: Oral: 400 mg twice daily for 7-21 days depending on infection

Dosage Forms

Solution, ophthalmic: 0.3% [3 mg/mL] (5 mL)

Tablet: 400 mg

Norgesic™ *see* orphenadrine, aspirin, and caffeine *on page 418*

Norgesic™ Forte *see* orphenadrine, aspirin, and caffeine *on page 418*

norgestimate and ethinyl estradiol *see* ethinyl estradiol and norgestimate *on page 225*

norgestrel (nor JES trel)

U.S./Canadian Brand Names Ovrette®

Therapeutic Category Contraceptive, Progestin Only

Use Prevention of pregnancy; treatment of hypermenorrhea, endometriosis, female hypogonadism

Usual Dosage Oral: Administer daily, starting the first day of menstruation, administer one tablet at the same time each day, every day of the year. If one dose is missed, administer as soon as remembered, then next tablet at regular time; if two doses are missed, administer one tablet and discard the other, then administer daily at usual time; if three doses are missed, use an additional form of birth control until menses or pregnancy is ruled out

Dosage Forms Tablet: 0.075 mg

norgestrel and ethinyl estradiol *see* ethinyl estradiol and norgestrel *on page 225*

Norinyl® 1+35 *see* ethinyl estradiol and norethindrone *on page 224*

Norinyl® 1+50 *see* mestranol and norethindrone *on page 359*

Noritate® (Can) *see* metronidazole *on page 372*

Norlutate® ***(Discontinued)*** *see page 700*

Norlutin® ***(Discontinued)*** *see page 700*

normal saline *see* sodium chloride *on page 526*

Normiflo® *see* ardeparin *on page 46*

Normodyne® *see* labetalol *on page 323*

Noroxin® Oral *see* norfloxacin *on this page*

Norpace® *see* disopyramide *on page 189*

Norpace® CR *see* disopyramide *on page 189*

Norplant® Implant *see* levonorgestrel *on page 332*

Norpramin® *see* desipramine *on page 165*

NOR-QD® *see* norethindrone *on previous page*

Nor-tet® Oral *see* tetracycline *on page 555*

North American coral snake antivenin *see* antivenin (*Micrurus fulvius*) *on page 42*

North and South American antisnake-bite serum *see* antivenin (*Crotalidae*) polyvalent *on page 41*

nortriptyline (nor TRIP ti leen)

U.S./Canadian Brand Names Aventyl® Hydrochloride; Pamelor®

Therapeutic Category Antidepressant, Tricyclic (Secondary Amine)

Use Treatment of various forms of depression, often in conjunction with psychotherapy; nocturnal enuresis

Usual Dosage Oral:

Adults: 25 mg 3-4 times/day up to 150 mg/day

Adolescents and Elderly: 30-50 mg/day in divided doses

Dosage Forms Nortriptyline hydrochloride:

Capsule: 10 mg, 25 mg, 50 mg, 75 mg

Solution: 10 mg/5 mL (473 mL)

Norvasc® *see* amlodipine *on page 29*

Norvir® *see* ritonavir *on page 507*

Nōstrilla® [OTC] *see* oxymetazoline *on page 423*

Nostril® Nasal Solution [OTC] *see* phenylephrine *on page 445*

Novacet® Topical *see* sulfur and sulfacetamide *on page 544*

Novafed® *(Discontinued)* *see page 700*

Novahistine® (Can) *see* phenylephrine *on page 445*

Novahistine DH® Liquid *(Discontinued)* *see page 700*

Novahistine DMX® Liquid *(Discontinued)* *see page 700*

Novahistine® Elixir *(Discontinued)* *see page 700*

Novahistine® Expectorant *(Discontinued)* *see page 700*

Novamoxin® (Can) *see* amoxicillin *on page 31*

Novantrone® *see* mitoxantrone *on page 378*

Nova Rectal® (Can) *see* pentobarbital *on page 437*

Novasen (Can) *see* aspirin *on page 49*

Novo-Aloprazol® (Can) *see* alprazolam *on page 19*

Novo-Atenol® (Can) *see* atenolol *on page 51*

Novo-AZT® (Can) *see* zidovudine *on page 610*

Novo-Butamide® (Can) *see* tolbutamide *on page 570*

Novocain® *see* procaine *on page 475*

Novo-Captopril® (Can) *see* captopril *on page 96*

Novo-Carbamaz® (Can) *see* carbamazepine *on page 97*

Novo-Chlorhydrate® (Can) *see* chloral hydrate *on page 115*

Novo-Chlorpromazine® (Can) *see* chlorpromazine *on page 127*

Novo-Cimetidine® (Can) *see* cimetidine *on page 131*

Novo-Clobetasol (Can) *see* clobetasol *on page 137*

Novo-Clonidine® (Can) *see* clonidine *on page 139*

Novo-Clopate® (Can) *see* clorazepate *on page 140*

Novo-Cloxin® (Can) *see* cloxacillin *on page 141*

Novo-Cromolyn® (Can) *see* cromolyn sodium *on page 150*

Novo-Cycloprine® (Can) *see* cyclobenzaprine *on page 153*

Novo-Difenac® (Can) *see* diclofenac *on page 175*

Novo-Difenac-SR® (Can) *see* diclofenac *on page 175*

Novo-Prazin® (Can) *see* prazosin *on page 470*

Novo-Prednisolone® (Can) *see* prednisolone (systemic) *on page 471*

Novo-Prednisone® (Can) *see* prednisone *on page 472*

Novo-Profen® (Can) *see* ibuprofen *on page 300*

Novo-Propamide® (Can) *see* chlorpropamide *on page 127*

Novo-Propoxyn® (Can) *see* propoxyphene *on page 482*

Novo-purol® (Can) *see* allopurinol *on page 19*

Novo-Pyrazone (Can) *see* sulfinpyrazone *on page 543*

Novo-Ranidine® (Can) *see* ranitidine hydrochloride *on page 497*

Novo-Reserpine® (Can) *see* reserpine *on page 500*

Novo-Ridazine® (Can) *see* thioridazine *on page 563*

Novo-Rythro Encap (Can) *see* erythromycin (systemic) *on page 215*

Novo-Salmol® (Can) *see* albuterol *on page 15*

Novo-Secobarb® (Can) *see* secobarbital *on page 517*

Novo-Selegiline (Can) *see* selegiline *on page 518*

Novo-Semide® (Can) *see* furosemide *on page 255*

Novo-Seven® *see* factor VIIa, recombinant *on page 230*

Novo-Soxazole® (Can) *see* sulfisoxazole *on page 543*

Novo-Spiroton® (Can) *see* spironolactone *on page 534*

Novo-Sucralate® (Can) *see* sucralfate *on page 538*

Novo-Sundac® (Can) *see* sulindac *on page 544*

Novo-Tamoxifen (Can) *see* tamoxifen *on page 547*

Novo-Terfenadine® (Can) *see* terfenadine *on page 551*

Novo-Tetra® (Can) *see* tetracycline *on page 555*

Novo-Thalidone® (Can) *see* chlorthalidone *on page 128*

Novo-Timol® (Can) *see* timolol *on page 567*

Novo-Tolmetin® (Can) *see* tolmetin *on page 571*

Novo-Triamzide (Can) *see* hydrochlorothiazide and triamterene *on page 287*

Novo-Trimel® (Can) *see* co-trimoxazole *on page 149*

Novo-Triolam® (Can) *see* triazolam *on page 579*

Novo-Tripramine (Can) *see* trimipramine *on page 583*

Novo-Tryptin® (Can) *see* amitriptyline *on page 28*

Novo-Veramil® (Can) *see* verapamil *on page 598*

Novo-Zolamide® (Can) *see* acetazolamide *on page 7*

NP-27® [OTC] *see* tolnaftate *on page 571*

NPH Iletin® I *see* insulin preparations *on page 307*

NPH Insulin *see* insulin preparations *on page 307*

NPH-N *see* insulin preparations *on page 307*

NTG *see* nitroglycerin *on page 404*

NTZ® Long Acting Nasal Solution [OTC] *see* oxymetazoline *on page 423*

Nu-Alprax® (Can) *see* alprazolam *on page 19*

Nu-Amoxi (Can) *see* amoxicillin *on page 31*

Nu-Ampi (Can) *see* ampicillin *on page 34*

Nu-Atenol® (Can) *see* atenolol *on page 51*

Nubain® *see* nalbuphine *on page 388*

Nu-Capto® (Can) *see* captopril *on page 96*

Nu-Carbamazepine® (Can) *see* carbamazepine *on page 97*

Nu-Cephalex® (Can) *see* cephalexin *on page 111*

Nu-Cimet® (Can) *see* cimetidine *on page 131*

Nu-Clonidine® (Can) *see* clonidine *on page 139*

Nu-Cloxi® (Can) *see* cloxacillin *on page 141*

Nucofed® *see* guaifenesin, pseudoephedrine, and codeine *on page 272*

Nucofed® Pediatric Expectorant *see* guaifenesin, pseudoephedrine, and codeine *on page 272*

Nu-Cotrimox® (Can) *see* co-trimoxazole *on page 149*

Nucotuss® *see* guaifenesin, pseudoephedrine, and codeine *on page 272*

Nu-Diclo® (Can) *see* diclofenac *on page 175*

Nu-Diflunisal (Can) *see* diflunisal *on page 179*

Nu-Diltiaz® (Can) *see* diltiazem *on page 182*

Nu-Doxycycline® (Can) *see* doxycycline *on page 197*

Nu-Famotidine® (Can) *see* famotidine *on page 231*

Nu-Flurprofen® (Can) *see* flurbiprofen *on page 248*

Nu-Gemfibrozil (Can) *see* gemfibrozil *on page 259*

Nu-Glyburide (Can) *see* glyburide *on page 263*

Nu-Hydral® (Can) *see* hydralazine *on page 284*

Nu-Ibuprofen® (Can) *see* ibuprofen *on page 300*

Nu-Indo® (Can) *see* indomethacin *on page 305*

Nu-Iron® [OTC] *see* polysaccharide-iron complex *on page 460*

Nu-Ketoprofen (Can) *see* ketoprofen *on page 321*

Nu-Ketoprofen-E (Can) *see* ketoprofen *on page 321*

Nullo® [OTC] *see* chlorophyll *on page 118*

Nu-Loraz® (Can) *see* lorazepam *on page 340*

NuLYTELY® *see* polyethylene glycol-electrolyte solution *on page 459*

Nu-Medopa® (Can) *see* methyldopa *on page 367*

Nu-Metop (Can) *see* metoprolol *on page 371*

Numorphan® *see* oxymorphone *on page 424*

Numzitdent® [OTC] *see* benzocaine *on page 66*

Numzit Teething® [OTC] *see* benzocaine *on page 66*

Nu-Naprox® (Can) *see* naproxen *on page 391*

Nu-Nifedin® (Can) *see* nifedipine *on page 402*

Nu-Pen-VK® (Can) *see* penicillin V potassium *on page 435*

Nupercainal® [OTC] *see* dibucaine *on page 175*

Nu-Pindol (Can) *see* pindolol *on page 452*

Nu-Pirox® (Can) *see* piroxicam *on page 454*

Nu-Prazo® (Can) *see* prazosin *on page 470*

Nuprin® [OTC] *see* ibuprofen *on page 300*

Nu-Prochlor® (Can) *see* prochlorperazine *on page 476*

Nu-Propranolol® (Can) *see* propranolol *on page 483*

Nu-Ranit® (Can) *see* ranitidine hydrochloride *on page 497*

Nuromax® *see* doxacurium *on page 195*

Nursoy® *(Discontinued)* *see page 700*

Nu-Sulfinpyrazone (Can) *see* sulfinpyrazone *on page 543*

Nu-Tears® II Solution [OTC] *see* artificial tears *on page 47*

Nu-Tears® Solution [OTC] *see* artificial tears *on page 47*

Nu-Tetra® (Can) *see* tetracycline *on page 555*

Nu-Timolol® (Can) *see* timolol *on page 567*

Nutracort® Topical *see* hydrocortisone (topical) *on page 292*

Nutraplus® Topical [OTC] *see* urea *on page 591*

Nu-Triazide (Can) *see* hydrochlorothiazide and triamterene *on page 287*

Nu-Triazo® (Can) *see* triazolam *on page 579*

Nutrilipid® *see* fat emulsion *on page 231*

Nu-Trimipramine® (Can) *see* trimipramine *on page 583*

Nutrisource™ (Can) *see* enteral nutritional products *on page 208*

Nutropin® *see* human growth hormone *on page 283*

Nutropin® AQ *see* human growth hormone *on page 283*

Nu-Verap® (Can) *see* verapamil *on page 598*

Nyaderm (Can) *see* nystatin *on this page*

Nydrazid® Injection *(Discontinued)* *see page 700*

nystatin (nye STAT in)

U.S./Canadian Brand Names Candistatin® (Can); Mestatin® (Can); Mycostatin®; Nadostine® (Can); Nilstat®; Nyaderm (Can); Nystat-Rx®; Nystex®; O-V Staticin®; PMS-Nystatin (Can)

Therapeutic Category Antifungal Agent

Use Treatment of susceptible cutaneous, mucocutaneous, oral cavity and vaginal fungal infections normally caused by the *Candida* species

Usual Dosage

Oral candidiasis:

Infants: 200,000 units 4 times/day or 100,000 units to each side of mouth 4 times/day

Children and Adults: 400,000-600,000 units 4 times/day; troche: 200,000-400,000 units 4-5 times/day

Cutaneous candidal infections: Children and Adults: Topical: Apply 3-4 times/day

Intestinal infections: Adults: Oral: 500,000-1,000,000 units every 8 hours

Vaginal infections: Adults: Vaginal tablets: Insert 1-2 tablets/day at bedtime for 2 weeks

Dosage Forms

Cream: 100,000 units/g (15 g, 30 g)

Ointment, topical: 100,000 units/g (15 g, 30 g)

Powder, for preparation of oral suspension: 50 million units, 1 billion units, 2 billion units, 5 billion units

Powder, topical: 100,000 units/g (15 g)

Suspension, oral: 100,000 units/mL (5 mL, 60 mL, 480 mL)

Tablet:

Oral: 500,000 units

Vaginal: 100,000 units (15 and 30/box with applicator)

Troche: 200,000 units

nystatin and triamcinolone (nye STAT in & trye am SIN oh lone)

Synonyms triamcinolone and nystatin

U.S./Canadian Brand Names Mycogen II Topical; Mycolog®-II Topical; Myconel® Topical; Myco-Triacet® II; Mytrex® F Topical; N.G.T.® Topical; Tri-Statin® II Topical

Therapeutic Category Antifungal/Corticosteroid

Use Treatment of cutaneous candidiasis

Usual Dosage Topical: Apply twice daily

Dosage Forms

Cream: Nystatin 100,000 units and triamcinolone acetonide 0.1% (15 g, 30 g, 45 g, 60 g, 240 g)

Ointment, topical: Nystatin 100,000 units and triamcinolone acetonide 0.1% (15 g, 30 g, 60 g, 120 g)

Nystat-Rx® *see* nystatin *on previous page*

Nystex® *see* nystatin *on previous page*

Nytol® Oral [OTC] *see* diphenhydramine *on page 185*

Obe-Nix® 30 *(Discontinued)* *see page 700*

Obephen® *(Discontinued)* *see page 700*

Obermine® *(Discontinued)* *see page 700*

Obestin-30® *(Discontinued)* *see page 700*

Occlucort® (Can) *see* betamethasone (topical) *on page 72*

Occlusal®-HP Liquid *see* salicylic acid *on page 513*

Ocean Nasal Mist [OTC] *see* sodium chloride *on page 526*

OCL® *see* polyethylene glycol-electrolyte solution *on page 459*

Octamide® *see* metoclopramide *on page 370*

Octicair® Otic *see* neomycin, polymyxin B, and hydrocortisone *on page 396*

Octocaine® *see* lidocaine and epinephrine *on page 334*

Octostim® (Can) *see* desmopressin acetate *on page 166*

octreotide (ok TREE oh tide)

U.S./Canadian Brand Names Sandostatin®; Sandostatin LAR®

Therapeutic Category Somatostatin Analog

Use Control of symptoms in patients with metastatic carcinoid and vasoactive intestinal peptide-secreting tumors (VIPomas); acromegaly, insulinomas, Zollinger-Ellison syndrome, pancreatic tumors, gastrinoma, postgastrectomy dumping syndrome, bleeding esophageal varices, small bowel fistulas, AIDS-associated secretory diarrhea, chemotherapy-induced diarrhea, GVHD-induced diarrhea, control of bleeding of esophageal varices; depot suspension is indicated for long term maintenance therapy in acromegalic patients for whom medical treatment is appropriate and who have been shown to respond to and can tolerate the injection

Usual Dosage Adults: S.C.: Initial: 50 mcg 1-2 times/day and titrate dose based on patient tolerance and response

Carcinoid: 100-600 mcg/day in 2-4 divided doses

VIPomas: 200-300 mcg/day in 2-4 divided doses

Diarrhea: Initial: I.V.: 50-100 mcg every 8 hours; increase by 100 mcg/dose at 48-hour intervals; maximum dose: 500 mcg every 8 hours

Dosage Forms

Injection: 0.05 mg/mL (1 mL); 0.1 mg/mL (1 mL); 0.2 mg/mL (5 mL); 0.5 mg/mL (1 mL); 1 mg/mL (5 mL)

Injection, suspension, depot: 10 mg (5 mL); 20 mg (5 mL); 30 mg (5 mL)

Ocu-Carpine® Ophthalmic *see* pilocarpine *on page 451*

OcuClear® Ophthalmic [OTC] *see* oxymetazoline *on page 423*

OcuCoat® Ophthalmic Solution [OTC] *see* artificial tears *on page 47*

OcuCoat® PF Ophthalmic Solution [OTC] *see* artificial tears *on page 47*

Ocufen® Ophthalmic *see* flurbiprofen *on page 248*

Ocuflox™ Ophthalmic *see* ofloxacin *on next page*

Ocugram® (Can) *see* gentamicin *on page 260*

Ocupress® Ophthalmic *see* carteolol *on page 102*

Ocusert Pilo-20® Ophthalmic *see* pilocarpine *on page 451*

Ocusert Pilo-40® Ophthalmic *see* pilocarpine *on page 451*

Ocutricin® Topical Ointment *see* bacitracin, neomycin, and polymyxin B *on page 59*

Ocuvite™ (Can) *see* vitamin, multiple (oral) *on page 604*

Oestrillin® (Can) *see* estrone *on page 220*

ofloxacin (oh FLOKS a sin)

U.S./Canadian Brand Names Floxin®; Ocuflox™ Ophthalmic

Therapeutic Category Antibiotic, Ophthalmic; Antibiotic, Otic; Quinolone

Use Quinolone antibiotic for skin and skin structure, lower respiratory and urinary tract infections, and sexually transmitted diseases; bacterial conjunctivitis caused by susceptible organisms; otitis externa in adults and pediatric ≥1 year of age caused by susceptible organisms; otitis media in patients ≥12 years of age with perforated tympanic membranes caused by susceptible organisms; acute otitis media in pediatric patients ≥1 year of age with tympanostomy tubes caused by susceptible organisms

Usual Dosage

Children >1 year and Adults: Ophthalmic: Instill 1-2 drops in affected eye(s) every 2-4 hours for the first 2 days, then use 4 times/day for an additional 5 days

Children >1 year to 12 years: Otic: Instill 5 drops in affected ear(s) twice daily for 10 days

Children ≥12 years: Otic: Instill 10 drops in affected ear(s) twice daily for 10 days

Adults: Oral, I.V.: 200-400 mg every 12 hours for 7-10 days for most infections or for 6 weeks for prostatitis

Dosage Forms

Injection: 200 mg (50 mL); 400 mg (10 mL, 20 mL, 100 mL)

Solution:

- Ophthalmic: 0.3% (5 mL)
- Otic: 0.3% (5 mL)

Tablet: 200 mg, 300 mg, 400 mg

Ogen® Oral *see* estropipate *on page 220*

Ogen® Vaginal *see* estropipate *on page 220*

OGMT *see* metyrosine *on page 373*

OKT3 *see* muromonab-CD3 *on page 385*

olanzapine (oh LAN za peen)

Synonyms LY170053

U.S./Canadian Brand Names Zyprexa™

Therapeutic Category Antipsychotic Agent

Use Treatment of schizophrenia

Usual Dosage Adults: Oral: Usual starting dose: 10 mg/day, up to a maximum of 20 mg/day

Dosage Forms Tablet: 2.5 mg, 5 mg, 7.5 mg, 10 mg

old tuberculin *see* tuberculin tests *on page 588*

oleovitamin A *see* vitamin A *on page 602*

oleum ricini *see* castor oil *on page 103*

olopatadine (oh LOP ah tah deen)

U.S./Canadian Brand Names Patanol®

Therapeutic Category Antihistamine

Use Allergic conjunctivitis

Usual Dosage Adults: Ophthalmic: 1 drop in affected eye(s) every 6-8 hours (twice daily)

Dosage Forms Solution, ophthalmic: 0.1% (5 mL)

olsalazine (ole SAL a zeen)

U.S./Canadian Brand Names Dipentum®

Therapeutic Category 5-Aminosalicylic Acid Derivative

Use Maintenance of remission of ulcerative colitis in patients intolerant to sulfasalazine

Usual Dosage Adults: Oral: 1 g daily in 2 divided doses

Dosage Forms Capsule, as sodium: 250 mg

omeprazole (oh ME pray zol)

U.S./Canadian Brand Names Losec® (Can); Prilosec™

Therapeutic Category Gastric Acid Secretion Inhibitor

Use Short-term (4-8 weeks) treatment of erosive esophagitis (grade 2 or above), diagnosed by endoscopy; maintain healing of erosive esophagitis; short-term treatment of symptomatic gastroesophageal reflux disease (GERD) poorly responsive to customary medical treatment; short-term treatment of active duodenal ulcer; long-term treatment of pathological hypersecretory conditions

Usual Dosage Adults: Oral:

Duodenal ulcer: 20 mg/day for 4-8 weeks

GERD or erosive esophagitis: 20 mg/day for 4-8 weeks

Maintenance of healing erosive esophagitis: 20 mg/day

Pathological hypersecretory conditions: 60 mg once daily initially; doses up to 120 mg 3 times/day have been administered; administer daily doses >80 mg in divided doses; patients with Zollinger-Ellison syndrome have been treated continuously for over 5 years

Dosage Forms Capsule, delayed release: 10 mg, 20 mg

Omnicef® *see* cefdinir *on page 105*

OmniHIB™ *see Haemophilus* B conjugate vaccine *on page 275*

Omnipaque® *see* radiological/contrast media (non-ionic) *on page 496*

Omnipen® *see* ampicillin *on page 34*

Omnipen®-N *see* ampicillin *on page 34*

OMS® Oral *see* morphine sulfate *on page 382*

Oncaspar® *see* pegaspargase *on page 432*

Oncet® *see* hydrocodone and homatropine *on page 289*

Oncovin® *see* vincristine *on page 600*

ondansetron (on DAN se tron)

U.S./Canadian Brand Names Zofran®; Zofran® ODT

Therapeutic Category Selective 5-HT_3 Receptor Antagonist

Use Prevention of nausea and vomiting associated with initial and repeat courses of emetogenic cancer chemotherapy and prevention of postoperative nausea and vomiting; prevent postoperative nausea/vomiting (I.M.)

Usual Dosage

Oral:

Children 4-11 years: 4 mg 30 minutes before chemotherapy; repeat 4 and 8 hours after initial dose

Children >11 years and Adults: 8 mg 30 minutes before chemotherapy; repeat 4 and 8 hours after initial dose or every 8 hours for a maximum of 48 hours

I.V.: Administer either three 0.15 mg/kg doses or a single 32 mg dose; with the 3-dose regimen, the initial dose is given 30 minutes prior to chemotherapy with subsequent doses administered 4 and 8 hours after the first dose. With the single-dose regimen 32 mg is infused over 15 minutes beginning 30 minutes before the start of emetogenic chemotherapy. Dosage should be calculated based on weight:

Children: Pediatric dosing should follow the manufacturer's guidelines for 0.15 mg/kg/dose administered 30 minutes prior to chemotherapy, 4 and 8 hours after the first dose. While not as yet FDA-approved, literature supports the day's total dose administered as a single dose 30 minutes prior to chemotherapy.

(Continued)

ondansetron *(Continued)*

Adults:
>80 kg: 12 mg IVPB
45-80 kg: 8 mg IVPB
<45 kg: 0.15 mg/kg/dose IVPB

Dosage Forms Ondansetron hydrochloride:
Injection: 2 mg/mL (2 mL, 20 mL); 32 mg (single-dose vials)
Tablet: 4 mg, 8 mg

Ontak® *see* denileukin deftitox *on page 163*

Ony-Clear® Nail *see* triacetin *on page 576*

Ony-Clear® Spray *see* miconazole *on page 373*

Onyvul® (Can) *see* urea *on page 591*

OPC-17116 *see* grepafloxacin *Withdrawn from U.S. market 10/27/99 on page 266*

OP-CCK *see* sincalide *on page 523*

Opcon® Ophthalmic *see* naphazoline *on page 390*

o,p′-DDD *see* mitotane *on page 378*

Operand® [OTC] *see* povidone-iodine *on page 467*

Ophthacet® *see* sulfacetamide *on page 540*

Ophthaine® ***(Discontinued)*** *see page 700*

Ophthalgan® Ophthalmic *see* glycerin *on page 263*

Ophthetic® *see* proparacaine *on page 481*

Ophthochlor® Ophthalmic *see* chloramphenicol *on page 116*

Ophthocort® ***(Discontinued)*** *see page 700*

Ophtho-tate® (Can) *see* prednisolone (ophthalmic) *on page 471*

opium alkaloids (OH pee um AL ka loyds)

U.S./Canadian Brand Names Pantopon®
Therapeutic Category Analgesic, Narcotic
Controlled Substance C-II
Use For relief of severe pain
Usual Dosage Adults: I.M., S.C.: 5-20 mg every 4-5 hours
Dosage Forms Injection: 20 mg/mL (1 mL)

opium and belladonna *see* belladonna and opium *on page 63*

opium tincture (OH pee um TINGK chur)

Synonyms deodorized opium tincture; DTO
Therapeutic Category Analgesic, Narcotic
Controlled Substance C-II
Use Treatment of diarrhea or relief of pain; **a 25-fold dilution with water** (final concentration 0.4 mg/mL morphine) can be used to treat neonatal abstinence syndrome (opiate withdrawal)
Usual Dosage Oral:
Children:
Diarrhea: 0.005-0.01 mL/kg/dose every 3-4 hours
Analgesia: 0.01-0.02 mL/kg/dose every 3-4 hours
Adults: 0.6 mL 4 times/day
Dosage Forms Liquid: 10% [0.6 mL equivalent to morphine 6 mg] with alcohol 19%

oprelvekin (oh PREL ve kin)

Synonyms IL-11; Interleukin-11; Recombinant Human Interleukin-11; Recombinant Interleukin-11; rhIL-11; rIL-11

U.S./Canadian Brand Names Neumega®

Therapeutic Category Platelet Growth Factor

Use Prevention and treatment of severe thrombocytopenia following myelosuppressive chemotherapy

Usual Dosage Refer to individual protocols

Children: 75-100 mcg/kg/day for 10-21 days (until platelet count >50,000/mm^3)

Adults: 50 mcg/kg/day for 10-21 days (until platelet count >50,000/mm^3)

Dosage Forms Powder for injection, lyophilized: 5 mg

Optho-Bunolol® (Can) *see* levobunolol *on page 330*

Optho-Dipivefrin™ (Can) *see* dipivefrin *on page 188*

Opticrom® *see* cromolyn sodium *on page 150*

Optifast® 900 (Can) *see* enteral nutritional products *on page 208*

Optigene® Ophthalmic [OTC] *see* tetrahydrozoline *on page 556*

Optimine® *see* azatadine *on page 55*

Optimoist® Solution [OTC] *see* saliva substitute *on page 514*

OptiPranolol® Ophthalmic *see* metipranolol *on page 370*

Optiray® *see* radiological/contrast media (non-ionic) *on page 496*

OPV *see* poliovirus vaccine, live, trivalent, oral *on page 459*

Orabase®-B [OTC] *see* benzocaine *on page 66*

Orabase® HCA Topical *see* hydrocortisone (topical) *on page 292*

Orabase®-O [OTC] *see* benzocaine *on page 66*

Orabase® Plain [OTC] *see* gelatin, pectin, and methylcellulose *on page 258*

Orabase® With Benzocaine [OTC] *see* benzocaine, gelatin, pectin, and sodium carboxymethylcellulose *on page 67*

Oradex-C® ***(Discontinued)*** *see page 700*

Oragrafin® Calcium *see* radiological/contrast media (ionic) *on page 495*

Oragrafin® Sodium *see* radiological/contrast media (ionic) *on page 495*

Orajel® Brace-Aid Oral Anesthetic [OTC] *see* benzocaine *on page 66*

Orajel® Maximum Strength [OTC] *see* benzocaine *on page 66*

Orajel® Mouth-Aid [OTC] *see* benzocaine *on page 66*

Orajel® Perioseptic® [OTC] *see* carbamide peroxide *on page 98*

Oramorph SR™ Oral *see* morphine sulfate *on page 382*

Orap™ *see* pimozide *on page 452*

Orasept® [OTC] *see* benzocaine *on page 66*

Orasol® [OTC] *see* benzocaine *on page 66*

Orasone® *see* prednisone *on page 472*

Oratect® ***(Discontinued)*** *see page 700*

Orazinc® Oral [OTC] *see* zinc sulfate *on page 612*

Orbenin® (Can) *see* cloxacillin *on page 141*

orciprenaline *see* metaproterenol *on page 359*

Ordrine AT® Extended Release Capsule *see* caramiphen and phenylpropanolamine *on page 97*

Oretic® *see* hydrochlorothiazide *on page 286*

Oreticyl® ***(Discontinued)*** *see page 700*

Oreton® Methyl *see* methyltestosterone *on page 369*

Orexin® [OTC] *see* vitamin B complex *on page 603*

Organidin® *(Discontinued)* *see page 700*

Organidin® NR *see* guaifenesin *on page 267*

Orgaran® *see* danaparoid *on page 158*

ORG NC 45 *see* vecuronium *on page 597*

Orifer® F (Can) *see* vitamin, multiple (oral) *on page 604*

Orimune® *see* poliovirus vaccine, live, trivalent, oral *on page 459*

Orinase® Diagnostic Injection *see* tolbutamide *on page 570*

Orinase® Oral *see* tolbutamide *on page 570*

ORLAAM® *see* levomethadyl acetate hydrochloride *on page 331*

orlistat (OR li stat)

U.S./Canadian Brand Names Xenical®

Therapeutic Category Lipase Inhibitor

Use Management of obesity, including weight loss and weight management when used in conjunction with a reduced-calorie diet; reduce the risk of weight regain after prior weight loss; indicated for obese patients with an initial body mass index (BMI) ≥30 kg/m^2 or ≥27 kg/m^2 in the presence of other risk factors

Usual Dosage Adults: Oral: 120 mg 3 times/day with each main meal containing fat (during or up to 1 hour after the meal); omit dose if meal is occasionally missed or contains no fat

Dosage Forms Capsule: 120 mg

Ormazine® *see* chlorpromazine *on page 127*

Ornade® Spansule® *see* chlorpheniramine and phenylpropanolamine *on page 122*

Ornex® No Drowsiness [OTC] *see* acetaminophen and pseudoephedrine *on page 5*

Ornidyl® *see* eflornithine *on page 204*

Oro-Clense (Can) *see* chlorhexidine gluconate *on page 117*

orphenadrine (or FEN a dreen)

U.S./Canadian Brand Names Norflex™

Therapeutic Category Skeletal Muscle Relaxant

Use Treatment of muscle spasm associated with acute painful musculoskeletal conditions; supportive therapy in tetanus

Usual Dosage Adults:

Oral: 100 mg twice daily

I.M., I.V.: 60 mg every 12 hours

Dosage Forms Orphenadrine citrate:

Injection: 30 mg/mL (2 mL, 10 mL)

Tablet: 100 mg

Tablet, sustained release: 100 mg

orphenadrine, aspirin, and caffeine (or FEN a dreen, AS pir in, & KAF een)

Synonyms aspirin, orphenadrine, and caffeine; caffeine, orphenadrine, and aspirin

U.S./Canadian Brand Names Norgesic™; Norgesic™ Forte

Therapeutic Category Analgesic, Non-narcotic; Skeletal Muscle Relaxant

Use Relief of discomfort associated with skeletal muscular conditions

Usual Dosage Oral: 1-2 tablets 3-4 times/day

Dosage Forms

Tablet: Orphenadrine citrate 25 mg, aspirin 385 mg, and caffeine 30 mg

Tablet (Norgesic® Forte): Orphenadrine citrate 50 mg, aspirin 770 mg, and caffeine 60 mg

Ortho® 0.5/35 (Can) *see* ethinyl estradiol and norethindrone *on page 224*

Ortho-Cept® *see* ethinyl estradiol and desogestrel *on page 222*

Ortho-Chloram® (Can) *see* chloramphenicol *on page 116*

Orthoclone® OKT3 *see* muromonab-CD3 *on page 385*

Ortho-Cyclen® *see* ethinyl estradiol and norgestimate *on page 225*

Ortho®-Dienestrol Vaginal *see* dienestrol *on page 177*

Ortho-Est® Oral *see* estropipate *on page 220*

Ortho-Novum® 1/35 *see* ethinyl estradiol and norethindrone *on page 224*

Ortho-Novum® 1/50 *see* mestranol and norethindrone *on page 359*

Ortho-Novum® 7/7/7 *see* ethinyl estradiol and norethindrone *on page 224*

Ortho-Novum® 10/11 *see* ethinyl estradiol and norethindrone *on page 224*

Ortho Tri-Cyclen® *see* ethinyl estradiol and norgestimate *on page 225*

Or-Tyl® Injection *see* dicyclomine *on page 177*

Orudis® *see* ketoprofen *on page 321*

Orudis® KT [OTC] *see* ketoprofen *on page 321*

Oruvail® *see* ketoprofen *on page 321*

Os-Cal® 500 [OTC] *see* calcium carbonate *on page 89*

oseltamivir (o sel TAM e veer)

U.S./Canadian Brand Names Tamiflu™

Therapeutic Category Antiviral Agent, Oral

Use Treatment of umcomplicated influenza in adults whose flu symptoms have not lasted more than two days; approved to treat Type A and B influenza

Usual Dosage Oral: Adults: 1 capsule (75 mg) twice daily for 5 days; may be taken with or without food

Dosage Forms Capsule, as phosphate: 75 mg

Osmitrol® Injection *see* mannitol *on page 347*

Osmoglyn® *see* glycerin *on page 263*

Osmolite® HN [OTC] *see* enteral nutritional products *on page 208*

Osteocalcin® *see* calcitonin *on page 88*

Ostoforte® (Can) *see* ergocalciferol *on page 212*

Otic-Care® Otic *see* neomycin, polymyxin B, and hydrocortisone *on page 396*

Otic Domeboro® *see* aluminum acetate and acetic acid *on page 21*

Otic Tridesilon® ***(Discontinued)*** *see page 700*

Otobiotic® Otic *see* polymyxin B and hydrocortisone *on page 460*

Otocalm® Ear *see* antipyrine and benzocaine *on page 41*

Otocort® Otic *see* neomycin, polymyxin B, and hydrocortisone *on page 396*

Otosporin® Otic *see* neomycin, polymyxin B, and hydrocortisone *on page 396*

Otrivin® Nasal [OTC] *see* xylometazoline *on page 608*

Ovcon® 35 *see* ethinyl estradiol and norethindrone *on page 224*

Ovcon® 50 *see* ethinyl estradiol and norethindrone *on page 224*

Ovide™ Topical *see* malathion *on page 347*

Ovol® (Can) *see* simethicone *on page 522*

Ovral® *see* ethinyl estradiol and norgestrel *on page 225*

Ovrette® *see* norgestrel *on page 407*

O-V Staticin® *see* nystatin *on page 412*

oxacillin (oks a SIL in)

Synonyms methylphenyl isoxazolyl penicillin

Therapeutic Category Penicillin

Use Treatment of bacterial infections such as osteomyelitis, septicemia, endocarditis, and CNS infections due to susceptible penicillinase-producing strains of *Staphylococcus*

Usual Dosage

Infants and Children:

I.M., I.V.: 150-200 mg/kg/day in divided doses every 6 hours; maximum dose: 12 g/day

Oral: 50-100 mg/kg/day divided every 6 hours

Adults:

Oral: 500-1000 mg every 4-6 hours for at least 5 days

I.M., I.V.: 250 mg to 2 g/dose every 4-6 hours

Dosage Forms Oxacillin sodium:

Capsule: 250 mg, 500 mg

Powder for injection: 250 mg, 500 mg, 1 g, 2 g, 4 g, 10 g

Powder for oral solution: 250 mg/5 mL (100 mL)

oxamniquine (oks AM ni kwin)

U.S./Canadian Brand Names Vansil™

Therapeutic Category Anthelmintic

Use Treat all stages of *Schistosoma mansoni* infection

Usual Dosage Oral:

Children <30 kg: 20 mg/kg in 2 divided doses of 10 mg/kg at 2- to 8-hour intervals

Adults: 12-15 mg/kg as a single dose

Dosage Forms Capsule: 250 mg

Oxandrin® *see* oxandrolone *on this page*

oxandrolone (oks AN droe lone)

U.S./Canadian Brand Names Oxandrin®

Therapeutic Category Androgen

Controlled Substance C-III

Use Treatment of catabolic or tissue-depleting processes

Usual Dosage Adults: Oral: 2.5 mg 2-4 times/day

Dosage Forms Tablet: 2.5 mg

oxaprozin (oks a PROE zin)

U.S./Canadian Brand Names Daypro™

Therapeutic Category Analgesic, Non-narcotic; Nonsteroidal Anti-inflammatory Drug (NSAID)

Use Acute and long-term use in the management of signs and symptoms of osteoarthritis and rheumatoid arthritis

Usual Dosage Adults: Oral (individualize the dosage to the lowest effective dose to minimize adverse effects):

Osteoarthritis: 600-1200 mg once daily

Rheumatoid arthritis: 1200 mg once daily

Maximum dose: 1800 mg/day or 26 mg/kg (whichever is lower) in divided doses

Dosage Forms Tablet: 600 mg

oxazepam (oks A ze pam)

U.S./Canadian Brand Names Apo-Oxazepam® (Can); Novo-Oxazepam® (Can); Oxpam® (Can); PMS-Oxazepam (Can); Serax®; Zapex® (Can)

Therapeutic Category Anticonvulsant; Benzodiazepine

Controlled Substance C-IV

Use Treatment of anxiety and management of alcohol withdrawal; may also be used as an anticonvulsant in management of simple partial seizures

Usual Dosage Oral:
Children: 1 mg/kg/day has been administered
Adults:
Anxiety: 10-30 mg 3-4 times/day
Alcohol withdrawal: 15-30 mg 3-4 times/day
Hypnotic: 15-30 mg

Dosage Forms
Capsule: 10 mg, 15 mg, 30 mg
Tablet: 15 mg

oxiconazole (oks i KON a zole)

U.S./Canadian Brand Names Oxistat® Topical
Therapeutic Category Antifungal Agent
Use Treatment of tinea pedis, tinea cruris, and tinea corporis
Usual Dosage Topical: Apply once daily to affected areas for 2 weeks to 1 month
Dosage Forms Oxiconazole nitrate:
Cream: 1% (15 g, 30 g, 60 g)
Lotion: 1% (30 mL)

oxilapine *see* loxapine *on page 341*

Oxistat® Topical *see* oxiconazole *on this page*

Oxpam® (Can) *see* oxazepam *on previous page*

oxpentifylline *see* pentoxifylline *on page 438*

oxprenolol *(Canada only)* (ox PREN oh lole)

U.S./Canadian Brand Names Trasicor® (Can)
Therapeutic Category Beta-Adrenergic Blocker
Use Treatment of mild to moderate hypertension
Usual Dosage Adults: Oral: Start with 20 mg three times/day, titrated upward to a maximum dose of 480 mg/day
Dosage Forms Tablet: 40 mg, 80 mg

Oxsoralen® Oral *(Discontinued)* *see page 700*

Oxsoralen-Ultra® *see* methoxsalen *on page 365*

oxtriphylline (oks TRYE fi lin)

Synonyms choline theophyllinate
Therapeutic Category Theophylline Derivative
Use Bronchodilator in symptomatic treatment of asthma and reversible bronchospasm
Usual Dosage Oral:
Children:
1-9 years: 6.2 mg/kg/dose every 6 hours
9-16 years: 4.7 mg/kg/dose every 6 hours
Adults: 4.7 mg/kg every 8 hours; sustained release: administer every 12 hours

Dosage Forms
Elixir: 100 mg/5 mL (5 mL, 10 mL, 473 mL)
Syrup: 50 mg/5 mL (473 mL)
Tablet: 100 mg, 200 mg
Sustained release: 400 mg, 600 mg

Oxy-5® Advanced Formula for Sensitive Skin [OTC] *see* benzoyl peroxide *on page 68*

Oxy-5® Tinted [OTC] *see* benzoyl peroxide *on page 68*

Oxy-10® Advanced Formula for Sensitive Skin [OTC] *see* benzoyl peroxide *on page 68*

Oxy 10® Wash [OTC] *see* benzoyl peroxide *on page 68*

oxybutynin (oks i BYOO ti nin)

U.S./Canadian Brand Names Ditropan®; Ditropan® XL

Therapeutic Category Antispasmodic Agent, Urinary

Use Relief of bladder spasms associated with voiding in patients with uninhibited and reflex neurogenic bladder

Usual Dosage Oral:

Children:

1-5 years: 0.2 mg/kg/dose 2-4 times/day

>5 years: 5 mg twice daily, up to 5 mg 3 times/day

Adults: 5 mg 2-3 times/day up to 5 mg 4 times/day maximum

Dosage Forms Oxybutynin chloride:

Syrup: 5 mg/5 mL (473 mL)

Tablet: 5 mg

Tablet, extended release: 5 mg, 10 mg

Oxycel® *see* cellulose, oxidized *on page 110*

oxychlorosene (oks i KLOR oh seen)

U.S./Canadian Brand Names Clorpactin® WCS-90

Therapeutic Category Antibiotic, Topical

Use Treating localized infections

Usual Dosage Topical (0.1% to 0.5% solutions): Apply by irrigation, instillation, spray, soaks, or wet compresses

Dosage Forms Powder for solution, as sodium: 2 g, 5 g

Oxycocet® (Can) *see* oxycodone and acetaminophen *on this page*

Oxycodan® (Can) *see* oxycodone and aspirin *on next page*

oxycodone (oks i KOE done)

Synonyms dihydrohydroxycodeinone

U.S./Canadian Brand Names OxyContin®; OxyIR™; Percolone™; Roxicodone™

Therapeutic Category Analgesic, Narcotic

Controlled Substance C-II

Use Management of moderate to severe pain, normally used in combination with non-narcotic analgesics

Usual Dosage Oral:

Children:

6-12 years: 1.25 mg every 6 hours as needed

>12 years: 2.5 mg every 6 hours as needed

Adults: 5 mg every 6 hours as needed

Dosage Forms

Capsule, as hydrochloride, immediate release (OxyIR™): 5 mg

Liquid, oral, as hydrochloride: 5 mg/5 mL (500 mL)

Solution, oral concentrate, as hydrochloride: 20 mg/mL (30 mL)

Tablet, as hydrochloride: 5 mg

Percolone™: 5 mg

Tablet, controlled release, as hydrochloride (OxyContin®): 10 mg, 20 mg, 40 mg, 80 mg

oxycodone and acetaminophen (oks i KOE done & a seet a MIN oh fen)

Synonyms acetaminophen and oxycodone

U.S./Canadian Brand Names Endocet® (Can); Oxycocet® (Can); Percocet®; Percocet®-Demi (Can); Roxicet® 5/500; Roxilox®; Tylox®

Therapeutic Category Analgesic, Narcotic

Controlled Substance C-II

Use Management of moderate to severe pain

Usual Dosage Oral (doses should be titrated to appropriate analgesic effects):

Children: Oxycodone: 0.05-0.15 mg/kg/dose to 5 mg/dose (maximum) every 4-6 hours as needed

Adults: 1-2 tablets every 4-6 hours as needed for pain
Maximum daily dose of acetaminophen: 4 g/day

Dosage Forms
Caplet: Oxycodone hydrochloride 5 mg and acetaminophen 500 mg
Capsule: Oxycodone hydrochloride 5 mg and acetaminophen 500 mg
Solution, oral: Oxycodone hydrochloride 5 mg and acetaminophen 325 mg per 5 mL (5 mL, 500 mL)
Tablet: Oxycodone hydrochloride 5 mg and acetaminophen 325 mg

oxycodone and aspirin (oks i KOE done & AS pir in)

Synonyms aspirin and oxycodone

U.S./Canadian Brand Names Codoxy®; Endodan® (Can); Oxycodan® (Can); Percodan®; Percodan®-Demi; Roxiprin®

Therapeutic Category Analgesic, Narcotic

Controlled Substance C-II

Use Relief of moderate to moderately severe pain

Usual Dosage Oral (based on oxycodone combined salts):
Children: 0.05-0.15 mg/kg/dose every 4-6 hours as needed; maximum: 5 mg/dose (1 tablet Percodan® or 2 tablets Percodan®-Demi/dose) **or**
Alternatively:
6-12 years: Percodan®-Demi: 1/4 tablet every 6 hours as needed for pain
>12 years: 1/2 tablet every 6 hours as needed for pain
Adults: Percodan®: 1 tablet every 6 hours as needed for pain or Percodan®-Demi: 1-2 tablets every 6 hours as needed for pain

Dosage Forms Tablet: Oxycodone hydrochloride 4.5 mg, oxycodone terephthalate 0.38 mg, and aspirin 325 mg; oxycodone hydrochloride 2.25 mg, oxycodone terephthalate 0.19 mg, and aspirin 325 mg

OxyContin® *see* oxycodone *on previous page*

Oxyderm™ 5%, 10%, 20% (Can) *see* benzoyl peroxide *on page 68*

OxyIR™ *see* oxycodone *on previous page*

oxymetazoline (oks i met AZ oh leen)

U.S./Canadian Brand Names Afrin® Children's Nose Drops [OTC]; Afrin® Nasal Solution [OTC]; Allerest® 12 Hour Nasal Solution [OTC]; Chlorphed®-LA Nasal Solution [OTC]; Dristan® Long Lasting Nasal Solution [OTC]; Drixoral® Nasal (Can); Duramist Plus® [OTC]; Duration® Nasal Solution [OTC]; Neo-Synephrine® 12 Hour Nasal Solution [OTC]; Nōstrilla® [OTC]; NTZ® Long Acting Nasal Solution [OTC]; OcuClear® Ophthalmic [OTC]; Sinarest® 12 Hour Nasal Solution; Sinex® Long-Acting [OTC]; Twice-A-Day® Nasal Solution [OTC]; Visine® L.R. Ophthalmic [OTC]; 4-Way® Long Acting Nasal Solution [OTC]

Therapeutic Category Adrenergic Agonist Agent

Use Symptomatic relief of nasal mucosal congestion associated with acute or chronic rhinitis, the common cold, sinusitis, hay fever, or other allergies

Usual Dosage
Intranasal:
Children 2-5 years: 0.025% solution: Instill 2-3 drops in each nostril twice daily
Children ≥6 years and Adults: 0.05% solution: Instill 2-3 drops or 2-3 sprays into each nostril twice daily
Ophthalmic: Adults: Instill 1-2 drops into affected eye(s) every 6 hours

Dosage Forms Oxymetazoline hydrochloride:
Ophthalmic solution (OcuClear®, Visine® L.R.): 0.025% (15 mL, 30 mL)
Solution, nasal:
Drops:
Afrin® Children's Nose Drops: 0.025% (20 mL)
Afrin®, NTZ® Long Acting Nasal Solution: 0.05% (15 mL, 20 mL)
(Continued)

oxymetazoline *(Continued)*

Spray: Afrin® Sinus, Allerest® 12 Hours, Chlorphed®-LA, Dristan® Long Lasting, Duration®, 4-Way® Long Acting, Genasal®, Nasal Relief®, Nōstrilla®, NTZ® Long Acting Nasal Solution, Sinex® Long-Acting, Twice-A-Day®: 0.05% (15 mL, 30 mL)

oxymetholone (oks i METH oh lone)

U.S./Canadian Brand Names Anadrol®; Anapolon® (Can)

Therapeutic Category Anabolic Steroid

Controlled Substance C-III

Use Anemias caused by the administration of myelotoxic drugs

Usual Dosage Erythropoietic effects: 1-5 mg/kg/day as a single dose; maximum: 100 mg/day

Dosage Forms Tablet: 50 mg

oxymorphone (oks i MOR fone)

U.S./Canadian Brand Names Numorphan®

Therapeutic Category Analgesic, Narcotic

Controlled Substance C-II

Use Management of moderate to severe pain and preoperatively as a sedative and a supplement to anesthesia

Usual Dosage Adults:

I.M., S.C.: Initial: 0.5 mg, then 1-1.5 mg every 4-6 hours as needed

I.V.: Initial: 0.5 mg

Rectal: 5 mg every 4-6 hours

Dosage Forms Oxymorphone hydrochloride:

Injection: 1 mg (1 mL); 1.5 mg/mL (1 mL, 10 mL)

Suppository, rectal: 5 mg

oxyphenbutazone (oks i fen BYOO ta zone)

Therapeutic Category Analgesic, Non-narcotic; Nonsteroidal Anti-inflammatory Drug (NSAID)

Use Management of inflammatory disorders, as an analgesic in the treatment of mild to moderate pain and as an antipyretic; I.V. form used as an alternate to surgery in management of patent ductus arteriosus in premature neonates; acute gouty arthritis

Usual Dosage Adults: Oral:

Rheumatoid arthritis: 100-200 mg 3-4 times/day until desired effect, then reduce dose to ≤400 mg/day

Acute gouty arthritis: Initial: 400 mg then 100 mg every 4 hours until acute attack subsides

Dosage Forms Tablet: 100 mg

oxytetracycline (oks i tet ra SYE kleen)

U.S./Canadian Brand Names Terramycin® I.M. Injection; Terramycin® Oral

Therapeutic Category Tetracycline Derivative

Use Treatment of susceptible bacterial infections; both gram-positive and gram-negative, as well as *Rickettsia* and *Mycoplasma* organisms

Usual Dosage

Oral:

Children: 40-50 mg/kg/day in divided doses every 6 hours (maximum: 2 g/24 hours)

Adults: 250-500 mg/dose every 6 hours

I.M.:

Children >8 years: 15-25 mg/kg/day (maximum: 250 mg/dose) in divided doses every 8-12 hours

Adults: 250-500 mg every 24 hours or 300 mg/day divided every 8-12 hours

Dosage Forms Oxytetracycline hydrochloride:

Capsule: 250 mg

Injection with lidocaine 2%: 5% [50 mg/mL] (2 mL, 10 mL); 12.5% [125 mg/mL] (2 mL)

oxytetracycline and hydrocortisone

(oks i tet ra SYE kleen & hye droe KOR ti sone)

Synonyms hydrocortisone and oxytetracycline

U.S./Canadian Brand Names Terra-Cortril® Ophthalmic Suspension

Therapeutic Category Antibiotic/Corticosteroid, Ophthalmic

Use Treatment of susceptible ophthalmic bacterial infections with associated inflammation

Usual Dosage Ophthalmic: Adults: Instill 1-2 drops in eye(s) every 3-4 hours

Dosage Forms Suspension, ophthalmic: Oxytetracycline hydrochloride 0.5% and hydrocortisone 0.5% (5 mL)

oxytetracycline and polymyxin B

(oks i tet ra SYE kleen & pol i MIKS in bee)

Synonyms polymyxin B and oxytetracycline

U.S./Canadian Brand Names Terak® Ophthalmic Ointment; Terramycin® Ophthalmic Ointment; Terramycin® w/Polymyxin B Ophthalmic Ointment

Therapeutic Category Antibiotic, Ophthalmic

Use Treatment of superficial ocular infections involving the conjunctiva and/or cornea

Usual Dosage Ophthalmic: Apply $\frac{1}{2}$" of ointment onto the lower lid of affected eye 2-4 times/day

Dosage Forms

Ointment, ophthalmic/otic: Oxytetracycline hydrochloride 5 mg and polymyxin B 10,000 units per g (3.5 g)

Tablet, vaginal: Oxytetracycline hydrochloride 100 mg and polymyxin B 100,000 units (10s)

oxytocin (oks i TOE sin)

Synonyms PIT

U.S./Canadian Brand Names Pitocin®; Toesen® (Can)

Therapeutic Category Oxytocic Agent

Use Induce labor at term; control postpartum bleeding

Usual Dosage Adults:

Induction of labor: I.V.: 0.001-0.002 unit/minute; increase by 0.001-0.002 units every 15-30 minutes until contraction pattern has been established

Postpartum bleeding: I.V.: 0.001-0.002 unit/minute as needed

Dosage Forms Injection: 10 units/mL (1 mL, 10 mL)

Oyst-Cal 500 [OTC] *see* calcium carbonate *on page 89*

Oystercal® 500 *see* calcium carbonate *on page 89*

P-071 *see* cetirizine *on page 113*

Pacerone® *see* amiodarone *on page 28*

Pacis™ (Can) *see* BCG vaccine *on page 61*

paclitaxel (PAK li taks el)

U.S./Canadian Brand Names Paxene®; Taxol®

Therapeutic Category Antineoplastic Agent

Use Treatment of metastatic carcinoma of the ovary after failure of first-line or subsequent chemotherapy; treatment for AIDS-related Kaposi's sarcoma

Usual Dosage Adults: I.V.: 135 mg/m^2 over 24 hours every 3 weeks

Dosage Forms Injection: 6 mg/mL (5 mL, 16.7 mL)

Palafer® (Can) *see* ferrous fumarate *on page 236*

palivizumab (pah li VIZ u mab)

U.S./Canadian Brand Names Synagis®

Therapeutic Category Monoclonal Antibody

(Continued)

palivizumab *(Continued)*

Use Prevention of serious lower respiratory tract disease caused by respiratory syncytial virus (RSV) in pediatric patients at high risk of RSV disease; safety and efficacy were established in infants with bronchopulmonary dysplasia (BPD) and infants with a history of prematurity ≤35 weeks gestational age

Usual Dosage Children: I.M.: 15 mg/kg of body weight, monthly throughout RSV season (First dose administered prior to commencement of RSV season)

Dosage Forms Injection, lyophilized: 100 mg

Palmitate-A® 5000 [OTC] *see* vitamin A *on page 602*

Palmocare® (Can) *see* enteral nutritional products *on page 208*

PALS® [OTC] *see* chlorophyll *on page 118*

2-PAM *see* pralidoxime *on page 468*

Pamelor® *see* nortriptyline *on page 408*

pamidronate (pa mi DROE nate)

U.S./Canadian Brand Names Aredia™

Therapeutic Category Bisphosphonate Derivative

Use Symptomatic treatment of Paget's disease; hypercalcemia associated with malignancy

Usual Dosage Drug must be diluted properly before administration and infused slowly (at least over 2 hours)

Adults: I.V.:

- Moderate cancer-related hypercalcemia (12-13 mg/dL): 60-90 mg administered as a slow infusion over 2-24 hours
- Severe cancer-related hypercalcemia (>13.5 mg/dL): 90 mg as a slow infusion over 2-24 hours
  - A period of 7 days should elapse before the use of second course; repeat infusions every 2-3 weeks have been suggested, however, could be administered every 2-3 months according to the degree and of severity of hypercalcemia and/or the type of malignancy
- Paget's disease: 60 mg as a single 2- to 24-hour infusion

Dosage Forms Powder for injection, lyophilized, as disodium: 30 mg, 60 mg, 90 mg

Pamine® *see* methscopolamine *on page 366*

Pamprin IB® [OTC] *see* ibuprofen *on page 300*

Panadol® [OTC] *see* acetaminophen *on page 3*

Panasal® 5/500 *see* hydrocodone and aspirin *on page 288*

Pan-B antibodies *see* rituximab *on page 507*

Pancrease® *see* pancrelipase *on next page*

Pancrease® MT *see* pancrelipase *on next page*

pancreatin (PAN kree a tin)

U.S./Canadian Brand Names Creon®; Digepepsin®; Donnazyme®; Hi-Vegi-Lip®

Therapeutic Category Enzyme

Use Replacement therapy in symptomatic treatment of malabsorption syndrome caused by pancreatic insufficiency

Usual Dosage Enteric coated microspheres: The following dosage recommendations are only an approximation for initial dosages. The actual dosage will depend on the digestive requirements of the individual patient.

Oral:

- Children:
  - <1 year: 2000 units of lipase with meals/feedings
  - 1-6 years: 4000-8000 units of lipase with meals and 4000 units with snacks

7-12 years: 4000-12,000 units of lipase with meals and snacks
Adults: 4000-16,000 units of lipase with meals and with snacks

Dosage Forms

Capsule, enteric coated microspheres (Creon®): Lipase 8000 units, amylase 30,000 units, protease 13,000 units and pancreatin 300 mg

Tablet:

Digepepsin®: Pancreatin 300 mg, pepsin 250 mg, and bile salts 150 mg

Donnazyme®: Lipase 1000 units, amylase 12,500 units, protease 12,500 units and pancreatin 500 mg

Hi-Vegi-Lip®: Lipase 4800 units, amylase 60,000 units, protease 60,000 units and pancreatin 2400 mg

Pancrecarb® *see* pancrelipase *on this page*

pancrelipase (pan kre LI pase)

Synonyms lipancreatin; lipase, protease, and amylase

U.S./Canadian Brand Names Cotazym®; Cotazym-S®; Creon® 10; Creon® 20; Digess®8000 (Can); Ilozyme®; Ku-Zyme® HP; Pancrease®; Pancrease® MT; Pancrecarb®; Protilase®; Ultrase® MT; Viokase®; Zymase®

Therapeutic Category Enzyme

Use Replacement therapy in symptomatic treatment of malabsorption syndrome caused by pancreatic insufficiency

Usual Dosage Oral:

Powder: Actual dose depends on the digestive requirements of the patient
Children <1 year: Start with 1/8 teaspoonful with feedings

Enteric coated microspheres and microtablets: The following dosage recommendations are only an approximation for initial dosages. The actual dosage will depend on the digestive requirements of the individual patient.

Children:
<1 year: 2000 units of lipase with meals/feedings
1-6 years: 4000-8000 units of lipase with meals and 4000 units with snacks
7-12 years: 4000-12,000 units of lipase with meals and snacks
Adults: 4000-16,000 units of lipase with meals and with snacks

Dosage Forms

Capsule:

Cotazym®: Lipase 8000 units, protease 30,000 units, amylase 30,000 units
Ku-Zyme® HP: Lipase 8000 units, protease 30,000 units, amylase 30,000 units
Ultrase® MT12: Lipase 12,000 units, protease 39,000 units, amylase 39,000 units
Ultrase® MT20: Lipase 20,000 units, protease 65,000 units, amylase 65,000 units
Enteric coated microspheres (Pancrease®): Lipase 4000 units, protease 25,000 units, amylase 20,000 units

Enteric coated microtablets:
Pancrease® MT 4: Lipase 4500 units, protease 12,000 units, amylase 12,000 units
Pancrease® MT 10: Lipase 10,000 units, protease 30,000 units, amylase 30,000 units
Pancrease® MT 16: Lipase 16,000 units, protease 48,000 units, amylase 48,000 units
Pancrease® MT 20: Lipase 20,000 units, protease 44,000 units, amylase 56,000 units

Enteric coated spheres:
Cotazym-S®: Lipase 5000 units, protease 20,000 units, amylase 20,000 units
Pancrelipase, Protilase®: Lipase 4000 units, protease 25,000 units, amylase 20,000 units
Zymase®: Lipase 12,000 units, protease 24,000 units, amylase 24,000 units

Delayed release:
Creon® 10: Lipase 10,000 units, protease 37,500 units, amylase 33,200 units
Creon® 20: Lipase 20,000 units, protease 75,000 units, amylase 66,400 units

Powder (Viokase®): Lipase 16,800 units, protease 70,000 units, amylase 70,000 units per 0.7 g

Tablet:
Ilozyme®: Lipase 11,000 units, protease 30,000 units, amylase 30,000 units
Viokase®: Lipase 8000 units, protease 30,000 units, amylase 30,000 units

pancuronium (pan kyoo ROE nee um)

U.S./Canadian Brand Names Pavulon®

Therapeutic Category Skeletal Muscle Relaxant

Use Produces skeletal muscle relaxation during surgery after induction of general anesthesia, increases pulmonary compliance during assisted mechanical respiration, facilitates endotracheal intubation

Usual Dosage Infants >1 month, Children, and Adults: I.V.: 0.04-0.1 mg/kg; maintenance dose: 0.02-0.1 mg/kg/dose every 30-60 minutes as needed

Dosage Forms Injection, as bromide: 1 mg/mL (10 mL); 2 mg/mL (2 mL, 5 mL)

Panhematin® *see* hemin *on page 278*

Panmycin® Oral *see* tetracycline *on page 555*

PanOxyl®-AQ *see* benzoyl peroxide *on page 68*

PanOxyl® Bar [OTC] *see* benzoyl peroxide *on page 68*

Panretin™ *see* alitretinoin *on page 18*

Panscol® Lotion [OTC] *see* salicylic acid *on page 513*

Panscol® Ointment [OTC] *see* salicylic acid *on page 513*

Panthoderm® Cream [OTC] *see* dexpanthenol *on page 169*

Pantoloc™ (Can) *see* pantoprazole *(Canada only) on this page*

Pantopon® *see* opium alkaloids *on page 416*

pantoprazole *(Canada only)* (pan TOE pra zole)

U.S./Canadian Brand Names Pantoloc™ (Can)

Therapeutic Category Proton Pump Inhibitor

Use Treatment of acute gastric and duodenal ulcer; severe gastroesophageal reflux disease (GERD)

Usual Dosage Adults: Oral: 40 mg once daily in the morning

Dosage Forms Tablet, enteric coated: 40 mg

pantothenic acid (pan toe THEN ik AS id)

Synonyms calcium pantothenate; vitamin B_5

Therapeutic Category Vitamin, Water Soluble

Use Pantothenic acid deficiency

Usual Dosage Adults: Oral: Recommended daily dose: 4-7 mg/day

Dosage Forms Tablet: 25 mg, 50 mg, 100 mg, 218 mg, 250 mg, 500 mg, 545 mg, 1000 mg

pantothenyl alcohol *see* dexpanthenol *on page 169*

Panwarfarin® ***(Discontinued)*** *see page 700*

papaverine (pa PAV er een)

U.S./Canadian Brand Names Genabid®; Pavabid®; Pavatine®

Therapeutic Category Vasodilator

Use Relief of peripheral and cerebral ischemia associated with arterial spasm

Investigational use: Prophylaxis of migraine headache

Usual Dosage Adults:

Oral: 100-300 mg 3-5 times/day

Oral, sustained release: 150-300 mg every 12 hours

Dosage Forms Papaverine hydrochloride:

Capsule, sustained release: 150 mg

Tablet: 30 mg, 60 mg, 100 mg, 150 mg, 200 mg, 300 mg

Tablet, timed release: 200 mg

Paplex® ***(Discontinued)*** *see page 700*

parabromdylamine *see* brompheniramine *on page 80*

paracetaldehyde *see* paraldehyde *on this page*

paracetamol *see* acetaminophen *on page 3*

parachlorometaxylenol (PAIR a klor oh met a ZYE le nol)

Synonyms PCMX

U.S./Canadian Brand Names Metasep® [OTC]

Therapeutic Category Antiseborrheic Agent, Topical

Use Aid in relief of dandruff and associated conditions

Usual Dosage Massage to a foamy lather, allow to remain on hair for 5 minutes, rinse thoroughly and repeat

Dosage Forms Shampoo: 2% with isopropyl alcohol 9%

Paradione® ***(Discontinued)*** *see page 700*

Paraflex® *see* chlorzoxazone *on page 128*

Parafon Forte™ DSC *see* chlorzoxazone *on page 128*

Para-Hist AT® ***(Discontinued)*** *see page 700*

Paral® *see* paraldehyde *on this page*

paraldehyde (par AL de hyde)

Synonyms paracetaldehyde

U.S./Canadian Brand Names Paral®

Therapeutic Category Anticonvulsant

Controlled Substance C-IV

Use Treatment of status epilepticus and tetanus-induced seizures; has been used as a sedative/hypnotic and in the treatment of alcohol withdrawal symptoms

Usual Dosage Dilute in milk or iced fruit juice to mask taste and odor

Oral, rectal:
- Children: 0.15-0.3 mL/kg
- Adults:
  - Hypnotic: 10-30 mL
  - Sedative: 5-10 mL

Rectal: Mix paraldehyde 2:1 with oil (cottonseed or olive)

Dosage Forms Liquid, oral or rectal: 1 g/mL (30 mL)

paramethasone acetate (par a METH a sone AS e tate)

U.S./Canadian Brand Names Haldrone®; Stemex®

Therapeutic Category Adrenal Corticosteroid

Use Treatment of variety of diseases including those of hematologic, allergic, inflammatory, neoplastic, and autoimmune in origin

Usual Dosage Oral: 2-24 mg/day

Dosage Forms Tablet: 1 mg

Paraplatin® *see* carboplatin *on page 100*

Parathar™ *see* teriparatide *on page 551*

Par Decon® *see* chlorpheniramine, phenyltoloxamine, phenylpropanolamine, and phenylephrine *on page 125*

Paredrine® *see* hydroxyamphetamine *on page 294*

paregoric (par e GOR ik)

Synonyms camphorated tincture of opium

Therapeutic Category Analgesic, Narcotic

Controlled Substance C-III

Use Treatment of diarrhea or relief of pain; neonatal abstinence syndrome (neonatal opiate withdrawal)

(Continued)

paregoric *(Continued)*

Usual Dosage Oral:

Neonatal opiate withdrawal: 3-6 drops every 3-6 hours as needed, or initially 0.2 mL every 3 hours; increase dosage by approximately 0.05 mL every 3 hours until withdrawal symptoms are controlled; it is rare to exceed 0.7 mL/dose. Stabilize withdrawal symptoms for 3-5 days, then gradually decrease dosage over a 2- to 4-week period.

Children: 0.25-0.5 mL/kg 1-4 times/day

Adults: 5-10 mL 1-4 times/day

Dosage Forms Liquid: 2 mg morphine equivalent/5 mL [equivalent to 20 mg opium powder] (5 mL, 60 mL, 473 mL, 4000 mL)

Paremyd® Ophthalmic *see* hydroxyamphetamine and tropicamide *on page 295*

Parepectolin® *see* kaolin and pectin with opium *on page 319*

Pargen Fortified® ***(Discontinued)*** *see page 700*

Par Glycerol® ***(Discontinued)*** *see page 700*

pargyline and methyclothiazide *see* methyclothiazide and pargyline *on page 366*

paricalcitol (par eh CAL ci tol)

U.S./Canadian Brand Names Zemplar™

Therapeutic Category Vitamin D Analog

Use Prevention and treatment of secondary hyperparathyroidism associated with chronic renal failure

Usual Dosage Adults: I.V.: 0.04-0.1 mcg/kg (2.8-7 mcg) given as a bolus dose no more frequently than every other day at any time during dialysis; doses as high as 0.24 mcg/kg (16.8 mcg) have been administered safely

Dosage Forms Injection: 5 mcg/mL (1 mL, 2 mL, 5 mL)

pariprazole *see* rabeprazole *on page 494*

Parlodel® *see* bromocriptine *on page 79*

Parmine® ***(Discontinued)*** *see page 700*

Parnate® *see* tranylcypromine *on page 574*

paromomycin (par oh moe MYE sin)

U.S./Canadian Brand Names Humatin®

Therapeutic Category Amebicide

Use Treatment of acute and chronic intestinal amebiasis due to susceptible *Entamoeba histolytica* (not effective in the treatment of extraintestinal amebiasis); tapeworm infestations; adjunctive management of hepatic coma; treatment of cryptosporidial diarrhea

Usual Dosage Oral:

Intestinal amebiasis: Children and Adults: 25-35 mg/kg/day in 3 divided doses for 5-10 days

Tapeworm (fish, dog, bovine, porcine):

- Children: 11 mg/kg every 15 minutes for 4 doses
- Adults: 1 g every 15 minutes for 4 doses

Hepatic coma: Adults: 4 g/day in 2-4 divided doses for 5-6 days

Dwarf tapeworm: Children and Adults: 45 mg/kg/dose every day for 5-7 days

Dosage Forms Capsule, as sulfate: 250 mg

paroxetine (pa ROKS e teen)

U.S./Canadian Brand Names Paxil™

Therapeutic Category Antidepressant, Selective Serotonin Reuptake Inhibitor

Use Treatment of depression, obsessive compulsive disorder (OCD) and panic disorder (PD)

Usual Dosage Adults: Oral: 20 mg once daily, preferably in the morning

Dosage Forms

Suspension, oral: 10 mg/5 mL
Tablet: 10 mg, 20 mg, 30 mg, 40 mg

Parsidol® *(Discontinued)* *see page 700*

Partuss® LA *see* guaifenesin and phenylpropanolamine *on page 270*

Parvolex® (Can) *see* acetylcysteine *on page 8*

PAS *see* aminosalicylate sodium *on page 28*

Patanol® *see* olopatadine *on page 414*

Pathilon® *see* tridihexethyl *on page 579*

Pathocil® *see* dicloxacillin *on page 176*

Pavabid® *see* papaverine *on page 428*

Pavabid HP® *(Discontinued)* *see page 700*

Pavasule® *(Discontinued)* *see page 700*

Pavatine® *see* papaverine *on page 428*

Pavatym® *(Discontinued)* *see page 700*

Paveral Stanley Syrup With Codeine Phosphate (Can) *see* codeine *on page 143*

Pavesed® *(Discontinued)* *see page 700*

Pavulon® *see* pancuronium *on page 428*

Paxene® *see* paclitaxel *on page 425*

Paxil™ *see* paroxetine *on previous page*

Paxipam® *see* halazepam *on page 275*

PBZ® *see* tripelennamine *on page 584*

PBZ® Elixir *(Discontinued)* *see page 700*

PBZ-SR® *see* tripelennamine *on page 584*

PCE® *see* erythromycin (systemic) *on page 215*

PCMX *see* parachlorometaxylenol *on page 429*

pectin and kaolin *see* kaolin and pectin *on page 318*

pectin with opium and kaolin *see* kaolin and pectin with opium *on page 319*

Pedameth® *see* methionine *on page 363*

PediaCare® Oral *see* pseudoephedrine *on page 486*

Pediacof® *see* chlorpheniramine, phenylephrine, and codeine *on page 123*

Pediaflor® *see* fluoride *on page 244*

Pedialyte® [OTC] *see* enteral nutritional products *on page 208*

PediaPatch Transdermal Patch [OTC] *see* salicylic acid *on page 513*

Pediapred® Oral *see* prednisolone (systemic) *on page 471*

Pedia-Profen™ *see* ibuprofen *on page 300*

Pediasure™ (Can) *see* enteral nutritional products *on page 208*

Pediatric Triban® *see* trimethobenzamide *on page 582*

Pediatrix® (Can) *see* acetaminophen *on page 3*

Pediazole® *see* erythromycin and sulfisoxazole *on page 214*

Pedi-Boro® [OTC] *see* aluminum acetate and calcium acetate *on page 22*

Pedi-Cort V® Creme *see* clioquinol and hydrocortisone *on page 137*

Pedi-Dent™ (Can) *see* fluoride *on page 244*

Pediotic® Otic *see* neomycin, polymyxin B, and hydrocortisone *on page 396*

Pedi-Pro Topical [OTC] *see* undecylenic acid and derivatives *on page 590*

Pedituss® *see* chlorpheniramine, phenylephrine, and codeine *on page 123*

PedTE-PAK-4® *see* trace metals *on page 573*

Pedtrace-4® *see* trace metals *on page 573*

PedvaxHIB™ *see Haemophilus* B conjugate vaccine *on page 275*

pegademase (bovine) (peg A de mase BOE vine)

U.S./Canadian Brand Names Adagen™

Therapeutic Category Enzyme

Use Enzyme replacement therapy for adenosine deaminase (ADA) deficiency in patients with severe combined immunodeficiency disease (SCID) who can not benefit from bone marrow transplant

Usual Dosage Children: I.M.: Dose administered every 7 days, 10 units/kg the first dose, 15 units/kg the second dose, and 20 units/kg the third; maintenance dose: 20 units/kg/week is recommended depending on patient's ADA level

Dosage Forms Injection: 250 units/mL (1.5 mL)

Peganone® *see* ethotoin *on page 226*

pegaspargase (peg AS par jase)

Synonyms PEG-L-asparaginase

U.S./Canadian Brand Names Oncaspar®

Therapeutic Category Antineoplastic Agent

Use Induction treatment of acute lymphoblastic leukemia in combination with other chemotherapeutic agents in patients who have developed hypersensitivity to native forms of asparaginase derived from *E. coli* and/or *Erwinia chrysanthem*, treatment of lymphoma

Usual Dosage **Refer to individual protocols**; I.M. administration may decrease the risk of anaphylaxis; dose must be individualized based upon clinical response and tolerance of the patient

I.M., I.V.: 2000 units/m^2 every 14 days

Dosage Forms Injection, preservative free: 750 units/mL

PEG-ES *see* polyethylene glycol-electrolyte solution *on page 459*

PEG-L-asparaginase *see* pegaspargase *on this page*

Peglyte™ (Can) *see* polyethylene glycol-electrolyte solution *on page 459*

pemoline (PEM oh leen)

Synonyms phenylisohydantoin; PIO

U.S./Canadian Brand Names Cylert®

Therapeutic Category Central Nervous System Stimulant, Nonamphetamine

Controlled Substance C-IV

Use Treatment of attention-deficit/hyperactivity disorder (ADHD); narcolepsy

Usual Dosage Oral:

Children <6 years: Not recommended

Children ≥6 years and Adults: Initial: 37.5 mg administered once daily in the morning, increase by 18.75 mg/day at weekly intervals; effective dose range: 56.25-75 mg/day; maximum: 112.5 mg/day; dosage range: 0.5-3 mg/kg/24 hours

Dosage Forms

Tablet: 18.75 mg, 37.5 mg, 75 mg

Tablet, chewable: 37.5 mg

penbutolol (pen BYOO toe lole)

U.S./Canadian Brand Names Levatol®

Therapeutic Category Beta-Adrenergic Blocker

Use Treatment of mild to moderate arterial hypertension

Usual Dosage Adults: Oral: Initial: 20 mg once daily, full effect of a 20 or 40 mg dose is seen by the end of a 2-week period, doses of 40-80 mg have been tolerated but have shown little additional antihypertensive effects

Dosage Forms Tablet, as sulfate: 20 mg

penciclovir (pen SYE kloe veer)

U.S./Canadian Brand Names Denavir™

Therapeutic Category Antiviral Agent

Use Antiviral cream for the treatment of recurrent herpes labialis (cold sores) in adults

Usual Dosage Apply cream at the first sign or symptom of cold sore (eg, tingling, swelling); apply every 2 hours during waking hours for 4 days

Dosage Forms Cream: 1% [10 mg/g] (2 g)

Penecort® Topical *see* hydrocortisone (topical) *on page 292*

Penetrex™ *see* enoxacin *on page 207*

penicillamine (pen i SIL a meen)

Synonyms d-3-mercaptovaline; β,β-dimethylcysteine; d-penicillamine

U.S./Canadian Brand Names Cuprimine®; Depen®

Therapeutic Category Chelating Agent

Use Treatment of Wilson's disease, cystinuria, adjunct in the treatment of severe rheumatoid arthritis; lead poisoning, primary biliary cirrhosis

Usual Dosage Oral:

Rheumatoid arthritis:

Children: Initial: 3 mg/kg/day (≤250 mg/day) for 3 months, then 6 mg/kg/day (≤500 mg/day) in divided doses twice daily for 3 months to a maximum of 10 mg/kg/day in 3-4 divided doses

Adults: 125-250 mg/day, may increase dose at 1- to 3-month intervals up to 1-1.5 g/day

Wilson's disease (doses titrated to maintain urinary copper excretion >1 mg/day):

Infants <6 months: 250 mg/dose once daily

Children <12 years: 250 mg/dose 2-3 times/day

Adults: 250 mg 4 times/day

Cystinuria:

Children: 30 mg/kg/day in 4 divided doses

Adults: 1-4 g/day in divided doses every 6 hours

Lead poisoning (continue until blood lead level is <60 mcg/dL):

Children: 25-40 mg/kg/day in 3 divided doses

Adults: 250 mg/dose every 8-12 hours

Primary biliary cirrhosis: 250 mg/day to start, increase by 250 mg every 2 weeks up to a maintenance dose of 1 g/day, usually administered 250 mg 4 times/day

Arsenic poisoning: Children: 100 mg/kg/day in divided doses every 6 hours for 5 days; maximum: 1 g/day

Dosage Forms

Capsule: 125 mg, 250 mg

Tablet: 250 mg

penicillin G benzathine (pen i SIL in jee BENZ a theen)

Synonyms benzathine benzylpenicillin; benzathine penicillin G; benzylpenicillin benzathine

U.S./Canadian Brand Names Bicillin® L-A; Megacillin® Susp (Can); Permapen®

Therapeutic Category Penicillin

Use Active against most gram-positive organisms and some spirochetes; used only for the treatment of mild to moderately severe infections (ie, *Streptococcus* pharyngitis) caused by organisms susceptible to low concentrations of penicillin G, or for prophylaxis of infections caused by these organisms such as rheumatic fever prophylaxis

Usual Dosage I.M.: Administer undiluted injection, very slowly released from site of injection, providing uniform levels over 2-4 weeks; higher doses result in more sustained

(Continued)

penicillin G benzathine *(Continued)*

rather than higher levels. Use a penicillin G benzathine-penicillin G procaine combination to achieve early peak levels in acute infections

Infants and Children:

Group A streptococcal upper respiratory infection: 25,000 units/kg as a single dose; maximum: 1.2 million units

Prophylaxis of recurrent rheumatic fever: 25,000 units/kg every 3-4 weeks; maximum: 1.2 million units/dose

Early syphilis: 50,000 units/kg as a single injection; maximum: 2.4 million units

Syphilis of more than 1-year duration: 50,000 units/kg every week for 3 doses; maximum: 2.4 million units/dose

Adults:

Group A streptococcal upper respiratory infection: 1.2 million units as a single dose

Prophylaxis of recurrent rheumatic fever: 1.2 million units every 3-4 weeks or 600,000 units twice monthly; a single dose of 600,000 to 1,2000,000 units is effective in the prevention of rheumatic fever secondary to streptococcal pharyngitis

Early syphilis: 2.4 million units as a single dose

Syphilis of more than 1-year duration: 2.4 million units once weekly for 3 doses

Dosage Forms Injection: 300,000 units/mL (10 mL); 600,000 units/mL (1 mL, 2 mL, 4 mL)

penicillin G benzathine and procaine combined

(pen i SIL in jee BENZ a theen & PROE kane KOM bined)

Synonyms penicillin G procaine and benzathine combined

U.S./Canadian Brand Names Bicillin® C-R; Bicillin® C-R 900/300

Therapeutic Category Penicillin

Use Active against most gram-positive organisms, mostly streptococcal and pneumococcal

Usual Dosage I.M.:

Children:

<30 lb: 600,000 units in a single dose

30-60 lb: 900,000 units to 1.2 million units in a single dose

Children >60 lb and Adults: 2.4 million units in a single dose

Dosage Forms

Injection:

300,000 units [150,000 units each of penicillin G benzathine and penicillin G procaine] (10 mL)

600,000 units [300,000 units each penicillin G benzathine and penicillin G procaine] (1 mL)

1,200,000 units [600,000 units each penicillin G benzathine and penicillin G procaine] (2 mL)

2,400,000 units [1,200,000 units each penicillin G benzathine and penicillin G procaine] (4 mL)

Injection: Penicillin G benzathine 900,000 units and penicillin G procaine 300,000 units per dose (2 mL)

penicillin G, parenteral, aqueous

(pen i SIL in jee, pa REN ter al, AYE kwee us)

Synonyms benzylpenicillin; crystalline penicillin

U.S./Canadian Brand Names Pfizerpen®

Therapeutic Category Penicillin

Use Active against most gram-positive organisms except *Staphylococcus aureus*; some gram-negative such as *Neisseria gonorrhoeae* and some anaerobes and spirochetes; although ceftriaxone is now the drug of choice for Lyme disease and gonorrhea

Usual Dosage I.M., I.V.:

Infants and Children (sodium salt is preferred in children): 100,000-250,000 units/kg/day in divided doses every 4 hours; maximum: 4.8 million units/24 hours

Severe infections: Up to 400,000 units/kg/day in divided doses every 4 hours; maximum dose: 24 million units/day

Adults: 2-24 million units/day in divided doses every 4 hours

Dosage Forms Injection:

Penicillin G potassium:

Frozen premixed: 1 million units, 2 million units, 3 million units

Powder: 1 million units, 5 million units, 10 million units, 20 million units

Penicillin G sodium: 5 million units

penicillin G procaine (pen i SIL in jee PROE kane)

Synonyms APPG; aqueous procaine penicillin G; procaine benzylpenicillin; procaine penicillin G

U.S./Canadian Brand Names Ayercillin® (Can); Crysticillin® A.S.; Wycillin®

Therapeutic Category Penicillin

Use Moderately severe infections due to *Neisseria gonorrhoeae*, *Treponema pallidum*, and other penicillin G-sensitive microorganisms that are susceptible to low but prolonged serum penicillin concentrations

Usual Dosage I.M.:

Newborns: 50,000 units/kg/day administered every day (avoid using in this age group since sterile abscesses and procaine toxicity occur more frequently with neonates than older patients)

Children: 25,000-50,000 units/kg/day in divided doses 1-2 times/day; not to exceed 4.8 million units/24 hours

Gonorrhea: 100,000 units/kg one time (in 2 injection sites) along with probenecid 25 mg/kg (maximum: 1 g) orally 30 minutes prior to procaine penicillin

Adults: 0.6-4.8 million units/day in divided doses 1-2 times/day

Uncomplicated gonorrhea: 1 g probenecid orally, then 4.8 million units procaine penicillin divided into 2 injection sites 30 minutes later. When used in conjunction with an aminoglycoside for the treatment of endocarditis caused by susceptible *S. viridans*: 1.2 million units every 6 hours for 2-4 weeks

Dosage Forms Injection, suspension: 300,000 units/mL (10 mL); 500,000 units/mL (1.2 mL); 600,000 units/mL (1 mL, 2 mL, 4 mL)

penicillin G procaine and benzathine combined *see* penicillin G benzathine and procaine combined *on previous page*

penicillin V potassium (pen i SIL in vee poe TASS ee um)

Synonyms pen VK; phenoxymethyl penicillin

U.S./Canadian Brand Names Apo®-Pen VK (Can); Beepen-VK®; Nadopen-V® (Can); Novo-Pen-VK® (Can); Nu-Pen-VK® (Can); Pen-Vee® (Can); Pen.Vee® K; PVF® K (Can); Veetids®

Therapeutic Category Penicillin

Use Treatment of mild to moderately severe susceptible bacterial infections involving the upper respiratory tract, skin, and urinary tract; prophylaxis of pneumococcal infections and rheumatic fever

Usual Dosage Oral:

Systemic infections:

Children <12 years: 25-50 mg/kg/day in divided doses every 6-8 hours; maximum dose: 3 g/day

Children >12 years and Adults: 125-500 mg every 6-8 hours

Prophylaxis of pneumococcal infections:

Children <5 years: 125 mg twice daily

Children ≥5 years: 250 mg twice daily

Prophylaxis of recurrent rheumatic fever:

Children <5 years: 125 mg

Children ≥5 years and Adults: 250 mg twice daily

Dosage Forms

Powder for oral solution: 125 mg/5 mL (3 mL, 100 mL, 150 mL, 200 mL); 250 mg/5 mL (100 mL, 150 mL, 200 mL)

Tablet: 125 mg, 250 mg, 500 mg

penicilloyl-polylysine *see* benzylpenicilloyl-polylysine *on page 70*

Penta/3B® Plus (Can) *see* vitamin, multiple (oral) *on page 604*

Pentacarinat® Injection *see* pentamidine *on this page*

pentaerythritol tetranitrate (pen ta er ITH ri tole te tra NYE trate)

Synonyms PETN

U.S./Canadian Brand Names Duotrate®; Peritrate®; Peritrate® SA

Therapeutic Category Vasodilator

Use Prophylactic long-term management of angina pectoris

Usual Dosage Adults: Oral: 10-20 mg 4 times/day (160 mg/day) up to 40 mg 4 times/day before or after meals and at bedtime; administer sustained-release preparation every 12 hours; maximum daily dose: 240 mg

Dosage Forms

Capsule: sustained release: 15 mg, 30 mg

Tablet: 10 mg, 20 mg, 40 mg

Sustained release: 80 mg

pentagastrin (pen ta GAS trin)

U.S./Canadian Brand Names Peptavlon®

Therapeutic Category Diagnostic Agent

Use Evaluate gastric acid secretory function in pernicious anemia, gastric carcinoma; in suspected duodenal ulcer or Zollinger-Ellison tumor

Usual Dosage Adults: S.C.: 6 mcg/kg

Dosage Forms Injection: 0.25 mg/mL (2 mL)

Pentam-300® Injection *see* pentamidine *on this page*

pentamidine (pen TAM i deen)

U.S./Canadian Brand Names NebuPent™ Inhalation; Pentacarinat® Injection; Pentam-300® Injection

Therapeutic Category Antiprotozoal

Use Treatment and prevention of pneumonia caused by *Pneumocystis carinii* in patients who cannot tolerate co-trimoxazole or who fail to respond to this drug; treatment of African trypanosomiasis; treatment of visceral leishmaniasis caused by *L. donovani*

Usual Dosage

Children:

Treatment: I.M., I.V. (I.V. preferred): 4 mg/kg/day once daily for 14-21 days

Prevention:

I.M., I.V.: 4 mg/kg monthly or biweekly

Inhalation (aerosolized pentamidine in children $\geq$5 years): 300 mg/dose administered every 3 weeks or monthly via Respirgard® II inhaler (8 mg/kg dose has also been used in children <5 years)

Treatment of trypanosomiasis: I.V.: 4 mg/kg/day once daily for 10 days

Adults:

Treatment: I.M., I.V. (I.V. preferred): 4 mg/kg/day once daily for 14 days

Prevention: Inhalation: 300 mg every 4 weeks via Respirgard® II nebulizer

Dosage Forms Pentamidine isethionate:

Inhalation: 300 mg

Powder for injection, lyophilized: 300 mg

Pentamycetin® (Can) *see* chloramphenicol *on page 116*

Pentasa® Oral *see* mesalamine *on page 358*

Pentaspan® *see* pentastarch *on this page*

pentastarch (PEN ta starch)

U.S./Canadian Brand Names Pentaspan®

Therapeutic Category Blood Modifiers

Use Adjunct in leukapheresis to improve the harvesting and increase the yield of leukocytes by centrifugal means

Usual Dosage 250-700 mL to which citrate anticoagulant has been added is administered by adding to the input line of the centrifugation apparatus at a ratio of 1:8-1:13 to venous whole blood

Dosage Forms Injection, in NS: 10%

pentazocine (pen TAZ oh seen)

U.S./Canadian Brand Names Talwin®; Talwin® NX

Therapeutic Category Analgesic, Narcotic

Controlled Substance C-IV

Use Relief of moderate to severe pain; a sedative prior to surgery; supplement to surgical anesthesia

Usual Dosage

Children: I.M., S.C.:

5-8 years: 15 mg

8-14 years: 30 mg

Children >12 years and Adults: Oral: 50 mg every 3-4 hours; may increase to 100 mg/dose if needed, but should not exceed 600 mg/day

Adults:

I.M., S.C.: 30-60 mg every 3-4 hours, not to exceed total daily dose of 360 mg

I.V.: 30 mg every 3-4 hours

Dosage Forms

Injection, as lactate: 30 mg/mL (1 mL, 1.5 mL, 2 mL, 10 mL)

Tablet: Pentazocine hydrochloride 50 mg and naloxone hydrochloride 0.5 mg

pentazocine compound (pen TAZ oh seen KOM pownd)

U.S./Canadian Brand Names Talacen®; Talwin® Compound

Therapeutic Category Analgesic, Narcotic

Use Relief of moderate to severe pain; has also been used as a sedative prior to surgery and as a supplement to surgical anesthesia

Usual Dosage Adults: Oral: 2 tablets 3-4 times/day

Dosage Forms Tablet:

Talacen®: Pentazocine hydrochloride 25 mg and acetaminophen 650 mg

Talwin® Compound: Pentazocine hydrochloride 12.5 mg and aspirin 325 mg

Penthrane® *see* methoxyflurane *on page 365*

Pentids® (all Forms) ***(Discontinued)*** *see page 700*

pentobarbital (pen toe BAR bi tal)

U.S./Canadian Brand Names Nembutal®; Nova Rectal® (Can)

Therapeutic Category Barbiturate

Controlled Substance C-II

Use Short-term treatment of insomnia; preoperative sedation; high-dose barbiturate coma for treatment of increased intracranial pressure or status epilepticus unresponsive to other therapy

Usual Dosage

Children:

Sedative: Oral: 2-6 mg/kg/day divided in 3 doses; maximum: 100 mg/day

Hypnotic: I.M.: 2-6 mg/kg; maximum: 100 mg/dose

Rectal:

2 months to 1 year (10-20 lb): 30 mg

1-4 years (20-40 lb): 30-60 mg

5-12 years (40-80 lb): 60 mg

12-14 years (80-110 lb): 60-120 mg **or**

<4 years: 3-6 mg/kg/dose

>4 years: 1.5-3 mg/kg/dose

(Continued)

pentobarbital *(Continued)*

Preoperative/preprocedure sedation: ≥6 months:
Oral, I.M., rectal: 2-6 mg/kg; maximum: 100 mg/dose
I.V.: 1-3 mg/kg to a maximum of 100 mg until asleep
Children 5-12 years: Conscious sedation prior to a procedure: I.V.: 2 mg/kg 5-10 minutes before procedures, may repeat one time
Adolescents: Conscious sedation: Oral, I.V.: 100 mg prior to a procedure

Children and Adults: Barbiturate coma in head injury patients: I.V.:
Loading dose: 5-10 mg/kg administered slowly over 1-2 hours; monitor blood pressure and respiratory rate
Maintenance infusion: Initial: 1 mg/kg/hour; may increase to 2-3 mg/kg/hour; maintain burst suppression on EEG
Adults:
Hypnotic:
Oral: 100-200 mg at bedtime or 20 mg 3-4 times/day for daytime sedation
I.M.: 150-200 mg
I.V.: Initial: 100 mg, may repeat every 1-3 minutes up to 200-500 mg total dose
Rectal: 120-200 mg at bedtime
Preoperative sedation: I.M.: 150-200 mg

Dosage Forms Pentobarbital sodium:
Capsule (C-II): 50 mg, 100 mg
Elixir (C-II): 18.2 mg/5 mL (473 mL, 4000 mL)
Injection (C-II): 50 mg/mL (1 mL, 2 mL, 20 mL, 50 mL)
Suppository, rectal (C-III): 30 mg, 60 mg, 120 mg, 200 mg

pentosan polysulfate sodium (PEN toe san pol i SUL fate SOW dee um)

Synonyms PPS
U.S./Canadian Brand Names Elmiron®
Therapeutic Category Analgesic, Urinary
Use Bladder pain relief or discomfort associated with interstitial cystitis
Usual Dosage Adults: Oral: 100 mg capsule 3 times/day; administer with water at least 1 hour before meals or 2 hours after meals
Dosage Forms Capsule: 100 mg

pentostatin (PEN toe stat in)

Synonyms DCF; 2′-deoxycoformycin
U.S./Canadian Brand Names Nipent™
Therapeutic Category Antineoplastic Agent
Use Treatment of adult patients with alpha-interferon-refractory hairy cell leukemia; significant antitumor activity in various lymphoid neoplasms has been demonstrated; pentostatin also is known as 2′-deoxycoformycin; it is a purine analogue capable of inhibiting adenosine deaminase
Usual Dosage Refractory hairy cell leukemia: Adults: I.V.: 4 mg/m^2 every other week
Dosage Forms Powder for injection: 10 mg/vial

Pentothal® Sodium *see* thiopental *on page 562*

pentoxifylline (pen toks I fi leen)

Synonyms oxpentifylline
U.S./Canadian Brand Names Trental®
Therapeutic Category Blood Viscosity Reducer Agent
Use Symptomatic management of peripheral vascular disease, mainly intermittent claudication

Investigational use: AIDS patients with increased tumor necrosis factor, cerebrovascular accidents, cerebrovascular diseases, new onset type I diabetes mellitus, diabetic atherosclerosis, diabetic neuropathy, gangrene, cutaneous polyarteritis nodosa, hemodialysis shunt thrombosis, cerebral malaria, septic shock, sepsis in premature neonates, sickle cell syndromes, vasculitis, Kawasaki disease, Raynaud's syndrome, cystic fibrosis, and persistent pulmonary hypertension of the newborn (case report)

Usual Dosage Adults: Oral: 400 mg 3 times/day with meals; may reduce to 400 mg twice daily if GI or CNS side effects occur

Dosage Forms Tablet, controlled release: 400 mg

Pentrax® [OTC] *see* coal tar *on page 141*

Pen-Vee® (Can) *see* penicillin V potassium *on page 435*

Pen.Vee® K *see* penicillin V potassium *on page 435*

pen VK *see* penicillin V potassium *on page 435*

Pepcid® *see* famotidine *on page 231*

Pepcid® AC Acid Controller [OTC] *see* famotidine *on page 231*

Pepcid RPD® *see* famotidine *on page 231*

Peptavlon® *see* pentagastrin *on page 436*

Pepto-Bismol® [OTC] *see* bismuth subsalicylate *on page 75*

Pepto® Diarrhea Control [OTC] *see* loperamide *on page 339*

Peptol® (Can) *see* cimetidine *on page 131*

Perchloracap® *see* radiological/contrast media (ionic) *on page 495*

Percocet® *see* oxycodone and acetaminophen *on page 422*

Percocet®-Demi (Can) *see* oxycodone and acetaminophen *on page 422*

Percodan® *see* oxycodone and aspirin *on page 423*

Percodan®-Demi *see* oxycodone and aspirin *on page 423*

Percogesic® [OTC] *see* acetaminophen and phenyltoloxamine *on page 5*

Percolone™ *see* oxycodone *on page 422*

Perdiem® Plain [OTC] *see* psyllium *on page 488*

Perfectoderm® Gel [OTC] *see* benzoyl peroxide *on page 68*

pergolide (PER go lide)

U.S./Canadian Brand Names Permax®

Therapeutic Category Anti-Parkinson's Agent; Dopaminergic Agent (Anti-Parkinson's); Ergot Alkaloid and Derivative

Use Adjunctive treatment to levodopa/carbidopa in the management of Parkinson's Disease

Usual Dosage Adults: Oral: Initial: 0.05 mg/day for 2 days, then increase dosage by 0.1 or 0.15 mg/day every 3 days over next 12 days, increase dose by 0.25 mg/day every 3 days until optimal therapeutic dose is achieved

Dosage Forms Tablet, as mesylate: 0.05 mg, 0.25 mg, 1 mg

Pergonal® *see* menotropins *on page 354*

Periactin® *see* cyproheptadine *on page 155*

Peri-Colace® [OTC] *see* docusate and casanthranol *on page 191*

pericyazine *(Canada only)* (per ee CYE ah zeen)

Therapeutic Category Phenothiazine Derivative

Use As adjunctive medication in some psychotic patients, for the control of residual prevailing hostility, impulsiveness and aggressiveness

Usual Dosage Oral:

Children and adolescents (5 years of age and over): 2.5-10 mg in the morning and 5-30 mg in the evening. These dosages approximate a daily dosage range of 1-3 mg/year of age.

Adults: 5-20 mg in the morning and 10-40 mg in the evening. For maintenance therapy, the dosage should be reduced to the minimum effective dose. Lower doses of 2.5-15

(Continued)

pericyazine *(Canada only)* *(Continued)*

mg in the morning, and 5-30 mg in the evening have been suggested. For elderly patients the initial total daily dosage should be in the order of 5 mg and increased gradually as tolerated, until an adequate response is obtained. A daily dosage of more than 30 mg will rarely be needed. Children and adolescents (5 years of age and over): 2.5-10 mg in the morning and 5-30 mg in the evening. These dosages approximate a daily dosage range of 1-3 mg/year of age.

Dosage Forms

Capsule: 5 mg, 10 mg, 20 mg

Drops, oral: 10 mg/mL (100 mL)

Peridex® *see* chlorhexidine gluconate *on page 117*

Peridol (Can) *see* haloperidol *on page 276*

perindopril erbumine (per IN doe pril er BYOO meen)

U.S./Canadian Brand Names Aceon®; Coversyl® (Can)

Therapeutic Category Miscellaneous Product

Use Treatment of hypertension

Usual Dosage Adults: Oral: 4 mg once daily; usual range: 4-8 mg/day; maximum: 16 mg/day

Dosage Forms Tablet: 2 mg, 4 mg, 8 mg

Periochip® *see* chlorhexidine gluconate *on page 117*

PerioGard® *see* chlorhexidine gluconate *on page 117*

Peritrate® *see* pentaerythritol tetranitrate *on page 436*

Peritrate® SA *see* pentaerythritol tetranitrate *on page 436*

Permapen® *see* penicillin G benzathine *on page 433*

Permax® *see* pergolide *on previous page*

permethrin (per METH rin)

U.S./Canadian Brand Names Acticin® Cream; Elimite™ Cream; Nix™ Creme Rinse

Therapeutic Category Scabicides/Pediculicides

Use Single application treatment of infestation with *Pediculus humanus capitis* (head louse) and its nits, or *Sarcoptes scabiei* (scabies)

Usual Dosage

Head lice: Children >2 months and Adults: Topical: After hair has been washed with shampoo, rinsed with water and towel-dried, apply a sufficient volume to saturate the hair and scalp. Leave on hair for 10 minutes before rinsing off with water; remove remaining nits.

Scabies: Apply cream from head to toe; leave on for 8-14 hours before washing off with water

Dosage Forms

Cream: 5% (60 g)

Creme rinse: 1% (60 mL with comb)

Permitil® Oral *see* fluphenazine *on page 247*

Pernox® [OTC] *see* sulfur and salicylic acid *on page 543*

Peroxin A5® *see* benzoyl peroxide *on page 68*

Peroxin A10® *see* benzoyl peroxide *on page 68*

perphenazine (per FEN a zeen)

U.S./Canadian Brand Names Trilafon®

Therapeutic Category Phenothiazine Derivative

Use Symptomatic management of psychotic disorders, as well as severe nausea and vomiting

Usual Dosage
Children:
Psychoses: Oral:
1-6 years: 4-6 mg/day in divided doses
6-12 years: 6 mg/day in divided doses
>12 years: 4-16 mg 2-4 times/day
I.M.: 5 mg every 6 hours
Nausea/vomiting: I.M.: 5 mg every 6 hours
Adults:
Psychoses:
Oral: 4-16 mg 2-4 times/day not to exceed 64 mg/day
I.M.: 5 mg every 6 hours up to 15 mg/day in ambulatory patients and 30 mg/day in hospitalized patients
Nausea/vomiting:
Oral: 8-16 mg/day in divided doses up to 24 mg/day
I.M.: 5-10 mg every 6 hours as necessary up to 15 mg/day in ambulatory patients and 30 mg/day in hospitalized patients
I.V. (severe): 1 mg at 1- to 2-minute intervals up to a total of 5 mg

Dosage Forms
Concentrate, oral: 16 mg/5 mL (118 mL)
Injection: 5 mg/mL (1 mL)
Tablet: 2 mg, 4 mg, 8 mg, 16 mg

perphenazine and amitriptyline *see* amitriptyline and perphenazine *on page 29*

Persa-Gel® *see* benzoyl peroxide *on page 68*

Persantine® *see* dipyridamole *on page 188*

Pertussin® CS [OTC] *see* dextromethorphan *on page 171*

Pertussin® ES [OTC] *see* dextromethorphan *on page 171*

pethidine *see* meperidine *on page 355*

PETN *see* pentaerythritol tetranitrate *on page 436*

PFA *see* foscarnet *on page 253*

Pfizerpen® *see* penicillin G, parenteral, aqueous *on page 434*

Pfizerpen-AS® ***(Discontinued)*** *see page 700*

PGE_1 *see* alprostadil *on page 20*

PGE_2 *see* dinoprostone *on page 184*

$PGF_{2\alpha}$ *see* dinoprost tromethamine *on page 184*

Phanatuss® Cough Syrup [OTC] *see* guaifenesin and dextromethorphan *on page 268*

Pharmacal® (Can) *see* calcium carbonate *on page 89*

Pharmaflur® *see* fluoride *on page 244*

Phazyme® [OTC] *see* simethicone *on page 522*

Phenadex® Senior [OTC] *see* guaifenesin and dextromethorphan *on page 268*

Phenahist-TR® *see* chlorpheniramine, phenylephrine, phenylpropanolamine, and belladonna alkaloids *on page 124*

Phenameth® DM *see* promethazine and dextromethorphan *on page 479*

phenantoin *see* mephenytoin *on page 356*

Phenaphen®/Codeine #4 ***(Discontinued)*** *see page 700*

Phenaphen® ***(Discontinued)*** *see page 700*

Phenaseptic® ***(Discontinued)*** *see page 700*

Phenazine® Injection *see* promethazine *on page 478*

Phenazo (Can) *see* phenazopyridine *on next page*

phenazopyridine (fen az oh PEER i deen)

Synonyms phenylazo diamino pyridine hydrochloride

U.S./Canadian Brand Names Azo-Standard®; Baridium®; Geridium®; Phenazo (Can); Prodium® [OTC]; Pyridiate®; Pyridium®; Pyronium® (Can); Urodine®; Urogesic®; Vito Reins® (Can)

Therapeutic Category Analgesic, Urinary

Use Symptomatic relief of urinary burning, itching, frequency and urgency in association with urinary tract infection, or following urologic procedures

Usual Dosage Oral:

Children 6-12 years: 12 mg/kg/day in 3 divided doses administered after meals for 2 days

Adults: 100-200 mg 3-4 times/day for 2 days

Dosage Forms Phenazopyridine hydrochloride: Tablet:

Azo-Standard®, Prodium®: 95 mg

Baridium®, Geridium®, Pyridiate®, Pyridium®, Urodine®, Urogesic®: 100 mg

Geridium®, Phenazodine®, Pyridium®, Urodine®: 200 mg

phenazopyridine and sulfamethoxazole *see* sulfamethoxazole and phenazopyridine *on page 542*

phenazopyridine and sulfisoxazole *see* sulfisoxazole and phenazopyridine *on page 543*

Phencen-50® ***(Discontinued)*** *see page 700*

Phenchlor® S.H.A. *see* chlorpheniramine, phenylephrine, phenylpropanolamine, and belladonna alkaloids *on page 124*

phendimetrazine (fen dye ME tra zeen)

Synonyms phendimetrazine tartrate

U.S./Canadian Brand Names Bontril PDM®; Bontril® Slow-Release; Dital®; Dyrexan-OD®; Melfiat-105® Unicelles®; Plegine®; Prelu-2®; Rexigen Forte®

Therapeutic Category Anorexiant

Controlled Substance C-III

Use Appetite suppressant during the first few weeks of dieting to help establish new eating habits; its effectiveness lasts only for short periods 3-12 weeks

Usual Dosage Adults: Oral:

Regular capsule or tablet: 35 mg 2-3 times/day one hour before meals

Sustained release: 105 mg once daily in the morning before breakfast

Dosage Forms

Capsule, as tartrate: 35 mg

Capsule, as tartrate, sustained release (Adipost®, Bontril® Slow-Release, Dital®, Dyrexan-OD®, Melfiat-105® Unicelles®, Prelu-2®; Rexigen Forte®): 105 mg

Tablet, as tartrate (Bontril PDM®, Plegine®): 35 mg

phendimetrazine tartrate *see* phendimetrazine *on this page*

Phendry® Oral [OTC] *see* diphenhydramine *on page 185*

phenelzine (FEN el zeen)

U.S./Canadian Brand Names Nardil®

Therapeutic Category Antidepressant, Monoamine Oxidase Inhibitor

Use Symptomatic treatment of atypical, nonendogenous or neurotic depression

Usual Dosage Adults: Oral: 15 mg 3 times/day; may increase to 60-90 mg/day during early phase of treatment, then reduce to dose for maintenance therapy slowly after maximum benefit is obtained; takes 2-4 weeks for a significant response to occur

Dosage Forms Tablet, as sulfate: 15 mg

Phenerbel-S® *see* belladonna, phenobarbital, and ergotamine tartrate *on page 63*

Phenerbel-S® *see* ergotamine *on page 213*

Phenergan® Injection *see* promethazine *on page 478*

Phenergan® Oral *see* promethazine *on page 478*

Phenergan® Rectal *see* promethazine *on page 478*

Phenergan® VC Syrup *see* promethazine and phenylephrine *on page 479*

Phenergan® VC With Codeine *see* promethazine, phenylephrine, and codeine *on page 479*

Phenergan® With Codeine *see* promethazine and codeine *on page 479*

Phenergan® With Dextromethorphan *see* promethazine and dextromethorphan *on page 479*

Phenetron® ***(Discontinued)*** *see page 700*

Phenhist® Expectorant *see* guaifenesin, pseudoephedrine, and codeine *on page 272*

phenindamine (fen IN dah meen)

U.S./Canadian Brand Names Nolahist® [OTC]

Therapeutic Category Antihistamine

Use Treatment of perennial and seasonal allergic rhinitis and chronic urticaria

Usual Dosage Oral:

Children <6 years: As directed by physician

Children 6 to <12 years: 12.5 mg every 4-6 hours, up to 75 mg/24 hours

Adults: 25 mg every 4-6 hours, up to 150 mg/24 hours

Dosage Forms Tablet, as tartrate: 25 mg

pheniramine and naphazoline *see* naphazoline and pheniramine *on page 391*

pheniramine, phenylpropanolamine, and pyrilamine

(fen EER a meen, fen il proe pa NOLE a meen, & peer IL a meen)

U.S./Canadian Brand Names Triaminic® Oral Infant Drops

Therapeutic Category Antihistamine/Decongestant Combination

Use Symptomatic relief of nasal congestion and postnasal drip as well as allergic rhinitis

Usual Dosage Infants <1 year: Drops: 0.05 mL/kg/dose 4 times/day

Dosage Forms Drops: Pheniramine maleate 10 mg, phenylpropanolamine hydrochloride 20 mg, and pyrilamine maleate 10 mg per mL (15 mL)

phenobarbital (fee noe BAR bi tal)

Synonyms phenobarbitone; phenylethylmalonylurea

U.S./Canadian Brand Names Barbilixir® (Can); Barbita®; Luminal®; Solfoton®

Therapeutic Category Anticonvulsant; Barbiturate

Controlled Substance C-IV

Use Management of generalized tonic-clonic (grand mal) and partial seizures; neonatal seizures; febrile seizures in children; sedation; may also be used for prevention and treatment of neonatal hyperbilirubinemia and lowering of bilirubin in chronic cholestasis

Usual Dosage

Children:

Sedation: Oral: 2 mg/kg 3 times/day

Hypnotic: I.M., I.V., S.C.: 3-5 mg/kg at bedtime

Hyperbilirubinemia: <12 years: Oral: 3-8 mg/kg/day in 2-3 divided doses; doses up to 12 mg/kg/day have been used

Preoperative sedation: Oral, I.M., I.V.: 1-3 mg/kg 1-1.5 hours before procedure

Adults:

Sedation: Oral, I.M.: 30-120 mg/day in 2-3 divided doses

Hypnotic: Oral, I.M., I.V., S.C.: 100-320 mg at bedtime

Hyperbilirubinemia: Oral: 90-180 mg/day in 2-3 divided doses

Preoperative sedation: I.M.: 100-200 mg 1-1½ hours before procedure

(Continued)

phenobarbital *(Continued)*

Anticonvulsant: Status epilepticus: **Loading dose:** I.V.:
Infants, Children, and Adults: 15-18 mg/kg in a single or divided dose; usual maximum loading dose: 20 mg/kg; in select patients may administer additional 5 mg/kg/dose every 15-30 minutes until seizure is controlled or a total dose of 30 mg/kg is reached
Anticonvulsant: Maintenance dose: Oral, I.V.:
Infants: 5-6 mg/kg/day in 1-2 divided doses
Children:
1-5 years: 6-8 mg/kg/day in 1-2 divided doses
5-12 years: 4-6 mg/kg/day in 1-2 divided doses
Children >12 years and Adults: 1-3 mg/kg/day in divided doses

Dosage Forms Phenobarbital sodium:
Capsule: 16 mg
Elixir: 15 mg/5 mL (5 mL, 10 mL, 20 mL); 20 mg/5 mL (3.75 mL, 5 mL, 7.5 mL, 120 mL, 473 mL, 946 mL, 4000 mL)
Injection: 30 mg/mL (1 mL); 60 mg/mL (1 mL); 65 mg/mL (1 mL); 130 mg/mL (1 mL)
Powder for injection: 120 mg
Tablet: 8 mg, 15 mg, 16 mg, 30 mg, 32 mg, 60 mg, 65 mg, 100 mg

phenobarbital, belladonna, and ergotamine tartrate *see* belladonna, phenobarbital, and ergotamine tartrate *on page 63*

phenobarbital, hyoscyamine, atropine, and scopolamine *see* hyoscyamine, atropine, scopolamine, and phenobarbital *on page 298*

phenobarbital, theophylline, and ephedrine *see* theophylline, ephedrine, and phenobarbital *on page 559*

phenobarbitone *see* phenobarbital *on previous page*

phenol (FEE nol)

Synonyms carbolic acid

U.S./Canadian Brand Names Baker's P&S Topical [OTC]; Cēpastat® [OTC]; Chloraseptic® Oral [OTC]; Ulcerease® [OTC]

Therapeutic Category Pharmaceutical Aid

Use Relief of sore throat pain, mouth, gum, and throat irritations

Usual Dosage Oral: Allow to dissolve slowly in mouth; may be repeated every 2 hours as needed

Dosage Forms
Liquid:
Oral, sugar free (Ulcerease®): 6% with glycerin (180 mL)
Topical (Baker's P&S): 1% with sodium chloride, liquid paraffin oil and water (120 mL, 240 mL)
Lozenge:
Cēpastat®: 1.45% with menthol and eucalyptus oil
Cēpastat® Cherry: 0.72% with menthol and eucalyptus oil
Chloraseptic®: 32.5 mg total phenol, sugar, corn syrup
Mouthwash (Chloraseptic®): 1.4% with thymol, sodium borate, menthol, and glycerin (180 mL)
Solution (Liquified Phenol): 88% [880 mg/mL]
Aqueous: 6% [60 mg/mL]

phenol red *see* phenolsulfonphthalein *on this page*

phenolsulfonphthalein (fee nol sul fon THAY leen)

Synonyms phenol red; PSP

Therapeutic Category Diagnostic Agent

Use Evaluation of renal blood flow to aid in the determination of renal function

Usual Dosage I.M., I.V.: 6 mg

Dosage Forms Injection: 6 mg/mL (1 mL)

Phenoxine® [OTC] *see* phenylpropanolamine *on page 447*

phenoxybenzamine (fen oks ee BEN za meen)

U.S./Canadian Brand Names Dibenzyline®

Therapeutic Category Alpha-Adrenergic Blocking Agent

Use Symptomatic management of hypertension and sweating in patients with pheochromocytoma

Usual Dosage Oral:

Children: Initial: 0.2 mg/kg (maximum: 10 mg) once daily, increase by 0.2 mg/kg increments; usual maintenance dose: 0.4-1.2 mg/kg/day every 6-8 hours, maximum single dose: 10 mg

Adults: 10-40 mg every 8-12 hours

Dosage Forms Capsule, as hydrochloride: 10 mg

phenoxymethyl penicillin *see* penicillin V potassium *on page 435*

phensuximide (fen SUKS i mide)

U.S./Canadian Brand Names Milontin®

Therapeutic Category Anticonvulsant

Use Control of absence (petit mal) seizures

Usual Dosage Children and Adults: Oral: 0.5-1 g 2-3 times/day

Dosage Forms Capsule: 500 mg

phentolamine (fen TOLE a meen)

U.S./Canadian Brand Names Regitine®; Rogitine® (Can)

Therapeutic Category Alpha-Adrenergic Blocking Agent; Diagnostic Agent

Use Diagnosis of pheochromocytoma; treatment of hypertension associated with pheochromocytoma or other causes of excess sympathomimetic amines; local treatment of dermal necrosis after extravasation of drugs with alpha-adrenergic effects (dobutamine, dopamine, epinephrine, metaraminol, norepinephrine, phenylephrine)

Usual Dosage

Treatment of extravasation: Infiltrate area S.C. with small amount of solution made by diluting 5-10 mg in 10 mL 0.9% NaCl within 12 hours of extravasation; for children, use 0.1-0.2 mg/kg up to a maximum of 10 mg

Children: I.M., I.V.:

- Diagnosis of pheochromocytoma: 0.05-0.1 mg/kg/dose, maximum single dose: 5 mg
- Hypertension: 0.05-0.1 mg/kg/dose administered 1-2 hours before procedure; repeat as needed until hypertension is controlled; maximum single dose: 5 mg

Adults: I.M., I.V.:

- Diagnosis of pheochromocytoma: 5 mg
- Hypertension: 5 mg administered 1-2 hours before procedure

Dosage Forms Injection, as mesylate: 5 mg/mL (1 mL)

Phentrol® ***(Discontinued)*** *see page 700*

Phenurone® ***(Discontinued)*** *see page 700*

phenylalanine mustard *see* melphalan *on page 354*

phenylazo diamino pyridine hydrochloride *see* phenazopyridine *on page 442*

Phenyldrine® [OTC] *see* phenylpropanolamine *on page 447*

phenylephrine (fen il EF rin)

U.S./Canadian Brand Names AK-Dilate® Ophthalmic Solution; AK-Nefrin® Ophthalmic Solution; Alconefrin® Nasal Solution [OTC]; Dionephrine (Can); Doktors® Nasal Solution [OTC]; I-Phrine® Ophthalmic Solution; Isopto® Frin Ophthalmic Solution; Mydfrin® Ophthalmic Solution; Neo-Synephrine® Nasal Solution [OTC]; Neo-Synephrine® Ophthalmic Solution; Nostril® Nasal Solution [OTC]; Novahistine® (Can); Prefrin® Liquifilm® (Can); Prefrin™ Ophthalmic Solution; Relief® Ophthalmic Solution; Rhinall® Nasal

(Continued)

phenylephrine *(Continued)*

Solution [OTC]; Sinarest® Nasal Solution [OTC]; St. Joseph® Measured Dose Nasal Solution [OTC]; Vicks® Sinex® Nasal Solution [OTC]

Therapeutic Category Adrenergic Agonist Agent

Use Treatment of hypotension and vascular failure in shock; supraventricular tachycardia; as a vasoconstrictor in regional analgesia; symptomatic relief of nasal and nasopharyngeal mucosal congestion; as a mydriatic in ophthalmic procedures and treatment of wide-angle glaucoma

Usual Dosage

Ophthalmic procedures:

Infants <1 year: Instill 1 drop of 2.5% 15-30 minutes before procedures

Children and Adults: Instill 1 drop of 2.5% or 10% solution, may repeat in 10-60 minutes as needed

Nasal decongestant:

Children:

2-6 years: Instill 1 drop every 2-4 hours of 0.125% solution as needed

6-12 years: Instill 1-2 sprays or instill 1-2 drops every 4 hours of 0.25% solution as needed

Children >12 years and Adults: Instill 1-2 sprays or instill 1-2 drops every 4 hours of 0.25% to 0.5% solution as needed; 1% solution may be used in adult in cases of extreme nasal congestion; do not use nasal solutions more than 3 days

Hypotension/shock:

Children:

I.M., S.C.: 0.1 mg/kg/dose every 1-2 hours as needed (maximum: 5 mg)

I.V. bolus: 5-20 mcg/kg/dose every 10-15 minutes as needed

I.V. infusion: 0.1-0.5 mcg/kg/minute; the concentration and rate of infusion can be calculated using the following formulas: Dilute 0.6 mg x weight (kg) to 100 mL; then the dose in mcg/kg/minute = 0.1 x the infusion rate in mL/hour

Adults:

I.M., S.C.: 2-5 mg/dose every 1-2 hours as needed (initial dose should not exceed 5 mg)

I.V. bolus: 0.1-0.5 mg/dose every 10-15 minutes as needed (initial dose should not exceed 0.5 mg)

I.V. infusion: 10 mg in 250 mL D_5W or NS (1:25,000 dilution) (40 mcg/mL); start at 100-180 mcg/minute (2-5 mL/minute; 50-90 drops/minute) initially. When blood pressure is stabilized, maintenance rate: 40-60 mcg/minute (20-30 drops/minute)

Paroxysmal supraventricular tachycardia: I.V.:

Children: 5-10 mcg/kg/dose over 20-30 seconds

Adults: 0.25-0.5 mg/dose over 20-30 seconds

Dosage Forms

Phenylephrine hydrochloride:

Injection (Neo-Synephrine®): 1% [10 mg/mL] (1 mL)

Nasal solution:

Drops:

Neo-Synephrine®: 0.125% (15 mL)

Alconefrin® 12: 0.16% (30 mL)

Alconefrin® 25, Neo-Synephrine®, Children's Nostril®, Rhinall®: 0.25% (15 mL, 30 mL, 40 mL)

Alconefrin®, Neo-Synephrine®: 0.5% (15 mL, 30 mL)

Spray:

Alconefrin® 25, Neo-Synephrine®, Rhinall®: 0.25% (15 mL, 30 mL, 40 mL)

Neo-Synephrine®, Nostril®, Sinex®: 0.5% (15 mL, 30 mL)

Neo-Synephrine®: 1% (15 mL)

Ophthalmic solution:

AK-Nefrin®, Isopto® Frin, Prefrin™ Liquifilm®, Relief®: 0.12% (0.3 mL, 15 mL, 20 mL)

AK-Dilate®, Mydfrin®, Neo-Synephrine®, Phenoptic®: 2.5% (2 mL, 3 mL, 5 mL, 15 mL)

AK-Dilate®, Neo-Synephrine®, Neo-Synephrine® Viscous: 10% (1 mL, 2 mL, 5 mL, 15 mL)

phenylephrine and chlorpheniramine *see* chlorpheniramine and phenylephrine *on page 121*

phenylephrine and cyclopentolate *see* cyclopentolate and phenylephrine *on page 153*

phenylephrine and guaifenesin *see* guaifenesin and phenylephrine *on page 269*

phenylephrine and isoproterenol *see* isoproterenol and phenylephrine *on page 315*

phenylephrine and promethazine *see* promethazine and phenylephrine *on page 479*

phenylephrine and scopolamine (fen il EF rin & skoe POL a meen)

Synonyms scopolamine and phenylephrine

U.S./Canadian Brand Names Murocoll-2® Ophthalmic

Therapeutic Category Anticholinergic/Adrenergic Agonist

Use Mydriasis, cycloplegia and to break posterior synechiae in iritis

Usual Dosage Ophthalmic: Instill 1-2 drops into eye(s); repeat in 5 minutes

Dosage Forms Solution, ophthalmic: Phenylephrine hydrochloride 10% and scopolamine hydrobromide 0.3% (7.5 mL)

phenylephrine and sulfacetamide *see* sulfacetamide and phenylephrine *on page 540*

phenylephrine and zinc sulfate (fen il EF rin & zingk SUL fate)

U.S./Canadian Brand Names Zincfrin® Ophthalmic [OTC]

Therapeutic Category Adrenergic Agonist Agent

Use Soothe, moisturize, and remove redness due to minor eye irritation

Usual Dosage Ophthalmic: Instill 1-2 drops in eye(s) 2-4 times/day as needed

Dosage Forms Solution, ophthalmic: Phenylephrine hydrochloride 0.12% and zinc sulfate 0.25% (15 mL)

phenylephrine, chlorpheniramine, phenylpropanolamine, and belladonna alkaloids *see* chlorpheniramine, phenylephrine, phenylpropanolamine, and belladonna alkaloids *on page 124*

phenylephrine, guaifenesin, and phenylpropanolamine *see* guaifenesin, phenylpropanolamine, and phenylephrine *on page 272*

phenylephrine, hydrocodone, chlorpheniramine, acetaminophen, and caffeine *see* hydrocodone, chlorpheniramine, phenylephrine, acetaminophen, and caffeine *on page 290*

phenylephrine, promethazine, and codeine *see* promethazine, phenylephrine, and codeine *on page 479*

phenylethylmalonylurea *see* phenobarbital *on page 443*

Phenylfenesin® L.A. *see* guaifenesin and phenylpropanolamine *on page 270*

phenylisohydantoin *see* pemoline *on page 432*

phenylpropanolamine (fen il proe pa NOLE a meen)

Synonyms *dl*-norephedrine; PPA

U.S./Canadian Brand Names Acutrim® 16 Hours [OTC]; Acutrim® II, Maximum Strength [OTC]; Acutrim® Late Day [OTC]; Control® [OTC]; Dexatrim® Pre-Meal [OTC]; Maximum Strength Dex-A-Diet® [OTC]; Maximum Strength Dexatrim® [OTC]; Phenoxine® [OTC]; Phenyldrine® [OTC]; Propagest® [OTC]; Unitrol® [OTC]

Therapeutic Category Adrenergic Agonist Agent

Use Anorexiant and nasal decongestant

Usual Dosage Oral:

Children: Decongestant:

2-6 years: 6.25 mg every 4 hours

(Continued)

phenylpropanolamine *(Continued)*

6-12 years: 12.5 mg every 4 hours not to exceed 75 mg/day
Adults:
Decongestant: 25 mg every 4 hours or 50 mg every 8 hours, not to exceed 150 mg/day
Anorexic: 25 mg 3 times/day 30 minutes before meals or 75 mg (timed release) once daily in the morning
Precision release: 75 mg after breakfast

Dosage Forms Phenylpropanolamine hydrochloride:
Capsule: 37.5 mg
Capsule, timed release: 25 mg, 75 mg
Tablet: 25 mg, 50 mg
Tablet:
Precision release: 75 mg
Timed release: 75 mg

phenylpropanolamine and brompheniramine *see* brompheniramine and phenylpropanolamine *on page 81*

phenylpropanolamine and caramiphen *see* caramiphen and phenylpropanolamine *on page 97*

phenylpropanolamine and chlorpheniramine *see* chlorpheniramine and phenylpropanolamine *on page 122*

phenylpropanolamine and guaifenesin *see* guaifenesin and phenylpropanolamine *on page 270*

phenylpropanolamine and hydrocodone *see* hydrocodone and phenylpropanolamine *on page 289*

phenylpropanolamine, brompheniramine, and codeine *see* brompheniramine, phenylpropanolamine, and codeine *on page 82*

phenylpropanolamine, chlorpheniramine, phenylephrine, and belladonna alkaloids *see* chlorpheniramine, phenylephrine, phenylpropanolamine, and belladonna alkaloids *on page 124*

phenylpropanolamine, guaifenesin, and dextromethorphan *see* guaifenesin, phenylpropanolamine, and dextromethorphan *on page 271*

phenylpropanolamine, guaifenesin, and phenylephrine *see* guaifenesin, phenylpropanolamine, and phenylephrine *on page 272*

phenyltoloxamine, phenylpropanolamine, and acetaminophen

(fen il tol OKS a meen, fen il proe pa NOLE a meen, & a seet a MIN oh fen)

U.S./Canadian Brand Names Sinubid®

Therapeutic Category Antihistamine/Decongestant/Analgesic

Use Intermittent symptomatic treatment of nasal congestion in sinus or other frontal headache; allergic rhinitis, vasomotor rhinitis, coryza; facial pain and pressure of acute and chronic sinusitis

Usual Dosage Oral:
Children 6-12 years: ½ tablet every 12 hours (twice daily)
Adults: 1 tablet every 12 hours (twice daily)

Dosage Forms Tablet: Phenyltoloxamine citrate 22 mg, phenylpropanolamine hydrochloride 25 mg, and acetaminophen 325 mg

phenyltoloxamine, phenylpropanolamine, pyrilamine, and pheniramine

(fen il tol OKS a meen, fen il proe pa NOLE a meen, peer IL a meen, & fen IR a meen)

U.S./Canadian Brand Names Poly-Histine-D® Capsule

Therapeutic Category Cold Preparation

Use Treatment of nasal congestion

Usual Dosage Adults: Oral: 1 capsule every 8-12 hours

Dosage Forms Capsule: Phenyltoloxamine citrate 16 mg, phenylpropanolamine hydrochloride 50 mg, pyrilamine maleate 16 mg, and pheniramine maleate 16 mg

phenytoin (FEN i toyn)

Synonyms diphenylhydantoin; DPH

U.S./Canadian Brand Names Dilantin®; Diphenylan Sodium®; Tremytoine® (Can)

Therapeutic Category Antiarrhythmic Agent, Class I-B; Hydantoin

Use Management of generalized tonic-clonic (grand mal), simple partial and complex partial seizures; prevention of seizures following head trauma/neurosurgery; ventricular arrhythmias, including those associated with digitalis intoxication, prolonged Q-T interval and surgical repair of congenital heart diseases in children; epidermolysis bullosa

Usual Dosage

Status epilepticus: I.V.:

Infants and Children: Loading dose: 15-18 mg/kg in a single or divided dose; maintenance, anticonvulsant: Initial: 5 mg/kg/day in 2 divided doses, usual doses:

6 months to 3 years: 8-10 mg/kg/day

4-6 years: 7.5-9 mg/kg/day

7-9 years: 7-8 mg/kg/day

10-16 years: 6-7 mg/kg/day, some patients may require every 8 hours dosing

Adults: Loading dose: 15-18 mg/kg in a single or divided dose; maintenance, anticonvulsant: usual: 300 mg/day or 5-6 mg/kg/day in 3 divided doses or 1-2 divided doses using extended release

Anticonvulsant: Children and Adults: Oral: Loading dose: 15-20 mg/kg; based on phenytoin serum concentrations and recent dosing history; administer oral loading dose in 3 divided doses administered every 2-4 hours to decrease GI adverse effects and to ensure complete oral absorption; maintenance dose: same as I.V.

Arrhythmias:

Children and Adults: Loading dose: I.V.: 1.25 mg/kg IVP every 5 minutes may repeat up to total loading dose: 15 mg/kg

Children: Maintenance dose: Oral, I.V.: 5-10 mg/kg/day in 2 divided doses

Adults: Maintenance dose: Oral: 250 mg 4 times/day for 1 day, 250 mg twice daily for 2 days, then maintenance at 300-400 mg/day in divided doses 1-4 times/day

Dosage Forms Phenytoin sodium:

Capsule, extended release: 30 mg, 100 mg

Capsule, prompt: 30 mg, 100 mg

Injection: 50 mg/mL (2 mL, 5 mL)

Suspension, oral: 125 mg/5 mL (5 mL, 240 mL)

Tablet, chewable: 50 mg

Pherazine® VC w/ Codeine *see* promethazine, phenylephrine, and codeine *on page 479*

Pherazine® w/DM *see* promethazine and dextromethorphan *on page 479*

Pherazine® With Codeine *see* promethazine and codeine *on page 479*

Phicon® [OTC] *see* pramoxine *on page 469*

Phillips'® Milk of Magnesia [OTC] *see* magnesium hydroxide *on page 345*

pHisoHex® *see* hexachlorophene *on page 281*

Phos-Ex® 62.5 ***(Discontinued)*** *see page 700*

Phos-Ex® 125 ***(Discontinued)*** *see page 700*

Phos-Ex® 167 ***(Discontinued)*** *see page 700*

Phos-Ex® 250 ***(Discontinued)*** *see page 700*

Phos-Flur® *see* fluoride *on page 244*

PhosLo® *see* calcium acetate *on page 89*

pHos-pHaid® ***(Discontinued)*** *see page 700*

Phosphaljel® ***(Discontinued)*** *see page 700*

Phospholine Iodide® Ophthalmic *see* echothiophate iodide *on page 202*

phosphonoformic acid *see* foscarnet *on page 253*

phosphorated carbohydrate solution

(FOS for ate ed kar boe HYE drate soe LOO shun)

Synonyms dextrose, levulose and phosphoric acid; levulose, dextrose and phosphoric acid; phosphoric acid, levulose and dextrose

U.S./Canadian Brand Names Emecheck® [OTC]; Emetrol® [OTC]; Naus-A-Way® [OTC]; Nausetrol® [OTC]

Therapeutic Category Antiemetic

Use Relief of nausea associated with upset stomach that occurs with intestinal flu, pregnancy, food indiscretions, and emotional upsets

Usual Dosage Oral:

Morning sickness: 15-30 mL on arising; repeat every 3 hours or when nausea threatens

Motion sickness and vomiting due to drug therapy: 5 mL doses for young children; 15 mL doses for older children and adults

Regurgitation in infants: 5 or 10 mL, 10-15 minutes before each feeding; in refractory cases: 10-15 mL, 30 minutes before each feeding

Vomiting due to psychogenic factors:

Children: 5-10 mL; repeat dose every 15 minutes until distress subsides; do not take for more than 1 hour

Adults: 15-30 mL; repeat dose every 15 minutes until distress subsides; do not take for more than 1 hour

Dosage Forms Liquid, oral: Fructose, dextrose, and orthophosphoric acid (120 mL, 480 mL, 4000 mL)

phosphoric acid, levulose and dextrose *see* phosphorated carbohydrate solution *on this page*

Photofrin® *see* porfimer *on page 461*

Phrenilin® *see* butalbital compound and acetaminophen *on page 85*

Phrenilin® Forte *see* butalbital compound and acetaminophen *on page 85*

***p*-hydroxyampicillin** *see* amoxicillin *on page 31*

Phyllocontin® *see* aminophylline *on page 27*

phylloquinone *see* phytonadione *on next page*

physostigmine (fye zoe STIG meen)

U.S./Canadian Brand Names Antilirium®

Therapeutic Category Cholinesterase Inhibitor

Use Reverse toxic CNS and cardiac effects caused by anticholinergics and tricyclic antidepressants; ophthalmic solution is used to treat open-angle glaucoma

Usual Dosage

Children: Reserve for life-threatening situations only: I.V.: 0.01-0.03 mg/kg/dose; may repeat after 15-20 minutes to a maximum total dose of 2 mg

Adults:

I.M., I.V., S.C.: 0.5-2 mg to start, repeat every 20 minutes until response occurs or adverse effect occurs

I.M., I.V. to reverse the anticholinergic effects of atropine or scopolamine administered as preanesthetic medications: Administer twice the dose, on a weight basis of the anticholinergic drug

Ophthalmic: 1-2 drops of 0.25% or 0.5% solution every 4-8 hours (up to 4 times/day); the ointment can be instilled at night

Dosage Forms

Injection, as salicylate: 1 mg/mL (2 mL)

Ointment, ophthalmic, as sulfate: 0.25% (3.5 g, 3.7 g)

phytomenadione *see* phytonadione *on next page*

phytonadione (fye toe na DYE one)

Synonyms methylphytyl napthoquinone; phylloquinone; phytomenadione; vitamin K_1

U.S./Canadian Brand Names AquaMEPHYTON® Injection; Konakion® Injection; Mephyton® Oral

Therapeutic Category Vitamin, Fat Soluble

Use Prevention and treatment of hypoprothrombinemia caused by vitamin K deficiency or anticoagulant-induced hypoprothrombinemia; hemorrhagic disease of the newborn

Usual Dosage I.V. route should be restricted for emergency use only

Hemorrhagic disease of the newborn:

Prophylaxis: I.M., S.C.: 0.5-1 mg within 1 hour of birth

Treatment: I.M., S.C.: 1-2 mg/dose/day

Oral anticoagulant overdose:

Infants: I.M., I.V., S.C.: 1-2 mg/dose every 4-8 hours

Children and Adults: Oral, I.M., I.V., S.C.: 2.5-10 mg/dose; rarely up to 25-50 mg has been used; may repeat in 6-8 hours if administered by I.M., I.V., S.C. route; may repeat 12-48 hours after oral route

Vitamin K deficiency: Due to drugs, malabsorption or decreased synthesis of vitamin K

Infants and Children:

Oral: 2.5-5 mg/24 hours

I.M., I.V.: 1-2 mg/dose as a single dose

Adults:

Oral: 5-25 mg/24 hours

I.M., I.V.: 10 mg

Minimum daily requirement: Not well established

Infants: 1-5 mcg/kg/day

Adults: 0.03 mcg/kg/day

Dosage Forms

Injection:

Aqueous colloidal: 2 mg/mL (0.5 mL); 10 mg/mL (1 mL, 2.5 mL, 5 mL)

Aqueous (I.M. only): 2 mg/mL (0.5 mL); 10 mg/mL (1 mL)

Tablet: 5 mg

Pilagan® Ophthalmic *see* pilocarpine *on this page*

Pilocar® Ophthalmic *see* pilocarpine *on this page*

pilocarpine (pye loe KAR peen)

U.S./Canadian Brand Names Adsorbocarpine® Ophthalmic; Akarpine® Ophthalmic; Diocarpine (Can); Isopto® Carpine Ophthalmic; Minims® Pilocarpine (Can); Miocarpine® (Can); Ocu-Carpine® Ophthalmic; Ocusert Pilo-20® Ophthalmic; Ocusert Pilo-40® Ophthalmic; Pilagan® Ophthalmic; Pilocar® Ophthalmic; Pilopine HS® Ophthalmic; Piloptic® Ophthalmic; Pilostat® Ophthalmic; Salagen® Oral

Therapeutic Category Cholinergic Agent

Use

Ophthalmic: Management of chronic simple glaucoma, chronic and acute angle-closure glaucoma; counter effects of cycloplegics

Oral: Symptomatic treatment of xerostomia caused by salivary gland hypofunction resulting from radiotherapy for cancer of the head and neck

Usual Dosage Adults:

Oral: 5 mg 3 times/day, titration up to 10 mg 3 times/day may be considered for patients who have not responded adequately

Ophthalmic:

Nitrate solution: Shake well before using; instill 1-2 drops 2-4 times/day

Hydrochloride solution:

Instill 1-2 drops up to 6 times/day; adjust the concentration and frequency as required to control elevated intraocular pressure

To counteract the mydriatic effects of sympathomimetic agents: Instill 1 drop of a 1% solution in the affected eye

Gel: Instill 0.5" ribbon into lower conjunctival sac once daily at bedtime

(Continued)

pilocarpine *(Continued)*

Ocular systems: Systems are labeled in terms of mean rate of release of pilocarpine over 7 days; begin with 20 mcg/hour at night and adjust based on response

Dosage Forms

Ocular therapeutic system (Ocusert® Pilo): Releases 20 or 40 mcg/hour for 1 week (8s)
Tablet: 5 mg

Pilocarpine hydrochloride:
Gel, ophthalmic (Pilopine HS®): 4% (3.5 g)
Solution, ophthalmic (Adsorbocarpine®, Akarpine®, Isopto® Carpine, Pilagan®, Pilocar®, Piloptic®, Pilostat®): 0.25% (15 mL); 0.5% (15 mL, 30 mL); 1% (1 mL, 2 mL, 15 mL, 30 mL); 2% (1 mL, 2 mL, 15 mL, 30 mL); 3% (15 mL, 30 mL); 4% (1 mL, 2 mL, 15 mL, 30 mL); 5% (15 mL); 6% (15 mL, 30 mL); 8% (2 mL); 10% (15 mL)
Pilocarpine nitrate: Solution, ophthalmic (Pilagan®): 1% (15 mL); 2% (15 mL); 4% (15 mL)

pilocarpine and epinephrine (pye loe KAR peen & ep i NEF rin)

Synonyms epinephrine and pilocarpine
U.S./Canadian Brand Names E-Pilo-x® Ophthalmic; P_xE_x® Ophthalmic
Therapeutic Category Cholinergic Agent
Use Treatment of glaucoma; counter effect of cycloplegics
Usual Dosage Ophthalmic: Instill 1-2 drops up to 6 times/day
Dosage Forms Solution, ophthalmic: Epinephrine bitartrate 1% and pilocarpine hydrochloride 1%, 2%, 3%, 4%, 6% (15 mL)

Pilopine HS® Ophthalmic *see* pilocarpine *on previous page*

Piloptic® Ophthalmic *see* pilocarpine *on previous page*

Pilostat® Ophthalmic *see* pilocarpine *on previous page*

Pima® *see* potassium iodide *on page 466*

pimaricin *see* natamycin *on page 392*

pimozide (PI moe zide)

U.S./Canadian Brand Names Orap™
Therapeutic Category Neuroleptic Agent
Use Suppression of severe motor and phonic tics in patients with Tourette's disorder
Usual Dosage Children >12 years and Adults: Oral: Initial: 1-2 mg/day, then increase dosage as needed every other day; range: 7-16 mg/day, maximum dose: 20 mg/day or 0.3 mg/kg/day should not be exceeded
Dosage Forms Tablet: 2 mg

pinaverium *(Canada only)* (pin ah VEER ee um)

U.S./Canadian Brand Names Dicetel® (Can)
Therapeutic Category Calcium Antagonist; Gastrointestinal Agent, Miscellaneous
Use For the treatment and relief of symptoms associated with irritable bowel syndrome (IBS): abdominal pain, bowel disturbances and intestinal discomfort; treatment of symptoms related to functional disorders of the biliary tract
Usual Dosage Adults: Oral: Three 50 mg tablets (1 tablet 3 times a day). In exceptional cases, the dosage may be increased up to 6 tablets a day (2 tablets 3 times/day). It is recommended that the tablet be taken with a glass of water during meals or snacks. The tablet should not be swallowed when in the lying position or just before bedtime.
Dosage Forms Tablet, as bromide: 50 mg

Pindac® ***(Discontinued)*** *see page 700*

pindolol (PIN doe lole)

U.S./Canadian Brand Names Apo-Pindol® (Can); Gen-Pindolol (Can); Novo-Pindol (Can); Nu-Pindol (Can); Syn-Pindol® (Can); Visken®

Therapeutic Category Beta-Adrenergic Blocker
Use Management of hypertension
Usual Dosage Oral: 5 mg twice daily
Dosage Forms Tablet: 5 mg, 10 mg

Pin-Rid® [OTC] *see* pyrantel pamoate *on page 488*

Pin-X® [OTC] *see* pyrantel pamoate *on page 488*

PIO *see* pemoline *on page 432*

pioglitazone (pye oh GLI ta zone)

U.S./Canadian Brand Names Actos™
Therapeutic Category Antidiabetic Agent; Thiazolidinedione Derivative
Use
Type 2 diabetes, monotherapy: Adjunct to diet and exercise, to improve glycemic control
Type 2 diabetes, combination therapy with sulfonylurea, metformin, or insulin: When diet, exercise, and a single agent alone does not result in adequate glycemic control
Usual Dosage Adults: Oral:
Monotherapy: Initial: 15-30 mg once daily; if response is inadequate, the dosage may be increased in increments up to 45 mg once daily; maximum recommended dose: 45 mg once daily
Combination therapy:
With sulfonylureas: Initial: 15-30 mg once daily; dose of sulfonylurea should be reduced if the patient reports hypoglycemia
With metformin: Initial: 15-30 mg once daily; it is unlikely that the dose of metformin will need to be reduced due to hypoglycemia
With insulin: Initial: 15-30 mg once daily; dose of insulin should be reduced by 10% to 25% if the patient reports hypoglycemia or if the plasma glucose falls to below 100 mg/dL. Doses greater than 30 mg/day have not been evaluated in combination regimens.
A 1-week washout period is recommended in patients with normal liver enzymes who are changed from troglitazone to pioglitazone therapy.
Dosage Forms Tablet: 15 mg, 30 mg, 45 mg

pipecuronium (pi pe kur OH nee um)

U.S./Canadian Brand Names Arduan®
Therapeutic Category Skeletal Muscle Relaxant
Use Adjunct to general anesthesia, to provide skeletal muscle relaxation during surgery and to provide skeletal muscle relaxation for endotracheal intubation; recommended only for procedures anticipated to last 90 minutes or longer
Usual Dosage I.V.:
Children:
3 months to 1 year: Adult dosage
1-14 years: May be less sensitive to effects
Adults: Dose is individualized based on ideal body weight, ranges are 85-100 mcg/kg initially to a maintenance dose of 5-25 mcg/kg
Dosage Forms Injection, as bromide: 10 mg (10 mL)

piperacillin (pi PER a sil in)

U.S./Canadian Brand Names Pipracil®
Therapeutic Category Penicillin
Use Treatment of serious infections caused by susceptible strains of gram-positive, gram-negative, and anaerobic bacilli; mixed aerobic-anaerobic bacterial infections or empiric antibiotic therapy in granulocytopenic patients. Its primary use is in the treatment of serious carbenicillin-resistant or ticarcillin-resistant *Pseudomonas aeruginosa* infections susceptible to piperacillin.
Usual Dosage
Infants and Children: I.M., I.V.: 200-300 mg/kg/day in divided doses every 4-6 hours; maximum dose: 24 g/day
(Continued)

piperacillin *(Continued)*

Higher doses have been used in cystic fibrosis: 350-500 mg/kg/day in divided doses every 4 hours

Adults:

I.M.: 2-3 g/dose every 6-12 hours I.M.; maximum 24 g/24 hours

I.V.: 3-4 g/dose every 4-6 hours; maximum 24 g/24 hours

Dosage Forms Powder for injection, as sodium: 2 g, 3 g, 4 g, 40 g

piperacillin and tazobactam sodium

(pi PER a sil in & ta zoe BAK tam SOW dee um)

Synonyms tazobactam and piperacillin

U.S./Canadian Brand Names Tacozin® (Can); Zosyn™

Therapeutic Category Penicillin

Use Treatment of infections caused by piperacillin-resistant, beta-lactamase-producing strains that are piperacillin/tazobactam susceptible involving the lower respiratory tract, urinary tract, skin and skin structures, gynecologic, intra-abdominal, and septicemia. Tazobactam expands activity of piperacillin to include beta-lactamase producing strains of *S. aureus*, *H. influenzae*, *B. fragilis*, *Klebsiella*, *E. coli*, and *Acinetobacter*.

Usual Dosage Adults: I.V.: 3.375 g (3 g piperacillin/0.375 g tazobactam) every 6 hours

Dosage Forms Injection: Piperacillin sodium 2 g and tazobactam sodium 0.25 g; piperacillin sodium 3 g and tazobactam sodium 0.375 g; piperacillin sodium 4 g and tazobactam sodium 0.5 g (vials at an 8:1 ratio of piperacillin sodium to tazobactam sodium)

piperazine estrone sulfate *see* estropipate *on page 220*

pipobroman (pi poe BROE man)

Therapeutic Category Antineoplastic Agent

Use Treat polycythemia vera; chronic myelocytic leukemia

Usual Dosage Children >15 years and Adults: Oral:

Polycythemia: 1 mg/kg/day for 30 days; may increase to 1.5-3 mg/kg until hematocrit reduced to 50% to 55%; maintenance: 0.1-0.2 mg/kg/day

Myelocytic leukemia: 1.5-2.5 mg/kg/day until WBC drops to 10,000 mm^3 then start maintenance 7-175 mg/day; stop if WBC falls below 3000/mm^3 or platelets fall below 150,000/mm^3

Dosage Forms Tablet: 25 mg

Pipracil® *see* piperacillin *on previous page*

pirbuterol (peer BYOO ter ole)

U.S./Canadian Brand Names Maxair™ Inhalation Aerosol

Therapeutic Category Adrenergic Agonist Agent

Use Prevention and treatment of reversible bronchospasm including asthma

Usual Dosage Children >12 years and Adults: 2 inhalations every 4-6 hours for prevention; 2 inhalations at an interval of at least 1-3 minutes, followed by a third inhalation in treatment of bronchospasm, not to exceed 12 inhalations/day

Dosage Forms

Aerosol, oral, as acetate: 0.2 mg per actuation (25.6 g (300 inhalations))

Autohaler™: 0.2 mg per actuation (2.8 g (80 inhalations); 14 g (400 inhalations))

piroxicam (peer OKS i kam)

U.S./Canadian Brand Names Apo®-Piroxicam (Can); Feldene®; Novo-Piroxicam® (Can); Nu-Pirox® (Can); Pro-Piroxicam® (Can)

Therapeutic Category Analgesic, Non-narcotic; Nonsteroidal Anti-inflammatory Drug (NSAID)

Use Management of inflammatory disorders; symptomatic treatment of acute and chronic rheumatoid arthritis, osteoarthritis, and ankylosing spondylitis; also used to treat sunburn; dysmenorrhea

Usual Dosage Oral:

Children: 0.2-0.3 mg/kg/day once daily; maximum dose: 15 mg/day

Adults: 10-20 mg/day once daily; although associated with increases in GI adverse effects, doses >20 mg/day have been used (ie, 30-40 mg/day)

Therapeutic efficacy of the drug should not be assessed for at least 2 weeks after initiation of therapy or adjustment of dosage

Dosage Forms Capsule: 10 mg, 20 mg

p-isobutylhydratropic acid *see* ibuprofen *on page 300*

PIT *see* oxytocin *on page 425*

Pitocin® *see* oxytocin *on page 425*

Pitressin® *see* vasopressin *on page 597*

Pitrex® (Can) *see* tolnaftate *on page 571*

pit vipers antivenin *see* antivenin (*Crotalidae*) polyvalent *on page 41*

pivampicillin *(Canada only)* (piv am pi SIL in)

U.S./Canadian Brand Names Pondocillin® (Can)

Therapeutic Category Antibiotic, Penicillin

Use For the treatment of respiratory tract infections (including acute bronchitis, acute exacerbations of chronic bronchitis and pneumonia); ear, nose and throat infections; gynecological infections; urinary tract infections (including acute uncomplicated gonococcal urethritis) when caused by nonpenicillinase-producing susceptible strains of the following organisms: gram-positive organisms, ie, streptococci, pneumococci and staphylococci; gram-negative organisms, ie, *H. influenzae, N. gonorrhoeae, E. coli, P. mirabilis.*

Usual Dosage Oral

Suspension:

Infants 3 to 12 months: 40-60 mg/kg body weight daily divided into 2 equal doses

Children:

1 to 3 years: 5 mL (175 mg) twice daily

4 to 6 years: 7.5 mL (262.5 mg) twice daily

7 to 10 years: 10 mL (350 mg) twice daily

In children 10 years of age or less the dosage range is 25 to 35 mg/kg/day and should not exceed the recommended adult dose of 500 mg twice daily

Children over 10 years and adults: 15 mL (525 mg) twice daily. For severe infections: Dosage may be doubled.

Tablet: Adults and children over 10 years: 500 mg twice daily; double in severe infections

In gonococcal urethritis: 1.5 g as a single dose with 1 g probenecid concurrently

Dosage Forms

Suspension, oral: 35 mg/5 mL (100 mL, 150 mL, 200 mL)

Tablet: 500 mg (equivalent to ampicillin 377 mg)

pix carbonis *see* coal tar *on page 141*

Placidyl® *see* ethchlorvynol *on page 222*

plague vaccine (plaig vak SEEN)

Therapeutic Category Vaccine, Inactivated Bacteria

Use Vaccination of persons at high risk exposure to plaque

Usual Dosage Three I.M. doses: First dose 1 mL, second dose (0.2 mL) 1 month later, third dose (0.2 mL) 5 months after the second dose; booster doses (0.2 mL) at 1- to 2-year intervals if exposure continues

Dosage Forms Injection: 2 mL, 20 mL

plantago seed *see* psyllium *on page 488*

plantain seed *see* psyllium *on page 488*

Plaquenil® *see* hydroxychloroquine *on page 295*

Plasbumin® *see* albumin *on page 15*

Plasmanate® *see* plasma protein fraction *on this page*

Plasma-Plex® *see* plasma protein fraction *on this page*

plasma protein fraction (PLAS mah PROE teen FRAK shun)

U.S./Canadian Brand Names Plasmanate®; Plasma-Plex®; Plasmatein®; Protenate®

Therapeutic Category Blood Product Derivative

Use Plasma volume expansion and maintenance of cardiac output in the treatment of certain types of shock or impending shock

Usual Dosage I.V.: 250-1500 mL/day

Dosage Forms Injection: 5% (50 mL, 250 mL, 500 mL)

Plasmatein® *see* plasma protein fraction *on this page*

Platinol® *see* cisplatin *on page 133*

Platinol®-AQ *see* cisplatin *on page 133*

Plavix® *see* clopidogrel *on page 139*

Plegine® *see* phendimetrazine *on page 442*

Plendil® *see* felodipine *on page 233*

Pletal® *see* cilostazol *on page 131*

plicamycin (plye kay MYE sin)

Synonyms mithramycin

U.S./Canadian Brand Names Mithracin®

Therapeutic Category Antidote; Antineoplastic Agent

Use Malignant testicular tumors; treatment of hypercalcemia and hypercalciuria of malignancy not responsive to conventional treatment; chronic myelogenous leukemia in blast phase; Paget's disease

Usual Dosage Refer to individual protocols. Adults: I.V. (dose based on ideal body weight):

Testicular cancer: 25-50 mcg/kg/day or every other day for 5-10 days

Blastic chronic granulocytic leukemia: 25 mcg/kg over 2-4 hours every other day for 3 weeks

Paget's disease: 15 mcg/kg/day once daily for 10 days

Hypercalcemia:

25 mcg/kg single dose which may be repeated in 48 hours if no response occurs

or 25 mcg/kg/day for 3-4 days

or 25-50 mcg/kg/dose every other day for 3-8 doses

Dosage Forms Powder for injection: 2.5 mg

PMS-Amantadine (Can) *see* amantadine *on page 24*

PMS-Baclofen (Can) *see* baclofen *on page 59*

PMS-Benztropine (Can) *see* benztropine *on page 69*

PMS-Bethanechol Chloride (Can) *see* bethanechol *on page 73*

PMS-Bisacodyl (Can) *see* bisacodyl *on page 74*

PMS-Carbamazepine (Can) *see* carbamazepine *on page 97*

PMS-Chloral Hydrate (Can) *see* chloral hydrate *on page 115*

PMS-Cholestyramine (Can) *see* cholestyramine resin *on page 129*

PMS-Clonazepam (Can) *see* clonazepam *on page 138*

PMS-Cyproheptadine (Can) *see* cyproheptadine *on page 155*

PMS-Desipramine (Can) *see* desipramine *on page 165*

PMS-Diazepam (Can) *see* diazepam *on page 173*

PMS-Dimenhydrinate (Can) *see* dimenhydrinate *on page 182*

PMS-Docusate Calcium (Can) *see* docusate *on page 191*

PMS-Erythromycin (Can) *see* erythromycin (systemic) *on page 215*

PMS-Ferrous Sulfate (Can) *see* ferrous sulfate *on page 237*

PMS-Flupam (Can) *see* flurazepam *on page 248*

PMS-Fluphenazine (Can) *see* fluphenazine *on page 247*

PMS-Hydromorphone (Can) *see* hydromorphone *on page 293*

PMS-Hydroxyzine (Can) *see* hydroxyzine *on page 297*

PMS-Imipramine (Can) *see* imipramine *on page 302*

PMS-Isoniazid (Can) *see* isoniazid *on page 314*

PMS-Ketoprofen (Can) *see* ketoprofen *on page 321*

PMS-Lactulose (Can) *see* lactulose *on page 325*

PMS-Levothyroxine Sodium (Can) *see* levothyroxine *on page 332*

PMS-Lidocaine Viscous (Can) *see* lidocaine *on page 333*

PMS-Lindane (Can) *see* lindane *on page 335*

PMS-Loperamine (Can) *see* loperamide *on page 339*

PMS-Lorazepam (Can) *see* lorazepam *on page 340*

PMS-Methylphenidate (Can) *see* methylphenidate *on page 368*

PMS-Nystatin (Can) *see* nystatin *on page 412*

PMS-Opium & Beladonna (Can) *see* belladonna and opium *on page 63*

PMS-Oxazepam (Can) *see* oxazepam *on page 420*

PMS-Prochlorperazine (Can) *see* prochlorperazine *on page 476*

PMS-Procyclidine (Can) *see* procyclidine *on page 477*

PMS-Progesterone (Can) *see* progesterone *on page 477*

PMS-Pseudoephedrine (Can) *see* pseudoephedrine *on page 486*

PMS-Pyrazinamide (Can) *see* pyrazinamide *on page 489*

PMS-Sodium Cromoglycate (Can) *see* cromolyn sodium *on page 150*

PMS-Sulfasalazine (Can) *see* sulfasalazine *on page 542*

PMS-Thioridazine (Can) *see* thioridazine *on page 563*

PMS-Trihexyphenidyl (Can) *see* trihexyphenidyl *on page 581*

pneumococcal polysaccharide vaccine *see* pneumococcal vaccine *on this page*

pneumococcal vaccine (noo moe KOK al vak SEEN)

Synonyms pneumococcal polysaccharide vaccine

U.S./Canadian Brand Names Pneumovax® 23; Pnu-Imune® 23

Therapeutic Category Vaccine, Inactivated Bacteria

Use Immunity to pneumococcal lobar pneumonia and bacteremia in individuals ≥2 years of age who are at high risk of morbidity and mortality from pneumococcal infection

Usual Dosage Children >2 years and Adults: I.M., S.C.: 0.5 mL

Revaccination should be considered if ≥6 years since initial vaccination; revaccination is recommended in patients who received 14-valent pneumococcal vaccine and are at highest risk (asplenic) for fatal infection, or at ≥6 years in patients with nephrotic syndrome, renal failure, or transplant recipients, or 3-5 years in children with nephrotic syndrome, asplenia, or sickle cell disease

Dosage Forms Injection: 25 mcg each of 23 polysaccharide isolates/0.5 mL dose (0.5 mL, 1 mL, 5 mL)

Pneumomist® *see* guaifenesin *on page 267*

Pneumovax® 23 *see* pneumococcal vaccine *on this page*

Pnu-Imune® 23 *see* pneumococcal vaccine *on previous page*

Pod-Ben-25® *see* podophyllum resin *on this page*

Podocon-25® *see* podophyllum resin *on this page*

Podofilm® (Can) *see* podophyllum resin *on this page*

podofilox (po do FIL oks)

U.S./Canadian Brand Names Condylox®

Therapeutic Category Keratolytic Agent

Use Treatment of external genital warts

Usual Dosage Adults: Topical: Apply twice daily (morning and evening) for 3 consecutive days, then withhold use for 4 consecutive days; cycle may be repeated up to 4 times until there is no visible wart tissue

Dosage Forms Solution, topical: 0.5% (3.5 mL)

Podofin® *see* podophyllum resin *on this page*

podophyllin and salicylic acid (po DOF fil um & sal i SIL ik AS id)

Synonyms salicylic acid and podophyllin

U.S./Canadian Brand Names Verrex-C&M®

Therapeutic Category Keratolytic Agent

Use Topical treatment of benign growths including external genital and perianal warts, papillomas, fibroids

Usual Dosage Topical: Apply daily with applicator, allow to dry; remove necrotic tissue before each application

Dosage Forms Solution, topical: Podophyllum 10% and salicylic acid 30% with penederm 0.5% (7.5 mL)

podophyllum resin (po DOF fil um REZ in)

Synonyms mandrake; may apple

U.S./Canadian Brand Names Pod-Ben-25®; Podocon-25®; Podofilm® (Can); Podofin®

Therapeutic Category Keratolytic Agent

Use Topical treatment of benign growths including external genital and perianal warts (condylomata acuminata), papillomas, fibroids

Usual Dosage Topical:

Children and Adults: 10% to 25% solution in compound benzoin tincture; apply drug to dry surface, use 1 drop at a time allowing drying between drops until area is covered; total volume should be limited to <0.5 mL per treatment session

Condylomata acuminatum: 25% solution is applied daily; use a 10% solution when applied to or near mucous membranes

Verrucae: 25% solution is applied 3-5 times/day directly to the wart

Dosage Forms Liquid, topical: 25% in benzoin tincture (5 mL, 7.5 mL, 30 mL)

Point-Two® *see* fluoride *on page 244*

Poladex® *see* dexchlorpheniramine *on page 169*

Polaramine® *see* dexchlorpheniramine *on page 169*

Polargen® ***(Discontinued)*** *see page 700*

poliomyelitis vaccine *see* poliovirus vaccine, inactivated *on this page*

Poliovax® Injection ***(Discontinued)*** *see page 700*

poliovirus vaccine, inactivated

(POE lee oh VYE rus vak SEEN, in ak ti VAY ted)

Synonyms IPV; poliomyelitis vaccine; Salk vaccine

U.S./Canadian Brand Names IPOL™

Therapeutic Category Vaccine, Live Virus and Inactivated Virus

Use Active immunization for the prevention of poliomyelitis

Usual Dosage

S.C.: 3 doses of 0.5 mL; the first 2 doses should be administered at an interval of 8 weeks; the third dose should be administered at least 6 and preferably 12 months after the second dose

Booster dose: All children who have received the 3 dose primary series in infancy and early childhood should receive a booster dose of 0.5 mL before entering school. However, if the third dose of the primary series is administered on or after the fourth birthday, a fourth (booster) dose is not required at school entry.

Dosage Forms Injection, Suspension: Three types of poliovirus (Types 1, 2, and 3) grown in monkey kidney cell cultures (0.5 mL)

poliovirus vaccine, live, trivalent, oral

(POE lee oh VYE rus vak SEEN, live, try VAY lent, OR al)

Synonyms OPV; Sabin vaccine; TOPV

U.S./Canadian Brand Names Orimune®

Therapeutic Category Vaccine, Live Virus

Use Poliovirus immunization

Usual Dosage Oral:

Infants: 0.5 mL dose at age 2 months, 4 months, and 18 months; optional dose may be administered at 6 months in areas where poliomyelitis is endemic

Older Children, Adolescents and Adults: Two 0.5 mL doses 8 weeks apart; third dose of 0.5 mL 6-12 months after second dose; a reinforcing dose of 0.5 mL should be administered before entry to school, in children who received the third primary dose before their fourth birthday

Dosage Forms Solution, oral: Mixture of type 1, 2, and 3 viruses in monkey kidney tissue (0.5 mL)

Polocaine® *see* mepivacaine *on page 356*

Polycillin-N® Injection *(Discontinued)* *see page 700*

Polycillin® Oral *(Discontinued)* *see page 700*

Polycillin-PRB® *(Discontinued)* *see page 700*

Polycitra® *see* sodium citrate and potassium citrate mixture *on page 527*

Polycitra®-K *see* potassium citrate and citric acid *on page 465*

Polycose® [OTC] *see* glucose polymers *on page 262*

Polydine® [OTC] *see* povidone-iodine *on page 467*

polyestradiol (pol i es tra DYE ole)

Therapeutic Category Estrogen Derivative

Use Palliative treatment of advanced, inoperable carcinoma of the prostate

Usual Dosage Adults: I.M.: 40 mg every 2-4 weeks or less frequently

Dosage Forms Powder for injection, as phosphate: 40 mg

polyethylene glycol-electrolyte solution

(pol i ETH i leen GLY kol ee LEK troe lite soe LOO shun)

Synonyms electrolyte lavage solution; PEG-ES

U.S./Canadian Brand Names Co-Lav®; Colovage®; CoLyte®; CoLyte®-Flavored; Go-Evac®; GoLYTELY®; Klean-Prep® (Can); NuLYTELY®; OCL®; Peglyte™ (Can)

Therapeutic Category Laxative

Use For bowel cleansing prior to GI examination

Usual Dosage The recommended dose for adults is 4 L of solution prior to gastrointestinal examination, as ingestion of this dose produces a satisfactory preparation in >95% of patients. The solution is usually administered orally, but may be administered via nasogastric tube to patients who are unwilling or unable to drink the solution.

Children: Oral: 25-40 mL/kg/hour for 4-10 hours

(Continued)

polyethylene glycol-electrolyte solution *(Continued)*

Adults:

Oral: At a rate of 240 mL (8 oz) every 10 minutes, until 4 liters are consumed or the rectal effluent is clear; rapid drinking of each portion is preferred to drinking small amounts continuously

Nasogastric tube: At the rate of 20-30 mL/minute (1.2-1.8 L/hour); the first bowel movement should occur approximately one hour after the start of administration

Dosage Forms Powder, for oral solution: PEG 3350 236 g, sodium sulfate 22.74 g, sodium bicarbonate 6.74 g, sodium chloride 5.86 g and potassium chloride 2.97 g (2000 mL, 4000 mL, 4800 mL, 6000 mL)

Polyflex® Tablet *(Discontinued)* *see page 700*

Polygam® Injection *(Discontinued)* *see page 700*

Polygam® S/D *see* immune globulin, intravenous *on page 303*

Poly-Histine CS® *see* brompheniramine, phenylpropanolamine, and codeine *on page 82*

Poly-Histine-D® Capsule *see* phenyltoloxamine, phenylpropanolamine, pyrilamine, and pheniramine *on page 448*

Polymox® *(Discontinued)* *see page 700*

polymyxin B and bacitracin *see* bacitracin and polymyxin B *on page 58*

polymyxin B and hydrocortisone

(pol i MIKS in bee & hye droe KOR ti sone)

Synonyms hydrocortisone and polymyxin B

U.S./Canadian Brand Names Otobiotic® Otic

Therapeutic Category Antibiotic/Corticosteroid, Otic

Use Treatment of superficial bacterial infections of external ear canal

Usual Dosage Otic: Instill 4 drops 3-4 times/day

Dosage Forms Solution, otic: Polymyxin B sulfate 10,000 units and hydrocortisone 0.5% [5 mg/mL] per mL (10 mL, 15 mL)

polymyxin B and neomycin *see* neomycin and polymyxin B *on page 395*

polymyxin B and oxytetracycline *see* oxytetracycline and polymyxin B *on page 425*

polymyxin B and trimethoprim *see* trimethoprim and polymyxin B *on page 583*

polymyxin B, bacitracin, and neomycin *see* bacitracin, neomycin, and polymyxin B *on page 59*

polymyxin B, bacitracin, neomycin, and hydrocortisone *see* bacitracin, neomycin, polymyxin B, and hydrocortisone *on page 59*

polymyxin B, neomycin, and dexamethasone *see* neomycin, polymyxin B, and dexamethasone *on page 396*

polymyxin B, neomycin, and gramicidin *see* neomycin, polymyxin B, and gramicidin *on page 396*

polymyxin B, neomycin, and hydrocortisone *see* neomycin, polymyxin B, and hydrocortisone *on page 396*

polymyxin B, neomycin, and prednisolone *see* neomycin, polymyxin B, and prednisolone *on page 397*

Poly-Pred® Ophthalmic Suspension *see* neomycin, polymyxin B, and prednisolone *on page 397*

polysaccharide-iron complex (pol i SAK a ride-EYE ern KOM pleks)

U.S./Canadian Brand Names Hytinic® [OTC]; Niferex® [OTC]; Nu-Iron® [OTC]

Therapeutic Category Electrolyte Supplement, Oral

Use Prevention and treatment of iron deficiency anemias

Usual Dosage Oral:

Children: 3 mg/kg 3 times/day

Adults: 200 mg 3-4 times/day

Dosage Forms

Capsule: Elemental iron 150 mg

Elixir: Elemental iron 100 mg/5 mL (240 mL)

Tablet: Elemental iron 50 mg

Polysporin® Ophthalmic *see* bacitracin and polymyxin B *on page 58*

Polysporin® Topical *see* bacitracin and polymyxin B *on page 58*

Polytar® [OTC] *see* coal tar *on page 141*

polythiazide (pol i THYE a zide)

U.S./Canadian Brand Names Renese®

Therapeutic Category Diuretic, Thiazide

Use Adjunctive therapy in treatment of edema and hypertension

Usual Dosage Adults: Oral: 1-4 mg/day

Dosage Forms Tablet: 1 mg, 2 mg, 4 mg

polythiazide and prazosin *see* prazosin and polythiazide *on page 470*

Polytopic® (Can) *see* bacitracin and polymyxin B *on page 58*

Polytracin® (Can) *see* bacitracin and polymyxin B *on page 58*

Polytrim® Ophthalmic *see* trimethoprim and polymyxin B *on page 583*

Poly-Vi-Flor® *see* vitamin, multiple (pediatric) *on page 606*

polyvinyl alcohol *see* artificial tears *on page 47*

Poly-Vi-Sol® [OTC] *see* vitamin, multiple (pediatric) *on page 606*

Pondimin® ***(Discontinued)*** *see page 700*

Pondocillin® (Can) *see* pivampicillin *(Canada only) on page 455*

Ponstan® (Can) *see* mefenamic acid *on page 353*

Ponstel® *see* mefenamic acid *on page 353*

Pontocaine® *see* tetracaine *on page 555*

Pontocaine® With Dextrose *see* tetracaine and dextrose *on page 555*

Porcelana® [OTC] *see* hydroquinone *on page 294*

Porcelana® Sunscreen [OTC] *see* hydroquinone *on page 294*

porfimer (POR fi mer)

U.S./Canadian Brand Names Photofrin®

Therapeutic Category Antineoplastic Agent

Use Esophageal cancer: Photodynamic therapy (PDT) with porfimer for palliation of patients with completely obstructing esophageal cancer, or of patients with partially obstructing esophageal cancer who cannot be satisfactorily treated with Nd:YAG laser therapy; early-stage lung cancer (endobronchial microinvasive nonsmall cell)

Usual Dosage I.V. (refer to individual protocols):

Children: Safety and efficacy have not been established

Adults: I.V.: 2 mg/kg over 3-5 minutes

Photodynamic therapy is a two-stage process requiring administration of both drug and light. The first stage of PDT is the I.V. injection of porfimer. Illumination with laser light 40-50 hours following the injection with porfimer constitutes the second stage of therapy. A second laser light application may be administered 90-120 hours after injection, preceded by gentle debridement of residual tumor.

Patients may receive a second course of PDT a minimum of 30 days after the initial therapy; up to three courses of PDT (each separated by a minimum of 30 days) can be

(Continued)

porfimer *(Continued)*

given. Before each course of treatment, evaluate patients for the presence of a tracheoesophageal or bronchoesophageal fistula.

Dosage Forms Powder for injection, as sodium: 75 mg

Pork NPH *see* insulin preparations *on page 307*

Pork Regular Iletin® II *see* insulin preparations *on page 307*

Portagen® [OTC] *see* enteral nutritional products *on page 208*

Posicor® *(Discontinued)* *see page 700*

Posture® [OTC] *see* calcium phosphate, dibasic *on page 93*

Potasalan® *see* potassium chloride *on page 464*

potassium acetate (poe TASS ee um AS e tate)

Therapeutic Category Electrolyte Supplement, Oral

Use Potassium deficiency, treatment of hypokalemia, correction of metabolic acidosis through conversion of acetate to bicarbonate

Usual Dosage I.V. infusion:

Children: Not to exceed 3 mEq/kg/day

Adults: Up to 150 mEq/day administered at a rate up to 20 mEq/hour; maximum concentration: 40 mEq/L

Dosage Forms Injection: 2 mEq/mL (20 mL, 50 mL, 100 mL); 4 mEq/mL (50 mL)

potassium acetate, potassium bicarbonate, and potassium citrate

(poe TASS ee um AS e tate, poe TASS ee um bye KAR bun ate, & poe TASS ee um SIT rate)

U.S./Canadian Brand Names Tri-K®

Therapeutic Category Electrolyte Supplement, Oral

Use Treatment or prevention of hypokalemia

Usual Dosage Oral:

Children: 1-4 mEq/kg/24 hours in divided doses as required to maintain normal serum potassium

Adults:

Prevention: 16-24 mEq/day in 2-4 divided doses

Treatment: 40-100 mEq/day in 2-4 divided doses

Dosage Forms Solution, oral: 45 mEq/15 mL from potassium acetate 1500 mg, potassium bicarbonate 1500 mg, and potassium citrate 1500 mg per 15 mL

potassium acid phosphate (poe TASS ee um AS id FOS fate)

U.S./Canadian Brand Names K-Phos® Original

Therapeutic Category Urinary Acidifying Agent

Use Acidify the urine and lower urinary calcium concentration; reduces odor and rash caused by ammoniacal urine

Usual Dosage Adults: Oral: 1000 mg dissolved in 6-8 oz of water 4 times/day with meals and at bedtime

Dosage Forms Tablet, sodium free: 500 mg [potassium 3.67 mEq]

potassium bicarbonate (poe TASS ee um bye KAR bun ate)

U.S./Canadian Brand Names K+ Care® Effervescent; K-Electrolyte® Effervescent; K-Gen® Effervescent; K-Lyte® Effervescent

Therapeutic Category Electrolyte Supplement, Oral

Use Potassium deficiency, hypokalemia

Usual Dosage Oral:

Normal daily requirements:

Children: 2-3 mEq/kg/day

Adults: 40-80 mEq/day

Prevention during diuretic therapy:

Children: 1-2 mEq/kg/day in 1-2 divided doses

Adults: 20-40 mEq/day in 1-2 divided doses

Treatment of hypokalemia: Children: 1-2 mEq/kg initially, then as needed based on frequently obtained lab values. If deficits are severe or ongoing losses are great, I.V. route should be considered.

Treatment of hypokalemia: Adults:

Potassium >2.5 mEq/L: 60-80 mEq/day plus additional amounts if needed

Potassium <2.5 mEq/L: Up to 40-60 mEq initial dose, followed by further doses based on lab values; deficits at a plasma level of 2 mEq/L may be as high as 400-800 mEq of potassium

Dosage Forms

Tablet for oral solution, effervescent: 6.5 mEq, 25 mEq

K+ Care® Effervescent; K-Electrolyte® Effervescent; K-Gen® Effervescent; K-Ide®; Klor-Con®/EF; K-Lyte® Effervescent: 25 mEq

potassium bicarbonate and potassium chloride, effervescent

(poe TASS ee um bye KAR bun ate & poe TASS ee um KLOR ide, ef er VES ent)

U.S./Canadian Brand Names Klorvess® Effervescent; K/Lyte/CL®

Therapeutic Category Electrolyte Supplement, Oral

Use Treatment or prevention of hypokalemia

Usual Dosage Oral:

Children: 1-4 mEq/kg/24 hours in divided doses as required to maintain normal serum potassium

Adults:

Prevention: 16-24 mEq/day in 2-4 divided doses

Treatment: 40-100 mEq/day in 2-4 divided doses

Dosage Forms

Granules for oral solution, effervescent (Klorvess®): 20 mEq per packet

Tablet for oral solution, effervescent

Klorvess®: 20 mEq per packet

K/Lyte/Cl®: 25 mEq, 50 mEq per packet

potassium bicarbonate and potassium citrate, effervescent

(poe TASS ee um bye KAR bun ate & poe TASS ee um SIT rate, ef er VES ent)

Synonyms potassium citrate and potassium bicarbonate, effervescent

U.S./Canadian Brand Names Effer-K™; K-Ide®; Klor-con®/EF; K-Lyte®; K-Vescent®

Therapeutic Category Electrolyte Supplement, Oral

Use Treatment or prevention of hypokalemia

Usual Dosage Oral:

Children: 1-4 mEq/kg/24 hours as required to maintain normal serum potassium

Adults:

Prevention: 16-24 mEq/day in 2-4 divided doses

Treatment: 40-100 mEq/day in 2-4 divided doses

Dosage Forms

Capsule, extended release: 8 mEq, 10 mEq

Powder for oral solution: 15 mEq/packet; 20 mEq/packet; 25 mEq/packet

Tablet, effervescent: 25 mEq, 50 mEq

potassium bicarbonate, potassium chloride, and potassium citrate

(poe TASS ee um bye KAR bun ate, poe TASS ee um KLOR ide & poe TASS ee um SIT rate)

U.S./Canadian Brand Names Kaochlor-Eff®

Therapeutic Category Electrolyte Supplement, Oral

Use Treatment or prevention of hypokalemia

(Continued)

potassium bicarbonate, potassium chloride, and potassium citrate *(Continued)*

Usual Dosage Oral:

Children: 1-4 mEq/kg/24 hours in divided doses as required to maintain normal serum potassium

Adults:

Prevention: 16-24 mEq/day in 2-4 divided doses

Treatment: 40-100 mEq/day in 2-4 divided doses

Dosage Forms Tablet for oral solution: 20 mEq from potassium bicarbonate 1 g, potassium chloride 600 mg, and potassium citrate 220 mg

potassium chloride (poe TASS ee um KLOR ide)

Synonyms KCl

U.S./Canadian Brand Names Cena-K®; Gen-K®; K+ 10®; Kaochlor®; Kaochlor® SF; Kaon-Cl®; Kaon-Cl-10®; Kay Ciel®; K+ Care®; K-Dur® 10; K-Dur® 20; K-Lease®; K-Lor™; Klor-Con®; Klor-Con® 8; Klor-Con® 10; Klor-Con®/25; Klorvess®; Klotrix®; K-Lyte®/Cl; K-Norm®; K-Tab®; Micro-K® 10; Micro-K® 10 Extencaps®; Micro-K® LS; Potasalan®; Rum-K®; Slow-K®; Ten-K®

Therapeutic Category Electrolyte Supplement, Oral

Use Potassium deficiency, treatment or prevention of hypokalemia

Usual Dosage I.V. doses should be incorporated into the patient's maintenance I.V. fluids, intermittent I.V. potassium administration should be reserved for severe depletion situations in patients undergoing EKG monitoring.

Normal daily requirement: Oral, I.V.:

Newborns: 2-6 mEq/kg/day

Children: 2-3 mEq/kg/day

Adults: 40-80 mEq/day

Prevention during diuretic therapy: Oral:

Children: 1-2 mEq/kg/day in 1-2 divided doses

Adults: 20-40 mEq/day in 1-2 divided doses

Treatment: Oral, I.V.:

Children: 2-3 mEq/kg/day

Adults: 40-100 mEq/day

I.V. intermittent infusion:

Children: Dose should not exceed 0.5 mEq/kg/hour, not to exceed 20 mEq/hour

Adults: 10-20 mEq/hour, not to exceed 40 mEq/hour and 150 mEq/day

Dosage Forms

Capsule, controlled release (microcapsulated): 600 mg [8 mEq]; 750 mg [10 mEq]

Micro-K® Extencaps®: 600 mg [8 mEq]

K-Lease®, K-Norm®, Micro-K® 10: 750 mg [10 mEq]

Crystals for oral suspension, extended release (Micro-K® LS®): 20 mEq per packet

Infusion, concentrate: 0.1 mEq/mL, 0.2 mEq/mL, 0.3 mEq/mL, 0.4 mEq/mL

Injection, concentrate: 1.5 mEq/mL, 2 mEq/mL, 3 mEq/mL

Liquid: 10% [20 mEq/15 mL] (480 mL, 4000 mL); 20% [40 mEq/15 mL] (480 mL, 4000 mL)

Cena-K®, Kaochlor®, Kaochlor® SF, Kay Ciel®, Klorvess®, Potasalan®: 10% [20 mEq/15 mL] (480 mL, 4000 mL)

Rum-K®: 15% [30 mEq/15 mL] (480 mL, 4000 mL)

Cena-K®, Kaon-Cl® 20%: 20% [40 mEq/15 mL]

Powder: 20 mEq per packet (30s, 100s)

K+ Care®, K-Lor™: 15 mEq per packet (30s, 100s)

Gen-K®, Kay Ciel®, K+ Care®, K-Lor™, Klor-Con®: 20 mEq per packet (30s, 100s)

K+ Care®, Klor-Con/25®: 25 mEq per packet (30s, 100s)

K-Lyte/Cl®: 25 mEq per dose (30s)

Tablet, controlled release (microencapsulated)

K-Dur® 10, Ten-K®: 750 mg [10 mEq]

K-Dur® 20: 1500 mg [20 mEq]

Tablet, controlled release (wax matrix): 600 mg [8 mEq]; 750 mg [10 mEq]

Kaon-Cl®: 500 mg [6.7 mEq]
Klor-Con® 8, Slow-K®: 600 mg [8 mEq]
K+ 10®, Kaon-Cl-10®, Klor-Con® 10, Klotrix®, K-Tab®: 750 mg [10 mEq]

potassium chloride and potassium gluconate

(poe TASS ee um KLOR ide & poe TASS ee um GLOO coe nate)

Therapeutic Category Electrolyte Supplement, Oral

Use Treatment or prevention of hypokalemia

Usual Dosage Oral:

Children: 1-4 mEq/kg/24 hours in divided doses as required to maintain normal serum potassium

Adults:

Prevention: 16-24 mEq/day in 2-4 divided doses

Treatment: 40-100 mEq/day in 2-4 divided doses

Dosage Forms Solution, oral: Potassium 20 mEq/15 mL

potassium citrate (poe TASS ee um SIT rate)

U.S./Canadian Brand Names Urocit®-K

Therapeutic Category Alkalinizing Agent

Use Prevention of uric acid nephrolithiasis; prevention of calcium renal stones in patients with hypocitraturia; urinary alkalinizer when sodium citrate is contraindicated

Usual Dosage Adults: Oral: 10-20 mEq 3 times/day with meals, up to 100 mEq/day

Dosage Forms Tablet: 540 mg [5 mEq], 1080 mg [10 mEq]

potassium citrate and citric acid (poe TASS ee um SIT rate & SI trik AS id)

Synonyms citric acid and potassium citrate

U.S./Canadian Brand Names Polycitra®-K

Therapeutic Category Alkalinizing Agent

Use Treatment of metabolic acidosis; alkalinizing agent in conditions where long-term maintenance of an alkaline urine is desirable

Usual Dosage Oral:

Mild to moderate hypocitraturia: 10 mEq 3 times/day with meals

Severe hypocitraturia: Initial: 20 mEq 3 times/day or 15 mEq 4 times/day with meals or within 30 minutes after meals; do not exceed 100 mEq/day

Dosage Forms

Crystals for reconstitution: Potassium citrate 3300 mg and citric acid 1002 mg per packet

Solution, oral: Potassium citrate 1100 mg and citric acid 334 mg per 5 mL

potassium citrate and potassium bicarbonate, effervescent *see* potassium bicarbonate and potassium citrate, effervescent *on page 463*

potassium citrate and potassium gluconate

(poe TASS ee um SIT rate & poe TASS ee um GLOO coe nate)

U.S./Canadian Brand Names Twin-K®

Therapeutic Category Electrolyte Supplement, Oral

Use Treatment or prevention of hypokalemia

Usual Dosage Oral:

Children: 1-4 mEq/kg/24 hours in divided doses as required to maintain normal serum potassium

Adults:

Prevention: 16-24 mEq/day in 2-4 divided doses

Treatment: 40-100 mEq/day in 2-4 divided doses

Dosage Forms Solution, oral: 20 mEq/5 mL from potassium citrate 170 mg and potassium gluconate 170 mg per 5 mL

potassium gluconate (poe TASS ee um GLOO coe nate)

U.S./Canadian Brand Names Kaon®; K-G®

Therapeutic Category Electrolyte Supplement, Oral

(Continued)

potassium gluconate *(Continued)*

Use Treatment or prevention of hypokalemia

Usual Dosage Oral:

Normal daily requirement:
- Children: 2-3 mEq/kg/day
- Adults: 40-80 mEq/day

Prevention during diuretic therapy:
- Children: 1-2 mEq/kg/day in 1-2 divided doses
- Adults: 20-40 mEq/day in 1-2 divided doses

Treatment of hypokalemia:
- Children: 2-3 mEq/kg/day in 2-4 divided doses
- Adults: 40-100 mEq/day in 2-4 divided doses

Dosage Forms

Elixir: 20 mEq/15 mL
- K-G®, Kaon®, Kaylixir®: 20 mEq/15 mL

Tablet:
- Glu-K®: 2 mEq
- Kaon®: 5 mEq

potassium iodide (poe TASS ee um EYE oh dide)

Synonyms KI; Lugol's solution; strong iodine solution

U.S./Canadian Brand Names Pima®; SSKI®; Thyro-Block®

Therapeutic Category Antithyroid Agent; Expectorant

Use Facilitate bronchial drainage and cough; to reduce thyroid vascularity prior to thyroidectomy and management of thyrotoxic crisis; block thyroidal uptake of radioactive isotopes of iodine in a radiation emergency

Usual Dosage Oral:

Adults RDA: 130 mcg

Expectorant:
- Children: 60-250 mg every 6-8 hours; maximum single dose: 500 mg
- Adults: 300-1000 mg 2-3 times/day, may increase to 1-1.5 g 3 times/day

Preoperative thyroidectomy: Children and Adults: 50-250 mg 3 times/day (2-6 drops strong iodine solution); administer for 10 days before surgery

Thyrotoxic crisis:
- Infants <1 year: ½ adult dosage
- Children and Adults: 300 mg = 6 drops SSKI® every 8 hours

Graves' disease in neonates: 1 drop of Lugol's solution every 8 hours

Sporotrichosis:
- Initial:
  - Preschool: 50 mg/dose 3 times/day
  - Children: 250 mg/dose 3 times/day
  - Adults: 500 mg/dose 3 times/day
- Oral increase 50 mg/dose daily
- Maximum dose:
  - Preschool: 500 mg/dose 3 times/day
  - Children and Adults: 1-2 g/dose 3 times/day
  - Continue treatment for 4-6 weeks after lesions have completely healed

Dosage Forms

Solution, oral:
- SSKI®: 1 g/mL (30 mL, 240 mL, 473 mL)
- Lugol's solution, strong iodine: 100 mg/mL with iodine 50 mg/mL (120 mL)

Syrup: 325 mg/5 mL

Tablet: 130 mg

potassium phosphate (poe TASS ee um FOS fate)

U.S./Canadian Brand Names Neutra-Phos®-K

Therapeutic Category Electrolyte Supplement, Oral

Use Treatment and prevention of hypophosphatemia

Usual Dosage I.V. doses should be incorporated into the patient's maintenance I.V. fluids; intermittent I.V. infusion should be reserved for severe depletion situations and requires continuous cardiac monitoring. It is difficult to determine total body phosphorus deficit, the following dosages are empiric guidelines: **Note:** Doses listed as mmol of **phosphate**:

Replacement intermittent infusion: I.V.:

Children:

Low dose: 0.08 mmol/kg over 6 hours; use if recent losses and uncomplicated

Intermediate dose: 0.16-0.24 mmol/kg over 4-6 hours; use if serum phosphorus level 0.5-1 mg/dL

High dose: 0.36 mmol/kg over 6 hours; use if serum phosphorus <0.5 mg/dL

Adults: Varying dosages: 0.15-0.3 mmol/kg/dose over 12 hours; may repeat as needed to achieve desired serum level **or**

15 mmol/dose over 2 hours; use if serum phosphorus <2 mg/dL **or**

Low dose: 0.16 mmol/kg over 4-6 hours; use if serum phosphorus level 2.3-3 mg/dL

Intermediate dose: 0.32 mmol/kg over 4-6 hours; use if serum phosphorus level 1.6-2.2 mg/dL

High dose: 0.64 mmol/kg over 8-12 hours; use if serum phosphorus <1.5 mg/dL

Maintenance:

Children: 0.5-1.5 mmol/kg/24 hours I.V. or 2-3 mmol/kg/24 hours orally in divided doses

Adults: 50-70 mmol/24 hours I.V. or 50-150 mmol/24 hours orally in divided doses

Dosage Forms

Capsule: Neutra-Phos®-K: Phosphorus 250 mg [8 mmol] and potassium 556 mg [14.25 mEq] per capsule

Injection: Potassium phosphate monobasic anhydrous 224 mg and potassium phosphate dibasic anhydrous 236 mg per mL; [phosphorus 3 mmol and potassium 4.4 mEq per mL] (15 mL)

Powder: Neutra-Phos®-K: Phosphorus 250 mg [8 mmol] and potassium 556 mg [14.25 mEq] per packet

potassium phosphate and sodium phosphate

(poe TASS ee um FOS fate & SOW dee um FOS fate)

Synonyms sodium phosphate and potassium phosphate

U.S./Canadian Brand Names K-Phos® Neutral; Uro-KP-Neutral®

Therapeutic Category Electrolyte Supplement, Oral

Use Treatment of conditions associated with excessive renal phosphate loss or inadequate GI absorption of phosphate

Usual Dosage All dosage forms to be mixed in 6-8 oz of water prior to administration

Children: 2-3 mmol phosphate/kg/24 hours administered 4 times/day

Adults: 100-150 mmol phosphate/24 hours in divided doses after meals and at bedtime; 1-8 tablets or capsules/day, administered 4 times/day

Dosage Forms

Capsule (Neutra-Phos®): Phosphorus 8 mmol, potassium 14.25 mEq

Powder, concentrate: Phosphate 8 mmol, sodium 7.125 mEq, and potassium 7.125 mEq per 75 mL when reconstituted

Tablet: Phosphate 8 mmol, sodium 13 mEq, and potassium 1.1 mEq (114 mg of phosphorus)

povidone-iodine (POE vi done EYE oh dyne)

U.S./Canadian Brand Names ACU-dyne® [OTC]; Aerodine® [OTC]; Betadine® [OTC]; Betadine® 5% Sterile Ophthalmic Prep Solution; Betagan® [OTC]; Biodine [OTC]; Efodine® [OTC]; Iodex® [OTC]; Iodex-p® [OTC]; Mallisol® [OTC]; Massengill® Medicated Douche w/Cepticin [OTC]; Minidyne® [OTC]; Operand® [OTC]; Polydine® [OTC]; Summer's Eve® Medicated Douche [OTC]; Yeast-Gard® Medicated Douche

Therapeutic Category Antibacterial, Topical

Use External antiseptic with broad microbicidal spectrum against bacteria, fungi, viruses, protozoa, and yeasts

(Continued)

povidone-iodine *(Continued)*

Usual Dosage Apply as needed for treatment and prevention of susceptible microbial infections

Dosage Forms

Aerosol: 5% (90 mL)
Cleanser, topical: 7.5% (30 mL, 120 mL)
Concentrate:
 Whirlpool: 10% (3840 mL)
 Perineal wash: 10% (240 mL)
Douche: 10% [0.3% when reconstituted]
Foam, topical: 10% (250 g)
Gel, vaginal: 10% (3 oz)
Mouthwash: 0.5% (180 mL)
Ointment, topical: 10% (0.9 g foil packet, 0.94 g, 28 g, 480 g)
Pads, antiseptic gauze: 10% (3" x 9", 5" x 9")
Scrub, surgical: 7.5% (480 mL, 946 mL)
Shampoo: 7.5% (120 mL)
Solution:
 Ophthalmic, sterile prep: 5% (50 mL)
  Swab aid: 10% (100s)
  Swabsticks, 4": 10%
 Topical: 10% (240 mL, 480 mL, 946 mL)
Suppository, vaginal: 10%

PPA *see* phenylpropanolamine *on page 447*

PPD *see* tuberculin tests *on page 588*

PPL *see* benzylpenicilloyl-polylysine *on page 70*

PPS *see* pentosan polysulfate sodium *on page 438*

pralidoxime (pra li DOKS eem)

Synonyms 2-PAM; 2-pyridine aldoxime methochloride

U.S./Canadian Brand Names Protopam® Injection

Therapeutic Category Antidote

Use Reverse muscle paralysis associated with toxic exposure to organophosphate anticholinesterase pesticides and chemicals; control of overdosage by anticholinesterase drugs used to treat myasthenia gravis

Usual Dosage Poisoning: I.V.:

Children: 20-50 mg/kg/dose; repeat in 1-2 hours if muscle weakness has not been relieved, then at 10- to 12-hour intervals if cholinergic signs recur

Adults: 1-2 g; repeat in 1-2 hours if muscle weakness has not been relieved, then at 10- to 12-hour intervals if cholinergic signs recur

Dosage Forms

Injection: 20 mL vial containing 1 g each pralidoxime chloride with one 20 mL ampul diluent, disposable syringe, needle, and alcohol swab
Pralidoxime chloride:
 Injection: 300 mg/mL (2 mL)

PrameGel® [OTC] *see* pramoxine *on next page*

Pramet® FA *see* vitamin, multiple (prenatal) *on page 606*

Pramilet® FA *see* vitamin, multiple (prenatal) *on page 606*

pramipexole (pra mi PEX ole)

U.S./Canadian Brand Names Mirapex®

Therapeutic Category Dopaminergic Agent (Anti-Parkinson's)

Use Treatment of the signs and symptoms of idiopathic Parkinson's Disease

Usual Dosage Adults: Oral: Initial: 0.375 mg/day given in 3 divided doses, increase gradually by 0.125 mg/dose every 5-7 days; range: 1.5-4.5 mg/day

Dosage Forms Tablet: 0.125 mg, 0.25 mg, 1 mg, 1.5 mg

Pramosone® *see* pramoxine and hydrocortisone *on this page*

pramoxine (pra MOKS een)

U.S./Canadian Brand Names Anusol® Ointment [OTC]; Fleet® Pain Relief [OTC]; Itch-X® [OTC]; Phicon® [OTC]; PrameGel® [OTC]; Prax® [OTC]; ProctoFoam® NS [OTC]; Tronolane® [OTC]

Therapeutic Category Local Anesthetic

Use Temporary relief of pain and itching associated with anogenital pruritus or irritation; dermatosis, minor burns or hemorrhoids

Usual Dosage Apply as directed, usually every 3-4 hours

Dosage Forms Pramoxine hydrochloride:

Aerosol foam (ProctoFoam® NS): 1% (15 g)

Cream:

Prax®: 1% (30 g, 113.4 g, 454 g)

Tronolane®: 1% (30 g, 60 g)

Tronothane® HCl: 1% (28.4 g)

Gel, topical:

Itch-X®: 1% (35.4 g)

PrameGel®: 1% (118 g)

Lotion (Prax®): 1% (15 mL, 120 mL, 240 mL)

Ointment (Anusol®): 1% (30 g)

Pads (Fleet® Pain Relief): 1% (100s)

Spray (Itch-X®): 1% (60 mL)

pramoxine and hydrocortisone (pra MOKS een & hye droe KOR ti sone)

Synonyms hydrocortisone and pramoxine

U.S./Canadian Brand Names Enzone®; Pramosone®; Proctofoam®-HC; Zone-A Forte®

Therapeutic Category Anesthetic/Corticosteroid

Use Treatment of severe anorectal or perianal inflammation

Usual Dosage Apply to affected areas 3-4 times/day

Dosage Forms

Cream, topical: Pramoxine hydrochloride 1% and hydrocortisone acetate 0.5% (30 g); pramoxine hydrochloride 1% and hydrocortisone acetate 1%

Foam, rectal: Pramoxine hydrochloride 1% and hydrocortisone acetate 1% (10 g)

Lotion, topical: Pramoxine hydrochloride 1% and hydrocortisone 0.25%; pramoxine hydrochloride 1% and hydrocortisone 2.5%; pramoxine hydrochloride 2.5% and hydrocortisone 1% (37.5 mL, 120 mL, 240 mL)

Prandin™ *see* repaglinide *on page 500*

Pravachol® *see* pravastatin *on this page*

pravastatin (PRA va stat in)

U.S./Canadian Brand Names Pravachol®

Therapeutic Category HMG-CoA Reductase Inhibitor

Use Adjunct to diet for the reduction of elevated total and LDL-cholesterol levels in patients with hypercholesterolemia (Type IIa and IIb)

Usual Dosage Adults: Oral: 10-20 mg once daily at bedtime

Dosage Forms Tablet, as sodium: 10 mg, 20 mg, 40 mg

Prax® [OTC] *see* pramoxine *on this page*

praziquantel (pray zi KWON tel)

U.S./Canadian Brand Names Biltricide®

Therapeutic Category Anthelmintic

(Continued)

praziquantel *(Continued)*

Use Treatment of all stages of schistosomiasis caused by *Schistosoma* species pathogenic to humans; also active in the treatment of clonorchiasis, opisthorchiasis, cysticercosis, and many intestinal tapeworm infections and trematode

Usual Dosage Children and Adults: Oral:

Schistosomiasis: 20 mg/kg/dose 2-3 times/day for 1 day at 4- to 6-hour intervals

Flukes: 25 mg/kg/dose every 8 hours for 1-2 days

Cysticercosis: 50 mg/kg/day divided every 8 hours for 14 days

Tapeworms: 10-20 mg/kg as a single dose (25 mg/kg for *H. nana*)

Dosage Forms Tablet, tri-scored: 600 mg

prazosin (PRA zoe sin)

Synonyms furazosin

U.S./Canadian Brand Names Apo®-Prazo (Can); Minipress®; Novo-Prazin® (Can); Nu-Prazo® (Can)

Therapeutic Category Alpha-Adrenergic Blocking Agent

Use Hypertension, severe congestive heart failure (in conjunction with diuretics and cardiac glycosides)

Unlabeled use: Symptoms of benign prostatic hyperplasia

Usual Dosage Oral:

Children: Initial: 5 mcg/kg/dose (to assess hypotensive effects); usual dosing interval every 6 hours; increase dosage gradually up to maintenance of 25-150 mcg/kg/day divided every 6 hours

Adults: Initial: 1 mg/dose 2-3 times/day; usual maintenance dose: 3-15 mg/day in divided doses 2-4 times/day; maximum daily dose: 20 mg

Dosage Forms Capsule, as hydrochloride: 1 mg, 2 mg, 5 mg

prazosin and polythiazide (PRA zoe sin & pol i THYE a zide)

Synonyms polythiazide and prazosin

U.S./Canadian Brand Names Minizide®

Therapeutic Category Antihypertensive Agent, Combination

Use Management of mild to moderate hypertension

Usual Dosage Adults: Oral: 1 capsule 2-3 times/day

Dosage Forms Capsule:

1: Prazosin 1 mg and polythiazide 0.5 mg

2: Prazosin 2 mg and polythiazide 0.5 mg

5: Prazosin 5 mg and polythiazide 0.5 mg

Precose® *see* acarbose *on page 2*

Predaject-50® ***(Discontinued)*** *see page 700*

Predalone® ***(Discontinued)*** *see page 700*

Pred Forte® Ophthalmic *see* prednisolone (ophthalmic) *on next page*

Pred-G® Ophthalmic *see* prednisolone and gentamicin *on next page*

Predicort-50® ***(Discontinued)*** *see page 700*

Pred Mild® Ophthalmic *see* prednisolone (ophthalmic) *on next page*

prednicarbate (PRED ni kar bate)

U.S./Canadian Brand Names Dermatop®

Therapeutic Category Corticosteroid, Topical

Use Relief of the inflammatory and pruritic manifestations of corticosteroid-responsive dermatoses

Usual Dosage Adults: Topical: Apply a thin film to affected area twice daily

Dosage Forms Cream: 0.1% (15 g, 60 g)

Prednicen-M® *see* prednisone *on page 472*

prednisolone and chloramphenicol *see* chloramphenicol and prednisolone *on page 116*

prednisolone and gentamicin (pred NIS oh lone & jen ta MYE sin)

Synonyms gentamicin and prednisolone

U.S./Canadian Brand Names Pred-G® Ophthalmic

Therapeutic Category Antibiotic/Corticosteroid, Ophthalmic

Use Treatment of steroid responsive inflammatory conditions and superficial ocular infections due to strains of microorganisms susceptible to gentamicin such as *Staphylococcus, E. coli, H. influenzae, Klebsiella, Neisseria, Pseudomonas, Proteus,* and *Serratia* species

Usual Dosage Children and Adults: Ophthalmic: 1 drop 2-4 times/day; during the initial 24-48 hours, the dosing frequency may be increased if necessary

Dosage Forms

Ointment, ophthalmic: Prednisolone acetate 0.6% and gentamicin sulfate 0.3% (3.5 g)

Suspension, ophthalmic: Prednisolone acetate 1% and gentamicin sulfate 0.3% (2 mL, 5 mL, 10 mL)

prednisolone and sulfacetamide *see* sulfacetamide and prednisolone *on page 540*

prednisolone, neomycin, and polymyxin B *see* neomycin, polymyxin B, and prednisolone *on page 397*

prednisolone (ophthalmic) (pred NIS oh lone)

Synonyms deltahydrocortisone; metacortandralone

U.S./Canadian Brand Names AK-Pred® Ophthalmic; Econopred® Ophthalmic; Econopred® Plus Ophthalmic; Inflamase® Forte Ophthalmic; Inflamase® Mild Ophthalmic; Metreton® Ophthalmic; Ophtho-tate® (Can); Pred Forte® Ophthalmic; Pred Mild® Ophthalmic

Therapeutic Category Adrenal Corticosteroid

Use Treatment of palpebral and bulbar conjunctivitis; corneal injury from chemical, radiation, thermal burns, or foreign body penetration

Usual Dosage Adults: Ophthalmic: 1-2 drops into conjunctival sac every hour during day, every 2 hours at night until favorable response is obtained, then use 1 drop every 4 hours

Dosage Forms

Solution, ophthalmic, as sodium phosphate: 0.125% (5 mL, 10 mL, 15 mL); 1% (5 mL, 10 mL, 15 mL)

Suspension, ophthalmic, as acetate: 0.12% (5 mL, 10 mL); 0.125% (5 mL, 10 mL, 15 mL); 1% (1 mL, 5 mL, 10 mL, 15 mL)

prednisolone (systemic) (pred NIS oh lone)

Synonyms deltahydrocortisone; metacortandralone

U.S./Canadian Brand Names Delta-Cortef® Oral; Key-Pred® Injection; Key-Pred-SP® Injection; Novo-Prednisolone® (Can); Pediapred® Oral; Prednisol® TBA Injection; Prelone® Oral

Therapeutic Category Adrenal Corticosteroid

Use Treatment of endocrine disorders, rheumatic disorders, collagen diseases, dermatologic diseases, allergic states, ophthalmic diseases, respiratory diseases, hematologic disorders, neoplastic diseases, edematous states, and gastrointestinal diseases

Usual Dosage Dose depends upon condition being treated and response of patient; dosage for infants and children should be based on severity of the disease and response of the patient rather than on strict adherence to dosage indicated by age, weight, or body surface area. Consider alternate day therapy for long-term therapy. Discontinuation of long-term therapy requires gradual withdrawal by tapering the dose.

Children:

Acute asthma:

Oral: 1-2 mg/kg/day in divided doses 1-2 times/day for 3-5 days

I.V.: 2-4 mg/kg/day divided 3-4 times/day

(Continued)

prednisolone (systemic) *(Continued)*

Anti-inflammatory or immunosuppressive dose: Oral, I.V.: 0.1-2 mg/kg/day in divided doses 1-4 times/day

Nephrotic syndrome: Oral: Initial: 2 mg/kg/day (maximum: 80 mg/day) in divided doses 3-4 times/day until urine is protein free for 5 days (maximum: 28 days); if proteinuria persists, use 4 mg/kg/dose every other day for an additional 28 days (maximum: 120 mg/day); maintenance: 2 mg/kg/dose every other day for 28 days (maximum: 80 mg/dose); then taper over 4-6 weeks

Adults:

Oral, I.V.: 5-60 mg/day

Dosage Forms

Injection, as acetate (for I.M., intralesional, intra-articular, or soft tissue administration only): 25 mg/mL (10 mL, 30 mL); 50 mg/mL (30 mL)

Injection, as sodium phosphate (for I.M., I.V., intra-articular, intralesional, or soft tissue administration): 20 mg/mL (2 mL, 5 mL, 10 mL)

Injection, as tebutate (for intra-articular, intralesional, soft tissue administration only): 20 mg/mL (1 mL, 5 mL, 10 mL)

Liquid, oral, as sodium phosphate: 5 mg/5 mL (120 mL)

Syrup: 15 mg/5 mL (240 mL)

Tablet: 5 mg

Prednisol® TBA Injection *see* prednisolone (systemic) *on previous page*

prednisone (PRED ni sone)

Synonyms deltacortisone; deltadehydrocortisone

U.S./Canadian Brand Names Apo®-Prednisone (Can); Deltasone®; Jaa-Prednisone® (Can); Liquid Pred®; Meticorten®; Novo-Prednisone® (Can); Orasone®; Prednicen-M®; Winpred (Can)

Therapeutic Category Adrenal Corticosteroid

Use Management of adrenocortical insufficiency; used for its anti-inflammatory or immunosuppressant effects

Usual Dosage Dose depends upon condition being treated and response of patient; dosage for infants and children should be based on severity of the disease and response of the patient rather than on strict adherence to dosage indicated by age, weight, or body surface area. Consider alternate day therapy for long-term therapy. Discontinuation of long-term therapy requires gradual withdrawal by tapering the dose.

Children: Oral: 0.05-2 mg/kg/day (anti-inflammatory or immunosuppressive dose) divided 1-4 times/day

Acute asthma: Oral: 1-2 mg/kg/day in divided doses 1-2 times/day for 3-5 days

Nephrotic syndrome: Oral: Initial: 2 mg/kg/day (maximum: of 80 mg/day) in divided doses 3-4 times/day until urine is protein free for 5 days (maximum: 28 days); if proteinuria persists, use 4 mg/kg/dose every other day (maximum: 120 mg/day) for an additional 28 days; maintenance: 2 mg/kg/dose every other day for 28 days (maximum: 80 mg/day); then taper over 4-6 weeks

Children and Adults: Physiologic replacement: 4-5 mg/m^2/day

Adults: Oral: 5-60 mg/day in divided doses 1-4 times/day

Dosage Forms

Solution:

Concentrate: 5 mg/mL (5 mL, 30 mL)

Oral: 5 mg/5 mL (10 mL, 20 mL, 500 mL)

Syrup: 5 mg/5 mL (120 mL, 240 mL)

Tablet: 1 mg, 2.5 mg, 5 mg, 10 mg, 20 mg, 50 mg

Prefrin® Liquifilm® (Can) *see* phenylephrine *on page 445*

Prefrin™ Ophthalmic Solution *see* phenylephrine *on page 445*

Pregestimil® [OTC] *see* enteral nutritional products *on page 208*

pregnenedione *see* progesterone *on page 477*

Pregnyl® *see* chorionic gonadotropin *on page 130*

Prelone® Oral *see* prednisolone (systemic) *on page 471*

Prelu-2® *see* phendimetrazine *on page 442*

Preludin® ***(Discontinued)*** *see page 700*

Premarin® *see* estrogens, conjugated (equine) *on page 219*

Premarin® Vaginal Cream ***(Discontinued)*** *see page 700*

Premarin® With Methyltestosterone *see* estrogens and methyltestosterone *on page 219*

Premphase™ *see* estrogens and medroxyprogesterone *on page 218*

Prempro™ *see* estrogens and medroxyprogesterone *on page 218*

prenatal vitamins *see* vitamin, multiple (prenatal) *on page 606*

Prenavite® [OTC] *see* vitamin, multiple (prenatal) *on page 606*

Prenavite® Forte (Can) *see* vitamin, multiple (oral) *on page 604*

Prepcat® *see* radiological/contrast media (ionic) *on page 495*

Pre-Pen® *see* benzylpenicilloyl-polylysine *on page 70*

Prepidil® Vaginal Gel *see* dinoprostone *on page 184*

Prepulsid® (Can) *see* cisapride *on page 133*

Prescription Strength Desenex® [OTC] *see* miconazole *on page 373*

Pressyn® (Can) *see* vasopressin *on page 597*

PreSun® 29 [OTC] *see* methoxycinnamate and oxybenzone *on page 365*

Pretz® [OTC] *see* sodium chloride *on page 526*

Pretz-D® [OTC] *see* ephedrine *on page 208*

Prevacid® *see* lansoprazole *on page 326*

Prevalite® *see* cholestyramine resin *on page 129*

Preven™ *see* ethinyl estradiol and levonorgestrel *on page 223*

Preveon® *see* adefovir *on page 12*

Prevex™ Baby Diaper Rash (Can) *see* zinc oxide *on page 612*

Prevex™ HC (Can) *see* hydrocortisone (topical) *on page 292*

Prevident® *see* fluoride *on page 244*

Priftin® *see* rifapentine *on page 505*

prilocaine (PRIL oh kane)

U.S./Canadian Brand Names Citanest® Forte; Citanest® Plain

Therapeutic Category Local Anesthetic

Use In dentistry for infiltration anesthesia and for nerve block anesthesia

Usual Dosage Dose varies with procedure, desired depth, and duration of anesthesia, desired muscle relaxation, vascularity of tissues, physical condition, and age of patient

Dosage Forms Injection:

Citanest® Plain: 4% (1.8 mL)

Citanest® Forte: 4% with epinephrine bitartrate 1:200,000 (1.8 mL)

prilocaine and lidocaine *see* lidocaine and prilocaine *on page 334*

Prilosec™ *see* omeprazole *on page 415*

primaclone *see* primidone *on next page*

Primacor® *see* milrinone *on page 376*

primaquine (PRIM a kween FOS fate)

Synonyms prymaccone

Therapeutic Category Aminoquinoline (Antimalarial)

(Continued)

primaquine *(Continued)*

Use In conjunction with a blood schizonticidal agent to provide radical cure of *P. vivax* or *P. ovale* malaria after a clinical attack has been confirmed by blood smear or serologic titer; prevention of relapse of *P. ovale* or *P. vivax* malaria; malaria postexposure prophylaxis

Usual Dosage Oral:

Children: 0.3 mg base/kg/day once daily for 14 days not to exceed 15 mg/day or 0.9 mg base/kg once weekly for 8 weeks not to exceed 45 mg base/week

Adults: 15 mg/day (base) once daily for 14 days or 45 mg base once weekly for 8 weeks

Dosage Forms Tablet, as phosphate: 26.3 mg [15 mg base]

primaquine and chloroquine *see* chloroquine and primaquine *on page 118*

Primatene® Mist [OTC] *see* epinephrine *on page 209*

Primaxin® *see* imipenem and cilastatin *on page 302*

primidone (PRI mi done)

Synonyms desoxyphenobarbital; primaclone

U.S./Canadian Brand Names Apo®-Primidone (Can); Mysoline®; Sertan® (Can)

Therapeutic Category Anticonvulsant; Barbiturate

Use Management of generalized tonic-clonic (grand mal), complex partial and simple partial (focal) seizures

Usual Dosage Oral:

Children <8 years: Initial: 50-125 mg/day given at bedtime; increase by 50-125 mg/day increments every 3-7 days; usual dose: 10-25 mg/kg/day in divided doses 3-4 times/day

Children >8 years and Adults: Initial: 125-250 mg/day at bedtime; increase by 125-250 mg/day every 3-7 days; usual dose: 750-1500 mg/day in divided doses 3-4 times/day with maximum dosage of 2 g/day

Dosage Forms

Suspension, oral: 250 mg/5 mL (240 mL)

Tablet: 50 mg, 250 mg

Principen® *see* ampicillin *on page 34*

Prinivil® *see* lisinopril *on page 337*

Prinzide® *see* lisinopril and hydrochlorothiazide *on page 337*

Priscoline® *see* tolazoline *on page 570*

pristinamycin *see* quinupristin and dalfopristin *on page 493*

Privine® Nasal [OTC] *see* naphazoline *on page 390*

ProAmatine *see* midodrine *on page 376*

Pro-Amox® (Can) *see* amoxicillin *on page 31*

Proampacin® ***(Discontinued)*** *see page 700*

Pro-Ampi® (Can) *see* ampicillin *on page 34*

Pro-Banthine® *see* propantheline *on page 480*

probenecid (proe BEN e sid)

U.S./Canadian Brand Names Benemid® (Can); Benuryl™ (Can)

Therapeutic Category Uricosuric Agent

Use Prevention of gouty arthritis; hyperuricemia; prolong serum levels of penicillin/cephalosporin

Usual Dosage Oral:

Children:

<2 years: Not recommended

2-14 years: Prolong penicillin serum levels: 25 mg/kg starting dose, then 40 mg/kg/day administered 4 times/day

Gonorrhea: <45 kg: 25 mg/kg x 1 (maximum: 1 g/dose) 30 minutes before penicillin, ampicillin or amoxicillin

Adults:

Hyperuricemia with gout: 250 mg twice daily for one week; increase to 500 mg 2 times/day; may increase by 500 mg/month, if needed, to maximum of 2-3 g/day (dosages may be decreased by 500 mg every 6 months if serum urate concentrations are controlled)

Prolong penicillin serum levels: 500 mg 4 times/day

Gonorrhea: 1 g 30 minutes before penicillin, ampicillin or amoxicillin

Dosage Forms Tablet: 500 mg

probenecid and colchicine *see* colchicine and probenecid *on page 144*

procainamide (proe kane A mide)

Synonyms procaine amide hydrochloride

U.S./Canadian Brand Names Apo®-Procainamide (Can); Procanbid™; Procan™ SR (Can); Pronestyl®; Pronestyl-SR®

Therapeutic Category Antiarrhythmic Agent, Class I-A

Use Ventricular tachycardia, premature ventricular contractions, paroxysmal atrial tachycardia, and atrial fibrillation; to prevent recurrence of ventricular tachycardia, paroxysmal supraventricular tachycardia, atrial fibrillation or flutter

Usual Dosage Must be titrated to patient's response

Children:

Oral: 15-50 mg/kg/24 hours divided every 3-6 hours; maximum 4 g/24 hours

I.M.: 20-30 mg/kg/24 hours divided every 4-6 hours in divided doses; maximum 4 g/24 hours

I.V.: Load: 3-6 mg/kg/dose over 5 minutes not to exceed 100 mg/dose; may repeat every 5-10 minutes to maximum of 15 mg/kg/load; maintenance as continuous I.V. infusion: 20-80 mcg/kg/minute; maximum: 2 g/24 hours

Adults:

Oral: 250-500 mg/dose every 3-6 hours or 500 mg to 1 g every 6 hours sustained release; usual dose: 50 mg/kg/24 hours or 2-4 g/24 hours

I.V.: Load: 50-100 mg/dose, repeated every 5-10 minutes until patient controlled; or load with 15-18 mg/kg, maximum loading dose: 1-1.5 g; maintenance: 2-6 mg/minute continuous I.V. infusion, usual maintenance: 3-4 mg/minute

Dosage Forms Procainamide hydrochloride:

Capsule: 250 mg, 375 mg, 500 mg

Injection: 100 mg/mL (10 mL); 500 mg/mL (2 mL)

Tablet: 250 mg, 375 mg, 500 mg

Sustained release: 250 mg, 500 mg, 750 mg, 1000 mg

Sustained release (Procanbid™): 500 mg, 1000 mg

procaine (PROE kane)

U.S./Canadian Brand Names Novocain®

Therapeutic Category Local Anesthetic

Use Produce spinal anesthesia and epidural and peripheral nerve block by injection and infiltration methods

Usual Dosage Dose varies with procedure, desired depth and duration of anesthesia, desired muscle relaxation, vascularity of tissues, physical condition, and age of patient

Dosage Forms Injection, as hydrochloride: 1% [10 mg/mL] (2 mL, 6 mL, 30 mL, 100 mL); 2% [20 mg/mL] (30 mL, 100 mL); 10% (2 mL)

procaine amide hydrochloride *see* procainamide *on this page*

procaine benzylpenicillin *see* penicillin G procaine *on page 435*

procaine penicillin G *see* penicillin G procaine *on page 435*

Pro-Cal-Sof® [OTC] *see* docusate *on page 191*

Procanbid™ *see* procainamide *on this page*

Procan™ SR (Can) *see* procainamide *on previous page*

Procan SR® *(Discontinued)* *see page 700*

procarbazine (proe KAR ba zeen)

Synonyms ibenzmethyzin; MIH; n-methylhydrazine

U.S./Canadian Brand Names Matulane®; Natulan® (Can)

Therapeutic Category Antineoplastic Agent

Use Treatment of Hodgkin's disease, non-Hodgkin's lymphoma, brain tumor, bronchogenic carcinoma

Usual Dosage Refer to individual protocols. Oral:

Children: 50-100 mg/m^2/day in a single dose; doses as high as 100-200 mg/m^2/day once daily have been used for neuroblastoma and medulloblastoma

Adults: Initial: 2-4 mg/kg/day in single or divided doses for 7 days then increase dose to 4-6 mg/kg/day until response is obtained or leukocyte count decreased <4000/mm^3 or the platelet count decreased <100,000/mm^3; maintenance: 1-2 mg/kg/day

Dosage Forms Capsule, as hydrochloride: 50 mg

Procardia® *see* nifedipine *on page 402*

Procardia XL® *see* nifedipine *on page 402*

procetofene *see* fenofibrate *on page 233*

prochlorperazine (proe klor PER a zeen)

U.S./Canadian Brand Names Compazine®; Nu-Prochlor® (Can); PMS-Prochlorperazine (Can); Prorazin® (Can); Stemetil® (Can)

Therapeutic Category Phenothiazine Derivative

Use Management of nausea and vomiting; acute and chronic psychoses

Usual Dosage

Children: Oral, rectal:

>10 kg: 0.4 mg/kg/24 hours in 3-4 divided doses; **or**

9-14 kg: 2.5 mg every 12-24 hours as needed; maximum: 7.5 mg/day

14-18 kg: 2.5 mg every 8-12 hours as needed; maximum: 10 mg/day

18-39 kg: 2.5 mg every 8 hours or 5 mg every 12 hours as needed; maximum: 15 mg/day

I.M.: 0.1-0.15 mg/kg/dose; usual: 0.13 mg/kg/dose; change to oral as soon as possible

I.V.: Not recommended

Adults:

Oral: 5-10 mg 3-4 times/day; usual maximum: 40 mg/day; doses up to 150 mg/day may be required in some patients

I.M.: 5-10 mg every 3-4 hours; usual maximum: 40 mg/day; doses up to 10-20 mg every 4-6 hours may be required in some patients

I.V.: 2.5-10 mg; maximum 10 mg/dose or 40 mg/day; may repeat dose every 3-4 hours as needed

Rectal: 25 mg twice daily

Dosage Forms

Suppository, rectal: 2.5 mg, 5 mg, 25 mg (12/box)

Prochlorperazine edisylate:

Injection: 5 mg/mL (2 mL, 10 mL)

Syrup: 5 mg/5 mL (120 mL)

Prochlorperazine maleate:

Capsule, sustained action: 10 mg, 15 mg, 30 mg

Tablet: 5 mg, 10 mg, 25 mg

Procrit® *see* epoetin alfa *on page 211*

Proctocort™ Rectal *see* hydrocortisone (rectal) *on page 291*

proctofene *see* fenofibrate *on page 233*

Proctofoam®-HC *see* pramoxine and hydrocortisone *on page 469*

ProctoFoam® NS [OTC] *see* pramoxine *on page 469*

Procyclid® (Can) *see* procyclidine *on this page*

procyclidine (proe SYE kli deen)

U.S./Canadian Brand Names Kemadrin®; PMS-Procyclidine (Can); Procyclid® (Can)

Therapeutic Category Anticholinergic Agent; Anti-Parkinson's Agent

Use Relief of symptoms of Parkinsonian syndrome and drug-induced extrapyramidal symptoms

Usual Dosage Adults: Oral: 2-2.5 mg 3 times/day after meals; if tolerated, gradually increase dose to 4-5 mg 3 times/day

Dosage Forms Tablet, as hydrochloride: 5 mg

Procytox® (Can) *see* cyclophosphamide *on page 153*

Prodiem® Plain (Can) *see* psyllium *on page 488*

Prodium® [OTC] *see* phenazopyridine *on page 442*

Profasi® HP *see* chorionic gonadotropin *on page 130*

Profenal® Ophthalmic *see* suprofen *on page 545*

Profen II® *see* guaifenesin and phenylpropanolamine *on page 270*

Profen II DM® *see* guaifenesin, phenylpropanolamine, and dextromethorphan *on page 271*

Profen LA® *see* guaifenesin and phenylpropanolamine *on page 270*

Profilate-HP® ***(Discontinued)*** *see page 700*

Profilate® OSD *see* antihemophilic factor (human) *on page 39*

Profilate® SD *see* antihemophilic factor (human) *on page 39*

Profilnine® SD *see* factor IX complex (human) *on page 230*

Progestaject® Injection ***(Discontinued)*** *see page 700*

Progestasert® *see* progesterone *on this page*

progesterone (proe JES ter one)

Synonyms pregnenedione; progestin

U.S./Canadian Brand Names Crinone™; PMS-Progesterone (Can); Progestasert®; Progesterone Oil (Can)

Therapeutic Category Progestin

Use

Gel: Progesterone supplementation or replacement as part of an assisted reproductive technology treatment for infertile women with progesterone deficiency

Reservoir: Endometrial carcinoma or renal carcinoma as well as secondary amenorrhea or abnormal uterine bleeding due to hormonal imbalance

Usual Dosage Adults:

Amenorrhea: I.M.: 5-10 mg/day for 6-8 consecutive days

Functional uterine bleeding: I.M.: 5-10 mg/day for 6 doses

Contraception: Female: Intrauterine device: Insert a single system into the uterine cavity; contraceptive effectiveness is retained for 1 year and system must be replaced 1 year after insertion

Dosage Forms

Gel, single use: 8% (90 mg applicator)

Intrauterine system, reservoir: 38 mg in silicone fluid

Progesterone Oil (Can) *see* progesterone *on this page*

progestin *see* progesterone *on this page*

Proglycem® Oral *see* diazoxide *on page 174*

Prograf® *see* tacrolimus *on page 546*

ProHIBiT® *see Haemophilus* B conjugate vaccine *on page 275*

Pro-Indo® (Can) *see* indomethacin *on page 305*

Prokine® Injection *(Discontinued)* *see page 700*

Prolamine® *(Discontinued)* *see page 700*

Prolastin® *see* alpha$_1$-proteinase inhibitor *on page 19*

Proleukin® *see* aldesleukin *on page 16*

Prolixin Decanoate® Injection *see* fluphenazine *on page 247*

Prolixin Enanthate® Injection *see* fluphenazine *on page 247*

Prolixin® Injection *see* fluphenazine *on page 247*

Prolixin® Oral *see* fluphenazine *on page 247*

Proloid® *(Discontinued)* *see page 700*

Prolopa® (Can) *see* benserazide and levodopa *(Canada only) on page 65*

Proloprim® *see* trimethoprim *on page 583*

Pro-Lorazepam® (Can) *see* lorazepam *on page 340*

promazine (PROE ma zeen)

U.S./Canadian Brand Names Sparine®

Therapeutic Category Phenothiazine Derivative

Use Treatment of psychoses

Usual Dosage Oral, I.M.:

Children >12 years: Antipsychotic: 10-25 mg every 4-6 hours

Adults:

- Psychosis: 10-200 mg every 4-6 hours not to exceed 1000 mg/day
- Antiemetic: 25-50 mg every 4-6 hours as needed

Dosage Forms Promazine hydrochloride:

Injection: 25 mg/mL (10 mL); 50 mg/mL (1 mL, 2 mL, 10 mL)

Tablet: 25 mg, 50 mg, 100 mg

Prometa® *see* metaproterenol *on page 359*

promethazine (proe METH a zeen)

U.S./Canadian Brand Names Histantil (Can); Phenazine® Injection; Phenergan® Injection; Phenergan® Oral; Phenergan® Rectal; Prorex® Injection

Therapeutic Category Antiemetic; Phenothiazine Derivative

Use Symptomatic treatment of various allergic conditions and motion sickness; sedative and an antiemetic

Usual Dosage

Children:

- Antihistamine: Oral: 0.1 mg/kg/dose every 6 hours during the day and 0.5 mg/kg/dose at bedtime as needed
- Antiemetic: Oral, I.M., I.V., rectal: 0.25-1 mg/kg 4-6 times/day as needed
- Motion sickness: Oral: 0.5 mg/kg 30 minutes to 1 hour before departure, then every 12 hours as needed
- Sedation: Oral, I.M., I.V., rectal: 0.5-1 mg/kg/dose every 6 hours as needed

Adults:

- Antihistamine:
  - Oral: 25 mg at bedtime or 12.5 mg 3 times/day
  - I.M., I.V., rectal: 25 mg, may repeat in 2 hours
- Antiemetic: Oral, I.M., I.V., rectal: 12.5-25 mg every 4 hours as needed
- Motion sickness: Oral: 25 mg 30 minutes to 1 hour before departure, then every 12 hours as needed
- Sedation: Oral, I.M., I.V., rectal: 25-50 mg/dose

Dosage Forms Promethazine hydrochloride:

Injection: 25 mg/mL (1 mL, 10 mL); 50 mg/mL (1 mL, 10 mL)

Suppository, rectal: 12.5 mg, 25 mg, 50 mg

Syrup: 6.25 mg/5 mL (5 mL, 120 mL, 240 mL, 480 mL, 4000 mL); 25 mg/5 mL (120 mL, 480 mL, 4000 mL)

Tablet: 12.5 mg, 25 mg, 50 mg

promethazine and codeine (proe METH a zeen & KOE deen)

Synonyms codeine and promethazine

U.S./Canadian Brand Names Phenergan® With Codeine; Pherazine® With Codeine; Prothazine-DC®

Therapeutic Category Antihistamine/Antitussive

Controlled Substance C-V

Use Temporary relief of coughs and upper respiratory symptoms associated with allergy or the common cold

Usual Dosage Oral (in terms of codeine):

Children: 1-1.5 mg/kg/day every 4 hours as needed; maximum: 30 mg/day **or**

2-6 years: 1.25-2.5 mL every 4-6 hours or 2.5-5 mg/dose every 4-6 hours as needed; maximum: 30 mg codeine/day

6-12 years: 2.5-5 mL every 4-6 hours as needed or 5-10 mg/dose every 4-6 hours as needed; maximum: 60 mg codeine/day

Adults: 10-20 mg/dose every 4-6 hours as needed; maximum: 120 mg codeine/day; or 5-10 mL every 4-6 hours as needed

Dosage Forms Syrup: Promethazine hydrochloride 6.25 mg and codeine phosphate 10 mg per 5 mL (120 mL, 180 mL, 473 mL)

promethazine and dextromethorphan

(proe METH a zeen & deks troe meth OR fan)

Synonyms dextromethorphan and promethazine

U.S./Canadian Brand Names Phenameth® DM; Phenergan® With Dextromethorphan; Pherazine® w/DM

Therapeutic Category Antihistamine/Antitussive

Use Temporary relief of coughs and upper respiratory symptoms associated with allergy or the common cold

Usual Dosage Oral:

Children:

2-6 years: 1.25-2.5 mL every 4-6 hours up to 10 mL in 24 hours

6-12 years: 2.5-5 mL every 4-6 hours up to 20 mL in 24 hours

Adults: 5 mL every 4-6 hours up to 30 mL in 24 hours

Dosage Forms Syrup: Promethazine hydrochloride 6.25 mg and dextromethorphan hydrobromide 15 mg per 5 mL with alcohol 7% (120 mL, 480 mL, 4000 mL)

promethazine and meperidine *see* meperidine and promethazine *on page 355*

promethazine and phenylephrine (proe METH a zeen & fen il EF rin)

Synonyms phenylephrine and promethazine

U.S./Canadian Brand Names Phenergan® VC Syrup; Promethazine VC Plain Syrup; Promethazine VC Syrup; Prometh VC Plain Liquid

Therapeutic Category Antihistamine/Decongestant Combination

Use Temporary relief of upper respiratory symptoms associated with allergy or the common cold

Usual Dosage Oral:

Children:

2-6 years: 1.25 mL every 4-6 hours, not to exceed 7.5 mL in 24 hours

6-12 years: 2.5 mL every 4-6 hours, not to exceed 15 mL in 24 hours

Children >12 years and Adults: 5 mL every 4-6 hours, not to exceed 30 mL in 24 hours

Dosage Forms Liquid: Promethazine hydrochloride 6.25 mg and phenylephrine hydrochloride 5 mg per 5 mL (120 mL, 240 mL, 473 mL)

promethazine, phenylephrine, and codeine

(proe METH a zeen, fen il EF rin, & KOE deen)

Synonyms codeine, promethazine, and phenylephrine; phenylephrine, promethazine, and codeine

(Continued)

promethazine, phenylephrine, and codeine *(Continued)*

U.S./Canadian Brand Names Phenergan® VC With Codeine; Pherazine® VC w/ Codeine; Promethist® With Codeine; Prometh® VC With Codeine

Therapeutic Category Antihistamine/Decongestant/Antitussive

Controlled Substance C-V

Use Temporary relief of coughs and upper respiratory symptoms including nasal congestion

Usual Dosage Oral:

Children (expressed in terms of codeine dosage): 1-1.5 mg/kg/day every 4 hours, maximum: 30 mg/day **or**
- <2 years: Not recommended
- 2 to 6 years:
  - Weight 25 lb: 1.25-2.5 mL every 4-6 hours, not to exceed 6 mL/24 hours
  - Weight 30 lb: 1.25-2.5 mL every 4-6 hours, not to exceed 7 mL/24 hours
  - Weight 35 lb: 1.25-2.5 mL every 4-6 hours, not to exceed 8 mL/24 hours
  - Weight 40 lb: 1.25-2.5 mL every 4-6 hours, not to exceed 9 mL/24 hours
- 6 to <12 years: 2.5-5 mL every 4-6 hours, not to exceed 15 mL/24 hours

Adults: 5 mL every 4-6 hours, not to exceed 30 mL/24 hours

Dosage Forms Liquid: Promethazine hydrochloride 6.25 mg, phenylephrine hydrochloride 5 mg, and codeine phosphate 10 mg per 5 mL with alcohol 7% (120 mL, 240 mL, 480 mL, 4000 mL)

Promethazine VC Plain Syrup *see* promethazine and phenylephrine *on previous page*

Promethazine VC Syrup *see* promethazine and phenylephrine *on previous page*

Prometh® *(Discontinued)* *see page 700*

Promethist® With Codeine *see* promethazine, phenylephrine, and codeine *on previous page*

Prometh VC Plain Liquid *see* promethazine and phenylephrine *on previous page*

Prometh® VC With Codeine *see* promethazine, phenylephrine, and codeine *on previous page*

Promit® *see* dextran 1 *on page 170*

Pronestyl® *see* procainamide *on page 475*

Pronestyl-SR® *see* procainamide *on page 475*

Pronto® Shampoo [OTC] *see* pyrethrins *on page 489*

Propac™ [OTC] *see* enteral nutritional products *on page 208*

Propacet® *see* propoxyphene and acetaminophen *on page 482*

Propaderm® (Can) *see* beclomethasone *on page 62*

propafenone (proe pa FEEN one)

U.S./Canadian Brand Names Rythmol®

Therapeutic Category Antiarrhythmic Agent, Class I-C

Use Life-threatening ventricular arrhythmias; an oral sodium channel blocker similar to encainide and flecainide; in clinical trials was used effectively to treat atrial flutter, atrial fibrillation and other arrhythmias, but are not labeled indications; can worsen or even cause new ventricular arrhythmias (proarrhythmic effect)

Usual Dosage Adults: Oral: 150 mg every 8 hours, up to 300 mg every 8 hours

Dosage Forms Tablet, as hydrochloride: 150 mg, 225 mg, 300 mg

Propagest® [OTC] *see* phenylpropanolamine *on page 447*

Propanthel™ (Can) *see* propantheline *on this page*

propantheline (proe PAN the leen)

U.S./Canadian Brand Names Pro-Banthine®; Propanthel™ (Can)

Therapeutic Category Anticholinergic Agent

Use Adjunctive treatment of peptic ulcer, irritable bowel syndrome, pancreatitis, ureteral and urinary bladder spasm; to reduce duodenal motility during diagnostic radiologic procedures

Usual Dosage Oral:

Antisecretory:

Children: 1-2 mg/kg/day in 3-4 divided doses

Elderly patients: 7.5 mg 3 times/day before meals and at bedtime

Antispasmodic:

Children: 2-3 mg/kg/day in divided doses every 4-6 hours and at bedtime

Adults: 15 mg 3 times/day before meals or food and 30 mg at bedtime

Dosage Forms Tablet, as bromide: 7.5 mg, 15 mg

proparacaine (proe PAR a kane)

Synonyms proxymetacaine

U.S./Canadian Brand Names AK-Taine®; Alcaine®; Diocaine(Can); I-Paracaine®; Ophthetic®

Therapeutic Category Local Anesthetic

Use Local anesthesia for tonometry, gonioscopy; suture removal from cornea; removal of corneal foreign body; cataract extraction, glaucoma surgery; short operative procedure involving the cornea and conjunctiva

Usual Dosage Children and Adults:

Ophthalmic surgery: Instill 1 drop of 0.5% solution in eye every 5-10 minutes for 5-7 doses

Tonometry, gonioscopy, suture removal: Instill 1-2 drops 0.5% solution in eye just prior to procedure

Dosage Forms Ophthalmic, solution, as hydrochloride: 0.5% (2 mL, 15 mL)

proparacaine and fluorescein (proe PAR a kane & FLURE e seen)

U.S./Canadian Brand Names Fluoracaine® Ophthalmic

Therapeutic Category Diagnostic Agent; Local Anesthetic

Use Anesthesia for tonometry, gonioscopy; suture removal from cornea; removal of corneal foreign body; cataract extraction, glaucoma surgery

Usual Dosage

Tonometry, gonioscopy, suture removal: Adults: Instill 1-2 drops 0.5% solution in eye just prior to procedure

Ophthalmic surgery: Children and Adults: Instill 1 drop of 0.5% solution in eye every 5-10 minutes for 5-7 doses

Dosage Forms Solution: Proparacaine hydrochloride 0.5% and fluorescein sodium 0.25% (2 mL, 5 mL)

Propine® *see* dipivefrin *on page 188*

propiomazine (proe pee OH ma zeen)

Therapeutic Category Phenothiazine Derivative

Use Relief of restlessness, nausea and apprehension before and during surgery or during labor

Usual Dosage I.M., I.V.:

Children: 0.55-1.1 mg/kg

Adults: 10-40 mg prior to procedure, additional may be repeated at 3-hour intervals

Dosage Forms Injection, as hydrochloride: 20 mg/mL (1 mL)

Pro-Piroxicam® (Can) *see* piroxicam *on page 454*

Proplex® SX-T Injection *(Discontinued)* *see page 700*

Proplex® T *see* factor IX complex (human) *on page 230*

propofol (PROE po fole)

U.S./Canadian Brand Names Diprivan®

Therapeutic Category General Anesthetic

(Continued)

propofol *(Continued)*

Use Induction or maintenance of anesthesia; sedation

Usual Dosage Dosage must be individualized and titrated to the desired clinical effect; however, as a general guideline:

No pediatric dose has been established

Induction: I.V.:

Adults ≤55 years, and/or ASA I or II patients: 2-2.5 mg/kg of body weight (approximately 40 mg every 10 seconds until onset of induction)

Elderly, debilitated, hypovolemic, and/or ASA III or IV patients: 1-1.5 mg/kg of body weight (approximately 20 mg every 10 seconds until onset of induction)

Maintenance: I.V. infusion:

Adults ≤55 years, and/or ASA I or II patients: 0.1-0.2 mg/kg of body weight/minute (6-12 mg/kg of body weight/hour)

Elderly, debilitated, hypovolemic, and/or ASA III or IV patients: 0.05-0.1 mg/kg of body weight/minute (3-6 mg/kg of body weight/hour)

I.V. intermittent: 25-50 mg increments, as needed

Dosage Forms Injection: 10 mg/mL (20 mL, 50 mL, 100 mL)

propoxyphene (proe POKS i feen)

Synonyms dextropropoxyphene

U.S./Canadian Brand Names 642® (Can); Darvon®; Darvon-N®; Dolene®; Novo-Propoxyn® (Can)

Therapeutic Category Analgesic, Narcotic

Controlled Substance C-IV

Use Management of mild to moderate pain

Usual Dosage Adults: Oral:

Hydrochloride: 65 mg every 3-4 hours as needed for pain; maximum: 390 mg/day

Napsylate: 100 mg every 4 hours as needed for pain; maximum: 600 mg/day

Dosage Forms

Capsule, as hydrochloride: 65 mg

Tablet, as napsylate: 100 mg

propoxyphene and acetaminophen

(proe POKS i feen & a seet a MIN oh fen)

Synonyms acetaminophen and propoxyphene

U.S./Canadian Brand Names Darvocet-N®; Darvocet-N® 100; Propacet®; Wygesic®

Therapeutic Category Analgesic, Narcotic

Controlled Substance C-IV

Use Management of mild to moderate pain

Usual Dosage Adults: Oral:

Darvocet-N®: 1-2 tablets every 4 hours as needed; maximum: 600 mg propoxyphene napsylate/day

Darvocet-N® 100: 1 tablet every 4 hours as needed; maximum: 600 mg propoxyphene napsylate/day

Dosage Forms Tablet:

Darvocet-N®: Propoxyphene napsylate 50 mg and acetaminophen 325 mg

Darvocet-N® 100: Propoxyphene napsylate 100 mg and acetaminophen 650 mg

Genagesic®, Wygesic®: Propoxyphene hydrochloride 65 mg and acetaminophen 650 mg

propoxyphene and aspirin (proe POKS i feen & AS pir in)

Synonyms aspirin and propoxyphene

U.S./Canadian Brand Names Bexophene®; Darvon® Compound-65 Pulvules®

Therapeutic Category Analgesic, Narcotic

Controlled Substance C-IV

Use Management of mild to moderate pain

Usual Dosage Oral: 1-2 capsules every 4 hours as needed

Dosage Forms

Capsule: Propoxyphene hydrochloride 65 mg and aspirin 389 mg with caffeine 32.4 mg

Tablet (Darvon-N® with A.S.A.): Propoxyphene napsylate 100 mg and aspirin 325 mg

propranolol (proe PRAN oh lole)

U.S./Canadian Brand Names Apo®-Propranolol (Can); Betachron®; Detensol® (Can); Inderal®; Inderal® LA; Nu-Propranolol® (Can)

Therapeutic Category Antiarrhythmic Agent, Class II; Beta-Adrenergic Blocker

Use Management of hypertension, angina pectoris, pheochromocytoma, essential tremor, tetralogy of Fallot cyanotic spells, and arrhythmias (such as atrial fibrillation and flutter, A-V nodal re-entrant tachycardias, and catecholamine-induced arrhythmias); prevention of myocardial infarction, migraine headache; symptomatic treatment of hypertrophic subaortic stenosis; short-term adjunctive therapy of thyrotoxicosis

Usual Dosage

Tachyarrhythmias:

Oral:

Children: Initial: 0.5-1 mg/kg/day in divided doses every 6-8 hours; titrate dosage upward every 3-7 days; usual dose: 2-4 mg/kg/day; higher doses may be needed; do not exceed 16 mg/kg/day or 60 mg/day

Adults: 10-80 mg/dose every 6-8 hours

I.V.:

Children: 0.01-0.1 mg/kg slow IVP over 10 minutes; maximum dose: 1 mg

Adults: 1 mg/dose slow IVP; repeat every 5 minutes up to a total of 5 mg

Hypertension: Oral:

Children: Initial: 0.5-1 mg/kg/day in divided doses every 6-12 hours; increase gradually every 3-7 days; maximum: 2 mg/kg/24 hours

Adults: Initial: 40 mg twice daily or 60-80 mg once daily as sustained release capsules; increase dosage every 3-7 days; usual dose: ≤320 mg divided in 2-3 doses/day or once daily as sustained release; maximum daily dose: 640 mg

Migraine headache prophylaxis: Oral:

Children: 0.6-1.5 mg/kg/day **or**

≤35 kg: 10-20 mg 3 times/day

>35 kg: 20-40 mg 3 times/day

Adults: Initial: 80 mg/day divided every 6-8 hours; increase by 20-40 mg/dose every 3-4 weeks to a maximum of 160-240 mg/day administered in divided doses every 6-8 hours; if satisfactory response not achieved within 6 weeks of starting therapy, drug should be withdrawn gradually over several weeks

Tetralogy spells: Children: Oral: 1-2 mg/kg/day every 6 hours as needed, may increase by 1 mg/kg/day to a maximum of 5 mg/kg/day, or if refractory may increase slowly to a maximum of 10-15 mg/kg/day

Thyrotoxicosis:

Adolescents and Adults: Oral: 10-40 mg/dose every 6 hours

Adults: I.V.: 1-3 mg/dose slow IVP as a single dose

Adults: Oral:

Angina: 80-320 mg/day in doses divided 2-4 times/day or 80-160 mg of sustained release once daily

Pheochromocytoma: 30-60 mg/day in divided doses

Myocardial infarction prophylaxis: 180-240 mg/day in 3-4divided doses

Hypertrophic subaortic stenosis: 20-40 mg 3-4 times/day

Essential tremor: 40 mg twice daily initially; maintenance doses: usually 120-320 mg/day

Dosage Forms Propranolol hydrochloride:

Capsule, sustained action: 60 mg, 80 mg, 120 mg, 160 mg

Injection: 1 mg/mL (1 mL)

Solution, oral (strawberry-mint flavor): 4 mg/mL (5 mL, 500 mL); 8 mg/mL (5 mL, 500 mL)

Solution, oral, concentrate: 80 mg/mL (30 mL)

Tablet: 10 mg, 20 mg, 40 mg, 60 mg, 80 mg, 90 mg

propranolol and hydrochlorothiazide

(proe PRAN oh lole & hye droe klor oh THYE a zide)

Synonyms hydrochlorothiazide and propranolol

U.S./Canadian Brand Names Inderide®

Therapeutic Category Antihypertensive Agent, Combination

Use Management of hypertension

Usual Dosage Dose is individualized

Dosage Forms

Capsule, long-acting (Inderide® LA):

80/50 Propranolol hydrochloride 80 mg and hydrochlorothiazide 50 mg

120/50 Propranolol hydrochloride 120 mg and hydrochlorothiazide 50 mg

160/50 Propranolol hydrochloride 160 mg and hydrochlorothiazide 50 mg

Tablet (Inderide®):

40/25 Propranolol hydrochloride 40 mg and hydrochlorothiazide 25 mg

80/25 Propranolol hydrochloride 80 mg and hydrochlorothiazide 25 mg

Propulsid® *see* cisapride *on page 133*

propylene glycol and salicylic acid *see* salicylic acid and propylene glycol *on page 514*

propylhexedrine (proe pil HEKS e dreen)

U.S./Canadian Brand Names Benzedrex® [OTC]

Therapeutic Category Adrenergic Agonist Agent

Use Topical nasal decongestant

Usual Dosage Inhale through each nostril while blocking the other

Dosage Forms Inhaler: 250 mg

2-propylpentanoic acid *see* valproic acid and derivatives *on page 594*

propylthiouracil (proe pil thye oh YOOR a sil)

Synonyms PTU

U.S./Canadian Brand Names Propyl-Thyracil® (Can)

Therapeutic Category Antithyroid Agent

Use Palliative treatment of hyperthyroidism, adjunct to ameliorate hyperthyroidism in preparation for surgical treatment or radioactive iodine therapy, management of thyrotoxic crisis

Usual Dosage Oral:

Children: Initial: 5-7 mg/kg/day in divided doses every 8 hours or

6-10 years: 50-150 mg/day

>10 years: 150-300 mg/day

Maintenance: ⅓ to ⅔ of the initial dose in divided doses every 8-12 hours

Adults: Initial: 300-450 mg/day in divided doses every 8 hours; maintenance: 100-150 mg/day in divided doses every 8-12 hours

Dosage Forms Tablet: 50 mg

Propyl-Thyracil® (Can) *see* propylthiouracil *on this page*

2-propylvaleric acid *see* valproic acid and derivatives *on page 594*

Prorazin® (Can) *see* prochlorperazine *on page 476*

Prorex® Injection *see* promethazine *on page 478*

Proscar® *see* finasteride *on page 239*

Pro-Sof® *(Discontinued)* *see page 700*

Pro-Sof® Plus [OTC] *see* docusate and casanthranol *on page 191*

ProSom™ *see* estazolam *on page 216*

prostaglandin E_1 *see* alprostadil *on page 20*

prostaglandin E_2 *see* dinoprostone *on page 184*

prostaglandin F_2 alpha *see* dinoprost tromethamine *on page 184*

Prostaphlin® *(Discontinued)* *see page 700*

ProStep® Patch *see* nicotine *on page 401*

Prostigmin® *see* neostigmine *on page 397*

Prostin E_2® Vaginal Suppository *see* dinoprostone *on page 184*

Prostin F_2 Alpha® *see* dinoprost tromethamine *on page 184*

Prostin VR Pediatric® Injection *see* alprostadil *on page 20*

protamine sulfate (PROE ta meen SUL fate)

Therapeutic Category Antidote

Use Treatment of heparin overdosage; neutralize heparin during surgery or dialysis procedures

Usual Dosage Children and Adults: I.V.: 1 mg of protamine neutralizes 90 USP units of heparin (lung) and 115 USP units of heparin (intestinal); heparin neutralization occurs within 5 minutes following I.V. injection; administer 1 mg for each 100 units of heparin administered in preceding 3-4 hours up to a maximum dose of 50 mg

Dosage Forms Injection: 10 mg/mL (5 mL, 10 mL, 25 mL)

Protenate® *see* plasma protein fraction *on page 456*

Prothazine-DC® *see* promethazine and codeine *on page 479*

Protilase® *see* pancrelipase *on page 427*

protirelin (proe TYE re lin)

Synonyms lopremone

U.S./Canadian Brand Names Combantrin® (Can); Relefact® TRH; Thypinone®; Thyrel® TRH

Therapeutic Category Diagnostic Agent

Use Adjunct in the diagnostic assessment of thyroid function, and an adjunct to other diagnostic procedures in assessment of patients with pituitary or hypothalamic dysfunction; also causes release of prolactin from the pituitary and is used to detect defective control of prolactin secretion.

Usual Dosage I.V.:

- Children: 7 mcg/kg to a maximum dose of 500 mcg
- Adults: 500 mcg (range: 200-500 mcg)

Dosage Forms Injection: 500 mcg/mL (1 mL)

Protopam® Injection *see* pralidoxime *on page 468*

Protopam® Tablet *(Discontinued)* *see page 700*

Protostat® Oral *see* metronidazole *on page 372*

Pro-Trin® (Can) *see* co-trimoxazole *on page 149*

protriptyline (proe TRIP ti leen)

U.S./Canadian Brand Names Triptil® (Can); Vivactil®

Therapeutic Category Antidepressant, Tricyclic (Secondary Amine)

Use Treatment of various forms of depression, often in conjunction with psychotherapy

Usual Dosage Oral:

- Adolescents: 15-20 mg/day
- Adults: 15-60 mg in 3-4 divided doses
- Elderly: 15-20 mg/day

Dosage Forms Tablet, as hydrochloride: 5 mg, 10 mg

Protropin® *see* human growth hormone *on page 283*

Provatene® *(Discontinued)* *see page 700*

Proventil® *see* albuterol *on page 15*

Proventil® HFA *see* albuterol *on page 15*

Provera® Oral *see* medroxyprogesterone acetate *on page 352*

Provigil® *see* modafinil *on page 379*

Provocholine® *see* methacholine *on page 361*

Proxigel® Oral [OTC] *see* carbamide peroxide *on page 98*

proxymetacaine *see* proparacaine *on page 481*

Prozac® *see* fluoxetine *on page 246*

PRP-D *see* *Haemophilus* B conjugate vaccine *on page 275*

prymaccone *see* primaquine *on page 473*

Pseudo-Car® DM *see* carbinoxamine, pseudoephedrine, and dextromethorphan *on page 99*

pseudoephedrine (soo doe e FED rin)

Synonyms *d*-isoephedrine

U.S./Canadian Brand Names Actifed® Allergy Tablet (Day) [OTC]; Afrinol® [OTC]; Balminil® Decongestant (Can); Cenafed® [OTC]; Children's Silfedrine® [OTC]; Decofed® Syrup [OTC]; Drixoral® Non-Drowsy [OTC]; Efidac/24® [OTC]; Eltor® (Can); Neofed® [OTC]; PediaCare® Oral; PMS-Pseudoephedrine (Can); Robidrine® (Can); Sudafed® [OTC]; Sudafed® 12 Hour [OTC]; Sufedrin® [OTC]; Triaminic® AM Decongestant Formula [OTC]

Therapeutic Category Adrenergic Agonist Agent

Use Temporary symptomatic relief of nasal congestion due to common cold, upper respiratory allergies, and sinusitis; also promotes nasal or sinus drainage

Usual Dosage Oral:

Children:
- <2 years: 4 mg/kg/day in divided doses every 6 hours
- 2-5 years: 15 mg every 6 hours; maximum: 60 mg/24 hours
- 6-12 years: 30 mg every 6 hours; maximum: 120 mg/24 hours

Adults: 60 mg every 6 hours; maximum: 240 mg/24 hours

Dosage Forms

Pseudoephedrine hydrochloride:
- Capsule: 60 mg
- Capsule, timed release: 120 mg
- Drops, oral: 7.5 mg/0.8 mL (15 mL)
- Liquid: 15 mg/5 mL (120 mL); 30 mg/5 mL (120 mL, 240 mL, 473 mL)
- Syrup: 15 mg/5 mL (118 mL)
- Tablet: 30 mg, 60 mg
- Tablet, timed release: 120 mg

Pseudoephedrine sulfate:
- Extended release: 120 mg, 240 mg

pseudoephedrine, acetaminophen, and dextromethorphan *see* acetaminophen, dextromethorphan, and pseudoephedrine *on page 6*

pseudoephedrine and acetaminophen *see* acetaminophen and pseudoephedrine *on page 5*

pseudoephedrine and acrivastine *see* acrivastine and pseudoephedrine *on page 10*

pseudoephedrine and azatadine *see* azatadine and pseudoephedrine *on page 55*

pseudoephedrine and carbinoxamine *see* carbinoxamine and pseudoephedrine *on page 99*

pseudoephedrine and chlorpheniramine *see* chlorpheniramine and pseudoephedrine *on page 122*

pseudoephedrine and dexbrompheniramine *see* dexbrompheniramine and pseudoephedrine *on page 168*

pseudoephedrine and dextromethorphan

(soo doe e FED rin & deks troe meth OR fan)

U.S./Canadian Brand Names Drixoral® Cough & Congestion Liquid Caps [OTC]; Vicks® 44D Cough & Head Congestion; Vicks® 44 Non-Drowsy Cold & Cough Liqui-Caps [OTC]

Therapeutic Category Antitussive/Decongestant

Use Temporary symptomatic relief of nasal congestion due to common cold, upper respiratory allergies, and sinusitis; also promotes nasal or sinus drainage; symptomatic relief of coughs caused by minor viral upper respiratory tract infections or inhaled irritants; most effective for a chronic nonproductive cough

Usual Dosage Adults: Oral: 1 capsule every 6 hours

Dosage Forms

Capsule: Pseudoephedrine hydrochloride 60 mg and dextromethorphan hydrobromide 30 mg

Liquid: Pseudoephedrine hydrochloride 20 mg and dextromethorphan hydrobromide 10 mg per 5 mL

pseudoephedrine and guaifenesin *see* guaifenesin and pseudoephedrine *on page 270*

pseudoephedrine and ibuprofen (soo doe e FED rin & eye byoo PROE fen)

U.S./Canadian Brand Names Advil® Cold & Sinus Caplets [OTC]; Dimetapp® Sinus Caplets [OTC]; Dristan® Sinus Caplets [OTC]; Motrin® IB Sinus [OTC]; Sine-Aid® IB [OTC]

Therapeutic Category Decongestant/Analgesic

Use Temporary symptomatic relief of nasal congestion due to common cold, upper respiratory allergies, and sinusitis; also promotes nasal or sinus drainage; sinus headaches and pains

Usual Dosage Adults: Oral: 1-2 caplets every 4-6 hours

Dosage Forms Caplet: Pseudoephedrine hydrochloride 30 mg and ibuprofen 200 mg

pseudoephedrine and loratadine *see* loratadine and pseudoephedrine *on page 339*

pseudoephedrine and triprolidine *see* triprolidine and pseudoephedrine *on page 584*

pseudoephedrine, dextromethorphan, and acetaminophen *see* acetaminophen, dextromethorphan, and pseudoephedrine *on page 6*

pseudoephedrine, dextromethorphan, and guaifenesin *see* guaifenesin, pseudoephedrine, and dextromethorphan *on page 273*

pseudoephedrine, guaifenesin, and codeine *see* guaifenesin, pseudoephedrine, and codeine *on page 272*

pseudoephedrine, hydrocodone, and guaifenesin *see* hydrocodone, pseudoephedrine, and guaifenesin *on page 290*

Pseudo-Gest Plus® Tablet [OTC] *see* chlorpheniramine and pseudoephedrine *on page 122*

pseudomonic acid A *see* mupirocin *on page 384*

Psorcon™ *see* diflorasone *on page 179*

psoriGel® [OTC] *see* coal tar *on page 141*

Psorion® Topical *see* betamethasone (topical) *on page 72*

PSP *see* phenolsulfonphthalein *on page 444*

P&S® Shampoo [OTC] *see* salicylic acid *on page 513*

psyllium (SIL i yum)

Synonyms plantago seed; plantain seed

U.S./Canadian Brand Names Effer-Syllium® [OTC]; Fiberall® Powder [OTC]; Fiberall® Wafer [OTC]; Fibrepur® (Can); Hydrocil® [OTC]; Konsyl® [OTC]; Konsyl-D® [OTC]; Metamucil® [OTC]; Metamucil® Instant Mix [OTC]; Modane® Bulk [OTC]; Novo-Mucilax® (Can); Perdiem® Plain [OTC]; Prodiem® Plain (Can); Reguloid® [OTC]; Serutan® [OTC]; Syllact® [OTC]; V-Lax® [OTC]

Therapeutic Category Laxative

Use Treatment of chronic atonic or spastic constipation and in constipation associated with rectal disorders; management of irritable bowel syndrome

Usual Dosage Oral:

Children 6-11 years: ½ to 1 rounded teaspoonful 1-3 times/day

Adults: 1-2 rounded teaspoonfuls or 1-2 packets 1-4 times/day

Dosage Forms

Granules: 4.03 g per rounded teaspoon (100 g, 250 g); 2.5 g per rounded teaspoon

Powder: Psyllium 50% and dextrose 50% (6.5 g, 325 g, 420 g, 480 g, 500 g)

Powder:

Effervescent: 3 g/dose (270 g, 480 g); 3.4 g/dose (single-dose packets)

Psyllium hydrophilic: 3.4 g per rounded teaspoon (210 g, 300 g, 420 g, 630 g)

Squares, chewable: 1.7 g, 3.4 g

Wafers: 3.4 g

P.T.E.-4® *see* trace metals *on page 573*

P.T.E.-5® *see* trace metals *on page 573*

pteroylglutamic acid *see* folic acid *on page 251*

PTU *see* propylthiouracil *on page 484*

Pulmicort® Turbuhaler® *see* budesonide *on page 82*

Pulmozyme® *see* dornase alfa *on page 194*

Puralube® Tears Solution [OTC] *see* artificial tears *on page 47*

Purge® [OTC] *see* castor oil *on page 103*

Puri-Clens™ [OTC] *see* methylbenzethonium chloride *on page 366*

purified protein derivative *see* tuberculin tests *on page 588*

Purinethol® *see* mercaptopurine *on page 357*

Purinol® (Can) *see* allopurinol *on page 19*

PVF® K (Can) *see* penicillin V potassium *on page 435*

P-V-Tussin® *see* hydrocodone, phenylephrine, pyrilamine, phenindamine, chlorpheniramine, and ammonium chloride *on page 290*

P_xE_x® Ophthalmic *see* pilocarpine and epinephrine *on page 452*

pyrantel pamoate (pi RAN tel PAM oh ate)

U.S./Canadian Brand Names Antiminth® [OTC]; Pin-Rid® [OTC]; Pin-X® [OTC]; Reese's® Pinworm Medicine [OTC]

Therapeutic Category Anthelmintic

Use Roundworm (*Ascaris lumbricoides*), pinworm (*Enterobius vermicularis*), and hookworm (*Ancylostoma duodenale* and *Necator americanus*) infestations, and trichostrongyliasis

Usual Dosage Children and Adults: Oral:

Roundworm, pinworm, or trichostrongyliasis: 11 mg/kg administered as a single dose; maximum dose is 1 g; dosage should be repeated in 2 weeks for pinworm infection

Hookworm: 11 mg/kg/day once daily for 3 days

Dosage Forms

Capsule: 180 mg

Liquid: 50 mg/mL (30 mL); 144 mg/mL (30 mL)

Suspension, oral (caramel-currant flavor): 50 mg/mL (60 mL)

pyrazinamide (peer a ZIN a mide)

Synonyms pyrazinoic acid amide

U.S./Canadian Brand Names PMS-Pyrazinamide (Can); Tebrazid (Can)

Therapeutic Category Antitubercular Agent

Use In combination with other antituberculosis agents in the treatment of *Mycobacterium* tuberculosis infection (especially useful in disseminated and meningeal tuberculosis); CDC currently recommends a 3 or 4 multidrug regimen which includes pyrazinamide, rifampin, INH, and at times ethambutol or streptomycin for the treatment of tuberculosis

Usual Dosage Oral:

Children: 15-30 mg/kg/day in divided doses every 12-24 hours; daily dose not to exceed 2 g

Adults: 15-30 mg/kg/day in 3-4 divided doses; maximum daily dose: 2 g/day

Dosage Forms Tablet: 500 mg

pyrazinamide, rifampin, and isoniazid *see* rifampin, isoniazid, and pyrazinamide *on page 505*

pyrazinoic acid amide *see* pyrazinamide *on this page*

pyrethrins (pye RE thrins)

U.S./Canadian Brand Names A-200™ Shampoo [OTC]; Barc™ Liquid [OTC]; End Lice® Liquid [OTC]; Lice-Enz® Shampoo [OTC]; Pronto® Shampoo [OTC]; Pyrinex® Pediculicide Shampoo [OTC]; Pyrinyl II® Liquid [OTC]; Pyrinyl Plus® Shampoo [OTC]; R & C® Shampoo [OTC]; RID® Shampoo [OTC]; Tisit® Blue Gel [OTC]; Tisit® Liquid [OTC]; Tisit® Shampoo [OTC]; Triple X® Liquid [OTC]

Therapeutic Category Scabicides/Pediculicides

Use Treatment of *Pediculus humanus* infestations

Usual Dosage Application of pyrethrins: Topical:

Apply enough solution to completely wet infested area, including hair
Allow to remain on area for 10 minutes
Wash and rinse with large amounts of warm water
Use fine-toothed comb to remove lice and eggs from hair
Shampoo hair to restore body and luster
Treatment may be repeated if necessary once in a 24-hours period
Repeat treatment in 7-10 days to kill newly hatched lice

Dosage Forms

Gel, topical: 0.3% (30 g, 480 g)
Liquid, topical: 0.18% (60 mL); 0.2% (60 mL, 120 mL); 0.3% (60 mL, 120 mL, 240 mL)
Shampoo: 0.3% (60 mL, 118 mL); 0.33% (60 mL, 120 mL)

Pyridiate® *see* phenazopyridine *on page 442*

2-pyridine aldoxime methochloride *see* pralidoxime *on page 468*

Pyridium® *see* phenazopyridine *on page 442*

Pyridium Plus® ***(Discontinued)*** *see page 700*

pyridostigmine (peer id oh STIG meen)

U.S./Canadian Brand Names Mestinon® Injection; Mestinon® Oral; Regonol® Injection

Therapeutic Category Cholinergic Agent

Use Symptomatic treatment of myasthenia gravis by improving muscle strength; reversal of effects of nondepolarizing neuromuscular blocking agents

Usual Dosage Normally, sustained release dosage form is used at bedtime for patients who complain of morning weakness

Myasthenia gravis:

Oral:

Children: 7 mg/kg/day in 5-6 divided doses

Adults: Initial: 60 mg 3 times/day with maintenance dose ranging from 60 mg to 1.5 g/day; sustained release formulation should be dosed at least every 6 hours (usually 12-24 hours)

(Continued)

pyridostigmine *(Continued)*

I.M., I.V.:

Children: 0.05-0.15 mg/kg/dose (maximum single dose: 10 mg)

Adults: 2 mg every 2-3 hours or 1/30th of oral dose

Reversal of nondepolarizing neuromuscular blocker: I.M., I.V.:

Children: 0.1-0.25 mg/kg/dose preceded by atropine

Adults: 10-20 mg preceded by atropine

Dosage Forms Pyridostigmine bromide:

Injection: 5 mg/mL (2 mL, 5 mL)

Syrup (raspberry flavor): 60 mg/5 mL (480 mL)

Tablet: 60 mg

Tablet, sustained release: 180 mg

pyridoxine (peer i DOKS een)

Synonyms vitamin B_6

U.S./Canadian Brand Names Nestrex®

Therapeutic Category Vitamin, Water Soluble

Use Prevent and treat vitamin B_6 deficiency, pyridoxine-dependent seizures in infants, treatment of drug-induced deficiency (eg, isoniazid or hydralazine)

Usual Dosage

Pyridoxine-dependent Infants:

Oral: 2-100 mg/day

I.M., I.V.: 10-100 mg

Dietary deficiency: Oral:

Children: 5-10 mg/24 hours for 3 weeks

Adults: 10-20 mg/day for 3 weeks

Drug-induced neuritis (eg, isoniazid, hydralazine, penicillamine, cycloserine): Oral treatment:

Children: 10-50 mg/24 hours; prophylaxis: 1-2 mg/kg/24 hours

Adults: 100-200 mg/24 hours; prophylaxis: 10-100 mg/24 hours

For the treatment of seizures and/or coma from acute isoniazid toxicity, a dose of pyridoxine hydrochloride equal to the amount of INH ingested can be administered I.M./I.V. in divided doses together with other anticonvulsants

Dosage Forms Pyridoxine hydrochloride:

Injection: 100 mg/mL (10 mL, 30 mL)

Tablet: 25 mg, 50 mg, 100 mg

Tablet, extended release: 100 mg

pyrimethamine (peer i METH a meen)

U.S./Canadian Brand Names Daraprim®

Therapeutic Category Folic Acid Antagonist (Antimalarial)

Use Prophylaxis of malaria due to susceptible strains of plasmodia; used in conjunction with quinine and sulfadoxine for the treatment of uncomplicated attacks of chloroquine-resistant *P. falciparum* malaria; used in conjunction with fast-acting schizonticide to initiate transmission control and suppression cure; synergistic combination with sulfadiazine in treatment of toxoplasmosis

Usual Dosage Oral:

Malaria chemoprophylaxis:

Children: 0.5 mg/kg once weekly; not to exceed 25 mg/dose **or**

Children:

<4 years: 6.25 mg once weekly

4-10 years: 12.5 mg once weekly

Children >10 years and Adults: 25 mg once weekly

Dosage should be continued for all age groups for at least 6-10 weeks after leaving endemic areas

Chloroquine-resistant *P. falciparum* malaria (when used in conjunction with quinine and sulfadiazine):
Children:
<10 kg: 6.25 mg/day once daily for 3 days
10-20 kg: 12.5 mg/day once daily for 3 days
20-40 kg: 25 mg/day once daily for 3 days
Adults: 25 mg twice daily for 3 days
Toxoplasmosis (with sulfadiazine or trisulfapyrimidines):
Children: 1 mg/kg/day divided into 2 equal daily doses; decrease dose after 2-4 days by 50%, continue for about 1 month; used with 100 mg sulfadiazine/kg/day divided every 6 hours; **or** 2 mg/kg/day divided every 12 hours for 3 days followed by 1 mg/kg/day once daily for 4 weeks
Adults: 50-75 mg/day together with 1-4 g of a sulfonamide for 1-3 weeks depending on patient's tolerance and response

Dosage Forms Tablet: 25 mg

Pyrinex® Pediculicide Shampoo [OTC] *see* pyrethrins *on page 489*

Pyrinyl II® Liquid [OTC] *see* pyrethrins *on page 489*

Pyrinyl Plus® Shampoo [OTC] *see* pyrethrins *on page 489*

pyrithione zinc (peer i THYE one zingk)

U.S./Canadian Brand Names DHS Zinc® [OTC]; Head & Shoulders® [OTC]; Theraplex Z® [OTC]; Zincon® Shampoo [OTC]; ZNP® Bar [OTC]

Therapeutic Category Antiseborrheic Agent, Topical

Use Relieves the itching, irritation and scalp flaking associated with dandruff and/or seborrheal dermatitis of the scalp

Usual Dosage Topical: Shampoo hair twice weekly, wet hair, apply to scalp and massage vigorously, rinse and repeat

Dosage Forms
Bar: 2% (119 g)
Shampoo: 1% (120 mL); 2% (120 mL, 180 mL, 240 mL, 360 mL)

Pyronium® (Can) *see* phenazopyridine *on page 442*

quazepam (KWAY ze pam)

U.S./Canadian Brand Names Doral®

Therapeutic Category Benzodiazepine

Controlled Substance C-IV

Use Short-term treatment of insomnia

Usual Dosage Adults: Oral: Initial: 15 mg at bedtime; in some patients the dose may be reduced to 7.5 mg after a few nights

Dosage Forms Tablet: 7.5 mg, 15 mg

Quelicin® *see* succinylcholine *on page 537*

Questran® *see* cholestyramine resin *on page 129*

Questran® Light *see* cholestyramine resin *on page 129*

Questran® Tablet *(Discontinued)* *see page 700*

quetiapine (kwe TYE a peen)

U.S./Canadian Brand Names Seroquel®

Therapeutic Category Antipsychotic Agent

Use Management of psychotic disorders; this antipsychotic drug belongs to a new chemical class, the dibenzothiazepine derivatives

Usual Dosage Adults: Oral: 25-100 mg 2-3 times/day

Dosage Forms Tablet, as fumarate: 25 mg, 100 mg, 200 mg

Quibron® *see* theophylline and guaifenesin *on page 559*

Quibron®-T *see* theophylline *on page 557*

Quibron®-T/SR *see* theophylline *on page 557*

Quiess® Injection *see* hydroxyzine *on page 297*

Quinaglute® Dura-Tabs® *see* quinidine *on this page*

Quinalan® *see* quinidine *on this page*

quinalbarbitone *see* secobarbital *on page 517*

Quinamm® ***(Discontinued)*** *see page 700*

quinapril (KWIN a pril)

U.S./Canadian Brand Names Accupril®

Therapeutic Category Angiotensin-Converting Enzyme (ACE) Inhibitor

Use Treatment of hypertension, either alone or in combination with other antihypertensive agents

Usual Dosage Adults: Oral: Initial: 10 mg once daily, adjust according to blood pressure response at peak and trough blood levels; in general, the normal dosage range is 40-80 mg/day

Dosage Forms Tablet, as hydrochloride: 5 mg, 10 mg, 20 mg, 40 mg

quinapril and hydrochlorothiazide *(Canada only)*

(KWIN a pril & hye droe klor oh THYE a zide)

U.S./Canadian Brand Names Accuretic® (Can)

Therapeutic Category Angiotensin-Converting Enzyme (ACE) Inhibitor; Diuretic, Thiazide

Use Treatment of essential hypertension when combination therapy is appropriate

Usual Dosage Dosage must be individualized; the fixed combination is not for initial therapy; the dose should be determined by titration of the individual components

Dosage Forms Tablet: Quinapril hydrochloride 10 mg and hydrochlorothiazide 12.5 mg; quinapril hydrochloride 20 mg and hydrochlorothiazide 12.5 mg

quinethazone (kwin ETH a zone)

U.S./Canadian Brand Names Hydromox®

Therapeutic Category Diuretic, Thiazide

Use Adjunctive therapy in treatment of edema and hypertension

Usual Dosage Adults: Oral: 50-100 mg once daily up to a maximum of 200 mg/day

Dosage Forms Tablet: 50 mg

Quinidex® Extentabs® *see* quinidine *on this page*

quinidine (KWIN i deen)

U.S./Canadian Brand Names Biquin® Durules® (Can); Cardioquin®; Quinaglute® Dura-Tabs®; Quinalan®; Quinidex® Extentabs®; Quinora®

Therapeutic Category Antiarrhythmic Agent, Class I-A

Use Prophylaxis after cardioversion of atrial fibrillation and/or flutter to maintain normal sinus rhythm; also used to prevent reoccurrence of paroxysmal supraventricular tachycardia, paroxysmal A-V junctional rhythm, paroxysmal ventricular tachycardia, paroxysmal atrial fibrillation, and atrial or ventricular premature contractions; also has activity against *Plasmodium falciparum* malaria

Usual Dosage Note: Dosage expressed in terms of the salt: 267 mg of quinidine gluconate = 275 mg of quinidine polygalacturonate = 200 mg of quinidine sulfate

Children: Test dose for idiosyncratic reaction (sulfate, oral or gluconate, I.M.): 2 mg/kg or 60 mg/m^2

Oral (quinidine sulfate): 15-60 mg/kg/day in 4-5 divided doses or 6 mg/kg every 4-6 hours (AMA 1991); usual 30 mg/kg/day or 900 mg/m^2/day administered in 5 daily doses

I.V. **not** recommended (quinidine gluconate): 2-10 mg/kg/dose every 3-6 hours as needed

Adults: Test dose: 200 mg administered several hours before full dosage (to determine possibility of idiosyncratic reaction)

Oral (sulfate): 100-600 mg/dose every 4-6 hours; begin at 200 mg/dose and titrate to desired effect

Oral (gluconate): 324-972 mg every 8-12 hours

Oral (polygalacturonate): 275 mg every 8-12 hours

I.M.: 400 mg/dose every 4-6 hours

I.V.: 200-400 mg/dose diluted and administered at a rate ≤10 mg/minute

Dosage Forms

Quinidine gluconate:

Injection: 80 mg/mL (10 mL)

Tablet, sustained release: 324 mg

Quinidine polygalacturonate:

Tablet: 275 mg

Quinidine sulfate:

Tablet: 200 mg, 300 mg

Tablet, sustained action: 300 mg

quinine (KWYE nine)

U.S./Canadian Brand Names Formula Q®

Therapeutic Category Antimalarial Agent

Use Suppression or treatment of chloroquine-resistant *P. falciparum* malaria (inactive against sporozoites, pre-erythrocytic or exoerythrocytic forms of plasmodia); treatment of *Babesia microti* infection

Usual Dosage Oral (parenteral dosage form may be obtained from Centers for Disease Control if needed):

Children: Chloroquine-resistant malaria and babesiosis: 25 mg/kg/day in divided doses every 8 hours for 7 days; maximum: 650 mg/dose

Adults:

Chloroquine-resistant malaria: 650 mg every 8 hours for 7 days in conjunction with another agent

Babesiosis: 650 mg every 6-8 hours for 7 days

Dosage Forms Quinine sulfate:

Capsule: 64.8 mg, 65 mg, 200 mg, 300 mg, 325 mg

Tablet: 162.5 mg, 260 mg

quinol *see* hydroquinone *on page 294*

Quinora® *see* quinidine *on previous page*

quinupristin and dalfopristin (kwi NYOO pris tin & dal FOE pris tin)

Synonyms pristinamycin; RP59500

U.S./Canadian Brand Names Synercid®

Therapeutic Category Antibiotic, Streptogramin

Use Treatment of serious or life-threatening infections associated with vancomycin-resistant *Enterococcus faecium* bacteremia; treatment of complicated skin and skin structure infections caused by methcillin-susceptible *Staphylococcus aureus* or *Streptococcus pyogenes*

Investigational use: Has been studied in the treatment of a variety of infections caused by *Enterococcus faecium* (not *E. fecalis*) including vancomycin-resistant strains. May also be effective in the treatment of serious infections caused by *Staphylococcus* species including those resistant to methicillin.

Usual Dosage Adults: I.V.:

Vancomycin-resistant *Enterococcus faecium:* 7.5 mg/kg every 8 hours

Complicated skin and skin structure infection: 7.5 mg/kg every 12 hours

Dosage adjustment in renal impairment: No adjustment required in renal failure, hemodialysis or peritoneal dialysis

(Continued)

quinupristin and dalfopristin *(Continued)*

Dosage adjustment in hepatic impairment: Pharmacokinetic data suggest dosage adjustment may be necessary, however, specific recommendations have not been proposed

Elderly: No dosage adjustment is required

Dosage Forms Powder for injection: 500 mg (350 mg dalfopristin and 150 mg quinupristin)

Quiphile® ***(Discontinued)*** *see page 700*

Q-vel® ***(Discontinued)*** *see page 700*

rabeprazole (ra BE pray zole)

Synonyms pariprazole

U.S./Canadian Brand Names Aciphex™

Therapeutic Category Gastric Acid Secretion Inhibitor

Use Short-term (4-8 weeks) treatment of erosive or ulcerative gastroesophageal reflux disease (GERD); maintenance therapy in erosive or ulcerative GERD; short-term (up to 4 weeks) treatment of duodenal ulcers; long-term treatment of pathological hypersecretory conditions, including Zollinger-Ellison syndrome

Usual Dosage Adults and Elderly:

GERD: 20 mg once daily for 4-8 weeks; maintenance: 20 mg once daily

Duodenal ulcer: 20 mg/day after breakfast for 4 weeks

Hypersecretory conditions: 60 mg once daily; dose may need to be adjusted as necessary. Doses as high as 100 mg and 60 mg twice daily have been used.

Dosage Forms Tablet, delayed release: 20 mg

rabies immune globulin (human)

(RAY beez i MYUN GLOB yoo lin, HYU man)

Synonyms RIG

U.S./Canadian Brand Names Hyperab®; Imogam®

Therapeutic Category Immune Globulin

Use Passive immunity to rabies for postexposure prophylaxis of individuals exposed to the virus

Usual Dosage Children and Adults: I.M.: 20 units/kg in a single dose (RIG should always be administered in conjunction with rabies vaccine (HDCV)) (infiltrate $^1/_2$ of the dose locally around the wound; administer the remainder I.M.)

Dosage Forms Injection: 150 units/mL (2 mL, 10 mL)

rabies virus vaccine (RAY beez VYE rus vak SEEN)

Synonyms HDCV; HDRS

U.S./Canadian Brand Names Imovax® Rabies I.D. Vaccine; Imovax® Rabies Vaccine

Therapeutic Category Vaccine, Inactivated Virus

Use Pre-exposure rabies immunization for high risk persons; postexposure antirabies immunization along with local treatment and immune globulin

Usual Dosage

Pre-exposure prophylaxis: Two 1 mL doses I.M. or I.D. one week apart, third dose 3 weeks after second dose. If exposure continues, booster doses can be administered every 2 years, or an antibody titer determined and a booster dose administered if the titer is inadequate.

Postexposure prophylaxis: All postexposure treatment should begin with immediate cleansing of the wound with soap and water. Persons not previously immunized as above: Rabies immune globulin 20 units/kg body weight, half infiltrated at bite site if possible, remainder I.M.; and 5 doses of rabies vaccine, 1 mL I.M., one each on days 0, 3, 7, 14, 28.

Persons who have previously received postexposure prophylaxis with rabies vaccine, received a recommended I.M. or I.D. pre-exposure series of rabies vaccine or have a previously documented rabies antibody titer considered adequate: Two doses of rabies vaccine, 1 mL I.M., one each on days 0 and 3

Dosage Forms Injection:

I.M. (HDCV): Rabies antigen 2.5 units/mL (1 mL)

Intradermal: Rabies antigen 0.25 units/mL (1 mL)

radiological/contrast media (ionic)

U.S./Canadian Brand Names Anatrast®; Angio Conray®; Angiovist®; Baricon®; Barobag®; Baro-CAT®; Baroflave®; Barosperse®; Bar-Test®; Bilopaque®; Cholebrine®; Cholografin® Meglumine; Conray®; Cystografin®; Dionosil Oily®; Enecat®; Entrobar®; Epi-C®; Ethiodol®; Flo-Coat®; Gastrografin®; HD 85®; HD 200 Plus®; Hexabrix™; Hypaque-Cysto®; Hypaque® Meglumine; Hypaque® Sodium; Liquid Barosperse®; Liquipake®; Lymphazurin®; Magnevist®; MD-Gastroview®; Oragrafin® Calcium; Oragrafin® Sodium; Perchloracap®; Prepcat®; Reno-M-30®; Reno-M-60®; Reno-M-Dip®; Renovue®-65; Renovue®-DIP; Sinografin®; Telepaque®; Tomocat®; Tonopaque®; Urovist Cysto®; Urovist® Meglumine; Urovist® Sodium 300; Vascoray®

Therapeutic Category Radiopaque Agents

Dosage Forms

Oral cholecystographic agents:

Iocetamic acid: Tablet (Cholebrine®): 750 mg

Iopanoic acid: Tablet (Telepaque®): 500 mg

Ipodate calcium: Granules for oral suspension (Oragrafin® Calcium): 3 g

Ipodate sodium: Capsule (Bilivist®, Oragrafin® Sodium): 500 mg

Tyropanoate sodium: Capsule (Bilopaque®): 750 mg

GI contrast agents: **Barium sulfate**:

Paste (Anatrast®): 100% (500 g)

Powder:

Baroflave®: 100%

Baricon®, HD 200 Plus®: 98%

Barosperse®, Tonopaque®: 95%

Suspension:

Baro-CAT®, Prepcat®: 1.5%

Enecat®, Tomocat®: 5%

Entrobar®: 50%

Liquid Barasperse®: 60%

HD 85®: 85%

Barobag®: 97%

Flo-Coat®, Liquipake®: 100%

Epi-C®: 150%

Tablet (Bar-Test®): 650 mg

Parenteral agents: Injection:

Diatrizoate meglumine:

Hypaque® Meglumine

Reno-M-DIP®

Urovist® Meglumine

Angiovist® 282

Hypaque® Meglumine

Reno-M-60®

Diatrizoate sodium:

Hypaque® Sodium

Hypaque® Sodium

Urovist® Sodium 300

Gadopentetate dimeglumine: Magnevist®

Iodamide meglumine:

Renovue®-DIP

Renovue®-65

Iodipamide meglumine: Cholografin® meglumine

(Continued)

radiological/contrast media (ionic) *(Continued)*

Iothalamate meglumine:
Conray® 30
Conray® 43
Conray®
Iothalamate sodium:
Angio Conray®
Conray® 325
Conray® 400
Diatrizoate meglumine and diatrizoate sodium:
Angiovist® 292
Angiovist® 370
Hypaque-76®
Hypaque-M®, 75%
Hypaque-M®, 90%
MD-60®
MD-76®
Renografin-60®
Renografin-76®
Renovist® II
Renovist®
Iothalamate meglumine and iothalamate sodium:
Vascoray®
Hexabrix™

Miscellaneous agents: (**NOT** for intravascular use, for instillation into various cavities)
Diatrizoate meglumine: Urogenital solution, sterile:
Crystografin®
Crystografin® Dilute
Hypaque-Cysto®
Reno-M-30®
Urovist Cysto®
Diatrizoate meglumine and diatrizoate sodium: Solution, oral or rectal:
Gastrografin®
MD-Gastroview®
Diatrizoate sodium:
Solution, oral or rectal (Hypaque® sodium oral)
Solution, urogenital (Hypaque® sodium 20%)
Iothalamate meglumine: Solution, urogenital:
Cysto-Conray®
Cysto-Conray® II

Diatrizoate meglumine and iodipamide meglumine:
Injection, urogenital for intrauterine instillation (Sinografin®)
Ethiodized oil: Injection (Ethiodol®)
Propyliodone: Suspension (Dionosil Oily®)
Isosulfan blue: Injection (Lymphazurin® 1%)
Potassium perchlorate: Capsule (Perchloracap®): 200 mg

radiological/contrast media (non-ionic)

U.S./Canadian Brand Names Amipaque®; Isovue®; Omnipaque®; Optiray®
Therapeutic Category Radiopaque Agents
Dosage Forms **Parenteral agents**: Injection:
Iohexol: Omnipaque®: 140 mg/mL; 180 mg/mL; 210 mg/mL; 240 mg/mL; 300 mg/mL; 350 mg/mL
Iopamidol:
Isovue-128®
Isovue-200®
Isovue-M 200®
Isovue-300®

Isovue-M 300®
Isovue-370®
Ioversol:
Optiray® 160
Optiray® 240
Optiray® 320
Metrizamide: Amipaque®

Radiostol® (Can) *see* ergocalciferol *on page 212*

R-albuterol *see* levalbuterol *on page 329*

raloxifene (ral OX i feen)

U.S./Canadian Brand Names Evista®
Therapeutic Category Selective Estrogen Receptor Modulator (SERM)
Use Prevention of osteoporosis in postmenopausal women
Usual Dosage Adults: Oral: 1 tablet daily, may be administered any time of the day without regard to meals
Dosage Forms Tablet, as hydrochloride: 60 mg

ramipril (ra MI pril)

U.S./Canadian Brand Names Altace™
Therapeutic Category Angiotensin-Converting Enzyme (ACE) Inhibitor
Use Treatment of hypertension, alone or in combination with thiazide diuretics; congestive heart failure immediately after myocardial infarction
Usual Dosage Adults: Oral: 2.5-5 mg once daily
Dosage Forms Capsule: 1.25 mg, 2.5 mg, 5 mg, 10 mg

Ramses® [OTC] *see* nonoxynol 9 *on page 406*

ranitidine bismuth citrate (ra NI ti deen BIZ muth SIT rate)

Synonyms RBC
U.S./Canadian Brand Names Tritec®
Therapeutic Category Gastrointestinal Agent, Gastric or Duodenal Ulcer Treatment
Use In combination with clarithromycin for the treatment of active duodenal ulcer associated with *H. pylori* infection; not to be used alone for the treatment of active duodenal ulcer
Usual Dosage Adults: Oral: 400 mg twice daily for 4 weeks (28 days) in conjunction with clarithromycin 500 mg 3 times/day for first 2 weeks
Dosage Forms Tablet: 400 mg (ranitidine 162 mg, trivalent bismuth 128 mg, and citrate 110 mg)

ranitidine hydrochloride (ra NI ti deen hye droe KLOR ide)

U.S./Canadian Brand Names Apo®-Ranitidine (Can); Novo-Ranidine® (Can); Nu-Ranit® (Can); Zantac®; Zantac® 75 [OTC]
Therapeutic Category Histamine H_2 Antagonist
Use Short-term treatment of active duodenal ulcers and benign gastric ulcers; long-term prophylaxis of duodenal ulcer and gastric hypersecretory states; gastroesophageal reflux (GER)
Usual Dosage
Children:
Oral: 1.5-2 mg/kg/dose every 12 hours
I.M., I.V.: 0.75-1.5 mg/kg/dose every 6-8 hours, maximum daily dose: 400 mg
Continuous infusion: 0.1-0.25 mg/kg/hour (preferred for stress ulcer prophylaxis in patients with concurrent maintenance I.V.s or TPNs)
Adults:
Short-term treatment of ulceration: 150 mg/dose twice daily or 300 mg at bedtime
Prophylaxis of recurrent duodenal ulcer: 150 mg at bedtime
Gastric hypersecretory conditions: Oral: 150 mg twice daily, up to 600 mg /day
(Continued)

ranitidine hydrochloride *(Continued)*

I.M., I.V.: 50 mg/dose every 6-8 hours (dose not to exceed 400 mg/day)

Dosage Forms Ranitidine hydrochloride:

Capsule (GELdose™): 150 mg, 300 mg

Granules, effervescent (EFFERdose™): 150 mg

Infusion, preservative free, in NaCl 0.45%: 1 mg/mL (50 mL)

Injection: 25 mg/mL (2 mL, 10 mL, 40 mL)

Syrup (peppermint flavor): 15 mg/mL (473 mL)

Tablet: 75 mg [OTC]; 150 mg, 300 mg

Tablet, effervescent (EFFERdose™): 150 mg

rapacuronium (ra pa kyoo ROE nee um)

U.S./Canadian Brand Names Raplon™

Therapeutic Category Neuromuscular Blocker Agent, Nondepolarizing

Use Adjunct to general anesthesia to facilitate tracheal intubation; to provide skeletal muscle relaxation during surgical procedures

Usual Dosage I.V. (do not administer I.M.):

Children 1 month to 12 years: Initial: 2 mg/kg. Repeat dosing is not recommended in pediatric patients.

Children 13-17 years: Clinicians should consider the physical maturity, height and weight of the patient in determining the dose. Adults (1.5 mg/kg), pediatric (2 mg/kg) and Cesarean section (2.5 mg/kg) dosing recommendations may serve as a general guideline in determining an intubating dose in this age group.

Adults: Tracheal Intubation:

Initial: Short surgical procedures: 1.5 mg/kg; Cesarean section: 2.5 mg/kg

Repeat dosing: Up to three maintenance doses of 0.5 mg/kg, administered at 25% recovery of control T1 may be administered. **Note:** The duration of neuromuscular blockade increases with each additional dose.

Elderly: No dosing adjustment is recommended in geriatric patients

Dosage Forms Powder for injection: 100 mg (5 mL); 200 mg (10 mL)

Rapamune® *see* sirolimus *on page 523*

Raplon™ *see* rapacuronium *on this page*

Raudixin® *see Rauwolfia serpentina on this page*

Rauverid® *see Rauwolfia serpentina on this page*

Rauwolfia serpentina (rah WOOL fee a ser pen TEEN ah)

Synonyms whole root rauwolfia

U.S./Canadian Brand Names Raudixin®; Rauverid®; Wolfina®

Therapeutic Category Rauwolfia Alkaloid

Use Mild essential hypertension; relief of agitated psychotic states

Usual Dosage Adults: Oral: 200-400 mg/day in 2 divided doses

Dosage Forms Tablet: 50 mg, 100 mg

Raxar® *see* grepafloxacin *Withdrawn from U.S. market 10/27/99 on page 266*

RBC *see* ranitidine bismuth citrate *on previous page*

R & C® Shampoo [OTC] *see* pyrethrins *on page 489*

Reactine™ (Can) *see* cetirizine *on page 113*

Rea-Lo® [OTC] *see* urea *on page 591*

Rebetron™ *see* interferon alfa-2b and ribavirin combination pack *on page 308*

recombinant human deoxyribonuclease *see* dornase alfa *on page 194*

Recombinant Human Interleukin-11 *see* oprelvekin *on page 416*

Recombinant Interleukin-11 *see* oprelvekin *on page 416*

recombinant plasminogen activator *see* reteplase *on page 501*

Recombinate® *see* antihemophilic factor (recombinant) *on page 40*

Recombivax HB® *see* hepatitis B vaccine *on page 280*

Rectacort® Suppository *(Discontinued)* *see page 700*

Rectocort (Can) *see* hydrocortisone (rectal) *on page 291*

Red Away® (Can) *see* naphazoline *on page 390*

Redisol® *see* cyanocobalamin *on page 152*

Redoxon® (Can) *see* ascorbic acid *on page 48*

Redutemp® [OTC] *see* acetaminophen *on page 3*

Redux® *(Discontinued)* *see page 700*

Reese's® Pinworm Medicine [OTC] *see* pyrantel pamoate *on page 488*

Refludan® *see* lepirudin *on page 328*

Refresh® Ophthalmic Solution [OTC] *see* artificial tears *on page 47*

Refresh® Plus Ophthalmic Solution [OTC] *see* artificial tears *on page 47*

Regitine® *see* phentolamine *on page 445*

Reglan® *see* metoclopramide *on page 370*

Regonol® Injection *see* pyridostigmine *on page 489*

Regranex® *see* becaplermin *on page 62*

Regulace® [OTC] *see* docusate and casanthranol *on page 191*

Regular Iletin® I *see* insulin preparations *on page 307*

Regular [Concentrated] Iletin® II U-500 *see* insulin preparations *on page 307*

Regular Insulin *see* insulin preparations *on page 307*

Regular Purified Pork Insulin *see* insulin preparations *on page 307*

Regulax SS® [OTC] *see* docusate *on page 191*

Regulex® (Can) *see* docusate *on page 191*

Reguloid® [OTC] *see* psyllium *on page 488*

Regutol® *(Discontinued)* *see page 700*

Relafen® *see* nabumetone *on page 387*

Relefact® TRH *see* protirelin *on page 485*

Relenza® *see* zanamivir *on page 610*

Relief® Ophthalmic Solution *see* phenylephrine *on page 445*

Remeron® *see* mirtazapine *on page 377*

Remicade® *see* infliximab *on page 305*

remifentanil (rem i FEN ta nil)

U.S./Canadian Brand Names Ultiva™

Therapeutic Category Analgesic, Narcotic

Use Analgesic for use during general anesthesia for continued analgesia

Usual Dosage Adults: I.V. continuous infusion:

During induction: 0.5-1 mcg/kg/minute

During maintenance:

With nitrous oxide (66%): 0.4 mcg/kg/minute (range: 0.1-2 mcg/kg/min)

With isoflurane: 0.25 mcg/kg/minute (range: 0.05-2 mcg/kg/min)

With propofol: 0.25 mcg/kg/minute (range: 0.05-2 mcg/kg/min)

Continuation as an analgesic in immediate postoperative period: 0.1 mcg/kg/minute (range: 0.025-0.2 mcg/kg/min)

Dosage Forms Powder for injection, lyophilized: 1 mg/3 mL vial, 2 mg/5 mL vial, 5 mg/10 mL vial

Renacidin® *see* citric acid bladder mixture *on page 134*

Renagel® *see* sevelamer *on page 520*

Renese® *see* polythiazide *on page 461*

Reno-M-30® *see* radiological/contrast media (ionic) *on page 495*

Reno-M-60® *see* radiological/contrast media (ionic) *on page 495*

Reno-M-Dip® *see* radiological/contrast media (ionic) *on page 495*

Renoquid® *see* sulfacytine *on page 541*

Renormax® *see* spirapril *on page 533*

Renovue®-65 *see* radiological/contrast media (ionic) *on page 495*

Renovue®-DIP *see* radiological/contrast media (ionic) *on page 495*

Rentamine® *see* chlorpheniramine, ephedrine, phenylephrine, and carbetapentane *on page 123*

ReoPro® *see* abciximab *on page 2*

repaglinide (re PAG li nide)

U.S./Canadian Brand Names Prandin™

Therapeutic Category Hypoglycemic Agent, Oral

Use As an adjunct to diet and exercise to lower blood glucose on noninsulin-dependent (Type II) diabetes patients

Usual Dosage Oral: Adults: 0.5-4 mg before each meal

Oral hypoglycemic-naive individuals or those with HbA1c levels <8%: Initial: 0.5 mg before each meal; for other patients, the starting dose is 1-2 mg before each meal

Dose can be adjusted (by prescribers) up to 4 mg before each meal. If a meal is skipped, the patient should also skip the repaglinide dose.

Dosage Forms Tablet: 0.5 mg, 1 mg, 2 mg

Repan® *see* butalbital compound and acetaminophen *on page 85*

Replasyn® (Can) *see* sodium hyaluronate *on page 527*

Reposans-10® Oral *see* chlordiazepoxide *on page 116*

Rep-Pred® ***(Discontinued)*** *see page 700*

Repronex™ *see* menotropins *on page 354*

Requip™ *see* ropinirole *on page 510*

Resaid® *see* chlorpheniramine and phenylpropanolamine *on page 122*

Rescaps-D® S.R. Capsule *see* caramiphen and phenylpropanolamine *on page 97*

Rescon Liquid [OTC] *see* chlorpheniramine and phenylpropanolamine *on page 122*

Rescriptor® *see* delavirdine *on page 162*

Resectisol® Irrigation Solution *see* mannitol *on page 347*

reserpine (re SER peen)

U.S./Canadian Brand Names Novo-Reserpine® (Can); Serpalan®

Therapeutic Category Rauwolfia Alkaloid

Use Management of mild to moderate hypertension

Usual Dosage Adults: Oral: 0.1-0.5 mg/day in 1-2 doses

Dosage Forms Tablet: 0.1 mg, 0.25 mg

reserpine and chlorothiazide *see* chlorothiazide and reserpine *on page 120*

reserpine and hydrochlorothiazide *see* hydrochlorothiazide and reserpine *on page 286*

reserpine and hydroflumethiazide *see* hydroflumethiazide and reserpine *on page 293*

reserpine, hydralazine, and hydrochlorothiazide *see* hydralazine, hydrochlorothiazide, and reserpine *on page 285*

Resource® (Can) *see* enteral nutritional products *on page 208*

Respa-1st® *see* guaifenesin and pseudoephedrine *on page 270*

Respa-DM® *see* guaifenesin and dextromethorphan *on page 268*

Respa-GF® *see* guaifenesin *on page 267*

Respaire®-60 SR *see* guaifenesin and pseudoephedrine *on page 270*

Respaire®-120 SR *see* guaifenesin and pseudoephedrine *on page 270*

Respbid® *see* theophylline *on page 557*

RespiGam™ *see* respiratory syncytial virus immune globulin (intravenous) *on this page*

respiratory syncytial virus immune globulin (intravenous)

(RES peer rah tor ee sin SISH al VYE rus i MYUN GLOB yoo lin in tra VEE nus)

Synonyms RSV-IGIV

U.S./Canadian Brand Names RespiGam™

Therapeutic Category Immune Globulin

Use Prevention of serious lower respiratory infection caused by respiratory syncytial virus (RSV) in children <24 months of age with bronchopulmonary dysplasia (BPD) or a history of premature birth (≤35 weeks gestation)

Usual Dosage I.V.: 750 mg/kg/month according to the following infusion schedule: 1.5 mL/kg/hour for 15 minutes, then at 3 mL/kg/hour for the next 15 minutes if the clinical condition does not contraindicate a higher rate, and finally, administer at 6 mL/kg/hour until completion of dose

Dosage Forms Injection: 2500 mg RSV immunoglobulin/50 mL vial

Restoril® *see* temazepam *on page 549*

Retavase™ *see* reteplase *on this page*

reteplase (RE ta plase)

Synonyms recombinant plasminogen activator; r-PA

U.S./Canadian Brand Names Retavase™

Therapeutic Category Thrombolytic Agent

Use Management of acute myocardial infarction

Usual Dosage Adults: I.V.: Given as two (2) bolus doses of 10 units each over a period of 2 minutes (second dose given 30 minutes after the initiation of the first dose)

Dosage Forms Powder for injection, lyophilized: 10.8 units [reteplase 18.8 mg]

Retin-A™ *see* tretinoin (topical) *on page 576*

retinoic acid *see* tretinoin (topical) *on page 576*

Retinova™ (Can) *see* tretinoin (topical) *on page 576*

Retisol-A® (Can) *see* tretinoin (topical) *on page 576*

Retrovir® *see* zidovudine *on page 610*

Reversol® *see* edrophonium *on page 203*

Revex® *see* nalmefene *on page 389*

Rēv-Eyes™ *see* dapiprazole *on page 159*

ReVia® *see* naltrexone *on page 390*

Revitalose C-1000® (Can) *see* ascorbic acid *on page 48*

Rexigen Forte® *see* phendimetrazine *on page 442*

Rezulin® *see* troglitazone *on page 586*

rFVIIa *see* factor VIIa, recombinant *on page 230*

R-Gel® [OTC] *see* capsaicin *on page 96*

R-Gen® *(Discontinued)* *see page 700*

R-Gene® *see* arginine *on page 46*

RGM-CSF *see* sargramostim *on page 515*

Rheaban® [OTC] *see* attapulgite *on page 53*

Rheomacrodex® *see* dextran *on page 170*

Rhesonativ® Injection *(Discontinued)* *see page 700*

Rheumatrex® *see* methotrexate *on page 364*

rhIL-11 *see* oprelvekin *on page 416*

Rhinalar® (Can) *see* flunisolide *on page 243*

Rhinall® Nasal Solution [OTC] *see* phenylephrine *on page 445*

Rhinaris-F® (Can) *see* flunisolide *on page 243*

Rhinatate® Tablet *see* chlorpheniramine, pyrilamine, and phenylephrine *on page 126*

Rhindecon® *(Discontinued)* *see page 700*

Rhinocort® *see* budesonide *on page 82*

Rhinocort® Turbuhaler® (Can) *see* budesonide *on page 82*

Rhinolar® *(Discontinued)* *see page 700*

Rhinosyn-DMX® [OTC] *see* guaifenesin and dextromethorphan *on page 268*

Rhinosyn® Liquid [OTC] *see* chlorpheniramine and pseudoephedrine *on page 122*

Rhinosyn-PD® Liquid [OTC] *see* chlorpheniramine and pseudoephedrine *on page 122*

Rhinosyn-X® Liquid [OTC] *see* guaifenesin, pseudoephedrine, and dextromethorphan *on page 273*

Rh_o(D) immune globulin (intramuscular)

(ar aych oh (dee) i MYUN GLOB yoo lin)

U.S./Canadian Brand Names Gamulin® Rh; HypRho®-D; HypRho®-D Mini-Dose; MICRhoGAM™; Mini-Gamulin® Rh; RhoGAM™

Therapeutic Category Immune Globulin

Use Prevent isoimmunization in Rh-negative individuals exposed to Rh-positive blood during delivery of an Rh-positive infant, as a result of an abortion, following amniocentesis or abdominal trauma, or following a transfusion accident; to prevent hemolytic disease of the newborn if there is a subsequent pregnancy with an Rh-positive fetus

Usual Dosage Adults: I.M.:

Obstetrical usage: 1 vial (300 mcg) prevents maternal sensitization if fetal packed red blood cell volume that has entered the circulation is <15 mL; if it is more, administer additional vials. The number of vials = RBC volume of the calculated fetomaternal hemorrhage divided by 15 mL

Postpartum prophylaxis: 300 mcg within 72 hours of delivery

Antepartum prophylaxis: 300 mcg at approximately 26-28 weeks gestation; followed by 300 mcg within 72 hours of delivery if infant is Rh-positive

Following miscarriage, abortion, or termination of ectopic pregnancy at up to 13 weeks of gestation: 50 mcg ideally within 3 hours, but may be administered up to 72 hours after; if pregnancy has been terminated at 13 or more weeks of gestation, administer 300 mcg

Dosage Forms

Injection: Each package contains one single dose 300 mcg of Rh_o (D) immune globulin

Injection, microdose: Each package contains one single dose of microdose, 50 mcg of Rh_o (D) immune globulin

rh_o(D) immune globulin (intravenous-human)

(ar aych oh (dee) i MYUN GLOB yoo lin in tra VEE nus HYU man)

Synonyms RhoIGIV

U.S./Canadian Brand Names WinRho SD®; WinRho SDF®

Therapeutic Category Immune Globulin

Use

Prevention of Rh isoimmunization in nonsensitized Rho(D) antigen-negative women within 7 hours after spontaneous or induced abortion, amniocentesis, chorionic villus sampling, ruptured tubal pregnancy, abdominal trauma, transplacental hemorrhage, or in the normal course of pregnancy unless the blood type of the fetus or father is known to be Rho(D) antigen-negative

Suppression of Rh isoimmunization in Rho(D) antigen-negative female children and female adults in their childbearing years transfused with Rho(D) antigen-positive RBCs or blood components containing Rho(D) antigen-positive RBCs

Treatment of idiopathic thrombocytopenic purpura (ITP) in nonsplenectomized Rho(D) antigen-positive patients

Usual Dosage

Prevention of Rh isoimmunization:

I.V.: 1500 units (300 mcg) at 28 weeks gestation or immediately after amniocentesis if <34 weeks gestation or after chorionic villus sampling; repeat this dose every 12 weeks during the pregnancy, 600 units (120 mcg) at delivery (within 72 hours) and after invasive intrauterine procedures such as abortion, amniocentesis, or any other manipulation if at >34 weeks gestation. **Note:** If the Rh status of the baby is not known at 72 hours, administer Rho(D) immune globulin to the mother at 72 hours after delivery. If >72 hours have elapsed, do not withhold Rho(D) immune globulin, but administer as soon as possible, up to 28 days after delivery.

I.M.: Reconstitute vial with 1.25 mL and administer as above

Transfusion: Administer within 72 hours after exposure for treatment of incompatible blood transfusions or massive fetal hemorrhage as follows:

I.V.: 3000 units (600 mcg) every 8 hours until the total dose is administered (45 units [9 mcg] of Rh+ blood/mL blood; 90 units [18 mcg] Rh+ red cells/mL cells)

I.M.: 6000 units [1200 mcg] every 12 hours until the total dose is administered (60 units [12 mcg] of Rh+ blood/mL blood; 120 units [24 mcg] Rh+ red cells/mL cells)

Treatment of ITP: I.V.: Initial: 25-50 mcg/kg depending on the patient's Hg concentration; maintenance: 25-60 mcg/kg depending on the clinical response

Dosage Forms Injection: 600 units [120 mcg], 1500 units [300 mcg]

Rhodis® (Can) *see* ketoprofen *on page 321*

Rhodis-EC® (Can) *see* ketoprofen *on page 321*

RhoGAM™ *see* Rh_o(D) immune globulin (intramuscular) *on previous page*

RhoIGIV *see* rh_o(D) immune globulin (intravenous-human) *on this page*

Rhoprolene® (Can) *see* betamethasone (topical) *on page 72*

Rhoprosone® (Can) *see* betamethasone (topical) *on page 72*

Rhotral® (Can) *see* acebutolol *on page 3*

Rhotrimine® (Can) *see* trimipramine *on page 583*

RHUEPO-α *see* epoetin alfa *on page 211*

Rhulicaine® [OTC] *see* benzocaine *on page 66*

Rhuli® Cream *(Discontinued)* *see page 700*

ribavirin (rye ba VYE rin)

Synonyms RTCA; tribavirin

U.S./Canadian Brand Names Virazole® Aerosol

Therapeutic Category Antiviral Agent

Use Treatment of patients with respiratory syncytial virus (RSV) infections; specially indicated for treatment of severe lower respiratory tract RSV infections in patients with an

(Continued)

ribavirin *(Continued)*

underlying compromising condition (prematurity, bronchopulmonary dysplasia and other chronic lung conditions, congenital heart disease, immunodeficiency, immunosuppression), and recent transplant recipients; may also be used in other viral infections including influenza A and B and adenovirus

Usual Dosage Infants, Children, and Adults:

Aerosol inhalation: Use with Viratek® small particle aerosol generator (SPAG-2) at a concentration of 20 mg/mL (6 g reconstituted with 300 mL of sterile water without preservatives)

Aerosol only: 12-18 hours/day for 3 days, up to 7 days in length

Dosage Forms Powder for aerosol: 6 g (100 mL)

riboflavin (RYE boe flay vin)

Synonyms lactoflavin; vitamin B_2; vitamin G

U.S./Canadian Brand Names Riobin®

Therapeutic Category Vitamin, Water Soluble

Use Prevent riboflavin deficiency and treat ariboflavinosis

Usual Dosage Oral:

Riboflavin deficiency:

Children: 2.5-10 mg/day in divided doses

Adults: 5-30 mg/day in divided doses

Required daily allowance: Adults:

Male: 1.4-4.8 mg

Female: 1.2-1.3 mg

Dosage Forms Tablet: 25 mg, 50 mg, 100 mg

Rid-A-Pain® [OTC] *see* benzocaine *on page 66*

Ridaura® *see* auranofin *on page 54*

Ridenol® [OTC] *see* acetaminophen *on page 3*

RID® Shampoo [OTC] *see* pyrethrins *on page 489*

rifabutin (rif a BYOO tin)

Synonyms ansamycin

U.S./Canadian Brand Names Mycobutin®

Therapeutic Category Antibiotic, Miscellaneous

Use Prevention of disseminated *Mycobacterium avium* complex (MAC) in patients with advanced HIV infection; utilized in multiple drug regimens for treatment of MAC

Usual Dosage Oral:

Children: Efficacy and safety of rifabutin have not been established in children; a limited number of HIV-positive children with MAC (n=22) have been given rifabutin for MAC prophylaxis; doses of 5 mg/kg/day have been useful

Adults: 300 mg once daily; for patients who experience gastrointestinal upset, rifabutin can be administered 150 mg twice daily with food

Dosage Forms Capsule: 150 mg

Rifadin® Injection *see* rifampin *on this page*

Rifadin® Oral *see* rifampin *on this page*

Rifamate® *see* rifampin and isoniazid *on next page*

rifampicin *see* rifampin *on this page*

rifampin (RIF am pin)

Synonyms rifampicin

U.S./Canadian Brand Names Rifadin® Injection; Rifadin® Oral; Rimactane® Oral; Rofact™ (Can)

Therapeutic Category Antibiotic, Miscellaneous

Use In combination with other antitubercular drugs for the treatment of active tuberculosis; eliminate meningococci from asymptomatic carriers; prophylaxis in contacts of patients with *Haemophilus influenzae* type B infection; used in combination with other anti-infectives in the treatment of staphylococcal infections

Usual Dosage Oral (I.V. infusion dose is the same as for the oral route):

Tuberculosis:

Children: 10-20 mg/kg/day in divided doses every 12-24 hours

Adults: 10 mg/kg/day; maximum: 600 mg/day

American Thoracic Society and CDC currently recommend twice weekly therapy as part of a short-course regimen which follows 1-2 months of daily treatment of uncomplicated pulmonary tuberculosis in the compliant patient

Children: 10-20 mg/kg/dose (up to 600 mg) twice weekly under supervision to ensure compliance

Adults: 10 mg/kg (up to 600 mg) twice weekly

H. influenzae prophylaxis:

Infants and Children: 20 mg/kg/day every 24 hours for 4 days

Adults: 600 mg every 24 hours for 4 days

Meningococcal prophylaxis:

<1 month: 10 mg/kg/day in divided doses every 12 hours

Infants and Children: 20 mg/kg/day in divided doses every 12 hours for 2 days

Adults: 600 mg every 12 hours for 2 days

Nasal carriers of *Staphylococcus aureus*: Adults: 600 mg/day for 5-10 days in combination with other antibiotics

Dosage Forms

Capsule: 150 mg, 300 mg

Powder for injection: 600 mg (contains a sulfite)

rifampin and isoniazid (RIF am pin & eye soe NYE a zid)

Synonyms isoniazid and rifampin

U.S./Canadian Brand Names Rifamate®

Therapeutic Category Antibiotic, Miscellaneous

Use Management of active tuberculosis; see individual monographs for additional information

Usual Dosage Oral: 2 capsules/day

Dosage Forms Capsule: Rifampin 300 mg and isoniazid 150 mg

rifampin, isoniazid, and pyrazinamide

(RIF am pin , eye soe NYE a zid, & peer a ZIN a mide)

Synonyms isoniazid, rifampin, and pyrazinamide; pyrazinamide, rifampin, and isoniazid

U.S./Canadian Brand Names Rifater®

Therapeutic Category Antibiotic, Miscellaneous

Use Management of active tuberculosis

Usual Dosage Adults: Oral: Patients weighing:

≤44 kg: 4 tablets

45-54 kg: 5 tablets

≥55 kg: 6 tablets

Doses should be administered in a single daily dose

Dosage Forms Tablet: Rifampin 120 mg, isoniazid 50 mg, and pyrazinamide 300 mg

rifapentine (RIF a pen teen)

U.S./Canadian Brand Names Priftin®

Therapeutic Category Antitubercular Agent

Use Treatment of pulmonary tuberculosis (indication is based on the 6-month follow-up treatment outcome observed in controlled clinical trial). Rifapentine must always be used in conjunction with at least one other antituberculosis drug to which the isolate is susceptible; it may also be necessary to add a third agent (either streptomycin or ethambutol) until susceptibility is known.

(Continued)

rifapentine *(Continued)*

Usual Dosage

Children: No dosing information available

Adults: **Rifapentine should not be used alone**; initial phase should include a 3- to 4-drug regimen

Intensive phase of short-term therapy: 600 mg (four 150 mg tablets) given weekly (every 72 hours); following the intensive phase, treatment should continue with rifapentine 600 mg once weekly for 4 months in combination with INH or appropriate agent for susceptible organisms

Dosage Forms Tablet, film-coated: 150 mg

Rifater® *see* rifampin, isoniazid, and pyrazinamide *on previous page*

rIFN-A *see* interferon alfa-2a *on page 308*

RIG *see* rabies immune globulin (human) *on page 494*

rIL-11 *see* oprelvekin *on page 416*

Rilutek® *see* riluzole *on this page*

riluzole (RIL yoo zole)

Synonyms 2-amino-6-trifluoromethoxy-benzothiazole; RP54274

U.S./Canadian Brand Names Rilutek®

Therapeutic Category Miscellaneous Product

Use Treatment of amyotrophic lateral sclerosis (ALS), also known as Lou Gehrig's disease

Usual Dosage Adults: Oral: 50 mg twice daily

Dosage Forms Tablet: 50 mg

Rimactane® Oral *see* rifampin *on page 504*

rimantadine (ri MAN ta deen)

U.S./Canadian Brand Names Flumadine®

Therapeutic Category Antiviral Agent

Use Prophylaxis (adults and children) and treatment (adults) of influenza A viral infection

Usual Dosage Oral:

Prophylaxis:

Children <10 years: 5 mg/kg administered once daily

Children >10 years and Adults: 100 mg twice daily

Treatment: Adults: 100 mg twice daily

Dosage Forms Rimantadine hydrochloride:

Syrup: 50 mg/5 mL (60 mL, 240 mL, 480 mL)

Tablet: 100 mg

rimexolone (ri MEKS oh lone)

U.S./Canadian Brand Names Vexol® Ophthalmic Suspension

Therapeutic Category Adrenal Corticosteroid

Use Treatment of inflammation after ocular surgery and the treatment of anterior uveitis

Usual Dosage Children >2 years and Adults: Ophthalmic: Instill 1-2 drops into conjunctival sac every hour during day, every 2 hours at night until favorable response is obtained, then use 1 drop every 4 hours; for mild to moderate inflammation, instill 1-2 drops into conjunctival sac 2-4 times/day

Dosage Forms Suspension, ophthalmic: 1% (5 mL, 10 mL)

Rimso®-50 *see* dimethyl sulfoxide *on page 183*

Riobin® *see* riboflavin *on page 504*

Riopan® [OTC] *see* magaldrate *on page 344*

Riopan Plus® [OTC] *see* magaldrate and simethicone *on page 344*

risedronate (ris ED roe nate)

U.S./Canadian Brand Names Actonel®

Therapeutic Category Bisphosphonate Derivative

Use Treatment of hypercalcemia associated with malignancy, osteolytic bone lesions of multiple myeloma; also used in postmenopausal osteoporosis; primary hyperparathyroidism and Paget's disease (moderate to severe)

Usual Dosage Adults: Oral: 30 mg once daily for 2 months

Dosage Forms Tablet: 30 mg

Risperdal® *see* risperidone *on this page*

risperidone (ris PER i done)

U.S./Canadian Brand Names Risperdal®

Therapeutic Category Antipsychotic Agent, Benzisoxazole

Use Management of psychotic disorders (eg, schizophrenia)

Usual Dosage Oral: Recommended starting dose: 1 mg twice daily; slowly increase to the optimum range of 4-8 mg/day; daily dosages >10 mg does not appear to confer any additional benefit, and the incidence of extrapyramidal reactions is higher than with lower doses

Dosage Forms

Solution, oral: 1 mg/mL

Tablet: 1 mg, 2 mg, 3 mg, 4 mg

Ritalin® *see* methylphenidate *on page 368*

Ritalin-SR® *see* methylphenidate *on page 368*

ritodrine (RI toe dreen)

U.S./Canadian Brand Names Yutopar®

Therapeutic Category Adrenergic Agonist Agent

Use Inhibit uterine contraction in preterm labor

Usual Dosage Adults:

Oral: Start 30 minutes before stopping I.V. infusion; 10 mg every 2 hours for 24 hours, then 10-20 mg every 4-6 hours up to 120 mg/day. Continue treatment as long as it is desirable to prolong pregnancy.

I.V.: 50-100 mcg/minute; increase by 50 mcg/minute every 10 minutes; continue for 12 hours after contractions have stopped

Dosage Forms Ritodrine hydrochloride:

Injection: 10 mg/mL (5 mL); 15 mg/mL (10 mL)

Tablet: 10 mg

ritonavir (rye TON a veer)

U.S./Canadian Brand Names Norvir®

Therapeutic Category Antiviral Agent

Use Treatment of HIV, especially advanced cases; usually is used as part of triple or double therapy with other nucleoside and protease inhibitors

Usual Dosage Adults: Oral: 600 mg twice daily with meals

Dosage Forms

Capsule: 100 mg

Solution: 80 mg/mL (240 mL)

Rituxan® *see* rituximab *on this page*

rituximab (ri TUK si mab)

Synonyms anti-CD20 monoclonal antibodies; C2B8 monoclonal antibody; Pan-B antibodies

U.S./Canadian Brand Names Rituxan®

Therapeutic Category Antineoplastic Agent

(Continued)

rituximab *(Continued)*

Use Treatment of patients with relapsed or refractory low-grade or follicular, CD20 positive, B-cell non-Hodgkin's lymphoma

Usual Dosage Adults: I.V.: 375 mg/m^2 given as an I.V. infusion once weekly for 4 doses (days 1, 8, 15, and 22); may be administered in an outpatient setting; **do not administer as an intravenous push or bolus**

Dosage Forms Injection: 100 mg (10 mL); 500 mg (10 mL)

Rivotril® (Can) *see* clonazepam *on page 138*

rizatriptan (rye za TRIP tan)

U.S./Canadian Brand Names Maxalt®; Maxalt-MLT™

Therapeutic Category Antimigraine Agent; Serotonin Agonist

Use Acute treatment of migraine with or without aura

Usual Dosage Oral: 10-20 mg, repeat after 2 hours if significant relief is not attained

Dosage Forms Tablet, as benzoate:

Maxalt®: 5 mg, 10 mg

Maxalt-MLT™ (orally disintegrating): 5 mg, 10 mg

rLFN-α2 *see* interferon alfa-2b *on page 308*

RMS® Rectal *see* morphine sulfate *on page 382*

Robafen® AC *see* guaifenesin and codeine *on page 268*

Robafen® CF [OTC] *see* guaifenesin, phenylpropanolamine, and dextromethorphan *on page 271*

Robafen DM® [OTC] *see* guaifenesin and dextromethorphan *on page 268*

Robaxin® *see* methocarbamol *on page 363*

Robaxisal® *see* methocarbamol and aspirin *on page 363*

Robicillin® Tablet *(Discontinued)* *see page 700*

Robidrine® (Can) *see* pseudoephedrine *on page 486*

Robinul® *see* glycopyrrolate *on page 264*

Robinul® Forte *see* glycopyrrolate *on page 264*

Robitet® *(Discontinued)* *see page 700*

Robitet® Oral *see* tetracycline *on page 555*

Robitussin® [OTC] *see* guaifenesin *on page 267*

Robitussin® A-C *see* guaifenesin and codeine *on page 268*

Robitussin-CF® [OTC] *see* guaifenesin, phenylpropanolamine, and dextromethorphan *on page 271*

Robitussin® Cough Calmers [OTC] *see* dextromethorphan *on page 171*

Robitussin®-DAC *see* guaifenesin, pseudoephedrine, and codeine *on page 272*

Robitussin®-DM [OTC] *see* guaifenesin and dextromethorphan *on page 268*

Robitussin-PE® [OTC] *see* guaifenesin and pseudoephedrine *on page 270*

Robitussin® Pediatric [OTC] *see* dextromethorphan *on page 171*

Robitussin® Severe Congestion Liqui-Gels® [OTC] *see* guaifenesin and pseudoephedrine *on page 270*

Rocaltrol® *see* calcitriol *on page 89*

Rocephin® *see* ceftriaxone *on page 109*

rocuronium (roe kyoor OH nee um)

U.S./Canadian Brand Names Zemuron™

Therapeutic Category Skeletal Muscle Relaxant

Use Produces skeletal muscle relaxation during surgery after induction of general anesthesia, increases pulmonary compliance during assisted mechanical respiration, facilitates endotracheal intubation

Usual Dosage I.V.:

Children:

Initial: 0.6 mg/kg under halothane anesthesia produce excellent to good intubating conditions within 1 minute and will provide a median time of 41 minutes of clinical relaxation in children 3 months to 1 year of age, and 27 minutes in children 1-12 years

Maintenance: 0.075-0.125 mg/kg administered upon return of T_1 to 25% of control provides clinical relaxation for 7-10 minutes

Adults:

Tracheal intubation:

Initial: 0.6 mg/kg is expected to provide approximately 31 minutes of clinical relaxation under opioid/nitrous oxide/oxygen anesthesia with neuromuscular block sufficient for intubation attained in 1-2 minutes; lower doses (0.45 mg/kg) may be used to provide 22 minutes of clinical relaxation with median time to neuromuscular block of 1-3 minutes; maximum blockade is achieved in <4 minutes

Maximum: 0.9-1.2 mg/kg may be administered during surgery under opioid/nitrous oxide/oxygen anesthesia without adverse cardiovascular effects and is expected to provide 58-67 minutes of clinical relaxation; neuromuscular blockade sufficient for intubation is achieved in <2 minutes with maximum blockade in <3 minutes

Maintenance: 0.1, 0.15, and 0.2 mg/kg administered at 25% recovery of control T_1 (defined as 3 twitches of train-of-four) provides a median of 12, 17, and 24 minutes of clinical duration under anesthesia

Rapid sequence intubation: 0.6-1.2 mg/kg in appropriately premedicated and anesthetized patients with excellent or good intubating conditions within 2 minutes

Continuous infusion: Initial: 0.01-0.012 mg/kg/minute only after early evidence of spontaneous recovery of neuromuscular function is evident

Dosage Forms Injection, as bromide: 10 mg/mL

Rofact™ (Can) *see* rifampin *on page 504*

rofecoxib (roe fe COX ib)

U.S./Canadian Brand Names Vioxx®

Therapeutic Category Selective Cyclooxygenase-2 Inhibitor

Use Relief of the signs and symptoms of osteoarthritis; management of acute pain in adults; treatment of primary dysmenorrhea

Usual Dosage Adult: Oral:

Osteoarthritis: 12.5 mg once daily; may be increased to a maximum of 25 mg once daily

Acute pain and management of dysmenorrhea: 50 mg once daily as needed (use for longer than 5 days is not recommended)

Dosage Forms

Suspension, oral: 12.5 mg/5 mL (150 mL); 25 mg/5 mL (150 mL)

Tablets: 12.5 mg, 25 mg

Roferon-A® *see* interferon alfa-2a *on page 308*

Rogaine® Topical *see* minoxidil *on page 377*

Rogitine® (Can) *see* phentolamine *on page 445*

Rolaids® [OTC] *see* dihydroxyaluminum sodium carbonate *on page 181*

Rolaids® Calcium Rich [OTC] *see* calcium carbonate *on page 89*

Rolatuss® Plain Liquid *see* chlorpheniramine and phenylephrine *on page 121*

Romazicon® *see* flumazenil *on page 242*

Romycin® Solution *(Discontinued)* *see page 700*

Rondamine-DM® Drops *see* carbinoxamine, pseudoephedrine, and dextromethorphan *on page 99*

Rondec®-DM *see* carbinoxamine, pseudoephedrine, and dextromethorphan *on page 99*

Rondec® Drops *see* carbinoxamine and pseudoephedrine *on page 99*

Rondec® Filmtab® *see* carbinoxamine and pseudoephedrine *on page 99*

Rondec® Syrup *see* carbinoxamine and pseudoephedrine *on page 99*

Rondec-TR® *see* carbinoxamine and pseudoephedrine *on page 99*

Rondomycin® Capsule *(Discontinued)* *see page 700*

ropinirole (roe PIN i role)

U.S./Canadian Brand Names Requip™

Therapeutic Category Anti-Parkinson's Agent

Use Treatment of idiopathic Parkinson's disease; in patients with early Parkinson's disease who were not receiving concomitant levodopa therapy as well as in patients with advanced disease on concomitant levodopa

Usual Dosage Adults: Oral: Dosage should be increased to achieve a maximum therapeutic effect, balanced against the principal side effects of nausea, dizziness, somnolence, and dyskinesia

Recommended starting dose: 0.25 mg 3 times/day; based on individual patient response, the dosage should be titrated with weekly increments

Week 1: 0.25 mg 3 times/day; total daily dose: 0.75 mg

Week 2: 0.5 mg 3 times/day; total daily dose: 1.5 mg

Week 3: 0.75 mg 3 times/day; total daily dose: 2.25 mg

Week 4: 1 mg 3 times/day; total daily dose: 3 mg

After week 4, if necessary, daily dosage may be increased by 1.5 mg/day on a weekly basis up to a dose of 9 mg/day, and then by up to 3 mg/day weekly to a total of 24 mg/day

Dosage Forms Tablet, as hydrochloride: 0.25 mg, 0.5 mg, 1 mg, 2 mg, 5 mg

ropivacaine (roe PIV a kane)

U.S./Canadian Brand Names Naropin™

Therapeutic Category Local Anesthetic

Use Production of local or regional anesthesia for surgery, postoperative pain management and obstetrical procedures by infiltration anesthesia and nerve block anesthesia

Usual Dosage Administer the smallest dose and concentration required to produce the desired result

Dosage Forms Ropivacaine hydrochloride:

Infusion: 2 mg/mL (100 mL, 200 mL)

Injection: (single dose): 2 mg/mL (20 mL); 5 mg/mL (30 mL); 7.5 mg/mL (10 mL, 20 mL); 10 mg/mL (10 mL, 20 mL)

rosiglitazone (roe si GLI ta zone)

U.S./Canadian Brand Names Avandia®

Therapeutic Category Hypoglycemic Agent, Oral; Thiazolidinedione Derivative

Use

Type II diabetes, monotherapy: Improve glycemic control as an adjunct to diet and exercise

Type II diabetes, combination therapy: In combination with metformin when diet, exercise and metformin alone or diet, exercise and rosiglitazone alone do not result in adequate glycemic control.

Usual Dosage Adults: Oral: Initial: 4 mg daily as a single daily dose or in divided doses twice daily. If response is inadequate after 12 weeks of treatment, the dosage may be increased to 8 mg daily as a single daily dose or in divided doses twice daily.

Dosage Forms Tablet: 2 mg, 4 mg

RotaShield® *see* rotavirus vaccine *on next page*

rotavirus vaccine (RO ta vye rus vak SEEN)

U.S./Canadian Brand Names RotaShield®

Therapeutic Category Vaccine

Use Prevention of gastroenteritis caused by the rotavirus serotypes responsible for the majority of disease in infants and children in the U.S. (serotypes G 1,2,3 and 4)

Usual Dosage **For oral administration only**

Children: Three 2.5 mL doses are administered. The recommended schedule for immunization is at 2, 4, and 6 months of age. The first dose may be administered as early as 6 weeks of age, with subsequent doses at least 3 weeks apart. The third dose has been administered to infants up to 33 weeks of age with no increase in adverse reactions. Initiation of vaccination after the age of 6 months is not currently recommended due to an increased risk of fever. RotaShield® does not diminish the efficacy of OPV, DTP, or Hib when administered concurrently. Repeat dosing of vaccine is not recommended if an infant should regurgitate a dose.

Adults: Not approved for administration to adults

Dosage Forms Powder, lyophilized, for oral solution: 2.5 mL diluent (Dispette®); specialized diluent contains citric acid and sodium bicarbonate

Roubac® (Can) *see* co-trimoxazole *on page 149*

Rovamycine® (Can) *see* spiramycin *(Canada only) on page 533*

Rowasa® Rectal *see* mesalamine *on page 358*

Roxanol™ Oral *see* morphine sulfate *on page 382*

Roxanol SR™ Oral *see* morphine sulfate *on page 382*

Roxicet® 5/500 *see* oxycodone and acetaminophen *on page 422*

Roxicodone™ *see* oxycodone *on page 422*

Roxilox® *see* oxycodone and acetaminophen *on page 422*

Roxiprin® *see* oxycodone and aspirin *on page 423*

RP54274 *see* riluzole *on page 506*

RP59500 *see* quinupristin and dalfopristin *on page 493*

r-PA *see* reteplase *on page 501*

RSV-IGIV *see* respiratory syncytial virus immune globulin (intravenous) *on page 501*

R-Tannamine® Tablet *see* chlorpheniramine, pyrilamine, and phenylephrine *on page 126*

R-Tannate® Tablet *see* chlorpheniramine, pyrilamine, and phenylephrine *on page 126*

RTCA *see* ribavirin *on page 503*

rubella and measles vaccines, combined *see* measles and rubella vaccines, combined *on page 350*

rubella and mumps vaccines, combined

(rue BEL a & mumpz vak SEENS, kom BINED)

U.S./Canadian Brand Names Biavax® II

Therapeutic Category Vaccine, Live Virus

Use Promote active immunity to rubella and mumps by inducing production of antibodies

Usual Dosage Children >12 months and Adults: 1 vial in outer aspect of the upper arm

Dosage Forms Injection (mixture of 2 viruses):

1. Wistar RA 27/3 strain of rubella virus
2. Jeryl Lynn (B level) mumps strain grown cell cultures of chick embryo

rubella virus vaccine, live (rue BEL a VYE rus vak SEEN, live)

Synonyms german measles vaccine

U.S./Canadian Brand Names Meruvax® II

(Continued)

rubella virus vaccine, live *(Continued)*

Therapeutic Category Vaccine, Live Virus

Use Provide vaccine-induced immunity to rubella

Usual Dosage S.C.: 1000 $TCID_{50}$ of rubella

Dosage Forms Injection, single dose: 1000 $TCID_{50}$ (Wistar RA 27/3 Strain)

rubeola vaccine *see* measles virus vaccine, live *on page 350*

Rubex® *see* doxorubicin *on page 196*

rubidomycin *see* daunorubicin hydrochloride *on page 160*

Rubramin® (Can) *see* cyanocobalamin *on page 152*

Rubramin-PC® *see* cyanocobalamin *on page 152*

Rufen® ***(Discontinued)*** *see page 700*

Rum-K® *see* potassium chloride *on page 464*

Ru-Tuss® *see* chlorpheniramine, phenylephrine, phenylpropanolamine, and belladonna alkaloids *on page 124*

Ru-Tuss® DE *see* guaifenesin and pseudoephedrine *on page 270*

Ru-Tuss® Expectorant [OTC] *see* guaifenesin, pseudoephedrine, and dextromethorphan *on page 273*

Ru-Tuss® Liquid *see* chlorpheniramine and phenylephrine *on page 121*

Ru-Vert-M® *see* meclizine *on page 351*

Rymed® *see* guaifenesin and pseudoephedrine *on page 270*

Rymed-TR® *see* guaifenesin and phenylpropanolamine *on page 270*

Ryna-C® Liquid *see* chlorpheniramine, pseudoephedrine, and codeine *on page 126*

Rynacrom® (Can) *see* cromolyn sodium *on page 150*

Ryna-CX® *see* guaifenesin, pseudoephedrine, and codeine *on page 272*

Ryna® Liquid [OTC] *see* chlorpheniramine and pseudoephedrine *on page 122*

Rynatan® *see* azatadine and pseudoephedrine *on page 55*

Rynatan® Pediatric Suspension *see* chlorpheniramine, pyrilamine, and phenylephrine *on page 126*

Rynatan® Tablet *see* chlorpheniramine, pyrilamine, and phenylephrine *on page 126*

Rynatuss® Pediatric Suspension *see* chlorpheniramine, ephedrine, phenylephrine, and carbetapentane *on page 123*

Rythmodan®, -LA (Can) *see* disopyramide *on page 189*

Rythmol® *see* propafenone *on page 480*

Sabin vaccine *see* poliovirus vaccine, live, trivalent, oral *on page 459*

Sabulin® (Can) *see* albuterol *on page 15*

sacrosidase (sak RO se dase)

U.S./Canadian Brand Names Sucraid™

Therapeutic Category Enzyme

Use An enzyme replacement therapy for the treatment of the genetically determined sucrase deficiency, which is part of congenital sucrase-isomaltase deficiency (CSID)

Usual Dosage Oral:

<15 kg: 1 mL [8500 int. units] (one full measuring scoop or 22 drops) per meal or snack

>15 kg: 2 mL [17,000 int. units] (two full measuring scoops or 44 drops) per meal or snack

It is recommended that approximately half of the dosage be taken at the beginning of each meal or snack, and the remainder be taken at the end of each meal or snack.

The beverage or infant formula should be served cold or at room temperature; the beverage or infant formula should not be warmed or heated before or after addition of sacrosidase

Dosage Forms Solution, oral: 8500 int. units/mL (118 mL)

Safe Tussin® 30 [OTC] *see* guaifenesin and dextromethorphan *on page 268*

Saizen® *see* human growth hormone *on page 283*

Salac™ (Can) *see* salicylic acid *on this page*

Salacid® Ointment *see* salicylic acid *on this page*

Sal-Acid® Plaster *see* salicylic acid *on this page*

Salagen® Oral *see* pilocarpine *on page 451*

Salazopyrin® (Can) *see* sulfasalazine *on page 542*

Salazopyrin EN-Tabs® (Can) *see* sulfasalazine *on page 542*

salbutamol *see* albuterol *on page 15*

Saleto-200® [OTC] *see* ibuprofen *on page 300*

Saleto-400® *see* ibuprofen *on page 300*

Salflex® *see* salsalate *on page 515*

Salgesic® *see* salsalate *on page 515*

salicylazosulfapyridine *see* sulfasalazine *on page 542*

salicylic acid (sal i SIL ik AS id)

U.S./Canadian Brand Names Acnex® (Can); Acnomel® (Can); Clear Away® Disc [OTC]; Duoforte® 27 (Can); Freezone® Solution [OTC]; Gordofilm® Liquid; Mediplast® Plaster [OTC]; Occlusal®-HP Liquid; Panscol® Lotion [OTC]; Panscol® Ointment [OTC]; PediaPatch Transdermal Patch [OTC]; P&S® Shampoo [OTC]; Salac™ (Can); Salacid® Ointment; Sal-Acid® Plaster; Sebcur® (Can); Soluver® (Can); Trans-Plantar® (Can); Trans-Plantar® Transdermal Patch [OTC]; Trans-Ver-Sal® Transdermal Patch [OTC]; Vergogel® Gel [OTC]; Verukan® Solution; X-Seb™ (Can)

Therapeutic Category Keratolytic Agent

Use Topically for its keratolytic effect in controlling seborrheic dermatitis or psoriasis of body and scalp, dandruff, and other scaling dermatoses; to remove warts, corns, calluses; also used in the treatment of acne

Usual Dosage

Shampoo: Apply to scalp and allow to remain for a few minutes, then rinse, initially use every day or every other day; 2 treatments/week are usually sufficient to maintain control

Topical: Apply to affected area and place under occlusion at night; hydrate skin for at least 5 minutes before use

Dosage Forms

Cream: 2% (30 g)
Disk: 40%
Gel: 5% (60 g); 6% (30 g); 17% (7.5 g)
Liquid: 13.6% (9.3 mL); 17% (9.3 mL, 13.5 mL, 15 mL); 16.7% (15 mL)
Lotion: 3% (120 mL)
Ointment: 3% (90 g)
Patch, transdermal: 15% (20 mm); 40% (20 mm)
Plaster: 40%
Soap: 2% (97.5 g)
Strip: 40%

salicylic acid and benzoic acid *see* benzoic acid and salicylic acid *on page 67*

salicylic acid and lactic acid (sal i SIL ik AS id & LAK tik AS id)

Synonyms lactic acid and salicylic acid

U.S./Canadian Brand Names Duofilm® Solution

Therapeutic Category Keratolytic Agent

Use Treatment of benign epithelial tumors such as warts

Usual Dosage Topical: Apply a thin layer directly to wart once daily (may be useful to apply at bedtime and wash off in morning)

Dosage Forms Solution, topical: Salicylic acid 16.7% and lactic acid 16.7% in flexible collodion (15 mL)

salicylic acid and podophyllin *see* podophyllin and salicylic acid *on page 458*

salicylic acid and propylene glycol
(sal i SIL ik AS id & PROE pi leen GLYE cole)

Synonyms propylene glycol and salicylic acid

U.S./Canadian Brand Names Keralyt® Gel

Therapeutic Category Keratolytic Agent

Use Removal of excessive keratin in hyperkeratotic skin disorders, including various ichthyosis, keratosis palmaris and plantaris and psoriasis; may be used to remove excessive keratin in dorsal and plantar hyperkeratotic lesions

Usual Dosage Topical: Apply to area at night after soaking region for at least 5 minutes to hydrate area, and place under occlusion; medication is washed off in morning

Dosage Forms Gel, topical: Salicylic acid 6% and propylene glycol 60% in ethyl alcohol 19.4% with hydroxypropyl methylcellulose and water (30 g)

salicylic acid and sulfur *see* sulfur and salicylic acid *on page 543*

Saline from Otrivin® (Can) *see* sodium chloride *on page 526*

SalineX® [OTC] *see* sodium chloride *on page 526*

Salivart® Solution [OTC] *see* saliva substitute *on this page*

saliva substitute (sa LYE va SUB stee tute)

U.S./Canadian Brand Names Entertainer's Secret® Spray [OTC]; Moi-Stir® Solution [OTC]; Moi-Stir® Swabsticks [OTC]; Mouthkote® Solution [OTC]; Optimoist® Solution [OTC]; Salivart® Solution [OTC]; Salix® Lozenge [OTC]

Therapeutic Category Gastrointestinal Agent, Miscellaneous

Use Relief of dry mouth and throat in xerostomia

Usual Dosage Use as needed

Dosage Forms

Lozenge: 100s

Solution: 60 mL, 75 mL, 120 mL, 180 mL, 240 mL

Swabstix: 3s

Salix® Lozenge [OTC] *see* saliva substitute *on this page*

Salk vaccine *see* poliovirus vaccine, inactivated *on page 458*

salmeterol (sal ME te role)

U.S./Canadian Brand Names Serevent®; Serevent® Diskus®

Therapeutic Category Adrenergic Agonist Agent

Use Maintenance treatment of asthma; prevention of bronchospasm in patients >12 years of age with reversible obstructive airway disease, including patients with symptoms of nocturnal asthma who require regular treatment with inhaled, short-acting $beta_2$ agonists; prevention of exercise-induced bronchospasm

Usual Dosage

Inhalation: 42 mcg (2 puffs) twice daily (12 hours apart) for maintenance and prevention of symptoms of asthma

Prevention of exercise-induced asthma: 42 mcg (2 puffs) 30-60 minutes prior to exercise; additional doses should not be used for 12 hours

Dosage Forms Aerosol, oral, as xinafoate: 21 mcg/spray [60 inhalations] (6.5 g), [120 inhalations] (13 g)

Salmonine® *see* calcitonin *on page 88*

salsalate (SAL sa late)

Synonyms disalicylic acid

U.S./Canadian Brand Names Argesic®-SA; Artha-G®; Disalcid®; Marthritic®; Mono-Gesic®; Salflex®; Salgesic®; Salsitab®

Therapeutic Category Analgesic, Non-narcotic; Antipyretic; Nonsteroidal Anti-inflammatory Drug (NSAID)

Use Treatment of minor pain or fever; rheumatoid arthritis, osteoarthritis, and related inflammatory conditions

Usual Dosage Adults: Oral: 1 g 2-4 times/day

Dosage Forms

Capsule: 500 mg

Tablet: 500 mg, 750 mg

Salsitab® *see* salsalate *on this page*

salt *see* sodium chloride *on page 526*

Saluron® *see* hydroflumethiazide *on page 293*

Salutensin® *see* hydroflumethiazide and reserpine *on page 293*

Sandimmune® *see* cyclosporine *on page 154*

Sandoglobulin® *see* immune globulin, intravenous *on page 303*

Sandosource™ Peptide (Can), Sustacal® (Can) *see* enteral nutritional products *on page 208*

Sandostatin® *see* octreotide *on page 413*

Sandostatin LAR® *see* octreotide *on page 413*

SangCya™ *see* cyclosporine *on page 154*

Sani-Supp® Suppository [OTC] *see* glycerin *on page 263*

Sanorex® *see* mazindol *on page 349*

Sansert® *see* methysergide *on page 370*

Santyl® *see* collagenase *on page 146*

saquinavir (sa KWIN a veer)

U.S./Canadian Brand Names Fortovase®; Invirase®

Therapeutic Category Antiviral Agent

Use Treatment of advanced HIV infection, used in combination with older nucleoside analog medications

Usual Dosage Adults: Oral:

Fortovase®: Six 200 mg (1200 mg) capsules 3 times/day within 2 hours after a meal

Invirase®: Three 200 mg (600 mg) capsules 3 times/day within 2 hours after a full meal

Dosage Forms

Capsule (hard) as mesylate (Invirase®): 200 mg

Capsule (soft) (Fortovase®): 200 mg

sargramostim (sar GRAM oh stim)

Synonyms GM-CSF; granulocyte-macrophage colony-stimulating factor; RGM-CSF

U.S./Canadian Brand Names Leukine™

Therapeutic Category Colony-Stimulating Factor

Use Myeloid reconstitution after autologous bone marrow transplantation; to accelerate myeloid recovery in patients with non-Hodgkin's lymphoma, Hodgkin's lymphoma, and

(Continued)

sargramostim *(Continued)*

acute lymphoblastic leukemia undergoing autologous BMT; following induction chemotherapy in patients with acute myelogenous leukemia to shorten time to neutrophil recovery

Usual Dosage

Children and Adults (may also administer S.C.):

Bone marrow transplant: I.V.: 250 mcg/m^2/day over at least 2 hours to begin 2-4 hours after the marrow infusion on day 0 of autologous bone marrow transplant or not <24 hours after chemotherapy or 12 hours after last dose of radiotherapy. If significant adverse effects or "first dose" reaction is seen at this dose, discontinue the drug until toxicity resolves, then restart at a reduced dose of 125 mcg/m^2/day

Cancer chemotherapy recovery: I.V.: 3-15 mcg/kg/day over at least 2 hours for 14-21 days; maximum daily dose is 15 mcg/kg/day due to dose-related adverse effects

Discontinue therapy if the ANC count is >20,000/mm^3.

Excessive blood counts return to normal or baseline levels within 3-7 days following cessation of therapy.

Length of therapy: Bone marrow transplant patients: GM-CSF should be administered daily for up to 30 days or until the ANC has reached 1000/mm^3 for 3 consecutive days following the expected chemotherapy-induced neutrophil-nadir.

Dosage Forms Injection: 250 mcg, 500 mcg

Sarna [OTC] *see* camphor, menthol, and phenol *on page 94*

S.A.S™ (Can) *see* sulfasalazine *on page 542*

SAStid® Plain Therapeutic Shampoo and Acne Wash [OTC] *see* sulfur and salicylic acid *on page 543*

Scabene® ***(Discontinued)*** *see page 700*

Scalpicin® Topical *see* hydrocortisone (topical) *on page 292*

Sclavo - PPD® Solution ***(Discontinued)*** *see page 700*

Sclavo Test - PPD® ***(Discontinued)*** *see page 700*

Scleromate™ *see* morrhuate sodium *on page 383*

Scopace® Tablet *see* scopolamine *on this page*

scopolamine (skoe POL a meen)

Synonyms hyoscine

U.S./Canadian Brand Names Isopto® Hyoscine; Scopace® Tablet; Transdermal-V® (Can); Transderm Scop®

Therapeutic Category Anticholinergic Agent

Use Preoperative medication to produce amnesia and decrease salivary and respiratory secretions; to produce cycloplegia and mydriasis; treatment of iridocyclitis; prevention of motion sickness; prevention of nausea/vomiting associated with anesthesia or opiate analgesia (patch)

Usual Dosage

Preoperatively:

Children: I.M., S.C.: 6 mcg/kg/dose (maximum: 0.3 mg/dose) or 0.2 mg/m^2 may be repeated every 6-8 hours **or** alternatively:

4-7 months: 0.1 mg

7 months to 3 years: 0.15 mg

3-8 years: 0.2 mg

8-12 years: 0.3 mg

Adults: I.M., I.V., S.C.: 0.3-0.65 mg; may be repeated every 4-6 hours

Motion sickness: Transdermal: Children >12 years and Adults: Apply 1 disc behind the ear at least 4 hours prior to exposure and every 3 days as needed

Ophthalmic:

Refraction:

Children: Instill 1 drop of 0.25% to eye(s) twice daily for 2 days before procedure

Adults: Instill 1-2 drops of 0.25% to eye(s) 1 hour before procedure

Iridocyclitis:
Children: Instill 1 drop of 0.25% to eye(s) up to 3 times/day
Adults: Instill 1-2 drops of 0.25% to eye(s) up to 4 times/day

Dosage Forms
Disc, transdermal: 1.5 mg/disc (4's)
Injection, as hydrobromide: 0.3 mg/mL (1 mL); 0.4 mg/mL (0.5 mL, 1 mL); 0.86 mg/mL (0.5 mL); 1 mg/mL (1 mL)
Solution, ophthalmic, as hydrobromide: 0.25% (5 mL, 15 mL)
Tablet: 0.4 mg

scopolamine and phenylephrine *see* phenylephrine and scopolamine *on page 447*

scopolamine, hyoscyamine, atropine, and phenobarbital *see* hyoscyamine, atropine, scopolamine, and phenobarbital *on page 298*

Scot-Tussin® [OTC] *see* guaifenesin *on page 267*

Scot-Tussin DM® Cough Chasers [OTC] *see* dextromethorphan *on page 171*

Scot-Tussin® Senior Clear [OTC] *see* guaifenesin and dextromethorphan *on page 268*

SeaMist® [OTC] *see* sodium chloride *on page 526*

Sebcur® (Can) *see* salicylic acid *on page 513*

Sebulex® *(Discontinued)* *see page 700*

Sebulon® *(Discontinued)* *see page 700*

secobarbital (see koe BAR bi tal)

Synonyms quinalbarbitone
U.S./Canadian Brand Names Novo-Secobarb® (Can); Seconal™ Injection
Therapeutic Category Barbiturate
Controlled Substance C-II
Use Short-term treatment of insomnia and as preanesthetic agent
Usual Dosage Hypnotic:
Children: I.M.: 3-5 mg/kg/dose; maximum: 100 mg/dose
Adults:
I.M.: 100-200 mg/dose
I.V.: 50-250 mg/dose
Dosage Forms Injection, as sodium: 50 mg/mL (2 mL)

secobarbital and amobarbital *see* amobarbital and secobarbital *on page 31*

Seconal™ Injection *see* secobarbital *on this page*

Seconal™ Oral *(Discontinued)* *see page 700*

Secran® *see* vitamin, multiple (oral) *on page 604*

secretin (SEE kre tin)

U.S./Canadian Brand Names Secretin-Ferring Powder
Therapeutic Category Diagnostic Agent
Use Diagnosis of Zollinger-Ellison syndrome, chronic pancreatic dysfunction, and some hepatobiliary diseases such as obstructive jaundice resulting from cancer or stones in the biliary tract
Usual Dosage I.V.:
Pancreatic function: 1 CU/kg slow I.V. injection over 1 minute
Zollinger-Ellison: 2 CU/kg slow I.V. injection over 1 minute
Dosage Forms Powder for injection: 75 units (10 mL)

Secretin-Ferring Powder *see* secretin *on this page*

Sectral® *see* acebutolol *on page 3*

Sedapap-10® *see* butalbital compound and acetaminophen *on page 85*

Selax® (Can) *see* docusate *on page 191*

Seldane® *see* terfenadine *on page 551*

Seldane-D® ***(Discontinued)*** *see page 700*

Seldane® ***(Discontinued)*** *see page 700*

Selecor® ***(Discontinued)*** *see page 700*

selegiline (seh LEDGE ah leen)

Synonyms deprenyl; *l*-deprenyl

U.S./Canadian Brand Names Eldepryl®; Novo-Selegiline (Can)

Therapeutic Category Anti-Parkinson's Agent; Dopaminergic Agent (Anti-Parkinson's)

Use Adjunct in the management of Parkinsonian patients in which levodopa/carbidopa therapy is deteriorating

Unlabeled uses: Early Parkinson's disease, Alzheimer's disease

Usual Dosage Adults: Oral: 5 mg twice daily

Dosage Forms

Capsule, as hydrochloride (Eldepryl®): 5 mg

Tablet: 5 mg

selenium sulfide (se LEE nee um SUL fide)

U.S./Canadian Brand Names Exsel® Shampoo; Selsun Blue® Shampoo [OTC]; Selsun® Shampoo; Versel™ (Can)

Therapeutic Category Antiseborrheic Agent, Topical

Use Treat itching and flaking of the scalp associated with dandruff; to control scalp seborrheic dermatitis; treatment of tinea versicolor

Usual Dosage Topical:

Dandruff, seborrhea: Massage 5-10 mL into wet scalp, leave on scalp 2-3 minutes, rinse thoroughly and repeat application; shampoo twice weekly for 2 weeks initially, then use once every 1-4 weeks as indicated depending upon control

Tinea versicolor: Apply the 2.5% lotion to affected area and lather with small amounts of water; leave on skin for 10 minutes, then rinse thoroughly; apply every day for 7 days

Dosage Forms Shampoo: 1% (120 mL, 210 mL, 240 mL, 330 mL); 2.5% (120 mL)

Sele-Pak® *see* trace metals *on page 573*

Selepen® *see* trace metals *on page 573*

Selestoject® (Can) *see* betamethasone (systemic) *on page 71*

Selestoject® ***(Discontinued)*** *see page 700*

Selsun Blue® Shampoo [OTC] *see* selenium sulfide *on this page*

Selsun® Shampoo *see* selenium sulfide *on this page*

Semicid® [OTC] *see* nonoxynol 9 *on page 406*

Semprex®-D *see* acrivastine and pseudoephedrine *on page 10*

senna (SEN na)

U.S./Canadian Brand Names Black Draught® [OTC]; Glysennid® (Can); Senna-Gen® [OTC]; Senokot® [OTC]; X-Prep® Liquid [OTC]

Therapeutic Category Laxative

Use Short-term treatment of constipation; evacuate the colon for bowel or rectal examinations

Usual Dosage

Children:

Oral:

>6 years: 10-20 mg/kg/dose at bedtime; maximum daily dose: 872 mg

6-12 years, >27 kg: 1 tablet at bedtime, up to 4 tablets/day **or** ½ teaspoonful of granules (326 mg/tsp) at bedtime (up to 2 teaspoonfuls/day)

Liquid:

2-5 years: 5-10 mL at bedtime

6-15 years: 10-15 mL at bedtime
Suppository: 1/2 at bedtime
Syrup:
1 month to 1 year: 1.25-2.5 mL at bedtime up to 5 mL/day
1-5 years: 2.5-5 mL at bedtime up to 10 mL/day
5-10 years: 5-10 mL at bedtime up to 20 mL/day
Adults:
Granules (326 mg/teaspoon): 1 teaspoonful at bedtime, not to exceed 2 teaspoonfuls twice daily
Liquid: 15-30 mL with meals and at bedtime
Suppository: 1 at bedtime, may repeat once in 2 hours
Syrup: 2-3 teaspoonfuls at bedtime, not to exceed 30 mL/day
Tablet: 187 mg: 2 tablets at bedtime, not to exceed 8 tablets/day
Tablet: 374 mg: 1 at bedtime, up to 4/day; 600 mg: 2 tablets at bedtime, up to 3 tablets/day

Dosage Forms
Granules: 326 mg/teaspoonful
Liquid: 7% [70 mg/mL] (130 mL, 360 mL); 6.5% [65 mg/mL] (75 mL, 150 mL)
Suppository, rectal: 652 mg
Syrup: 218 mg/5 mL (60 mL, 240 mL)
Tablet: 187 mg, 217 mg, 600 mg

Senna-Gen® [OTC] *see* senna *on previous page*

Senokot® [OTC] *see* senna *on previous page*

Senolax® ***(Discontinued)*** *see page 700*

Sensorcaine® *see* bupivacaine *on page 83*

Sensorcaine®-MPF *see* bupivacaine *on page 83*

Septa® Topical Ointment [OTC] *see* bacitracin, neomycin, and polymyxin B *on page 59*

Septisol® *see* hexachlorophene *on page 281*

Septra® *see* co-trimoxazole *on page 149*

Septra® DS *see* co-trimoxazole *on page 149*

Ser-Ap-Es® *see* hydralazine, hydrochlorothiazide, and reserpine *on page 285*

Serax® *see* oxazepam *on page 420*

Serc® (Can) *see* betahistine *(Canada only) on page 71*

Serentil® *see* mesoridazine *on page 358*

Serevent® *see* salmeterol *on page 514*

Serevent® Diskus® *see* salmeterol *on page 514*

sermorelin acetate (ser moe REL in AS e tate)

U.S./Canadian Brand Names Geref®
Therapeutic Category Diagnostic Agent
Use Evaluate ability of the somatotroph of the pituitary gland to secrete growth hormone
Usual Dosage I.V. (in a single dose in the morning following an overnight fast):
Children or subjects <50 kg: Draw venous blood samples for GH determinations 15 minutes before and immediately prior to administration, then administer 1 mcg/kg followed by a 3 mL normal saline flush, draw blood samples again for GH determinations
Adults or subjects >50 kg: Determine the number of ampules needed based on a dose of 1 mcg/kg, draw venous blood samples for GH determinations 15 minutes before and immediately prior to administration, then administer 1 mcg/kg followed by a 3 mL normal saline flush, draw blood samples again for GH determinations
Dosage Forms Powder for injection, lyophilized: 50 mcg

Seromycin® Pulvules® *see* cycloserine *on page 154*

Serophene® *see* clomiphene *on page 138*

Seroquel® *see* quetiapine *on page 491*

Serostim® *see* human growth hormone *on page 283*

Serpalan® *see* reserpine *on page 500*

Serpasil® ***(Discontinued)*** *see page 700*

Sertan® **(Can)** *see* primidone *on page 474*

sertraline (SER tra leen)

U.S./Canadian Brand Names Zoloft™

Therapeutic Category Antidepressant, Selective Serotonin Reuptake Inhibitor

Use Treatment of major depression; pediatric obsessive-compulsive disorder; also being studied for use in obesity

Usual Dosage Oral: Initial: 50 mg/day as a single dose, dosage may be increased at intervals of at least 1 week to a maximum recommended dosage of 200 mg/day

Dosage Forms Tablet, as hydrochloride: 25 mg, 50 mg, 100 mg

Serutan® **[OTC]** *see* psyllium *on page 488*

Serzone® *see* nefazodone *on page 393*

sevelamer (se VEL a mer)

U.S./Canadian Brand Names Renagel®

Therapeutic Category Phosphate Binder

Use Reduction of serum phosphorous in patients with end-stage renal disease

Usual Dosage Adults: Oral: 2-4 capsules 3 times/day with meals; the initial dose may be based on serum phosphorous:

(Phosphorous: Initial dose)

>6.0 and <7.5: 2 capsules 3 times/day

>7.5 and <9.0: 3 capsules 3 times/day

≥ 9.0: 4 capsules 3 times/day

Dosage should be adjusted based on serum phosphorous concentration, with a goal of lowering to <6.0 mg/dL; maximum daily dose studied was 30 capsules/day

Dosage Forms Capsule: 403 mg

sevoflurane (see voe FLOO rane)

U.S./Canadian Brand Names Ultane®

Therapeutic Category General Anesthetic

Use General induction and maintenance of anesthesia (inhalation)

Usual Dosage Surgical levels of anesthesia can usually be obtained with concentrations of 0.5% to 3%

Dosage Forms Liquid for inhalation: 250 mL

Shur-Seal® **[OTC]** *see* nonoxynol 9 *on page 406*

Siblin® ***(Discontinued)*** *see page 700*

sibutramine (si BYOO tra meen)

U.S./Canadian Brand Names Meridia™

Therapeutic Category Anorexiant

Use Management of obesity, including weight loss and maintenance of weight loss, and should be used in conjunction with a reduced calorie diet

Usual Dosage Adults ≥16 years: Initial: 10 mg once daily; after 4 weeks may titrate up to 15 mg once daily as needed and tolerated

Dosage Forms Capsule, as hydrochloride monohydrate: 5 mg, 10 mg, 15 mg

Silace-C® **[OTC]** *see* docusate and casanthranol *on page 191*

Siladryl® **Oral [OTC]** *see* diphenhydramine *on page 185*

Silafed® Syrup [OTC] *see* triprolidine and pseudoephedrine *on page 584*

Silain® [OTC] *see* simethicone *on next page*

Silaminic® Cold Syrup [OTC] *see* chlorpheniramine and phenylpropanolamine *on page 122*

Silaminic® Expectorant [OTC] *see* guaifenesin and phenylpropanolamine *on page 270*

Silapap® [OTC] *see* acetaminophen *on page 3*

sildenafil (sil DEN a fil)

Synonyms UK 92480

U.S./Canadian Brand Names Viagra®

Therapeutic Category Phosphodiesterase Enzyme Inhibitor

Use Effective in most men with erectile dysfunction (ED), the medical term for impotence, which is associated with a broad range of physical or psychological medical conditions.

Usual Dosage Oral: Adults: 50 mg taken one hour before sexual activity; individuals may need more (100 mg) or less (25 mg) and dosing should be determined by a physician depending on effectiveness and side effects. The drug should not be used more than once daily.

Dosage Forms Tablet, as citrate: 25 mg, 50 mg, 100 mg

Sildicon-E® [OTC] *see* guaifenesin and phenylpropanolamine *on page 270*

Silphen® Cough [OTC] *see* diphenhydramine *on page 185*

Silphen DM® [OTC] *see* dextromethorphan *on page 171*

Siltussin® [OTC] *see* guaifenesin *on page 267*

Siltussin-CF® [OTC] *see* guaifenesin, phenylpropanolamine, and dextromethorphan *on page 271*

Siltussin DM® [OTC] *see* guaifenesin and dextromethorphan *on page 268*

Silvadene® *see* silver sulfadiazine *on next page*

silver nitrate (SIL ver NYE trate)

Synonyms $AgNO_3$

U.S./Canadian Brand Names Dey-Drop® Ophthalmic Solution

Therapeutic Category Topical Skin Product

Use Prevention of gonococcal ophthalmia neonatorum; cauterization of wounds and sluggish ulcers, removal of granulation tissue and warts

Usual Dosage

Neonates: Ophthalmic: Instill 2 drops immediately after birth into conjunctival sac of each eye as a single dose; do not irrigate eyes following instillation of eye drops

Children and Adults:

Sticks: Apply to mucous membranes and other moist skin surfaces only on area to be treated 2-3 times/week for 2-3 weeks

Topical solution: Apply a cotton applicator dipped in solution on the affected area 2-3 times/week for 2-3 weeks

Dosage Forms

Applicator, topical: 75% with potassium nitrate 25% (6")

Ointment, topical: 10% (30 g)

Solution:

Ophthalmic: 1% (wax ampuls)

Topical: 10% (30 mL); 25% (30 mL); 50% (30 mL)

silver protein, mild (SIL ver PRO teen mild)

Therapeutic Category Antibiotic, Topical

Use Stain and coagulate mucus in eye surgery which is then removed by irrigation; eye infections

(Continued)

silver protein, mild *(Continued)*

Usual Dosage

Preop in eye surgery: Place 2-3 drops into eye(s), then rinse out with sterile irrigating solution

Eye infections: 1-3 drops into the affected eye(s) every 3-4 hours for several days

Dosage Forms Solution, ophthalmic: 20% (15 mL, 30 mL)

silver sulfadiazine (SIL ver sul fa DYE a zeen)

U.S./Canadian Brand Names Dermazin™ (Can); Flamazine® (Can); Silvadene®; SSD® AF; SSD® Cream; Thermazene®

Therapeutic Category Antibacterial, Topical

Use Adjunct in the prevention and treatment of infection in second and third degree burns

Usual Dosage Children and Adults: Topical: Apply once or twice daily with a sterile gloved hand; apply to a thickness of $^1/_{16}$"; burned area should be covered with cream at all times

Dosage Forms Cream, topical: 1% [10 mg/g] (20 g, 50 g, 100 g, 400 g, 1000 g)

simethicone (sye METH i kone)

Synonyms activated dimethicone; activated methylpolysiloxane

U.S./Canadian Brand Names Degas® [OTC]; Flatulex® [OTC]; Gas-X® [OTC]; Maalox Anti-Gas® [OTC]; Mylanta Gas® [OTC]; Mylicon® [OTC]; Ovol® (Can); Phazyme® [OTC]; Silain® [OTC]

Therapeutic Category Antiflatulent

Use Relieve flatulence, functional gastric bloating, and postoperative gas pains

Usual Dosage Oral:

Infants: 20 mg 4 times/day

Children <12 years: 40 mg 4 times/day

Children >12 years and Adults: 40-120 mg after meals and at bedtime as needed, not to exceed 500 mg/day

Dosage Forms

Capsule: 125 mg

Drops, oral: 40 mg/0.6 mL (30 mL)

Tablet: 50 mg, 60 mg, 95 mg

Chewable: 40 mg, 80 mg, 125 mg

simethicone and calcium carbonate *see* calcium carbonate and simethicone *on page 90*

simethicone and magaldrate *see* magaldrate and simethicone *on page 344*

Simron® [OTC] *see* ferrous gluconate *on page 236*

Simulect® *see* basiliximab *on page 61*

simvastatin (SIM va stat in)

U.S./Canadian Brand Names Zocor®

Therapeutic Category HMG-CoA Reductase Inhibitor

Use Adjunct to dietary therapy to decrease elevated serum total and LDL cholesterol concentrations in primary hypercholesterolemia; lowering elevated triglyceride levels

Usual Dosage Adults: Oral: Start with 5-10 mg/day as a single bedtime dose; starting dose of 5 mg/day should be considered for patients with LDL-C of ≤190 mg/dL and for the elderly; patients with LDL-C levels >190 mg/dL should be started on 10 mg/day; adjustments of dosage should be made at intervals of 4 weeks or more; maximum recommended dose: 40 mg/day

Dosage Forms Tablet: 5 mg, 10 mg, 20 mg, 40 mg

Sinarest® 12 Hour Nasal Solution *see* oxymetazoline *on page 423*

Sinarest® Nasal Solution [OTC] *see* phenylephrine *on page 445*

Sinarest®, No Drowsiness [OTC] *see* acetaminophen and pseudoephedrine *on page 5*

sincalide (SIN ka lide)

Synonyms C8-CCK; OP-CCK

U.S./Canadian Brand Names Kinevac®

Therapeutic Category Diagnostic Agent

Use Postevacuation cholecystography; gallbladder bile sampling; stimulate pancreatic secretion for analysis

Usual Dosage Adults: I.V.:

Contraction of gallbladder: 0.02 mcg/kg over 30 seconds to 1 minute, may repeat in 15 minutes a 0.04 mcg/kg dose

Pancreatic function: 0.02 mcg/kg over 30 minutes

Dosage Forms Injection: 5 mcg

Sine-Aid® IB [OTC] *see* pseudoephedrine and ibuprofen *on page 487*

Sine-Aid®, Maximum Strength [OTC] *see* acetaminophen and pseudoephedrine *on page 5*

Sinemet® *see* levodopa and carbidopa *on page 331*

Sine-Off® Maximum Strength No Drowsiness Formula [OTC] *see* acetaminophen and pseudoephedrine *on page 5*

Sinequan® Oral *see* doxepin *on page 195*

Sinex® Long-Acting [OTC] *see* oxymetazoline *on page 423*

Singulair® *see* montelukast *on page 381*

Sinografin® *see* radiological/contrast media (ionic) *on page 495*

Sintrom® (Can) *see* nicoumalone *(Canada only) on page 401*

Sinubid® *see* phenyltoloxamine, phenylpropanolamine, and acetaminophen *on page 448*

Sinufed® Timecelles® *see* guaifenesin and pseudoephedrine *on page 270*

Sinumist®-SR Capsulets® *see* guaifenesin *on page 267*

Sinupan® *see* guaifenesin and phenylephrine *on page 269*

Sinus Excedrin® Extra Strength [OTC] *see* acetaminophen and pseudoephedrine *on page 5*

Sinus-Relief® [OTC] *see* acetaminophen and pseudoephedrine *on page 5*

Sinutab® Tablets [OTC] *see* acetaminophen, chlorpheniramine, and pseudoephedrine *on page 6*

Sinutab® Without Drowsiness [OTC] *see* acetaminophen and pseudoephedrine *on page 5*

sirolimus (sir OH li mus)

U.S./Canadian Brand Names Rapamune®

Therapeutic Category Immunosuppressant Agent

Use Prophylaxis of organ rejection in patients receiving renal transplants, in combination with cyclosporin and corticosteroids

Usual Dosage Oral:

Adults ≥40 kg: Loading dose: For *de novo* transplant recipients, a loading dose of 3 times the daily maintenance dose should be administered on day 1 of dosing. Maintenance dose: 2 mg/day. Doses should be taken 4 hours after cyclosporine, and should be taken consistently either with or without food.

Children ≥13 years or Adults <40 kg: Loading dose: 3 mg/m^2 (day 1); followed by a maintenance of 1 mg/m^2/day.

Dosage Forms Solution, oral: 1 mg/mL (1 mL, 2 mL, 5 mL, 60 mL, 150 mL)

SK *see* streptokinase *on page 535*

Skelaxin® *see* metaxalone *on page 360*

Skelex® ***(Discontinued)*** *see page 700*

Skelid® *see* tiludronate *on page 566*

SKF 104864 *see* topotecan *on page 572*

skin test antigens, multiple (skin test AN tee gens, MUL ti pul)

U.S./Canadian Brand Names Multitest CMI®

Therapeutic Category Diagnostic Agent

Use Detection of nonresponsiveness to antigens by means of delayed hypersensitivity skin testing

Usual Dosage Select only test sites that permit sufficient surface area and subcutaneous tissue to allow adequate penetration of all 8 points, avoid hairy areas

Press loaded unit into the skin with sufficient pressure to puncture the skin and allow adequate penetration of all points, maintain firm contact for at least five seconds, during application the device should not be "rocked" back and forth and side to side without removing any of the test heads from the skin sites

If adequate pressure is applied it will be possible to observe:

1. The puncture marks of the nine tines on each of the eight test heads
2. An imprint of the circular platform surrounding each test head
3. Residual antigen and glycerin at each of the eight sites

If any of the above three criteria are not fully followed, the test results may not be reliable

Reading should be done in good light, read the test sites at both 24 and 48 hours, the largest reaction recorded from the two readings at each test site should be used; if two readings are not possible, a single 48 hour is recommended

A positive reaction from any of the seven delayed hypersensitivity skin test antigens is **induration of ≥2 mm** providing there is no induration at the negative control site; the size of the induration reactions with this test may be smaller than those obtained with other intradermal procedures

Dosage Forms Individual carton containing one preloaded skin test antigen for cellular hypersensitivity

Sleep-eze 3® Oral [OTC] *see* diphenhydramine *on page 185*

Sleepinal® [OTC] *see* diphenhydramine *on page 185*

Sleepwell 2-nite® [OTC] *see* diphenhydramine *on page 185*

Slim-Mint® [OTC] *see* benzocaine *on page 66*

Slo-bid™ *see* theophylline *on page 557*

Slo-Niacin® [OTC] *see* niacin *on page 399*

Slo-Phyllin® *see* theophylline *on page 557*

Slo-Phyllin® GG *see* theophylline and guaifenesin *on page 559*

Slo-Salt® *(Discontinued)* *see page 700*

Slow FE® [OTC] *see* ferrous sulfate *on page 237*

Slow-K® *see* potassium chloride *on page 464*

Slow-Mag® [OTC] *see* magnesium chloride *on page 344*

smelling salts *see* ammonia spirit, aromatic *on page 30*

SMX-TMP *see* co-trimoxazole *on page 149*

snake (pit vipers) antivenin *see* antivenin (*Crotalidae*) polyvalent *on page 41*

Snaplets-EX® [OTC] *see* guaifenesin and phenylpropanolamine *on page 270*

Snaplets-FR® Granules [OTC] *see* acetaminophen *on page 3*

sodium 2-mercaptoethane sulfonate *see* mesna *on page 358*

sodium acetate (SOW dee um AS e tate)

Therapeutic Category Alkalinizing Agent; Electrolyte Supplement, Oral

Use Sodium salt replacement; correction of acidosis through conversion of acetate to bicarbonate

Usual Dosage Sodium acetate is metabolized to bicarbonate on an equimolar basis outside the liver; administer in large volume I.V. fluids as a sodium source. Refer to sodium bicarbonate monograph.

Maintenance electrolyte requirements of sodium in parenteral nutrition solutions:
- Daily requirements: 3-4 mEq/kg/24 hours or 25-40 mEq/1000 kcal/24 hours
- Maximum: 100-150 mEq/24 hours

Dosage Forms Injection: 2 mEq/mL (20 mL, 50 mL); 4 mEq/mL (50 mL)

sodium acid carbonate *see* sodium bicarbonate *on this page*

sodium ascorbate (SOW dee um a SKOR bate)

U.S./Canadian Brand Names Cenolate®

Therapeutic Category Vitamin, Water Soluble

Use Prevention and treatment of scurvy and to acidify the urine; large doses may decrease the severity of "colds"

Usual Dosage Oral, I.V.:

Children:
- Scurvy: 100-300 mg/day in divided doses for at least 2 weeks
- Urinary acidification: 500 mg every 6-8 hours
- Dietary supplement: 35-45 mg/day

Adults:
- Scurvy: 100-250 mg 1-2 times/day for at least 2 weeks
- Urinary acidification: 4-12 g/day in divided doses
- Dietary supplement: 50-60 mg/day
- Prevention and treatment of cold: 1-3 g/day

Dosage Forms
- Crystals: 1020 mg per 1/4 teaspoonful [ascorbic acid 900 mg]
- Injection: 250 mg/mL [ascorbic acid 222 mg/mL] (30 mL); 562.5 mg/mL [ascorbic acid 500 mg/mL] (1 mL, 2 mL)
- Tablet: 585 mg [ascorbic acid 500 mg]

sodium benzoate and caffeine *see* caffeine and sodium benzoate *on page 87*

sodium bicarbonate (SOW dee um bye KAR bun ate)

Synonyms baking soda; $NaHCO_3$; sodium acid carbonate; sodium hydrogen carbonate

U.S./Canadian Brand Names Neut®

Therapeutic Category Alkalinizing Agent; Antacid; Electrolyte Supplement, Oral

Use Management of metabolic acidosis; antacid; alkalinize urine; stabilization of acid base status in cardiac arrest, and treatment of life-threatening hyperkalemia

Usual Dosage

Cardiac arrest (patient should be adequately ventilated before administering $NaHCO_3$):
- Infants: Use 1:1 dilution of 1 mEq/mL $NaHCO_3$ or use 0.5 mEq/mL $NaHCO_3$ at a dose of 1 mEq/kg slow IVP initially; may repeat with 0.5 mEq/kg in 10 minutes one time or as indicated by the patient's acid-base status. Rate of administration should not exceed 10 mEq/minute.
- Children and Adults: IVP: 1 mEq/kg initially; may repeat with 0.5 mEq/kg in 10 minutes one time or as indicated by the patient's acid-base status

Metabolic acidosis: Dosage should be based on the following formula if blood gases and pH measurements are available:
- Infants and Children: HCO_3-(mEq) = 0.3 x weight (kg) x base deficit (mEq/L) **or** HCO_3-(mEq) = 0.5 x weight (kg) x (24 - serum HCO_3-) (mEq/L)

Adults: HCO_3-(mEq) = 0.2 x weight (kg) x base deficit (mEq/L) **or** HCO_3-(mEq) = 0.5 x weight (kg) x (24 - serum HCO_3-) (mEq/L)
- If acid-base status is not available: Dose for older Children and Adults: 2-5 mEq/kg I.V. infusion over 4-8 hours; subsequent doses should be based on patient's acid-base status

Chronic renal failure: Oral: Children: 1-3 mEq/kg/day

(Continued)

sodium bicarbonate *(Continued)*

Renal tubular acidosis: Oral:
Distal:
Children: 2-3 mEq/kg/day
Adults: 1 mEq/kg/day
Proximal: Children: Initial: 5-10 mEq/kg/day; maintenance: Increase as required to maintain serum bicarbonate in the normal range
Urine alkalinization: Oral:
Children: 1-10 mEq (84-840 mg)/kg/day in divided doses; dose should be titrated to desired urinary pH
Adults: Initial: 48 mEq (4 g), then 12-24 mEq (1-2 g) every 4 hours; dose should be titrated to desired urinary pH; doses up to 16 g/day have been used

Dosage Forms

Injection: 4% [40 mg/mL = 2.4 mEq/5 mL] (5 mL); 4.2% [42 mg/mL = 5 mEq/10 mL] (10 mL); 7.5% [75 mg/mL = 8.92 mEq/10 mL] (10 mL, 50 mL); 8.4% [84 mg/mL = 10 mEq/10 mL] (10 mL, 50 mL)
Powder: 120 g, 480 g
Tablet: 300 mg [3.6 mEq]; 325 mg [3.8 mEq]; 520 mg [6.3 mEq]; 600 mg [7.3 mEq]; 650 mg [7.6 mEq]

sodium cellulose phosphate *see* cellulose sodium phosphate *on page 110*

sodium chloride (SOW dee um KLOR ide)

Synonyms NaCl; normal saline; salt

U.S./Canadian Brand Names Adsorbonac® Ophthalmic [OTC]; Afrin® Saline Mist [OTC]; AK-NaCl® [OTC]; Ayr® Nasal [OTC]; Breathe Free® [OTC]; Dristan® Saline Spray [OTC]; HuMist® Nasal Mist [OTC]; Muro 128® Ophthalmic [OTC]; Muroptic-5® [OTC]; NaSal™ [OTC]; Nasal Moist® [OTC]; Ocean Nasal Mist [OTC]; Pretz® [OTC]; Saline from Otrivin® (Can); SalineX® [OTC]; SeaMist® [OTC]

Therapeutic Category Electrolyte Supplement, Oral; Lubricant, Ocular

Use Prevention of muscle cramps and heat prostration; restoration of sodium ion in hyponatremia; restore moisture to nasal membranes; reduction of corneal edema

Usual Dosage

Newborn electrolyte requirement:
Premature: 2-8 mEq/kg/24 hours
Term:
0-48 hours: 0-2 mEq/kg/24 hours
>48 hours: 1-4 mEq/kg/24 hours
Children: I.V.: Hypertonic solutions (>0.9%) should only be used for the initial treatment of acute serious symptomatic hyponatremia; maintenance: 3-4 mEq/kg/day; maximum: 100-150 mEq/day; dosage varies widely depending on clinical condition
Replacement: Determined by laboratory determinations mEq
Sodium deficiency (mEq/kg) = [% dehydration (L/kg)/100 x 70 (mEq/L) = [0.6 (L/kg) x (140 - serum sodium) (mEq/L)]
Nasal: Use as often as needed
Adults:
GI irrigant: 1-3 L/day by intermittent irrigation
Heat cramps: Oral: 0.5-1 g with full glass of water, up to 4.8 g/day
Replacement I.V.: Determined by laboratory determinations mEq
Sodium deficiency (mEq/kg) = [% dehydration (L/kg)/100 x 70 (mEq/L)] + [0.6 (L/kg) x (140 - serum sodium) (mEq/L)]

To correct acute, serious hyponatremia: mEq sodium = (desired sodium (mEq/L) - actual sodium (mEq/L) x 0.6 x wt (kg)); for acute correction use 125 mEq/L as the desired serum sodium; acutely correct serum sodium in 5 mEq/L/dose increments; more gradual correction in increments of 10 mEq/L/day is indicated in the asymptomatic patient
Chloride maintenance electrolyte requirement in parenteral nutrition: 2-4 mEq/kg/24 hours or 25-40 mEq/1000 kcals/24 hours; maximum: 100-150 mEq/24 hours

Sodium maintenance electrolyte requirement in parenteral nutrition: 3-4 mEq/kg/24 hours or 25-40 mEq/1000 kcals/24 hours; maximum: 100-150 mEq/24 hours.
Nasal: Use as often as needed
Ophthalmic:
Ointment: Apply once daily or more often
Solution: Instill 1-2 drops into affected eye(s) every 3-4 hours
Abortifacient: 20% (250 mL) administered by transabdominal intra-amniotic instillation

Dosage Forms
Drops, nasal: 0.9% with dropper
Injection: 0.2% (3 mL); 0.45% (3 mL, 5 mL, 500 mL, 1000 mL); 0.9% (1 mL, 2 mL, 3 mL, 4 mL, 5 mL, 10 mL, 20 mL, 25 mL, 30 mL, 50 mL, 100 mL, 130 mL, 150 mL, 250 mL, 500 mL, 1000 mL); 3% (500 mL); 5% (500 mL); 20% (250 mL); 23.4% (30 mL, 100 mL)
Injection:
Admixtures: 50 mEq (20 mL); 100 mEq (40 mL); 625 mEq (250 mL)
Bacteriostatic: 0.9% (30 mL)
Concentrated: 14.6% (20 mL, 40 mL, 200 mL); 23.4% (10 mL, 20 mL, 30 mL)
Irrigation: 0.45% (500 mL, 1000 mL, 1500 mL); 0.9% (250 mL, 500 mL, 1000 mL, 1500 mL, 2000 mL, 3000 mL, 4000 mL)
Ointment, ophthalmic (Muro 128®): 5% (3.5 g)
Solution:
Irrigation: 0.9% (1000 mL, 2000 mL)
Nasal: 0.4% (15 mL, 50 mL); 0.6% (15 mL); 0.65% (20 mL, 45 mL, 50 mL)
Ophthalmic (Adsorbonac®): 2% (15 mL); 5% (15 mL, 30 mL)
Tablet: 650 mg, 1 g, 2.25 g
Enteric coated: 1 g
Slow release: 600 mg

sodium citrate and potassium citrate mixture

(SOW dee um SIT rate & poe TASS ee um SIT rate MIKS chur)

U.S./Canadian Brand Names Polycitra®

Therapeutic Category Alkalinizing Agent

Use Conditions where long-term maintenance of an alkaline urine is desirable as in control and dissolution of uric acid and cystine calculi of the urinary tract

Usual Dosage Oral:
Children: 5-15 mL diluted in water after meals and at bedtime
Adults: 15-30 mL diluted in water after meals and at bedtime

Dosage Forms Syrup: Sodium citrate 500 mg, potassium citrate 550 mg, with citric acid 334 mg per 5 mL [sodium 1 mEq, potassium 1 mEq, bicarbonate 2 mEq]

sodium edetate *see* edetate disodium *on page 203*

sodium ethacrynate *see* ethacrynic acid *on page 221*

sodium etidronate *see* etidronate disodium *on page 227*

Sodium Fusidate *see* fusidic acid *(Canada only) on page 255*

sodium hyaluronate (SOW dee um hye al yoor ON nate)

Synonyms hyaluronic acid

U.S./Canadian Brand Names AMO Vitrax®; Amvisc®; Amvisc® Plus; Healon®; Healon® GV; Replasyn® (Can)

Therapeutic Category Ophthalmic Agent, Viscoelastic

Use Surgical aid in cataract extraction, intraocular implantation, corneal transplant, glaucoma filtration, and retinal attachment surgery

Usual Dosage Depends upon procedure (slowly introduce a sufficient quantity into eye)

Dosage Forms Injection, intraocular:
Healon®: 10 mg/mL (0.4 mL, 0.55 mL, 0.85 mL, 2 mL)
Amvisc®: 12 mg/mL (0.5 mL, 0.8 mL)
Healon® GV: 14 mg/mL (0.55 mL, 0.85 mL)
Amvisc® Plus: 16 mg/mL (0.5 mL, 8 mL)
AMO Vitrax®: 30 mg/mL (0.65 mL)

sodium hyaluronate-chrondroitin sulfate *see* chondroitin sulfate-sodium hyaluronate *on page 130*

sodium hydrogen carbonate *see* sodium bicarbonate *on page 525*

sodium hypochlorite solution

(SOW dee um hye poe KLOR ite soe LOO shun)

Synonyms Dakin's solution; modified Dakin's solution

Therapeutic Category Disinfectant

Use Treatment of athlete's foot (0.5%); wound irrigation (0.5%); to disinfect utensils and equipment (5%)

Usual Dosage Topical irrigation

Dosage Forms

Solution: 5% (4000 mL)

Modified Dakin's solution:

Full strength: 0.5% (1000 mL)

Half strength: 0.25% (1000 mL)

Quarter strength: 0.125% (1000 mL)

sodium lactate (SOW dee um LAK tate)

Therapeutic Category Alkalinizing Agent

Use Source of bicarbonate for prevention and treatment of mild to moderate metabolic acidosis

Usual Dosage Dosage depends on degree of acidosis

Dosage Forms Injection:

1.87 g/100 mL [sodium 16.7 mEq and lactate 16.7 mEq per 100 mL] (1000 mL)

560 mg/mL [sodium 5 mEq sodium and lactate 5 mEq per mL] (10 mL)

sodium nitroferricyanide *see* nitroprusside *on page 405*

Sodium P.A.S.® *(Discontinued)* *see page 700*

sodium-pca and lactic acid *see* lactic acid and sodium-PCA *on page 324*

sodium phenylacetate and sodium benzoate

(SOW dee um fen il AS e tate & SOW dee um BENZ oh ate)

U.S./Canadian Brand Names Ucephan®

Therapeutic Category Ammonium Detoxicant

Use Adjunctive therapy to prevent/treat hyperammonemia in patients with urea cycle enzymopathy involving partial or complete deficiencies of carbamoyl-phosphate synthetase, ornithine transcarbamoylase or argininosuccinate synthetase

Usual Dosage Infants and Children: Oral: 2.5 mL (250 mg sodium benzoate and 250 mg sodium phenylacetate)/kg/day divided 3-6 times/day; total daily dose should not exceed 100 mL

Dosage Forms Solution: Sodium phenylacetate 100 mg and sodium benzoate 100 mg per mL (100 mL)

sodium phenylbutyrate (SOW dee um fen il BYOO ti rate)

Synonyms ammonapse

U.S./Canadian Brand Names Buphenyl®

Therapeutic Category Miscellaneous Product

Use Adjunctive therapy in the chronic management of patients with urea cycle disorder involving deficiencies of carbamoylphosphate synthetase, ornithine transcarbamylase, or argininosuccinic acid synthetase

Usual Dosage

Powder: Patients weighing <20 kg: 450-600 mg/kg/day or 9.9-13 g/m^2/day, administered in equally divided amounts with each meal or feeding, 4-6 times/day; safety and efficacy of doses >20 g/day have not been established

Tablet: Children >20 kg and Adults: 450-600 mg/kg/day or 9.9-13 g/m²/day, administered in equally divided amounts with each meal; safety and efficacy of doses >20 g/day have not been established

Dosage Forms

Powder: 3.2 g [sodium phenylbutyrate 3 g] per teaspoon (500 mL, 950 mL); 9.1 g [sodium phenylbutyrate 8.6 g] per **tablespoon** (500 mL, 950 mL)

Tablet: 500 mg

sodium phosphate and potassium phosphate *see* potassium phosphate and sodium phosphate *on page 467*

sodium phosphates (SOW dee um FOS fate)

U.S./Canadian Brand Names Enemol™ (Can); Fleet® Enema [OTC]; Fleet® Phospho®-Soda [OTC]

Therapeutic Category Electrolyte Supplement, Oral; Laxative

Use Source of phosphate in large volume I.V. fluids; short-term treatment of constipation (oral/rectal) and to evacuate the colon for rectal and bowel exams; treatment and prevention of hypophosphatemia

Usual Dosage

Normal requirements elemental phosphate: Oral:

0-6 months: 240 mg

6-12 months: 360 mg

1-10 years: 800 mg

>10 years: 1200 mg

Pregnancy lactation: Additional 400 mg/day

Treatment:

It is difficult to provide concrete guidelines for the treatment of severe hypophosphatemia because the extent of total body deficits and response to therapy are difficult to predict. Aggressive doses of phosphate may result in a transient serum elevation followed by redistribution into intracellular compartments or bone tissue. It is recommended that repletion of severe hypophosphatemia (<1 mg/dL in adults) be done I.V. because large doses of oral phosphate may cause diarrhea and intestinal absorption may be unreliable

Pediatric I.V. phosphate repletion:

Children: 0.25-0.5 mmol/kg **administer over 4-6 hours and repeat if symptomatic hypophosphatemia persists**; to assess the need for further phosphate administration: obtain serum inorganic phosphate after administration of the first dose and base further doses on serum levels and clinical status

Adult I.V. phosphate repletion:

Initial dose: 0.08 mmol/kg if recent uncomplicated hypophosphatemia

Initial dose: 0.16 mmol/kg if prolonged hypophosphatemia with presumed total body deficits; increase dose by 25% to 50% if patient symptomatic with severe hypophosphatemia

Severe hypophosphatemia:

High-dose = 0.36 mmol/kg over 6 hours; use if serum PO_4 <0.5 mg/dL

Adults: 0.15-0.3 mmol/kg/dose over 12 hours, may repeat as needed to achieve desired serum level

With orders for I.V. phosphate, there is considerable confusion associated with the use of millimoles (mmol) versus milliequivalents (mEq) to express the phosphate requirement. Because inorganic phosphate exists as monobasic and dibasic anions, with the mixture of valences is dependent on pH, ordering by mEq amounts is unreliable and may lead to large dosing errors. In addition, I.V. phosphate is available in the sodium and potassium salt; therefore, the content of these cations must be considered when ordering phosphate. The most reliable method of ordering I.V. phosphate is by millimoles, then specifying the potassium or sodium salt. For example, an order for 15 mmol of phosphate as potassium phosphate in one liter of normal saline would also provide 22 mEq of potassium.

Phosphate maintenance electrolyte requirement in parenteral nutrition: 2 mmol/kg/24 hours or 35 mmol/kcal/24 hours; Maximum: 15-30 mmol/24 hours

(Continued)

sodium phosphates *(Continued)*

Maintenance:

Children: 0.5-1.5 mmol/kg/24 hours I.V. **or** 2-3 mmol/kg/24 hours orally in divided doses

Adults: 15-30 mmol/24 hours I.V. **or** 50-150 mmol/24 hours orally in divided doses

Laxative (Fleet®): Rectal:

Children 2-12 years: 67.5 mL (1/2 bottle) as a single dose, may repeat

Children ≥12 years and Adults: 133 mL enema as a single dose, may repeat

Laxative (Fleet® Phospho®-Soda): Oral:

Children:

5-9 years: 5 mL as a single dose

10-12 years: 10 mL as a single dose

Children ≥12 years and Adults: 20-30 mL as a single dose

Dosage Forms

Enema: Sodium phosphate 6 g and sodium biphosphate 16 g/100 mL (67.5 mL pediatric enema unit, 135 mL adult enema unit)

Injection: Phosphate 3 mmol and sodium 4 mEq per mL (5 mL, 10 mL, 15 mL, 30 mL, 50 mL)

Solution, oral: Sodium phosphate 18 g and sodium biphosphate 48 g/100 mL (45 mL, 90 mL, 273 mL)

See table.

	Phosphate (mmol)	Sodium (mEq)	Potassium (mEq)
Oral			
Whole cow's milk	0.29/mL	0.025/mL	0.035/mL
Fleet® Phospho®-Soda	4.15/mL	4.8/mL	None
Intravenous			
Sodium phosphate	3/mL	4/mL	None

sodium polystyrene sulfonate (SOW dee um pol ee STYE reen SUL fon ate)

U.S./Canadian Brand Names Kayexalate®; Kionex®; SPS®

Therapeutic Category Antidote

Use Treatment of hyperkalemia

Usual Dosage

Children:

Oral: 1 g/kg/dose every 6 hours

Rectal: 1 g/kg/dose every 2-6 hours (In small children and infants employ lower doses by using the practical exchange ratio of 1 mEq potassium/g of resin as the basis for calculation)

Adults:

Oral: 15 g (60 mL) 1-4 times/day

Rectal: 30-50 g every 6 hours

Dosage Forms Oral or rectal:

Powder for suspension: 454 g

Suspension: 1.25 g/5 mL with sorbitol 33% and alcohol 0.3% (60 mL, 120 mL, 200 mL, 500 mL)

sodium salicylate (SOW dee um sa LIS i late)

U.S./Canadian Brand Names Uracel®

Therapeutic Category Analgesic, Non-narcotic; Antipyretic

Use Treatment of minor pain or fever; arthritis

Usual Dosage Adults: Oral: 325-650 mg every 4 hours

Dosage Forms Tablet, enteric coated: 325 mg, 650 mg

Sodium Sulamyd® *see* sulfacetamide *on page 540*

sodium tetradecyl (SOW dee um tetra DEK il)

U.S./Canadian Brand Names Sotradecol®; Trombovar® (Can)

Therapeutic Category Sclerosing Agent

Use Treatment of small, uncomplicated varicose veins of the lower extremities; endoscopic sclerotherapy in the management of bleeding esophageal varices

Usual Dosage I.V.: 0.5-2 mL of 1% (5-20 mg) for small veins; 0.5-2 mL of 3% (15-60 mg) for medium or large veins

Dosage Forms Injection, as sulfate: 1% [10 mg/mL] (2 mL); 3% [30 mg/mL] (2 mL)

sodium thiosulfate (SOW dee um thye oh SUL fate)

U.S./Canadian Brand Names Tinver® [OTC]; Versiclear™

Therapeutic Category Antidote; Antifungal Agent

Use

Parenteral: Used alone or with sodium nitrite or amyl nitrite in cyanide poisoning or arsenic poisoning; reduce the risk of nephrotoxicity associated with cisplatin therapy; local infiltration (in diluted form) of selected chemotherapy extravasation

Topical: Treatment of tinea versicolor

Usual Dosage I.V.:

Cyanide and nitroprusside antidote:

Children <25 kg: 50 mg/kg after receiving 4.5-10 mg/kg sodium nitrite; a half dose of each may be repeated if necessary

Children >25 kg and Adults: 12.5 g after 300 mg of sodium nitrite; a half dose of each may be repeated if necessary

Cyanide poisoning: Dose should be based on determination as with nitrite, at rate of 2.5-5 mL/minute to maximum of 50 mL

Dosage Forms

Injection: 100 mg/mL (10 mL); 250 mg/mL (50 mL)

Lotion: 25% with salicylic acid 1% and isopropyl alcohol 10% (120 mL, 180 mL)

Sofarin® *(Discontinued)* *see page 700*

Soflax™ (Can) *see* docusate *on page 191*

Solaquin® [OTC] *see* hydroquinone *on page 294*

Solaquin Forte® *see* hydroquinone *on page 294*

Solarcaine® [OTC] *see* benzocaine *on page 66*

Solarcaine® Topical *see* lidocaine *on page 333*

Solatene® *(Discontinued)* *see page 700*

Solfoton® *see* phenobarbital *on page 443*

Solganal® *see* aurothioglucose *on page 54*

Solium® (Can) *see* chlordiazepoxide *on page 116*

soluble fluorescein *see* fluorescein sodium *on page 244*

Solu-Cortef® Injection *see* hydrocortisone (systemic) *on page 291*

Solugel® 4, 8 (Can) *see* benzoyl peroxide *on page 68*

Solu-Medrol® Injection *see* methylprednisolone *on page 368*

Solurex L.A.® *see* dexamethasone (systemic) *on page 167*

Soluver® (Can) *see* salicylic acid *on page 513*

Soma® *see* carisoprodol *on page 101*

Soma® Compound *see* carisoprodol and aspirin *on page 101*

Soma® Compound w/Codeine *see* carisoprodol, aspirin, and codeine *on page 101*

somatrem *see* human growth hormone *on page 283*

somatropin *see* human growth hormone *on page 283*

Sominex® Oral [OTC] *see* diphenhydramine *on page 185*

Somnol® (Can) *see* flurazepam *on page 248*

Som Pam® (Can) *see* flurazepam *on page 248*

Sonata® *see* zaleplon *on page 609*

Sopalamine/3B Plus C (Can) *see* vitamin, multiple (oral) *on page 604*

Sopamycetin® (Can) *see* chloramphenicol *on page 116*

sorbitol (SOR bi tole)

Therapeutic Category Genitourinary Irrigant; Laxative

Use Humectant; sweetening agent; hyperosmotic laxative; facilitate the passage of sodium polystyrene sulfonate or a charcoal-toxin complex through the intestinal tract

Usual Dosage Hyperosmotic laxative (as single dose, at infrequent intervals):

Children 2-11 years:
- Oral: 2 mL/kg (as 70% solution)
- Rectal enema: 30-60 mL as 25% to 30% solution

Children >12 years and Adults:
- Oral: 30-150 mL (as 70% solution)
- Rectal enema: 120 mL as 25% to 30% solution
- Adjunct to sodium polystyrene sulfonate: 15 mL as 70% solution orally until diarrhea occurs (10-20 mL/2 hours) or 20-100 mL as an oral vehicle for the sodium polystyrene sulfonate resin

When administered with charcoal: Oral:
- Children: 4.3 mL/kg of 35% sorbitol with 1 g/kg of activated charcoal
- Adults: 4.3 mL/kg of 70% sorbitol with 1 g/kg of activated charcoal

Dosage Forms

Solution: 70%

Solution, genitourinary irrigation: 3% (1500 mL, 3000 mL); 3.3% (2000 mL)

Sorbitrate® *see* isosorbide dinitrate *on page 315*

Soriatane™ *see* acitretin *on page 9*

Sotacor® (Can) *see* sotalol *on this page*

sotalol (SOE ta lole)

U.S./Canadian Brand Names Betapace®; Sotacor® (Can)

Therapeutic Category Antiarrhythmic Agent, Class II; Antiarrhythmic Agent, Class III

Use Treatment of ventricular arrhythmias

Usual Dosage Adults: Oral: Initial: 80 mg twice daily; may be increased to 240-320 mg/day and up to 480-640 mg/day in patients with life-threatening refractory ventricular arrhythmias

Dosage Forms Tablet, as hydrochloride: 80 mg, 120 mg, 160 mg, 240 mg

Sotradecol® *see* sodium tetradecyl *on previous page*

Soyacal® *see* fat emulsion *on page 231*

Soyalac® [OTC] *see* enteral nutritional products *on page 208*

Span-FF® [OTC] *see* ferrous fumarate *on page 236*

sparfloxacin (spar FLOKS a sin)

U.S./Canadian Brand Names Zagam®

Therapeutic Category Quinolone

Use Treatment of adult patients with community acquired pneumonia caused by susceptible strains of *Chlamydia pneumoniae, Haemophilus influenzae, Haemophilus parainfluenzae, Moraxella catarrhalis, Mycoplasma pneumoniae*, or *Streptococcus pneumoniae* and acute bacterial exacerbations of acute bronchitis caused by susceptible strains of *Chlamydia pneumoniae, Enterobacter cloacae, Haemophilus influenzae, Haemophilus parainfluenzae, Klebsiella pneumoniae, Moraxella catarrhalis, Staphylococcus aureus*, or *Streptococcus pneumoniae*

Usual Dosage Adults: Oral: 400 mg on day 1, then 200 mg/day for the next 9 days (11 tablets total). In patients with creatinine clearance <50 mL/minute, administer 400 mg on day 1, then begin 200 mg every 48 hours on day 3 for a total of 9 days (6 tablets total).

Dosage Forms Tablet: 200 mg

Sparine® *see* promazine *on page 478*

Spasmoject® *(Discontinued)* *see page 700*

Spasmolin® *see* hyoscyamine, atropine, scopolamine, and phenobarbital *on page 298*

Spec-T® [OTC] *see* benzocaine *on page 66*

Spectazole™ *see* econazole *on page 202*

spectinomycin (spek ti noe MYE sin)

U.S./Canadian Brand Names Trobicin®

Therapeutic Category Antibiotic, Miscellaneous

Use Treatment of uncomplicated gonorrhea (ineffective against syphilis)

Usual Dosage I.M.:

Children:

<45 kg: 40 mg/kg/dose 1 time

≥45 kg: See adult dose

Children >8 years who are allergic to penicillins/cephalosporins may be treated with oral tetracycline

Adults: 2 g deep I.M. or 4 g where antibiotic resistance is prevalent 1 time; 4 g (10 mL) dose should be administered as 2-5 mL injections

Dosage Forms Injection, as hydrochloride: 2 g, 4 g

Spectrobid® Oral Suspension *(Discontinued)* *see page 700*

Spectrobid® Tablet *see* bacampicillin *on page 57*

Spectrum™ Forte 29 (Can) *see* vitamin, multiple (oral) *on page 604*

Spherulin® *see* coccidioidin skin test *on page 143*

spiramycin *(Canada only)* (speer a MYE sin)

U.S./Canadian Brand Names Rovamycine® (Can)

Therapeutic Category Antibiotic, Macrolide

Use The treatment of infections of the respiratory tract, buccal cavity, skin and soft tissues due to susceptible organisms. *N. gonorrheae*: as an alternate choice of treatment for gonorrhea in patients allergic to the penicillins. Before treatment of gonorrhea, the possibility of concomitant infection due to *T. pallidum* should be excluded.

Usual Dosage Oral:

Children: The usual daily dosage is based on 150,000 units/kg body weight in 2 or 3 divided doses Adults: Oral: 6,000,000-9,000,000 units per 24 hours, in 2 divided doses. In severe infections, the daily dosage may be increased to 12,000,000-15,000,000 units per day

Gonorrhea: 12,000,000-13,500000 units in a single dose.

Dosage Forms Capsule: 250 [750,000 units]; 500 [1,500,000 units]

spirapril (SPYE ra pril)

U.S./Canadian Brand Names Renormax®

Therapeutic Category Angiotensin-Converting Enzyme (ACE) Inhibitor

Use Management of mild to severe hypertension

Usual Dosage Adults: Oral: 12 mg/day in 1-2 divided doses

Dosage Forms Tablet: 3 mg, 6 mg, 12 mg, 24 mg

Spironazide® *see* hydrochlorothiazide and spironolactone *on page 286*

spironolactone (speer on oh LAK tone)

U.S./Canadian Brand Names Aldactone®; Novo-Spiroton® (Can)

Therapeutic Category Diuretic, Potassium Sparing

Use Management of edema associated with excessive aldosterone excretion; hypertension; primary hyperaldosteronism; hypokalemia; treatment of hirsutism

Usual Dosage Oral:

Children: 1.5-3.5 mg/kg/day in divided doses every 6-24 hours

Diagnosis of primary aldosteronism: 125-375 mg/m^2/day in divided doses

Vaso-occlusive disease: 7.5 mg/kg/day in divided doses twice daily (non-FDA approved dose)

Adults:

Edema, hypertension, hypokalemia: 25-200 mg/day in 1-2 divided doses

Diagnosis of primary aldosteronism: 100-400 mg/day in 1-2 divided doses

Dosage Forms Tablet: 25 mg, 50 mg, 100 mg

spironolactone and hydrochlorothiazide *see* hydrochlorothiazide and spironolactone *on page 286*

Spirozide® *see* hydrochlorothiazide and spironolactone *on page 286*

Sporanox® *see* itraconazole *on page 317*

Sportscreme® [OTC] *see* triethanolamine salicylate *on page 580*

SPS® *see* sodium polystyrene sulfonate *on page 530*

S-P-T *see* thyroid *on page 564*

SRC® Expectorant *see* hydrocodone, pseudoephedrine, and guaifenesin *on page 290*

SSD® AF *see* silver sulfadiazine *on page 522*

SSD® Cream *see* silver sulfadiazine *on page 522*

SSKI® *see* potassium iodide *on page 466*

Stadol® *see* butorphanol *on page 86*

Stadol® NS *see* butorphanol *on page 86*

Stagesic® *see* hydrocodone and acetaminophen *on page 287*

Stahist® *see* chlorpheniramine, phenylephrine, phenylpropanolamine, and belladonna alkaloids *on page 124*

stanozolol (stan OH zoe lole)

U.S./Canadian Brand Names Winstrol®

Therapeutic Category Anabolic Steroid

Controlled Substance C-III

Use Prophylactic use against angioedema

Usual Dosage

Children: Acute attacks:

<6 years: 1 mg/day

6-12 years: 2 mg/day

Adults: Oral: Initial: 2 mg 3 times/day, may then reduce to a maintenance dose of 2 mg/day or 2 mg every other day after 1-3 months

Dosage Forms Tablet: 2 mg

Staphcillin® ***(Discontinued)*** *see page 700*

Statex® (Can) *see* morphine sulfate *on page 382*

Staticin® Topical *see* erythromycin (ophthalmic/topical) *on page 214*

Statobex® ***(Discontinued)*** *see page 700*

stavudine (STAV yoo deen)

Synonyms d4T

U.S./Canadian Brand Names Zerit®

Therapeutic Category Antiviral Agent

Use Treatment of advanced HIV infection in patients who experience intolerance, toxicity, resistance, or HIV disease progression with either zidovudine or didanosine therapy; active against most zidovudine-resistant strains; in adults, stavudine used alone in patients with 50-500 CD4 cells/mm^3 and at least 6 months previous treatment with zidovudine was more effective than continued zidovudine in preventing disease progression and death

Usual Dosage Oral:

Children 7 months to 15 years: 1-2 mg/kg/day divided twice daily

Adults: 0.5-1 mg/kg/day **or**

<60 kg: 30 mg every 12 hours

≥60 kg: 40 mg every 12 hours

If peripheral neuropathy or elevations in liver enzymes occur, stavudine should be discontinued; once adverse effects resolve, reinitiate therapy at a lower dose of 20 mg every 12 hours (for ≥60 kg patients) or 15 mg every 12 hours (for <60 kg patients)

Dosage Forms

Capsule: 15 mg, 20 mg, 30 mg, 40 mg

Powder for oral solution: 1 mg/mL (200 mL)

S-T Cort® Topical *see* hydrocortisone (topical) *on page 292*

Stelazine® *see* trifluoperazine *on page 580*

Stemetil® (Can) *see* prochlorperazine *on page 476*

Stemex® *see* paramethasone acetate *on page 429*

Sterapred® *(Discontinued)* *see page 700*

Stieva-A® (Can) *see* tretinoin (topical) *on page 576*

Stieva-A® Forte (Can) *see* tretinoin (topical) *on page 576*

stilbestrol *see* diethylstilbestrol *on page 178*

Stilphostrol® *see* diethylstilbestrol *on page 178*

Stimate® *see* desmopressin acetate *on page 166*

St. Joseph® Cough Suppressant [OTC] *see* dextromethorphan *on page 171*

St. Joseph® Measured Dose Nasal Solution [OTC] *see* phenylephrine *on page 445*

Stop® [OTC] *see* fluoride *on page 244*

Streptase® *see* streptokinase *on this page*

streptokinase (strep toe KYE nase)

Synonyms SK

U.S./Canadian Brand Names Kabikinase®; Streptase®

Therapeutic Category Thrombolytic Agent

Use Thrombolytic agent used in treatment of recent severe or massive deep vein thrombosis, pulmonary emboli, myocardial infarction, and occluded arteriovenous cannulas

Usual Dosage I.V.:

Children: Safety and efficacy not established; limited studies have used: 3500-4000 units/kg over 30 minutes followed by 1000-1500 units/kg/hour; clotted catheter: 25,000 units, clamp for 2 hours then aspirate contents and flush with normal saline

Adults (best results are realized if used within 5-6 hours of myocardial infarction; antibodies to streptokinase remain for 3-6 months after initial dose, use another thrombolytic enzyme, ie, urokinase, if thrombolytic therapy is indicated):

Guidelines for Acute Myocardial Infarction (AMI):

1.5 million units infused over 60 minutes. Monitor for the first few hours for signs of anaphylaxis or allergic reaction. **Infusion should be slowed if lowering of 25 mm**

(Continued)

streptokinase *(Continued)*

Hg in blood pressure or terminated if asthmatic symptoms appear. Begin heparin 5000-10,000 unit bolus followed by 1000 units/hour approximately 3-4 hours after completion of streptokinase infusion or when PTT is <100 seconds.

Guidelines for Acute Pulmonary Embolism (APE):

3 million unit dose; administer 250,000 units over 30 minutes followed by 100,000 units/hour for 24 hours. Monitor for the first few hours for signs of anaphylaxis or allergic reaction. **Infusion should be slowed if blood pressure is lowered by 25 mm Hg or if asthmatic symptoms appear**. Begin heparin 1000 units/hour approximately 3-4 hours after completion of streptokinase infusion or when PTT is <100 seconds.

Thromboses: 250,000 units to start, then 100,000 units/hour for 24-72 hours depending on location

Cannula occlusion: 250,000 units into cannula, clamp for 2 hours, then aspirate contents and flush with normal saline

Dosage Forms Powder for injection: 250,000 units (5 mL, 6.5 mL); 600,000 units (5 mL); 750,000 units (6 mL, 6.5 mL); 1,500,000 units (6.5 mL, 10 mL, 50 mL)

streptomycin (strep toe MYE sin)

Therapeutic Category Antibiotic, Aminoglycoside; Antitubercular Agent

Use Combination therapy of active tuberculosis; used in combination with other agents for treatment of streptococcal or enterococcal endocarditis, mycobacterial infections, plague, tularemia, and brucellosis. Streptomycin is indicated for persons from endemic areas of drug-resistant *Mycobacterium tuberculosis* or who are HIV infected.

Usual Dosage Intramuscular (may also be given intravenous piggyback):

Tuberculosis therapy: **Note:** A four-drug regimen (isoniazid, rifampin, pyrazinamide and either streptomycin or ethambutol) is preferred for the initial, empiric treatment of TB. When the drug susceptibility results are available, the regimen should be altered as appropriate.

Patients with TB and without HIV infection:

OPTION 1:

Isoniazid resistance rate <4%: Administer daily isoniazid, rifampin, and pyrazinamide for 8 weeks followed by isoniazid and rifampin daily or directly observed therapy (DOT) 2-3 times/week for 16 weeks

If isoniazid resistance rate is not documented, ethambutol or streptomycin should also be administered until susceptibility to isoniazid or rifampin is demonstrated. Continue treatment for at least 6 months or 3 months beyond culture conversion.

OPTION 2: Administer daily isoniazid, rifampin, pyrazinamide, and either streptomycin or ethambutol for 2 weeks followed by DOT 2 times/week administration of the same drugs for 6 weeks, and subsequently, with isoniazid and rifampin DOT 2 times/week administration for 16 weeks

OPTION 3: Administer isoniazid, rifampin, pyrazinamide, and either ethambutol or streptomycin by DOT 3 times/week for 6 months

Patients with TB and with HIV infection: Administer any of the above OPTIONS 1, 2 or 3, however, treatment should be continued for a total of 9 months and at least 6 months beyond culture conversion

Note: Some experts recommend that the duration of therapy should be extended to 9 months for patients with disseminated disease, miliary disease, disease involving the bones or joints, or tuberculosis lymphadenitis

Children:

Daily therapy: 20-30 mg/kg/day (maximum: 1 g/day)

Directly observed therapy (DOT): Twice weekly: 25-30 mg/kg (maximum: 1.5 g)

DOT: 3 times/week: 25-30 mg/kg (maximum: 1 g)

Adults:

Daily therapy: 15 mg/kg/day (maximum: 1 g)

Directly observed therapy (DOT): Twice weekly: 25-30 mg/kg (maximum: 1.5 g)

DOT: 3 times/week: 25-30 mg/kg (maximum: 1 g)

Enterococcal endocarditis: 1 g every 12 hours for 2 weeks, 500 mg every 12 hours for 4 weeks in combination with penicillin

Streptococcal endocarditis: 1 g every 12 hours for 1 week, 500 mg every 12 hours for 1 week

Tularemia: 1-2 g/day in divided doses for 7-10 days or until patient is afebrile for 5-7 days

Plague: 2-4 g/day in divided doses until the patient is afebrile for at least 3 days

Elderly: 10 mg/kg/day, not to exceed 750 mg/day; dosing interval should be adjusted for renal function; some authors suggest not to give more than 5 days/week or give as 20-25 mg/kg/dose twice weekly

Dosage Forms Injection, as sulfate: 400 mg/mL (2.5 mL)

Streptomycin® *(Discontinued)* *see page 700*

streptozocin (strep toe ZOE sin)

U.S./Canadian Brand Names Zanosar®

Therapeutic Category Antineoplastic Agent

Use Treat metastatic islet cell carcinoma of the pancreas, carcinoid tumor and syndrome, Hodgkin's disease, palliative treatment of colorectal cancer

Usual Dosage Children and Adults: I.V.: 500 mg/m^2 for 5 days every 6 weeks until optimal benefit or toxicity occurs; or may be administered in single dose 1000 mg/m^2 at weekly intervals for 2 doses, then increased to 1500 mg/m^2 weekly; the median total dose to onset of response is about 2000 mg/m^2 and the median total dose to maximum response is about 4000 mg/m^2

Dosage Forms Injection: 1 g

Stresstabs® 600 Advanced Formula Tablets [OTC] *see* vitamin, multiple (oral) *on page 604*

Stromectol® *see* ivermectin *on page 317*

strong iodine solution *see* potassium iodide *on page 466*

strontium-89 (STRON shee um atey nine)

U.S./Canadian Brand Names Metastron®

Therapeutic Category Radiopharmaceutical

Use Relief of bone pain in patients with skeletal metastases

Usual Dosage Adults: I.V.: 148 megabecquerel (4 millicurie) administered by slow I.V. injection over 1-2 minutes or 1.5-2.2 megabecquerel (40-60 microcurie)/kg; repeated doses are generally not recommended at intervals <90 days

Dosage Forms Injection, as chloride: 10.9-22.6 mg/mL [148 megabecquerel, 4 millicurie] (10 mL)

Stuartnatal® 1 + 1 *see* vitamin, multiple (prenatal) *on page 606*

Stuart Prenatal® [OTC] *see* vitamin, multiple (prenatal) *on page 606*

Sublimaze® Injection *see* fentanyl *on page 235*

succimer (SUKS i mer)

U.S./Canadian Brand Names Chemet®

Therapeutic Category Chelating Agent

Use Treatment of lead poisoning in children with blood levels >45 mcg/dL. It is not indicated for prophylaxis of lead poisoning in a lead-containing environment.

Usual Dosage Children and Adults: Oral: 30 mg/kg/day in divided doses every 8 hours for an additional 5 days followed by 20 mg/kg/day for 14 days

Dosage Forms Capsule: 100 mg

succinate mafenide acetate *see* mafenide *on page 343*

succinylcholine (suks in il KOE leen)

Synonyms suxamethonium

U.S./Canadian Brand Names Anectine® Chloride; Anectine® Flo-Pack®; Quelicin®

(Continued)

succinylcholine *(Continued)*

Therapeutic Category Skeletal Muscle Relaxant

Use Produces skeletal muscle relaxation in procedures of short duration such as endotracheal intubation or endoscopic exams

Usual Dosage I.M., I.V.:

Children: 1-2 mg/kg

Intermittent: Initial: 1 mg/kg/dose one time; maintenance: 0.3-0.6 mg/kg every 5-10 minutes as needed

Adults: 0.6 mg/kg (range: 0.3-1.1 mg/kg) over 10-30 seconds, up to 150 mg total dose

Maintenance: 0.04-0.07 mg/kg every 5-10 minutes as needed

Continuous infusion: 2.5 mg/minute (or 0.5-10 mg/minute); dilute to concentration of 1-2 mg/mL in D_5W or NS

Note: Pretreatment with atropine may reduce occurrence of bradycardia

Dosage Forms Succinylcholine chloride:

Injection: 20 mg/mL (10 mL); 50 mg/mL (10 mL); 100 mg/mL (5 mL, 10 mL, 20 mL)

Powder for injection: 100 mg, 500 mg, 1 g

Sucostrin® *(Discontinued)* *see page 700*

Sucraid™ *see* sacrosidase *on page 512*

sucralfate (soo KRAL fate)

Synonyms aluminum sucrose sulfate, basic

U.S./Canadian Brand Names Carafate®; Novo-Sucralate® (Can); Sulcrate® (Can); Sulcrate® Suspension Plus (Can)

Therapeutic Category Gastrointestinal Agent, Gastric or Duodenal Ulcer Treatment

Use Short-term management of duodenal ulcers; gastric ulcers; suspension may be used topically for treatment of stomatitis due to cancer chemotherapy or other causes of esophageal and gastric erosions

Usual Dosage

Children: Dose not established, doses of 40-80 mg/kg/day divided every 6 hours have been used

Stomatitis: Oral: 2.5-5 mL (1 g/10 mL suspension), swish and spit or swish and swallow 4 times/day

Adults:

Duodenal ulcer treatment: Oral: 1 g 4 times/day, 1 hour before meals or food and at bedtime for 4-8 weeks, or alternatively 2 g twice daily

Duodenal ulcer maintenance therapy: Oral: 1 g twice daily

Stomatitis: Oral: 1 g/10 mL suspension, swish and spit or swish and swallow 4 times/day

Dosage Forms

Suspension, oral: 1 g/10 mL (420 mL)

Tablet: 1 g

Sucrets® [OTC] *see* dyclonine *on page 201*

Sucrets® Cough Calmers [OTC] *see* dextromethorphan *on page 171*

Sucrets® Sore Throat [OTC] *see* hexylresorcinol *on page 281*

Sudafed® [OTC] *see* pseudoephedrine *on page 486*

Sudafed® 12 Hour [OTC] *see* pseudoephedrine *on page 486*

Sudafed® Children *(Discontinued)* *see page 700*

Sudafed® Cold & Cough Liquid Caps [OTC] *see* guaifenesin, pseudoephedrine, and dextromethorphan *on page 273*

Sudafed® Cough *(Discontinued)* *see page 700*

Sudafed Plus® Liquid *(Discontinued)* *see page 700*

Sudafed® Plus Tablet [OTC] *see* chlorpheniramine and pseudoephedrine *on page 122*

Sudafed® Severe Cold [OTC] *see* acetaminophen, dextromethorphan, and pseudoephedrine *on page 6*

Sufedrin® [OTC] *see* pseudoephedrine *on page 486*

Sufenta® *see* sufentanil *on this page*

sufentanil (soo FEN ta nil)

U.S./Canadian Brand Names Sufenta®

Therapeutic Category Analgesic, Narcotic; General Anesthetic

Controlled Substance C-II

Use Analgesia; analgesia adjunct; anesthetic agent

Usual Dosage I.V.:

Children <12 years: 10-25 mcg/kg with 100% O_2, maintenance: 25-50 mcg as needed (total dose of up to 1-2 mcg/kg)

Adults: Dose should be based on body weight. **Note:** In obese patients (ie, >20% above ideal body weight), use lean body weight to determine dosage

- 1-2 mcg/kg with N_2O/O_2 for endotracheal intubation; maintenance: 10-25 mcg as needed
- 2-8 mcg/kg with N_2O/O_2 more complicated major surgical procedures; maintenance: 10-50 mcg as needed
- 8-30 mcg/kg with 100% O_2 and muscle relaxant produces sleep; at doses of ≥8 mcg/kg maintains a deep level of anesthesia; maintenance: 10-50 mcg as needed

Dosage Forms Injection, as citrate: 50 mcg/mL (1 mL, 2 mL, 5 mL)

Sular® *see* nisoldipine *on page 403*

sulbactam and ampicillin *see* ampicillin and sulbactam *on page 35*

sulconazole (sul KON a zole)

U.S./Canadian Brand Names Exelderm® Topical

Therapeutic Category Antifungal Agent

Use Treatment of superficial fungal infections of the skin, including tinea cruris, tinea corporis, tinea versicolor and possibly tinea pedis

Usual Dosage Topical: Apply once or twice daily for 4-6 weeks

Dosage Forms Sulconazole nitrate:

Cream: 1% (15 g, 30 g, 60 g)

Solution, topical: 1% (30 mL)

Sulcrate® (Can) *see* sucralfate *on previous page*

Sulcrate® Suspension Plus (Can) *see* sucralfate *on previous page*

Sulf-10® *see* sulfacetamide *on next page*

sulfabenzamide, sulfacetamide, and sulfathiazole

(sul fa BENZ a mide, sul fa SEE ta mide & sul fa THYE a zole)

Synonyms sulfacetamide, sulfabenzamide, and sulfathiazole; sulfathiazole, sulfacetamide, and sulfabenzamide; triple sulfa

U.S./Canadian Brand Names Femguard®; Gyne-Sulf®; Sulfa-Gyn®; Sulfa-Trip®; Sultrin™; Trysul®; V.V.S.®

Therapeutic Category Antibiotic, Vaginal

Use Treatment of *Haemophilus vaginalis* vaginitis

Usual Dosage Adults: Vaginal:

Cream: Insert 1 applicatorful in vagina twice daily for 4-6 days; dosage may then be decreased to 1/2 to 1/4 of an applicatorful twice daily

Tablet: Insert 1 intravaginally twice daily for 10 days

Dosage Forms

Cream, vaginal: Sulfabenzamide 3.7%, sulfacetamide 2.86%, and sulfathiazole 3.42% (78 g with applicator, 90 g, 120 g)

Tablet, vaginal: Sulfabenzamide 184 mg, sulfacetamide 143.75 mg, and sulfathiazole 172.5 mg (20 tablets/box with vaginal applicator)

sulfacetamide (sul fa SEE ta mide)

U.S./Canadian Brand Names AK-Sulf®; Bleph®-10; Cetamide®; I-Sulfacet®; Ophthacet®; Sodium Sulamyd®; Sulf-10®; Sulfair®; Sulfex® 10% (Can)

Therapeutic Category Antibiotic, Ophthalmic

Use Treatment and prophylaxis of conjunctivitis, corneal ulcers, and other superficial ocular infections due to susceptible organisms; adjunctive treatment with systemic sulfonamides for therapy of trachoma

Usual Dosage Children >2 months and Adults: Ophthalmic:

Ointment: Apply to lower conjunctival sac 1-4 times/day and at bedtime

Solution: 1-2 drops every 2-3 hours in the lower conjunctival sac during the waking hours and less frequently at night

Dosage Forms Sulfacetamide sodium:

Lotion: 10% (85 g)

Ointment, ophthalmic: 10% (3.5 g)

Solution, ophthalmic: 10% (1 mL, 2 mL, 2.5 mL, 5 mL, 15 mL); 15% (5 mL, 15 mL); 30% (15 mL)

sulfacetamide and phenylephrine (sul fa SEE ta mide & fen il EF rin)

Synonyms phenylephrine and sulfacetamide

U.S./Canadian Brand Names Vasosulf® Ophthalmic

Therapeutic Category Antibiotic, Ophthalmic

Use Treatment of conjunctivitis, corneal ulcer, and other superficial ocular infections due to susceptible microorganisms; adjunctive in systemic sulfonamide therapy

Usual Dosage Ophthalmic: Instill 1-3 drops in lower conjunctival sac every 3-4 hours

Dosage Forms Solution, ophthalmic: Sulfacetamide sodium 15% and phenylephrine hydrochloride 0.125% (5 mL, 15 mL)

sulfacetamide and prednisolone (sul fa SEE ta mide & pred NIS oh lone)

Synonyms prednisolone and sulfacetamide

U.S./Canadian Brand Names AK-Cide® Ophthalmic; Blephamide® Ophthalmic; Cetapred® Ophthalmic; Isopto® Cetapred® Ophthalmic; Metimyd® Ophthalmic; Vasocidin® Ophthalmic

Therapeutic Category Antibiotic/Corticosteroid, Ophthalmic

Use Steroid-responsive inflammatory ocular conditions where infection is present or there is a risk of infection; ophthalmic suspension may be used as an otic preparation

Usual Dosage Children >2 and Adults: Ophthalmic:

Ointment: Apply to lower conjunctival sac 1-4 times/day

Solution: Instill 1-3 drops every 2-3 hours while awake

Dosage Forms

Ointment, ophthalmic:

- AK-Cide®, Metimyd®, Vasocidin®: Sulfacetamide sodium 10% and prednisolone acetate 0.5% (3.5 g)
- Blephamide®: Sulfacetamide sodium 10% and prednisolone acetate 0.2% (3.5 g)
- Cetapred®: Sulfacetamide sodium 10% and prednisolone acetate 0.25% (3.5 g)

Suspension, ophthalmic: Sulfacetamide sodium 10% and prednisolone sodium phosphate 0.25% (5 mL)

Suspension, ophthalmic:

- AK-Cide®, Metimyd®: Sulfacetamide sodium 10% and prednisolone acetate 0.5% (5 mL)
- Blephamide®: Sulfacetamide sodium 10% and prednisolone acetate 0.2% (2.5 mL, 5 mL, 10 mL)
- Isopto® Cetapred®: Sulfacetamide sodium 10% and prednisolone acetate 0.25% (5 mL, 15 mL)
- Vasocidin®: Sulfacetamide sodium 10% and prednisolone sodium phosphate: 0.25% (5 mL, 10 mL)

sulfacetamide and sulfur *see* sulfur and sulfacetamide *on page 544*

sulfacetamide sodium and fluorometholone

(sul fa SEE ta mide & flure oh METH oh lone)

Synonyms fluorometholone and sulfacetamide

U.S./Canadian Brand Names FML-S® Ophthalmic Suspension

Therapeutic Category Antibiotic/Corticosteroid, Ophthalmic

Use Steroid-responsive inflammatory ocular conditions where infection is present or there is a risk of infection

Usual Dosage Children >2 months and Adults: Ophthalmic: Instill 1-3 drops every 2-3 hours while awake

Dosage Forms Suspension, ophthalmic: Sulfacetamide sodium 10% and fluorometholone 0.1% (5 mL, 10 mL)

sulfacetamide, sulfabenzamide, and sulfathiazole *see* sulfabenzamide, sulfacetamide, and sulfathiazole *on page 539*

Sulfacet-R® Topical *see* sulfur and sulfacetamide *on page 544*

sulfacytine (sul fa SYE teen)

U.S./Canadian Brand Names Renoquid®

Therapeutic Category Sulfonamide

Use Treatment of urinary tract infections

Usual Dosage Adults: Oral: Initial: 500 mg, then 250 mg every 4 hours for 10 days

Dosage Forms Tablet: 250 mg

sulfadiazine (sul fa DYE a zeen)

U.S./Canadian Brand Names Coptin® (Can)

Therapeutic Category Sulfonamide

Use Adjunctive treatment in toxoplasmosis; treatment of urinary tract infections and nocardiosis; rheumatic fever prophylaxis in penicillin-allergic patient; uncomplicated attack of malaria

Usual Dosage Oral:

Congenital toxoplasmosis:

Newborns and Children <2 months: 100 mg/kg/day divided every 6 hours in conjunction with pyrimethamine 1 mg/kg/day once daily and supplemental folinic acid 5 mg every 3 days for 6 months

Children >2 months: 25-50 mg/kg/dose 4 times/day

Toxoplasmosis:

Children: 120-150 mg/kg/day, maximum dose: 6 g/day; divided every 6 hours in conjunction with pyrimethamine 2 mg/kg/day divided every 12 hours for 3 days followed by 1 mg/kg/day once daily (maximum: 25 mg/day) with supplemental folinic acid

Adults: 2-8 g/day divided every 6 hours in conjunction with pyrimethamine 25 mg/day and with supplemental folinic acid

Dosage Forms Tablet: 500 mg

sulfadiazine, sulfamethazine, and sulfamerazine

(sul fa DYE a zeen, sul fa METH a zeen & sul fa MER a zeen)

Synonyms multiple sulfonamides; trisulfapyrimidines

Therapeutic Category Sulfonamide

Use Treatment of toxoplasmosis

Usual Dosage Adults: Oral: 2-4 g to start, then 2-4 g/day in 3-6 divided doses

Dosage Forms Tablet: Sulfadiazine 167 mg, sulfamethazine 167 mg, and sulfamerazine 167 mg

Sulfa-Gyn® *see* sulfabenzamide, sulfacetamide, and sulfathiazole *on page 539*

Sulfair® *see* sulfacetamide *on previous page*

Sulfalax® [OTC] *see* docusate *on page 191*

Sulfamethoprim® *see* co-trimoxazole *on page 149*

sulfamethoxazole (sul fa meth OKS a zole)

U.S./Canadian Brand Names Apo®-Sulfamethoxazole (Can); Gantanol®; Urobak®

Therapeutic Category Sulfonamide

Use Treatment of urinary tract infections, nocardiosis, chlamydial infections, toxoplasmosis, acute otitis media, and acute exacerbations of chronic bronchitis due to susceptible organisms

Usual Dosage Oral:

Children >2 months: 50-60 mg/kg/day divided every 12 hours; maximum: 3 g/24 hours or 75 mg/kg/day

Adults: 2 g stat, 1 g 2-3 times/day; maximum: 3 g/24 hours

Dosage Forms

Suspension, oral (cherry flavor): 500 mg/5 mL (480 mL)

Tablet: 500 mg

sulfamethoxazole and phenazopyridine

(sul fa meth OKS a zole & fen az oh PEER i deen)

Synonyms phenazopyridine and sulfamethoxazole

Therapeutic Category Sulfonamide

Use Treatment of urinary tract infections complicated with pain

Usual Dosage Oral: Initial: 4 tablets, then 2 tablets twice daily for up to 2 days, then switch to sulfamethoxazole only

Dosage Forms Tablet: Sulfamethoxazole 500 mg and phenazopyridine 100 mg

sulfamethoxazole and trimethoprim *see* co-trimoxazole *on page 149*

Sulfamylon® Topical *see* mafenide *on page 343*

sulfanilamide (sul fa NIL a mide)

U.S./Canadian Brand Names AVC™ Cream; AVC™ Suppository; Vagitrol®

Therapeutic Category Antifungal Agent

Use Treatment of vulvovaginitis caused by *Candida albicans*

Usual Dosage Vaginal: 1 applicatorful once or twice daily continued through 1 complete menstrual cycle

Dosage Forms

Cream, vaginal (AVC™, Vagitrol®): 15% [150 mg/g] (120 g with applicator)

Suppository, vaginal (AVC™): 1.05 g (16s)

sulfasalazine (sul fa SAL a zeen)

Synonyms salicylazosulfapyridine

U.S./Canadian Brand Names Apo®-Sulfasalazine (Can); Azulfidine®; Azulfidine® EN-tabs®; PMS-Sulfasalazine (Can); Salazopyrin® (Can); Salazopyrin EN-Tabs® (Can); S.A.S™ (Can)

Therapeutic Category 5-Aminosalicylic Acid Derivative

Use Management of ulcerative colitis; treatment of active Crohn's disease

Usual Dosage Oral:

Children >2 years:

Initial: 40-60 mg/kg/day divided every 4-6 hour

Maintenance dose: 20-30 mg/kg/day divided every 6 hours, up to a maximum of 2 g/day

Adults:

Initial: 3-4 g/day divided every 4-6 hours

Maintenance dose: 2 g/day divided every 6 hours

Dosage Forms

Tablet: 500 mg

Tablet, enteric coated: 500 mg

sulfathiazole, sulfacetamide, and sulfabenzamide *see* sulfabenzamide, sulfacetamide, and sulfathiazole *on page 539*

Sulfatrim® *see* co-trimoxazole *on page 149*

Sulfatrim® DS *see* co-trimoxazole *on page 149*

Sulfa-Trip® *see* sulfabenzamide, sulfacetamide, and sulfathiazole *on page 539*

Sulfex® 10% (Can) *see* sulfacetamide *on page 540*

sulfinpyrazone (sul fin PEER a zone)

U.S./Canadian Brand Names Antazone® (Can); Anturan® (Can); Anturane®; Apo-Sulfinpyrazone® (Can); Novo-Pyrazone (Can); Nu-Sulfinpyrazone (Can)

Therapeutic Category Uricosuric Agent

Use Treatment of chronic gouty arthritis and intermittent gouty arthritis

Usual Dosage Oral: 200 mg twice daily

Dosage Forms

Capsule: 200 mg

Tablet: 100 mg

sulfisoxazole (sul fi SOKS a zole)

Synonyms sulphafurazole

U.S./Canadian Brand Names Gantrisin®; Novo-Soxazole® (Can); Sulfizole® (Can)

Therapeutic Category Sulfonamide

Use Treatment of uncomplicated urinary tract infections, otitis media, *Chlamydia*; nocardiosis; treatment of acute pelvic inflammatory disease in prepubertal children

Usual Dosage

Children >2 months: Oral: 75 mg/kg stat, 120-150 mg/kg/day in divided doses every 4-6 hours; not to exceed 6 g/day

Pelvic inflammatory disease: 100 mg/kg/day in divided doses every 6 hours; used in combination with ceftriaxone

Chlamydia trachomatis: 100 mg/kg/day divided every 6 hours

Adults: Oral: 2-4 g stat, 4-8 g/day in divided doses every 4-6 hours

Dosage Forms

Suspension, oral, pediatric, as acetyl (raspberry flavor): 500 mg/5 mL (480 mL)

Tablet: 500 mg

sulfisoxazole and erythromycin *see* erythromycin and sulfisoxazole *on page 214*

sulfisoxazole and phenazopyridine

(sul fi SOKS a zole & fen az oh PEER i deen)

Synonyms phenazopyridine and sulfisoxazole

Therapeutic Category Sulfonamide

Use Treatment of urinary tract infections and nocardiosis

Usual Dosage Oral: 4-6 tablets to start, then 2 tablets 4 times/day for 2 days, then continue with sulfisoxazole only

Dosage Forms Tablet: Sulfisoxazole 500 mg and phenazopyridine 50 mg

Sulfizole® (Can) *see* sulfisoxazole *on this page*

sulfur and salicylic acid (SUL fur & sal i SIL ik AS id)

Synonyms salicylic acid and sulfur

U.S./Canadian Brand Names Aveeno® Cleansing Bar [OTC]; Fostex® [OTC]; Pernox® [OTC]; SAStid® Plain Therapeutic Shampoo and Acne Wash [OTC]

Therapeutic Category Antiseborrheic Agent, Topical

Use Therapeutic shampoo for dandruff and seborrheal dermatitis; acne skin cleanser

Usual Dosage Children and Adults: Topical:

Shampoo: Initial: Use daily or every other day; 1-2 treatments/week will usually maintain control

Soap: Use daily or every other day

Dosage Forms

Cake: Sulfur 2% and salicylic acid 2% (123 g)

(Continued)

sulfur and salicylic acid *(Continued)*

Cleanser: Sulfur 2% and salicylic acid 1.5% (60 mL, 120 mL)
Shampoo: Micropulverized sulfur 2% and salicylic acid 2% (120 mL, 240 mL)
Soap: Micropulverized sulfur 2% and salicylic acid 2% (113 g)
Wash: Sulfur 1.6% and salicylic acid 1.6% (75 mL)

sulfur and sulfacetamide (SUL fur & sul fa SEE ta mide)

Synonyms sulfacetamide and sulfur
U.S./Canadian Brand Names Novacet® Topical; Sulfacet-R® Topical
Therapeutic Category Antiseborrheic Agent, Topical
Use Aid in the treatment of acne vulgaris, acne rosacea and seborrheic dermatitis
Usual Dosage Topical: Apply in a thin film 1-3 times/day
Dosage Forms Lotion, topical: Sulfur colloid 5% and sulfacetamide sodium 10% (30 mL)

sulindac (sul IN dak)

U.S./Canadian Brand Names Apo®-Sulin (Can); Clinoril®; Novo-Sundac® (Can)
Therapeutic Category Analgesic, Non-narcotic; Nonsteroidal Anti-inflammatory Drug (NSAID)
Use Management of inflammatory disease, rheumatoid disorders; acute gouty arthritis
Usual Dosage Oral:
Children: Dose not established
Adults: 150-200 mg twice daily; not to exceed 400 mg/day
Dosage Forms Tablet: 150 mg, 200 mg

sulphafurazole *see* sulfisoxazole *on previous page*

Sultrin™ *see* sulfabenzamide, sulfacetamide, and sulfathiazole *on page 539*

Sumacal® [OTC] *see* glucose polymers *on page 262*

sumatriptan succinate (SOO ma trip tan SUKS i nate)

U.S./Canadian Brand Names Imitrex®
Therapeutic Category Antimigraine Agent
Use Acute treatment of migraine with or without aura
Unlabeled use: Cluster headaches
Usual Dosage Adults:
Oral: 25 mg (taken with fluids); maximum recommended dose is 100 mg. If a satisfactory response has not been obtained at 2 hours, a second dose of up to 100 mg may be given. Efficacy of this second dose has not been examined. If a headache returns, additional doses may be taken at intervals of at least 2 hours up to a daily maximum of 300 mg. There is no evidence that an initial dose of 100 mg provides substantially greater relief than 25 mg.
Intranasal: Single dose of 5, 10, or 20 mg administered in one nostril; a 10 mg dose may be achieved by administration of a single 5 mg dose in each nostril; if headache returns, the dose may be repeated once after 2 hours, not to exceed a total daily dose of 40 mg
S.C.: 6 mg; a second injection may be administered at least 1 hour after the initial dose, but not more than two injections in a 24-hour period
Dosage Forms
Injection: 12 mg/mL (0.5 mL, 2 mL)
Spray, nasal: 5 mg (100 mcL); 20 mg (100 mcL)
Tablet: 25 mg, 50 mg

Summer's Eve® Medicated Douche [OTC] *see* povidone-iodine *on page 467*

Sumycin® Oral *see* tetracycline *on page 555*

sunscreen (paba-free) *see* methoxycinnamate and oxybenzone *on page 365*

Superchar® ***(Discontinued)*** *see page 700*

Superchar® With Sorbitol ***(Discontinued)*** *see page 700*

Supprelin™ *see* histrelin *on page 282*

Suppress® [OTC] *see* dextromethorphan *on page 171*

Supracaine® (Can) *see* tetracaine *on page 555*

Suprane® *see* desflurane *on page 165*

Suprax® *see* cefixime *on page 105*

suprofen (soo PROE fen)

U.S./Canadian Brand Names Profenal® Ophthalmic

Therapeutic Category Nonsteroidal Anti-inflammatory Drug (NSAID)

Use Inhibition of intraoperative miosis

Usual Dosage Ophthalmic: On day of surgery, instill 2 drops in conjunctival sac at 3, 2, and 1 hour prior to surgery; or 2 drops in sac every 4 hours, while awake, the day preceding surgery

Dosage Forms Solution, ophthalmic: 1% (2.5 mL)

Surbex® [OTC] *see* vitamin B complex *on page 603*

Surbex-T® Filmtabs® [OTC] *see* vitamin B complex with vitamin C *on page 603*

Surbex® With C Filmtabs® [OTC] *see* vitamin B complex with vitamin C *on page 603*

Surfak® [OTC] *see* docusate *on page 191*

Surgam® (Can) *see* tiaprofenic acid *(Canada only) on page 565*

Surgam® SR (Can) *see* tiaprofenic acid *(Canada only) on page 565*

Surgicel® *see* cellulose, oxidized *on page 110*

Surital® ***(Discontinued)*** *see page 700*

Surmontil® *see* trimipramine *on page 583*

Survanta® *see* beractant *on page 70*

Sus-Phrine® *see* epinephrine *on page 209*

Sustaire® *see* theophylline *on page 557*

Sustiva™ *see* efavirenz *on page 204*

suxamethonium *see* succinylcholine *on page 537*

Sween Cream® [OTC] *see* methylbenzethonium chloride *on page 366*

Swim-Ear® Otic [OTC] *see* boric acid *on page 77*

Syllact® [OTC] *see* psyllium *on page 488*

Symadine® *see* amantadine *on page 24*

Symmetrel® Capsule ***(Discontinued)*** *see page 700*

Symmetrel® Syrup *see* amantadine *on page 24*

Synacol® CF [OTC] *see* guaifenesin and dextromethorphan *on page 268*

Synacort® Topical *see* hydrocortisone (topical) *on page 292*

synacthen *see* cosyntropin *on page 149*

Synacthen® Depot (Can) *see* cosyntropin *on page 149*

Synagis® *see* palivizumab *on page 425*

Synalar-HP® Topical *see* fluocinolone *on page 243*

Synalar® Topical *see* fluocinolone *on page 243*

Synalgos®-DC *see* dihydrocodeine compound *on page 180*

Synarel® *see* nafarelin *on page 387*

Syn-Captopril® (Can) *see* captopril *on page 96*

Syn-Diltiazem® (Can) *see* diltiazem *on page 182*

Synemol® Topical *see* fluocinolone *on page 243*

Synercid® *see* quinupristin and dalfopristin *on page 493*

Synflex® (Can) *see* naproxen *on page 391*

Syn-Flunisolide® (Can) *see* flunisolide *on page 243*

Synkayvite® *(Discontinued)* *see page 700*

Syn-Minocycline® (Can) *see* minocycline *on page 377*

Syn-Nadolol® (Can) *see* nadolol *on page 387*

Synphasic® (Can) *see* ethinyl estradiol and norethindrone *on page 224*

Syn-Pindol® (Can) *see* pindolol *on page 452*

synthetic lung surfactant *see* colfosceril palmitate *on page 145*

Synthroid® *see* levothyroxine *on page 332*

Syntocinon® Nasal *(Discontinued)* *see page 700*

Syprine® *see* trientine *on page 580*

Syracol-CF® [OTC] *see* guaifenesin and dextromethorphan *on page 268*

Sytobex® *see* cyanocobalamin *on page 152*

t_3/t_4 liotrix *see* liotrix *on page 336*

t_3 thyronine *see* liothyronine *on page 335*

t_4 thyroxine *see* levothyroxine *on page 332*

Tabron® *(Discontinued)* *see page 700*

Tac™-3 Injection *see* triamcinolone (systemic) *on page 577*

Tac™-40 Injection *see* triamcinolone (systemic) *on page 577*

Tacaryl® *(Discontinued)* *see page 700*

TACE® *see* chlorotrianisene *on page 120*

Tacozin® (Can) *see* piperacillin and tazobactam sodium *on page 454*

tacrine (TAK reen)

Synonyms tetrahydroaminoacrine; THA

U.S./Canadian Brand Names Cognex®

Therapeutic Category Acetylcholinesterase Inhibitor

Use Treatment of Alzheimer's disease

Usual Dosage Adults: Oral: 40 mg/day

Dosage Forms Capsule, as hydrochloride: 10 mg, 20 mg, 30 mg, 40 mg

tacrolimus (ta KROE li mus)

Synonyms FK506

U.S./Canadian Brand Names Prograf®

Therapeutic Category Immunosuppressant Agent

Use Potent immunosuppressive drug used in liver, kidney, heart, lung, or small bowel transplant recipients

Usual Dosage

Initial: I.V. continuous infusion: 0.1 mg/kg/day until the tolerance of oral intake

Oral: Usually 3-4 times the I.V. dose, or 0.3 mg/kg/day in divided doses every 12 hours

Dosage Forms

Capsule: 1 mg, 5 mg

Injection, with alcohol and surfactant: 5 mg/mL (1 mL)

Tagamet® *see* cimetidine *on page 131*

Tagamet-HB® [OTC] *see* cimetidine *on page 131*

Talacen® *see* pentazocine compound *on page 437*

Talwin® *see* pentazocine *on page 437*

Talwin® Compound *see* pentazocine compound *on page 437*

Talwin® NX *see* pentazocine *on page 437*

Tambocor™ *see* flecainide *on page 240*

Tamiflu™ *see* oseltamivir *on page 419*

Tamine® [OTC] *see* brompheniramine and phenylpropanolamine *on page 81*

Tamofen® (Can) *see* tamoxifen *on this page*

Tamone® (Can) *see* tamoxifen *on this page*

tamoxifen (ta MOKS i fen)

U.S./Canadian Brand Names Alpha-Tamoxifen® (Can); Apo-Tamox® (Can); Nolvadex®; Novo-Tamoxifen (Can); Tamofen® (Can); Tamone® (Can)

Therapeutic Category Antineoplastic Agent

Use Palliative or adjunctive treatment of advanced breast cancer in postmenopausal women

Usual Dosage Oral: 10-20 mg twice daily

Dosage Forms Tablet, as citrate: 10 mg, 20 mg

tamsulosin (tam SOO loe sin)

U.S./Canadian Brand Names Flomax®

Therapeutic Category Alpha-Adrenergic Blocking Agent

Use Treatment of signs and symptoms of benign prostatic hyperplasia (BPH)

Usual Dosage Oral: Adults: 0.4 mg once daily approximately 30 minutes after the same meal each day

Dosage Forms Capsule, as hydrochloride: 0.4 mg

Tanac® [OTC] *see* benzocaine *on page 66*

Tanoral® Tablet *see* chlorpheniramine, pyrilamine, and phenylephrine *on page 126*

Tantaphen® (Can) *see* acetaminophen *on page 3*

Tao® *see* troleandomycin *on page 586*

Tapanol® [OTC] *see* acetaminophen *on page 3*

Tapazole® *see* methimazole *on page 363*

Tarabine® PFS *see* cytarabine *on page 156*

Taractan® *(Discontinued)* *see page 700*

Tarka® *see* trandolapril and verapamil *on page 574*

Taro-Ampicillin® (Can) *see* ampicillin *on page 34*

Taro-Atenol® (Can) *see* atenolol *on page 51*

Taro-Cloxacillin® (Can) *see* cloxacillin *on page 141*

Taro-Sone® (Can) *see* betamethasone (topical) *on page 72*

Tasmar® *see* tolcapone *on page 571*

TAT *see* tetanus antitoxin *on page 553*

Tavist® *see* clemastine *on page 135*

Tavist®-1 [OTC] *see* clemastine *on page 135*

Tavist-D® *see* clemastine and phenylpropanolamine *on page 136*

Taxol® *see* paclitaxel *on page 425*

Taxotere® *see* docetaxel *on page 190*

tazarotene (taz AR oh teen)

U.S./Canadian Brand Names Tazorac®

Therapeutic Category Keratolytic Agent

Use Topical treatment of facial acne vulgaris; topical treatment of stable plaque psoriasis of up to 20% body surface area involvement

Usual Dosage Children >12 years and Adults: Topical:

(Continued)

tazarotene *(Continued)*

Acne: Cleanse the face gently. After the skin is dry, apply a thin film of tazarotene (2 mg/ cm^2) once daily, in the evening, to the skin where the acne lesions appear. Use enough to cover the entire affected area. Tazarotene was investigated ≤12 weeks during clinical trials for acne.

Psoriasis: Apply tazarotene once daily, in the evening, to psoriatic lesions using enough (2 mg/cm^2) to cover only the lesion with a thin film to no more than 20% of body surface area. If a bath or shower is taken prior to application, dry the skin before applying the gel. Because unaffected skin may be more susceptible to irritation, avoid application of tazarotene to these areas. Tazarotene was investigated for up to 12 months during clinical trials for psoriasis.

Dosage Forms Gel: 0.05% (30 g, 100 g); 0.1% (30 g, 100 g)

Tazicef® *see* ceftazidime *on page 108*

Tazidime® *see* ceftazidime *on page 108*

tazobactam and piperacillin *see* piperacillin and tazobactam sodium *on page 454*

Tazorac® *see* tazarotene *on previous page*

3TC *see* lamivudine *on page 325*

T-Caine® Lozenge *(Discontinued)* *see page 700*

3TC® (Can) *see* lamivudine *on page 325*

TCN *see* tetracycline *on page 555*

Td *see* diphtheria and tetanus toxoid *on page 186*

Tear Drop® Solution [OTC] *see* artificial tears *on page 47*

TearGard® Ophthalmic Solution [OTC] *see* artificial tears *on page 47*

Teargen® Ophthalmic Solution [OTC] *see* artificial tears *on page 47*

Tearisol® Solution [OTC] *see* artificial tears *on page 47*

Tears Naturale® Free Solution [OTC] *see* artificial tears *on page 47*

Tears Naturale® II Solution [OTC] *see* artificial tears *on page 47*

Tears Naturale® Solution [OTC] *see* artificial tears *on page 47*

Tears Plus® Solution [OTC] *see* artificial tears *on page 47*

Tears Renewed® Solution [OTC] *see* artificial tears *on page 47*

Tebamide® *see* trimethobenzamide *on page 582*

Tebrazid (Can) *see* pyrazinamide *on page 489*

Teczem® *see* enalapril and diltiazem *on page 206*

Tedral® *see* theophylline, ephedrine, and phenobarbital *on page 559*

Teejel® (Can) *see* choline salicylate *on page 129*

Tega-Vert® Oral *see* dimenhydrinate *on page 182*

Tegison® *see* etretinate *on page 229*

Tegopen® *(Discontinued)* *see page 700*

Tegretol® *see* carbamazepine *on page 97*

Tegretol®-XR *see* carbamazepine *on page 97*

Tegrin®-HC Topical [OTC] *see* hydrocortisone (topical) *on page 292*

Telachlor® Oral *see* chlorpheniramine *on page 120*

Teladar® Topical *see* betamethasone (topical) *on page 72*

Teldrin® Oral [OTC] *see* chlorpheniramine *on page 120*

Telepaque® *see* radiological/contrast media (ionic) *on page 495*

Teline® *(Discontinued)* *see page 700*

telmisartan (tel mi SAR tan)

U.S./Canadian Brand Names Micardis®

Therapeutic Category Angiotensin II Antagonist

Use Treatment of hypertension alone or in combination with other antihypertensives

Usual Dosage Adults: Oral: The usual starting dose is 40 mg once daily. Blood pressure response is dose-related over the range of 20 mg-80 mg/day; when additional antihypertensive effects are needed beyond that achieved with 80 mg/day, a diuretic may be added.

Dosage Forms Tablet: 40 mg, 80 mg

Temaril® ***(Discontinued)*** *see page 700*

temazepam (te MAZ e pam)

U.S./Canadian Brand Names Restoril®

Therapeutic Category Benzodiazepine

Controlled Substance C-IV

Use Treatment of anxiety and as an adjunct in the treatment of depression; also may be used in the management of panic attacks; transient insomnia and sleep latency

Usual Dosage Adults: Oral: 15-30 mg at bedtime

Dosage Forms Capsule: 7.5 mg, 15 mg, 30 mg

Temazin® Cold Syrup [OTC] *see* chlorpheniramine and phenylpropanolamine *on page 122*

Temodar® *see* temozolomide *on this page*

Temovate® *see* clobetasol *on page 137*

temozolomide (te mo ZOLE oh mide)

U.S./Canadian Brand Names Temodar®

Therapeutic Category Antineoplastic Agent, Alkylating Agent

Use Treatment of adult patients with refractory (first relapse) anaplastic astrocytoma who have experienced disease progression on nitrosourea and procarbazine

Unlabeled use: Glioma, first relapse/advanced metastatic malignant melanoma

Usual Dosage The dosage is adjusted according to nadir neutrophil and platelet counts of previous cycle and counts at the time of the next cycle.

Adults: Initial dose: 150 mg/m^2 once daily for 5 consecutive days per 28-day treatment cycle

Measure day 22 ANC and platelets. Measure day 29 ANC and platelets. Based on lowest counts at either day 22 or day 29:

On day 22 or day 29, if ANC <1,000/μL or the platelet count is <50,000/μL, postpone therapy until ANC >1,500/μL and platelet count >100,000/μL. Reduce dose by 50 mg/m^2 for subsequent cycle.

If ANC 1,000-1,500/μL or platelets 50,000-100,000/μL, postpone therapy until ANC >1,500/μL and platelet count >100,000/μL; maintain initial dose.

If ANC >1,500/μL (on day 22 and day 29) and platelet count >100,000/μL, increase dose to, or maintain dose at 200 mg/m^2/day for 5 for subsequent cycle.

Dosage Forms Capsule: 5 mg, 20 mg, 100 mg, 250 mg

Tempra® [OTC] *see* acetaminophen *on page 3*

Tenex® *see* guanfacine *on page 274*

teniposide (ten i POE side)

Synonyms EPT; VM-26

U.S./Canadian Brand Names Vumon

Therapeutic Category Antineoplastic Agent

Use Treatment of Hodgkin's and non-Hodgkin's lymphomas, acute lymphocytic leukemia, bladder carcinoma and neuroblastoma

(Continued)

teniposide *(Continued)*

Usual Dosage I.V.:

Children: 130 mg/m^2/week, increasing to 150 mg/m^2 after 3 weeks and to 180 mg/m^2 after 6 weeks

Adults: 50-180 mg/m^2 once or twice weekly for 4-6 weeks

Dosage Forms Injection: 10 mg/mL (5 mL)

Ten-K® *see* potassium chloride *on page 464*

Tenoretic® *see* atenolol and chlorthalidone *on page 51*

Tenormin® *see* atenolol *on page 51*

Tensilon® *see* edrophonium *on page 203*

Tenuate® *see* diethylpropion *on page 178*

Tenuate® Dospan® *see* diethylpropion *on page 178*

Tepanil® ***(Discontinued)*** *see page 700*

Tepanil® TenTabs® ***(Discontinued)*** *see page 700*

Terak® Ophthalmic Ointment *see* oxytetracycline and polymyxin B *on page 425*

Terazol® Vaginal *see* terconazole *on next page*

terazosin (ter AY zoe sin)

U.S./Canadian Brand Names Hytrin®

Therapeutic Category Alpha-Adrenergic Blocking Agent

Use Management of mild to moderate hypertension; considered a step 2 drug in stepped approach to hypertension; benign prostate hypertrophy

Usual Dosage Adults: Oral: 1 mg; slowly increase dose to achieve desired blood pressure, up to 20 mg/day

Dosage Forms

Capsule: 1 mg, 2 mg, 5 mg, 10 mg

Tablet: 1 mg, 2 mg, 5 mg, 10 mg

terbinafine, oral (TER bin a feen, OR al)

U.S./Canadian Brand Names Lamisil® Oral

Therapeutic Category Antifungal Agent

Use Treatment of onychomycosis infections of the toenail or fingernail

Usual Dosage Adults: Oral:

Fingernail onychomycosis: 250 mg once daily for 6 weeks

Toenail onychomycosis: 250 mg once daily for 12 weeks

Dosage Forms Tablet: 250 mg

terbinafine, topical (TER bin a feen, TOP i kal)

U.S./Canadian Brand Names Lamisil® Cream

Therapeutic Category Antifungal Agent

Use Topical antifungal for the treatment of tinea pedis (athlete's foot), tinea cruris (jock itch), and tinea corporis (ring worm); tinea versicolor (lotion)

Unlabeled use: Cutaneous candidiasis

Usual Dosage Adults: Topical:

Athlete's foot: Apply to affected area twice daily for at least 1 week, not to exceed 4 weeks

Ringworm and jock itch: Apply to affected area once or twice daily for at least 1 week, not to exceed 4 weeks

Dosage Forms

Cream: 1% (15 g, 30 g)

Lotion: 1%

terbutaline (ter BYOO ta leen)

U.S./Canadian Brand Names Brethaire®; Brethine®; Bricanyl®

Therapeutic Category Adrenergic Agonist Agent

Use Bronchodilator in reversible airway obstruction and bronchial asthma

Usual Dosage

Children <6 years:

Oral: Initial: 0.05 mg/kg/dose 3 times/day, increased gradually as required; maximum: 0.15 mg/kg/dose 3-4 times/day or a total of 5 mg/24 hours

S.C.: 0.005-0.01 mg/kg/dose to a maximum of 0.3 mg/dose every 15-20 minutes for 3 doses

Inhalation nebulization dose: 0.06 mg/kg; maximum: 8 mg

Inhalation: 0.3 mg/kg/dose up to maximum of 10 mg/dose every 4-6 hours

Children >6 years and Adults:

Oral:

6-15 years: 2.5 mg every 6 hours 3 times/day; not to exceed 7.5 mg in 24 hours

>15 years: 5 mg/dose every 6 hours 3 times/day; if side effects occur, reduce dose to 2.5 mg every 6 hours; not to exceed 15 mg in 24 hours

S.C.: 0.25 mg/dose repeated in 15-30 minutes for one time only; a total dose of 0.5 mg should not be exceeded within a 4-hour period

Nebulization: 0.01-0.03 mL/kg (1 mg = 1 mL); minimum dose: 0.1 mL; maximum dose: 2.5 mL diluted with 1-2 mL normal saline

Inhalation: 2 inhalations every 4-6 hours; wait 1 minute between inhalations

Dosage Forms Terbutaline sulfate:

Aerosol, oral: 0.2 mg/actuation (10.5 g)

Injection: 1 mg/mL (1 mL)

Tablet: 2.5 mg, 5 mg

terconazole (ter KONE a zole)

Synonyms triaconazole

U.S./Canadian Brand Names Terazol® Vaginal

Therapeutic Category Antifungal Agent

Use Local treatment of vulvovaginal candidiasis

Usual Dosage Vaginal: 1 applicatorful in vagina at bedtime for 7 consecutive days

Dosage Forms

Cream, vaginal: 0.4% (45 g); 0.8% (20 g)

Suppository, vaginal: 80 mg (3s)

terfenadine (ter FEN a deen)

U.S./Canadian Brand Names Apo®-Terfenadine (Can); Novo-Terfenadine® (Can); Seldane®

Therapeutic Category Antihistamine

Use Perennial and seasonal allergic rhinitis and other allergic symptoms including urticaria

Usual Dosage Oral:

Children:

3-6 years: 15 mg twice daily

6-12 years: 30 mg twice daily

Children >12 years and Adults: 60 mg twice daily

Dosage Forms Tablet: 60 mg

teriparatide (ter i PAR a tide)

U.S./Canadian Brand Names Parathar™

Therapeutic Category Diagnostic Agent

Use Diagnosis of hypocalcemia in either hypoparathyroidism or pseudohypoparathyroidism

Usual Dosage I.V.:

Children ≥3 years: 3 units/kg up to 200 units

Adults: 200 units over 10 minutes

Dosage Forms Powder for injection: 200 units hPTH activity (10 mL)

terpin hydrate (TER pin HYE drate)

Therapeutic Category Expectorant

Use Symptomatic relief of cough

Usual Dosage Adults: Oral: 5-10 mL every 4-6 hours as needed

Dosage Forms Elixir: 85 mg/5 mL (120 mL)

terpin hydrate and codeine (TER pin HYE drate & KOE deen)

Synonyms ETH and C

Therapeutic Category Antitussive/Expectorant

Controlled Substance C-V

Use Symptomatic relief of cough

Usual Dosage Based on codeine content: Oral:

Children (not recommended): 1-1.5 mg/kg/24 hours divided every 4 hours; maximum: 30 mg/24 hours

2-6 years: 1.25-2.5 mL every 4-6 hours as needed

6-12 years: 2.5-5 mL every 4-6 hours as needed

Adults: 10-20 mg/dose every 4-6 hours as needed

Dosage Forms Elixir: Terpin hydrate 85 mg and codeine 10 mg per 5 mL with alcohol 42.5%

Terra-Cortril® Ophthalmic Suspension *see* oxytetracycline and hydrocortisone *on page 425*

Terramycin® I.M. Injection *see* oxytetracycline *on page 424*

Terramycin® Ophthalmic Ointment *see* oxytetracycline and polymyxin B *on page 425*

Terramycin® Oral *see* oxytetracycline *on page 424*

Terramycin® w/Polymyxin B Ophthalmic Ointment *see* oxytetracycline and polymyxin B *on page 425*

Tesamone® Injection *see* testosterone *on this page*

Teslac® *see* testolactone *on this page*

TESPA *see* thiotepa *on page 563*

Tessalon® Perles *see* benzonatate *on page 68*

Tes-Tape® ***(Discontinued)*** *see page 700*

Testoderm® Transdermal System *see* testosterone *on this page*

testolactone (tes toe LAK tone)

U.S./Canadian Brand Names Teslac®

Therapeutic Category Androgen

Use Palliative treatment of advanced disseminated breast carcinoma

Usual Dosage Adults: Females: Oral: 250 mg 4 times/day for at least 3 months; desired response may take as long as 3 months

Dosage Forms Tablet: 50 mg

Testopel® Pellet *see* testosterone *on this page*

testosterone (tes TOS ter one)

Synonyms aqueous testosterone

U.S./Canadian Brand Names Androderm® Transdermal System; Andro-L.A.® Injection; Andropository® Injection; Delatest® Injection; Delatestryl® Injection; depAndro® Injection; Depotest® Injection; Depo®-Testosterone Injection; Duratest® Injection; Durathate® Injection; Everone® Injection; Histerone® Injection; Tesamone® Injection; Testoderm® Transdermal System; Testopel® Pellet

Therapeutic Category Androgen

Controlled Substance C-III

Use Androgen replacement therapy in the treatment of delayed male puberty; male hypogonadism

Usual Dosage I.M.:

- Delayed puberty: Children: 40-50 mg/m^2/dose (cypionate or enanthate) monthly for 6 months
- Male hypogonadism: 50-400 mg every 2-4 weeks
  - Initiation of pubertal growth: 40-50 mg/m^2/dose (cypionate or enanthate) monthly until the growth rate falls to prepubertal levels (~5 cm/year)
  - During terminal growth phase: 100 mg/m^2/dose (cypionate or enanthate) monthly until growth ceases
  - Maintenance virilizing dose: 100 mg/m^2/dose (cypionate or enanthate) twice monthly or 50-400 mg/dose every 2-4 weeks
- Inoperable breast cancer: Adults: 200-400 mg every 2-4 weeks
- Hypogonadism: Adults:
  - Testosterone or testosterone propionate: 10-25 mg 2-3 times/week
  - Testosterone cypionate or enanthate: 50-400 mg every 2-4 weeks
  - Postpubertal cryptorchism: Testosterone or testosterone propionate: 10-25 mg 2-3 times/week
- Transdermal system: Males: Place the patch on clean, dry, scrotal skin; dry-shaved scrotal hair for optimal skin contact, do not use chemical depilatories; patients should start therapy with 6 mg/day system applied daily; if scrotal area is inadequate, use a 4 mg/day system; the system should be worn for 22-24 hours

Dosage Forms

- Injection:
  - Aqueous suspension: 25 mg/mL (10 mL, 30 mL); 50 mg/mL (10 mL, 30 mL); 100 mg/mL (10 mL, 30 mL)
  - In oil, as cypionate: 100 mg/mL (1 mL, 10 mL); 200 mg/mL (1 mL, 10 mL)
  - In oil, as enanthate: 100 mg/mL (5 mL, 10 mL); 200 mg/mL (5 mL, 10 mL)
  - In oil, as propionate: 50 mg/mL (10 mL, 30 mL); 100 mg/mL (10 mL, 30 mL)
- Pellet: 75 mg (1 pellet per vial)
- Transdermal system: 2.5 mg/day; 4 mg/day; 5 mg/day; 6 mg/day

Testred® *see* methyltestosterone *on page 369*

tetanus and diphtheria toxoid *see* diphtheria and tetanus toxoid *on page 186*

tetanus antitoxin (TET a nus an tee TOKS in)

Synonyms TAT

Therapeutic Category Antitoxin

Use Tetanus prophylaxis or treatment of active tetanus only when tetanus immune globulin (TIG) is not available

Usual Dosage

- Prophylaxis: I.M., S.C.:
  - Children <30 kg: 1500 units
  - Children and Adults >30 kg: 3000-5000 units
- Treatment: Children and Adults: Inject 10,000-40,000 units into wound; administer 40,000-100,000 units I.V.

Dosage Forms Injection, equine: Not less than 400 units/mL (12.5 mL, 50 mL)

tetanus immune globulin (human)

(TET a nus i MYUN GLOB yoo lin, HYU man)

Synonyms TIG

U.S./Canadian Brand Names Hyper-Tet®

Therapeutic Category Immune Globulin

Use Passive immunization against tetanus; tetanus immune globulin is preferred over tetanus antitoxin for treatment of active tetanus; part of the management of an unclean, nonminor wound in a person whose history of previous receipt of tetanus toxoid is unknown or who has received less than three doses of tetanus toxoid

(Continued)

tetanus immune globulin (human) *(Continued)*

Usual Dosage I.M.:

Prophylaxis of tetanus:

Children: 4 units/kg; some recommend administering 250 units to small children

Adults: 250 units

Treatment of tetanus:

Children: 500-3000 units; some should infiltrate locally around the wound

Adults: 3000-6000 units

Dosage Forms Injection: 250 units/mL

tetanus toxoid (adsorbed) (TET a nus TOKS oyd, ad SORBED)

Therapeutic Category Toxoid

Use Active immunization against tetanus

Usual Dosage Adults: I.M.:

Primary immunization: 0.5 mL; repeat 0.5 mL at 4-8 weeks after first dose and at 6-12 months after second dose

Routine booster doses are recommended only every 5-10 years

Dosage Forms Injection, adsorbed:

Tetanus 5 Lf units per 0.5 mL dose (0.5 mL, 5 mL)

Tetanus 10 Lf units per 0.5 mL dose (0.5 mL, 5 mL)

tetanus toxoid (fluid) (TET a nus TOKS oyd FLOO id)

Synonyms tetanus toxoid plain

Therapeutic Category Toxoid

Use Active immunization against tetanus in adults and children

Usual Dosage Inject 3 doses of 0.5 mL I.M. or S.C. at 4- to 8-week intervals with fourth dose administered only 6-12 months after third dose

Dosage Forms Injection, fluid:

Tetanus 4 Lf units per 0.5 mL dose (7.5 mL)

Tetanus 5 Lf units per 0.5 mL dose (0.5 mL, 7.5 mL)

tetanus toxoid plain *see* tetanus toxoid (fluid) *on this page*

tetrabenazine *(Canada only)* (tet ra BENZ a zeen)

U.S./Canadian Brand Names Nitoman® (Can)

Therapeutic Category Monoamine Depleting Agent

Use Treatment of hyperkinetic movement disorders such as Huntington's chorea, hemiballismus, senile chorea, tic and Gilles de la Tourette syndrome and tardive dyskinesia; not indicated for the treatment of levodopa-induced dyskinetic/choreiform movements; should only be used by (or in consultation with) physicians who are experienced in the treatment of hyperkinetic movement diso

Usual Dosage Oral:

Children: No adequately controlled clinical studies have been performed in children. Limited clinical experience suggests that treatment should be started at approximately half the adult dose, and titrated slowly and carefully according to tolerance and individual response.

Adults: An initial starting dose of 12.5 mg two to three times a day is recommended. This can be increased by 12.5 mg a day every three to five days until the maximal tolerated and effective dose is reached for the individual, and may have to be up/down titrated depending on individual tolerance. In most cases the maximal tolerated dose will be 25 mg three times/day. In very rare cases, a 200 mg dose has been reached (the maximum recommended dose in some publications). If there is no improvement at the maximal tolerated dose in seven days, it is unlikely that Nitoman® will be of benefit to the patient, either by increasing the dose or by extending the duration of treatment.

Elderly and debilitated patients: No adequately controlled clinical studies have been performed in the elderly and/or debilitated patients. Clinical experience suggests that a reduced initial and maintenance dose should be used. Parkinsonian-like adverse reactions are relatively common in these patients and may be dose-limiting.

Dosage Forms Tablet: 25 mg

tetracaine (TET ra kane)

Synonyms amethocaine

U.S./Canadian Brand Names Pontocaine®; Supracaine® (Can)

Therapeutic Category Local Anesthetic

Use Local anesthesia in the eye for various diagnostic and examination purposes; spinal anesthesia; topical anesthesia for local skin disorders; local anesthesia for mucous membranes

Usual Dosage

Children: Safety and efficacy have not been established

Adults:

Ophthalmic (not for prolonged use):

Ointment: Apply ½" to 1" to lower conjunctival fornix

Solution: Instill 1-2 drops

Spinal anesthesia 1% solution:

Subarachnoid injection: 5-20 mg

Saddle block: 2-5 mg; a 1% solution should be diluted with equal volume of CSF before administration

Topical mucous membranes (2% solution): Apply as needed; dose should not exceed 20 mg

Topical for skin: Apply to affected areas as needed

Dosage Forms Tetracaine hydrochloride:

Cream: 1% (28 g)

Injection: 1% [10 mg/mL] (2 mL)

Injection, with dextrose 6%: 0.2% [2 mg/mL] (2 mL); 0.3% [3 mg/mL] (5 mL)

Ointment:

Ophthalmic: 0.5% [5 mg/mL] (3.75 g)

Topical: 0.5% [5 mg/mL] (28 g)

Powder for injection: 20 mg

Solution:

Ophthalmic: 0.5% [5 mg/mL] (1 mL, 2 mL, 15 mL, 59 mL)

Topical: 2% [20 mg/mL] (30 mL, 118 mL)

tetracaine and dextrose (TET ra kane & DEKS trose)

U.S./Canadian Brand Names Pontocaine® With Dextrose

Therapeutic Category Local Anesthetic

Use Spinal anesthesia (saddle block)

Usual Dosage Dose varies with procedure, depth of anesthesia, duration desired, and physical condition of patient

Dosage Forms Injection: Tetracaine hydrochloride 0.2% and dextrose 6% (2 mL); tetracaine hydrochloride 0.3% and dextrose 6% (5 mL)

tetracaine hydrochloride, benzocaine, butyl aminobenzoate, and benzalkonium chloride *see* benzocaine, butyl aminobenzoate, tetracaine, and benzalkonium chloride *on page 67*

Tetracap® Oral *see* tetracycline *on this page*

tetracosactide *see* cosyntropin *on page 149*

tetracycline (tet ra SYE kleen)

Synonyms TCN

U.S./Canadian Brand Names Achromycin® Ophthalmic; Achromycin® Topical; Apo®-Tetra (Can); Nor-tet® Oral; Novo-Tetra® (Can); Nu-Tetra® (Can); Panmycin® Oral; Robitet® Oral; Sumycin® Oral; Tetracap® Oral; Tetracyn® (Can); Topicycline® Topical

Therapeutic Category Antibiotic, Ophthalmic; Antibiotic, Topical; Tetracycline Derivative

(Continued)

tetracycline *(Continued)*

Use

Children, Adolescents, and Adults: Treatment of Rocky mountain spotted fever caused by susceptible Rickettsia or brucellosis

Adolescents and Adults: Presumptive treatment of chlamydial infection in patients with gonorrhea

Older Children, Adolescents, and Adults: Treatment of Lyme disease, mycoplasmal disease or *Legionella*

Usual Dosage

Children >8 years:

Oral: 25-50 mg/kg/day in divided doses every 6 hours; not to exceed 3 g/day

Ophthalmic:

Suspension: Instill 1-2 drops 2-4 times/day or more often as needed

Ointment: Instill every 2-12 hours

Adults:

Oral: 250-500 mg/dose every 6 hours

Ophthalmic:

Suspension: Instill 1-2 drops 2-4 times/day or more often as needed

Ointment: Instill every 2-12 hours

Topical: Apply to affected areas 1-4 times/day

Dosage Forms Tetracycline hydrochloride:

Capsule: 100 mg, 250 mg, 500 mg

Ointment:

Ophthalmic: 1% [10 mg/mL] (3.5 g)

Topical: 3% [30 mg/mL] (14.2 g, 30 g)

Solution, topical: 2.2 mg/mL (70 mL)

Suspension:

Ophthalmic: 1% [10 mg/mL] (0.5 mL, 1 mL, 4 mL)

Oral: 125 mg/5 mL (60 mL, 480 mL)

Tablet: 250 mg, 500 mg

Tetracyn® (Can) *see* tetracycline *on previous page*

tetrahydroaminoacrine *see* tacrine *on page 546*

tetrahydrocannabinol *see* dronabinol *on page 198*

tetrahydrozoline (tet ra hye DROZ a leen)

Synonyms tetryzoline

U.S./Canadian Brand Names Collyrium Fresh® Ophthalmic [OTC]; Eyesine® Ophthalmic [OTC]; Geneye® Ophthalmic [OTC]; Mallazine® Eye Drops [OTC]; Murine® Plus Ophthalmic [OTC]; Optigene® Ophthalmic [OTC]; Tetrasine® Extra Ophthalmic [OTC]; Tetrasine® Ophthalmic [OTC]; Tyzine® Nasal; Visine® Extra Ophthalmic [OTC]

Therapeutic Category Adrenergic Agonist Agent

Use Symptomatic relief of nasal congestion and conjunctival congestion

Usual Dosage

Nasal congestion:

Children 2-6 years: Instill 2-3 drops of 0.05% solution every 4-6 hours as needed

Children >6 years and Adults: Instill 2-4 drops or 0.1% spray nasal mucosa every 4-6 hours as needed

Conjunctival congestion: Adults: Instill 1-2 drops in each eye 2-3 times/day

Dosage Forms Solution, as hydrochloride:

Nasal: 0.05% (15 mL), 0.1% (30 mL, 473 mL)

Ophthalmic: 0.05% (15 mL)

Tetralan® ***(Discontinued)*** *see page 700*

Tetram® ***(Discontinued)*** *see page 700*

Tetramune® *see* diphtheria, tetanus toxoids, whole-cell pertussis, and *Haemophilus* B conjugate vaccine *on page 187*

Tetrasine® Extra Ophthalmic [OTC] *see* tetrahydrozoline *on previous page*

Tetrasine® Ophthalmic [OTC] *see* tetrahydrozoline *on previous page*

tetryzoline *see* tetrahydrozoline *on previous page*

Texacort® Topical *see* hydrocortisone (topical) *on page 292*

TG *see* thioguanine *on page 561*

6-TG *see* thioguanine *on page 561*

T/Gel® [OTC] *see* coal tar *on page 141*

T-Gen® *see* trimethobenzamide *on page 582*

T-Gesic® *see* hydrocodone and acetaminophen *on page 287*

THA *see* tacrine *on page 546*

thalidomide (tha LI doe mide)

U.S./Canadian Brand Names Contergan®; Distaval®; Kevadon®; Thalomid®

Therapeutic Category Immunosuppressant Agent

Use Treatment or prevention of graft-versus-host reactions after bone marrow transplantation; in aphthous ulceration in HIV-positive patients; reactional lepromatous or erythema nodosum leprosy; Langerhans cell histiocytosis, Behçet's syndrome; hypnotic agent; also may be effective in rheumatoid arthritis, discoid lupus, and erythema multiforme; useful in type 2 lepra reactions, but not type 1; can assist in healing mouth ulcers in AIDS patients

Usual Dosage

Leprosy: Up to 400 mg/day; usual maintenance dose: 50-100 mg/day

Behçet's syndrome: 100-400 mg/day

Graft-vs-host reactions:

Children: 3 mg/kg 4 times/day

Adults: 100-1600 mg/day; usual initial dose: 200 mg 4 times/day for use up to 700 days

AIDS-related aphthous stomatitis: 200 mg twice daily for 5 days, then 200 mg/day for up to 8 weeks

Discoid lupus erythematosus: 100-400 mg/day; maintenance dose: 25-50 mg

Dosage Forms Capsule: 50 mg

Thalitone® *see* chlorthalidone *on page 128*

Thalomid® *see* thalidomide *on this page*

THAM® *see* tromethamine *on page 586*

THAM-E® *see* tromethamine *on page 586*

THC *see* dronabinol *on page 198*

Theelin® Aqueous Injection *(Discontinued)* *see page 700*

Theo-24® *see* theophylline *on this page*

Theobid® *see* theophylline *on this page*

Theobid® Jr Duracaps® *(Discontinued)* *see page 700*

Theochron® *see* theophylline *on this page*

Theoclear-80® *see* theophylline *on this page*

Theoclear® L.A. *see* theophylline *on this page*

Theo-Dur® *see* theophylline *on this page*

Theo-Dur® Sprinkle® *(Discontinued)* *see page 700*

Theolair™ *see* theophylline *on this page*

Theo-Organidin® *(Discontinued)* *see page 700*

theophylline (thee OF i lin)

U.S./Canadian Brand Names Aerolate III®; Aerolate JR®; Aerolate SR®; Aquaphyllin®; Asmalix®; Elixomin®; Elixophyllin®; Quibron®-T; Quibron®-T/SR; Respbid®; Slo-bid™; Slo-

(Continued)

theophylline *(Continued)*

Phyllin®; Sustaire®; Theo-24®; Theobid®; Theochron®; Theoclear-80®; Theoclear® L.A.; Theo-Dur®; Theolair™; Theo-Sav®; Theospan®-SR; Theostat-80®; Theovent®; Theo-X®; T-Phyl®; Uni-Dur®; Uniphyl®

Therapeutic Category Theophylline Derivative

Use Treatment of symptoms and reversible airway obstruction due to chronic asthma, chronic bronchitis, or COPD; for treatment of idiopathic apnea of prematurity in neonates

Usual Dosage

Apnea: Dosage should be determined by plasma level monitoring; each 0.5 mg/kg of theophylline administered as a loading dose will result in a 1 mcg/mL increase in serum theophylline concentration

Loading dose: 5 mg/kg; dilute dose in 1-hour I.V. fluid via syringe pump over 1 hour

Maintenance: 2 mg/kg every 8-12 hours or 1-3 mg/kg/dose every 8-12 hours; administer I.V. push 1 mL/minute (2 mg/minute)

Treatment of acute bronchospasm in older patients: (>6 months of age): Loading dose (in patients not currently receiving theophylline): 6 mg/kg (based on aminophylline) administered I.V. over 20-30 minutes; 4.7 mg/kg (based on theophylline) administered I.V. over 20-30 minutes; administration rate should not exceed 20 mg (1 mL)/minute (theophylline) or 25 mg (1 mL)/minute (aminophylline)

Approximate maintenance dosage for treatment of acute bronchospasm:

Children:

6 months to 9 years: 1.2 mg/kg/hour (aminophylline); 0.95 mg/kg/hour (theophylline)

9-16 years and young adult smokers: 1 mg/kg/hour (aminophylline); 0.79 mg/kg/hour (theophylline)

Adults (healthy, nonsmoking): 0.7 mg/kg/hour (aminophylline); 0.55 mg/kg/hour (theophylline)

Older patients and patients with cor pulmonale: 0.6 mg/kg/hour (aminophylline); 0.47 mg/kg/hour (theophylline)

Patients with CHF or liver failure: 0.5 mg/kg/hour (aminophylline); 0.39 mg/kg/hour (theophylline)

Chronic therapy: Slow clinical titration is generally preferred

Initial dose: 16 mg/kg/24 hours or 400 mg/24 hours, whichever is less

Increasing dose: The above dosage may be increased in ~25% increments at 2- to 3-day intervals so long as the drug is tolerated or until the maximum dose is reached; monitor serum levels

Exercise caution in younger children who cannot complain of minor side effects, older adults, and those with cor pulmonale; CHF or liver disease may have unusually low dosage requirements

Dosage Forms

Capsule:

Immediate release (Bronkodyl®, Elixophyllin®): 100 mg, 200 mg

Timed release:

8-12 hours (Aerolate®): 65 mg [III]; 130 mg [JR], 260 mg [SR]

8-12 hours (Slo-bid™): 50 mg, 75 mg, 100 mg, 125 mg, 200 mg, 300 mg

8-12 hours (Slo-Phyllin® Gyrocaps®): 60 mg, 125 mg, 250 mg

12 hours (Theobid® Duracaps®): 260 mg

12 hours (Theoclear® L.A.): 130 mg, 260 mg

12 hours (Theospan®-SR): 130 mg, 260 mg

12 hours (Theovent®): 125 mg, 250 mg

24 hours (Theo-24®): 100 mg, 200 mg, 300 mg

Elixir (Asmalix®, Elixomin®, Elixophyllin®, Lanophyllin®): 80 mg/15 mL (15 mL, 30 mL, 480 mL, 4000 mL)

Infusion, in D_5W: 0.4 mg/mL (1000 mL); 0.8 mg/mL (500 mL, 1000 mL); 1.6 mg/mL (250 mL, 500 mL); 2 mg/mL (100 mL); 3.2 mg/mL (250 mL); 4 mg/mL (50 mL, 100 mL);

Solution, oral:

Theolair™: 80 mg/15 mL (15 mL, 18.75 mL, 30 mL, 480 mL)

Syrup:

Aquaphyllin®, Slo-Phyllin®, Theoclear-80®, Theostat-80®: 80 mg/15 mL (15 mL, 30 mL, 500 mL)

Accurbron®: 150 mg/15 mL (480 mL)
Tablet: Immediate release:
Slo-Phyllin®: 100 mg, 200 mg
Theolair™: 125 mg, 250 mg
Quibron®-T: 300 mg
Tablet:
Controlled release (Theo-X®): 100 mg, 200 mg, 300 mg
Timed release:
12-24 hours: 100 mg, 200 mg, 300 mg, 450 mg
8-12 hours (Quibron®-T/SR): 300 mg
8-12 hours (Respbid®): 250 mg, 500 mg
8-12 hours (Sustaire®): 100 mg, 300 mg
8-12 hours (T-Phyl®): 200 mg
12-24 hours (Theochron®): 100 mg, 200 mg, 300 mg
8-24 hours (Theo-Dur®): 100 mg, 200 mg, 300 mg, 450 mg
8-24 hours (Theo-Sav®): 100 mg, 200 mg, 300 mg
24 hours (Theolair™-SR): 200 mg, 250 mg, 300 mg, 500 mg
24 hours (Uni-Dur®, Uniphyl®): 400 mg, 600 mg

theophylline and guaifenesin (thee OF i lin & gwye FEN e sin)

Synonyms guaifenesin and theophylline
U.S./Canadian Brand Names Bronchial®; Glycerol-T®; Quibron®; Slo-Phyllin® GG
Therapeutic Category Theophylline Derivative
Use Symptomatic treatment of bronchospasm associated with bronchial asthma, chronic bronchitis and pulmonary emphysema
Usual Dosage Adults: Oral: 1-2 capsules every 6-8 hours
Dosage Forms
Capsule: Theophylline 150 mg and guaifenesin 90 mg; theophylline 300 mg and guaifenesin 180 mg
Elixir: Theophylline 150 mg and guaifenesin 90 mg per 15 mL (480 mL)

theophylline, ephedrine, and hydroxyzine
(thee OF i lin, e FED rin, & hye DROKS i zeen)

Synonyms ephedrine, theophylline, and hydroxyzine; hydroxyzine, theophylline, and ephedrine
U.S./Canadian Brand Names Hydrophed®; Marax®
Therapeutic Category Theophylline Derivative
Use Possibly effective for controlling bronchospastic disorders
Usual Dosage Oral:
Children:
2-5 years: 1/2 tablet 2-4 times/day or 2.5 mL 3-4 times/day
>5 years: 1/2 tablet 2-4 times/day or 5 mL 3-4 times/day
Adults: 1 tablet 2-4 times/day
Dosage Forms
Syrup, dye free: Theophylline 32.5 mg, ephedrine 6.25 mg, and hydroxyzine 2.5 mg per 5 mL
Tablet: Theophylline 130 mg, ephedrine 25 mg, and hydroxyzine 10 mg

theophylline, ephedrine, and phenobarbital
(thee OF i lin, e FED rin, & fee noe BAR bi tal)

Synonyms ephedrine, theophylline, and phenobarbital; phenobarbital, theophylline, and ephedrine
U.S./Canadian Brand Names Tedral®
Therapeutic Category Theophylline Derivative
Use Prevention and symptomatic treatment of bronchial asthma; relief of asthmatic bronchitis and other bronchospastic disorders
Usual Dosage Oral:
Children >60 lb: 1 tablet or 5 mL every 4 hours
(Continued)

theophylline, ephedrine, and phenobarbital *(Continued)*

Adults: 1-2 tablets or 10-20 mL every 4 hours

Dosage Forms

Suspension: Theophylline 65 mg, ephedrine sulfate 12 mg, and phenobarbital 4 mg per 5 mL

Tablet: Theophylline 118 mg, ephedrine sulfate 25 mg, and phenobarbital 11 mg; theophylline 130 mg, ephedrine sulfate 24 mg, and phenobarbital 8 mg

theophylline ethylenediamine *see* aminophylline *on page 27*

Theo-Sav® *see* theophylline *on page 557*

Theospan®-SR *see* theophylline *on page 557*

Theostat-80® *see* theophylline *on page 557*

Theovent® *see* theophylline *on page 557*

Theo-X® *see* theophylline *on page 557*

Therabid® [OTC] *see* vitamin, multiple (oral) *on page 604*

Thera-Combex® H-P Kapseals® [OTC] *see* vitamin B complex with vitamin C *on page 603*

TheraCys® *see* BCG vaccine *on page 61*

Theraflu® Non-Drowsy Formula Maximum Strength [OTC] *see* acetaminophen, dextromethorphan, and pseudoephedrine *on page 6*

Thera-Flur® *see* fluoride *on page 244*

Thera-Flur-N® *see* fluoride *on page 244*

Theragran® [OTC] *see* vitamin, multiple (oral) *on page 604*

Theragran® Hematinic® *see* vitamin, multiple (oral) *on page 604*

Theragran® Liquid [OTC] *see* vitamin, multiple (oral) *on page 604*

Theragran-M® [OTC] *see* vitamin, multiple (oral) *on page 604*

Thera-Hist® Syrup [OTC] *see* chlorpheniramine and phenylpropanolamine *on page 122*

Theramine® Expectorant *(Discontinued)* *see page 700*

Theraplex Z® [OTC] *see* pyrithione zinc *on page 491*

Thermazene® *see* silver sulfadiazine *on page 522*

Theroxide® Wash [OTC] *see* benzoyl peroxide *on page 68*

thiabendazole (thye a BEN da zole)

Synonyms tiabendazole

U.S./Canadian Brand Names Mintezol®

Therapeutic Category Anthelmintic

Use Treatment of strongyloidiasis, cutaneous larva migrans, visceral larva migrans, dracunculosis, trichinosis, and mixed helminthic infections

Usual Dosage Children and Adults: Oral: 50 mg/kg/day divided every 12 hours (maximum dose: 3 g/day)

Strongyloidiasis: For 2 consecutive days

Cutaneous larva migrans: For 2-5 consecutive days

Visceral larva migrans: For 5-7 consecutive days

Trichinosis: For 2-4 consecutive days

Dracunculosis: 50-75 mg/kg/day divided every 12 hours for 3 days

Dosage Forms

Suspension, oral: 500 mg/5 mL (120 mL)

Tablet, chewable (orange flavor): 500 mg

Thiacide® *(Discontinued)* *see page 700*

thiamazole *see* methimazole *on page 363*

thiamine (THYE a min)

Synonyms aneurine; thiaminium; vitamin B_1

U.S./Canadian Brand Names Betalin®S; Betaxin® (Can); Bewon® (Can)

Therapeutic Category Vitamin, Water Soluble

Use Treatment of thiamine deficiency including beriberi, Wernicke's encephalopathy syndrome, and peripheral neuritis associated with pellagra; alcoholic patients with altered sensorium; various genetic metabolic disorders

Usual Dosage Dietary supplement (depends on caloric or carbohydrate content of the diet):

Infants: 0.3-0.5 mg/day
Children: 0.5-1 mg/day
Adults: 1-2 mg/day
Note: The above doses can be found as a combination in multivitamin preparations

Children:
- Noncritically ill thiamine deficiency: Oral: 10-50 mg/day in divided doses every day for 2 weeks followed by 5-10 mg/day for one month
- Beriberi: I.M.: 10-25 mg/day for 2 weeks, then 5-10 mg orally every day for one month (oral as therapeutic multivitamin)

Adults:
- Wernicke's encephalopathy: I.M., I.V.: 50 mg as a single dose, then 50 mg I.M. every day until normal diet resumed
- Noncritically ill thiamine deficiency: Oral: 10-50 mg/day in divided doses
- Beriberi: I.M., I.V.: 10-30 mg 3 times/day for 2 weeks, then switch to 5-10 mg orally every day for one month (oral as therapeutic multivitamin)

Dosage Forms Thiamine hydrochloride:
Injection: 100 mg/mL (1 mL, 2 mL, 10 mL, 30 mL); 200 mg/mL (30 mL)
Tablet: 50 mg, 100 mg, 250 mg, 500 mg
Tablet, enteric coated: 20 mg

thiaminium *see* thiamine *on this page*

thiethylperazine (thye eth il PER a zeen)

Therapeutic Category Phenothiazine Derivative

Use Relief of nausea and vomiting

Usual Dosage Children >12 years and Adults:
Oral, I.M., rectal: 10 mg 1-3 times/day as needed
I.V. and S.C. routes of administration are not recommended

Dosage Forms Thiethylperazine maleate:
Injection: 5 mg/mL (2 mL)
Tablet: 10 mg

thimerosal (thye MER oh sal)

U.S./Canadian Brand Names Aeroaid® [OTC]; Mersol® [OTC]; Merthiolate® [OTC]

Therapeutic Category Antibacterial, Topical

Use Organomercurial antiseptic with sustained bacteriostatic and fungistatic activity

Usual Dosage Apply 1-3 times/day

Dosage Forms
Ointment, ophthalmic: 0.02% [0.2 mg/mL] (3.5 g)
Solution, topical: 0.1% [1 mg/mL = 1:1000] (120 mL, 480 mL, 4000 mL)
Spray, antiseptic: 0.1% [1 mg/mL = 1:1000] with alcohol 2% (90 mL)
Tincture: 0.1% [1 mg/mL = 1:1000] with alcohol 50% (120 mL, 480 mL, 4000 mL)

thioguanine (thye oh GWAH neen)

Synonyms 2-amino-6-mercaptopurine; TG; 6-TG; 6-thioguanine; tioguanine

U.S./Canadian Brand Names Lanvis® (Can)

Therapeutic Category Antineoplastic Agent

Use Remission induction in acute myelogenous (nonlymphocytic) leukemia; treatment of chronic myelogenous leukemia and acute lymphocytic leukemia

(Continued)

thioguanine *(Continued)*

Usual Dosage Refer to individual protocols. Oral:

Infants <3 years: Combination drug therapy for acute nonlymphocytic leukemia: 3.3 mg/kg/day in divided doses twice daily for 4 days

Children and Adults: 2-3 mg/kg/day calculated to nearest 20 mg or 75-200 mg/m^2/day in 1-2 divided doses for 5-7 days or until remission is attained

Dosage Forms Tablet, scored: 40 mg

6-thioguanine *see* thioguanine *on previous page*

Thiola™ *see* tiopronin *on page 568*

thiopental (thye oh PEN tal)

U.S./Canadian Brand Names Pentothal® Sodium

Therapeutic Category Barbiturate

Controlled Substance C-III

Use Induction of anesthesia; adjunct for intubation in head injury patients; control of convulsive states; treatment of elevated intracranial pressure

Usual Dosage I.V.:

Induction anesthesia:

- Infants: 5-8 mg/kg
- Children 1-12 years: 5-6 mg/kg
- Adults: 3-5 mg/kg

Maintenance anesthesia:

- Children: 1 mg/kg as needed
- Adults: 25-100 mg as needed

Increased intracranial pressure: Children and Adults: 1.5-5 mg/kg/dose; repeat as needed to control intracranial pressure

Seizures:

- Children: 2-3 mg/kg/dose, repeat as needed
- Adults: 75-250 mg/dose, repeat as needed

Rectal administration: (Patient should be NPO for no less than 3 hours prior to administration)

Suggested initial doses of thiopental rectal suspension are:

<3 months: 15 mg/kg/dose

>3 months: 25 mg/kg/dose

Note: The age of a premature infant should be adjusted to reflect the age that the infant would have been if full-term (eg, an infant, now age 4 months, who was 2 months premature should be considered to be a 2-month old infant).

Doses should be rounded downward to the nearest 50 mg increment to allow for accurate measurement of the dose

Inactive or debilitated patients and patients recently medicated with other sedatives, (eg, chloral hydrate, meperidine, chlorpromazine, and promethazine), may require smaller doses than usual

If the patient is not sedated within 15-20 minutes, a single repeat dose of thiopental can be administered; the single repeat doses are:

<3 months of age: <7.5 mg/kg/dose

>3 months of age: 15 mg/kg/dose

Adults weighing >90 kg should not receive >3 g as a total dose (initial plus repeat doses)

Children weighing >34 kg should not receive >1 g as a total dose (initial plus repeat doses)

Neither adults nor children should receive more than one course of thiopental rectal suspension (initial dose plus repeat dose) per 24-hour period

Dosage Forms Thiopental sodium:

Injection: 250 mg, 400 mg, 500 mg, 1 g, 2.5 g, 5 g

Suspension, rectal: 400 mg/g (2 g)

Thioplex® *see* thiotepa *on next page*

thioridazine (thye oh RID a zeen)

U.S./Canadian Brand Names Apo®-Thioridazine (Can); Mellaril®; Mellaril-S®; Novo-Ridazine® (Can); PMS-Thioridazine (Can)

Therapeutic Category Phenothiazine Derivative

Use Management of psychotic disorders; depressive neurosis; dementia in elderly; severe behavioral problems in children

Usual Dosage Oral:

Children >2 years: Range: 0.5-3 mg/kg/day in 2-3 divided doses; usual: 1 mg/kg/day; maximum: 3 mg/kg/day

Behavior problems: Initial: 10 mg 2-3 times/day, increase gradually

Severe psychoses: Initial: 25 mg 2-3 times/day, increase gradually

Adults:

Psychoses: Initial: 50-100 mg 3 times/day with gradual increments as needed and tolerated; maximum daily dose: 800 mg/day in 2-4 divided doses

Depressive disorders, dementia: Initial: 25 mg 3 times/day; maintenance dose: 20-200 mg/day

Dosage Forms Thioridazine hydrochloride:

Concentrate, oral, as hydrochloride: 30 mg/mL (120 mL); 100 mg/mL (3.4 mL, 120 mL)

Suspension, oral, as hydrochloride: 25 mg/5 mL (480 mL); 100 mg/5 mL (480 mL)

Tablet, as hydrochloride: 10 mg, 15 mg, 25 mg, 50 mg, 100 mg, 150 mg, 200 mg

thiotepa (thye oh TEP a)

Synonyms TESPA; triethylenethiophosphoramide; TSPA

U.S./Canadian Brand Names Thioplex®

Therapeutic Category Antineoplastic Agent

Use Treatment of superficial tumors of the bladder; palliative treatment of adenocarcinoma of breast or ovary; lymphomas and sarcomas; meningeal neoplasms; control pleural, pericardial or peritoneal effusions caused by metastatic tumors; high-dose regimens with autologous bone marrow transplantation

Usual Dosage Refer to individual protocols

Children: Sarcomas: I.V.: 25-65 mg/m^2 as a single dose every 21 days

Adults:

I.M., I.V., S.C.: 8 mg/m^2 daily for 5 days or 30-60 mg/m^2 once per week

High-dose therapy for bone marrow transplant: I.V.: 500 mg/m^2

Intracavitary: 0.6-0.8 mg/kg or 60 mg in 60 mL SWI instilled into the bladder at 1- to 4-week intervals

Intrathecal: Doses of 1-10 mg/m^2 administered 1-2 times/week

Dosage Forms Powder for injection: 15 mg

thiothixene (thye oh THIKS een)

Synonyms tiotixene

U.S./Canadian Brand Names Navane® Capsule

Therapeutic Category Thioxanthene Derivative

Use Management of psychotic disorders

Usual Dosage

Children <12 years: Oral: Not well established; 0.25 mg/kg/24 hours in divided doses

Children >12 years and Adults:

Oral: Initial: 2 mg 3 times/day, up to 20-30 mg/day; maximum: 60 mg/day

I.M. (administer undiluted injection): 4 mg 2-4 times/day, increase dose gradually; usual: 16-20 mg/day; maximum: 30 mg/day; change to oral dose as soon as able

Dosage Forms

Capsule: 1 mg, 2 mg, 5 mg, 10 mg, 20 mg

Concentrate, as hydrochloride: 5 mg/mL

Thorazine® *see* chlorpromazine *on page 127*

Thrombate III™ *see* antithrombin III *on page 41*

Thrombinar® *see* thrombin, topical *on next page*

thrombin, topical (THROM bin, TOP i kal)

U.S./Canadian Brand Names Thrombinar®; Thrombogen®; Thrombostat®

Therapeutic Category Hemostatic Agent

Use Hemostasis whenever minor bleeding from capillaries and small venules is accessible

Usual Dosage Use 1000-2000 units/mL of solution where bleeding is profuse; apply powder directly to the site of bleeding or on oozing surfaces; use 100 units/mL for bleeding from skin or mucosal surfaces

Dosage Forms Powder: 1000 units, 5000 units, 10,000 units, 20,000 units, 50,000 units

Thrombogen® *see* thrombin, topical *on this page*

Thrombostat® *see* thrombin, topical *on this page*

Thypinone® *see* protirelin *on page 485*

Thyrar® *see* thyroid *on this page*

Thyrel® TRH *see* protirelin *on page 485*

Thyro-Block® *see* potassium iodide *on page 466*

Thyrogen® *see* thyrotropin alpha *on this page*

thyroid (THYE royd)

Synonyms desiccated thyroid; thyroid extract

U.S./Canadian Brand Names Armour® Thyroid; S-P-T; Thyrar®; Thyroid Strong®

Therapeutic Category Thyroid Product

Use Replacement or supplemental therapy in hypothyroidism

Usual Dosage Adults: Oral: Start at 30 mg/day and titrate by 30 mg/day in increments of 2- to 3-week intervals; usual maintenance dose: 60-120 mg/day

Dosage Forms

Capsule, pork source in soybean oil (S-P-T): 60 mg, 120 mg, 180 mg, 300 mg

Tablet:

- Armour® Thyroid: 15 mg, 30 mg, 60 mg, 90 mg, 120 mg, 180 mg, 240 mg, 300 mg
- Thyrar® (bovine source): 30 mg, 60 mg, 120 mg
- Thyroid Strong® (60 mg is equivalent to 90 mg thyroid USP):
  - Regular: 30 mg, 60 mg, 120 mg
  - Sugar coated: 30 mg, 60 mg, 120 mg, 180 mg
- Thyroid USP: 15 mg, 30 mg, 60 mg, 120 mg, 180 mg, 300 mg

thyroid extract *see* thyroid *on this page*

thyroid-stimulating hormone *see* thyrotropin *on this page*

Thyroid Strong® *see* thyroid *on this page*

Thyrolar® *see* liotrix *on page 336*

thyrotropin (thye roe TROE pin)

Synonyms thyroid-stimulating hormone; TSH

U.S./Canadian Brand Names Thytropar®

Therapeutic Category Diagnostic Agent

Use Diagnostic aid to determine subclinical hypothyroidism or decreased thyroid reserve, to differentiate between primary and secondary hypothyroidism and between primary hypothyroidism and euthyroidism in patients receiving thyroid replacement

Usual Dosage I.M., S.C.: 10 units/day for 1-3 days; follow by a radioiodine study 24 hours past last injection, no response in thyroid failure, substantial response in pituitary failure

Dosage Forms Injection: 10 units

thyrotropin alpha (thye roe TROE pin AL fa)

Synonyms human thyroid-stimulating hormone; TSH

U.S./Canadian Brand Names Thyrogen®

Therapeutic Category Diagnostic Agent

Use As an adjunctive diagnostic tool for serum thyroglobulin (Tg) testing with or without radioiodine imaging in the follow-up of patients with well-differentiated thyroid cancer

Potential clinical uses:

1. Patients with an undetectable Tg on thyroid hormone suppressive therapy to exclude the diagnosis of residual or recurrent thyroid cancer
2. Patients requiring serum Tg testing and radioiodine imaging who are unwilling to undergo thyroid hormone withdrawal testing and whose treating physician believes that use of a less sensitive test is justified
3. Patients who are either unable to mount an adequate endogenous TSH response to thyroid hormone withdrawal or in whom withdrawal is medically contraindicated

Usual Dosage Children >16 years and Adults: I.M.: 0.9 mg every 24 hours for 2 doses or every 72 hours for 3 doses. For radioiodine imaging, radioiodine administration should be given 24 hours following the final Thyrogen® injection. Scanning should be performed 48 hours after radioiodine administration (72 hours after the final injection of Thyrogen®).

Dosage Forms Kits containing two 1.1 mg vials (>4 int. units) of thyrogen® and two 10 mL vials of sterile water for injection

Thytropar® *see* thyrotropin *on previous page*

tiabendazole *see* thiabendazole *on page 560*

tiagabine (tye AG a bene)

U.S./Canadian Brand Names Gabitril®

Therapeutic Category Anticonvulsant

Use Adjunctive therapy in adults and children 12 years and older in the treatment of partial seizures

Usual Dosage Children >12 years and Adults: Oral: Initial: 4 mg, once daily; the total daily dose may be increased in 4 mg increments beginning the second week of therapy; thereafter, the daily dose may be increased by 4-8 mg/day until clinical response is achieved, up to a maximum of 32 mg/day; the total daily dose at higher levels should be given in divided doses, 2-4 times/day

Dosage Forms Tablet, as hydrochloride: 4 mg, 12 mg, 16 mg, 20 mg

Tiamate® *see* diltiazem *on page 182*

Tiamol® (Can) *see* fluocinonide *on page 243*

tiaprofenic acid *(Canada only)* (tye ah PRO fen ik AS id)

U.S./Canadian Brand Names Surgam® (Can); Surgam® SR (Can)

Therapeutic Category Nonsteroidal Anti-Inflammatory Agent (NSAID)

Use Relief of signs and symptoms of rheumatoid arthritis and osteoarthritis (degenerative joint disease)

Usual Dosage Adults: Oral:

Tablet:

Rheumatoid arthritis: Usual initial and maintenance dose: 600 mg/day in 3 divided doses; some patients may do well on 300 mg twice daily; maximum daily dose: 600 mg.

Osteoarthritis: Usual initial and maintenance dose: 600 mg/day in 2 or 3 divided doses; in rare instances patients may be maintained on 300 mg daily in divided doses; maximum daily dose: 600 mg

Extended release capsule:

Rheumatoid arthritis or osteoarthritis: Initial and maintenance dose: 2 sustained release capsules of 300 mg once daily. Surgam® SR capsules should be swallowed whole

Dosage Forms

Capsule, sustained release: 300 mg

Tablet: 200 mg, 300 mg

Tiazac® *see* diltiazem *on page 182*

Ticar® *see* ticarcillin *on next page*

ticarcillin (tye kar SIL in)

U.S./Canadian Brand Names Ticar®

Therapeutic Category Penicillin

Use Treatment of infections such as septicemia, acute and chronic respiratory tract infections, skin and soft tissue infections, and urinary tract infections due to susceptible strains of *Pseudomonas*, *Proteus*, *Escherichia coli*, and *Enterobacter*

Usual Dosage I.V. (ticarcillin is generally administered I.M. only for the treatment of uncomplicated urinary tract infections):

Infants and Children: 200-300 mg/kg/day in divided doses every 4-6 hours; maximum dose: 24 g/day

Adults: 1-4 g every 4-6 hours

Dosage Forms Powder for injection, as disodium: 1 g, 3 g, 6 g, 20 g, 30 g

ticarcillin and clavulanate potassium

(tye kar SIL in & klav yoo LAN ate poe TASS ee um)

Synonyms clavulanic acid and ticarcillin; ticarcillin and clavulanic acid

U.S./Canadian Brand Names Timentin®

Therapeutic Category Penicillin

Use Treatment of infections caused by susceptible organisms involving the lower respiratory tract, urinary tract, skin and skin structures, bone and joint, and septicemia. Clavulanate expands activity of ticarcillin to include beta-lactamase-producing strains of *S. aureus*, *H. influenzae*, *Moraxella catarrhalis*, *B. fragilis*, *Klebsiella*, and *Proteus* species

Usual Dosage I.V.:

Children: 200-300 mg of ticarcillin/kg/day in divided doses every 4-6 hours

Adults: 3.1 g (ticarcillin 3 g plus clavulanic acid 0.1 g) every 4-6 hours; maximum: 18-24 g/day; for urinary tract infections: 3.1 g every 6-8 hours

Dosage Forms

Infusion, premixed (frozen): Ticarcillin disodium 3 g and clavulanate potassium 0.1 g (100 mL)

Powder for injection: Ticarcillin disodium 3 g and clavulanate potassium 0.1 g (3.1 g, 31 g)

ticarcillin and clavulanic acid *see* ticarcillin and clavulanate potassium *on this page*

TICE® BCG *see* BCG vaccine *on page 61*

Ticlid® *see* ticlopidine *on this page*

ticlopidine (tye KLOE pi deen)

U.S./Canadian Brand Names Ticlid®

Therapeutic Category Antiplatelet Agent

Use Platelet aggregation inhibitor that reduces the risk of thrombotic stroke in patients who have had a stroke or stroke precursors

Usual Dosage Adults: Oral: 1 tablet twice daily with food

Dosage Forms Tablet, as hydrochloride: 250 mg

Ticon® *see* trimethobenzamide *on page 582*

TIG *see* tetanus immune globulin (human) *on page 553*

Tigan® *see* trimethobenzamide *on page 582*

Tiject-20® ***(Discontinued)*** *see page 700*

Tilade® Inhalation Aerosol *see* nedocromil *on page 393*

tiludronate (tye LOO droe nate)

Synonyms tiludronic acid

U.S./Canadian Brand Names Skelid®

Therapeutic Category Bisphosphonate Derivative

Use Paget's disease of the bone

Usual Dosage Adults: Oral: 400 mg/day (2 tablets) [tiludronic acid]

Dosage Forms Tablet, as disodium: 240 mg [tiludronic acid 200 mg]; dosage is expressed in terms of tiludronic acid.

tiludronic acid *see* tiludronate *on previous page*

Tim-AK (Can) *see* timolol *on this page*

Timecelles® [OTC] *see* ascorbic acid *on page 48*

Timentin® *see* ticarcillin and clavulanate potassium *on previous page*

timolol (TYE moe lole)

U.S./Canadian Brand Names Apo®-Timol (Can); Apo®-Timop (Can); Beta-Tim® (Can); Blocadren® Oral; Gen-Timolol® (Can); Novo-Timol® (Can); Nu-Timolol® (Can); Tim-AK (Can); Timoptic® Ophthalmic; Timoptic-XE® Ophthalmic

Therapeutic Category Beta-Adrenergic Blocker

Use Ophthalmic dosage form used to treat elevated intraocular pressure such as glaucoma or ocular hypertension; orally for treatment of hypertension and angina and for prevention of myocardial infarction and migraine headaches

Usual Dosage

Children and Adults: Ophthalmic: Initial: 0.25% solution, instill 1 drop twice daily; increase to 0.5% solution if response not adequate; decrease to 1 drop/day if controlled; do not exceed 1 drop twice daily of 0.5% solution

Adults: Oral:

Hypertension: Initial: 10 mg twice daily, increase gradually every 7 days, usual dosage: 20-40 mg/day in 2 divided doses; maximum: 60 mg/day

Prevention of myocardial infarction: 10 mg twice daily initiated within 1-4 weeks after infarction

Migraine headache: Initial: 10 mg twice daily, increase to maximum of 30 mg/day

Dosage Forms

Timolol hemihydrate:

Solution, ophthalmic (Betimol®): 0.25% (2.5 mL, 5 mL, 10 mL, 15 mL); 0.5% (2.5 mL, 5 mL, 10 mL, 15 mL)

Timolol maleate:

Gel, ophthalmic (Timoptic-XE®): 0.25% (2.5 mL, 5 mL); 0.5% (2.5 mL, 5 mL)

Solution, ophthalmic (Timoptic®): 0.25% (2.5 mL, 5 mL, 10 mL, 15 mL); 0.5% (2.5 mL, 5 mL, 10 mL, 15 mL)

Solution, ophthalmic, preservative free, single use (Timoptic® OcuDose®): 0.25%, 0.5%

Tablet (Blocadren®): 5 mg, 10 mg, 20 mg

Timoptic® Ophthalmic *see* timolol *on this page*

Timoptic-XE® Ophthalmic *see* timolol *on this page*

Tinactin® [OTC] *see* tolnaftate *on page 571*

TinBen® [OTC] *see* benzoin *on page 68*

TinCoBen® [OTC] *see* benzoin *on page 68*

Tindal® *(Discontinued)* *see page 700*

Tine Test PPD *see* tuberculin tests *on page 588*

Tinver® [OTC] *see* sodium thiosulfate *on page 531*

tinzaparin *(Canada only)* (tin ZA pa rin)

U.S./Canadian Brand Names Innohep® (Can)

Therapeutic Category Anticoagulant

Use Prevention of postoperative venous thromboembolism in patients undergoing orthopedic surgery; may be used in the management of the prevention of postoperative venous thromboembolism in patients undergoing general surgery who are at high risk of developing postoperative venous thromboembolism; postoperative administration does not preclude other prophylactic modalities including physical and mechanical methods of adjunct therapy

(Continued)

tinzaparin *(Canada only)* *(Continued)*

Usual Dosage Adults: S.C.: Postoperative venous thromboembolism in general surgery patients: 3500 anti-Xa int. units 2 hours before surgery followed by 3500 anti-Xa int. units once daily for 7 to 10 days

Dosage Forms Injection, as sodium:

Syringe: 10,000 anti-Xa int. units/mL (0.35 mL, 0.45 mL); 20,000 anti-Xa int. units/mL (0.5 mL, 0.7 mL, 0.9 mL)

Vial: 10,000 anti-Xa int. units/mL (2 mL); 20,000 anti-Xa int. units/mL (2 mL)

tioconazole (tye oh KONE a zole)

U.S./Canadian Brand Names Vagistat®-1 Vaginal [OTC]

Therapeutic Category Antifungal Agent

Use Local treatment of vulvovaginal candidiasis

Usual Dosage Vaginal: Insert 1 applicatorful in vagina, just prior to bedtime, as a single dose

Dosage Forms Cream, vaginal: 6.5% with applicator (4.6 g)

tioguanine *see* thioguanine *on page 561*

tiopronin (tye oh PROE nin)

U.S./Canadian Brand Names Thiola™

Therapeutic Category Urinary Tract Product

Use Prevention of kidney stone (cystine) formation in patients with severe homozygous cystinuric who have urinary cystine >500 mg/day who are resistant to treatment with high fluid intake, alkali, and diet modification, or who have had adverse reactions to penicillamine

Usual Dosage Adults: Initial: 800 mg/day; average dose: 1000 mg/day

Dosage Forms Tablet: 100 mg

tiotixene *see* thiothixene *on page 563*

tirofiban (tye roe FYE ban)

U.S./Canadian Brand Names Aggrastat®

Therapeutic Category Antiplatelet Agent

Use In combination with heparin, is indicated for the treatment of acute coronary syndrome, including patients who are to be managed medically and those undergoing PTCA or atherectomy. In this setting, it has been shown to decrease the rate of a combined endpoint of death, new myocardial infarction or refractory ischemia/repeat cardiac procedure.

Usual Dosage Adults: I.V.: Initial rate of 0.4 mcg/kg/minute for 30 minutes and then continued at 0.1 mcg/kg/minute

Dosage Forms Injection: 50 mcg/mL (500 mL); 250 mcg/mL (50 mL)

Ti-Screen® [OTC] *see* methoxycinnamate and oxybenzone *on page 365*

Tisit® Blue Gel [OTC] *see* pyrethrins *on page 489*

Tisit® Liquid [OTC] *see* pyrethrins *on page 489*

Tisit® Shampoo [OTC] *see* pyrethrins *on page 489*

tissue plasminogen activator, recombinant *see* alteplase *on page 21*

Titralac® Plus Liquid [OTC] *see* calcium carbonate and simethicone *on page 90*

tizanidine (tye ZAN i deen)

U.S./Canadian Brand Names Zanaflex®

Therapeutic Category Alpha$_2$-Adrenergic Agonist Agent

Use Intermittent management of increased muscle tone associated with spasticity (eg, multiple sclerosis, spinal cord injury)

Usual Dosage Adults: Oral: Initial: 4 mg every 6-8 hours, not to exceed 3 doses/day or 36 mg in a 24-hour period; doses may be increased at 2 mg or 4 mg increments with single doses not exceeding 12 mg

Dosage Forms Tablet, as hydrochloride: 4 mg

TMP *see* trimethoprim *on page 583*

TMP-SMX *see* co-trimoxazole *on page 149*

TOBI™ Inhalation Solution *see* tobramycin *on this page*

TobraDex® Ophthalmic *see* tobramycin and dexamethasone *on this page*

tobramycin (toe bra MYE sin)

U.S./Canadian Brand Names AKTob® Ophthalmic; Nebcin® Injection; TOBI™ Inhalation Solution; Tobrex® Ophthalmic

Therapeutic Category Aminoglycoside (Antibiotic); Antibiotic, Ophthalmic

Use Treatment of documented or suspected infections caused by susceptible gram-negative bacilli including *Pseudomonas aeruginosa*; infection with a nonpseudomonal enteric bacillus which is more sensitive to tobramycin than gentamicin based on susceptibility tests; susceptible organisms in lower respiratory tract infections, septicemia; intra-abdominal, skin, bone, and urinary tract infections; empiric therapy in cystic fibrosis and immunocompromised patients; used topically to treat superficial ophthalmic infections caused by susceptible bacteria

Usual Dosage Dosage should be based on an estimate of ideal body weight

Infants and Children: I.M., I.V.: 2.5 mg/kg/dose every 8 hours

Note: Some patients may require larger or more frequent doses if serum levels document the need (ie, cystic fibrosis or febrile granulocytopenic patients)

Adults: I.M., I.V.: 3-5 mg/kg/day in 3 divided doses

Children and Adults:

Renal dysfunction: 2.5 mg/kg (2-3 serum level measurements should be obtained after the initial dose to measure the half-life in order to determine the frequency of subsequent doses)

Ophthalmic: 1-2 drops every 4 hours; apply ointment 2-3 times/day; for severe infections apply ointment every 3-4 hours, or 2 drops every 30-60 minutes initially, then reduce to less frequent intervals

Dosage Forms Tobramycin sulfate:

Injection, (Nebcin®): 10 mg/mL (2 mL); 40 mg/mL (1.5 mL, 2 mL)

Ointment, ophthalmic (Tobrex®): 0.3% (3.5 g)

Powder for injection (Nebcin®): 40 mg/mL (1.2 g vials)

Solution, ophthalmic: 0.3% (5 mL)

AKTob®, Tobrex®: 0.3% (5 mL)

tobramycin and dexamethasone (toe bra MYE sin & deks a METH a sone)

Synonyms dexamethasone and tobramycin

U.S./Canadian Brand Names TobraDex® Ophthalmic

Therapeutic Category Antibiotic/Corticosteroid, Ophthalmic

Use Treatment of external ocular infection caused by susceptible gram-negative bacteria and steroid responsive inflammatory conditions of the palpebral and bulbar conjunctiva, lid, cornea, and anterior segment of the globe

Usual Dosage Ophthalmic: Adults:

Ointment: Apply 1.25 cm (½") every 3-4 hours to 2-3 times/day

Suspension: Instill 1-2 drops every 4-6 hours (first 24-48 hours may increase frequency to every 2 hours until signs of clinical improvement are seen); apply every 30-60 minutes for severe infections

Dosage Forms

Ointment, ophthalmic: Tobramycin 0.3% and dexamethasone 0.1% (3.5 g)

Suspension, ophthalmic: Tobramycin 0.3% and dexamethasone 0.1% (2.5 mL, 5 mL)

Tobrex® Ophthalmic *see* tobramycin *on this page*

tocainide (toe KAY nide)

U.S./Canadian Brand Names Tonocard®

Therapeutic Category Antiarrhythmic Agent, Class I-B

Use Suppress and prevent symptomatic ventricular arrhythmias

Usual Dosage Adults: Oral: 1200-1800 mg/day in 3 divided doses

Dosage Forms Tablet, as hydrochloride: 400 mg, 600 mg

tocophersolan (toe kof er SOE lan)

Synonyms TPGS

U.S./Canadian Brand Names Liqui-E®

Therapeutic Category Vitamin, Fat Soluble

Use Treatment of vitamin E deficiency resulting from malabsorption due to prolonged cholestatic hepatobiliary disease

Usual Dosage Dietary supplement: Oral: 15 mg (400 units) every day

Dosage Forms Liquid: 26.6 units/mL

Toesen® (Can) *see* oxytocin *on page 425*

Tofranil® *see* imipramine *on page 302*

Tofranil-PM® *see* imipramine *on page 302*

tolazamide (tole AZ a mide)

U.S./Canadian Brand Names Tolinase®

Therapeutic Category Antidiabetic Agent, Oral

Use Adjunct to diet for the management of mild to moderately severe, stable, noninsulin-dependent (type II) diabetes mellitus

Usual Dosage Adults: Oral: 100-1000 mg/day

Dosage Forms Tablet: 100 mg, 250 mg, 500 mg

tolazoline (tole AZ oh leen)

Synonyms benzazoline

U.S./Canadian Brand Names Priscoline®

Therapeutic Category Alpha-Adrenergic Blocking Agent

Use Persistent pulmonary hypertension of the newborn (PPHN), also known as persistent fetal circulation (PFC); peripheral vasospastic disorders

Usual Dosage

Neonates: Initial: I.V.: 1-2 mg/kg over 10-15 minutes via scalp vein or upper extremity; maintenance: 1-2 mg/kg/hour; use lower maintenance doses in patients with decreased renal function. Also used in neonates for acute vasospasm “cath toes” at 0.25 mg/kg/hour (no load)

Adults: Peripheral vasospastic disorder: I.M., I.V., S.C.: 10-50 mg 4 times/day

Dosage Forms Injection, as hydrochloride: 25 mg/mL (4 mL)

tolbutamide (tole BYOO ta mide)

U.S./Canadian Brand Names Apo-Tolbutamide® (Can); Mobenol® (Can); Novo-Butamide® (Can); Orinase® Diagnostic Injection; Orinase® Oral

Therapeutic Category Antidiabetic Agent, Oral

Use Adjunct to diet for the management of mild to moderately severe, stable, noninsulin-dependent (type II) diabetes mellitus

Usual Dosage Adults:

Oral: 250-2000 mg/day

I.V. bolus: 20 mg/kg

Dosage Forms Tolbutamide sodium:

Injection, diagnostic: 1 g (20 mL)

Tablet: 250 mg, 500 mg

tolcapone (TOLE ka pone)

U.S./Canadian Brand Names Tasmar®

Therapeutic Category Anti-Parkinson's Agent

Use Adjunct to levodopa and carbidopa for the treatment of signs and symptoms of idiopathic Parkinson's disease

Usual Dosage Adults: Oral: Initial: 100 mg 3 times/day, may increase to 200 mg 3 times/day

Dosage Forms Tablet: 100 mg, 200 mg

Tolectin® *see* tolmetin *on this page*

Tolectin® DS *see* tolmetin *on this page*

Tolerex® (Can) *see* enteral nutritional products *on page 208*

Tolinase® *see* tolazamide *on previous page*

tolmetin (TOLE met in)

U.S./Canadian Brand Names Novo-Tolmetin® (Can); Tolectin®; Tolectin® DS

Therapeutic Category Analgesic, Non-narcotic; Nonsteroidal Anti-inflammatory Drug (NSAID)

Use Treatment of inflammatory and rheumatoid disorders, including juvenile rheumatoid arthritis

Usual Dosage Oral:

Children ≥2 years: Anti-inflammatory: Initial: 20 mg/kg/day in 3 divided doses, then 15-30 mg/kg/day in 3 divided doses; maximum dose: 30 mg/kg/day

Adults: 400 mg 3 times/day; usual dose: 600 mg to 1.8 g/day; maximum: 2 g/day

Dosage Forms Tolmetin sodium:

Capsule (Tolectin® DS): 400 mg

Tablet (Tolectin®): 200 mg, 600 mg

tolnaftate (tole NAF tate)

U.S./Canadian Brand Names Absorbine® Antifungal [OTC]; Absorbine® Jock Itch [OTC]; Absorbine Jr.® Antifungal [OTC]; Aftate® [OTC]; Desenex® [OTC]; Genaspor® [OTC]; NP-27® [OTC]; Pitrex® (Can); Tinactin® [OTC]; Zeasorb-AF® [OTC]

Therapeutic Category Antifungal Agent

Use Treatment of tinea pedis, tinea cruris, tinea corporis, tinea manuum caused by *Trichophyton rubrum*, *T. mentagrophytes*, *T. tonsurans*, *M. canis*, *M. audouinii*, and *E. floccosum*; also effective in the treatment of tinea versicolor infections due to *Malassezia furfur*

Usual Dosage Children and Adults: Topical: Wash and dry affected area; apply 1-2 drops of solution or a small amount of cream or powder and rub into the affected areas twice daily for 2-4 weeks

Dosage Forms

Aerosol, topical:

Liquid: 1% (59.2 mL, 90 mL, 120 mL)

Powder: 1% (56.7 g, 100 g, 105 g, 150 g)

Cream: 1% (15 g, 30 g)

Gel, topical: 1% (15 g)

Powder, topical: 1% (45 g, 90 g)

Solution, topical: 1% (10 mL)

tolterodine (tole TER oh dine)

U.S./Canadian Brand Names Detrol™

Therapeutic Category Anticholinergic Agent

Use Treatment of patients with an overactive bladder with symptoms of urinary frequency, urgency, or urge incontinence

Usual Dosage Adults: Oral: 2 mg twice daily, dose may be reduced to 1 mg twice daily

Dosage Forms Tablet, as tartrate: 1 mg, 2 mg

Tolu-Sed® DM [OTC] *see* guaifenesin and dextromethorphan *on page 268*

Tomocat® *see* radiological/contrast media (ionic) *on page 495*

Tonocard® *see* tocainide *on page 570*

Tonopaque® *see* radiological/contrast media (ionic) *on page 495*

Topactin® (Can) *see* fluocinonide *on page 243*

Topamax® *see* topiramate *on this page*

Topicort® *see* desoximetasone *on page 166*

Topicort®-LP *see* desoximetasone *on page 166*

Topicycline® Topical *see* tetracycline *on page 555*

Topilene® (Can) *see* betamethasone (topical) *on page 72*

topiramate (toe PYE ra mate)

U.S./Canadian Brand Names Topamax®

Therapeutic Category Anticonvulsant

Use Adjunctive therapy for partial onset seizures in adults

Usual Dosage Adults: Oral: 200 mg twice daily (400 mg/day)

Dosage Forms Tablet: 25 mg, 100 mg, 200 mg

Topisone® (Can) *see* betamethasone (topical) *on page 72*

Toposar® Injection *see* etoposide *on page 228*

topotecan (toe poe TEE kan)

Synonyms hycamptamine; SKF 104864

U.S./Canadian Brand Names Hycamtin™

Therapeutic Category Antineoplastic Agent

Use Metastatic carcinoma of the ovary after failure of initial or subsequent chemotherapy; experimentally in childhood solid tumors and leukemia resistant to standard therapies; treatment of small cell lung cancer sensitive disease after failure of first-line chemotherapy (sensitive disease is defined as disease responding to chemotherapy but subsequently progressing at least 60 days or at least 90 days after chemotherapy)

Usual Dosage

Children: A phase I study in pediatric patients by CCSG determined the recommended phase II dose to be 5.5 mg/m^2 as a 24-hour continuous infusion

Adults: Most phase II studies currently utilize topotecan at 1.5-2.0 mg/m^2/day for 5 days, repeated every 21-28 days. Alternative dosing regimens evaluated in phase I studies have included 21-day continuous infusion (recommended phase II dose: 0.53-0.7 mg/m^2/day) and weekly 24-hour infusions (recommended phase II dose: 1.5 mg/m^2/week).

Dose modifications: Dosage modification may be required for toxicity

Dosage Forms Powder for injection, as hydrochloride, lyophilized: 4 mg (base)

Toprol XL® *see* metoprolol *on page 371*

Topsyn® (Can) *see* fluocinonide *on page 243*

TOPV *see* poliovirus vaccine, live, trivalent, oral *on page 459*

Toradol® *see* ketorolac tromethamine *on page 321*

Torecan® Suppository *(Discontinued)* *see page 700*

toremifene (TORE em i feen)

Synonyms FC1157a

U.S./Canadian Brand Names Fareston®

Therapeutic Category Antineoplastic Agent

Use Treatment of advanced breast cancer; management of desmoid tumors and endometrial carcinoma

Usual Dosage Refer to individual protocols

Adults: Oral: 60 mg once daily, generally continued until disease progression is observed

Dosage Forms Tablet, as citrate: 60 mg

Tornalate® *see* bitolterol *on page 76*

torsemide (TOR se mide)

U.S./Canadian Brand Names Demadex®

Therapeutic Category Diuretic, Loop

Use Management of edema associated with congestive heart failure and hepatic or renal disease; used alone or in combination with antihypertensives in treatment of hypertension

Usual Dosage Adults:

Oral: 5-10 mg once daily; if ineffective, may double dose until desired effect is achieved

I.V.: 10-20 mg/dose repeated in 2 hours as needed with a doubling of the dose with each succeeding dose until desired diuresis is achieved

Continues to be effective in patients with cirrhosis, no apparent change in dose is necessary

Dosage Forms

Injection: 10 mg/mL (2 mL, 5 mL)

Tablet: 5 mg, 10 mg, 20 mg, 100 mg

Totacillin® *see* ampicillin *on page 34*

Totacillin-N® ***(Discontinued)*** *see page 700*

Touro Ex® *see* guaifenesin *on page 267*

Touro LA® *see* guaifenesin and pseudoephedrine *on page 270*

t-PA *see* alteplase *on page 21*

TPGS *see* tocophersolan *on page 570*

T-Phyl® *see* theophylline *on page 557*

Trace-4® *see* trace metals *on this page*

trace metals (trase MET als)

Synonyms chromium injection; copper injection; manganese injection; molybdenum injection; neonatal trace metals; zinc injection

U.S./Canadian Brand Names Chroma-Pak®; Iodopen®; Molypen®; M.T.E.-4®; M.T.E.-5®; M.T.E.-6®; MulTE-PAK-4®; MulTE-PAK-5®; Neotrace-4®; PedTE-PAK-4®; Pedtrace-4®; P.T.E.-4®; P.T.E.-5®; Sele-Pak®; Selepen®; Trace-4®; Zinca-Pak®

Therapeutic Category Trace Element

Use Prevent and correct trace metal deficiencies

Dosage Forms

Chromium: Injection: 4 mcg/mL, 20 mcg/mL

Copper: Injection: 0.4 mg/mL, 2 mg/mL

Manganese: Injection: 0.1 mg/mL (as chloride or sulfate salt)

Molybdenum: Injection: 25 mcg/mL

Selenium: Injection: 40 mcg/mL

Zinc: Injection: 1 mg/mL (sulfate); 1 mg/mL (chloride); 5 mg/mL (sulfate)

Tracrium® *see* atracurium *on page 52*

Tral® ***(Discontinued)*** *see page 700*

tramadol (TRA ma dole)

U.S./Canadian Brand Names Ultram®

Therapeutic Category Analgesic, Non-narcotic

Use Relief of moderate to moderately severe pain

Usual Dosage Adults: Oral: 50-100 mg every 4-6 hours, not to exceed 400 mg/day

Dosage Forms Tablet, as hydrochloride: 50 mg

Trandate® *see* labetalol *on page 323*

trandolapril (tran DOE la pril)

U.S./Canadian Brand Names Mavik®

Therapeutic Category Angiotensin-Converting Enzyme (ACE) Inhibitor

Use Management of hypertension alone or in combination with other antihypertensive agents

Unlabeled use: As a class, ACE inhibitors are recommended in the treatment of systolic congestive heart failure

Usual Dosage Adults:

Non-Black patients: 0.5-1 mg for those not receiving diuretics; increase dose at 0.5-1 mg increments at 1- to 2-week intervals; maximum dose: 4 mg/day

Black patients: Initiate doses of 1-2 mg; maximum dose: 4 mg/day

Dosage Forms Tablet: 1 mg, 2 mg, 4 mg

trandolapril and verapamil (tran DOE la pril & ver AP a mil)

U.S./Canadian Brand Names Tarka®

Therapeutic Category Antihypertensive Agent, Combination

Use Combination drug for the treatment of hypertension

Usual Dosage Dose is individualized

Dosage Forms Tablet:

Trandolapril 1 mg and verapamil hydrochloride 240 mg
Trandolapril 2 mg and verapamil hydrochloride 180 mg
Trandolapril 2 mg and verapamil hydrochloride 240 mg
Trandolapril 4 mg and verapamil hydrochloride 240 mg

tranexamic acid (tran eks AM ik AS id)

U.S./Canadian Brand Names Cyklokapron®

Therapeutic Category Antihemophilic Agent

Use Short-term use (2-8 days) in hemophilia patients during and following tooth extraction to reduce or prevent hemorrhage

Usual Dosage Children and Adults: I.V.: 10 mg/kg immediately before surgery, then 25 mg/kg/dose orally 3-4 times/day for 2-8 days

Alternatively:

Oral: 25 mg/kg 3-4 times/day beginning 1 day prior to surgery

I.V.: 10 mg/kg 3-4 times/day in patients who are unable to take oral

Dosage Forms

Injection: 100 mg/mL (10 mL)

Tablet: 500 mg

transamine *see* tranylcypromine *on this page*

Transdermal-NTG® Patch *see* nitroglycerin *on page 404*

Transdermal-V® (Can) *see* scopolamine *on page 516*

Transderm-Nitro® Patch *see* nitroglycerin *on page 404*

Transderm Scop® *see* scopolamine *on page 516*

Trans-Plantar® (Can) *see* salicylic acid *on page 513*

Trans-Plantar® Transdermal Patch [OTC] *see* salicylic acid *on page 513*

Trans-Ver-Sal® Transdermal Patch [OTC] *see* salicylic acid *on page 513*

Tranxene® *see* clorazepate *on page 140*

tranylcypromine (tran il SIP roe meen)

Synonyms transamine

U.S./Canadian Brand Names Parnate®

Therapeutic Category Antidepressant, Monoamine Oxidase Inhibitor

Use Symptomatic treatment of depressed patients refractory to or intolerant to tricyclic antidepressants or electroconvulsive therapy; has a more rapid onset of therapeutic effect than other MAO inhibitors, but causes more severe hypertensive reactions

Usual Dosage Adults: Oral: 10 mg twice daily, increase by 10 mg increments at 1- to 3-week intervals; maximum: 60 mg/day

Dosage Forms Tablet, as sulfate: 10 mg

Trasicor® (Can) *see* oxprenolol *(Canada only)* *on page 421*

trastuzumab (tras TU zoo mab)

U.S./Canadian Brand Names Herceptin®

Therapeutic Category Antineoplastic Agent

Use Treatment of patients with metastatic breast cancer whose tumors overexpress the HER2 protein

Usual Dosage Adults: I.V.:

Loading dose: 4 mg/kg over 90 minutes; do not administer as an I.V. bolus or I.V. push

Maintenance dose: 2 mg/kg once weekly (may be infused over 30 minutes if prior infusions are well tolerated)

Dosage Forms Powder for injection: 440 mg

Trasylol® *see* aprotinin *on page 45*

Travase® ***(Discontinued)*** *see page 700*

Travasol® (Can) *see* enteral nutritional products *on page 208*

Travel Aid® (Can) *see* dimenhydrinate *on page 182*

Travel Tabs (Can) *see* dimenhydrinate *on page 182*

trazodone (TRAZ oh done)

U.S./Canadian Brand Names Desyrel®

Therapeutic Category Antidepressant, Triazolopyridine

Use Treatment of depression

Usual Dosage Oral:

Adolescents: Initial: 25-50 mg/day; increase to 100-150 mg/day in divided doses

Adults: Initial: 150 mg/day in 3 divided doses (may increase by 50 mg/day every 3-7 days); maximum: 600 mg/day

Dosage Forms Tablet, as hydrochloride: 50 mg, 100 mg, 150 mg, 300 mg

Trecator®-SC *see* ethionamide *on page 226*

Tremytoine® (Can) *see* phenytoin *on page 449*

Trendar® [OTC] *see* ibuprofen *on page 300*

Trental® *see* pentoxifylline *on page 438*

tretinoin (oral) (TRET i noyn, oral)

Synonyms all-*trans*-retinoic acid

U.S./Canadian Brand Names Vesanoid®

Therapeutic Category Antineoplastic Agent

Use Acute promyelocytic leukemia (APL): Induction of remission in patients with APL, French American British (FAB) classification M3 (including the M3 variant), characterized by the presence of the t(15;17) translocation or the presence of the PML/RARα gene who are refractory to or who have relapsed from anthracycline chemotherapy, or for whom anthracycline-based chemotherapy is contraindicated. Tretinoin is for the induction of remission only. All patients should receive an accepted form of remission consolidation or maintenance therapy for APL after completion of induction therapy with tretinoin.

Usual Dosage Oral:

Children: There are limited clinical data on the pediatric use of tretinoin. Of 15 pediatric patients (age range: 1-16 years) treated with tretinoin, the incidence of complete remission was 67%. Safety and efficacy in pediatric patients <1 year of age have not been established. Some pediatric patients experience severe headache and pseudotumor cerebri, requiring analgesic treatment and lumbar puncture for relief. Increased caution

(Continued)

tretinoin (oral) *(Continued)*

is recommended. Consider dose reduction in children experiencing serious or intolerable toxicity; however, the efficacy and safety of tretinoin at doses <45 mg/m²/day have not been evaluated.

Adults: 45 mg/m²/day administered as two evenly divided doses until complete remission is documented. Discontinue therapy 30 days after achievement of complete remission or after 90 days of treatment, whichever occurs first. If after initiation of treatment the presence of the t(15;17) translocation is not confirmed by cytogenetics or by polymerase chain reaction studies and the patient has not responded to tretinoin, consider alternative therapy.

Note: Tretinoin is for the induction of remission only. Optimal consolidation or maintenance regimens have not been determined. All patients should, therefore, receive a standard consolidation or maintenance chemotherapy regimen for APL after induction therapy with tretinoin unless otherwise contraindicated.

Dosage Forms Capsule: 10 mg

tretinoin (topical) (TRET i noyn, TOP i kal)

Synonyms retinoic acid; vitamin A acid

U.S./Canadian Brand Names Retin-A™; Retinova™ (Can); Retisol-A® (Can); Stieva-A® (Can); Stieva-A® Forte (Can); Vitinoin™ (Can)

Therapeutic Category Retinoic Acid Derivative

Use Treatment of acne vulgaris, photodamaged skin, and some skin cancers

Usual Dosage Children >12 years and Adults: Topical: Apply once daily before retiring; if stinging or irritation develop, decrease frequency of application

Dosage Forms

Cream:
- Retin-A™: 0.025% (20 g, 45 g); 0.05% (20 g, 45 g); 0.1% (20 g, 45 g)
- Avita®: 0.025% (20 g, 45 g)

Gel, topical:
- Retin-A™: 0.01% (15 g, 45 g); 0.025% (15 g, 45 g)
- Retin-A™ Micro: 0.1% (20 g, 45 g)

Liquid, topical (Retin-A™): 0.05% (28 mL)

triacetin (trye a SEE tin)

Synonyms glycerol triacetate

U.S./Canadian Brand Names Ony-Clear® Nail

Therapeutic Category Antifungal Agent

Use Fungistat for athlete's foot and other superficial fungal infections

Usual Dosage Topical: Apply twice daily, cleanse areas with dilute alcohol or mild soap and water before application; continue treatment for 7 days after symptoms have disappeared

Dosage Forms

Cream: With cetylpyridinium chloride and chloroxylenol (30 g)

Liquid: With cetylpyridinium chloride and chloroxylenol (30 mL)

Solution: With cetylpyridinium chloride, chloroxylenol, and benzalkonium chloride in an oil base (15 mL)

Spray, aerosol: With cetylpyridinium chloride, chloroxylenol, and benzalkonium chloride (45 mL, 60 mL)

Triacet™ Topical *see* triamcinolone (topical) *on page 578*

triacetyloleandomycin *see* troleandomycin *on page 586*

Triacin-C® *see* triprolidine, pseudoephedrine, and codeine *on page 585*

triaconazole *see* terconazole *on page 551*

Triadapin® (Can) *see* doxepin *on page 195*

Triam-A® Injection *see* triamcinolone (systemic) *on next page*

triamcinolone and nystatin *see* nystatin and triamcinolone *on page 412*

triamcinolone (inhalation, nasal) (trye am SIN oh lone)

U.S./Canadian Brand Names Nasacort®; Nasacort® AQ

Therapeutic Category Corticosteroid, Topical

Use Symptoms of seasonal and perennial allergic rhinitis

Usual Dosage Children >12 years and Adults: Intranasal: 2 sprays in each nostril once daily; may increase after 4-7 days up to 4 sprays once daily or 1 spray 4 times/day in each nostril

Dosage Forms

Aerosol: Nasal: 55 mcg per actuation (15 mL)

Spray, nasal: 55 mcg per actuation in aqueous base (16.5 g)

triamcinolone (inhalation, oral) (trye am SIN oh lone)

U.S./Canadian Brand Names Azmacort™ Oral Inhaler

Therapeutic Category Adrenal Corticosteroid

Use Asthma

Usual Dosage

Children 6-12 years:

Inhalation: 1-2 inhalations 3-4 times/day, not to exceed 12 inhalations/day

Children >12 years and Adults:

Oral inhalation: 2 inhalations 3-4 times/day, not to exceed 16 inhalations/day

Dosage Forms Aerosol: Oral inhalation: 100 mcg/metered spray (2 oz)

triamcinolone (systemic) (trye am SIN oh lone)

U.S./Canadian Brand Names Amcort® Injection; Aristocort® Forte Injection; Aristocort® Intralesional Injection; Aristocort® Oral; Aristospan® Intra-articular Injection; Aristospan® Intralesional Injection; Atolone® Oral; Kenacort® Oral; Kenaject® Injection; Kenalog® Injection; Tac™-3 Injection; Tac™-40 Injection; Triam-A® Injection; Triam Forte® Injection; Triamonide® Injection; Tri-Kort® Injection; Trilog® Injection; Trilone® Injection; Trisoject® Injection

Therapeutic Category Adrenal Corticosteroid

Use Severe inflammation or immunosuppression

Usual Dosage In general, single I.M. dose of 4-7 times oral dose will control patient from 4-7 days up to 3-4 weeks

Children 6-12 years:

I.M.: Acetonide or hexacetonide: 0.03-0.2 mg/kg at 1- to 7-day intervals

Children >12 years and Adults:

Oral: 4-100 mg/day

I.M.: Acetonide or hexacetonide: 60 mg (of 40 mg/mL), additional 20-100 mg doses (usual: 40-80 mg) may be administered when signs and symptoms recur, best at 6-week intervals to minimize HPA suppression

Intra-articularly, intrasynovially, intralesionally: 2.5-40 mg as diacetate salt or acetonide salt, dose may be repeated when signs and symptoms recur

Intra-articularly: Hexacetonide: 2-20 mg every 3-4 weeks as hexacetonide salt

Intralesional (use 10 mg/mL): Diacetate or acetonide: 1 mg/injection site, may be repeated one or more times/week depending upon patients response; maximum; 30 mg at any one time; may use multiple injections if they are more than 1 cm apart

Intra-articular, intrasynovial, and soft-tissue injection (use 10 mg/mL or 40 mg/mL): Diacetate or acetonide: 2.5-40 mg depending upon location, size of joints, and degree of inflammation; repeat when signs and symptoms recur

Sublesionally (as acetonide): Up to 1 mg per injection site and may be repeated one or more times weekly; multiple sites may be injected if they are 1 cm or more apart, not to exceed 30 mg

Dosage Forms

Syrup: 2 mg/5 mL (120 mL); 4 mg/5 mL (120 mL)

Tablet: 1 mg, 2 mg, 4 mg, 8 mg

Triamcinolone acetonide:

Injection: 10 mg/mL (5 mL); 40 mg/mL (1 mL, 5 mL, 10 mL)

(Continued)

triamcinolone (systemic) *(Continued)*

Triamcinolone diacetate: Injection: 25 mg/mL (5 mL); 40 mg/mL (1 mL, 5 mL, 10 mL)

Triamcinolone hexacetonide: Injection: 5 mg/mL (5 mL); 20 mg/mL (1 mL, 5 mL)

triamcinolone (topical) (trye am SIN oh lone)

U.S./Canadian Brand Names Aristocort® A Topical; Aristocort® Topical; Delta-Tritex® Topical; Flutex® Topical; Kenalog® in Orabase®; Kenalog® Topical; Kenonel® Topical; Triacet™ Topical

Therapeutic Category Corticosteroid, Topical

Use Severe inflammation or immunosuppression; nasal spray for symptoms of seasonal and perennial allergic rhinitis

Usual Dosage Children >12 years and Adults: Topical: Apply a thin film 2-3 times/day

Dosage Forms

Ointment, oral: 0.1% (5 g)

Aerosol, topical: 0.2 mg/2 second spray (23 g, 63 g)

Cream: 0.025% (15 g, 60 g, 80 g, 240 g, 454 g); 0.1% (15 g, 30 g, 60 g, 80 g, 90 g, 120 g, 240 g); 0.5% (15 g, 20 g, 30 g, 240 g)

Lotion: 0.025% (60 mL); 0.1% (15 mL, 60 mL)

Ointment, topical: 0.025% (15 g, 30 g, 60 g, 80 g, 120 g, 454 g); 0.1% (15 g, 30 g, 60 g, 80 g, 120 g, 240 g, 454 g); 0.5% (15 g, 20 g, 30 g, 240 g)

Triam Forte® Injection *see* triamcinolone (systemic) *on previous page*

Triaminic® Allergy Tablet [OTC] *see* chlorpheniramine and phenylpropanolamine *on page 122*

Triaminic® AM Decongestant Formula [OTC] *see* pseudoephedrine *on page 486*

Triaminic® Cold Tablet [OTC] *see* chlorpheniramine and phenylpropanolamine *on page 122*

Triaminic DM (Can) *see* dextromethorphan *on page 171*

Triaminic® Expectorant [OTC] *see* guaifenesin and phenylpropanolamine *on page 270*

Triaminicol® Multi-Symptom Cold Syrup [OTC] *see* chlorpheniramine, phenylpropanolamine, and dextromethorphan *on page 125*

Triaminic® Oral Infant Drops *see* pheniramine, phenylpropanolamine, and pyrilamine *on page 443*

Triaminic® Syrup [OTC] *see* chlorpheniramine and phenylpropanolamine *on page 122*

Triamonide® Injection *see* triamcinolone (systemic) *on previous page*

triamterene (trye AM ter een)

U.S./Canadian Brand Names Dyrenium®

Therapeutic Category Diuretic, Potassium Sparing

Use Alone or in combination with other diuretics to treat edema and hypertension; decreases potassium excretion caused by kaliuretic diuretics

Usual Dosage Oral:

Children: 2-4 mg/kg/day in 1-2 divided doses; maximum: 300 mg/day

Adults: 100-300 mg/day in 1-2 divided doses; maximum: 300 mg/day

Dosage Forms Capsule: 50 mg, 100 mg

triamterene and hydrochlorothiazide *see* hydrochlorothiazide and triamterene *on page 287*

Triapin® *see* butalbital compound and acetaminophen *on page 85*

Triavil® *see* amitriptyline and perphenazine *on page 29*

triazolam (trye AY zoe lam)

U.S./Canadian Brand Names Apo®-Triazo (Can); Gen-Triazolam® (Can); Halcion®; Novo-Triolam® (Can); Nu-Triazo® (Can)

Therapeutic Category Benzodiazepine

Controlled Substance C-IV

Use Short-term treatment of insomnia

Usual Dosage Oral (onset of action is rapid, patient should be in bed when taking medication):

Children <18 years: Dosage not established

Adults: 0.125-0.25 mg at bedtime

Dosage Forms Tablet: 0.125 mg, 0.25 mg

Triban® *see* trimethobenzamide *on page 582*

tribavirin *see* ribavirin *on page 503*

Tri-Chlor® *see* trichloroacetic acid *on this page*

trichlormethiazide (trye klor meth EYE a zide)

U.S./Canadian Brand Names Metahydrin®; Naqua®

Therapeutic Category Diuretic, Thiazide

Use Management of mild to moderate hypertension; treatment of edema in congestive heart failure and nephrotic syndrome

Usual Dosage Oral:

Children >6 months: 0.07 mg/kg/24 hours or 2 mg/m^2/24 hours

Adults: 1-4 mg/day

Dosage Forms Tablet: 2 mg, 4 mg

trichloroacetaldehyde monohydrate *see* chloral hydrate *on page 115*

trichloroacetic acid (trye klor oh a SEE tik AS id)

U.S./Canadian Brand Names Tri-Chlor®

Therapeutic Category Keratolytic Agent

Use Debride callous tissue

Usual Dosage Apply to verruca, cover with bandage for 5-6 days, remove verruca, reapply as needed

Dosage Forms Liquid: 80% (15 mL)

***Trichophyton* skin test** (trye koe FYE ton skin test)

U.S./Canadian Brand Names Dermatophytin®

Therapeutic Category Diagnostic Agent

Use Assess cell-mediated immunity

Usual Dosage 0.1 mL intradermally, examine reaction site in 24-48 hours; induration of ≥5 mm in diameter is a positive reaction

Dosage Forms Injection:

Diluted: 1:30 V/V (5 mL)

Undiluted: 5 mL

Tri-Clear® Expectorant [OTC] *see* guaifenesin and phenylpropanolamine *on page 270*

TriCor™ *see* fenofibrate *on page 233*

Tridesilon® Topical *see* desonide *on page 166*

tridihexethyl (trye dye heks ETH il)

U.S./Canadian Brand Names Pathilon®

Therapeutic Category Anticholinergic Agent

Use Adjunctive therapy in peptic ulcer treatment

Usual Dosage Adults: Oral: 1-2 tablets 3-4 times/day before meals and 2 tablets at bedtime

(Continued)

tridihexethyl *(Continued)*

Dosage Forms Tablet, as chloride: 25 mg

Tridil® Injection *see* nitroglycerin *on page 404*

Tridione® Oral *see* trimethadione *on page 582*

Tridione® Suppository *(Discontinued)* *see page 700*

trientine (TRYE en teen)

U.S./Canadian Brand Names Syprine®

Therapeutic Category Chelating Agent

Use Treatment of Wilson's disease in patients intolerant to penicillamine

Usual Dosage Oral (administer on an empty stomach):

Children <12 years: 500-750 mg/day in divided doses 2-4 times/day; maximum: 1.5 g/day

Adults: 750-1250 mg/day in divided doses 2-4 times/day; maximum daily dose: 2 g

Dosage Forms Capsule, as hydrochloride: 250 mg

triethanolamine polypeptide oleate-condensate

(trye eth a NOLE a meen pol i PEP tide OH lee ate-KON den sate)

U.S./Canadian Brand Names Cerumenex® Otic

Therapeutic Category Otic Agent, Cerumenolytic

Use Removal of ear wax (cerumen)

Usual Dosage Children and Adults: Otic: Fill ear canal, insert cotton plug; allow to remain 15-30 minutes; flush ear with lukewarm water

Dosage Forms Solution, otic: 6 mL, 12 mL

triethanolamine salicylate (trye eth a NOLE a meen sa LIS i late)

U.S./Canadian Brand Names Myoflex® [OTC]; Sportscreme® [OTC]

Therapeutic Category Analgesic, Topical

Use Relief of pain of muscular aches, rheumatism, neuralgia, sprains, arthritis on intact skin

Usual Dosage Topical: Apply to area as needed

Dosage Forms Cream: 10% in a nongreasy base

triethylenethiophosphoramide *see* thiotepa *on page 563*

Trifed-C® *see* triprolidine, pseudoephedrine, and codeine *on page 585*

trifluoperazine (trye floo oh PER a zeen)

U.S./Canadian Brand Names Stelazine®

Therapeutic Category Phenothiazine Derivative

Use Treatment of psychoses and management of anxiety

Usual Dosage

Children 6-12 years: Psychoses:

Oral: Hospitalized or well supervised patients: Initial dose: 1 mg 1-2 times/day, gradually increase until symptoms are controlled or adverse effects become troublesome; maximum: 15 mg/day

I.M.: 1 mg twice daily

Adults:

Psychoses:

Outpatients: Oral: 1-2 mg twice daily

Hospitalized or well supervised patients: Initial dose: 2-5 mg twice daily with optimum response in the 15-20 mg/day range; do not exceed 40 mg/day

I.M.: 1-2 mg every 4-6 hours as needed up to 10 mg/24 hours maximum

Nonpsychotic anxiety: Oral: 1-2 mg twice daily; maximum: 6 mg/day; therapy for anxiety should not exceed 12 weeks; do not exceed 6 mg/day for longer than 12 weeks when treating anxiety; agitation, jitteriness or insomnia may be confused with original neurotic or psychotic symptoms

Dosage Forms Trifluoperazine hydrochloride:
Concentrate, oral: 10 mg/mL (60 mL)
Injection: 2 mg/mL (10 mL)
Tablet: 1 mg, 2 mg, 5 mg, 10 mg

trifluorothymidine *see* trifluridine *on this page*

triflupromazine (trye floo PROE ma zeen)

U.S./Canadian Brand Names Vesprin®
Therapeutic Category Phenothiazine Derivative
Use Treatment of psychoses, nausea, vomiting, and intractable hiccups
Usual Dosage
Children: I.M.: 0.2-0.25 mg/kg
Adults:
I.M.: 5-15 mg every 4 hours
I.V.: 1 mg
Dosage Forms Injection, as hydrochloride: 20 mg/mL (1 mL)

trifluridine (trye FLURE i deen)

Synonyms f_3t; trifluorothymidine
U.S./Canadian Brand Names Viroptic® Ophthalmic
Therapeutic Category Antiviral Agent
Use Treatment of primary keratoconjunctivitis and recurrent epithelial keratitis caused by herpes simplex virus types I and II
Usual Dosage Adults: Ophthalmic: Instill 1 drop into affected eye every 2 hours while awake, to a maximum of 9 drops/day, until re-epithelialization of corneal ulcer occurs; then use 1 drop every 4 hours for another 7 days; do **not** exceed 21 days of treatment
Dosage Forms Solution, ophthalmic: 1% (7.5 mL)

triglycerides, medium chain *see* medium chain triglycerides *on page 352*

Trihexy® *see* trihexyphenidyl *on this page*

Trihexyphen® (Can) *see* trihexyphenidyl *on this page*

trihexyphenidyl (trye heks ee FEN i dil)

Synonyms benzhexol
U.S./Canadian Brand Names Apo®-Trihex (Can); Artane®; Novo-Hexidyl® (Can); PMS-Trihexyphenidyl (Can); Trihexy®; Trihexyphen® (Can)
Therapeutic Category Anticholinergic Agent; Anti-Parkinson's Agent
Use Adjunctive treatment of Parkinson's disease; also used in treatment of drug-induced extrapyramidal effects and acute dystonic reactions
Usual Dosage Oral:
Parkinsonism: Initial: Administer 1-2 mg the first day; increase by 2 mg increments at intervals of 3-5 days, until a total of 6-10 mg is administered daily. Many patients derive maximum benefit from a total daily dose of 6-10 mg; however, postencephalitic patients may require a total daily dose of 12-15 mg in 3-4 divided doses
Concomitant use with levodopa: 3-6 mg/day in divided doses is usually adequate
Drug-induced extrapyramidal disorders: Start with a single 1 mg dose; daily dosage usually ranges between 5-15 mg in 3-4 divided doses
Dosage Forms Trihexyphenidyl hydrochloride:
Capsule, sustained release: 5 mg
Elixir: 2 mg/5 mL (480 mL)
Tablet: 2 mg, 5 mg

Tri-Immunol® *see* diphtheria, tetanus toxoids, and whole-cell pertussis vaccine *on page 187*

Tri-K® *see* potassium acetate, potassium bicarbonate, and potassium citrate *on page 462*

TriKacide® (Can) *see* metronidazole *on page 372*

Tri-Kort® Injection *see* triamcinolone (systemic) *on page 577*

Trilafon® *see* perphenazine *on page 440*

Tri-Levlen® *see* ethinyl estradiol and levonorgestrel *on page 223*

Trilisate® *see* choline magnesium trisalicylate *on page 129*

Trilog® Injection *see* triamcinolone (systemic) *on page 577*

Trilone® Injection *see* triamcinolone (systemic) *on page 577*

Trimazide® *see* trimethobenzamide *on this page*

trimebutine *(Canada only)* (trye me BYOO teen)

U.S./Canadian Brand Names Modulon® (Can)

Therapeutic Category Antispasmodic Agent, Gastrointestinal

Use For the treatment and relief of symptoms associated with the irritable bowel syndrome (spastic colon). In postoperative paralytic ileus in order to accelerate the resumption of the intestinal transit following abdominal surgery.

Usual Dosage Adults:

Parenteral: Dosage should be individually tailored according to response, but the total parenteral daily dose should not exceed 300 mg. The usual adult dose is 50-100 mg 3 times daily, administered as an I.M. injection, as a 3 minute I.V. injection, or as a 60 minute I.V. infusion (in D_5W or NS), until resumption of intestinal motility.

Tablets: Up to 600 mg daily in divided doses. It may be administered as two 100 mg tablets 3 times daily before meals or one 200 mg tablet 3 times daily before meals.

Dosage Forms

Injection, as maleate: 10 mg/mL (5 mL)

Tablet, as maleate: 100 mg, 200 mg

trimethadione (trye meth a DYE one)

Synonyms troxidone

U.S./Canadian Brand Names Tridione® Oral

Therapeutic Category Anticonvulsant

Use Control absence (petit mal) seizures refractory to other drugs

Usual Dosage Oral:

Children: Initial: 25-50 mg/kg/24 hours in 3-4 equally divided doses every 6-8 hours

Adults: Initial: 900 mg/day in 3-4 equally divided doses, increase by 300 mg/day at weekly intervals until therapeutic results or toxic symptoms appear

Dosage Forms

Capsule: 300 mg

Tablet, chewable: 150 mg

trimethobenzamide (trye meth oh BEN za mide)

U.S./Canadian Brand Names Arrestin®; Pediatric Triban®; Tebamide®; T-Gen®; Ticon®; Tigan®; Triban®; Trimazide®

Therapeutic Category Anticholinergic Agent; Antiemetic

Use Control of nausea and vomiting (especially for long term antiemetic therapy)

Usual Dosage Rectal use: Contraindicated in neonates and premature infants

Children:

Oral, rectal: 15-20 mg/kg/day or 400-500 mg/m²/day divided into 3-4 doses

I.M.: Not recommended

Adults:

Oral: 250 mg 3-4 times/day

I.M., rectal: 200 mg 3-4 times/day

Dosage Forms Trimethobenzamide hydrochloride:

Capsule: 100 mg, 250 mg

Injection: 100 mg/mL (2 mL, 20 mL)

Suppository, rectal: 100 mg, 200 mg

trimethoprim (trye METH oh prim)

Synonyms TMP

U.S./Canadian Brand Names Proloprim®; Trimpex®

Therapeutic Category Antibiotic, Miscellaneous

Use Treatment and prophylaxis of urinary tract infections; in combination with other agents for treatment of *Pneumocystis carinii* pneumonia

Usual Dosage Adults: Oral: 100 mg every 12 hours or 200 mg every 24 hours

Dosage Forms Tablet: 100 mg, 200 mg

trimethoprim and polymyxin B (trye METH oh prim & pol i MIKS in bee)

Synonyms polymyxin B and trimethoprim

U.S./Canadian Brand Names Polytrim® Ophthalmic

Therapeutic Category Antibiotic, Ophthalmic

Use Treatment of surface ocular bacterial conjunctivitis and blepharoconjunctivitis

Usual Dosage Ophthalmic: Instill 1-2 drops in eye(s) every 4-6 hours

Dosage Forms Solution, ophthalmic: Trimethoprim sulfate 1 mg and polymyxin B sulfate 10,000 units per mL (10 mL)

trimethoprim and sulfamethoxazole *see* co-trimoxazole *on page 149*

trimethylpsoralen *see* trioxsalen *on next page*

trimetrexate glucuronate (tri me TREKS ate gloo KYOOR oh nate)

U.S./Canadian Brand Names Neutrexin®

Therapeutic Category Antibiotic, Miscellaneous

Use Alternative therapy for the treatment of moderate-to-severe *Pneumocystis carinii* pneumonia (PCP) in immunocompromised patients, including patients with acquired immunodeficiency syndrome (AIDS), who are intolerant of, or are refractory to, co-trimoxazole therapy or for whom co-trimoxazole is contraindicated

Usual Dosage Adults: I.V.: 45 mg/m^2 once daily over 60 minutes for 21 days; it is necessary to reduce the dose in patients with liver dysfunction, although no specific recommendations exist

Dosage Forms Powder for injection: 25 mg

trimipramine (trye MI pra meen)

U.S./Canadian Brand Names Apo-Trimip® (Can); Novo-Tripramine (Can); Nu-Trimipramine® (Can); Rhotrimine® (Can); Surmontil®

Therapeutic Category Antidepressant, Tricyclic (Tertiary Amine)

Use Treatment of various forms of depression, often in conjunction with psychotherapy

Usual Dosage Oral: 50-150 mg/day as a single bedtime dose

Dosage Forms Capsule, as maleate: 25 mg, 50 mg, 100 mg

Trimox® *see* amoxicillin *on page 31*

Trimox® 500 mg *(Discontinued)* *see page 700*

Trimpex® *see* trimethoprim *on this page*

Trinalin® *see* azatadine and pseudoephedrine *on page 55*

Tri-Nefrin® Extra Strength Tablet [OTC] *see* chlorpheniramine and phenylpropanolamine *on page 122*

Tri-Norinyl® *see* ethinyl estradiol and norethindrone *on page 224*

Triofed® Syrup [OTC] *see* triprolidine and pseudoephedrine *on next page*

Triostat™ Injection *see* liothyronine *on page 335*

Triotann® Tablet *see* chlorpheniramine, pyrilamine, and phenylephrine *on page 126*

trioxsalen (trye OKS a len)

Synonyms trimethylpsoralen

U.S./Canadian Brand Names Trisoralen®

Therapeutic Category Psoralen

Use In conjunction with controlled exposure to ultraviolet light or sunlight for repigmentation of idiopathic vitiligo; increasing tolerance to sunlight with albinism; enhance pigmentation

Usual Dosage Children >12 years and Adults: Oral: 10 mg/day as a single dose, 2-4 hours before controlled exposure to UVA or sunlight

Dosage Forms Tablet: 5 mg

Tripedia® *see* diphtheria, tetanus toxoids, and acellular pertussis vaccine *on page 187*

tripelennamine (tri pel EN a meen)

U.S./Canadian Brand Names PBZ®; PBZ-SR®

Therapeutic Category Antihistamine

Use Perennial and seasonal allergic rhinitis and other allergic symptoms including urticaria

Usual Dosage Oral:

Infants and Children: 5 mg/kg/day in 4-6 divided doses, up to 300 mg/day maximum

Adults: 25-50 mg every 4-6 hours, extended release tablets 100 mg morning and evening up to 100 mg every 8 hours

Dosage Forms Tripelennamine hydrochloride:

Tablet: 25 mg, 50 mg

Tablet, extended release: 100 mg

Triphasil® *see* ethinyl estradiol and levonorgestrel *on page 223*

Tri-Phen-Chlor® *see* chlorpheniramine, phenyltoloxamine, phenylpropanolamine, and phenylephrine *on page 125*

Triphenyl® Expectorant [OTC] *see* guaifenesin and phenylpropanolamine *on page 270*

Triphenyl® Syrup [OTC] *see* chlorpheniramine and phenylpropanolamine *on page 122*

Triple Antibiotic® Topical *see* bacitracin, neomycin, and polymyxin B *on page 59*

triple sulfa *see* sulfabenzamide, sulfacetamide, and sulfathiazole *on page 539*

Triple X® Liquid [OTC] *see* pyrethrins *on page 489*

Triposed® Syrup [OTC] *see* triprolidine and pseudoephedrine *on this page*

Triposed® Tablet [OTC] *see* triprolidine and pseudoephedrine *on this page*

triprolidine and pseudoephedrine (trye PROE li deen & soo doe e FED rin)

Synonyms pseudoephedrine and triprolidine

U.S./Canadian Brand Names Actagen® Syrup [OTC]; Actagen® Tablet [OTC]; Allercon® Tablet [OTC]; Allerfrin® Syrup [OTC]; Allerfrin® Tablet [OTC]; Allerphed® Syrup [OTC]; Aprodine® Syrup [OTC]; Aprodine® Tablet [OTC]; Cenafed® Plus Tablet [OTC]; Genac® Tablet [OTC]; Silafed® Syrup [OTC]; Triofed® Syrup [OTC]; Triposed® Syrup [OTC]; Triposed® Tablet [OTC]

Therapeutic Category Antihistamine/Decongestant Combination

Use Temporary relief of nasal congestion, running nose, sneezing, itching of nose or throat and itchy, watery eyes due to common cold, hay fever or other upper respiratory allergies

Usual Dosage May dose according to **pseudoephedrine** component (4 mg/kg/day in divided doses 3-4 times/day) Oral:

Children:

4 months to 2 years: 1.25 mL 3-4 times/day

2-4 years: 2.5 mL 3-4 times/day

4-6 years: 3.75 mL 3-4 times/day
6-12 years: 5 mL or ½ tablet 3-4 times/day, not to exceed 2 tablets/day
Children >12 years and Adults: 10 mL or 1 tablet 3-4 times/day, not to exceed 4 tablets/day

Dosage Forms
Capsule: Triprolidine hydrochloride 2.5 mg and pseudoephedrine hydrochloride 60 mg
Extended release: Triprolidine hydrochloride 5 mg and pseudoephedrine hydrochloride 120 mg
Syrup: Triprolidine hydrochloride 1.25 mg and pseudoephedrine hydrochloride 30 mg per 5 mL
Tablet: Triprolidine hydrochloride 2.5 mg and pseudoephedrine hydrochloride 60 mg

triprolidine, pseudoephedrine, and codeine

(trye PROE li deen, soo doe e FED rin, & KOE deen)

U.S./Canadian Brand Names Actagen-C®; Allerfrin® w/Codeine; Aprodine® w/C; Triacin-C®; Trifed-C®

Therapeutic Category Antihistamine/Decongestant/Antitussive

Controlled Substance C-V

Use Symptomatic relief of cough

Usual Dosage Oral:
Children:
2-6 years: 2.5 mL 4 times/day
7-12 years: 5 mL 4 times/day
Children >12 years and Adults: 10 mL 4 times/day

Dosage Forms Syrup: Triprolidine hydrochloride 1.25 mg, pseudoephedrine hydrochloride 30 mg, and codeine phosphate 10 mg per 5 mL with alcohol 4.3%

Triptil® (Can) *see* protriptyline *on page 485*

TripTone® Caplets® [OTC] *see* dimenhydrinate *on page 182*

tris buffer *see* tromethamine *on next page*

tris(hydroxymethyl)aminomethane *see* tromethamine *on next page*

Trisoject® Injection *see* triamcinolone (systemic) *on page 577*

Trisoralen® *see* trioxsalen *on previous page*

Tri-Statin® II Topical *see* nystatin and triamcinolone *on page 412*

Trisulfa® (Can) *see* co-trimoxazole *on page 149*

trisulfapyrimidines *see* sulfadiazine, sulfamethazine, and sulfamerazine *on page 541*

Trisulfa-S® (Can) *see* co-trimoxazole *on page 149*

Tri-Tannate Plus® *see* chlorpheniramine, ephedrine, phenylephrine, and carbetapentane *on page 123*

Tri-Tannate® Tablet *see* chlorpheniramine, pyrilamine, and phenylephrine *on page 126*

Tritec® *see* ranitidine bismuth citrate *on page 497*

Tri-Vi-Flor® *see* vitamin, multiple (pediatric) *on page 606*

Tri-Vi-Sol® [OTC] *see* vitamin, multiple (pediatric) *on page 606*

Trobicin® *see* spectinomycin *on page 533*

Trocaine® [OTC] *see* benzocaine *on page 66*

Trocal® [OTC] *see* dextromethorphan *on page 171*

Trofan® *(Discontinued)* *see page 700*

Trofan DS® *(Discontinued)* *see page 700*

troglitazone (TROE gli to zone)

U.S./Canadian Brand Names Rezulin®

Therapeutic Category Thiazolidinedione Derivative

Use Troglitazone is indicated for the following:

In combination with a sulfonylurea drug together with metformin for patients who are not adequately controlled with the combination of a sulfonylurea and metformin

In combination with a sulfonylurea drug for patients who are not adequately controlled with a sulfonylurea alone

In combination with insulin in patients who are not adequately controlled on insulin alone

Rezulin® is **not indicated for monotherapy**

Usual Dosage Adults: Oral: 200 mg once daily with a meal; for patients on insulin therapy continue current insulin dose; dose may be increased to 400 mg/day after 2-4 weeks in those who are not responding adequately; maximum recommended dose: 600 mg/day. It is recommended that the insulin dose should be reduced by 10% to 25% when fasting plasma glucose concentrations decrease to <120 mg/dL in those patients receiving concomitant insulin.

Dosage Forms Tablet: 200 mg, 400 mg

troleandomycin (troe lee an doe MYE sin)

Synonyms triacetyloleandomycin

U.S./Canadian Brand Names Tao®

Therapeutic Category Macrolide (Antibiotic)

Use Adjunct in the treatment of severe corticosteroid-dependent asthma due to its steroid-sparing properties; obsolete antibiotic with spectrum of activity similar to erythromycin

Usual Dosage Oral:

Children: 25-40 mg/kg/day divided every 6 hours

Adjunct in corticosteroid-dependent asthma: 14 mg/kg/day in divided doses every 6-12 hours not to exceed 250 mg every 6 hours; dose is tapered to once daily then alternate day dosing

Adults: 250-500 mg 4 times/day

Dosage Forms Capsule: 250 mg

Trombovar® (Can) *see* sodium tetradecyl *on page 531*

tromethamine (troe METH a meen)

Synonyms tris buffer; tris(hydroxymethyl)aminomethane

U.S./Canadian Brand Names THAM®; THAM-E®

Therapeutic Category Alkalinizing Agent

Use Correction of metabolic acidosis associated with cardiac bypass surgery or cardiac arrest; to correct excess acidity of stored blood that is preserved with acid citrate dextrose (ACD); to prime the pump-oxygenator during cardiac bypass surgery; indicated in severe metabolic acidosis in patients in whom sodium or carbon dioxide elimination is restricted [eg, infants needing alkalinization after receiving maximum sodium bicarbonate (8-10 mEq/kg/24 hours)]

Usual Dosage Dose depends on buffer base deficit; when deficit is known: tromethamine mL of 0.3 M solution = body weight (kg) x base deficit (mEq/L); when base deficit is not known: 3-6 mL/kg/dose I.V. (1-2 mEq/kg/dose)

Metabolic acidosis with cardiac arrest:

I.V.: 3.5-6 mL/kg (1-2 mEq/kg/dose) into large peripheral vein; 500-1000 mL if needed in adults

I.V. continuous drip: Infuse slowly by syringe pump over 3-6 hours

Excess acidity of ACD priming blood: 14-70 mL of 0.3 molar solution added to each 500 mL of blood

Dosage Forms Injection:

Tham®: 18 g [0.3 molar] (500 mL)

Tham-E®: 36 g with sodium 30 mEq, potassium 5 mEq, and chloride 35 mEq (1000 mL)

Tronolane® [OTC] *see* pramoxine *on page 469*

Tropicacyl® *see* tropicamide *on this page*

tropicamide (troe PIK a mide)

Synonyms bistropamide

U.S./Canadian Brand Names Diotrope (Can); I-Picamide®; Mydriacyl®; Tropicacyl®

Therapeutic Category Anticholinergic Agent

Use Short-acting mydriatic used in diagnostic procedures; as well as preoperatively and postoperatively; treatment of some cases of acute iritis, iridocyclitis, and keratitis

Usual Dosage Children and Adults: Ophthalmic:

Cycloplegia: 1-2 drops (1%); may repeat in 5 minutes

Mydriasis: 1-2 drops (0.5%) 15-20 minutes before exam; may repeat every 30 minutes as needed

Dosage Forms Solution, ophthalmic: 0.5% (2 mL, 15 mL); 1% (2 mL, 3 mL, 15 mL)

trovafloxacin (TROE va flox a sin)

Synonyms alatrofloxacin; CP-99,219-27

U.S./Canadian Brand Names Trovan™

Therapeutic Category Antibiotic, Quinolone

Use Should be used only in life- or limb-threatening infections

Treatment of nosocomial pneumonia, community-acquired pneumonia, complicated intra-abdominal infections, gynecologic/pelvic infections, complicated skin and skin structure infections

Usual Dosage Adults:

Nosocomial pneumonia: I.V.: 300 mg single dose followed by 200 mg/day orally for a total duration of 10-14 days

Community-acquired pneumonia: Oral, I.V.: 200 mg/day for 7-14 days

Complicated intra-abdominal infections, including postsurgical infections/gynecologic and pelvic infections: I.V.: 300 mg as a single dose followed by 200 mg/day orally for a total duration of 7-14 days

Skin and skin structure infections, complicated, including diabetic foot infections: Oral, I.V.: 200 mg/day for 10-14 days

Dosage Forms

Injection, as mesylate (alatrofloxacin): 5 mg/mL (40 mL, 60 mL)

Tablet, as mesylate (trovafloxacin): 100 mg, 200 mg

Trovan™ *see* trovafloxacin *on this page*

troxidone *see* trimethadione *on page 582*

Truphylline® *see* aminophylline *on page 27*

Trusopt® *see* dorzolamide *on page 194*

trypsin, balsam Peru, and castor oil

(TRIP sin, BAL sam pe RUE , & KAS tor oyl)

U.S./Canadian Brand Names Granulex

Therapeutic Category Protectant, Topical

Use Treatment of decubitus ulcers, varicose ulcers, debridement of eschar, dehiscent wounds and sunburn

Usual Dosage Topical: Apply a minimum of twice daily or as often as necessary

Dosage Forms Aerosol, topical: Trypsin 0.1 mg, balsam Peru 72.5 mg, and castor oil 650 mg per 0.82 mL (60 g, 120 g)

Tryptacin® ***(Discontinued)*** *see page 700*

Trysul® *see* sulfabenzamide, sulfacetamide, and sulfathiazole *on page 539*

TSH *see* thyrotropin *on page 564*

TSH *see* thyrotropin alpha *on page 564*

TSPA *see* thiotepa *on page 563*

T-Stat® Topical *see* erythromycin (ophthalmic/topical) *on page 214*

Tubasal® (Can) *see* aminosalicylate sodium *on page 28*

tuberculin tests (too BER kyoo lin tests)

Synonyms Mantoux; old tuberculin; PPD; purified protein derivative

U.S./Canadian Brand Names Aplisol®; Aplitest®; Tine Test PPD; Tubersol®

Therapeutic Category Diagnostic Agent

Use Skin test in diagnosis of tuberculosis, to aid in assessment of cell-mediated immunity; routine tuberculin testing is recommended at 12 months of age and at every 1-2 years thereafter, before the measles vaccination

Usual Dosage Children and Adults: Intradermally: 0.1 mL approximately 4" below elbow; use 1/4" to 1/2" or 26- or 27-gauge needle; significant reactions are ≥5 mm in diameter

Dosage Forms Injection:

First test strength: 1 TU/0.1 mL (1 mL)
Intermediate test strength: 5 TU/0.1 mL (1 mL, 5 mL, 10 mL)
Second test strength: 250 TU/0.1 mL (1 mL)
Tine: 5 TU each test

Tubersol® *see* tuberculin tests *on this page*

tubocurarine (too boe kyoor AR een)

Synonyms *d*-tubocurarine

Therapeutic Category Skeletal Muscle Relaxant

Use Adjunct to anesthesia to induce skeletal muscle relaxation

Usual Dosage Children and Adults: I.V.: 0.2-0.4 mg/kg as a single dose; maintenance: 0.04-0.2 mg/kg/dose as needed to maintain paralysis

Alternative adult dose: 6-9 mg once daily, then 3-4.5 mg as needed to maintain paralysis

Dosage Forms Injection, as chloride: 3 mg/mL [3 units/mL] (5 mL, 10 mL, 20 mL)

Tucks® [OTC] *see* witch hazel *on page 607*

Tucks® Cream *(Discontinued)* *see page 700*

Tuinal® *see* amobarbital and secobarbital *on page 31*

Tums® [OTC] *see* calcium carbonate *on page 89*

Tums® E-X Extra Strength Tablet [OTC] *see* calcium carbonate *on page 89*

Tums® Extra Strength Liquid [OTC] *see* calcium carbonate *on page 89*

Tusal® *(Discontinued)* *see page 700*

Tusibron® [OTC] *see* guaifenesin *on page 267*

Tusibron-DM® [OTC] *see* guaifenesin and dextromethorphan *on page 268*

Tussafed® Drops *see* carbinoxamine, pseudoephedrine, and dextromethorphan *on page 99*

Tussafin® Expectorant *see* hydrocodone, pseudoephedrine, and guaifenesin *on page 290*

Tuss-Allergine® Modified T.D. Capsule *see* caramiphen and phenylpropanolamine *on page 97*

Tussar® SF Syrup *see* guaifenesin, pseudoephedrine, and codeine *on page 272*

Tuss-DM® [OTC] *see* guaifenesin and dextromethorphan *on page 268*

Tussigon® *see* hydrocodone and homatropine *on page 289*

Tussionex® *see* hydrocodone and chlorpheniramine *on page 288*

Tussi-Organidin® *(Discontinued)* *see page 700*

Tussi-Organidin® DM *(Discontinued)* *see page 700*

Tussi-Organidin® DM NR *see* guaifenesin and dextromethorphan *on page 268*

Tussi-Organidin® NR *see* guaifenesin and codeine *on page 268*

Tuss-LA® *see* guaifenesin and pseudoephedrine *on page 270*

Tusso-DM® *(Discontinued)* *see page 700*

Tussogest® Extended Release Capsule *see* caramiphen and phenylpropanolamine *on page 97*

Tuss-Ornade® *(Discontinued)* *see page 700*

Tusstat® Syrup *see* diphenhydramine *on page 185*

Twice-A-Day® Nasal Solution [OTC] *see* oxymetazoline *on page 423*

Twilite® Oral [OTC] *see* diphenhydramine *on page 185*

Twin-K® *see* potassium citrate and potassium gluconate *on page 465*

Two-Dyne® *see* butalbital compound and acetaminophen *on page 85*

Tylenol® [OTC] *see* acetaminophen *on page 3*

Tylenol® Cold Effervescent Medication Tablet [OTC] *see* chlorpheniramine, phenylpropanolamine, and acetaminophen *on page 125*

Tylenol® Cold No Drowsiness [OTC] *see* acetaminophen, dextromethorphan, and pseudoephedrine *on page 6*

Tylenol® Flu Maximum Strength [OTC] *see* acetaminophen, dextromethorphan, and pseudoephedrine *on page 6*

Tylenol® Sinus, Maximum Strength [OTC] *see* acetaminophen and pseudoephedrine *on page 5*

Tylenol® With Codeine *see* acetaminophen and codeine *on page 4*

Tylox® *see* oxycodone and acetaminophen *on page 422*

Ty-Pap [OTC] *see* acetaminophen *on page 3*

Typhim Vi® *see* typhoid vaccine *on this page*

typhoid vaccine (TYE foid vak SEEN)

Synonyms typhoid vaccine live oral Ty21a

U.S./Canadian Brand Names Typhim Vi®; Vivotif Berna™ Oral

Therapeutic Category Vaccine, Inactivated Bacteria

Use Promotes active immunity to typhoid fever for patients exposed to typhoid carrier or foreign travel to typhoid fever endemic area

Usual Dosage

Oral: Adults:

Primary immunization: 1 capsule on alternate days (day 1, 3, 5, and 7)

Booster immunization: Repeat full course of primary immunization every 5 years

S.C.:

Children 6 months to 10 years: 0.25 mL; repeat in ≥4 weeks (total immunization is 2 doses)

Children >10 years and Adults: 0.5 mL; repeat dose in ≥4 weeks (total immunization is 2 doses)

Booster: 0.25 mL every 3 years for children 6 months to 10 years and 0.5 mL every 3 years for adults and children >10 years

Dosage Forms

Capsule, enteric coated (Vivotif Berna™): Viable *S. typhi* Ty21a Colony-forming units 2-6 x 10^9 and nonviable *S. typhi* Ty21a Colony-forming units 50 x 10^9 with sucrose, ascorbic acid, amino acid mixture, lactose and magnesium stearate

Injection, suspension (H-P): Heat- and phenol-inactivated, killed Ty-2 strain of *S. typhi* organisms; provides 8 units/mL, ≤1 billion/mL and ≤35 mcg nitrogen/mL (5 mL, 10 mL)

Injection (Typhim Vi®): Purified Vi capsular polysaccharide 25 mcg/0.5 mL (0.5 mL)

Powder for suspension (AKD): 8 units/mL ≤1 billion/mL, acetone inactivated dried (50 doses)

typhoid vaccine live oral Ty21a *see* typhoid vaccine *on this page*

Tyrodone® Liquid *see* hydrocodone and pseudoephedrine *on page 289*

Tyzine® Nasal *see* tetrahydrozoline *on page 556*

U-90152S *see* delavirdine *on page 162*

UAD Otic® *see* neomycin, polymyxin B, and hydrocortisone *on page 396*

UCB-P071 *see* cetirizine *on page 113*

Ucephan® *see* sodium phenylacetate and sodium benzoate *on page 528*

U-Cort™ Topical *see* hydrocortisone (topical) *on page 292*

UK *see* urokinase *on page 592*

UK 92480 *see* sildenafil *on page 521*

Ulcerease® [OTC] *see* phenol *on page 444*

ULR-LA® *see* guaifenesin and phenylpropanolamine *on page 270*

Ultane® *see* sevoflurane *on page 520*

Ultiva™ *see* remifentanil *on page 499*

Ultralente® U *(Discontinued)* *see page 700*

Ultram® *see* tramadol *on page 573*

Ultra Mide® Topical *see* urea *on next page*

Ultramop™ (Can) *see* methoxsalen *on page 365*

Ultraquin™ (Can) *see* hydroquinone *on page 294*

Ultrase® MT *see* pancrelipase *on page 427*

Ultrase® MT24 *(Discontinued)* *see page 700*

Ultra Tears® Solution [OTC] *see* artificial tears *on page 47*

Ultravate™ *see* halobetasol *on page 276*

Unasyn® *see* ampicillin and sulbactam *on page 35*

undecylenic acid and derivatives (un de sil EN ik AS id & dah RIV ah tivs)

Synonyms zinc undecylenate

U.S./Canadian Brand Names Caldesene® Topical [OTC]; Fungoid® AF Topical Solution [OTC]; Pedi-Pro Topical [OTC]

Therapeutic Category Antifungal Agent

Use Treatment of athlete's foot (tinea pedis), ringworm (except nails and scalp), prickly heat, jock itch (tinea cruris), diaper rash and other minor skin irritations due to superficial dermatophytes

Usual Dosage Children and Adults: Topical: Apply as needed twice daily after cleansing the affected area for 2-4 weeks

Dosage Forms

Cream: Total undecylenate 20% (15 g, 82.5 g)

Foam, topical: Undecylenic acid 10% (42.5 g)

Liquid, topical: Undecylenic acid 10% (42.5 g)

Ointment, topical: Total undecylenate 22% (30 g, 60 g, 454 g); total undecylenate 25% (60 g, 454 g)

Powder, topical: Calcium undecylenate 10% (45 g, 60 g, 120 g); total undecylenate 22% (45 g, 54 g, 81 g, 90 g, 105 g, 165 g, 454 g)

Solution, topical: Undecylenic acid 25% (29.57 mL)

Unguentine® [OTC] *see* benzocaine *on page 66*

Uni-Ace® [OTC] *see* acetaminophen *on page 3*

Uni-Bent® Cough Syrup *see* diphenhydramine *on page 185*

Unicap® [OTC] *see* vitamin, multiple (oral) *on page 604*

Uni-Decon® *see* chlorpheniramine, phenyltoloxamine, phenylpropanolamine, and phenylephrine *on page 125*

Uni-Dur® *see* theophylline *on page 557*

Unipen® *(Discontinued)* *see page 700*

Uniphyl® *see* theophylline *on page 557*

Unipres® ***(Discontinued)*** *see page 700*

Uni-Pro® [OTC] *see* ibuprofen *on page 300*

Uniretic™ *see* moexipril and hydrochlorothiazide *on page 380*

Unitrol® [OTC] *see* phenylpropanolamine *on page 447*

Uni-tussin® [OTC] *see* guaifenesin *on page 267*

Uni-tussin® DM [OTC] *see* guaifenesin and dextromethorphan *on page 268*

Univasc® *see* moexipril *on page 379*

Unna's boot *see* zinc gelatin *on page 612*

Unna's paste *see* zinc gelatin *on page 612*

Urabeth® *see* bethanechol *on page 73*

Uracel® *see* sodium salicylate *on page 530*

uracil mustard (YOOR a sil MUS tard)

U.S./Canadian Brand Names Ursofalk® (Can)

Therapeutic Category Antineoplastic Agent

Use Palliative treatment in symptomatic chronic lymphocytic leukemia; non-Hodgkin's lymphomas

Usual Dosage Oral:

Children: 0.3 mg/kg in a single weekly dose for 4 weeks

Adults: 0.15 mg/kg in a single weekly dose for 4 weeks

Thrombocytosis: 1-2 mg/day for 14 days

Dosage Forms Capsule: 1 mg

Urasal® (Can) *see* methenamine *on page 362*

urea (yoor EE a)

Synonyms carbamide

U.S./Canadian Brand Names Amino-Cerv™ Vaginal Cream; Aquacare® Topical [OTC]; Carmol® Topical [OTC]; Gormel® Creme [OTC]; Lanaphilic® Topical [OTC]; Nutraplus® Topical [OTC]; Onyvul® (Can); Rea-Lo® [OTC]; Ultra Mide® Topical; Ureacin®-20 Topical [OTC]; Ureaphil® Injection; Uremol® (Can); Urisec® (Can); Velvelan® (Can)

Therapeutic Category Diuretic, Osmotic; Topical Skin Product

Use Reduce intracranial pressure and intraocular pressure (30%); promotes hydration and removal of excess keratin in hyperkeratotic conditions and dry skin; mild cervicitis

Usual Dosage

Children: I.V. slow infusion:

<2 years: 0.1-0.5 g/kg

>2 years: 0.5-1.5 g/kg

Adults:

I.V. infusion: 1-1.5 g/kg by slow infusion (1-2$^1/_2$ hours); maximum: 120 g/24 hours

Topical: Apply 1-3 times/day

Vaginal: 1 applicatorful in vagina at bedtime for 2-4 weeks

Dosage Forms

Cream:

Topical: 2% [20 mg/mL] (75 g); 10% [100 mg/mL] (75 g, 90 g, 454 g); 20% [200 mg/mL] (45 g, 75 g, 90 g, 454 g); 30% [300 mg/mL] (60 g, 454 g); 40% (30 g)

Vaginal: 8.34% [83.4 mg/g] (82.5 g)

Injection: 40 g/150 mL

Lotion: 2% (240 mL); 10% (180 mL, 240 mL, 480 mL); 15% (120 mL, 480 mL); 25% (180 mL)

urea and hydrocortisone (yoor EE a & hye droe KOR ti sone)

Synonyms hydrocortisone and urea

U.S./Canadian Brand Names Carmol-HC® Topical

(Continued)

urea and hydrocortisone *(Continued)*

Therapeutic Category Corticosteroid, Topical

Use Inflammation of corticosteroid-responsive dermatoses

Usual Dosage Topical: Apply thin film and rub in well 1-4 times/day

Dosage Forms Cream, topical: Urea 10% and hydrocortisone acetate 1% in a water-washable vanishing cream base (30 g)

Ureacin®-20 Topical [OTC] *see* urea *on previous page*

Ureacin®-40 Topical *(Discontinued)* *see page 700*

urea peroxide *see* carbamide peroxide *on page 98*

Ureaphil® Injection *see* urea *on previous page*

Urecholine® *see* bethanechol *on page 73*

Uremol® (Can) *see* urea *on previous page*

Urex® *see* methenamine *on page 362*

Uridon® (Can) *see* chlorthalidone *on page 128*

Urisec® (Can) *see* urea *on previous page*

Urispas® *see* flavoxate *on page 240*

Uri-Tet® *(Discontinued)* *see page 700*

Uritol® (Can) *see* furosemide *on page 255*

Urobak® *see* sulfamethoxazole *on page 542*

Urobiotic-25® *(Discontinued)* *see page 700*

Urocit®-K *see* potassium citrate *on page 465*

Urodine® *see* phenazopyridine *on page 442*

urofollitropin (yoor oh fol li TROE pin)

U.S./Canadian Brand Names Fertinex®; Metrodin®

Therapeutic Category Ovulation Stimulator

Use Induction of ovulation in patients with polycystic ovarian disease and to stimulate the development of multiple oocytes

Usual Dosage Adults: Female: S.C.: 75 units/day for 7-12 days, used with hCG may repeat course of treatment 2 more times

Dosage Forms Injection: 0.83 mg [75 units FSH activity] (2 mL); 1.66 mg [150 units FSH activity]

Urogesic® *see* phenazopyridine *on page 442*

urokinase (yoor oh KIN ase)

Synonyms UK

U.S./Canadian Brand Names Abbokinase®

Therapeutic Category Thrombolytic Agent

Use Treatment of recent severe or massive deep vein or arterial thrombosis, pulmonary emboli, and occluded arteriovenous cannulas

Usual Dosage

Children and Adults: Deep vein thrombosis: I.V.: Loading: 4400 units/kg over 10 minutes, then 4400 units/kg/hour for 12 hours

Adults:

Myocardial infarction: Intracoronary: 750,000 units over 2 hours (6000 units/minute over up to 2 hours)

Occluded I.V. catheters:

5000 units (use only Abbokinase® Open Cath) in each lumen over 1-2 minutes, leave in lumen for 1-4 hours, then aspirate; may repeat with 10,000 units in each lumen if 5000 units fails to clear the catheter; **do not infuse into the patient**; volume to instill into catheter is equal to the volume of the catheter

I.V. infusion: 200 units/kg/hour in each lumen for 12-48 hours at a rate of at least 20 mL/hour

Dialysis patients: 5000 units is administered in each lumen over 1-2 minutes; leave urokinase in lumen for 1-2 days, then aspirate

Clot lysis (large vessel thrombi): Loading: I.V.: 4400 units/kg over 10 minutes, increase to 6000 units/kg/hour; maintenance: 4400-6000 units/kg/hour adjusted to achieve clot lysis or patency of affected vessel; doses up to 50,000 units/kg/hour have been used. **Note:** Therapy should be initiated as soon as possible after diagnosis of thrombi and continued until clot is dissolved (usually 24-72 hours).

Acute pulmonary embolism: Three treatment alternatives: 3 million unit dosage

Alternative 1: 12-hour infusion: 4400 units/kg (2000 units/lb) bolus over 10 minutes followed by 4400 units/kg/hour (2000 units/lb); begin heparin 1000 units/hour approximately 3-4 hours after completion of urokinase infusion or when PTT is <100 seconds

Alternative 2: 2-hour infusion: 1 million unit bolus over 10 minutes followed by 2 million units over 110 minutes; begin heparin 1000 units/hour approximately 3-4 hours after completion of urokinase infusion or when PTT is <100 seconds

Alternative 3: Bolus dose only: 15,000 units/kg over 10 minutes; begin heparin 1000 units/hour approximately 3-4 hours after completion of urokinase infusion or when PTT is <100 seconds

Dosage Forms

Powder for injection: 250,000 units (5 mL)

Powder for injection, catheter clear: 5000 units (1 mL)

Uro-KP-Neutral® *see* potassium phosphate and sodium phosphate *on page 467*

Urolene Blue® *see* methylene blue *on page 367*

Uroplus® DS *see* co-trimoxazole *on page 149*

Uroplus® SS *see* co-trimoxazole *on page 149*

Urovist Cysto® *see* radiological/contrast media (ionic) *on page 495*

Urovist® Meglumine *see* radiological/contrast media (ionic) *on page 495*

Urovist® Sodium 300 *see* radiological/contrast media (ionic) *on page 495*

Urozide® (Can) *see* hydrochlorothiazide *on page 286*

Urso® *see* ursodiol *on this page*

ursodeoxycholic acid *see* ursodiol *on this page*

ursodiol (ER soe dye ole)

Synonyms ursodeoxycholic acid

U.S./Canadian Brand Names Actigall™; Urso®

Therapeutic Category Gallstone Dissolution Agent

Use Gallbladder stone dissolution

Usual Dosage Oral: 8-10 mg/kg/day in 2-3 divided doses

Dosage Forms Capsule: 300 mg

Ursofalk® (Can) *see* uracil mustard *on page 591*

Uticort® ***(Discontinued)*** *see page 700*

Vagistat®-1 Vaginal [OTC] *see* tioconazole *on page 568*

Vagitrol® *see* sulfanilamide *on page 542*

valacyclovir (val ay SYE kloe veer)

U.S./Canadian Brand Names Valtrex®

Therapeutic Category Antiviral Agent

Use Treatment of herpes zoster (shingles) in immunocompetent patients; once daily therapy for the suppression of genital herpes

Usual Dosage Adults: Oral: 1000 mg 3 times/day for 7 days

Dosage Forms Caplets: 500 mg

Valadol® *(Discontinued)* *see page 700*

Valergen® Injection *(Discontinued)* *see page 700*

Valertest No.1® *see* estradiol and testosterone *on page 218*

Valisone® Topical *see* betamethasone (topical) *on page 72*

Valium® Injection *see* diazepam *on page 173*

Valium® Oral *see* diazepam *on page 173*

Valmid® Capsule *(Discontinued)* *see page 700*

Valpin® 50 *(Discontinued)* *see page 700*

valproic acid and derivatives (val PROE ik AS id & dah RIV ah tives)

Synonyms dipropylacetic acid; DPA; 2-propylpentanoic acid; 2-propylvaleric acid

U.S./Canadian Brand Names Depacon®; Depakene®; Depakote®

Therapeutic Category Anticonvulsant

Use Management of simple and complex absence seizures; mixed seizure types; myoclonic and generalized tonic-clonic (grand mal) seizures; prevent migraine headaches in adults (Depakote®); mania associated with bipolar disorder; may be effective in partial seizures and infantile spasms; Depakote® can be used for the treatment of complex partial seizures; Depacon® is indicated as a temporary intravenous alternative when oral administration is not possible

Usual Dosage Children and Adults:

Oral: Initial: 10-15 mg/kg/day in 1-3 divided doses; increase by 5-10 mg/kg/day at weekly intervals until therapeutic levels are achieved; maintenance: 30-60 mg/kg/day in 2-3 divided doses

Children receiving more than one anticonvulsant (ie, polytherapy) may require doses up to 100 mg/kg/day in 3-4 divided doses

I.V.: Administer as a 60 minute infusion (≤20 mg/min) with the same frequency as oral products; switch patient to oral products as soon as possible

Rectal: Dilute syrup 1:1 with water for use as a retention enema; loading dose: 17-20 mg/kg one time; maintenance: 10-15 mg/kg/dose every 8 hours

Dosage Forms

Divalproex sodium:

Capsule, sprinkle (Depakote® Sprinkle®): 125 mg

Tablet, delayed release, as divalproex sodium (Depakote®): 125 mg, 250 mg, 500 mg

Valproic acid: Capsule (Depakene®): 250 mg

Valproate sodium:

Injection (Depacon®): 100 mg/mL (5 mL)

Syrup (Depakene®): 250 mg/5 mL (5 mL, 50 mL, 480 mL)

Valrelease® *(Discontinued)* *see page 700*

valrubicin (val ru BYE cin)

U.S./Canadian Brand Names Valstar™

Therapeutic Category Antineoplastic Agent

Use Intravesical therapy of BCG-refractory carcinoma *in situ* of the urinary bladder

Usual Dosage Adults: Intravesical: 800 mg once weekly for 6 weeks

Dosage Forms Injection: 200 mg/5 mL

valsartan (val SAR tan)

U.S./Canadian Brand Names Diovan™

Therapeutic Category Angiotensin II Antagonist

Use Treatment of hypertension alone or in combination with other antihypertensives

Usual Dosage Adults: Oral: 80 mg/day; may be increased to 160 mg if needed (maximal effects observed in 4-6 weeks)

Dosage Forms Capsule: 80 mg, 160 mg

valsartan and hydrochlorothiazide

(val SAR tan & hye droe klor oh THYE a zide)

U.S./Canadian Brand Names Diovan HCTZ™

Therapeutic Category Angiotensin II Antagonist; Diuretic, Thiazide

Use Treatment of hypertension

Usual Dosage Adults: Oral: Dose is individualized

Dosage Forms Tablet: Valsartan 80 mg and hydrochlorothiazide 12.5 mg; valsartan 160 mg and hydrochlorothiazide 12.5 mg

Valstar™ *see* valrubicin *on previous page*

Valtrex® *see* valacyclovir *on page 593*

Vamate® Oral *see* hydroxyzine *on page 297*

Vancenase® AQ 84 mcg *see* beclomethasone *on page 62*

Vancenase® AQ Inhaler *see* beclomethasone *on page 62*

Vancenase® Nasal Inhaler *see* beclomethasone *on page 62*

Vanceril® 84 mcg Double Strength *see* beclomethasone *on page 62*

Vanceril® Oral Inhaler *see* beclomethasone *on page 62*

Vancocin® CP (Can) *see* vancomycin *on this page*

Vancocin® Injection *see* vancomycin *on this page*

Vancocin® Oral *see* vancomycin *on this page*

Vancoled® Injection *see* vancomycin *on this page*

vancomycin (van koe MYE sin)

U.S./Canadian Brand Names Lyphocin® Injection; Vancocin® CP (Can); Vancocin® Injection; Vancocin® Oral; Vancoled® Injection

Therapeutic Category Antibiotic, Miscellaneous

Use Treatment of patients with the following infections or conditions: treatment of infections due to documented or suspected methicillin-resistant *S. aureus* or beta-lactam resistant coagulase negative *Staphylococcus*; treatment of serious or life-threatening infections (ie, endocarditis, meningitis, osteomyelitis) due to documented or suspected staphylococcal or streptococcal infections in patients who are allergic to penicillins and/or cephalosporins; empiric therapy of infections associated with central lines, VP shunts, hemodialysis shunts, vascular grafts, prosthetic heart valves; used orally for staphylococcal enterocolitis or for antibiotic-associated pseudomembranous colitis produced by *C. difficile*

Usual Dosage I.V. (initial dosage recommendation):

Infants >1 month and Children: 40 mg/kg/day in divided doses every 6 hours

Infants >1 month and Children with staphylococcal central nervous system infection: 60 mg/kg/day in divided doses every 6 hours

Adults: With normal renal function: 0.5 g every 6 hours or 1 g every 12 hours

Intrathecal:

Children: 5-20 mg/day

Adults: 20 mg/day

Oral:

Children: 10-50 mg/kg/day in divided doses every 6-8 hours; not to exceed 2 g/day

Adults: 0.5-2 g/day in divided doses every 6-8 hours

Pseudomembranous colitis produced by *C. difficile*:

Children: 40 mg/kg/day in divided doses, added to fluids

Adults: 500 mg to 2 g/day administered in 3 or 4 divided doses for 7-10 days

Dosage Forms Vancomycin hydrochloride:

Capsule: 125 mg, 250 mg

Powder for oral solution: 1 g, 10 g

Powder for injection: 500 mg, 1 g, 2 g, 5 g, 10 g

Vanex-LA® ***(Discontinued)*** *see page 700*

Vanoxide® [OTC] *see* benzoyl peroxide *on page 68*

Vanoxide-HC® *see* benzoyl peroxide and hydrocortisone *on page 69*

Vanseb-T® Shampoo *(Discontinued)* *see page 700*

Vansil™ *see* oxamniquine *on page 420*

Vantin® *see* cefpodoxime *on page 107*

Vapocet® (Can) *see* hydrocodone and acetaminophen *on page 287*

Vaponefrin® [OTC] *see* epinephrine *on page 209*

varicella virus vaccine (var i SEL a VYE rus vak SEEN)

Synonyms chicken pox vaccine; varicella-zoster virus (VZV) vaccine

U.S./Canadian Brand Names Varivax®

Therapeutic Category Vaccine, Live Virus

Use The American Association of Pediatrics recommends that the chickenpox vaccine should be given to all healthy children between 12 months and 18 years; children between 12 months and 13 years who have not been immunized or who have not had chickenpox should receive 1 vaccination while children 13-18 years of age require 2 vaccinations 4-8 weeks apart; the vaccine has been added to the childhood immunization schedule for infants 12-28 months of age and children 11-12 years of age who have not been vaccinated previously or who have not had the disease; it is recommended to be given with the measles, mumps, and rubella (MMR) vaccine

Usual Dosage S.C.:

Children 12 months to 12 years: 0.5 mL

Children 12 years to Adults: 2 doses of 0.5 mL separated by 4-8 weeks

Dosage Forms Powder for injection, lyophilized powder, preservative free: 1350 plaque forming units (PFU)/0.5 mL (0.5 mL single-dose vials)

varicella-zoster immune globulin (human)

(var i SEL a- ZOS ter i MYUN GLOB yoo lin HYU man)

Synonyms VZIG

Therapeutic Category Immune Globulin

Use Passive immunization of susceptible immunodeficient patients after exposure to varicella; most effective if begun within 96 hours of exposure

VZIG supplies are limited, restrict administration to those meeting the following criteria:

One of the following underlying illnesses or conditions:

Neoplastic disease (eg, leukemia or lymphoma)

Congenital or acquired immunodeficiency

Immunosuppressive therapy with steroids, antimetabolites or other immunosuppressive treatment regimens

Newborn of mother who had onset of chickenpox within 5 days before delivery or within 48 hours after delivery

Premature (≥28 weeks gestation) whose mother has no history of chickenpox

Premature (<28 weeks gestation or ≤1000 g VZIG) regardless of maternal history

One of the following types of exposure to chickenpox or zoster patient(s):

Continuous household contact

Playmate contact (>1 hour play indoors)

Hospital contact (in same 2-4 bedroom or adjacent beds in a large ward or prolonged face-to-face contact with an infectious staff member or patient)

Susceptible to varicella-zoster

Age of <15 years; administer to immunocompromised adolescents and adults and to other older patients on an individual basis

An acceptable alternative to VZIG prophylaxis is to treat varicella, if it occurs, with high-dose I.V. acyclovir

Usual Dosage High-risk susceptible patients who are exposed again more than 3 weeks after a prior dose of VZIG should receive another full dose; there is no evidence VZIG modifies established varicella-zoster infections.

I.M.: Administer by deep injection in the gluteal muscle or in another large muscle mass. Inject 125 units/10 kg (22 lb); maximum dose: 625 units (5 vials); minimum dose: 125 units; do not administer fractional doses. Do not inject I.V.

Dosage Forms Injection: 125 units of antibody in single dose vials

varicella-zoster virus (VZV) vaccine *see* varicella virus vaccine *on previous page*

Varivax® *see* varicella virus vaccine *on previous page*

Vascor® *see* bepridil *on page 70*

Vascoray® *see* radiological/contrast media (ionic) *on page 495*

Vaseretic® 10-25 *see* enalapril and hydrochlorothiazide *on page 206*

Vasocidin® Ophthalmic *see* sulfacetamide and prednisolone *on page 540*

VasoClear® Ophthalmic [OTC] *see* naphazoline *on page 390*

Vasocon-A® [OTC] Ophthalmic *see* naphazoline and antazoline *on page 391*

Vasocon Regular® Ophthalmic *see* naphazoline *on page 390*

Vasodilan® *see* isoxsuprine *on page 316*

vasopressin (vay soe PRES in)

Synonyms antidiuretic hormone (ADH); 8-arginine vasopressin

U.S./Canadian Brand Names Pitressin®; Pressyn® (Can)

Therapeutic Category Hormone, Posterior Pituitary

Use Treatment of diabetes insipidus; prevention and treatment of postoperative abdominal distention; differential diagnosis of diabetes insipidus; adjunct in the treatment of acute massive hemorrhage of GI tract or esophageal varices

Usual Dosage

Diabetes insipidus:

I.M., S.C.:

Children: 2.5-5 units 2-4 times/day as needed

Adults: 5-10 units 2-4 times/day as needed (dosage range 5-60 units/day)

Intranasal: Administer on cotton pledget or nasal spray

Abdominal distention Adults: I.M.: 5 mg stat, 10 mg every 3-4 hours

GI hemorrhage: I.V.: Administer in a peripheral vein; dilute aqueous in NS or D_5W to 0.1-1 unit/mL and infuse at 0.2-0.4 unit/minute and progressively increase to 0.9 unit/minute if necessary; I.V. infusion administration requires the use of an infusion pump and should be administered in a peripheral line to minimize adverse reactions on coronary arteries

Dosage Forms Injection, aqueous: 20 pressor units/mL (0.5 mL, 1 mL)

Vasosulf® Ophthalmic *see* sulfacetamide and phenylephrine *on page 540*

Vasotec® I.V. *see* enalapril *on page 206*

Vasotec® Oral *see* enalapril *on page 206*

Vasoxyl® *see* methoxamine *on page 365*

V-Cillin K® *(Discontinued)* *see page 700*

VCR *see* vincristine *on page 600*

V-Dec-M® *see* guaifenesin and pseudoephedrine *on page 270*

Vectrin® *see* minocycline *on page 377*

vecuronium (ve KYOO roe nee um)

Synonyms ORG NC 45

U.S./Canadian Brand Names Norcuron®

Therapeutic Category Skeletal Muscle Relaxant

Use Adjunct to anesthesia, to facilitate endotracheal intubation, and provide skeletal muscle relaxation during surgery or mechanical ventilation

(Continued)

vecuronium *(Continued)*

Usual Dosage I.V.:

Infants >7 weeks to 1 year: Initial: 0.08-0.1 mg/kg/dose; maintenance: 0.05-0.1 mg/kg/ every hour as needed

Children >1 year and Adults: Initial: 0.08-0.1 mg/kg/dose; maintenance: 0.05-0.1 mg/kg/ every hour as needed; may be administered as a continuous infusion at 0.1 mg/kg/hour

Note: Children may require slightly higher initial doses and slightly more frequent supplementation

Dosage Forms Powder for injection:

With diluent: 10 mg (10 mL)

Without diluent: 10 mg (10 mL); 20 mg (20 mL)

Veetids® *see* penicillin V potassium *on page 435*

Velban® *see* vinblastine *on page 600*

Velbe® (Can) *see* vinblastine *on page 600*

Velosef® *see* cephradine *on page 112*

Velosulin® *see* insulin preparations *on page 307*

Velsar® Injection *(Discontinued)* *see page 700*

Velvelan® (Can) *see* urea *on page 591*

venlafaxine (VEN la faks een)

U.S./Canadian Brand Names Effexor®; Effexor-XR®

Therapeutic Category Antidepressant, Phenethylamine

Use Treatment of depression

Usual Dosage Adults: Oral:

Capsule: One capsule daily

Tablet: 75 mg/day, administered in 2 or 3 divided doses, taken with food; dose may be increased in 75 mg/day increments at intervals of at least 4 days, up to 225-375 mg/day

Dosage Forms

Capsule, extended release: 37.5 mg, 75 mg, 150 mg

Tablet: 25 mg, 37.5 mg, 50 mg, 75 mg, 100 mg, 150 mg

Venoglobulin®-I *see* immune globulin, intravenous *on page 303*

Venoglobulin®-S *see* immune globulin, intravenous *on page 303*

Ventolin® *see* albuterol *on page 15*

Ventolin® Rotocaps® *see* albuterol *on page 15*

VePesid® *see* etoposide *on page 228*

verapamil (ver AP a mil)

Synonyms iproveratril

U.S./Canadian Brand Names Apo®-Verap (Can); Calan®; Calan® SR; Covera-HS®; Isoptin®; Isoptin® SR; Novo-Veramil® (Can); Nu-Verap® (Can); Verelan®

Therapeutic Category Antiarrhythmic Agent, Class IV; Calcium Channel Blocker

Use Angina, hypertension; I.V. for supraventricular tachyarrhythmias (PSVT, atrial fibrillation, atrial flutter)

Usual Dosage

Children: I.V.:

0-1 year: 0.1-0.2 mg/kg/dose, repeated after 30 minutes as needed

1-16 years: 0.1-0.3 mg/kg over 2-3 minutes; maximum: 5 mg/dose, may repeat dose once in 30 minutes if adequate response not achieved; maximum for second dose: 10 mg/dose

Children: Oral (dose not well established):

4-8 mg/kg/day in 3 divided doses **or** 1-5 years: 40-80 mg every 8 hours

>5 years: 80 mg every 6-8 hours

Adults:
Oral: 240-480 mg/24 hours divided 3-4 times/day
I.V.: 5-10 mg (0.075-0.15 mg/kg); may repeat 10 mg (0.15 mg/kg) 15-30 minutes after the initial dose if needed and if patient tolerated initial dose

Dosage Forms Verapamil hydrochloride:
Capsule, sustained release (Verelan®): 120 mg, 180 mg, 240 mg, 360 mg
Injection: 2.5 mg/mL (2 mL, 4 mL)
Isoptin®: 2.5 mg/mL (2 mL, 4 mL)
Tablet: 40 mg, 80 mg, 120 mg
Calan®, Isoptin®: 40 mg, 80 mg, 120 mg
Tablet sustained release: 180 mg, 240 mg
Calan® SR, Isoptin® SR: 120 mg, 180 mg, 240 mg
Covera-HS®: 180 mg, 240 mg

Verazinc® Oral [OTC] *see* zinc sulfate *on page 612*

Vercyte® ***(Discontinued)*** *see page 700*

Verelan® *see* verapamil *on previous page*

Vergogel® Gel [OTC] *see* salicylic acid *on page 513*

Vergon® [OTC] *see* meclizine *on page 351*

Vermox® *see* mebendazole *on page 350*

Verr-Canth® ***(Discontinued)*** *see page 700*

Verrex-C&M® *see* podophyllin and salicylic acid *on page 458*

Verrex® ***(Discontinued)*** *see page 700*

Verrusol® ***(Discontinued)*** *see page 700*

Versacaps® *see* guaifenesin and pseudoephedrine *on page 270*

Versed® *see* midazolam *on page 375*

Versel™ (Can) *see* selenium sulfide *on page 518*

Versiclear™ *see* sodium thiosulfate *on page 531*

Verukan® Solution *see* salicylic acid *on page 513*

Vesanoid® *see* tretinoin (oral) *on page 575*

Vesprin® *see* triflupromazine *on page 581*

Vexol® Ophthalmic Suspension *see* rimexolone *on page 506*

V-Gan® Injection ***(Discontinued)*** *see page 700*

Viagra® *see* sildenafil *on page 521*

Vibramycin® *see* doxycycline *on page 197*

Vibra-Tabs® *see* doxycycline *on page 197*

Vicks® 44D Cough & Head Congestion *see* pseudoephedrine and dextromethorphan *on page 487*

Vicks® 44E [OTC] *see* guaifenesin and dextromethorphan *on page 268*

Vicks® 44 Non-Drowsy Cold & Cough Liqui-Caps [OTC] *see* pseudoephedrine and dextromethorphan *on page 487*

Vicks Children's Chloraseptic® [OTC] *see* benzocaine *on page 66*

Vicks Chloraseptic® Sore Throat [OTC] *see* benzocaine *on page 66*

Vicks® DayQuil® Allergy Relief 4 Hour Tablet [OTC] *see* brompheniramine and phenylpropanolamine *on page 81*

Vicks® DayQuil® Sinus Pressure & Congestion Relief [OTC] *see* guaifenesin and phenylpropanolamine *on page 270*

Vicks Formula 44® [OTC] *see* dextromethorphan *on page 171*

Vicks Formula 44® Pediatric Formula [OTC] *see* dextromethorphan *on page 171*

Vicks® Pediatric Formula 44E [OTC] *see* guaifenesin and dextromethorphan *on page 268*

Vicks® Sinex® Nasal Solution [OTC] *see* phenylephrine *on page 445*

Vicks® Vatronol® *(Discontinued)* *see page 700*

Vicodin® *see* hydrocodone and acetaminophen *on page 287*

Vicodin® ES *see* hydrocodone and acetaminophen *on page 287*

Vicon-C® [OTC] *see* vitamin B complex with vitamin C *on page 603*

Vicon Forte® *see* vitamin, multiple (oral) *on page 604*

Vicon® Plus [OTC] *see* vitamin, multiple (oral) *on page 604*

Vicoprofen® *see* hydrocodone and ibuprofen *on page 289*

vidarabine (vye DARE a been)

Synonyms adenine arabinoside; ARA-A; arabinofuranosyladenine

U.S./Canadian Brand Names Vira-A® Ophthalmic

Therapeutic Category Antiviral Agent

Use Treatment of acute keratoconjunctivitis and epithelial keratitis due to herpes simplex virus; herpes simplex encephalitis; neonatal herpes simplex virus infections; disseminated varicella-zoster in immunosuppressed patients

Usual Dosage Children and Adults: Ophthalmic: Keratoconjunctivitis: ½" of ointment in lower conjunctival sac 5 times/day every 3 hours while awake until complete re-epithelialization has occurred, then twice daily for an additional 7 days

Dosage Forms Ointment, ophthalmic, as monohydrate: 3% [30 mg/mL = 28 mg/mL base] (3.5 g)

Vi-Daylin® [OTC] *see* vitamin, multiple (pediatric) *on page 606*

Vi-Daylin/F® *see* vitamin, multiple (pediatric) *on page 606*

Videx® *see* didanosine *on page 177*

vinblastine (vin BLAS teen)

Synonyms vincaleukoblastine; VLB

U.S./Canadian Brand Names Alkaban-AQ®; Velban®; Velbe® (Can)

Therapeutic Category Antineoplastic Agent

Use Palliative treatment of Hodgkin's disease; advanced testicular germinal-cell cancers; non-Hodgkin's lymphoma, histiocytosis, and choriocarcinoma

Usual Dosage Refer to individual protocol. Varies depending upon clinical and hematological response. Administer at intervals of at least 7 days and only after leukocyte count has returned to at least 4000/mm^3; maintenance therapy should be titrated according to leukocyte count. Dosage should be reduced in patients with recent exposure to radiation therapy or chemotherapy; single doses in these patients should not exceed 5.5 mg/m^2.

Children and Adults: I.V.: 4-12 mg/m^2 every 7-10 days **or** 5-day continuous infusion of 1.4-1.8 mg/m^2/day **or** 0.1-0.5 mg/kg/week

Dosage Forms Vinblastine sulfate:

Injection: 1 mg/mL (10 mL)

Powder for reconstitution: 10 mg

vincaleukoblastine *see* vinblastine *on this page*

Vincasar® PFS™ *see* vincristine *on this page*

vincristine (vin KRIS teen)

Synonyms LCR; leurocristine; VCR

U.S./Canadian Brand Names Oncovin®; Vincasar® PFS™

Therapeutic Category Antineoplastic Agent

Use Treatment of leukemias, Hodgkin's disease, neuroblastoma, malignant lymphomas, Wilms' tumor, and rhabdomyosarcoma

Usual Dosage Refer to individual protocol as dosages vary with protocol used. Adjustments are made depending upon clinical and hematological response and upon adverse reactions.

Children: I.V.:
$\leq$10 kg or BSA <1 m^2: 0.05 mg/kg once weekly
2 mg/m^2; may repeat every week
Adults: I.V.: 0.4-1.4 mg/m^2, up to 2 mg maximum; may repeat every week

Dosage Forms Injection, as sulfate: 1 mg/mL (1 mL, 2 mL, 5 mL)

vinorelbine (vi NOR el been)

Synonyms vinorelbine tartrate hydrochloride

U.S./Canadian Brand Names Navelbine®

Therapeutic Category Antineoplastic Agent

Use Treatment of nonsmall cell lung cancer (as a single agent or in combination with cisplatin)

Unlabeled use: Breast cancer, ovarian carcinoma (cisplatin-resistant), Hodgkin's disease

Usual Dosage Varies depending upon clinical and hematological response (refer to individual protocols)

Adults: I.V.: 30 mg/m^2 every 7 days

Dosage adjustment in hematological toxicity (based on granulocyte counts):
Granulocytes $\geq$1500 $cells/mm^3$ on day of treatment: Administer 30 mg/m^2
Granulocytes 1000-1499 $cells/mm^3$ on day of treatment: Administer 15 mg/m^2
Granulocytes <1000 $cells/mm^3$ on day of treatment: Do not administer. Repeat granulocyte count in one week; if 3 consecutive doses are held because granulocyte count is <1000 $cells/mm^3$, discontinue vinorelbine

For patients who, during treatment, have experienced fever or sepsis while granulocytopenic or had 2 consecutive weekly doses held due to granulocytopenia, subsequent doses of vinorelbine should be:
22.5 mg/m^2 for granulocytes $\geq$1,500 $cells/mm^3$
11.25 mg/m^2 for granulocytes 1000-1499 $cells/mm^3$

Dosage Forms Injection, as tartrate: 10 mg/mL (1 mL, 5 mL)

vinorelbine tartrate hydrochloride *see* vinorelbine *on this page*

Vioform® [OTC] *see* clioquinol *on page 137*

Vioform®-Hydrocortisone Topical *(Discontinued)* *see page 700*

Viokase® *see* pancrelipase *on page 427*

viosterol *see* ergocalciferol *on page 212*

Vioxx® *see* rofecoxib *on page 509*

Viprinex® (Can) *see* ancrod *on page 37*

Vira-A® Ophthalmic *see* vidarabine *on previous page*

Viracept® *see* nelfinavir *on page 393*

Viramune® *see* nevirapine *on page 399*

Virazole® Aerosol *see* ribavirin *on page 503*

Virilon® *see* methyltestosterone *on page 369*

Viroptic® Ophthalmic *see* trifluridine *on page 581*

Viscoat® *see* chondroitin sulfate-sodium hyaluronate *on page 130*

Visine® *(Discontinued)* *see page 700*

Visine® Extra Ophthalmic [OTC] *see* tetrahydrozoline *on page 556*

Visine® L.R. Ophthalmic [OTC] *see* oxymetazoline *on page 423*

Visken® *see* pindolol *on page 452*

Vistacon-50® Injection *see* hydroxyzine *on page 297*

Vistaject-25® *(Discontinued)* *see page 700*

Vistaject-50® *(Discontinued)* *see page 700*

Vistaquel® Injection *see* hydroxyzine *on page 297*

Vistaril® Injection *see* hydroxyzine *on page 297*

Vistaril® Oral *see* hydroxyzine *on page 297*

Vistazine® Injection *see* hydroxyzine *on page 297*

Vistide® *see* cidofovir *on page 131*

Vita-C® [OTC] *see* ascorbic acid *on page 48*

VitaCarn® Oral *see* levocarnitine *on page 330*

Vital HN® [OTC] *see* enteral nutritional products *on page 208*

vitamin A (VYE ta min aye)

Synonyms oleovitamin A

U.S./Canadian Brand Names Aquasol A®; Del-Vi-A®; Palmitate-A® 5000 [OTC]

Therapeutic Category Vitamin, Fat Soluble

Use Treatment and prevention of vitamin A deficiency; supplementation in patients with measles

Usual Dosage

RDA:
- 0-3 years: 400 mcg*
- 4-6 years: 500 mcg*
- 7-10 years: 700 mcg*
- >10 years: 800-1000 mcg*
- *mcg retinol equivalent (0.3 mcg retinol = 1 unit vitamin A)

Supplementation in measles: Children: Oral:
- <1 year: 100,000 units/day for 2 days
- >1 year: 200,000 units/day for 2 days

Severe deficiency with xerophthalmia:
- Children 1-8 years:
  - Oral: 5000-10,000 units/kg/day for 5 days or until recovery occurs
  - I.M.: 5000-15,000 units/day for 10 days
- Children >8 years and Adults:
  - Oral: 500,000 units/day for 3 days, then 50,000 units/day for 14 days, then 10,000-20,000 units/day for 2 months
  - I.M.: 50,000-100,000 units/day for 3 days, 50,000 units/day for 14 days

Deficiency (without corneal changes): Oral:
- Infants <1 year: 10,000 units/kg/day for 5 days, then 7500-15,000 units/day for 10 days
- Children 1-8 years: 5000-10,000 units/kg/day for 5 days, then 17,000-35,000 units/day for 10 days
- Children >8 years and Adults: 100,000 units/day for 3 days then 50,000 units/day for 14 days

Malabsorption syndrome (prophylaxis): Children >8 years and Adults: Oral: 10,000-50,000 units/day of water miscible product

Dietary supplement: Oral:
- Infants up to 6 months: 1500 units/day
- Children:
  - 6 months to 3 years: 1500-2000 units/day
  - 4-6 years: 2500 units/day
  - 7-10 years: 3300-3500 units/day
- Children >10 years and Adults: 4000-5000 units/day

Dosage Forms
- Capsule: 10,000 units [OTC], 25,000 units, 50,000 units
- Drops, oral (water miscible) [OTC]: 5000 units/0.1 mL (30 mL)
- Injection: 50,000 units/mL (2 mL)
- Tablet [OTC]: 5000 units

vitamin A acid *see* tretinoin (topical) *on page 576*

vitamin A and vitamin D (VYE ta min aye & VYE ta min dee)

Synonyms cod liver oil

U.S./Canadian Brand Names A and D™ Ointment [OTC]

Therapeutic Category Protectant, Topical

Use Temporary relief of discomfort due to chapped skin, diaper rash, minor burns, abrasions, as well as irritations associated with ostomy skin care

Usual Dosage

Oral, oil: Dietary supplement: 2.5 mL/day

Topical: Apply locally with gentle massage as needed

Dosage Forms Ointment, topical: In a lanolin-petrolatum base (60 g)

vitamin B_1 *see* thiamine *on page 561*

vitamin B_2 *see* riboflavin *on page 504*

vitamin B_3 *see* niacin *on page 399*

vitamin B_5 *see* pantothenic acid *on page 428*

vitamin B_6 *see* pyridoxine *on page 490*

vitamin B_{12} *see* cyanocobalamin *on page 152*

vitamin B_{12a} *see* hydroxocobalamin *on page 294*

vitamin B complex (VYE ta min bee KOM pleks)

U.S./Canadian Brand Names Apatate® [OTC]; Gevrabon® [OTC]; Lederplex® [OTC]; Lipovite® [OTC]; Mega B® [OTC]; Megaton™ [OTC]; Mucoplex® [OTC]; NeoVadrin® B Complex [OTC]; Orexin® [OTC]; Surbex® [OTC]

Therapeutic Category Vitamin, Water Soluble

Usual Dosage Dosage is usually 1 tablet or capsule/day; please refer to package insert

Dosage Forms

Capsule

Solution: 5 mL, 360 mL

vitamin B complex with vitamin C

(VYE ta min bee KOM pleks with VYE ta min see)

U.S./Canadian Brand Names Allbee® With C [OTC]; Surbex-T® Filmtabs® [OTC]; Surbex® With C Filmtabs® [OTC]; Thera-Combex® H-P Kapseals® [OTC]; Vicon-C® [OTC]

Therapeutic Category Vitamin, Water Soluble

Use Supportive nutritional supplementation in conditions in which water-soluble vitamins are required like GI disorders, chronic alcoholism, pregnancy, severe burns, and recovery from surgery

Usual Dosage Adults: Oral: 1 tablet/capsule daily

Dosage Forms Actual vitamin content may vary slightly depending on product used

Tablet/capsule: Vitamin B_1 10-15 mg, vitamin B_2 10 mg, vitamin B_3 100 mg, vitamin B_5 20 mg, vitamin B_6 2-5 mg, vitamin B_{12} 6-10 mg, vitamin C 300-500 mg

vitamin B complex with vitamin C and folic acid

(VYE ta min bee KOM pleks with VYE ta min see & FOE lik AS id)

U.S./Canadian Brand Names Berocca®; Nephrocaps®

Therapeutic Category Vitamin, Water Soluble

Use Supportive nutritional supplementation in conditions in which water-soluble vitamins are required like GI disorders, chronic alcoholism, pregnancy, severe burns, and recovery from surgery

Usual Dosage Adults: Oral: 1 capsule/day

Dosage Forms Capsule

vitamin C *see* ascorbic acid *on page 48*

Vitamin C Drops [OTC] *see* ascorbic acid *on page 48*

vitamin D_2 *see* ergocalciferol *on page 212*

vitamin E (VYE ta min ee)

Synonyms *d*-alpha tocopherol; *dl*-alpha tocopherol

U.S./Canadian Brand Names Amino-Opti-E® [OTC]; Aquasol E® [OTC]; E-Complex-600® [OTC]; E-Vitamin® [OTC]; Vita-Plus® E Softgels® [OTC]; Vitec® [OTC]; Vite E® Creme [OTC]

Therapeutic Category Vitamin, Fat Soluble; Vitamin, Topical

Use Prevention and treatment of vitamin E deficiency

Usual Dosage

RDA: Oral:

Premature Infants ≤3 months: 25 units/day

Infants:

≤6 months: 4.5 units/day

6-12 months: 6 units/day

Children:

1-3 years: 9 units/day

4-10 years: 10.5 units/day

Adults >11 years:

Female: 12 units/day

Male: 15 units/day

Prevention of vitamin E deficiency: Neonates, premature, low birthweight (results in normal levels within 1 week): Oral: 25-50 units/24 hours until 6-10 weeks of age or 125-150 units/kg total in 4 doses on days 1, 2, 7, and 8 of life

Vitamin E deficiency treatment: Adults: Oral: 50-200 units/24 hours for 2 weeks

Topical: Apply a thin layer over affected areas as needed

Dosage Forms

Capsule: 100 units, 200 units, 330 mg, 400 units, 500 units, 600 units, 1000 units

Capsule, water miscible: 73.5 mg, 147 mg, 165 mg, 330 mg, 400 units

Cream: 50 mg/g (15 g, 30 g, 60 g, 75 g, 120 g, 454 g)

Drops, oral: 50 mg/mL (12 mL, 30 mL)

Liquid, topical: 10 mL, 15 mL, 30 mL, 60 mL

Lotion: 120 mL

Oil: 15 mL, 30 mL, 60 mL

Ointment, topical: 30 mg/g (45 g, 60 g)

Tablet: 200 units, 400 units

vitamin G *see* riboflavin *on page 504*

vitamin K_1 *see* phytonadione *on page 451*

vitamin, multiple (injectable)

U.S./Canadian Brand Names M.V.C.® 9 + 3; M.V.I.®-12; M.V.I.® Concentrate; M.V.I.® Pediatric

Therapeutic Category Vitamin

Usual Dosage I.V.:

Children:

≤5 kg: 10 mL/1000 mL TPN (M.V.I.® Pediatric)

5.1 kg to 11 years: 5 mL/one TPN bag/day (M.V.I.® Pediatric)

Children >11 years and Adults: 5 mL of vials 1 and 2 (M.V.I.®-12)/one TPN bag/day

Dosage Forms See Multivitamins table.

vitamin, multiple (oral) (VYE ta mins, MUL ti pul)

U.S./Canadian Brand Names Becotin® Pulvules®; Cefol® Filmtab®; Eldercaps® [OTC]; Icaps® (Can); Infantol® (Can); Maltlevol® (Can); Materna® (Can); NeoVadrin® [OTC]; Niferex®-PN; Ocuvite™ (Can); Orifer® F (Can); Penta/3B® Plus (Can); Prenavite® Forte (Can); Secran®; Sopalamine/3B Plus C (Can); Spectrum™ Forte 29 (Can); Stresstabs® 600 Advanced Formula Tablets [OTC]; Therabid® [OTC]; Theragran® [OTC]; Theragran®

Multivitamin Products Available

Product	Content Given Per	A IU	D IU	E IU	C mg	FA mg	B_1 mg	B_2 mg	B_3 mg	B_6 mg	B_{12} mcg	Other
Theragran®	5 mL liquid	10,000	400		200		10	10	100	4.1	5	B_5 21.4 mg
Vi-Daylin®	1 mL drops	1500	400	4.1	35		0.5	0.6	8	0.4	1.5	Alcohol <0.5%
Vi-Daylin® Iron	1 mL	1500	400	4.1	35		0.5	0.6	8	0.4		Fe 10 mg
Albee® with C	tablet				300		15	10.2		5		Niacinamide 50 mg, pantothenic acid 10 mg
Vitamin B complex	tablet					400 mcg	1.5	1.7		2	6	Niacinamide 20 mg
Hexavitamin	cap/tab	5000	400		75		2	3	20			
Iberet-Folic-500®	tablet				500	0.8	6	6	30	5	25	B_5 10 mg, Fe 105 mg
Stuartnatal® 1+1	tablet	4000	400	11	120	1	1.5	3	20	10	12	Cu, Zn 25 mg, Fe 65 mg, Ca 200 mg
Theragran-M®	tablet	5000	400	30	90	0.4	3	3.4	30	3	9	Cl, Cr, I, K, B_5 10 mg, Mg, Mn, Mo, P, Se, Zn 15 mg, Fe 27 mg, biotin 30 mcg, beta-carotene 1250 IU
Vi-Daylin®	tablet	2500	400	15	60	0.3	1.05	1.2	13.5	1.05	4.5	
M.V.I.®-12 injection	5 mL	3300	200	10	100	0.4	3	3.6	40	4	5	B_5 15 mg, biotin 60 mcg
M.V.I.®-12 unit vial	20 mL											
M.V.I.® pediatric powder	5 mL	2300	400	7	80	0.14	1.2	1.4	17	1	1	B_5 5 mg, biotin 20 mcg, vitamin K 200 mcg

vitamin, multiple (oral) *(Continued)*

Hematinic®; Theragran® Liquid [OTC]; Theragran-M® [OTC]; Unicap® [OTC]; Vicon Forte®; Vicon® Plus [OTC]

Therapeutic Category Vitamin

Use Dietary supplement

Usual Dosage Adults: Oral: 1 tablet/day or 5 mL/day liquid

Dosage Forms See Multivitamins table.

vitamin, multiple (pediatric)

Synonyms children's vitamins; multivitamins/fluoride

U.S./Canadian Brand Names Adeflor®; ADEKs® Pediatric Drops; LKV-Drops® [OTC]; Multi Vit® Drops [OTC]; Poly-Vi-Flor®; Poly-Vi-Sol® [OTC]; Tri-Vi-Flor®; Tri-Vi-Sol® [OTC]; Vi-Daylin® [OTC]; Vi-Daylin/F®

Therapeutic Category Vitamin

Use Nutritional supplement, vitamin deficiency

Usual Dosage Oral: 0.6 mL or 1 mL/day; please refer to package insert

Dosage Forms See Multivitamins table.

vitamin, multiple (prenatal)

Synonyms prenatal vitamins

U.S./Canadian Brand Names Chromagen® OB [OTC]; Natabec® [OTC]; Natabec® FA [OTC]; Natabec® Rx; Natalins® [OTC]; Natalins® Rx; Pramet® FA; Pramilet® FA; Prenavite® [OTC]; Stuartnatal® 1 + 1; Stuart Prenatal® [OTC]

Therapeutic Category Vitamin

Use Nutritional supplement, vitamin deficiency

Usual Dosage Oral: 1 tablet or capsule daily; please refer to package insert

Vitaneed™ [OTC] *see* enteral nutritional products *on page 208*

Vita-Plus® E Softgels® [OTC] *see* vitamin E *on page 604*

Vitec® [OTC] *see* vitamin E *on page 604*

Vite E® Creme [OTC] *see* vitamin E *on page 604*

Vitinoin™ (Can) *see* tretinoin (topical) *on page 576*

Vito Reins® (Can) *see* phenazopyridine *on page 442*

Vitrasert® *see* ganciclovir *on page 257*

Vitravene™ *see* fomivirsen *on page 252*

Vivactil® *see* protriptyline *on page 485*

Viva-Drops® Solution [OTC] *see* artificial tears *on page 47*

Vivelle™ Transdermal *see* estradiol *on page 217*

Vivol® (Can) *see* diazepam *on page 173*

Vivonex® [OTC] *see* enteral nutritional products *on page 208*

Vivonex® Plus (Can) *see* enteral nutritional products *on page 208*

Vivonex® T.E.N. [OTC] *see* enteral nutritional products *on page 208*

Vivotif Berna™ Oral *see* typhoid vaccine *on page 589*

V-Lax® [OTC] *see* psyllium *on page 488*

VLB *see* vinblastine *on page 600*

VM-26 *see* teniposide *on page 549*

Volmax® (Can) *see* albuterol *on page 15*

Voltaren® Ophthalmic *see* diclofenac *on page 175*

Voltaren® Oral *see* diclofenac *on page 175*

Voltaren®-XR Oral *see* diclofenac *on page 175*

Vontrol® *(Discontinued)* *see page 700*

VōSol® HC Otic *see* acetic acid, propylene glycol diacetate, and hydrocortisone *on page 8*

VōSol® Otic *see* acetic acid *on page 7*

VP-16 *see* etoposide *on page 228*

Vumon *see* teniposide *on page 549*

V.V.S.® *see* sulfabenzamide, sulfacetamide, and sulfathiazole *on page 539*

Vytone® Topical *see* iodoquinol and hydrocortisone *on page 311*

VZIG *see* varicella-zoster immune globulin (human) *on page 596*

warfarin (WAR far in)

U.S./Canadian Brand Names Coumadin®; Warfilone® (Can)

Therapeutic Category Anticoagulant

Use Prophylaxis and treatment of venous thromboembolic disorders; prevention of arterial thromboembolism in patients with prosthetic heart valves or atrial fibrillation; prevention of death, venous thromboembolism, and recurrent MI after acute MI

Usual Dosage

Oral:

Infants and Children: 0.05-0.34 mg/kg/day; infants <12 months of age may require doses at or near the high end of this range; consistent anticoagulation may be difficult to maintain in children <5 years of age

Adults: 5-15 mg/day for 2-5 days, then adjust dose according to results of prothrombin time; usual maintenance dose ranges from 2-10 mg/day

I.V. (administer as a slow bolus injection): 2-5 mg/day

Dosage Forms Warfarin sodium:

Powder for injection, lyophilized: 2 mg, 5 mg

Tablet: 1 mg, 2 mg, 2.5 mg, 3 mg, 4 mg, 5 mg, 6 mg, 7.5 mg, 10 mg

Warfilone® (Can) *see* warfarin *on this page*

4-Way® Long Acting Nasal Solution [OTC] *see* oxymetazoline *on page 423*

Wehamine® Injection *(Discontinued)* *see page 700*

Wehdryl® *(Discontinued)* *see page 700*

Wellbutrin® *see* bupropion *on page 84*

Wellbutrin® SR *see* bupropion *on page 84*

Wellcovorin® *see* leucovorin *on page 328*

Wesprin® Buffered *(Discontinued)* *see page 700*

Westcort® Topical *see* hydrocortisone (topical) *on page 292*

Whitfield's Ointment [OTC] *see* benzoic acid and salicylic acid *on page 67*

whole root rauwolfia *see* *Rauwolfia serpentina* *on page 498*

Wigraine® *see* ergotamine *on page 213*

Winks® [OTC] *see* diphenhydramine *on page 185*

Winpred (Can) *see* prednisone *on page 472*

WinRho SD® *see* rh_o(D) immune globulin (intravenous-human) *on page 503*

WinRho SDF® *see* rh_o(D) immune globulin (intravenous-human) *on page 503*

Winstrol® *see* stanozolol *on page 534*

witch hazel (witch HAY zel)

Synonyms hamamelis water

U.S./Canadian Brand Names Tucks® [OTC]

Therapeutic Category Astringent

(Continued)

witch hazel *(Continued)*

Use After-stool wipe to remove most causes of local irritation; temporary management of vulvitis, pruritus ani and vulva; help relieve the discomfort of simple hemorrhoids, anorectal surgical wounds, and episiotomies

Usual Dosage Apply to anorectal area as needed

Dosage Forms

Gel: 50% with glycerin (19.8 g)

Pads: 50% with glycerin, water and methylparaben (40/jar)

Wolfina® *see Rauwolfia serpentina on page 498*

wood sugar *see* d-xylose *on page 201*

Wyamine® Sulfate *see* mephentermine *on page 356*

Wyamycin® S *see* erythromycin (systemic) *on page 215*

Wyamycin S® *(Discontinued)* *see page 700*

Wycillin® *see* penicillin G procaine *on page 435*

Wydase® *see* hyaluronidase *on page 284*

Wygesic® *see* propoxyphene and acetaminophen *on page 482*

Wymox® *see* amoxicillin *on page 31*

Wytensin® *see* guanabenz *on page 273*

Xalatan® *see* latanoprost *on page 327*

Xanax® *see* alprazolam *on page 19*

Xeloda™ *see* capecitabine *on page 95*

Xenical® *see* orlistat *on page 418*

Xopenex™ *see* levalbuterol *on page 329*

X-Prep® Liquid [OTC] *see* senna *on page 518*

X-Seb™ (Can) *see* salicylic acid *on page 513*

X-seb® T [OTC] *see* coal tar and salicylic acid *on page 142*

Xylocaine® HCl I.V. Injection for Cardiac Arrhythmias *see* lidocaine *on page 333*

Xylocaine® Oral *see* lidocaine *on page 333*

Xylocaine® Topical Ointment *see* lidocaine *on page 333*

Xylocaine® Topical Solution *see* lidocaine *on page 333*

Xylocaine® Topical Spray *see* lidocaine *on page 333*

Xylocaine® With Epinephrine *see* lidocaine and epinephrine *on page 334*

Xylocard® (Can) *see* lidocaine *on page 333*

xylometazoline (zye loe met AZ oh leen)

U.S./Canadian Brand Names Otrivin® Nasal [OTC]

Therapeutic Category Adrenergic Agonist Agent

Use Symptomatic relief of nasal and nasopharyngeal mucosal congestion

Usual Dosage

Children <12 years: 2-3 drops (0.05%) in each nostril every 8-10 hours

Children >12 years and Adults: 2-3 drops or sprays (0.1%) in each nostril every 8-10 hours

Dosage Forms Solution, nasal, as hydrochloride: 0.05% [0.5 mg/mL] (20 mL); 0.1% [1 mg/mL] (15 mL, 20 mL)

Xylo-Pfan® [OTC] *see* d-xylose *on page 201*

Yeast-Gard® Medicated Douche *see* povidone-iodine *on page 467*

yellow fever vaccine (YEL oh FEE ver vak SEEN)

U.S./Canadian Brand Names YF-VAX®

Therapeutic Category Vaccine, Live Virus

Use Active immunization against yellow fever

Usual Dosage Single-dose S.C.: 0.5 mL

Dosage Forms Injection: Not less than 5.04 Log_{10} Plaque Forming Units (PFU) per 0.5 mL

yellow mercuric oxide *see* mercuric oxide *on page 357*

YF-VAX® *see* yellow fever vaccine *on this page*

Yocon® *see* yohimbine *on this page*

Yodoxin® *see* iodoquinol *on page 310*

yohimbine (yo HIM bine)

U.S./Canadian Brand Names Aphrodyne™; Dayto Himbin®; Yocon®; Yohimex™

Therapeutic Category Miscellaneous Product

Use No FDA sanctioned indications

Usual Dosage Adults: Oral: 1 tablet 3 times/day

Dosage Forms Tablet, as hydrochloride: 5.4 mg

Yohimex™ *see* yohimbine *on this page*

Yutopar® *see* ritodrine *on page 507*

Zaditor™ *see* ketotifen *on page 321*

zafirlukast (za FIR loo kast)

Synonyms ICI 204, 219

U.S./Canadian Brand Names Accolate®

Therapeutic Category Leukotriene Receptor Antagonist

Use Prophylaxis and chronic treatment of asthma in adults and children ≥12 years

Usual Dosage Adults: Oral: 20 mg twice daily; administer 1 hour before food or 2 hours after food

Dosage Forms Tablet: 20 mg

Zagam® *see* sparfloxacin *on page 532*

zalcitabine (zal SITE a been)

Synonyms ddC; dideoxycytidine

U.S./Canadian Brand Names Hivid®

Therapeutic Category Antiviral Agent

Use Treatment of HIV infections as monotherapy (in patients intolerant to zidovudine or with disease progression while on zidovudine) or in combination with zidovudine in patients with advanced HIV disease (adult CD4 cell count of 150-300 cells/mm^3)

Usual Dosage Oral:

Safety and efficacy in children <13 years of age have not been established

Adults (dosed in combination with zidovudine): Daily dose: 0.750 mg every 8 hours, administered together with 200 mg of zidovudine (ie, total daily dose: 2.25 mg of zalcitabine and 600 mg of zidovudine)

Dosage Forms Tablet: 0.375 mg, 0.75 mg

zaleplon (ZAL e plon)

U.S./Canadian Brand Names Sonata®

Therapeutic Category Hypnotic, Nonbenzodiazepine (Pyrazolopyrimidine)

Use Short-term treatment of insomnia

Usual Dosage

Adults: Oral: 10 mg at bedtime (range: 5-20 mg)

Elderly: 5 mg at bedtime

(Continued)

zaleplon *(Continued)*

Dosage Forms Capsule: 5 mg, 10 mg

Zanaflex® *see* tizanidine *on page 568*

zanamivir (za NA mi veer)

U.S./Canadian Brand Names Relenza®

Therapeutic Category Antiviral Agent, Inhalation Therapy

Use Treatment of uncomplicated acute illness due to influenza virus in adults and adolescents 12 years of age or older. Treatment should only be initiated in patients who have been symptomatic for no more than 2 days.

Usual Dosage Adolescents ≥12 years and Adults: 2 Inhalations: (10 mg total) twice daily for 5 days. Two doses should be taken on the first day of dosing, regardless of interval, while doses should be spaced by approximately 12 hours on subsequent days.

Dosage Forms Powder, for inhalation: 5 mg per blister

Zanosar® *see* streptozocin *on page 537*

Zantac® *see* ranitidine hydrochloride *on page 497*

Zantac® 75 [OTC] *see* ranitidine hydrochloride *on page 497*

Zapex® (Can) *see* oxazepam *on page 420*

Zarontin® *see* ethosuximide *on page 226*

Zaroxolyn® *see* metolazone *on page 371*

Zartan® *see* cephalexin *on page 111*

Z-Chlopenthixol *see* zuclopenthixol *(Canada only)* *on page 613*

Zeasorb-AF® [OTC] *see* tolnaftate *on page 571*

Zeasorb-AF® Powder [OTC] *see* miconazole *on page 373*

Zebeta® *see* bisoprolol *on page 76*

Zebrax® *(Discontinued)* *see page 700*

Zefazone® *see* cefmetazole *on page 106*

Zemplar™ *see* paricalcitol *on page 430*

Zemuron™ *see* rocuronium *on page 508*

Zenapax® *see* daclizumab *on page 157*

Zephiran® [OTC] *see* benzalkonium chloride *on page 66*

Zephrex® *see* guaifenesin and pseudoephedrine *on page 270*

Zephrex LA® *see* guaifenesin and pseudoephedrine *on page 270*

Zerit® *see* stavudine *on page 535*

Zestoretic® *see* lisinopril and hydrochlorothiazide *on page 337*

Zestril® *see* lisinopril *on page 337*

Zetar® [OTC] *see* coal tar *on page 141*

Zetran® *(Discontinued)* *see page 700*

Ziac™ *see* bisoprolol and hydrochlorothiazide *on page 76*

Ziagen™ *see* abacavir *on page 2*

zidovudine (zye DOE vyoo deen)

Synonyms azidothymidine; AZT; compound S

U.S./Canadian Brand Names Apo®-Zidovudine (Can); Novo-AZT® (Can); Retrovir®

Therapeutic Category Antiviral Agent

Use Management of patients with HIV infections who have had at least one episode of *Pneumocystis carinii* pneumonia or who have CD4 cell counts (cells/mm^3) of ≤500 in children >6 years and adults, <750 in children 2-6 years, <1000 in children 1-2 years, and

<1750 for children <1 year; patients who have HIV-related symptoms or who are asymptomatic with abnormal laboratory values indicating HIV-related immunosuppression; prevention of maternal-fetal HIV transmission

Usual Dosage

Children 3 months to 12 years:

Oral: 90-180 mg/m²/dose every 6 hours; maximum: 200 mg every 6 hours

I.V. continuous infusion: 0.5-1.8 mg/kg/hour

I.V. intermittent infusion: 100 mg/m²/dose every 6 hours

Adults:

Oral:

Asymptomatic infection: 100 mg every 4 hours while awake (500 mg/day)

Symptomatic HIV infection: Initial: 200 mg every 4 hours (1200 mg/day), then after 1 month, 100 mg every 4 hours (600 mg/day)

I.V.: 1-2 mg/kg/dose every 4 hours

Dosage Forms

Capsule: 100 mg

Injection: 10 mg/mL (20 mL)

Syrup (strawberry flavor): 50 mg/5 mL (240 mL)

Tablet: 300 mg

zidovudine and lamivudine (zye DOE vyoo deen & la MI vyoo deen)

Synonyms AZT + 3TC

U.S./Canadian Brand Names Combivir®

Therapeutic Category Antiviral Agent

Use Combivir® given twice a day, provides an alternative regimen to lamivudine 150 mg twice a day plus zidovudine 600 mg per day in divided doses; this drug form reduces capsule/tablet intake for these two drugs to two per day instead of up to eight

Usual Dosage Children >12 years and Adults: Oral: One tablet twice daily

Dosage Forms Tablet: Zidovudine 300 mg and lamivudine 150 mg

Zilactin-B® Medicated [OTC] *see* benzocaine *on page 66*

zileuton (zye LOO ton)

U.S./Canadian Brand Names Zyflo™

Therapeutic Category 5-Lipoxygenase Inhibitor

Use Prophylaxis and chronic treatment of asthma in adults and children ≥12 years of age

Usual Dosage Children ≥12 years and Adults: Oral: 1 tablet 4 times/day, may be taken with meals and at bedtime

Dosage Forms Tablet: 600 mg

Zinacef® Injection *see* cefuroxime *on page 109*

Zinaderm (Can) *see* zinc oxide *on next page*

Zinca-Pak® *see* trace metals *on page 573*

Zincate® Oral *see* zinc sulfate *on next page*

zinc chloride (zingk KLOR ide)

Therapeutic Category Trace Element

Use Cofactor for replacement therapy to different enzymes helps maintain normal growth rates, normal skin hydration and senses of taste and smell

Usual Dosage Clinical response may not occur for up to 6-8 weeks

Supplemental to I.V. solutions:

Premature Infants <1500 g, up to 3 kg: 300 mcg/kg/day

Full-term Infants and Children ≤5 years: 100 mcg/kg/day

Adults:

Stable with fluid loss from small bowel: 12.2 mg zinc/liter TPN or 17.1 mg zinc/kg (added to 1000 mL I.V. fluids) of stool or ileostomy output

Metabolically stable: 2.5-4 mg/day, add 2 mg/day for acute catabolic states

(Continued)

zinc chloride *(Continued)*

Dosage Forms Injection: 1 mg/mL (10 mL)

Zincfrin® Ophthalmic [OTC] *see* phenylephrine and zinc sulfate *on page 447*

zinc gelatin (zingk JEL ah tin)

Synonyms Unna's boot; Unna's paste

U.S./Canadian Brand Names Gelucast®

Therapeutic Category Protectant, Topical

Use Protectant and to support varicosities and similar lesions of the lower limbs

Usual Dosage Apply externally as an occlusive boot

Dosage Forms Bandage: 3" x 10 yards, 4" x 10 yards

zinc injection *see* trace metals *on page 573*

Zincofax® (Can) *see* zinc oxide *on this page*

Zincon® Shampoo [OTC] *see* pyrithione zinc *on page 491*

zinc oxide (zingk OKS ide)

Synonyms Lassar's zinc paste

U.S./Canadian Brand Names Prevex™ Baby Diaper Rash (Can); Zinaderm (Can); Zincofax® (Can)

Therapeutic Category Topical Skin Product

Use Protective coating for mild skin irritations and abrasions; soothing and protective ointment to promote healing of chapped skin, diaper rash

Usual Dosage Infants, Children, and Adults: Topical: Apply several times daily to affected area

Dosage Forms

Ointment, topical: 20% in white ointment (480 g)

Paste, topical: 25% in white petrolatum (480 g)

zinc oxide, cod liver oil, and talc (zingk OKS ide, kod LIV er oyl, & talk)

U.S./Canadian Brand Names Desitin® [OTC]

Therapeutic Category Protectant, Topical

Use Relief of diaper rash, superficial wounds and burns, and other minor skin irritations

Usual Dosage Topical: Apply thin layer as needed

Dosage Forms Ointment, topical: Zinc oxide, cod liver oil and talc in a petrolatum and lanolin base (30 g, 60 g, 120 g, 240 g, 270 g)

zinc sulfate (zingk SUL fate)

U.S./Canadian Brand Names Eye-Sed® Ophthalmic [OTC]; Orazinc® Oral [OTC]; Verazinc® Oral [OTC]; Zincate® Oral

Therapeutic Category Electrolyte Supplement, Oral

Use Zinc supplement (oral and parenteral); may improve wound healing in those who are deficient

Usual Dosage

RDA: Oral:

- Birth to 6 months: 3 mg elemental zinc/day
- 6-12 months: 5 mg elemental zinc/day
- 1-10 years: 10 mg elemental zinc/day
- ≥11 years: 15 mg elemental zinc/day

Zinc deficiency: Oral:

- Infants and Children: 0.5-1 mg elemental zinc/kg/day divided 1-3 times/day; somewhat larger quantities may be needed if there is impaired intestinal absorption or an excessive loss of zinc
- Adults: 110-220 mg zinc sulfate (25-50 mg elemental zinc)/dose 3 times/day

Dosage Forms
Capsule: 110 mg [elemental zinc 25 mg]; 220 mg [elemental zinc 50 mg]
Injection: 1 mg/mL (10 mL, 30 mL); 4 mg/mL (10 mL); 5 mg/mL (5 mL, 10 mL, 50 mL)
Tablet: 66 mg [elemental zinc 15 mg]; 200 mg [elemental zinc 46 mg]

zinc undecylenate *see* undecylenic acid and derivatives *on page 590*

Zinecard® *see* dexrazoxane *on page 169*

Zithromax™ *see* azithromycin *on page 56*

ZNP® Bar [OTC] *see* pyrithione zinc *on page 491*

Zocor® *see* simvastatin *on page 522*

Zofran® *see* ondansetron *on page 415*

Zofran® ODT *see* ondansetron *on page 415*

Zoladex® Implant *see* goserelin *on page 266*

Zolicef® *see* cefazolin *on page 105*

zolmitriptan (zohl mi TRIP tan)

Synonyms 311C90
U.S./Canadian Brand Names Zomig®
Therapeutic Category Antimigraine Agent; Serotonin Agonist
Use Acute treatment of adult migraine, with or without auras.
Usual Dosage Adults: Oral: Single doses of 1, 2.5, or 5 mg are effective in reducing symptoms of a migraine attack. Patients should be started at a dose of 2.5 mg or lower since the incidence of side effects increases somewhat with dose. If the headache returns, the dose may be repeated after 2 hours but **not to exceed** 10 mg within a 24-hour period.
Dosage Forms Tablet: 2.5 mg, 5 mg

Zoloft™ *see* sertraline *on page 520*

zolpidem (zole PI dem)

U.S./Canadian Brand Names Ambien™
Therapeutic Category Hypnotic, Nonbarbiturate
Use Short-term treatment of insomnia
Usual Dosage Adults: Oral: 10 mg immediately before bedtime
Dosage Forms Tablet, as tartrate: 5 mg, 10 mg

Zolyse® ***(Discontinued)*** *see page 700*

Zomig® *see* zolmitriptan *on this page*

Zonalon® Topical Cream *see* doxepin *on page 195*

Zone-A Forte® *see* pramoxine and hydrocortisone *on page 469*

ZORprin® *see* aspirin *on page 49*

Zostrix® [OTC] *see* capsaicin *on page 96*

Zostrix®-HP [OTC] *see* capsaicin *on page 96*

Zosyn™ *see* piperacillin and tazobactam sodium *on page 454*

Zovia® *see* ethinyl estradiol and ethynodiol diacetate *on page 222*

Zovirax® *see* acyclovir *on page 11*

zuclopenthixol *(Canada only)* (zoo kloe pen THIX ol)

Synonyms Z-Chlopenthixol
U.S./Canadian Brand Names Clopixol-Acuphase® (Can); Clopixol® (Can); Clopixol® Depot (Can)
Therapeutic Category Antipsychotic Agent
Use Schizophrenia, bipolar disorder, psychoses; usually useful in agitated states

(Continued)

zuclopenthixol *(Canada only)* *(Continued)*

Usual Dosage

Oral: Zuclopenthixol hydrochloride: Initial: 20-30 mg/day in divided doses; usual maintenance dose: 20-75 mg/day; maximum daily dose: 150 mg

I.M.:

Zuclopenthixol acetate: 50-150 mg; may be repeated in 2-3 days; no more than 4 injections should be given in the course of treatment; maximum dose during course of treatment: 400 mg

Zuclopenthixol decanoate: 100 mg by deep I.M. injection; additional doses of 100-200 mg (I.M.) may be given over the following 1-4 weeks; maximum weekly dose: 600 mg

Dosage Forms

Injection:

Acuphase, as acetate: 50 mg/mL [zuclopenthixol 42.5 mg/mL] (1 mL, 2 mL)

Depot, as decanoate: 200 mg/mL [zuclopenthixol 144.4 mg/mL] (10 mL)

Tablet, as dihydrochloride: 10 mg, 25 mg, 40 mg

Zyban™ *see* bupropion *on page 84*

Zyban 100 mg *(Discontinued)* *see page 700*

Zydone® *see* hydrocodone and acetaminophen *on page 287*

Zyflo™ *see* zileuton *on page 611*

Zyloprim® *see* allopurinol *on page 19*

Zymase® *see* pancrelipase *on page 427*

Zyprexa™ *see* olanzapine *on page 414*

Zyrtec® *see* cetirizine *on page 113*

APPENDIX

ABBREVIATIONS & SYMBOLS COMMONLY USED IN MEDICAL ORDERS

Abbreviation	From	Meaning
μg		microgram
μmol		micromole
°C		degrees Celsius (Centigrade)
$<$		less than
$>$		greater than
$\leq$		less than or equal to
$\geq$		greater than or equal to
$\overline{aa}$, aa	ana	of each
ABG		arterial blood gas
ac	ante cibum	before meals or food
ACE		angiotensin-converting enzyme
ACLS		adult cardiac life support
ad	ad	to, up to
a.d.	aurio dextra	right ear
ADH		antidiuretic hormone
ad lib	ad libitum	at pleasure
AED		antiepileptic drug
a.l.	aurio laeva	left ear
ALL		acute lymphoblastic leukemia
ALT		alanine aminotransferase (was SGPT)
AM	ante meridiem	morning
AML		acute myeloblastic leukemia
amp		ampul
amt		amount
ANA		antinuclear antibodies
ANC		absolute neutrophil count
ANL		acute nonlymphoblastic leukemia
aq	aqua	water
aq. dest.	aqua destillata	distilled water
APTT		activated partial thromboplastin time
a.s.	aurio sinister	left ear
ASA (class I-IV)		classification of surgical patients according to their baseline health (eg, healthy ASA and II or increased severity of illness ASA III or IV)
ASAP		as soon as possible
AST		aspartate aminotransferase (was SGOT)
a.u.	aures utrae	each ear
A-V		atrial-ventricular
bid	bis in die	twice daily
bm		bowel movement
BMT		bone marrow transplant
bp		blood pressure
BSA		body surface area
BUN		blood urea nitrogen
c	cong	a gallon
$\bar{c}$	cum	with
cal		calorie
cAMP		cyclic adenosine monophosphate
cap	capsula	capsule
CBC		complete blood count
cc		cubic centimeter
CHF		congestive heart failure
CI		cardiac index
Cl_{cr}		creatinine clearance
cm		centimeter
CNS		central nervous system
comp	compositus	compound
cont		continue

(continued)

Abbreviation	From	Meaning
COPD		chronic obstructive pulmonary disease
CSF		cerebral spinal fluid
CT		computed tomography
CVA		cerebral vascular accident
CVP		central venous pressure
d	dies	day
D_5W		dextrose 5% in water
$D_{10}W$		dextrose 10% in water
d/c		discontinue
DIC		disseminated intravascular coagulation
dil	dilue	dilute
disp	dispensa	dispense
div	divide	divide
DNA		deoxyribonucleic acid
dtd	dentur tales doses	give of such a dose
DVT		deep vein thrombosis
EEG		electroencephalogram
EKG		electrocardiogram
elix, el	elixir	elixir
emp		as directed
ESR		erythrocyte sedimentation rate
E.T.		endotracheal
et	et	and
ex aq		in water
f, ft	fac, fiat, fiant	make, let be made
FDA		Food and Drug Administration
FEV_11		forced expiratory volume
FVC		forced vital capacity
g	gramma	gram
G-6-PD		glucose-6-phosphate dehydrogenase
GA		gestational age
GABA		gamma-aminobutyric acid
GE		gastroesophageal
GI		gastrointestinal
gr	granum	grain
gtt	gutta	a drop
GU		genitourinary
h	hora	hour
HIV		human immunodeficiency virus
HPLC		high performance liquid chromatography
hs	hora somni	at bedtime
IBW		ideal body weight
ICP		intracranial pressure
IgG		immune globulin G
I.M.		intramuscular
INR		international normalized ratio
I.O.		intraosseous
I & O		input and output
IOP		intraocular pressure
I.T.		intrathecal
I.V.		intravenous
IVH		intraventricular hemorrhage
IVP		intravenous push
JRA		juvenile rheumatoid arthritis
kcal		kilocalorie
kg		kilogram
L		liter
LDH		lactate dehydrogenase
LE		lupus erythematosus
liq	liquor	a liquor, solution
LP		lumbar puncture

(continued)

Abbreviation	From	Meaning
M	misce	mix
MAO		monoamine oxidase
MAP		mean arterial pressure
mcg		microgram
m. dict	more dictor	as directed
mEq		milliequivalent
mg		milligram
MI		myocardial infarction
min		minute
mixt	mixtura	a mixture
mL		milliliter
mm		millimeter
mo		month
mOsm		milliosmols
MRI		magnetic resonance image
ND		nasoduodenal
NF		National Formulary
ng		nanogram
no.	numerus	number
noc	nocturnal	in the night
non rep	non repetatur	do not repeat, no refills
NPO		nothing by mouth
NSAID		nonsteroidal anti-inflammatory drug
O, Oct	octarius	a pint
o.d.	oculus dexter	right eye
o.l.	oculus laevus	left eye
O.R.		operating room
o.s.	oculus sinister	left eye
OTC		over-the-counter (nonprescription)
o.u.	oculo uterque	each eye
PALS		pediatric advanced life support
pc, post cib	post cibos	after meals
PCA		postconceptional age
PCP		*Pneumocystis carinii* pneumonia
PCWP		pulmonary capillary wedge pressure
PDA		patent ductus arteriosus
per		through or by
PM	post meridiem	afternoon or evening
PNA		postnatal age
P.O.	per os	by mouth
P.R.	per rectum	rectally
prn	pro re nata	as needed
PSVT		paroxysmal supraventricular tachycardia
PT		prothrombin time
PTT		partial thromboplastin time
PUD		peptic ulcer disease
pulv	pulvis	a powder
PVC		premature ventricular contraction
q		every
qad	quoque alternis die	every other day
qd		every day
qh	quiaque hora	every hour
qid	quater in die	four times a day
qod		every other day
qs	quantum sufficiat	a sufficient quantity
qs ad		a sufficient quantity to make
qty		quantity
qv	quam volueris	as much as you wish
Rx	recipe	take, a recipe
RAP		right atrial pressure
rep	repetatur	let it be repeated

(continued)

Abbreviation	From	Meaning
$\bar{s}$	sine	without
S-A		sino-atrial
sa	secundum artem	according to art
sat	sataratus	saturated
S.C.		subcutaneous
S_{cr}		serum creatinine
SIADH		syndrome of inappropriate antidiuretic hormone
sig	signa	label, or let it be printed
S.L.		sublingual
SLE		systemic lupus erythematosus
sol	solutio	solution
solv		dissolve
$\overline{ss}$, ss	semis	one-half
sos	si opus sit	if there is need
stat	statim	at once, immediately
supp	suppositorium	suppository
SVR		systemic vascular resistance
SVT		supraventricular tachycardia
SWI		sterile water for injection
syr	syrupus	syrup
tab	tabella	tablet
tal		such
tid	ter in die	three times a day
tr, tinct	tincture	tincture
trit		triturate
tsp		teaspoonful
TT		thrombin time
u.d., ut dict	ut dictum	as directed
ung	unguentum	ointment
USAN		United States Adopted Names
USP		United States Pharmacopeia
UTI		urinary tract infection
V_d		volume of distribution
V_{dss}		volume of distribution at steady-state
v.o.		verbal order
w.a.		while awake
x3		3 times
x4		4 times
y		year

NORMAL LABORATORY VALUES FOR ADULTS*

CHEMISTRY

Test		Value
Chemistry, Routine		
Albumin		3.5-5.0 g/dL
Bilirubin, conjugated		0-0.2 mg/dL
Bilirubin, total		0.2-1.2 mg/dL
Blood urea nitrogen		8-23 mg/dL
Calcium		8.4-10.3 mg/dL
Creatinine		0.5-1.2 mg/dL
Glucose		65-110 mg/dL
Phosphorus		2.8-4.5 mg/dL
Protein, total		6.0-8.0 g/dL
Uric acid	male	3.5-7.2 mg/dL
	female	2.6-6.5 mg/dL
Electrolytes		
Chlorides		100-110 mEq/L
CO_2		23-31 mEq/L
Potassium		3.5-5.0 mEq/L
Sodium		136-146 mEq/L
Anion gap		5-14 mEq/L
Enzymes		
Alkaline phosphatase	male	34-110 units/L
	female	24-100 units/L
ALT		5-35 units/L
AST		5-35 units/L
CPK	male	0-206 units/L
	female	0-175 units/L
LDH		50-200 units/L
Thyroid Function		
FTI (free thyroxine index)		4.5-12.0
T_3 resin uptake		25%-35%
T_3 (tri-iodothyronine) by RIA		70-200 ng/dL
T_4 (thyroxine) by RIA		4.0-11.0 µg/dL
Others		
Ammonia, plasma		20-60 µg/dL
Amylase, serum		44-128 units/L
Calcium, ionized		4.6-5.2 mg/dL
Cholesterol		140-230 mg/dL
Iron, serum		50-170 µg/dL
Lactate, serum		1.4-3.9 mEq/L
Lipase		10-208 units/L
Magnesium		1.5-2.5 mg/dL
Oncotic pressure		22-28 mm Hg
Osmolality		280-300 mOsm/kg
Serum ferritin	male	25-400 ng/mL
	female	10-150 ng/mL
TIBC		270-390 µg/dL
Triglycerides		50-150 mg/dL

*The normal ranges for laboratory values vary with different age groups, and may change as new methodologies for the lab tests are used. These values are current for adults (age 17 years or older). **Note:** Normal laboratory values may differ according to laboratory, institution, and analytical technique.

HEMATOLOGY

Test		Value
Hematocrit	male	40%-52%
	female	35%-47%
Hemoglobin	male	13.5-17.5 g/dL
	female	11.5-16.0 g/dL
MCH		27-34 pg
MCV		82-100 fL
Platelet count		150-450 $10^3/mm^3$
RBC count	male	4.5-5.9 $10^6/mm^3$
	female	4.0-4.9 $10^6/mm^3$
Reticulocyte count		0.5%-1.5%
Sed rate (Westergren)	male	0-10 mm/h
	female	0-20 mm/h
WBC count		4.5-11.0 $10^3/mm^3$
WBC differential		
bands		2%-8%
basophils		0%-2%
eosinophils		0%-4%
lymphocytes		20%-45%
monocytes		2%-8%
neutrophils		40%-70%

BLOOD GASES

	Arterial	**Venous**
Base excess	-3.0 to +3.0 mEq/L	-5.0 to +5.0 mEq/L
HCO_3	18-25 mEq/L	18-25 mEq/L
O_2 saturation	90%-98%	60%-85%
pCO_2	34-45 mm Hg	35-52 mm Hg
pH	7.35-7.45	7.32-7.42
pO_2	80-95 mm Hg	30-48 mm Hg
TCO_2	23-29 mEq/L	24-30 mEq/L

Weight/Volume Equivalents

1 mg/dL = 10 µg/mL

1 mg/dL = 1 mg%

1 ppm = 1 mg/L

1 µg/mL = 1 mg/L

NORMAL LABORATORY VALUES FOR CHILDREN

CHEMISTRY

Test	Age	Value
Albumin	0-1 y	2-4 g/dL
	1 y - adult	3.5-5.5 g/dL
Ammonia	newborn	90-150 μg/dL
	child	40-120 μg/dL
	adult	18-54 μg/dL
Amylase	newborn	0-60 units/L
	adult	30-110 units/L
Bilirubin, conjugated, direct	newborn	<1.5 mg/dL
	1 mo - adult	0-0.5 mg/dL
Bilirubin, total	0-3 d	2-10 mg/dL
	1 mo - adult	0-1.5 mg/dL
Bilirubin, unconjugated, indirect		0.6-10.5 mg/dL
Calcium	newborn	7-12 mg/dL
	0-2 y	8.8-11.2 mg/dL
	2 y - adult	9-11 mg/dL
Calcium, ionized, whole blood		4.4-5.4 mg/dL
Carbon dioxide, total		23-33 mEq/L
Chloride		95-105 mEq/L
Cholesterol	newborn	45-170 mg/dL
	0-1 y	65-175 mg/dL
	1-20 y	120-230 mg/dL
Creatinine	0-1 y	≤0.6 mg/dL
	1 y - adult	0.5-1.5 mg/dL
Glucose	newborn	30-90 mg/dL
	0-2 y	60-105 mg/dL
	child - adult	70-110 mg/dL
Iron	newborn	110-270 μg/dL
	infant	30-70 μg/dL
	child	55-120 μg/dL
	adult	70-180 μg/dL
Iron binding	newborn	59-175 μg/dL
	infant	100-400 μg/dL
	adult	250-400 μg/dL
Lactic acid, lactate		2-20 mg/dL
Lead, whole blood		<30 μg/dL
Lipase	child	20-140 units/L
	adult	0-190 units/L
Magnesium		1.5-2.5 mEq/L
Osmolality, serum		275-296 mOsm/kg
Osmolality, urine		50-1400 mOsm/kg

Chemistry *(continued)*

Phosphorus	newborn	4.2-9 mg/dL
	0 wk - 19 mo	3.8-6.7 mg/dL
	18 mo - 3 y	2.9-5.9 mg/dL
	3-15 y	3.6-5.6 mg/dL
	>15 y	2.5-5 mg/dL
Potassium, plasma	newborn	4.5-7.2 mEq/L
	2 d - 3 mo	4-6.2 mEq/L
	3 mo - 1 y	3.7-5.6 mEq/L
	1-16 y	3.5-5 mEq/L
Protein, total	0-2 y	4.2-7.4 g/dL
	>2 y	6-8 g/dL
Sodium		136-145 mEq/L
Triglycerides	infant	0-171 mg/dL
	child	20-130 mg/dL
	adult	30-200 mg/dL
Urea nitrogen, blood	0-2 y	4-15 mg/dL
	2 y - adult	5-20 mg/dL
Uric acid	male	3-7 mg/dL
	female	2-6 mg/dL

ENZYMES

Alanine aminotransferase (ALT) (SGPT)	0-2 mo	8-78 units/L
	>2 mo	8-36 units/L
Alkaline phosphatase (ALKP)	newborn	60-130 units/L
	0-16 y	85-400 units/L
	>16 y	30-115 units/L
Aspartate aminotransferase (AST) (SGOT)	infant	18-74 units/L
	child	15-46 units/L
	adult	5-35 units/L
Creatine kinase (CK)	infant	20-200 units/L
	child	10-90 units/L
	adult male	0-206 units/L
	adult female	0-175 units/L
Lactate dehydrogenase (LDH)	newborn	290-501 units/L
	1 mo - 2 y	110-144 units/L
	>16 y	60-170 units/L

BLOOD GASES

	Arterial	Capillary	Venous
pH	7.35-7.45	7.35-7.45	7.32-7.42
pCO_2 (mm Hg)	35-45	35-45	38-52
pO_2 (mm Hg)	70-100	60-80	24-48
HCO_3 (mEq/L)	19-25	19-25	19-25
TCO_2 (mEq/L)	19-29	19-29	23-33
O_2 saturation (%)	90-95	90-95	40-70
Base excess (mEq/L)	-5 to +5	-5 to +5	-5 to +5

THYROID FUNCTION TESTS

Test	Age	Value
T_4 (thyroxine)	1-7 d	10.1-20.9 μg/dL
	8-14 d	9.8-16.6 μg/dL
	1 mo - 1 y	5.5-16 μg/dL
	>1 y	4-12 μg/dL
FTI	1-3 d	9.3-26.6
	1-4 wk	7.6-20.8
	1-4 mo	7.4-17.9
	4-12 mo	5.1-14.5
	1-6 y	5.7-13.3
	>6 y	4.8-14
T_3 by RIA	newborns	100-470 ng/dL
	1-5 y	100-260 ng/dL
	5-10 y	90-240 ng/dL
	10 y - adult	70-210 ng/dL
T_3 uptake		35%-45%
TSH	cord	3-22 μU/mL
	1-3 d	<40 μU/mL
	3-7 d	<25 μU/mL
	>7 d	0-10 μU/mL

HEMATOLOGY VALUES

Complete Blood Count

	Hgb (g/dL)	Hct (%)	MCV (fL)	MCH (pg)	MCHC (%)	RBC (x 10^6/mm^3)	RDW	PLTS (x 10^3/mm^3)
0-3 d	15.0-20.0	45-61	95-115	31-37	29-37	4.0-5.9	<18.0	250-450
1-2 wk	12.5-18.5	39-57	86-110	28-36	28-38	3.6-5.5	<17.0	250-450
1-6 mo	10.0-13.0	29-42	74-96	25-35	30-36	3.1-4.3	<16.5	300-700
7 mo - 2 y	10.5-13.0	33-38	70-84	23-30	31-37	3.7-4.9	<16.0	250-600
2-5 y	11.5-13.0	34-39	75-87	24-30	31-37	3.9-5.0	<15.0	250-550
5-8 y	11.5-14.5	35-42	77-95	25-33	31-37	4.0-4.9	<15.0	250-550
13-18 y	12.0-15.2	36-47	78-96	25-35	31-37	4.5-5.1	<14.5	150-450
Adult male	13.5-16.5	41-50	80-100	26-34	31-37	4.5-5.9	<14.5	150-450
Adult female	12.0-15.0	36-45	80-100	26-34	31-37	4.0-4.9	<14.5	150-450

WBC and Differential

	WBC (x 10^3/mm^3)	Segs	Bands	Eos	Basos	Lymphs	Atypical Lymphs	Monos	# of NRBCs
0-3 d	9.0-35.0	32-62	10-18	0-2	0-1	19-29	0-8	5-7	0-2
1-2 wk	5.0-20.0	14-34	6-14	0-2	0-1	36-45	0-8	6-10	0
1-6 mo	6.0-17.5	13-33	4-12	0-3	0-1	41-71	0-8	4-7	0
7 mo - 2 y	6.0-17.0	15-35	5-11	0-3	0-1	45-76	0-8	3-6	0
2-5 y	5.5-15.5	23-45	5-11	0-3	0-1	35-65	0-8	3-6	0
5-8 y	5.0-14.5	32-54	5-11	0-3	0-1	28-48	0-8	3-6	0
13-18 y	4.5-13.0	34-64	5-11	0-3	0-1	25-45	0-8	3-6	0
Adults	4.5-11.0	35-66	5-11	0-3	0-1	24-44	0-8	3-6	0

Sedimentation rate, Westergren	
Children	0-20 mm/h
Adult male	0-15 mm/h
Adult female	0-20 mm/h
Sedimentation rate, Wintrobe	
Children	0-13 mm/h
Adult male	0-10 mm/h
Adult female	0-15 mm/h
Reticulocyte count	
Newborn	2%-6%
1-6 months	0%-2.8%
Adults	0.5%-1.5%

APOTHECARY/METRIC CONVERSIONS

Liquid Measures

Basic equivalent: 1 fluid ounce = 30 mL

Examples:

1 gallon . . . . . 3800 mL
1 quart . . . . 960 mL
1 pint . . . . 480 mL
8 fluid oz . . . . . 240 mL

4 fluid oz . . . . 120 mL
15 minims . . . . 1 mL
10 minims . . . . 0.6 mL

1 gallon . . . . . . 128 fluid ounces
1 quart . . . . 32 fluid ounces
1 pint . . . . 16 fluid ounces

Approximate Household Equivalents

1 teaspoonful . . . . 5 mL
1 tablespoonful . . . 15 mL

Weights

Basic equivalents:

1 oz = 30 g
15 gr = 1 g

Examples:

4 oz . . . . 120 g
2 oz . . . . 60 g
10 gr . . . . 600 mg
7 $\frac{1}{2}$ gr . . . . 500 mg

1 gr . . . . 60 mg
$\frac{1}{100}$ gr . . . . 600 mcg
$\frac{1}{150}$ gr . . . . 400 mcg
$\frac{1}{200}$ gr . . . . 300 mcg

16 oz . . . . 1 pound

Metric Conversions

Basic equivalents:

1 g . . . . 1000 mg
1 mg . . . . 1000 mcg

Examples:

5 g . . . . 5000 mg
0.5 g . . . . 500 mg
0.05 g . . . . 50 mg

5 mg . . . . 5000 mcg
0.5 mg . . . . 500 mcg
0.05 mg . . . . 50 mcg

Exact Equivalents

1 g = 15.43 grains
1 milliliter (mL) = 16.23 minims
1 minim = 0.06 milliliter
1 gr = 64.8 milligrams
1 oz = 28.35 grams
1 lb = 453.6 grams
1 kg = 2.2 pounds

0.1 mg = 1/600 gr
0.12 mg = 1/500 gr
0.15 mg = 1/400 gr
0.2 mg = 1/300 gr
0.5 mg = 1/120 gr
0.8 mg = 1/80 gr
1 mg = 1/65 gr

Solids*

$\frac{1}{4}$ grain = 15 mg
$\frac{1}{2}$ grain = 30 mg
$1\frac{1}{2}$ grain = 100 mg
5 grains = 300 mg
10 grains = 600 mg

*Use exact equivalents for compounding and calculations requiring a high degree of accuracy.

POUNDS/KILOGRAMS CONVERSION

1 pound = 0.45359 kilograms
1 kilogram = 2.2 pounds

lb	= kg	lb	= kg	lb	= kg
1	0.45	70	31.75	140	63.50
5	2.27	75	34.02	145	65.77
10	4.54	80	36.29	150	68.04
15	6.80	85	38.56	155	70.31
20	9.07	90	40.82	160	72.58
25	11.34	95	43.09	165	74.84
30	13.61	100	45.36	170	77.11
35	15.88	105	47.63	175	79.38
40	18.14	110	49.90	180	81.65
45	20.41	115	52.16	185	83.92
50	22.68	120	54.43	190	86.18
55	24.95	125	56.70	195	88.45
60	27.22	130	58.91	200	90.72
65	29.48	135	61.24		

TEMPERATURE CONVERSION

Centigrade to Fahrenheit = (°C x 9/5) + 32 = °F
Fahrenheit to Centigrade = (°F - 32) x 5/9 = °C

°C	= °F	°C	= °F	°C	= °F
100.0	212.0	39.0	102.2	36.8	98.2
50.0	122.0	38.8	101.8	36.6	97.9
41.0	105.8	38.6	101.5	36.4	97.5
40.8	105.4	38.4	101.1	36.2	97.2
40.6	105.1	38.2	100.8	36.0	96.8
40.4	104.7	38.0	100.4	35.8	96.4
40.2	104.4	37.8	100.1	35.6	96.1
40.0	104.0	37.6	99.7	35.4	95.7
39.8	103.6	37.4	99.3	35.2	95.4
39.6	103.3	37.2	99.0	35.0	95.0
39.4	102.9	37.0	98.6	0	32.0
39.2	102.6				

ACQUIRED IMMUNODEFICIENCY SYNDROME (AIDS) — LAB TESTS AND APPROVED DRUGS FOR HIV INFECTION AND AIDS-RELATED CONDITIONS

This list of tests is not intended in any way to suggest patterns of physician's orders, nor is it complete. These tests may support possible clinical diagnoses or rule out other diagnostic possibilities. Each laboratory test relevant to AIDS is listed and weighted. Two symbols (**) indicate that the test is diagnostic, that is, documents the diagnosis if the expected is found. A single symbol (*) indicates a test frequently used in the diagnosis or management of the disease. The other listed tests are useful on a selective basis with consideration of clinical factors and specific aspects of the case.

Acid-Fast Stain
Acid-Fast Stain, Modified, *Nocardia* Species
Antimicrobial Susceptibility Testing, Fungi
Antimicrobial Susceptibility Testing, Mycobacteria
Arthropod Identification
Babesiosis Serological Test
Bacteremia Detection, Buffy Coat Micromethod
Bacterial Culture, Blood
Bacterial Culture, Bronchoscopy Specimen
Bacterial Culture, Sputum
Bacterial Culture, Stool
Bacterial Culture, Throat
Bacterial Culture, Urine, Clean Catch
$Beta_2$-Microglobulin
Blood and Fluid Precautions, Specimen Collection
Bronchial Washings Cytology
Bronchoalveolar Lavage Cytology
Brushings Cytology
Candida Antigen
Candidiasis Serologic Test
Cat Scratch Disease Serology
CD4/CD8 Enumeration
Cerebrospinal Fluid Cytology
Cryptococcal Antigen Titer
Cryptosporidium Diagnostic Procedures
Cytomegalic Inclusion Disease Cytology
Cytomegalovirus Antibody
Cytomegalovirus Antigen Detection
Cytomegalovirus Culture
Cytomegalovirus DNA Detection
Darkfield Examination, Syphilis
Electron Microscopy
Folic Acid, Serum
Fungal Culture, Biopsy or Body Fluid
Fungal Culture, Blood
Fungal Culture, Cerebrospinal Fluid
Fungal Culture, Sputum
Fungal Culture, Stool
Fungal Culture, Urine
Hemoglobin A_2
Hepatitis B Surface Antigen
Herpes Cytology
Herpes Simplex Virus Antigen Detection
Herpes Simplex Virus Culture
Histopathology

Histoplasmosis Antibody
Histoplasmosis Antigen
**HIV-1/HIV-2 Serology
HTLV-I/II Antibody
*Human Immunodeficiency Virus Culture
*Human Immunodeficiency Virus DNA Amplification
India Ink Preparation
Inhibitor, Lupus, Phospholipid Type
KOH Preparation
Leishmaniasis Serological Test
Leukocyte Immunophenotyping
Lymphocyte Transformation Test
Microsporidia Diagnostic Procedures
Mycobacteria by DNA Probe
Mycobacterial Culture, Biopsy or Body Fluid
Mycobacterial Culture, Cerebrospinal Fluid
Mycobacterial Culture, Cutaneous and Subcutaneous Tissue
Mycobacterial Culture, Sputum
Mycobacterial Culture, Stool
Neisseria gonorrhoeae Culture and Smear
Nocardia Culture
Ova and Parasites, Stool
*p24 Antigen
Platelet Count
Pneumocystis carinii Preparation
Pneumocystis Immunofluorescence
Polymerase Chain Reaction
Red Blood Cell Indices
Risks of Transfusion
Skin Biopsy
Sputum Cytology
Toxoplasmosis Serology
VDRL, Serum
Viral Culture
Viral Culture, Blood
Viral Culture, Body Fluid
Viral Culture, Central Nervous System Symptoms
Viral Culture, Dermatological Symptoms
Viral Culture, Tissue
Virus, Direct Detection by Fluorescent Antibody
White Blood Count

Approved Drugs for HIV/AIDS or AIDS-related Conditions

abacavir (Ziagen®)
Treatment of HIV-1 in adults and children
alitretinoin (Panretin™)
Topical treatment of lesions in patients with AIDS-related Kaposi's sarcoma
amphotericin B lipid complex (Abelcet®, Ambisome®)
Treatment of aspergillosis
amprenavir (Agenerase®)
Treatment of HIV-1 in adults and children
atovaquone (Mepron®)
Treatment of mild to moderate *Pneumocystis carinii* pneumonia in patients who are intolerant to Bactrim® or Septra®

azithromycin (Zithromax®)
Prevention of *Mycobacterium avium* complex (MAC) in persons with advanced HIV infection

cidofovir (Vistide®)
Treatment of AIDS-related cytomegalovirus retinitis

clarithromycin (Biaxin®, Klacid®)
Treatment of disseminated mycobacterial infections due to *Mycobacterium avium-intracellulare* complex (MAC); approved for prophylaxis of disseminated MAC in patients with advanced HIV infection

daunorubicin-liposomal (DaunoXome®)
Treatment of advanced HIV-related Kaposi's sarcoma

delavirdine mesylate (Rescriptor®)
In combination with appropriate antiretrovirals when therapy is warranted for treatment of HIV infection

didanosine (Videx®)
Treatment of adult and pediatric patients with advanced HIV who are intolerant to or deteriorating on AZT; approved for treatment of adult and pediatric patients with advanced HIV previously treated with AZT; approved for treatment of HIV infection when antiretroviral therapy is warranted

doxorubicin hydrochloride-liposomal (Doxil®)
Treatment of Kaposi's sarcoma in AIDS patients who are intolerant to or have disease progression on prior combination chemotherapy

dronabinol (Marinol®)
Treatment of anorexia associated with weight loss in patients with AIDS

efavirenz (Sustiva®)
Treatment of HIV and AIDS

erythropoietin (Epogen®, Procrit®)
Treatment of anemia related to AZT therapy in HIV infection

famciclovir (Famvir®)
Treatment of recurrent mucocutaneous herpes simplex infections in HIV-infected patients at a dose of 500 mg twice daily

filgrastim [G-CSF] (Neupogen®)
Treatment of neutropenia due to chemotherapy for cancers, including lymphomas and Kaposi's sarcoma

fluconazole (Diflucan®)
Treatment of oropharyngeal and esophageal candidiasis and for treatment of cryptococcal meningitis; approved for treatment of pediatric patients with cryptococcal meningitis and candida infections

fomivirsen sodium intravitreal injection (Vitravene®)
Local treatment of cytomegalovirus (CMV) retinitis in patients with AIDS who are intolerant of or have a contraindication to other treatment(s) for CMV retinitis or who were insufficiently responsive to previous treatment(s) for CMV retinitis

foscarnet (Foscavir®)
Treatment of CMV retinitis in patients with AIDS; approved for the treatment of acyclovir-resistant herpes simplex virus

ganciclovir - I.V., oral (Cytovene®)
Treatment of CMV retinitis in immunocompromised patients; oral approved for maintenance therapy for CMV retinitis in some patients; approved for prophylaxis of CMV disease

ganciclovir [DHPG] - implant (Vitrasert®)
Treatment of CMV retinitis in patients with AIDS

immune globulin - I.V. (Gamimune N®)
Prevention of bacterial infections in pediatric HIV infection

indinavir sulfate (Crixivan®)
For use alone or in combination with nucleoside analogues for treatment of HIV infection in adults

interferon alfa-2a (Roferon-A®)
Treatment of AIDS-related Kaposi's sarcoma in selected patients

interferon alfa-2b (Intron-A®)
Treatment of adult AIDS-related Kaposi's sarcoma in selected patients; approved for treatment of chronic non-A, non-B hepatitis

interferon alfa-n3 (Alferon N®)
Treatment of condyloma acuminata (genital warts)

itraconazole (Sporanox®)
Treatment of histoplasmosis, blastomycosis, and aspergillosis in immunocompromised and nonimmunocompromised patients

ketoconazole (Nizoral®)
Treatment of histoplasmosis, blastomycosis, and candidiasis

lamivudine [3TC] (Epivir®)
Combination use with AZT as a treatment option for HIV infection in adults and pediatric patients ≥3 months of age

megestrol acetate (Megace®, Ovaban®)
Treatment of anorexia, cachexia, or unexplained significant weight loss in patients with AIDS

nelfinavir mesylate (Viracept®)
Treatment of HIV infection when antiretroviral therapy is warranted in adults and pediatrics ≥2 years of age

nevirapine (Viramune®)
Combination use with nucleoside analogues for treatment of HIV-infected adults experiencing clinical and/or immunologic deterioration

pentamidine - I.M., I.V. (Pentam® 300)
Treatment of *Pneumocystis carinii* pneumonia

pentamidine - aerosolized (NebuPent®)
Prevention of *Pneumocystis carinii* pneumonia

pyrimethamine [with sulfonamide] (Daraprim®; Fansidar® when combined with sulfadoxine)
Treatment of toxoplasmosis

rifabutin (Ansamycin®, Mycobutin®)
Prevention of *Mycobacterium avium* complex in patients with advanced HIV

ritonavir (Norvir®)
For use alone or in combination with nucleoside analogues for treatment of HIV infection

saquinavir mesylate (Invirase®)
Combination use with nucleoside analogues for treatment of advanced HIV infection in selected patients

sargramostim [GM-CSF] (Leukine®)
Treatment of cancer patients with lymphomas or leukemia who are receiving bone marrow transplants

somatropin rDNA (Serostim®)
Treatment of AIDS-wasting and cachexia

stavudine [d4T] (Zerit®)
Treatment of adults with advanced HIV infection who are intolerant to or deteriorating on approved therapies; approved for treatment of adults with advanced HIV infection who have undergone prolonged treatment with AZT; approved for the treatment of pediatrics with HIV infection who have undergone prolonged prior AZT therapy

sulfamethoxazole (Bactrim® when combined with trimethoprim; Septra® when combined rimethoprim)
Treatment of *Pneumocystis carinii* pneumonia (PCP); approved for prevention of PCP

trimethoprim (Bactrim® when combined with sulfamethoxazole; Septra® when combined with ethoxazole)
Treatment of *Pneumocystis carinii* pneumonia (PCP); approved for prevention of PCP
trimetrexate (with leucovorin) [TMTX] (Neutrexin®)
Treatment of moderate to severe *Pneumocystis carinii* pneumonia when intolerant or refractory to TMP/SMX or when TMP/SMX is contraindicated
zalcitabine [ddC] (Hivid®)
Combination use with AZT for treatment of selected patients with advanced HIV disease; approved for monotherapy treatment of advanced HIV for patients ≥13 years of age who are intolerant to or have disease progression on AZT
zidovudine [AZT] (Retrovir®)
Treatment of adult AIDS or symptomatic HIV and CD4 ≤200; approved for treatment of adult HIV infection and CD4 ≤500; approved for treatment of pediatric HIV infection (3 months to 12 years of age); approved for prevention of perinatal transmission in HIV-positive pregnant women between 14 and 34 weeks gestation and in newborns of HIV-positive mothers
zidovudine and lamivudine (Combivir®)
Combination of AZT (zidovudine) and 3TC (lamivudine) for treating AIDS and HIV infection

Drugs Being Studied in HIV/AIDS Clinical Trials

A-007 [antineoplastic]
ABT-378 (new name: lopinavir) [protease inhibitor]
acetaminophen (Tylenol®, Panadol®) [analgesic, antipyretic]
acetylcysteine (Mucomyst®, Respaire®) [antiretroviral, mycolytic]
acitretin (Soriatane®) [antipsoriatic]
acyclovir (Zovirax®) [antiviral]
aldesleukin (Proleukin®) [immunomodulator, antineoplastic]
AL 721 [antiviral]
ALVAC-HIV gp 160 MN (vCP125) [vaccine]
ALVAC-HIV MN120TMG (vCP205) [vaccine]
ALVAC-HIV MN120TMGNP (vCP300) [vaccine]
ALVAC-RG rabies glycoprotein (vCP65) [vaccine]
allopurinol (Zyloprim®) [xanthine oxidase inhibitor]
aluminum hydroxide (Amphogel®) [adjuvant, immunostimulant]
alvircept sudotox (CD4-pseudomonas exotoxin) [immunomodulator, antiretroviral]
amikacin sulfate (Kanamycin®) [antibacterial]
aminosalicylic acid [antibacterial]
amitriptyline hydrochloride (Elavil®) [antidepressant, analgesic]
amoxicillin (Amoxil®) [antimicrobial]
amphotericin B (Fungizone®) [antifungal]
ampicillin (Omnipen®) [antimicrobial]
ampligen (Atvogen®) [antiretroviral, immunomodulator]
anti-HIV immune serum globulin (HIVIG®) [immunomodulator]
anti-Rh antibodies (Anti-D) [immunomodulator]
APL 400-003 [vaccine]
AS-101 (ammonium trichlorotellurate) [immunomodulator]
atevirdine mesylate (U-87201E) [antiretroviral]
azidodideoxyuridine (AzdU) [antiretroviral]
beclomethasone dipropionate (Beclovent®) [anti-inflammatory]
benztropine mesylate (Cogentin®) [anticholinergic, antiparkinsonian]
bis-POM PMEA [antiretroviral]
bleomycin (Blenoxane®) [antineoplastic]
BMS 232 [protease inhibitor]
butyldeoxynojirimicin (SC-48334) [antiretroviral]

calanolide A [antiviral]
capreomycin sulfate (Caprocin®) [antibacterial]
CD4 antigen [antiretroviral]
CD4-IgG [antiretroviral, immunomodulator]
ceftriaxone sodium (Rocephin®) [antimicrobial]
cefuroxime axetil (Ceftin®) [antibiotic]
chimeric anti-TNF monoclonal antibody (Chimeric A2) [immunomodulator]
chlorhexidine gluconate (Peridex®, Hibiclens®) [topical antibacterial, antimicrobial]
cimetidine (Tagamet®) [immunomodulator, histamine receptor antagonist]
ciprofloxacin (Cipro®) [antibacterial]
CI-0694 (Sulfasim®) [immunomodulator]
clavulanate potassium [antibacterial]
clindamycin (Cleocin®) [antibacterial]
clofazimine (Lamprene®) [antimicrobial, antileprotic]
clotrimazole (Lotrimin®, Mycelex®, Femcare®) [antifungal]
Cryptosporidium immune whey protein (bovine anticryptosporidium immunoglobulin) [antidiarrheal]
curdlan sulfate [antiviral]
cyclophosphamide (Cytoxan®) [antineoplastic, immunosuppressant]
cycloserine (Seromycin®) [antibacterial]
cysteamine (MEA; mercaptoethylamine) [antiretroviral, antiurolithic]
cytarabine (Cytosar-U®) [antimetabolite, antineoplastic, antiviral, immunosuppressant]
cytomegalovirus immune globulin intravenous (human) (CytoGam®) [immunomodulator]
dacarbazine [antineoplastic]
dapsone [antibacterial]
delavirdine mesylate (U-90152) [antiretroviral]
deoxy-fluorothymidine (FDT) [antiretroviral]
dexamethasone (Decadron®) [anti-inflammatory, immunomodulator, antineoplastic]
dextran sulfate [antiretroviral]
diclazuril [antiprotozoal]
dideoxyadenosine (ddA) [antiretroviral]
diethylhomospermine (DEHSPM) [antidiarrheal]
dinitrochlorobenzene (DNCB) [contact allergen, immunomodulator]
disulfiram (Antabuse®) [alcohol abuse deterrent, immunomodulator, antiretroviral]
ditiocarb sodium (Imuthiol®) [immunomodulator, chelator]
doxorubicin (Adriamycin®, Rubex®) [antineoplastic]
env 2-3 [vaccine]
ethambutol hydrochloride (Myambutol®) [antibacterial]
ethionamide [antibacterial]
etoposide (VePesid®) [antineoplastic]
F105 human monoclonal antibody [immunomodulator]
fiacitabine (FIAC) [antiviral]
fialuridine (FIAU) [antiviral]
flucytosine (Ancobon®) [antifungal]
fluorouracil (5-FU) [antineoplastic]
glutamic acid (Feracid®) [gastric acidifier]
gp-160 (MicroGeneSys®, VaxSyn®) [vaccine]
gp-160 vaccine (Immuno-AG) [vaccine]
guaifenesin (Robitussin®) [expectorant]
HBY 097 [antiretroviral]
hepatitis B vaccine (Engerix-B®, Recombivax HB®) [vaccine]
heptavalent pneumococcal conjugate vaccine [vaccine]
HIV p17/p24: Ty-VLP [vaccine]
HIV-1 C4-V3 polyvalent peptide vaccine [vaccine]
HIVAC-1e [vaccine]

hydroxyurea (Hydrea®) [anti-cancer drug]
hypericin (VIMRyxn®) [antiretroviral]
ibuprofen (Advil®; Motrin®; Nuprin®) [nonsteroidal anti-inflammatory]
ifosfamide [antineoplastic]
imipramine hydrochloride (Tofranil®) [antidepressant]
inosine pranobex (Isoprinosine®) [antiviral, immunostimulant, antiretroviral]
insulin-like growth factor (Somatomedin C®) [immunomodulator]
interferon alfa-n1 (Wellferon®) [antineoplastic, antiviral, immunomodulator]
interferon alfa-n3 (Alferon N®) [antineoplastic, antiviral, immunomodulator]
interferon beta (Betaseron®) [antineoplastic, antiviral, immunomodulator, antiretroviral]
interferon gamma (Actimmune®) [antineoplastic, antiviral, immunomodulator]
interleukin-3 (IL-3) [immunomodulator, hematopoietic]
interleukin-4 (IL-4) [immunomodulator, antineoplastic]
interleukin-10 (IL-10) [immunomodulator]
interleukin-12 (IL-12) [antiviral]
ISIS 2922 [antiviral]
isoniazid (INH) [antibacterial]
isotretinoin (Accutane®) [keratolytic]
ketoconazole (Nizoral®) [antifungal, antineoplastic, antiadrenal]
keyhole-limpet hemocyanin [immunomodulator]
kynostatin 272 (KNI-272®) [protease inhibitor, antiretroviral]
L-756,423 [protease inhibitor]
lentinan [immunomodulator, antineoplastic]
letrazuril [antiprotozoal]
leucovorin calcium (Wellcovorin®) [antianemic, antidote for folic acid antagonists]
levamisole [immunomodulator]
levocarnitine [antihyperlipoproteinemic]
levofloxacin [antimicrobial, antiretroviral]
liposome - encapsulated monophosphoryl lipid A [adjuvant, immunostimulant]
Liposyn® III (I.V. fat emulsion 2%) [nutritional support]
Liposyn® II (I.V. fat emulsion 20%) [nutritional support]
lobucavir [antiviral]
lodenosine (F-ddA) [nucleoside analog type drug similar to ddI]
lymphocytes, activated [immunomodulator]
L-697, 639 [antiretroviral]
L-697, 661 [antiretroviral]
magnesium sulfate [electrolyte replenisher, anticonvulsant, laxative]
MDL 28574 [antiretroviral]
methadone hydrochloride (Dolophine®) [detoxification maintenance, narcotic analgesic]
methotrexate (MTX) [antineoplastic, folic acid antagonist, anti-inflammatory]
methoxsalen (Oxsoralen-ultra®) [Photochemotherapeutic]
methylprednisolone (Medrol®) [anti-inflammatory, immunosuppressant]
mexiletine hydrochloride (Mexitil®) [analgesic, antiarrhythmic]
MF59 [adjuvant, immunostimulant]
microparticulate monovalent HIV-1 peptide vaccine [vaccine]
mitoguazone dihydrochloride (MGBG) [antineoplastic]
mitoxantrone hydrochloride (Novantrone®) [antineoplastic]
MKC-442 [antiviral-NNRTI]
monophosphoryl lipid A [adjuvant, immunostimulant]
MTP-PE/MF59 [immunostimulant, adjuvant emulsion]
multivalent HIV-1 peptide immunogen [vaccine]
nimodipine (Nimotop®) [calcium channel blocker, vasodilator]
nitazoxanide (NTZ) [antiparasitic]
nystatin (Mycostatin®) [antifungal]
octreotide acetate (Sandostatin®) [antidiarrheal]

OPC 14117 [antioxidant]
oxazepam (Serax®) [anxiolytic, minor tranquilizer]
P3C541b lipopeptide [vaccine]
paclitaxel (Taxol®) [antineoplastic]
paromomycin sulfate (Humatin®) [antibiotic, amebicidal, anthelmintic]
PCLUS [vaccine]
penicillin G [antibacterial]
pentosan polysulfate sodium [antineoplastic, antiviral, anticoagulant, anti-inflammatory,antiretroviral]
pentoxifylline (Trental®) [vasodilator, hemorrheologic]
peptide T [antiretroviral, immunomodulator]
piritrexim isethionate [antifolate, antineoplastic, antiproliferative, antiprotozoal]
PMEA [antiretroviral]
pneumococcal vaccine polyvalent [vaccine]
polyethylene glycolated IL-2 (PEG IL-2) [immunomodulator]
polymyxin B sulfate/bacitracin zinc ointment (Bacitracin®, Polysporin®) [antibacterial]
prednisone [glucocorticoid]
primaquine [antimalarial]
probenecid (Benemid®) [renal tubular blocker, uricosuric]
pseudoephedrine (Sudafed®) [decongestant, sympathomimetic]
pyrazinamide [antibacterial]
pyridoxine hydrochloride (vitamin B6) [vitamin (coenzyme)]
QS-21 [adjuvant, immunostimulant]
quinine [antimalarial, neuromuscular]
ranitidine hydrochloride (Zantac®) [histamine receptor antagonist, immunomodulator]
recombinant p24 vaccine [vaccine]
rgp 120/HIV-1IIIB [vaccine]
rgp 120/HIV-1MN [vaccine]
rgp 120/HIV 1MN monovalent octameric V3 peptide (SynVac®) [vaccine]
rgp 120/HIV-1SF2 [vaccine]
ribavirin (Virazole®) [antiviral, antiretroviral]
rifampin (Rifadin®, Rimactane®) [antibacterial]
RMP-7 [antifungal]
RO 24-7429 [antiretroviral, *tat* inhibitor]
saccharomyces boulardii [antidiarrheal]
SC-49483 [antiretroviral]
SC-52151 [protease inhibitor, antiretroviral]
SCH 39304 [antifungal]
selegiline hydrochloride (Deprenyl®) [MAO inhibitor, antidyskinetic, antiparkinsonian]
sevirumab (human monoclonal antibody to cytomegalovirus) [antiviral, immunomodulator]
smallpox vaccine (Dryvax®) [vaccine]
sorivudine (Brovavir®) [antiviral]
SP-303T [antiviral]
sparfloxacin (Zagam®) [antibacterial]
spiramycin [antibacterial, antiprotozoal]
streptomycin sulfate [antibacterial]
sulfadiazine [antibacterial]
sulfadoxine (Fansidar® when combined with pyrimethamine) [antibacterial]
syntex adjuvant formulation [adjuvant, immunostimulant]
T1249 [fusion inhibitor]
T20 [fusion inhibitor]
TBC-3B [vaccine]
tecogalan sodium (SP-PG) [angiogenesis inhibitor]
thalidomide (Synovir®) [immunomodulator, sedative, hypnotic]
thioctic acid [antioxidant]

threonyl muramyl dipeptide [adjuvant, immunostimulant]
thymic humoral factor (THF) [immunomodulator]
thymosin alpha 1 [immunomodulator]
thymopentin (Timunox®) [immunomodulator]
tipranavir [protease inhibitor]
TNP-470 [antineoplastic]
tretinoin (retinoic acid) [keratolytic]
trichosanthin (GLQ 223) [antiretroviral, immunosuppressant]
trifluridine (ophthalmic) [antiviral]
tuberculin purified protein derivative (PPD) [diagnostic aid]
tumor necrosis factor (TNF) [antineoplastic, antiretroviral]
tumor necrosis factor soluble receptor - immunoadhesion complex [immunomodulator]
valacyclovir hydrochloride (Valtrex®) [antiviral]
valproic acid (Depakene®) [anticonvulsant]
varicella virus vaccine live (Varivax®) [vaccine]
vesnarinone (OPC-8212) [antiretroviral, cardiotonic]
vidarabine [antiviral]
vinblastine sulfate (Velban®) [antineoplastic]
vincristine (Oncovin®) [antineoplastic]
WF10 [antiretroviral]
wobenzym [immunomodulator]
WR 6026 [antiprotozoal]
524W91 [antiretroviral]
882C87 [antiviral]
935U83 [antiretroviral]

CANCER CHEMOTHERAPY ACRONYMS

Acronyms	Used for
7 + 3	Leukemia — acute myeloid leukemia, induction
ABP	Lymphoma — non-Hodgkin's
ABC-P	Multiple myeloma
ABDIC	Lymphoma — Hodgkin's
ABVD	Lymphoma — Hodgkin's
AC	Sarcoma — bony sarcoma
AC	Breast cancer
AC (DC)	Multiple myeloma
ACE	Lung cancer — small cell
ACe	Breast cancer
ACMF	Breast cancer
ACOMLA	Lymphoma — non-Hodgkin's
ADOC	Thymoma (Malignant)
AVM	Breast cancer
m-BACOD	Lymphoma — non-Hodgkin's
BACOP	Lymphoma — non-Hodgkin's
BAP	Multiple myeloma
BAPP	Thymoma (Malignant)
BCDT	Malignant melanoma
BCNU-DAG	Brain tumors
B-CMF	Head and neck cancer
BCVM	Cervical cancer
BCP	Multiple myeloma
BEP	Genitourinary cancer — testicular, induction, good risk
BHD	Malignant melanoma Breast cancer
BMC	Head and neck cancer
B-MOPP	Lymphoma — Hodgkin's
BMVL	Head and neck cancer
BOMP	Cervical cancer
BVCPP	Lymphoma — Hodgkin's
CAF	Breast cancer
CAFVP	Breast cancer
CAM	Genitourinary cancer — prostate
CAMP	Lung cancer — non-small cell
CAP	Genitourinary cancer — bladder Head and neck cancer Lung cancer — non-small cell Adrenal cortical cancer Endometrial cancer
CAP-BOP	Lymphoma — non-Hodgkin's
CAP-M	Genitourinary cancer — bladder
CBM	Head and neck cancer
CC	Ovarian cancer — epithelial
CCCP	Multiple myeloma
CCNU-VP	Lymphoma — Hodgkin's
CCVPP	Lymphoma — Hodgkin's
CD	Leukemia — acute nonlymphoblastic, consolidation Ewing's sarcoma Genitourinary cancer — prostate
CDC	Ovarian cancer — epithelial
CDF	Genitourinary cancer — prostate

Acronyms	Used for
CE	Adrenal cortical cancer
CF	Head and neck cancer
CFM	Breast cancer
CFPT	Breast cancer
CHAP	Ovarian cancer — epithelial
CHL + PRED	Leukemia — chronic lymphocytic leukemia
CHOP	Lymphoma — non-Hodgkin's
CHOP-B (Yale)	Lymphoma — non-Hodgkin's
CHOP-Bleo	Lymphoma — non-Hodgkin's
CHOP (P)	Lymphoma — non-Hodgkin's
CHOR	Lung cancer — small cell
CISCA	Gastric cancer Genitourinary cancer — bladder
Cladribine (2-CdA)	Leukemia — chronic lymphocytic leukemia
CMB	Cervical cancer
CMC-High Dose	Lung cancer — small cell
CMF	Breast cancer
CMFP	Breast cancer
CMFVP (Cooper's)	Breast cancer
C-MOPP	Lymphoma — non-Hodgkin's
CMV	Genitourinary cancer — bladder
COB	Head and neck cancer
CODE	Lung cancer — small cell
COPE	Lung cancer — small cell
COLP	Thymoma (Malignant)
COM	Colon cancer
COMF	Colon cancer
COP-BLAM	Lymphoma — non-Hodgkin's
COP-BLAM III	Lymphoma — non-Hodgkin's
COP-BLAM IV	Lymphoma — non-Hodgkin's
COP	Lymphoma — non-Hodgkin's
COP-BLAM	Lymphoma — non-Hodgkin's
COPP (or "C" MOPP)	Lymphoma — non-Hodgkin's
CP	Ovarian cancer — epithelial
CV	Lung cancer — non-small cell
CVB	Esophageal cancer
CVI	Lung cancer — non-small cell
CVM	Gestational trophoblastic disease
CVP	Leukemia — chronic lymphocytic leukemia Lymphoma — non-Hodgkin's
CYADIC	Sarcoma — soft tissue
CYVADIC	Sarcoma — bony sarcoma Sarcoma — soft tissue
DAFS	Carcinoid (Malignant)
DAT	Leukemia — acute myeloid leukemia, induction Breast cancer
DC	Multiple myeloma
DHAP	Lymphoma — non-Hodgkin's
DMC	Gestational trophoblastic cancer
DS	Genitourinary cancer — prostate
DTIC-ACTD	Malignant melanoma
DVP	Leukemia — acute lymphoblastic, induction
DVPA	Leukemia — acute lymphoblastic, induction
ELF	Gastric cancer

Acronyms	Used for
EMA-CO	Gestational trophoblastic disease
FAC	Breast cancer
FAC-S	Carcinoid (Malignant)
FAM	Gastric cancer Lung cancer — non-small cell Pancreatic cancer
FAME	Gastric cancer
FAMTX	Gastric cancer
FAP	Gastric cancer
FAP-2	Pancreatic cancer
FCE	Gastric cancer
F-CL	Colon cancer
FDC	Gastric cancer
FL	Genitourinary cancer — prostate
FLe	Colon cancer
Fludarabine	Leukemia — chronic lymphocytic leukemia
FMS (SMF)	Pancreatic cancer
FMV	Colon cancer
FOAM	Breast cancer
FOMi	Lung cancer — non-small cell
FOMi/CAP	Lung cancer — non-small cell
5FU/LDLF	Colon cancer
FU/HU	Colon cancer
FU/LV	Colon cancer
5FU Hurt	Head and neck cancer
5FU/LV (Weekly)	Colon cancer
FL	Genitourinary cancer — prostate
HDAC	Leukemia — acute myeloid leukemia, induction
HDMTX	Sarcoma — bony sarcoma
IC	Leukemia — acute myeloid leukemia, induction
ID	Sarcoma — soft tissue
IMAC	Sarcoma — bony sarcoma
IMF	Breast cancer
IMVP-16	Lymphoma — non-Hodgkin's
LDAC	Leukemia — acute myeloid leukemia, induction
L-VAM	Genitourinary cancer — prostate
M-2	Multiple myeloma
MAC	Genitourinary cancer — bladder Endometrial cancer
MACC	Lung cancer — non-small cell
MACOP-B	Lymphoma — non-Hodgkin's
MAID	Sarcoma — soft tissue
MAP	Head and neck cancer
MBC (MBD)	Head and neck cancer Cervical cancer Esophageal cancer
MBD	Head and neck cancer
MC	Leukemia — acute myeloid leukemia, induction
MeCP	Multiple myeloma
MF	Head and neck cancer Esophageal cancer
MICE (ICE)	Lung cancer — small cell
MINE	Lymphoma — non-Hodgkin's
MM	Leukemia — acute lymphoblastic, maintenance
MMC (MTX + MP + CTX)	Leukemia — acute lymphoblastic, maintenance
MOF-STREP	Colon cancer
MOP-BAP	Lymphoma — Hodgkin's

Acronyms	Used for
MOPP	Lymphoma — Hodgkin's
MOPP/ABV Hybrid	Lymphoma — Hodgkin's
MP	Multiple myeloma
m-PFL	Genitourinary cancer — bladder
MS	Adrenal cortical cancer
MV	Leukemia — acute myeloid leukemia, induction
MVAC	Genitourinary cancer — bladder
MVPP	Lymphoma — Hodgkin's
NFL	Breast cancer
PAC (CAP)	Ovarian cancer — epithelial Endometrial cancer
PE	Genitourinary cancer — testicular, induction, good risk Lung cancer — small cell
PFL	Gastric cancer Head and neck cancer
PFL + IFV	Head and neck cancer
POCC	Lung cancer — small cell
Pro-MACE	Lymphoma — non-Hodgkin's
Pro-MACE-CytaBOM	Lymphoma — non-Hodgkin's
Pro-MACE-MOPP	Lymphoma — non-Hodgkin's
PT	Ovarian cancer — epithelial
SC	Carcinoid (Malignant)
SCAB	Lymphoma — Hodgkin's
SD	Pancreatic cancer
SF	Carcinoid (Malignant)
SMF	Pancreatic cancer
T-9	Ewing's sarcoma
VAB VI	Genitourinary cancer — testicular, induction, salvage
VAC	Ovarian cancer — germ cell Sarcoma — soft tissue Ewing's sarcoma
VAC (CAV) (Induction)	Lung cancer — small cell
VAD	Leukemia — acute lymphoblastic, induction Multiple myeloma
VADRIAC — High Dose	Sarcoma — bony sarcoma
VAIE	Sarcoma — bony sarcoma
VAM	Breast cancer
VAP	Multiple myeloma
VATH	Breast cancer
VBAP	Multiple myeloma
VBC	Malignant melanoma
VBP (PVB)	Genitourinary cancer — testicular, induction, salvage
VC	Lung cancer — small cell
VCAP	Multiple myeloma
VDCP	Endometrial cancer
VDP	Malignant melanoma
VIP	Genitourinary cancer — testicular, induction, poor risk
VIP (Einhorn)	Genitourinary cancer — testicular, induction, poor risk
VP	Leukemia — acute lymphoblastic, induction
VP-L-Asparaginase	Leukemia — acute lymphoblastic, induction
Wayne State	Head and neck cancer

CANCER CHEMOTHERAPY REGIMENS

ADULT REGIMENS

Adenocarcinoma – Unknown Primary

Carbo-Tax

Paclitaxel, I.V., 135 mg/m^2 over 24 hours, day 1, followed by
Carboplatin dose targeted by Calvert equation to AUC 7.5 I.V.

Repeat cycle every 21 days

EP

Cisplatin, I.V., 60-100 mg/m^2, day 1
Etoposide, I.V., 80-100 mg/m^2, days 1-3

Repeat cycle every 21 days

FAM

Fluorouracil, I.V., 600 mg/m^2, days 1, 8, 29, 36
Doxorubicin, I.V., 30 mg/m^2, days 1, 29
Mitomycin, I.V., 10 mg/m^2, day 1

Repeat cycle every 8 weeks

Paclitaxel/Carboplatin/Etoposide

Paclitaxel, I.V., 200 mg/m^2 over 1 hour, day 1, followed by
Carboplatin dose targeted by Calvert equation to AUC 6 I.V.
Etoposide, P.O., 50 mg/day alternated with 100 mg/day, days 1-10

Repeat cycle every 21 days

Breast Cancer

Standard adjuvant chemotherapy includes 4 cycles of AC or 6 cycles of CMF (d_1/d_8 variety)

AC

Doxorubicin, I.V., 60 mg/m^2, day 1
Cyclophosphamide, I.V., 400-600 mg/m^2, day 1

Repeat cycle every 21 days

ACe

Doxorubicin, I.V., 40 mg/m^2, day 1
Cyclophosphamide, P.O., 200 mg/m^2/day, days 1-3 or 3-6

Repeat cycle every 21-28 days

CAF

Cyclophosphamide, P.O., 100 mg/m^2, days 1-14 or 600 mg/m^2 I.V., day 1
Doxorubicin, I.V., 25 mg/m^2, days 1, 8 or 60 mg/m^2 I.V., day 1
Fluorouracil, I.V., 500-600 mg/m^2, days 1, 8

Repeat cycle every 28 days

or

Cyclophosphamide, I.V., 500 mg/m^2, day 1
Doxorubicin, I.V., 50 mg/m^2, day 1
Fluorouracil, I.V., 500 mg/m^2, day 1

Repeat cycle every 21 days

CFM

Cyclophosphamide, I.V., 500-600 mg/m^2, day 1
Fluorouracil, I.V., 500-600 mg/m^2, day 1
Mitoxantrone, I.V., 10-12 mg/m^2, day 1

Repeat cycle every 21 days

Breast Cancer *(continued)*

CFPT

Cyclophosphamide, I.V., 150 mg/m^2, days 1-5
Fluorouracil, I.V., 300 mg/m^2, days 1-5
Prednisone, P.O., 10 mg tid, days 1-7
Tamoxifen, P.O., 10 mg bid, days 1-42

Repeat cycle every 42 days

CMF

Cyclophosphamide, P.O., 100 mg/m^2, days 1-14 or 600 mg/m^2 I.V., days 1, 8
Methotrexate, I.V., 40 mg/m^2, days 1, 8
Fluorouracil, I.V., 600 mg/m^2, days 1, 8

Repeat cycle every 28 days

or

Cyclophosphamide, I.V., 600 mg/m^2, day 1
Methotrexate, I.V., 40 mg/m^2, day 1
Fluorouracil, I.V., 400-600 mg/m^2, day 1

Repeat cycle every 21 days

CMFP

Cyclophosphamide, P.O., 100 mg/m^2, days 1-14
Methotrexate, I.V., 40-60 mg/m^2, days 1, 8
Fluorouracil, I.V., 600-700 mg/m^2, days 1, 8
Prednisone, P.O., 40 mg (first 3 cycles only), days 1-14

Repeat cycle every 28 days

FAC

Fluorouracil, I.V., 500 mg/m^2, days 1, 8
Doxorubicin, I.V., 50 mg/m^2, day 1
Cyclophosphamide, I.V., 500 mg/m^2, day 1

Repeat cycle every 21 days

IMF

Ifosfamide, I.V., 1.5 g/m^2, days 1, 8
Mesna, I.V., 20% of ifosfamide dose, give immediately before and 4 and 8 hours after ifosfamide infusion, days 1, 8
Methotrexate, I.V., 40 mg/m^2, days 1, 8
Fluorouracil, I.V., 600 mg/m^2, days 1, 8

Repeat cycle every 28 days

NFL

Mitoxantrone, I.V., 12 mg/m^2, day 1
Fluorouracil, I.V., 350 mg/m^2, days 1-3, given after leucovorin calcium
Leucovorin calcium, I.V., 300 mg/m^2, days 1-3

or

Mitoxantrone, I.V., 10 mg/m^2, day 1
Fluorouracil, I.V., 1000 mg/m^2 continuous infusion, given after leucovorin calcium, days 1-3
Leucovorin calcium, I.V., 100 mg/m^2, days 1-3

Repeat cycle every 21 days

Sequential Dox-CMF

Doxorubicin, I.V., 75 mg/m^2, every 21 days for 4 cycles followed by 21- or 28-day CMF for 8 cycles

Vinorelbine/Doxorubicin

Vinorelbine, I.V., 25 mg/m^2, days 1, 8
Doxorubicin, I.V., 50 mg/m^2, day 1

Repeat cycle every 21 days

VATH

Vinblastine, I.V., 4.5 mg/m^2, day 1
Doxorubicin, I.V., 45 mg/m^2, day 1
Thiotepa, I.V., 12 mg/m^2, day 1
Fluoxymesterone, P.O., 10 mg tid, days 1-21

Repeat cycle every 21 days

Breast Cancer *(continued)*

Single-Agent Regimens

Anastrozole, P.O., 1 mg qd

Capecitabine, P.O., 2500 mg/m^2/day, bid regimen, days 1-14, repeat cycle every 21 days

Docetaxel, I.V., 60-100 mg/m^2 over 1 hour; patient must be premedicated with dexamethasone 8 mg bid P.O. for 5 days, start 1 day before docetaxel; repeat cycle every 3 weeks

Gemcitabine, I.V., 725 mg/m^2 over 30 minutes, weekly for 3 weeks, followed by 1-week rest, repeat cycle every 28 days

Letrozole, P.O., 2.5 mg qd

Megestrol, P.O., 40 mg qid

Paclitaxel, I.V., 175 mg/m^2 over 3 hours, every 21 days or 250 mg/m^2 over 3-24 hours, every 21 days
Patient must be premedicated with:
Dexamethasone 20 mg P.O., 12 and 6 hours prior
Diphenhydramine 50 mg I.V., 30 minutes prior
Cimetidine 300 mg I.V., or ranitidine 50 mg I.V., 30 minutes prior

Tamoxifen, P.O., 20 mg qd

Toremifene citrate, P.O., 60 mg qd

Vinorelbine, I.V., 30 mg/m^2, every 7 days

Cervical Cancer

CLD-BOMP

Bleomycin, I.V., 5 mg continuous infusion, days 1-7
Cisplatin, I.V., 10 mg/m^2, day 1, 22
Vincristine, I.V., 0.7 mg/m^2, day 7
Mitomycin-C. I.V., 7 mg/m^2, day 7

Repeat cycle every 21 days

MOBP

Bleomycin, I.V., 30 units/day continuous infusion, days 1, 4
Vincristine, I.V., 0.5 mg/m^2, days 1, 4
Mitomycin-C. I.V., 10 mg/m^2, day 1
Cisplatin, I.V., 50 mg/m^2, days 1, 22

Repeat cycle every 28 days

Single-Agent Regimen

Cisplatin, I.V., 50-100 mg/m^2, every 21 days

Colon Cancer

F-CL

Fluorouracil, I.V., 375 mg/m^2, days 1-5
Leucovorin calcium, I.V., 200 mg/m^2, days 1-5

Repeat cycle every 28 days

or

Fluorouracil, I.V., 500 mg/m^2/week 1 hour after initiating the calcium leucovorin infusion for 6 weeks
Leucovorin calcium, I.V., 500 mg/m^2, over 2 hours, weekly for 6 weeks

2-week break, then repeat cycle

FLe

Fluorouracil, I.V., 450 mg/m^2 for 5 days, then, after a pause of 4 weeks, 450 mg/m^2/week for 48 weeks
Levamisole, P.O., 50 mg tid for 3 days, repeated every 2 weeks for 1 year

Colon Cancer *(continued)*

FMV

Fluorouracil, I.V., 10 mg/kg/day, days 1-5
Methyl-CCNU, P.O., 175 mg/m^2, day 1
Vincristine, I.V., 1 mg/m^2 (max: 2 mg), day 1

Repeat cycle every 35 days

FU/LV

Fluorouracil, I.V., 370-400 mg/m^2/day, days 1-5
Leucovorin calcium, I.V., 200 mg/m^2/day, commence infusion 15 minutes prior to fluorouracil infusion, days 1-5

Repeat cycle every 21 days

or

Fluorouracil, I.V., 1000 mg/m^2/day by continuous infusion, days 1-4
Leucovorin calcium, I.V., 200 mg/m^2/day, days 1-4

Repeat cycle every 28 days

Weekly 5FU/LV

Fluorouracil, I.V., 600 mg/m^2 over 1 hour given after leucovorin, repeat weekly x 6 then 2-week rest period = 1 cycle, days 1, 8, 15, 22, 29, 36
Leucovorin calcium, I.V., 500 mg/m^2 over 2 hours, days 1, 8, 15, 22, 29, 36

Repeat cycle every 56 days

5FU/LDLF

Fluorouracil, I.V., 425 mg/m^2/day, days 1-5
Leucovorin calcium, I.V., 20-25 mg/m^2/day, days 1-5

Repeat cycle every 28 days

Single-Agent Regimens

5-FU, I.V., 1000 mg/m^2/day, continuous infusion, days 1-5

Repeat cycle every 21-28 days

Irinotecan, I.V., 125 mg/m^2 over 90 minutes every 7 days for 4 cycles or 350 mg/m^2 over 30 minutes

Repeat cycle every 21 days

Endometrial Cancer

AP

Doxorubicin, I.V., 60 mg/m^2, day 1
Cisplatin, I.V., 60 mg/m^2, day 1

Repeat cycle every 21 days

Single-Agent Regimens

Doxorubicin, I.V., 40-60 mg/m^2, day 1

Repeat cycle every 21-28 days

Medroxyprogesterone, P.O., 200 mg/day

Gastric Cancer

EAP

Etoposide, I.V., 120 mg/m^2, days 4, 5, 6
Doxorubicin, I.V., 20 mg/m^2, days 1, 7
Cisplatin, I.V., 40 mg/m^2, days 2, 8

Repeat cycle every 28 days

ELF

Leucovorin calcium, I.V., 300 mg/m^2, days 1-3 followed by
Etoposide, I.V., 120 mg/m^2, days 1-3 followed by
Fluorouracil, I.V., 500 mg/m^2, days 1-3

Repeat cycle every 21-28 days

Gastric Cancer *(continued)*

FAM

Fluorouracil, I.V., 600 mg/m^2, days 1, 8, 29, 36
Doxorubicin, I.V., 30 mg/m^2, days 1, 29
Mitomycin C, I.V., 10 mg/m^2, day 1

Repeat cycle every 8 weeks

FAME

Fluorouracil, I.V., 350 mg/m^2, days 1-5, 36-40
Doxorubicin, I.V., 40 mg/m^2, days 1, 36
Methyl-CCNU, P.O., 150 mg/m^2, day 1

Repeat cycle every 70 days

FAMTX

Methotrexate, IVPB, 1500 mg/m^2, day 1
Fluorouracil, IVPB, 1500 mg/m^2 1 hour after methotrexate, day 1
Leucovorin calcium, P.O., 15 mg/m^2 q6h x 48 hours, 24 hours after methotrexate, day 2
Doxorubicin, IVPB, 30 mg/m^2, day 15

Repeat cycle every 28 days

FCE

Fluorouracil, I.V., 900 mg/m^2/day continuous infusion, days 1-5
Cisplatin, I.V., 20 mg/m^2, days 1-5
Etoposide, I.V., 90 mg/m^2, days 1, 3, 5

Repeat cycle every 21 days

PFL

Cisplatin, I.V., 25 mg/m^2 continuous infusion, days 1-5
Fluorouracil, I.V., 800 mg/m^2 continuous infusion, days 2-5
Leucovorin calcium, I.V., 500 mg/m^2 continuous infusion, days 1-5

Repeat cycle every 28 days

Single-Agent Regimens

Irinotecan, I.V., over 90 minutes: 125 mg/m^2/week; repeat weekly for 4 weeks, then 2-week rest period

or

Irinotecan, I.V. over 30-90 minutes: 350 mg/m^2; repeat every 21 days

Genitourinary Cancer

Bladder

CAP

Cyclophosphamide, I.V., 400 mg/m^2, day 1
Doxorubicin, I.V., 40 mg/m^2, day 1
Cisplatin, I.V., 60 mg/m^2, day 1

Repeat cycle every 21 days

CISCA

Cisplatin, I.V., 70-100 mg/m^2, day 2
Cyclophosphamide, I.V., 650 mg/m^2, day 1
Doxorubicin, I.V., 50 mg/m^2, day 1

Repeat cycle every 21-28 days

CMV

Cisplatin, I.V., 100 mg/m^2 over 4 hours, start 12 hours after MTX, day 2
Methotrexate, I.V., 30 mg/m^2, days 1, 8
Vinblastine, I.V., 4 mg/m^2, days 1, 8

Repeat cycle every 21 days

Genitourinary Cancer — Bladder *(continued)*

m-PFL

Methotrexate, I.V., 60 mg/m^2, day 1
Cisplatin, I.V., 25 mg/m^2 continuous infusion, days 2-6
Fluorouracil, I.V., 800 mg/m^2 continuous infusion, days 2-6
Leucovorin calcium, I.V., 500 mg/m^2 continuous infusion, days 2-6

Repeat cycle every 28 days for 4 cycles

MVAC

Methotrexate, I.V., 30 mg/m^2, days 1, 15, 22
Vinblastine, I.V., 3 mg/m^2, days 2, 15, 22
Doxorubicin, I.V., 30 mg/m^2, day 2
Cisplatin, I.V., 70 mg/m^2, day 2

Repeat cycle every 28 days

PC

Paclitaxel, I.V., 200 mg/m^2 or 225 mg/m^2 over 3 hours, day 1
Carboplatin, I.V., dose targeted by Calvert equation to AUC 5 or 6 after paclitaxel, day 1

Repeat cycle every 21 days

Single-Agent Regimens

Gemcitabine, I.V., 1200 mg/m^2, days 1, 8, 15

Repeat cycle every 28 days

Paclitaxel, I.V., 250 mg/m^2 over 24 hours, day 1

Repeat cycle every 21 days

Ovarian, Epithelial

Carbo-Tax

Paclitaxel, I.V., 135 mg/m^2 over 24 hours, day 1

or

175 mg/m^2 over 3 hours, day 1, followed by
Carboplatin dose targeted by Calvert equation to AUC 7.5 I.V.

Repeat cycle every 21 days

CC

Carboplatin, I.V., dose targeted by Calvert equation to AUC 6-7
Cyclophosphamide, I.V., 600 mg/m^2, day 1

Repeat cycle every 28 days

CP

Cyclophosphamide, I.V., 750 mg/m^2, day 1
Cisplatin, I.V., 75 mg/m^2, day 1

Repeat cycle every 21 days

CT

Paclitaxel, I.V., 135 mg/m^2 over 24 hours, day 1

or

175 mg/m^2 over 3 hours, day 1, followed by
Cisplatin, I.V., 75 mg/m^2

Repeat cycle every 21 days

PAC (CAP)

Cisplatin, I.V., 50 mg/m^2, day 1
Doxorubicin, I.V., 50 mg/m^2, day 1
Cyclophosphamide, I.V., 750 mg/m^2, day 1

Repeat cycle every 21 days x 8 cycles

Genitourinary Cancer — Ovarian, Epithelial *(continued)*

Single-Agent Regimens

Altretamine, P.O., 260 mg/m^2/day, qid for 14-21 days

Repeat cycle every 28 days

Etoposide, I.V., 50-60 mg/m^2/day, days 1-21

Repeat cycle every 28 days

Liposomal doxorubicin, I.V., 50 mg/m^2, 1-hour infusion, day 1

Repeat cycle every 21 days

Paclitaxel, I.V., 135 mg/m^2, over 3 or 24 hours, day 1

Repeat cycle every 21 days

Topotecan, I.V., 1.5 mg/m^2, over 30 minutes, days 1-5

Repeat cycle every 21 days

Ovarian, Germ Cell

BEP

Bleomycin, I.V., 30 units, days 2, 9, 16
Etoposide, I.V., 100 mg/m^2, days 1-5
Cisplatin, I.V., 20 mg/m^2, days 1-5

VAC

Vincristine, I.V., 1.2-1.5 mg/m^2 (max: 2 mg) weekly for 10-12 weeks, or every 2 weeks for 12 doses
Dactinomycin, I.V., 0.3-0.4 mg/m^2, days 1-5
Cyclophosphamide, I.V., 150 mg/m^2, days 1-5

Repeat every 28 days

Prostate

EV

Estramustine, P.O., 200 mg tid, days 1-42
Vinblastine, I.V., 4 mg/m^2/week, begin day 1

Repeat cycle every 6 weeks

FL

Flutamide, P.O., 250 mg tid, days 1-28
Leuprolide acetate, S.C., 1 mg qd, days 1-28

Repeat cycle every 28 days

or

Flutamide, P.O., 250 mg tid, days 1-28
Leuprolide acetate depot, I.M., 7.5 mg, day 1

Repeat cycle every 28 days

FZ

Flutamide, P.O., 250 mg tid
Goserelin acetate, S.C., 3.6 mg implant, every 28 days or goserelin S.C., 10.8 mg depot every 12 weeks

L-VAM

Leuprolide acetate, S.C., 1 mg qd, days 1-28
Vinblastine, I.V., 1.5 mg/m^2/day continuous infusion, days 2-7
Doxorubicin, I.V., 50 mg/m^2 continuous infusion, day 1
Mitomycin C, I.V., 10 mg/m^2, day 2

Repeat cycle every 28 days

Mitoxantrone/Prednisone

Mitoxantrone, I.V., 12 mg/m^2, day 1
Prednisone, P.O., 5 mg bid

Repeat cycle every 21 days

No Known Acronym

Bicalutamide, P.O., 50 mg/day
Leuprolide acetate depot, I.M., 7.5 mg or goserelin S.C. 3.6 mg implant every 28 days

Genitourinary Cancer — Prostate *(continued)*

PE

Paclitaxel, I.V., 120 mg/m^2, days 1-4
Estramustine, P.O., 600 mg qd, 24 hours before paclitaxel

Repeat cycle every 21 days

Single-Agent Regimens

Estramustine, P.O., 14 mg/kg/day, tid or qid

Goserelin acetate implant, S.C., 3.6 mg every 28 days or 10.8 mg every 12 weeks

Nilutamide, P.O., 300 mg qd, days 1-30, then 150 mg qd in combination with surgical castration; begin on same day or day after castration

Prednisone, P.O., 5 mg bid

Renal

Interleukin-2 (rIL-2), S.C.
20 million units/m^2, days 3-5, weeks 1, 4
5 million units/m^2, days 1, 3, 5, weeks 2, 3, 5, 6

or

Interferon alfa (rIFNα2), S.C.
6 million units/m^2, day 1, weeks 1, 4;
6 million units/m^2, days 1, 3, 5, weeks 2, 3, 5, 6

Repeat cycle every 8 weeks

Single-Agent Regimen

Interleukin-2:
High dose: I.V. bolus over 15 minutes, 600,000-720,000 units/kg q8h until toxicity or 14 days; administer 2 courses separated by 7-10 days
Low dose: S.C., 18 million units/day for 5 days, then 9 million units/day for 2 days, then 18 million units/day 3 days/week for 6 weeks

or

3 million units/m^2/day for 5 days/week, every 2 weeks for 1 month, then every 4 weeks

Testicular

EP

Etoposide, I.V., 100 mg/m^2, days 1-5
Cisplatin, I.V., 20 mg/m^2, days 1-5

Repeat cycle every 21 days

Testicular, Induction, Good Risk

BEP

Bleomycin, I.V., 30 units, days 2, 9, 16
Etoposide, I.V., 100 mg/m^2, days 1-5
Cisplatin, I.V., 20 mg/m^2, days 1-5

Repeat cycle every 21 days

PVB

Cisplatin, I.V., 20 mg/m^2, days 1-5
Vinblastine, I.V., 0.15 mg/kg, days 1, 2
Bleomycin, I.V., 30 units, days 2, 9, 16

Repeat cycle every 21 days

Testicular, Induction, Poor Risk

VIP

Etoposide, I.V., 75 mg/m^2, days 1-5
Ifosfamide, I.V., 1.2 g/m^2, days 1-5
Cisplatin, I.V., 20 mg/m^2, days 1-5
Mesna, I.V., 400 mg/m^2, then 1200 mg/m^2/day continuous infusion, days 1-5

Repeat cycle every 21 days

Genitourinary Cancer — Testicular, Induction, Poor Risk *(continued)*

VIP (Einhorn)

Vinblastine, I.V., 0.11 mg/kg, days 1-2
Ifosfamide, I.V., 1200 mg/m^2, days 1-5
Cisplatin, I.V., 20 mg/m^2, days 1-5
Mesna, I.V., 400 mg/m^2, then 1200 mg/m^2/day continuous infusion, days 1-5

Repeat cycle every 21 days

Testicular, Induction, Salvage

VAB VI

Vinblastine, I.V., 4 mg/m^2, day 1
Dactinomycin, I.V., 1 mg/m^2, day 1
Bleomycin, I.V., 30 units push day 1, then 20 units/m^2/day continuous infusion, days 1-3
Cisplatin, I.V., 120 mg/m^2, day 4
Cyclophosphamide, I.V., 600 mg/m^2, day 1

Repeat cycle every 21 days

VBP (PVB)

Vinblastine, I.V., 6 mg/m^2, days 1, 2
Bleomycin, I.V., 30 units, days 1, 8, 15, (22)
Cisplatin, I.V., 20 mg/m^2, days 1-5

Repeat cycle every 21-28 days

Gestational Trophoblastic Cancer

DMC

Dactinomycin, I.V., 0.37 mg/m^2, days 1-5
Methotrexate, I.V., 11 mg/m^2, days 1-5
Cyclophosphamide, I.V., 110 mg/m^2, days 1-5

Repeat cycle every 21 days

Head and Neck Cancer

CAP

Cyclophosphamide, I.V., 500 mg/m^2, day 1
Doxorubicin, I.V., 50 mg/m^2, day 1
Cisplatin, I.V., 50 mg/m^2, day 1

Repeat cycle every 28 days

CF

Cisplatin, I.V., 100 mg/m^2, day 1
Fluorouracil, I.V., 1000 mg/m^2/day continuous infusion, days 1-5

Repeat cycle every 21-28 days

CF

Carboplatin, I.V., 400 mg/m^2, day 1
Fluorouracil, I.V., 1000 mg/m^2/day continuous infusion, days 1-5

Repeat cycle every 21-28 days

COB

Cisplatin, I.V., 100 mg/m^2, day 1
Vincristine, I.V., 1 mg/m^2, days 2, 5
Bleomycin, I.V., 30 units/day continuous infusion, days 2-5

Repeat cycle every 21 days

Head and Neck Cancer *(continued)*

5-FU HURT

Hydroxyurea, P.O., 1000 mg q12h x 11 doses; start PM of admission, give 2 hours prior to radiation therapy, days 0-5
Fluorouracil, I.V., 800 mg/m^2/day continuous infusion, start AM after admission, days 1-5
Paclitaxel, I.V., 5-25 mg/m^2/day continuous infusion, start AM after admission; dose escalation study – refer to protocol, days 1-5
G-CSF, S.C., 5 mcg/kg/day, days 6-12, start ≥12 hours after completion of 5-FU infusion

5-7 cycles may be administered

PFL

Cisplatin, I.V., 100 mg/m^2, day 1
Fluorouracil, I.V., 600-800 mg/m^2/day continuous infusion, days 1-5
Leucovorin calcium, I.V., 200-300 mg/m^2/day, days 1-5

Repeat cycle every 21 days

PFL+IFN

Cisplatin, I.V., 100 mg/m^2, day 1
Fluorouracil, I.V., 640 mg/m^2/day continuous infusion, days 1-5
Leucovorin calcium, P.O., 100 mg q4h, days 1-5
Interferon alfa-2b, S.C., 2 x 10^6 units/m^2, days 1-6

TIP

Paclitaxel, I.V., 175 mg/m^2 3-hour infusion, day 1
Ifosfamide, I.V., 1000 mg/m^2 2-hour infusion, days 1-3
Mesna, I.V., 400 mg/m^2 before ifosfamide and 200 mg/m^2 I.V., 4 hours after ifosfamide
Cisplatin, I.V., 60 mg/m^2, day 1

Repeat cycle every 21-28 days

Single-Agent Regimens

Carboplatin, I.V., 300-400 mg/m^2, over 2 hours every 21-28 days

Methotrexate, I.V., 40 mg/m^2, every week, escalating day 14 by 5 mg/m^2/week as tolerated

Cisplatin I.V., 100 mg/m^2, every 28 days divided into 1, 2, or 4 equal doses per month

Vinorelbine, I.V., 25-30 mg/m^2, repeat weekly

Leukemia

Acute Lymphoblastic, Induction

VAD

Vincristine, I.V., 0.4 mg continuous infusion, days 1-4
Doxorubicin, I.V., 12 mg/m^2 continuous infusion, days 1-4
Dexamethasone, P.O., 40 mg, days 1-4, 9-12, 17-20

VP

Vincristine, I.V., 2 mg/m^2/week for 4-6 weeks (max: 2 mg)
Prednisone, P.O., 60 mg/m^2/day in divided doses for 4 weeks, taper weeks 5-7

VP-L-Asparaginase

Vincristine, I.V., 2 mg/m^2/week for 4-6 weeks (max: 2 mg)
Prednisone, P.O., 60 mg/m^2/day for 4-6 weeks, then taper
L-asparaginase, I.V., 10,000 units/m^2/day

No Known Acronym

Cyclophosphamide, I.V., 1200 mg/m^2, day 1
Daunorubicin, I.V., 45 mg/m^2, days 1-3
Prednisone, P.O., 60 mg/m^2, days 1-21
Vincristine, I.V., 2 mg/m^2/week
L-asparaginase, I.V., 6000 units/m^2, 3 times/week

or

Pegaspargase, I.M./I.V., 2500 units/m^2, every 14 days if patient develops hypersensitivity to native L-asparaginase

Acute Lymphoblastic, Maintenance

MM

Mercaptopurine, P.O., 50-75 mg/m^2, days 1-7
Methotrexate, P.O./I.V., 20 mg/m^2, day 1

Repeat cycle every 7 days

MMC (MTX + MP + CTX)*

Methotrexate, I.V., 20 mg/m^2/week
Mercaptopurine, P.O., 50 mg/m^2/day
Cyclophosphamide, I.V., 200 mg/m^2/week

*Continue all 3 drugs until relapse of disease or after 3 years of remission.

Acute Lymphoblastic, Relapse

AVDP

Asparaginase, I.V., 15,000 units/m^2, days 1-5, 8-12, 15-19, 22-26
Vincristine, I.V., 2 mg/m^2 (max: 2 mg), days 8, 15, 22
Daunorubicin, I.V., 30-60 mg/m^2, days 8, 15, 22
Prednisone, P.O., 40 mg/m^2, days 8-12, 15-19, 22-26

Acute Myeloid Leukemia, Induction

7+3

Cytarabine, I.V., 100-200 mg/m^2/day continuous infusion, days 1-7

with

Daunorubicin, I.V., 45 mg/m^2, days 1-3

or

Idarubicin, I.V., 12 mg/m^2, days 1-3

or

Mitoxantrone, I.V., 12 mg/m^2, days 1-3

5+2*

Cytarabine, I.V., 100-200 mg/m^2/day continuous infusion, days 1-5

with

Daunorubicin, I.V., 45 mg/m^2, days 1-2

or

Mitoxantrone, I.V., 12 mg/m^2, days 1-2
*For reinduction

D-3+7

Daunorubicin, I.V., 45 mg/m^2, days 1-3
Cytarabine, I.V., 100-200 mg/m^2 continuous infusion, days 1-7

DAT/DCT

Daunorubicin, I.V., 60 mg/m^2/day, days 1-3
Cytarabine, I.V., 200 mg/m^2/day continuous infusion, days 1-5
Thioguanine, P.O., 100 mg/m^2 q12h, days 1-5

Modified DAT (considerations in elderly patients)

Daunorubicin, I.V., 50 mg/m^2, day 1
Cytarabine, S.C., 100 mg/m^2/day q12h, days 1-5
Thioguanine, P.O., 100 mg/m^2 q12h, days 1-5

EMA-86

Etoposide, I.V., 200 mg/m^2/day continuous infusion, days 8-10
Mitoxantrone, I.V., 12 mg/m^2, days 1-3
Cytarabine, I.V., 500 mg/m^2/day continuous infusion, days 1-3, 8-10

I-3+7

Idarubicin, I.V., 12 mg/m^2, days 1-3
Cytarabine, I.V., 100 mg/m^2 continuous infusion, days 1-7

IC

Idarubicin, I.V., 12 mg/m^2/day, days 1-3
Cytarabine, I.V., 100-200 mg/m^2/day continuous infusion, days 1-7

Leukemia — Acute Myeloid Leukemia, Induction *(continued)*

LDAC

Considerations in Elderly Patients

Cytarabine, S.C., 10 mg/m^2 bid, days 10-21

MC

Mitoxantrone, I.V., 12 mg/m^2/day, days 1-3

Cytarabine, I.V., 100-200 mg/m^2/day continuous infusion, days 1-7

Consolidation

Mitoxantrone, I.V., 12 mg/m^2, days 1-2

Cytarabine, I.V., 100 mg/m^2 continuous infusion, days 1-5

Repeat cycle every 28 days

MV

Mitoxantrone, I.V., 10 mg/m^2/day, days 1-5

Etoposide, I.V., 100 mg/m^2/day, days 1-3

Single-Agent Regimen

All transrelincic acid (ATRA), P.O., 45 mg/m^2/day (1 or 2 divided doses) with or without 7+3 induction regimen

Acute Myeloid Leukemia, Postremission

Single-Agent Regimens

Cytarabine, I.V., 100 mg/m^2/day continuous infusion, days 1-5*; repeat cycle every 28 days
*For patients]60 years of age

Cytarabine (HiDAC), I.V. 3000 mg/m^2 over 1-3 hours, every 12 hours, days 1-6

or

3000 mg/m^2 over 1-3 hours, every 12 hours, days 1, 3, 5. Administer with saline, methylcellulose, or steroid eyedrops OU, every 2-4 hours, beginning with cytarabine and continuing 48-72 hours after last cytarabine dose

Repeat cycle every 28 days

Acute Nonlymphoblastic, Consolidation

CD

Cytarabine, I.V., 3000 mg/m^2 q12h, days 1-6

Daunorubicin, I.V., 30 mg/m^2/day, days 7-9

Chronic Lymphocytic Leukemia

CHL + PRED

Chlorambucil, P.O., 0.4 mg/kg/day for 1 day every other week

Prednisone, P.O., 100 mg/day for 2 days every other week; adjust dosage according to blood counts every 2 weeks prior to therapy; increase initial dose of 0.4 mg/kg by 0.1 mg/kg every 2 weeks until toxicity or disease control is achieved

CVP

Cyclophosphamide, P.O., 400 mg/m^2/day, days 1-5

Vincristine, I.V., 1.4 mg/m^2 (max: 2 mg), day 1

Prednisone, P.O., 100 mg/m^2, days 1-5

Repeat cycle every 21 days

Leukemia — Chronic Lymphocytic Leukemia *(continued)*

Single-Agent Regimens

Chlorambucil, P.O., 0.1-0.2 mg/kg/day for 3-6 weeks

or

Chlorambucil, P.O., 20-30 mg/m^2, day 1

Repeat cycle every 14-28 days

Cladribine, I.V., 0.1 mg/kg/day continuous infusion, days 1-5 or 1-7

Repeat cycle every 28-35 days

Cyclophosphamide, P.O., 2-4 mg/kg, days 1-10

Repeat cycle every 21-28 days

Fludarabine, I.V., 25-30 mg/m^2, days 1-5

Repeat cycle every 28 days

Prednisone,* P.O., 30-60 mg/m^2, days 1-5 or 1-7

*Use if patient symptomatic with autoimmune thrombocytopenia or hemolytic anemia.

Chronic Myelogenous Leukemia

Single-Agent Regimens

Busulfan, P.O., 4-8 mg/day

Hydroxyurea, P.O., 2-5 g/day

Interferon alfa-2a, S.C., 3-5 million units/day

Hairy-Cell Leukemia

Single-Agent Regimens

Cladribine, I.V., 0.1 mg/kg/day continuous infusion, days 1-7

Administer one cycle

Interferon alfa-2a, S.C., 3 million units, 3 times/week

Pentostatin, I.V., 4 mg/m^2, day 1

Repeat cycle every 14 days

Lung Cancer

Small Cell

CAV/VAC

Cyclophosphamide, I.V., 750-1000 mg/m^2, day 1
Doxorubicin, I.V., 50 mg/m^2, day 1
Vincristine, I.V., 1.4 mg/m^2 (max: 2 mg), day 1

Repeat cycle every 3 weeks

CAVE

Cyclophosphamide, I.V., 750 mg/m^2, day 1
Doxorubicin, I.V., 50 mg/m^2, day 1
Vincristine, I.V., 1.4 mg/m^2 (max: 2 mg), day 1
Etoposide, I.V., 60-100 mg/m^2, days 1-3

Repeat cycle every 21 days

EC

Etoposide, I.V., 100-120 mg/m^2, days 1-3
Carboplatin, I.V., 325-400 mg/m^2, day 1

Repeat cycle every 28 days

EP/PE

Etoposide, I.V., 120 mg/m^2, days 1-3
Cisplatin, I.V., 60-120 mg/m^2, day 1

Repeat cycle every 21-28 days

Lung Cancer — Small Cell *(continued)*

Single-Agent Regimen

Etoposide, P.O., 50 mg/m^2, days 1-21

Repeat cycle every 28 days

Topotecan, I.V., 1.5 mg/m^2/day, over 30 minutes, days 1-5

Repeat cycle every 21 days

Nonsmall Cell

Carbo-Tax

Paclitaxel, I.V., 135 mg/m^2 over 24 hours, day 1 **or**
175 mg/m^2 over 3 hours, day 1, followed by
Carboplatin dose targeted by Calvert equation to AUC 7.5 I.V.

Repeat cycle every 21 days

EC

Etoposide, I.V., 100-120 mg/m^2, days 1-3

with

Carboplatin, I.V., 300-325 mg/m^2, day 1

Repeat cycle every 21-28 days

EP

Etoposide, I.V., 80 mg/m^2, days 1-3
Cisplatin, I.V., 60-100 mg/m^2, day 1

Repeat cycle every 21-28 days

Gemcitabine-Cis

Gemcitabine, I.V., 1000 mg/m^2, days 1, 8, 15
Cisplatin, I.V., 100 mg/m^2, day 2 or 15

Repeat cycle every 28 days

PC

Paclitaxel, I.V., 175 mg/m^2, 3-hour infusion, day 1
Cisplatin, I.V., 80 mg/m^2, day 1

Repeat cycle every 21 days

Vinorelbine-Cis

Vinorelbine, I.V., 30 mg/m^2, every 7 days
Cisplatin, I.V., 120 mg/m^2, day 1, 29, then every 6 weeks

Single-Agent Regimens

Topotecan, I.V., 1.5 mg/m^2/day, over 30 minutes, days 1-5

Repeat cycle every 21 days

Vinorelbine, I.V., 30 mg/m^2, every 7 days

Lymphoma

Hodgkin's

ABVD

Doxorubicin, I.V., 25 mg/m^2, days 1, 15
Bleomycin, I.V., 10 units/m^2, days 1, 15
Vinblastine, I.V., 6 mg/m^2, days 1, 15
Dacarbazine, I.V., 150 mg/m^2, days 1-5

or

Dacarbazine, I.V., 350-375 mg/m^2, days 1, 15

Repeat cycle every 28 days

Lymphoma — Hodgkin's *(continued)*

ChlVPP

Chlorambucil, P.O., 6 mg/m^2 (max: 10 mg/day), days 1-14
Vinblastine, I.V., 6 mg/m^2 (max: 10 mg dose), days 1, 8
Procarbazine, P.O., 100 mg/m^2 (max: 150 mg/day), days 1-14
Prednisone, P.O., 40 mg/day, days 1-14

Repeat cycle every 28 days

CVPP

Lomustine, P.O., 75 mg/m^2, day 1
Vinblastine, I.V., 4 mg/m^2, days 1, 8
Procarbazine, P.O., 100 mg/m^2, days 1-14
Prednisone, P.O., 30 mg/m^2, days 1-14 (cycles 1 and 4 only)

Repeat cycle every 28 days

DHAP

Dexamethasone, P.O./I.V., 40 mg, days 1-4
Cytarabine, I.V., 2 g/m^2, q12h for 2 doses, day 2
Cisplatin, I.V., 100 mg/m^2 continuous infusion, day 1

Repeat cycle every 3-4 weeks

EVA

Etoposide, I.V., 100 mg/m^2, days 1-3
Vinblastine, I.V., 6 mg/m^2, day 1
Doxorubicin, I.V., 50 mg/m^2, day 1

Repeat cycle every 28 days

MOPP

Mechlorethamine, I.V., 6 mg/m^2, days 1, 8
Vincristine, I.V., 1.4 mg/m^2 (max: 2.5 mg), days 1, 8
Procarbazine, P.O., 100 mg/m^2, days 1-14
Prednisone, P.O., 40 mg/m^2 (cycles 1 and 4 only), days 1-14

Repeat cycle every 28 days

MOPP/ABV Hybrid

Mechlorethamine, I.V., 6 mg/m^2, day 1
Vincristine, I.V., 1.4 mg/m^2 (max: 2 mg), day 1
Procarbazine, P.O., 100 mg/m^2, days 1-7
Prednisone, P.O., 40 mg/m^2, days 1-14
Doxorubicin, I.V., 35 mg/m^2, day 8
Bleomycin, I.V., 10 units/m^2, day 8
Vinblastine, I.V., 6 mg/m^2, day 8

Repeat cycle every 28 days

MVPP

Mechlorethamine, I.V., 6 mg/m^2, days 1, 8
Vinblastine, I.V., 6 mg/m^2, days 1, 8
Procarbazine, P.O., 100 mg/m^2, days 1-14
Prednisone, P.O., 40 mg/m^2, days 1-14

Repeat cycle every 42 days

NOVP

Mitoxantrone, I.V., 10 mg/m^2, day 1
Vincristine, I.V., 2 mg, day 8
Vinblastine, I.V., 6 mg/m^2, day 1
Prednisone, P.O., 100 mg/m^2, days 1-5

Repeat cycle every 21 days

Lymphoma — Hodgkin's *(continued)*

Stanford V*

Mechlorethamine, I.V., 6 mg/m^2, day 1
Doxorubicin, I.V., 25 mg/m^2, days 1, 15
Vinblastine, I.V., 6 mg/m^2, days 1, 15
Vincristine, I.V., 1.4 mg/m^2, days 8, 22
Bleomycin, I.V., 5 units/m^2, days 8, 22
Etoposide, I.V., 60 mg/m^2, days 15, 16
Prednisone, P.O., 40 mg/m^2/day, dose tapered over the last 15 days

Repeat cycle every 28 days

*In patients older than 50 years of age, vinblastine dose decreased to 4 mg/m^2 and vincristine dose decreased to 1 mg/m^2 on weeks 9-12. Concomitant trimethoprim/sulfamethoxazole DS P.O. bid; acyclovir 200 mg P.O. tid; ketoconazole 200 mg P.O. qd and stool softeners used.

Non-Hodgkin's

BACOP

Bleomycin, I.V., 5 units/m^2, days 15, 22
Doxorubicin, I.V., 25 mg/m^2, days 1, 8
Cyclophosphamide, I.V., 650 mg/m^2, days 1, 8
Vincristine, I.V., 1.4 mg/m^2 (max: 2 mg), days 1, 8
Prednisone, P.O., 60 mg/m^2, days 15-28

Repeat cycle every 28 days

CHOP

Cyclophosphamide, I.V., 750 mg/m^2, day 1
Doxorubicin, I.V., 50 mg/m^2, day 1
Vincristine, I.V., 1.4 mg/m^2 (max: 2 mg), day 1
Prednisone, P.O., 100 mg/m^2, days 1-5

Repeat cycle every 21 days

CHOP-Bleo

Cyclophosphamide, I.V., 750 mg/m^2, day 1
Doxorubicin, I.V., 50 mg/m^2, day 1
Vincristine, I.V., 2 mg, days 1, 5
Prednisone, P.O., 100 mg, days 1-5
Bleomycin, I.V., 15 units, days 1, 5

Repeat cycle every 21-28 days

CNOP

Cyclophosphamide, I.V., 750 mg/m^2, day 1
Mitoxantrone, I.V., 10 mg/m^2, day 1
Vincristine, I.V., 1.4 mg/m^2, day 1
Prednisone, P.O., 50 mg/m^2, days 1-5

Repeat cycle every 21 days

COMLA

Cyclophosphamide, I.V., 1500 mg/m^2, day 1
Vincristine, I.V., 1.4 mg/m^2 (max: 2.5 mg), days 1, 8, 15
Methotrexate, I.V., 120 mg/m^2, days 22, 29, 36, 43, 50, 57, 64, 71
Leucovorin calcium rescue, P.O., 25 mg/m^2, q6h for 4 doses, beginning 24 hours after each methotrexate dose
Cytarabine, I.V., 300 mg/m^2, days 22, 29, 36, 43, 50, 57, 64, 71

Repeat cycle every 21 days

COP

Cyclophosphamide, I.V., 800 mg/m^2, day 1
Vincristine, I.V., 1.4 mg/m^2 (max: 2 mg), day 1
Prednisone, P.O., 60 mg/m^2, days 1-5

Repeat cycle every 21 days

Lymphoma — Non-Hodgkin's *(continued)*

COP-BLAM

Cyclophosphamide, I.V., 400 mg/m^2, day 1
Vincristine, I.V., 1 mg/m^2, day 1
Prednisone, P.O., 40 mg/m^2, days 1-10
Bleomycin, I.V., 15 mg, day 14
Doxorubicin, I.V., 40 mg/m^2, day 1
Procarbazine, P.O., 100 mg/m^2, days 1-10

COPP (or "C" MOPP)

Cyclophosphamide, I.V., 400-650 mg/m^2, days 1, 8
Vincristine, I.V., 1.4-1.5 mg/m^2 (max: 2 mg), days 1, 8
Procarbazine, P.O., 100 mg/m^2, days 1-14
Prednisone, P.O., 40 mg/m^2, days 1-14

Repeat cycle every 28 days

CVP

Cyclophosphamide, P.O., 400 mg/m^2, days 1-5
Vincristine, I.V., 1.4 mg/m^2 (max: 2 mg), day 1
Prednisone, P.O., 100 mg/m^2, days 1-5

Repeat cycle every 21 days

DHAP*

Dexamethasone, I.V., 10 mg q6h, days 1-4
Cytarabine, I.V., 2 g/m^2 q12h x 2 doses, day 2
Cisplatin, I.V., 100 mg/m^2 continuous infusion, day 1

Repeat cycle every 21-28 days

*Administer with saline, methylcellulose, or steroid eyedrops OU, every 2-4 hours, beginning with cytarabine and continuing 48-72 hours after last cytarabine dose.

ESHAP*

Etoposide, I.V., 60 mg/m^2, days 1-4
Cisplatin, I.V., 25 mg/m^2 continuous infusion, days 1-4
Cytarabine, I.V., 2 g/m^2, immediately following completion of etoposide and cisplatin therapy
Methylprednisolone, I.V., 500 mg/day, days 1-4

Repeat cycle every 21-28 days

*Administer with saline, methylcellulose, or steroid eyedrops OU, every 2-4 hours, beginning with cytarabine and continuing 48-72 hours after last cytarabine dose.

IMVP-16

Ifosfamide, I.V., 4 g/m^2 continuous infusion over 24 hours, day 1
Mesna, I.V., 800 mg/m^2 bolus prior to ifosfamide, then 4 g/m^2 continuous infusion over 12 hours concurrent w/ifosfamide; then 2.4 g/m^2 continuous infusion over 12 hours after ifosfamide infusion, day 1
Methotrexate, I.V., 30 mg/m^2, days 3, 10
Etoposide, I.V., 100 mg/m^2, days 1-3

Repeat cycle every 21-28 days

MACOP-B

Methotrexate, I.V., 400 mg/m^2, weeks 2, 6, 10
Doxorubicin, I.V., 50 mg/m^2, weeks 1, 3, 5, 7, 9, 11
Cyclophosphamide, I.V., 350 mg/m^2, weeks 1, 3, 5, 7, 9, 11
Vincristine, I.V., 1.4 mg/m^2 (max: 2 mg), weeks 2, 4, 8, 10, 12
Bleomycin, I.V., 10 units/m^2, weeks 4, 8, 12
Prednisone, P.O., 75 mg/day tapered over 15 d, days 1-15
Leucovorin calcium, P.O., 15 mg/m^2, q6h x 6 doses 24 hours after methotrexate, weeks 2, 6, 10
Trimethoprim/sulfamethoxazole DS, P.O., tablet, bid, for 12 weeks
Ketoconazole, P.O., 200 mg/day

Administer one cycle

Lymphoma — Non-Hodgkin's *(continued)*

m-BACOD

Methotrexate, I.V., 200 mg/m^2, days 8, 15

Leucovorin calcium, P.O., 10 mg/m^2 q6h x 8 doses beginning 24 hours after each methotrexate dose, days 8, 15

Bleomycin, I.V., 4 units/m^2, day 1

Doxorubicin, I.V., 45 mg/m^2, day 1

Cyclophosphamide, I.V., 600 mg/m^2, day 1

Vincristine, I.V., 1 mg/m^2, day 1

Dexamethasone, P.O., 6 mg/m^2, days 1-5

Repeat cycle every 21 days

m-BACOS

Methotrexate, I.V., 1 g/m^2, day 2

Bleomycin, I.V., 10 units/m^2, day 1

Doxorubicin, I.V., 50 mg/m^2 continuous infusion, day 1

Cyclophosphamide, I.V., 750 mg/m^2, day 1

Vincristine, I.V., 1.4 mg/m^2 (max: 2 mg), day 1

Leucovorin calcium rescue, P.O., 15 mg q6h for 8 doses, starting 24 hours after methotrexate

Methylprednisolone, I.V., 500 mg, days 1-3

Repeat cycle every 21-25 days

MINE

Mesna, I.V., 1.33 g/m^2/day concurrent with ifosfamide dose, then 500 mg P.O. 4 hours after each ifosfamide infusion, days 1-3

Ifosfamide, I.V., 1.33 g/m^2/day, days 1-3

Mitoxantrone, I.V., 8 mg/m^2, day 1

Etoposide, I.V., 65 mg/m^2/day, days 1-3

Repeat cycle every 28 days

MINE-ESHAP

Mesna, I.V., 1.33 g/m^2, administered at same time as ifosfamide, then 500 mg P.O., 4 hours after ifosfamide, days 1-3

Ifosfamide, I.V., 1.33 g/m^2, over 1 hour, days 1-3

Mitoxantrone, I.V., 8 mg/m^2, day 1

Etoposide, I.V., 65 mg/m^2, days 1-3

Repeat cycle every 21 days for 6 cycles, followed by 3-6 cycles of ESHAP

NOVP

Mitoxantrone, I.V., 10 mg/m^2, day 1

Vinblastine, I.V., 6 mg/m^2, day 1

Prednisone, P.O., 100 mg, days 1-5

Vincristine, I.V., 2 mg, day 8

Repeat cycle every 21 days

Pro-MACE

Prednisone, P.O., 60 mg/m^2, days 1-14

Methotrexate, I.V., 1.5 g/m^2, day 14

Leucovorin calcium, I.V., 50 mg/m^2 q6h x 5 doses beginning 24 hours after methotrexate dose, day 14

Doxorubicin, I.V., 25 mg/m^2, days 1, 8

Cyclophosphamide, I.V., 650 mg/m^2, days 1, 8

Etoposide, I.V., 120 mg/m^2, days 1, 8

Repeat cycle every 28 days

Lymphoma — Non-Hodgkin's *(continued)*

Pro-MACE-CytaBOM

Prednisone, P.O., 60 mg/m^2, days 1-14
Doxorubicin, I.V., 25 mg/m^2, day 1
Cyclophosphamide, I.V., 650 mg/m^2, day 1
Etoposide, I.V., 120 mg/m^2, day 1
Cytarabine, I.V., 300 mg/m^2, day 8
Bleomycin, I.V., 5 units/m^2, day 8
Vincristine, I.V., 1.4 mg/m^2 (max: 2 mg), day 8
Methotrexate, I.V., 120 mg/m^2, day 8
Leucovorin calcium, P.O., 25 mg/m^2 q6h x 4 doses, day 9
Concomitant trimethoprim/sulfamethoxazole DS, P.O., bid

Repeat cycle every 21-28 days

Single-Agent Regimens

CDA cladribine, S.C., 0.1 mg/kg/day for 5 days or 0.1 mg/kg/day I.V., for 7 days

Repeat cycle every 28 days

Rituximab, I.V., 375 mg/m^2, days 1, 8, 15, 22

Malignant Melanoma

CVD

Cisplatin, I.V., 20 mg/m^2, days 1-5
Vinblastine, I.V., 1.6 mg/m^2, days 1-5
Dacarbazine, I.V., 800 mg/m^2, day 1

Repeat cycle every 21 days

CVD + IL-21

Cisplatin, I.V., 20 mg/m^2/day, days 1-4
Vinblastine, I.V., 1.6 mg/m^2/day, days 1-4
Dacarbazine, I.V., 800 mg/m^2, day 1
IL-2, I.V., 9 million units/m^2 continuous infusion, days 1-4
Interferon alfa, S.C., 5 million units/m^2, every day, days 1-5, 7, 9, 11, 13

Repeat cycle every 21 days

Dacarbazine/Tamoxifen

Dacarbazine, I.V., 250 mg/m^2, days 1-5, every 21 days
Tamoxifen,* P.O., 20 mg/day

No Known Acronym

Dacarbazine, I.V., 220 mg/m^2, days 1-3, every 21-28 days
Carmustine, I.V., 150 mg/m^2, day 1, every 42-56 days
Cisplatin, I.V., 25 mg/m^2, days 1-3, every 21-28 days
Tamoxifen,* P.O., 20 mg/day

*Use of tamoxifen is optional.

Single-Agent Regimens

Interferon alfa-2b adjuvant therapy, I.M., 20 million units/m^2, days 1-30, **then**

10 million units/m^2 S.C., 3 times/week for 48 weeks

Interferon alfa-2a, I.M., 20 million units/m^2 3 times/week for 12 weeks

Multiple Myeloma

EDAP

Etoposide, I.V., 100-200 mg/m^2, days 1-4
Dexamethasone, P.O./I.V., 40 mg/m^2, days 1-5
Cytarabine, 1000 mg, day 5
Cisplatin, I.V., 20 mg continuous infusion, days 1-4

Multiple Myeloma *(continued)*

MP

Melphalan, P.O., 8-10 mg/m^2, days 1-4
Prednisone, P.O., 40-60 mg/m^2/day, days 1-4

Repeat cycle every 28-42 days

M-2

Vincristine, I.V., 0.03 mg/kg (max: 2 mg), day 1
Carmustine, I.V., 0.5-1 mg/kg, day 1
Cyclophosphamide, I.V., 10 mg/kg, day 1
Melphalan, P.O., 0.25 mg/kg, days 1-4 or 0.1 mg/kg, days 1-7 or 1-10
Prednisone, P.O., 1 mg/kg/day, days 1-7

Repeat cycle every 35-42 days

VAD

Vincristine, I.V., 0.4 mg/day continuous infusion, days 1-4
Doxorubicin, I.V., 9 mg/m^2/day continuous infusion, days 1-4
Dexamethasone, P.O., 40 mg, days 1-4, 9-12, 17-20

Repeat cycle every 28-35 days

VAD induction therapy followed by maintenance
Interferon alfa, S.C., 3 million units/m^2, 3 times/week
Prednisone, P.O., 50 mg, 3 times/week, after interferon

VBAP

Vincristine, I.V., 1 mg, day 1
Carmustine, I.V., 30 mg/m^2, day 1
Doxorubicin, I.V., 30 mg/m^2, day 1
Prednisone, P.O., 100 mg, days 1-4

Repeat cycle every 21 days

VBMCP

Vincristine, I.V., 1.2 mg/m^2, day 1
Carmustine, I.V., 20 mg/m^2, day 1
Melphalan, P.O., 8 mg/m^2, days 1-4
Cyclophosphamide, I.V., 400 mg/m^2, day 1
Prednisone, P.O., 40 mg/m^2, days 1-7 all cycles, and 20 mg/m^2, days 8-14 first 3 cycles only

Repeat cycle every 35 days

VCAP

Vincristine, I.V., 1 mg, day 1
Cyclophosphamide, P.O., 100 mg/m^2, days 1-4
Doxorubicin, I.V., 25 mg/m^2, day 2
Prednisone, P.O., 60 mg/m^2, days 1-4

Repeat cycle every 28 days

Single-Agent Regimens

Aldesleukin, 600,000-700,000 int. units/kg every 8 hours x 14 doses

Repeat cycle every 14 days

Dexamethasone, P.O., 20 mg/m^2 for 4 days beginning on days 1-4, 9-12, and 17-20

Repeat cycle every 35 days

Interferon alfa-2b, S.C., 2 million units/m^2, 3 times/week for maintenance therapy in selected patients with significant response to initial chemotherapy treatment

Melphalan, I.V., 90-140 mg/m^2

Administer one cycle

Pancreatic Cancer

FAM

Fluorouracil, I.V., 600 mg/m^2, days 1, 8, 29, 36
Doxorubicin, I.V., 30 mg/m^2, days 1, 29
Mitomycin, I.V., 10 mg/m^2, day 1

Repeat cycle every 72 days

SMF

Streptozocin, I.V., 1000 mg/m^2, days 1, 8, 29, 36
Mitomycin, I.V., 10 mg/m^2, day 1
Fluorouracil, I.V., 600 mg/m^2, days 1, 8, 29, 36

Repeat cycle every 72 days

Single-Agent Regimens

Gemcitabine, I.V., 1000 mg/m^2 over 30 minutes once weekly for 7 weeks, followed by a 1-week rest period; subsequent cycles once weekly for 3 consecutive weeks out of every 4 weeks

Sarcoma

AC

Doxorubicin, I.V., 75-90 mg/m^2 96-hour continuous infusion
Cisplatin, I.A./I.V., 90-120 mg/m^2, 6 days

Repeat cycle every 28 days

AD

Doxorubicin, I.V., 22.5 mg/m^2/day continuous infusion, days 1-4
Dacarbazine, I.V., 225 mg/m^2/day continuous infusion, days 1-4

Repeat cycle every 21 days

CYVADIC

Cyclophosphamide, I.V., 500 mg/m^2, day 1
Vincristine, I.V., 1.4 mg/m^2, days 1, 5
Doxorubicin, I.V., 50 mg/m^2, day 1
Dacarbazine, I.V., 250 mg/m^2, days 1-5

Repeat cycle every 21 days

DI

Doxorubicin, I.V., 50 mg/m^2 bolus, day 1
Ifosfamide, I.V., 5000 mg/m^2/day continuous infusion, following doxorubicin, day 1
Mesna, I.V., 600 mg/m^2, bolus before ifosfamide, followed by 2500 mg/m^2/day, continuous infusion, for 36 hours

Repeat cycle every 21 days

HDMTX

Methotrexate, I.V., 8-12 g/m^2
Leucovorin calcium, P.O./I.V., 15-25 mg q6h for at least 10 doses beginning 24 hours after methotrexate dose; courses repeated weekly for 2-4 weeks, alternating with various cancer chemotherapy combination regimens

IE

Etoposide, I.V., 100 mg/m^2, days 1-5
Ifosfamide, I.V., 1800 mg/m^2, days 1-5
Mesna, I.V., at 20% of ifosfamide dose prior to and 4 and 8 hours after ifosfamide administration

Repeat cycle every 21-28 days

MAID

Mesna, I.V., 2500 mg/m^2/day continuous infusion, days 1-4
Doxorubicin, I.V., 15 mg/m^2/day continuous infusion, days 1-4
Ifosfamide, I.V., 2500 mg/m^2/day continuous infusion, days 1-3
Dacarbazine, I.V., 250 mg/m^2/day continuous infusion, days 1-4

Repeat cycle every 21-28 days

Sarcoma *(continued)*

VAC

Vincristine, I.V., 2 mg/m^2/week (max: 2 mg), during weeks 1-12
Dactinomycin, I.V., 0.015 mg/kg (max: 0.5 mg) every 3 months for 5-6 courses, days 1-5
Cyclophosphamide, P.O., 2.5 mg/kg/day for 2 years

Single-Agent Regimens

Doxorubicin, I.V., 75 mg/m^2, day 1

Repeat cycle every 21 days

PEDIATRIC REGIMENS

Small patients have a large body surface area relative to their kg weight and could possibly be overdosed if a m^2 dosing regimen is applied. Therefore, for calculating pediatric doses of chemotherapy agents, as a general rule a child who weighs 30 kg is ~1 m^2. **For children weighing <15 kg or with surface area <0.6 m^2**, the dose per m^2 of an agent listed herein should be divided by 30 and multiplied by the weight of the child (in kg) to obtain the correct dose.

ALL, Consolidation

IDMTX/6-MP

Methotrexate, I.V. push, 200 mg/m^2, then 800 mg/m^2 as a 24-hour infusion
Mercaptopurine, I.V., 200 mg/m^2 over 20 minutes, then 800 mg/m^2 as an 8-hour infusion
Leucovorin, P.O./I.V., 15 mg/m^2 q6h x 9; begin 24 hours after end of methotrexate

ALL, Continuation

MTX/6-MP

Methotrexate, I.M., 20 mg/m^2/week, during weeks 25-130
Mercaptopurine, P.O., 50 mg/m^2/day, during weeks 25-130

MTX/6-MP/VP

Methotrexate, P.O., 20 mg/m^2/week
Mercaptopurine, P.O., 75 mg/m^2/day
Vincristine, I.V., 1.5 mg/m^2 x 1 each month
Prednisone, P.O., 40 mg/m^2 x 5 days each month

ALL, Induction

PVD

Prednisone, P.O., 40 mg/m^2/day x 28 days
Vincristine, I.V., 1.5 mg/m^2/week x 4
Asparaginase, I.M., 5000 int. units/m^2 on days 2, 5, 8, 12, 15, 18

PVDA

Prednisone, P.O., 40 mg/m^2, days 1-28
Vincristine, I.V., 1.5 mg/m^2, days 2, 8, 15, 22
Daunorubicin, I.V., 25 mg/m^2, days 2, 8, 15, 22
Asparaginase, I.M., 5000 int. units/m^2 on days 2, 5, 8, 12, 15, 19

TIT (CNS Prophylaxis)

Methotrexate: 1 y: 10 mg; 2 y: 12.5 mg; ≥3 y: 15 mg
Cytarabine: 1 y: 20 mg; 2 y: 25 mg; ≥3 y: 30 mg
Hydrocortisone: 1 y: 10 mg; 2 y: 12.5 mg; ≥3 y: 15 mg

AML, Induction

CA

Cytarabine, I.V., 3 g/m^2, q12h for 4 doses
Asparaginase, I.M., 6000 int. units/m^2 3 hours after last dose of cytarabine

DA

Daunorubicin, I.V., 45 mg/m^2, days 1-3
Cytarabine, I.V., 100 mg/m^2/day, continuous infusion, days 1-7

DAT

Daunorubicin, I.V., 45 mg/m^2/day continuous infusion, days 1-3
Cytarabine, I.V., 100 mg/m^2/day continuous infusion, days 1-7
Thioguanine, P.O., 100 mg/m^2, days 1-7

DAV

Daunorubicin, I.V., 60 mg/m^2, days 3, 4, 5
Cytarabine, I.V., 100 mg/m^2 continuous infusion, days 1-2, then 30-minute infusion q12h on days 3-8
Etoposide, I.V., 150 mg/m^2, days 6, 7, 8

HI-CDAZE

Daunorubicin, I.V., 30 mg/m^2, days 1-3
Cytarabine, I.V., 3 g/m^2, q12h, days 1-4
Etoposide, I.V., 200 mg/m^2, days 1-3, 6-8
Azacytidine, I.V., 150 mg/m^2, days 3-5, 8-10

Brain Tumors

CDDP/VP

Cisplatin, I.V., 90 mg/m^2, day 1
Etoposide, I.V., 150 mg/m^2, days 3, 4

Repeat cycle every 21 days

CDDP/VP-16

Cisplatin, I.V., 90 mg/m^2, day 1
Etoposide, I.V., 150 mg/m^2, days 3, 4

Repeat cycle every 21 days

COPE or "Baby Brain I"

Cycle A:
Vincristine, I.V., 0.065 mg/kg (max: 1.5 mg), days 1, 8
Cyclophosphamide, I.V., 65 mg/kg, day 1
Cycle B:
Cisplatin, I.V., 4 mg/m^2, day 1
Etoposide, I.V., 6.5 mg/kg, days 3, 4

Regimens given in alternating 28-day cycles in the sequence AABAAB

MOP

Mechlorethamine (nitrogen mustard), I.V., 6 mg/m^2, days 1, 8
Vincristine, I.V., 1.4 mg/m^2, days 1, 8
Procarbazine, P.O., 100 mg/m^2, days 1-14

MOPP

Mechlorethamine (nitrogen mustard), I.V., 3 mg/m^2, days 1, 8
Vincristine, I.V., 1.4 mg/m^2, days 1, 8
Procarbazine, P.O., 50 mg on day 1, 100 mg on day 2, then 100 mg/m^2 on days 3-10
Prednisone, P.O., 40 mg/m^2, days 1-10

Repeat cycle every 28 days

PCV

Procarbazine, P.O., 60 mg/m^2, days 18-21
Methyl-CCNU, P.O., 110 mg/m^2, day 1
Vincristine, I.V., 1.4 mg/m^2, days 8 and 29

Brain Tumors *(continued)*

POC

Prednisone, P.O., 40 mg/m^2, days 1-14
CCNU, P.O., 100 mg/m^2, day 1
Vincristine, I.V., 1.5 mg/m^2, days 1, 8, 15

"8 in 1"

Methylprednisolone, P.O., 300 mg/m^2 for 3 doses q6h
Vincristine, I.V., 1.5 mg/m^2
Lomustine, P.O., 100 mg/m^2
Procarbazine, P.O., 75 mg/m^2
Hydroxyurea, P.O., 3000 mg/m^2
Cisplatin, I.V., 90 mg/m^2
Cytarabine, I.V., 300 mg/m^2
Dacarbazine, I.V., 150 mg/m^2

Repeat cycle every 14 days

Single-Agent Regimen

Carboplatin, I.V., 560 mg/m^2, every 4 weeks

Lymphoma

ABVD

Doxorubicin, I.V., 25 mg/m^2, days 1, 15
Bleomycin, I.V., 10 units/m^2, days 1, 15
Vinblastine, I.V., 6 mg/m^2, days 1, 15
Dacarbazine (DTIC), I.V., 375 mg/m^2, days 1, 15

Repeat cycle every 28 days

CHOP

Cyclophosphamide, I.V., 750 mg/m^2, days 1, 22
Doxorubicin, I.V., 40 mg/m^2, days 1, 22
Vincristine, I.V., 1.5 mg/m^2/week for 6 doses
Prednisone, P.O., 40 mg/m^2/day, for 28 days

COMP

Cyclophosphamide, I.V., 1.2 g/m^2, day 1
Vincristine, I.V., 2 mg/m^2, days 3, 10, 17, 24
Methotrexate, I.V., 300 mg/m^2, day 12
Prednisone, P.O., 60 mg/m^2, days 3-30, then taper for 7 days (max: 60 mg)

COPP

Cyclophosphamide, I.V., 500 mg/m^2, days 1, 8
Vincristine, I.V., 1.5 mg/m^2, days 1, 8
Procarbazine, P.O., 100 mg/m^2 (max: 150 mg), days 1-14
Prednisone, P.O., 40 mg/m^2, days 1-14

MOPP

Mechlorethamine (nitrogen mustard), I.V., 6 mg/m^2, days 1, 8
Vincristine, I.V., 1.4 mg/m^2, days 1, 8
Procarbazine, P.O., 50 mg, day 1, then 100 mg/m^2, days 2-14
Prednisone, P.O., 40 mg/m^2, days 1-14 in courses 1 and 4 only

OPA

Vincristine, I.V., 1.5 mg/m^2, days 1, 8, 15
Prednisone, P.O., 60 mg/m^2, days 1-15
Doxorubicin, I.V., 40 mg/m^2, days 1, 15

Lymphoma *(continued)*

OPPA

Vincristine, I.V., 1.5 mg/m^2, days 1, 8, 15
Procarbazine, P.O., 100 mg/m^2, days 1-15
Prednisone, P.O., 60 mg/m^2, days 1-15
Doxorubicin, I.V., 40 mg/m^2, days 1, 15

Repeat cycle every 28 days

Burkitt's Lymphoma

Advanced Stage Burkitt's/B-cell ALL

Methotrexate, I.T., 10 mg/m^2 at hour 0
Cytarabine, I.T., 50 mg/m^2 at hour 0
Cyclophosphamide, I.V., 300 mg/m^2 q12h x 6 at hours 0-60
Vincristine, I.V., 1.5 mg/m^2 at hour 72
Doxorubicin, I.V., 50 mg/m^2 at hour 72

Followed after hematopoietic recovery by:

Methotrexate, I.T., 12 mg/m^2 at hour 0
Methotrexate, I.V. push, 200 mg/m^2, then 800 mg/m^2 as a 24-hour infusion from hours 0-24
Cytarabine, I.T., 50 mg/m^2 at hour 24
Cytarabine, I.V., 400 mg/m^2 over 48 hours from hours 24-72, with escalating doses in succeeding courses
Leucovorin, I.V., 30 mg/m^2 at hours 36 and 42, then 3 mg/m^2 at hours 54, 66, 78

Neuroblastoma

Cy/A

Cyclophosphamide, P.O., 150 mg/m^2/day x 7 days
Doxorubicin, I.V., 35 mg/m^2 on day 8

Pt/VM

Cisplatin, I.V., 90 mg/m^2 over 6 hours
Teniposide, I.V., 100 mg/m^2, 48 hours after completion of cisplatin

Osteosarcoma

HDMTX

Methotrexate, I.V., 12 g/m^2/week for 2-12 weeks
Leucovorin calcium rescue, P.O./I.V., 15 mg/m^2 q6h for 10 doses beginning 30 hours after the beginning of the 4-hour methotrexate infusion (serum methotrexate levels must be monitored)

IFoVP

Ifosfamide, I.V., 1800 mg/m^2, days 1-5
Etoposide, I.V., 100 mg/m^2, days 1-5
Mesna uroprotection, I.V., 2880 mg/m^2, days 1-5

Repeat cycle every 21 days

MTX-CDDPAdr

Methotrexate, I.V., 12 g/m^2/week for 2 weeks
Leucovorin calcium rescue, I.V., 20 mg/m^2 q3h for 8 doses beginning 16 hours after completion of methotrexate, then q6h P.O. for 8 doses

alternating with

Cisplatin, I.V., 75 mg/m^2, day 15 of cycles 1-7, then 120 mg/m^2 for cycles 8-10
Doxorubicin, I.V., 25 mg/m^2, days 15, 16, 17 of cycles 1-7

Sarcoma (Bony and Soft Tissue)

ICE

Ifosfamide, I.V., 1500 mg/m^2, days 1-3 (with mesna uroprotection)
Carboplatin, I.V., 635 mg/m^2, day 3
Etoposide, I.V., 100 mg/m^2, days 1, 2, 3

Sarcoma (Bony and Soft Tissue) *(continued)*

Topo/CTX

Cyclophosphamide, I.V., 250 mg/m^2 on days 1-5, followed by
Topotecan, I.V., 0.75 mg/m^2 on days 1-5

VACAdr

Vincristine, I.V., 1.5 mg/m^2/week for 6 weeks
Cyclophosphamide, I.V., 500 mg/m^2/week for 6 weeks
Doxorubicin, I.V., 60 mg/m^2, week 6

6-week rest period, then

Dactinomycin, I.V., 15 mcg/kg/day, for 5 days, followed 9 days later by
Vincristine + cyclophosphamide as above, given weekly for 5 weeks, and with
Doxorubicin given with the last treatment

or

Vincristine, I.V., 1.4 mg/m^2, day 1
Doxorubicin, I.V., 50 mg/m^2, day 1
Cyclophosphamide, I.V., 750 mg/m^2, day 1

VAC

Vincristine, I.V., 2 mg/m^2, day 1
Dactinomycin, I.V., 1 mg/m^2, day 1
Cyclophosphamide, I.V., 600 mg/m^2, day 1

or

Vincristine, I.V., 1.5 mg/m^2, day 1
Dactinomycin, I.V., 25 mcg/kg, day 1
Cyclophosphamide, I.V., 1.5 g/m^2, day 1

Repeat cycle every 21 days

VACAdr-IfoVP

Vincristine, I.V., 1.5 mg/m^2 (max: 2 mg), weekly
Dactinomycin, I.V., 1.5 mg/m^2 (max: 2 mg), every other week
Doxorubicin, I.V., 60 mg/m^2 continuous infusion over 24 hours
Cyclophosphamide, I.V., 1-1.5 g/m^2
Ifosfamide, I.V., 1.6-2 g/m^2, days 1-5
Etoposide, I.V., 150 mg/m^2, days 1-5

VAdrC

Vincristine, I.V., 1.5 mg/m^2 (max: 2 mg)
Doxorubicin, I.V., 35-60 mg/m^2
Cyclophosphamide, I.V., 500-1500 mg/m^2

Wilms' Tumor

VAD

Vincristine, I.V., 1.5 mg/m^2/week for 10 weeks, then every 3 weeks
Dactinomycin, I.V., 1.5 mg/m^2, every 3 weeks, alternating with
Doxorubicin, I.V., 40 mg/m^2, every 3 weeks

or

Vincristine, I.V., 1.5 mg/m^2, every 6 weeks
Dactinomycin, I.V., 15 mcg/kg x 5

or

60 mcg/kg I.V. x 1 every 6 weeks ± (add if stage III or IV)
Doxorubicin, I.V., 20 mg/m^2, every 6 weeks

HERBS AND COMMON NATURAL AGENTS

The authors have chosen to include this list of natural products and proposed medical claims. However, due to limited scientific investigation to support these claims, this list is not intended to imply that these claims have been scientifically proven.

PROPOSED MEDICINAL CLAIMS

Herb	Medicinal Claim
Agrimony	Treat digestive disorders
Alfalfa	Source of carotene (vitamin A); contains natural fluoride
Aloe	Healing agent
Angelica root	Treat diseases of the lungs and heart; creates distaste for alcoholic beverages
Anise seed	Prevent gas
Arthritis tea	Treat osteoarthritis
Astragalus	Enhance energy reserves; used with ginseng
Barberry bark	Treat halitosis
Basil leaf	Treat vomiting
Bayberry bark	Relieve or prevent varicose veins
Bay leaf	Relieve cramps
Bee pollen	Renewal of enzymes, hormones, vitamins, amino acids, and others
Bergamot herb	Used as sedative
Bilberry leaf	Increases night vision, reduces eye fatigue
Birch bark	Treat urinary problems; used for rheumatism
Blackberry leaf	Treat diarrhea
Black cohosh	Relieve menstrual cramps; same effects as estrogen
Blessed thistle (Holy thistle)	Aids circulation to the brain
Blue Cohosh	Regulate menstrual flow; emergency remedy for allergic reactions to bee stings
Blue flag	Useful in the treatment of skin diseases and constipation
Blue violet	Relieve severe headaches
Boldo leaf	Stimulates digestion; treatment of gallstones
Boneset	Treatment of colds and flu
Borage leaf	Reduces high fevers
Bromelain	Fat melting enzyme; stimulates the metabolism
Buchu leaf	Diuretic; treatment of acute and chronic bladder and kidney disorders
Buckthorn bark	Expels worms and will remove warts
Burdock leaf and root	Treatment of severe skin problems and cases of arthritis
Butternut bark	Treat constipation
Calendula flower	Mending and healing of cuts or wounds
Capsicum (Cayenne)	Normalizes blood pressure; stops bleeding on contact
Caraway seed	Aids digestion
Cascara sagrada bark	Treatment for chronic constipation and gallstones
Catnip	Treat gas or stomach cramps
Celery leaf and seed	Treat incontinence
Centaury	Stimulates the salivary gland
Chamomile flower	Excellent for a nervous stomach; relieve cramping associated with the menstrual cycle
Chervil	Stimulant, mild diuretic, lowers blood pressure
Chickweed	Rich in vitamin C and minerals (calcium, magnesium, and potassium)
Chicory root	Effective in disorders of the kidneys, liver, and urinary canal
Cinnamon bark	Prevents infection and indigestion; helps break down fats during digestion

(continued)

Herb	Medicinal Claim
Cleavers	Treatment of kidney and bladder disorders; useful in obstructions of the urinary organ
Colombo root	Treat colon trouble
Coltsfoot herb and flower	Useful for asthma, bronchitis, and spasmodic cough
Coriander seed	Stomach tonic
Cornsilk	Treat prostate gland enlargement
Cranberry	Treat or prevents bladder or kidney infection
Cubeb berry	Treat chronic bladder trouble; increases flow of urine
Damiana leaf	Treatment for sexual impotency
Dandelion leaf and root	Detoxify poisons in the liver; beneficial in lowering blood pressure
Dong Quai root	Prevents and treat menstrual problems
Echinacea root	Treat strep throat, lymph glands
Fennel seed	Remedies for gas and acid stomach
Fenugreek seed	Treat allergies, coughs, digestion, emphysema, headaches, migraines, intestinal inflammation, ulcers, lungs, mucous membranes, and sore throat
Feverfew herb	Treat migraines; helps reduce inflammation in arthritis joints
Garlic capsules	"Nature's antibiotic"
Gentian	Treatment of digestive organs and improves circulation
Ginger root	Remedy for sore throat
Ginkgo biloba	Improves blood circulation to the brain
Ginseng root, Siberian	Resistance against stress; slows the aging process
Goldenseal	Treatment of bladder infections, cankers, mouth sores, mucous membranes, and ulcers
Gota kola	"Memory herb"; nerve tonic
Gravelroot (Queen of the Meadow)	Remedy for stones in the kidney and bladder
Green barley	Excellent antioxidant
Hawthorn	Strengthens and regulates the heart; relieve insomnia
Hibiscus flower	Stimulant for the intestines and kidneys
Holy thistle (Blessed thistle)	Remedy for migraine headaches
Hops flower	Treat insomnia; used to decrease the desire for alcohol
Horehound	Treat acute or chronic sore throat and coughs
Horsetail (Shavegrass)	Rich in minerals, especially silica; used to develop strong fingernails and hair, good for split ends
Ho shou wu	Rejuvenator
Hydrangea root	Treat backaches
Hyssop	Treat or prevents asthma
Juniper berry	Treat kidney ailments
Kava kava root	Induce sleep and help calm nervousness
Kelp	High contents of natural plant iodine, for proper function of the thyroid; high levels of natural calcium, potassium, and magnesium
Lavender flower	Flavor moderator
Lecithin	Break up cholesterol; prevent arteriosclerosis
Licorice root	Treatment of constipation
Ma-huang	Cleanses respiratory system
Malva flower	Soothes inflammation in the mouth and throat; helpful for earaches
Marjoram	Beneficial for a sour stomach or loss of appetite
Marshmallow leaf	Treat inflammation (anti-inflammatory)
Milk thistle herb	Liver detoxifier
Motherwort	Treat chest cold and nervousness
Mugwort	Used for treatment of rheumatism and gout
Mullein leaf	High in iron, magnesium, and potassium; sinuses; relieve swollen joints

(continued)

Herb	Medicinal Claim
Myrrh gum	Removes bad breath; sinus problems
Nettle leaf	In combination with seawrack, will bring splendid results in weight loss; remedy for dandruff
Nutmeg	Treat symptoms of gas
Oregano leaf	Settles the stomach after meals; helps treat colds
Oregon grape root	Treat rheumatism
Papaya leaf	Digestive stimulant; contains the enzyme papain
Paprika (sweet)	Stimulates the appetite and gastric secretions
Parsley leaf	High in iron
Passion flower	Mild sedative
Pau d'arco	Protects immune system
Pennyroyal	Relieve high fevers and brings on perspiration
Peppermint leaf	Treat headaches
Plantain leaf	Useful for infection, hemorrhoids, and inflammation
Pleurisy root	Treatment of a cold
Prickly ash bark	Increases circulation
Prince's pine	Diuretic; for rheumatism and chronic kidney problems
Psyllium seed	Treat constipation, lubricant to the intestinal tract
Red clover	Purify the blood
Red raspberry leaf	Eases menstrual cramps
Rhubarb root	Treat constipation, powerful laxative
Rose hips	High content of vitamin C
Safflower	Eliminates buildup of uric and lactic acid in the body, the leading cause of gout
Saffron	Natural digestive aid
Sanicle	Cleansing herb
Sarsaparilla root	Remedy for rheumatism and gout; acts as a diuretic; same effects on the body as the male hormone testosterone
Sassafras leaf and root	Stimulates the action of the liver to clear toxins from the body
Saw palmetto berry	Symptomatically treat mucus in the head and nose
Scullcap	Nerve sedative; hangover remedy
Seawrack (Bladderwrack)	Combat obesity
Senna leaf	Treat constipation, splendid laxative
Shepherd's purse	Remedy for diarrhea
Sheep sorrel	Remedy for kidney trouble
Slippery elm bark	Normalize bowel movement; beneficial for hemorrhoids and constipation
Solomon's seal root	Poultice for bruises
Speedwell	Used as a gargle for mouth and throat sores
Spikenard	Skin ailments such as acne, pimples, blackheads, rashes, and general skin problems
Star anise	Promotes appetite and relieve flatulence
St John's wort	Correct irregular menstruation
Strawberry leaf	Prevents diarrhea
Sumac berry and bark	Sores and cankers in the mouth
Summer savory leaf	Treat diarrhea, upset stomach, and sore throat
Thyme leaf	Relief of migraine headaches
Uva-ursi leaf	Digestive stimulant
Valerian root	Promotes sleep
Vervain	Remedy for fevers
White oak bark	Strong astringent
White willow bark	Used for minor aches and pains in the body
Wild alum root	Powerful astringent; used as rinse for sores in mouth and bleeding gums
Wild cherry	Prevent or treat asthma

(continued)

Herb	Medicinal Claim
Wild Oregon grape root	Chronic skin disease
Wild yam root	Helps expel gas
Wintergreen leaf	Valuable for colic and gas in the bowels
Witch hazel bark and leaf	Restores circulation; for stiff joints
Wood betony	Relieve pain in the face and head
Woodruff	Treatment of insomnia and hysteria
Wormwood	Aids bruises and sprains
Yarrow root	Unsurpasses for treatment of flu and fevers
Yerba santa	Treatment of bronchial congestion
Yohimbe	Treat impotency, natural aphrodisiac
Yucca root	Reduces inflammation of the joints

SOUND-ALIKE COMPARISON LIST

The following list contains over 1031 pairs of sound-alike drugs accompanied by a subjective pronunciation of each drug name. Any such list can only suggest possible pronunciation or enunciation miscues and is by no means meant to be exhaustive.

New or rarely used drugs are likely to cause the most problems related to interpretation. Healthcare workers should be made aware of the existence of both drugs in a sound-alike pair in order to avoid (or minimize) the potential for error. Drug companies attempt to avoid naming different drugs with similar-sounding names; however, mix-ups do occur. Reading current drug advertisements, professional literature, and drug handbooks is a good way to avert or surely lessen such sound-alike drug errors at all levels of the healthcare industry.

Drug Name	Pronunciation
Accolate®	(ak′ cue late)
Accutane®	(ak′ yu tane)
Accolate®	(ak′ cue late)
Accupril®	(ak′ yu pril)
Accubron®	(ak′ cue bron)
Accutane®	(ak′ yu tane)
Accupril®	(ak′ cue pril)
Accolate®	(ak′ cue late)
Accupril®	(ak′ cue pril)
Accutane®	(ak′ yu tane)
Accutane®	(ak′ yu tane)
Accubron®	(ak′ cue bron)
Accutane®	(ak′ yu tane)
Accolate®	(ak′ cue late)
Accutane®	(ak′ yu tane)
Accupril®	(ak′ cue pril)
Accutane®	(ak′ yu tane)
Acutrim®	(ak′ yu trim)
Acephen®	(a′ ce fen)
Aciphex™	(a′ si fecks)
acetazolamide	(a set a zole′ a mide)
acetohexamide	(a set o heks′ a mide)
acetohexamide	(a set o heks′ a mide)
acetazolamide	(a set a zole′ a mide)
Achromycin®	(ak roe mye′ sin)
Adriamycin™	(ade rya mye′ sin)
Achromycin®	(ak roe mye′ sin)
actinomycin	(ak ti noe mye′ sin)
Aciphex™	(a′ si fecks)
Acephen®	(a′ ce fen)
Acthar®	(ac′ thar)
Acular®	(ac′ yu lar)
Actidil®	(ak′ tee dill)
Actifed®	(ak′ tee fed)
Actidose®	(ac′ ti dose)
Actos®	(ac′ tose)
Actifed®	(ak′ tee fed)
Actidil®	(ak′ tee dill)
actinomycin	(ak ti noe mye′ sin)
Achromycin®	(ak roe mye′ sin)
Actos®	(ac′ tose)
Actidose®	(ac′ ti dose)
Actron®	(ak′ tron)
Acutrim®	(ak′ yu trim)
Acular®	(ac′ yu lar)
Acthar®	(ac′ thar)
Acutrim®	(ak′ yu trim)
Accutane®	(ak′ yu tane)
Acutrim®	(ak′ yu trim)
Actron®	(ak′ tron)
Adalat®	(ad′ da lat)
Adapin®	(ad′ da pin)
adapalene	(a dap′ a lene)
Adapin®	(ad′ a pin)
Adapin®	(ad′ da pin)
Adalat®	(ad′ da lat)
Adapin®	(ad′ a pin)
adapalene	(a dap′ a lene)
Adapin®	(ad′ da pin)
Adipex-P®	(ad′ di pex pea)
Adapin®	(ad′ da pin)
Ativan®	(at′ tee van)
Adderall®	(ad′ der all)
Inderal®	(in′ der al)
Adipex-P®	(ad′ di pex pea)
Adapin®	(ad′ da pin)
Adriamycin™	(ade rya mye′ sin)
Achromycin®	(ak roe mye′ sin)
Adriamycin™	(ade rya mye′ sin)
Idamycin®	(eye da mye′ sin)
Aerolone®	(air′ o lone)
Aralen®	(air′ a len)

Drug Name	Pronunciation
Afrin®	(aye′ frin or af′ rin)
aspirin	(as′ pir in)
Afrinol®	(af′ ree nol)
Arfonad®	(arr′ foe nad)
Agoral®	(ag′ a ral)
Argyrol®	(ar′ gee roll)
AK-Mycin®	(aye kay mye′ sin)
Akne-Mycin®	(ak nee mye′ sin)
Akne-Mycin®	(ak nee mye′ sin)
AK-Mycin®	(aye kay mye′ sin)
AKTob®	(ak′ tobe)
AK-Trol®	(aye′ kay trol)
AK-Trol®	(aye′ kay trol)
AKTob®	(ak′ tobe)
Alazide®	(al′ a zide)
Alazine®	(al′ a zine)
Alazine®	(al′ a zine)
Alazide®	(al′ a zide)
albuterol	(al byoo′ ter ole)
atenolol	(a ten′ oh lole)
Aldactazide®	(al dak′ ta zide)
Aldactone®	(al′ dak tone)
Aldactone®	(al′ dak tone)
Aldactazide®	(al dak′ ta zide)
Aldomet®	(al′ doe met)
Aldoril®	(al′ doe ril)
Aldomet®	(al′ doe met)
Anzemet®	(an′ ze met)
Aldoril®	(al′ doe ril)
Aldomet®	(al′ doe met)
Aldoril®	(al′ doe ril)
Elavil®	(el′ a vil)
Alesse®	(a less′)
Aleve®	(a leve′)
Aleve®	(a leve′)
Alesse®	(a less′)
Alfenta®	(al fen′ tah)
Sufenta®	(sue fen′ tah)
alfentanil	(al fen′ ta nill)
Anafranil®	(a naf′ ra nil)
alfentanil	(al fen′ ta nil)
remifentanil	(rem i fen′ ta nil)
alfentanil	(al fen′ ta nil)
sufentanil	(sue fen′ ta nil)
Alferon®	(al′ fer on)
Alkeran®	(al′ ker an)
Allegra®	(al leg′ ra)
Viagra®	(vye ag′ ra)

Drug Name	Pronunciation
Alkeran®	(al′ ker an)
Alferon®	(al′ fer on)
Allerfrin®	(al′ er frin)
Allergan®	(al′ er gan)
Allergan®	(al′ er gan)
Allerfrin®	(al′ er frin)
Allergan®	(al′ er gan)
Auralate®	(ahl′ a late)
alprazolam	(al pray′ zoe lam)
alprostadil	(al pros′ ta dil)
alprazolam	(al pray′ zoe lam)
triazolam	(trye ay′ zoe lam)
alprostadil	(al pros′ ta dil)
alprazolam	(al pray′ zoe lam)
Altace™	(al′ tase)
alteplase	(al′ te place)
alteplase	(al′ te place)
Altace™	(al′ tase)
alteplase	(al′ te place)
anistreplase	(a nis′ tre place)
Alupent®	(al′ yu pent)
Atrovent®	(at′ troe vent)
Alupent®	(al′ yu pent)
Atrovent®	(at′ troe vent)
amantadine	(a man′ ta deen)
rimantadine	(ri man′ to deen)
Amaryl®	(am′ ah ril)
Ambenyl®	(am′ ba nil)
Amaryl®	(am′ ah ril)
Amerge®	(a merge′)
Ambenyl®	(am′ ba nil)
Amaryl®	(am′ ah ril)
Ambenyl®	(am′ ba nil)
Aventyl®	(a ven′ til)
Ambi 10®	(am′ bee ten′)
Ambien™	(am′ bee en)
Ambien™	(am′ bee en)
Ambi 10®	(am′ bee ten′)
Amerge®	(a merge′)
Amaryl®	(am′ ah ril)
Amicar®	(am′ i car)
Amikin®	(am′ i kin)
Amikin®	(am′ i kin)
Amicar®	(am′ i car)
amiloride	(a mil′ o ride)
amiodarone	(a mee′ oh da rone)
amiloride	(a mil′ o ride)
amlodipine	(am lo′ di pine)

Drug Name	Pronunciation
aminophylline	(am in off′ I lin)
amitriptyline	(a mee′ trip ti leen)
amiodarone	(a mee′ oh da rone)
amiloride	(a mil′ o ride)
amiodarone	((a mee′ oh da rone)
amrinone	(am′ ri none)
amitriptyline	(a mee′ trip ti leen)
aminophylline	(am in off′ I lin)
amitriptyline	(a mee trip′ ti leen)
imipramine	(im ip′ ra meen)
amlodipine	(am lo′ di pine)
amiloride	(a mil′ o ride)
Amnipaque®	(am′ ne pak)
Omnipaque®	(om′ ne pak)
amoxapine	(a moks′ a peen)
amoxicillin	(a moks a sil′ in)
amoxicillin	(a moks a sil′ in)
amoxapine	(a moks′ a peen)
ampicillin	(am pi sil′ in)
bacampicillin hydrochloride	(ba kam pi sil′ in)
amrinone	(am′ ri none)
amiodarone	((a mee′ oh da rone)
Anafranil®	(a naf′ ra nil)
alfentanil	(al fen′ ta nill)
Anafranil®	(a naf′ ra nil)
enalapril	(e nal′ a pril)
Anaprox®	(an′ a prox)
Anaspaz®	(an′ a spaz)
Anaspaz®	(an′ a spaz)
Anaprox®	(an′ a prox)
Anaspaz®	(an′ a spaz)
Antispas®	(an′ te spaz)
Anatrast®	(an′ a trast)
Anatuss®	(an′ a tuss)
Anatuss®	(an′ a tuss)
Anatrast®	(an′ a trast)
Ancobon®	(an′ coe bon)
Oncovin®	(on′ coe vin)
anistreplase	(a nis′ tre place)
alteplase	(al′ te place)
Ansaid®	(an′ said)
Axid®	(aks′ id)
Antagon™	(an′ ta gon)
Auralgon®	(a ral′ gon)
Antispas®	(an′ te spaz)
Anaspaz®	(an′ a spaz)
Anturane®	(ann′ chu rane)
Artane®	(ar′ tane)
Anusol®	(an′ yu sol)
Aquasol®	(ah′ kwa sol)
Anzemet®	(an′ ze met)
Aldomet®	(al′ doe met)
Aplisol®	(ap′ lee sol)
A.P.L.®	(aye pee el′)
A.P.L.®	(aye pee el′)
Aplisol®	(ap′ lee sol)
Apresoline®	(aye press′ sow leen)
Priscoline®	(pris′ coe leen)
Aquasol®	(ah′ kwa sol)
Anusol®	(an′ yu sol)
AquaTar®	(ah′ kwa tar)
Aquatag®	(ah′ kwa tag)
Aquatag®	(ah′ kwa tag)
AquaTar®	(ah′ kwa tar)
ara-C	(a ra cee′)
Arasine®	(a ra seen′)
Aralen®	(air′ a len)
Aerolone®	(air′ o lone)
Aralen®	(air′ a len)
Arlidin®	(ar′ le din)
Aramine®	(air′ a meen)
Artane®	(ar′ tane)
Arasine®	(a ra seen′)
ara-C	(a ra cee′)
Arfonad®	(arr′ foe nad)
Afrinol®	(af′ ree nol)
Argyrol®	(ar′ gee roll)
Agoral®	(ag′ a ral)
Aricept®	(ar′ e cept)
Ascriptin®	(a crip′ tin)
Arlidin®	(ar′ le din)
Aralen®	(air′ a len)
Arrestin®	(aye res′ tin)
Aygestin®	(aye ges′ tin)
Artane®	(ar′ tane)
Anturane®	(an′ chu rane)
Artane®	(ar′ tane)
Aramine®	(air′ a meen)
Asacol®	(as′ a col)
Os-Cal®	(os′ cal)
Asbron®	(as′ bron)
aspirin	(as′ pir in)
Ascriptin®	(a crip′ tin)
Aricept®	(ar′ e cept)
aspirin	(as′ pir in)
Afrin®	(aye′ frin or af′ rin)

Drug Name	Pronunciation
aspirin	(as′ pir in)
Asbron®	(as′ bron)
Atarax®	(at′ a raks)
Ativan®	(at′ tee van)
Atarax®	(at′ a raks)
Marax®	(may′ raks)
atenolol	(a ten′ oh lole)
albuterol	(al byoo′ ter ole)
atenolol	(a ten′ oh lole)
Tylenol®	(tye′ le nole)
Atgam®	(at′ gam)
Ativan®	(at′ tee van)
Ativan®	(at′ tee van)
Adapin®	(add′ da pin)
Ativan®	(at′ tee van)
Atarax®	(at′ a raks)
Ativan®	(at′ tee van)
Atgam®	(at′ gam)
Ativan®	(at′ tee van)
ATnativ®	(aye tee nay′ tif)
Ativan®	(at′ tee van)
Avitene®	(aye′ va teen)
ATnativ®	(aye tee nay′ tif)
Ativan®	(at′ tee van)
Atrovent®	(at′ troe vent)
Alupent®	(al′ yu pent)
Augmentin®	(aug men′ tin)
Azulfidine®	(ay zul′ fi deen)
Auralate®	(ahl′ a late)
Allergan®	(al′ er gan)
Auralgon®	(a ral′ gon)
Antagon™	(an′ ta gon)
Auralgan®	(a ral′ gan)
Larylgan®	(la ril′ gan)
Auralgan®	(a ral′ gan)
Ophthalgan®	(opp thal′ gan)
Avalide®	(av′ a lide)
Avandia®	(a van′ de a)
Avandia®	(a van′ de a)
Avalide®	(av′ a lide)
Aventyl®	(a ven′ til)
Ambenyl®	(am′ ba nil)
Aventyl®	(a ven′ til)
Bentyl®	(ben′ till)
Avitene®	(aye′ va teen)
Ativan®	(at′ tee van)
Axid®	(aks′ id)
Ansaid®	(an′ said)

Drug Name	Pronunciation
Aygestin®	(aye ges′ tin)
Arrestin®	(aye res′ tin)
Azulfidine®	(ay zul′ fi deen)
Augmentin®	(aug men′ tin)
bacampicillin hydrochloride	(ba kam pi sil′ in)
ampicillin	(am pi sil′ in)
bacitracin	(bas i tray′ sin)
Bactrim®	(bac′ trim)
baclofen	(bak′ loe fen)
Bactroban®	(bak′ troe ban)
baclofen	(bak′ loe fen)
Beclovent®	(bec′ lo vent)
Bactocill®	(bak′ tow sill)
Pathocil®	(path′ o sill)
Bactrim®	(bac′ trim)
bacitracin	(bas i tray′ sin)
Bactroban®	(bak′ troe ban)
baclofen	(bak′ loe fen)
Banophen®	(ban′ o fen)
Barophen®	(bear′ o fen)
Banthine®	(ban′ theen)
Brethine®	(breath′ een)
Banthine®	(ban′ theen)
Pro-Banthine®	(pro ban′ theen)
Barophen®	(bear′ o fen)
Banophen®	(ban′ o fen)
Beclovent®	(bec′ lo vent)
baclofen	(bak′ loe fen)
Beconase®	(beck′ o nase)
Bexophene®	(beks′ o feen)
Beminal®	(bem′ eh nall)
Benemid®	(ben′ a mid)
Benadryl®	(ben′ a drill)
benazepril	(ban ay′ ze pril)
Benadryl®	(ben′ a drill)
Bentyl®	(ben′ till)
benazepril	(ban ay′ ze pril)
Benadryl®	(ben′ a drill)
Benemid®	(ben′ a mid)
Beminal®	(bem′ eh nall)
Benoxyl®	(ben ox′ ill)
Brevoxyl®	(brev ox′ il)
Bentyl®	(ben′ till)
Aventyl®	(a ven′ til)
Bentyl®	(ben′ till)
Benadryl®	(ben′ a drill)
Bentyl®	(ben′ till)
Cantil®	(can′ til)

Drug Name	Pronunciation
Bentyl®	(ben′ til)
Trental®	(tren′ tal)
Benylin®	(ben′ eh lin)
Ventolin®	(ven′ tow lin)
Benza®	(ben′ zah)
Benzac®	(ben′ zak)
Benzac®	(ben′ zak)
Benza®	(ben′ zah)
Bepridil®	(be′ pri dil)
Prepidil®	(pre′ pi dil)
Betadine®	(bay′ ta deen)
Betagan®	(bay′ ta gan)
Betagan®	(bay′ ta gan)
Betadine®	(bay′ ta deen)
Betapace®	(bay′ ta pace)
Betapen®	(bay′ ta pen)
Betapen®	(bay′ ta pen)
Betapace®	(bay′ ta pace)
Bexophene®	(beks′ o feen)
Beconase®	(beck′ o nase)
Bicillin®	(bye sil′ lin)
V-Cillin K®	(vee sil′ lin kay)
Bicillin®	(bye sil′ lin)
Wycillin®	(wye sil′ lin)
bleomycin	(blee o mye′ sin)
Cleocin®	(klee′ o sin)
Bleph®-10	(blef ten′)
Blephamide®	(blef′ a mide)
Blephamide®	(blef′ a mide)
Bleph®-10	(blef ten′)
Borofax®	(boroe′ faks)
Boropak®	(boroe′ pak)
Boropak®	(boroe′ pak)
Borofax®	(boroe′ faks)
Brethine®	(breath′ een)
Banthine®	(ban′ theen)
Bretylol®	(brett′ tee loll)
Brevital®	(brev′ i tall)
Brevital®	(brev′ i tall)
Bretylol®	(brett′ tee loll)
Brevoxyl®	(brev ox′ il)
Benoxyl®	(ben ox′ ill)
brimonidine	(bri moe′ ni deen)
bromocriptine	(broe moe krip′ teen)
Bromfed®	(brom′ fed)
Bromphen®	(brom′ fen)
bromocriptine	(broe moe krip′ teen)
brimonidine	(bri moe′ ni deen)

Drug Name	Pronunciation
Bromphen®	(brom′ fen)
Bromfed®	(brom′ fed)
bumetanide	(byoo met′ a nide)
Buminate®	(byoo′ mi nate)
Bumex®	(byoo′ mex)
Buprenex®	(byoo′ pre nex)
Buprenex®	(byoo′ pre nex)
Bumex®	(byoo′ mex)
Buminate®	(byoo′ mi nate)
bumetanide	(byoo met′ a nide)
bupivacaine	(byoo piv′ a kane)
mepivacaine	(me piv′ a kane)
busalfan	(byoo sul′ fan)
Butalan®	(byoo′ ta lan)
butabarbital	(byoo ta bar′ bi tal)
butalbital	(byoo tal′ bi tal)
Butalan®	(byoo′ ta lan)
busalfan	(byoo sul′ fan)
butalbital	(byoo tal′ bi tal)
butabarbital	(byoo ta bar′ bi tal)
Byclomine®	(bye′ clo meen)
Bydramine®	(bye′ dra meen)
Byclomine®	(bye′ clo meen)
Hycomine®	(hye′ coe meen)
Bydramine®	(bye′ dra meen)
Byclomine®	(bye′ clo meen)
Bydramine®	(bye′ dra meen)
Hydramyn®	(hye′ dra min)
Cepastat®	(sea′ pa stat)
Capastat®	(kap′ a stat)
Cankaid®	(kan′ kaid)
Enkaid®	(enn′ kaid)
Cantil®	(can′ til)
Bentyl®	(ben′ till)
Capastat®	(kap′ a stat)
Cepastat®	(sea′ pa stat)
Capital®	(kap′ i tal)
Capitrol®	(kap′ i trol)
Capitrol®	(kap′ i trol)
Capital®	(kap′ i tal)
Capitrol®	(kap′ i trol)
captopril	(kap′ toe pril)
captopril	(kap′ toe pril)
Capitrol®	(kap′ i trol)
carboplatin	(kar′ boe pla tin)
cisplatin	(sis′ pla tin)
Cardio-Green®	(kar′ dee yo green′)
Cardioquin®	(kar′ dee yo kwin)

Drug Name	Pronunciation
Cardioquin®	(kar′ dee yo kwin)
Cardio-Green®	(kar′ dee yo green′)
Cardura®	(kar dur′ ah)
Cordarone®	(kor da rone′)
Cardura®	(kar dur′ ah)
Cordran®	(kor′ dran)
Catapres®	(kat′ a pres)
Catarase®	(kat′ a race)
Catapres®	(kat′ a pres)
Combipres®	(kom′ bee pres)
Catapres®	(kat′ a pres)
Ser-Ap-Es®	(ser ap′ ess)
Catarase®	(kat′ a race)
Catapres®	(kat′ a pres)
cefazolin	(sef a′ zoe lin)
cephalexin	(sef a leks′ in)
cefazolin	(sef a′ zoe lin)
cephalothin	(sef a′ loe thin)
cefotaxime	(sef o taks′ eem)
cefoxitin	(se fox′ i tin)
cefoxitin	(se fox′ i tin)
cefotaxime	(sef o taks′ eem)
ceftizoxime	(sef ti zoks′ eem)
cefuroxime	(se fyoor ox′ eem)
cefuroxime	(se fyoor ox′ eem)
ceftizoxime	(sef ti zoks′ eem)
Cefzil®	(sef′ zil)
Kefzol®	(kef′ zol)
Celebrex®	(sel′ a brex)
Cerebyx®	(ser′ e bix)
Celexa®	(se lex′ a)
Zyprexa®	(zye preks′ a)
Cenestin®	(se nes′ tin)
Senexon®	(sen′ e son)
cephalexin	(sef a leks′ in)
cefazolin	(sef a′ zoe lin)
cephalothin	(sef a′ loe thin)
cefazolin	(sef a′ zoe lin)
cephapirin	(sef a pye′ rin)
cephradine	(sef′ ra deen)
cephradine	(sef′ ra deen)
cephapirin	(sef a pye′ rin)
Cerebyx®	(ser′ e bix)
Celebrex®	(sel′ a brex)
Cerebyx®	(ser′ e bix)
Cerezyme®	(ser′ e zime)
Cerezyme®	(ser′ e zime)
Cerebyx®	(ser′ e bix)

Drug Name	Pronunciation
chlorambucil	(klor am′ byoo sil)
Chloromycetin®	(klor oh my see′ tin)
Chloromycetin®	(klor oh my see′ tin)
chlorambucil	(klor am′ byoo sil)
chloroxine	(klor ox′ een)
Choloxin®	(koe lox′ in)
Choloxin®	(koe lox′ in)
chloroxine	(klor ox′ een)
chlorpropamide	(klor proe′ pa mide)
chlorpromazine	(klor proe′ ma zeen)
chlorpromazine	(klor proe′ ma zeen)
chlorpropamide	(klor proe′ pa mide)
Chorex®	(ko′ reks)
Chymex®	(kye′ meks)
Chymex®	(kye′ meks)
Chorex®	(ko′ reks)
Cidex®	(sy′ tecks)
Lidex®	(ly′ decks)
Ciloxan®	(sy loks′ an)
cinoxacin	(sin oks′ a sin)
Ciloxan®	(sy loks′ an)
Cytoxan®	(sy toks′ an)
cinoxacin	(sin oks′ a sin)
Ciloxan®	(sy loks′ an)
cisplatin	(sis′ pla tin)
carboplatin	(kar′ boe pla tin)
Citracal®	(sit′ tra cal)
Citrucel®	(sit′ tru cel)
Citrucel®	(sit′ tru cel)
Citracal®	(sit′ tra cal)
clarithromycin	(kla rith′ roe mye sin)
erythromycin	(er ith roe mye′ sin)
Cleocin®	(klee′ o sin)
bleomycin	(blee o mye′ sin)
Cleocin®	(klee′ o sin)
Lincocin®	(link′ o sin)
Clinoxide®	(klin ox′ ide)
Clipoxide®	(kleh pox′ ide)
Clipoxide®	(kleh pox′ ide)
Clinoxide®	(klin ox′ ide)
Clocort®	(klo′ kort)
Cloderm®	(klo′ derm)
Cloderm®	(klo′ derm)
Clocort®	(klo′ kort)
clofibrate	(kloe fye′ brate)
clorazepate	(klor az′ a pate)
clomiphene	(kloe′ mi feen)
clomipramine	(kloe mi′ pra meen)

Drug Name	Pronunciation
clomiphene	(kloe′ mi feen)
clonidine	(kloe′ ni deen)
clomipramine	(kloe mi′ pra meen)
clomiphene	(kloe′ mi feen)
clonidine	(kloe′ ni deen)
clomiphene	(kloe′ mi feen)
clonidine	(kloe′ ni deen)
clozapine	(kloe′ za peen)
clonidine	(kloe′ ni deen)
Klonopin™	(klon′ o pin)
clonidine	(kloe′ ni deen)
Loniten®	(lon′ eh ten)
clonidine	(kloe′ ni deen)
quinidine	(kwin′ i deen)
clorazepate	(klor az′ a pate)
clofibrate	(kloe fye′ brate)
clotrimazole	(kloe trim′ a zole)
co-trimoxazole	(koe-trye moks′ a zole)
Cloxapen®	(klox′ a pen)
clozapine	(kloe′ za peen)
clozapine	(kloe′ za peen)
clonidine	(kloe′ ni deen)
clozapine	(kloe′ za peen)
Cloxapen®	(klox′ a pen)
Co-Lav®	(koe′ lav)
Colax®	(koe′ laks)
co-trimoxazole	(koe-trye moks′ a zole)
clotrimazole	(kloe trim′ a zole)
CodAphen®	(kod′ a fen)
Codafed®	(kode′ a fed)
Codafed®	(kode′ a fed)
CodAphen®	(kod′ a fen)
codeine	(koe′ deen)
Cophene®	(koe′ feen)
codeine	(koe′ deen)
Cordran®	(kor′ dran)
codeine	(koe′ deen)
Lodine®	(low′ deen)
Colax®	(koe′ laks)
Co-Lav®	(koe′ lav)
Colestid®	(koe les′ tid)
colistin	(koe lis′ tin)
colistin	(koe lis′ tin)
Colestid®	(koe les′ tid)
Combipres®	(kom′ bee pres)
Catapres®	(kat′ a pres)
Combivent®	(kom′ bi vent)
Combivir®	(kom′ bi veer)

Drug Name	Pronunciation
Combivir®	(kom′ bi veer)
Combivent®	(kom′ bi vent)
Congestac®	(kon ges′ tin)
Congestant®	(kon ges′ tant)
Congestant®	(kon ges′ tant)
Congestac®	(kon ges′ tin)
Cophene®	(koe′ feen)
codeine	(koe′ deen)
Cordarone®	(kor da rone′)
Cardura®	(kar dur′ ah)
Cordarone®	(kor da rone′)
Cordran®	(kor′ dran)
Cordran®	(kor′ dran)
Cardura®	(kar dur′ ah)
Cordran®	(kor′ dran)
codeine	(koe′ deen)
Cordran®	(kor′ dran)
Cordarone®	(kor da rone′)
Cort-Dome®	(kort′ dome)
Cortone®	(kor′ tone)
cortisone	(kor′ ti sone)
Cortizone®	(kor′ ti sone)
Cortizone®	(kor′ ti sone)
cortisone	(kor′ ti sone)
Cortone®	(kor′ tone)
Cort-Dome®	(kort′ dome)
Coumadin®	(ku′ ma din)
Kemadrin®	(kem′ a drin)
Cozaar®	(koe′ zar)
Zocor®	(zoe′ cor)
Crysticillin®	(kris ta sil′ lin)
Crystodigin®	(kris toe dig′ in)
Crystodigin®	(kris toe dig′ in)
Crysticillin®	(kris ta sil′ lin)
cycloserine	(sye kloe ser′ een)
cyclosporine	(sye′ kloe spor een)
Cyclospasmol®	(sye kloe spas′ mol)
cyclosporine	(sye′ kloe spor een)
cyclosporine	(sye′ kloe spor een)
Cyclospasmol®	(sye kloe spas′ mol)
cyclosporine	(sye′ kloe spor een)
Cyklokapron®	(sye kloe kay′ pron)
cyclosporine	(sye′ kloe spor een)
cycloserine	(sye kloe ser′ een)
Cyklokapron®	(sye kloe kay′ pron)
cyclosporine	(sye′ kloe spor een)
cytarabine	(sye tare′ a been)
vidarabine	(vye dare′ a been)

Drug Name	Pronunciation
CytoGam®	(sy′ to gam)
Cytoxan®	(sy toks′ an)
Cytotec®	(sye′ toe tek)
Cytoxan®	(sye tox′ an)
Cytotec®	(sye′ toe tek)
Sytobex®	(sye′ toe beks)
Cytoxan®	(sy toks′ an)
Ciloxan®	(sy loks′ an)
Cytoxan®	(sy toks′ an)
CytoGam®	(sy′ to gam)
Cytoxan®	(sye tox′ an)
Cytotec®	(sye′ toe tek)
dacarbazine	(da kar′ ba zeen)
Dicarbosil®	(dye kar′ bow sil)
dacarbazine	(da kar′ ba zeen)
procarbazine	(proe kar′ ba zeen)
dactinomycin	(dak ti noe mye′ sin)
daunorubicin	(daw noe roo′ bi sin)
Dalmane®	(dal′ mane)
Demulen®	(dem′ yu len)
Dalmane®	(dal′ mane)
Dialume®	(dy′ a lume)
dapsone	(dap′ sone)
Diprosone®	(dip′ ro sone)
Daranide®	(dare′ a nide)
Daraprim®	(dare′ a prim)
Daraprim®	(dare′ a prim)
Daranide®	(dare′ a nide)
Daricon®	(dare′ eh kon)
Darvon®	(dar′ von)
Darvon®	(dar′ von)
Daricon®	(dare′ eh kon)
Darvon®	(dar′ von)
Devrom®	(dev′ rom)
Darvon®	(dar′ von)
Diovan®	(dye oh′ van)
daunorubicin	(daw noe roo′ bi sin)
dactinomycin	(dak ti noe mye′ sin)
daunorubicin	(daw noe roo′ bi sin)
doxorubicin	(dox o roo′ bi sin)
Daypro®	(day′ pro)
Deprol®	(deh′ prol)
Decadron®	(dek′ a dron)
Decholin®	(dek′ o lin)
Decadron®	(dek′ a dron)
Percodan®	(per′ coe dan)
Decholin®	(dek′ o lin)
Decadron®	(dek′ a dron)

Drug Name	Pronunciation
Deconal®	(dek′ o nal)
Deconsal®	(dek′ on sal)
Deconsal®	(dek′ on sal)
Deconal®	(dek′ o nal)
Delacort®	(del′ a kort)
Delcort®	(del′ kort)
Delcort®	(del′ kort)
Delacort®	(del′ a kort)
Delfen®	(del′ fen)
Delsym®	(del′ sim)
Delsym®	(del′ sim)
Delfen®	(del′ fen)
Demadex®	(dem′ a deks)
Denorex®	(den′ o reks)
Demerol®	(dem′ eh rol)
dicumarol	(dye koo′ ma role)
Demerol®	(dem′ eh rol)
Demulen®	(dem′ yu len)
Demerol®	(dem′ eh rol)
Dymelor®	(dye′ meh lo)
Demerol®	(dem′ eh rol)
Temaril®	(tem′ a ril)
Demulen®	(dem′ yu len)
Dalmane®	(dal′ mane)
Demulen®	(dem′ yu len)
Demerol®	(dem′ eh rol)
Denorex®	(den′ o reks)
Demadex®	(dem′ a deks)
Depakene®	(dep′ a keen)
Depakote®	(dep′ a kote)
Depakote®	(dep′ a kote)
Depakene®	(dep′ a keen)
DepoCyt®	(de′ po set)
Depoject®	(de′ po ject)
Depogen®	(dep′ o gen)
Depoject®	(dep′ o ject)
Depoject®	(de′ po ject)
DepoCyt®	(de′ po set)
Depoject®	(dep′ o ject)
Depogen®	(dep′ o gen)
Depo-Testadiol®	(dep o tes ta dye′ ol)
Depotestogen®	(dep o tes′ tow gen)
Depotestogen®	(dep o tes′ tow gen)
Depo-Testadiol®	(dep o tes ta dye′ ol)
Deprol®	(deh′ prol)
Daypro®	(day′ pro)
Dermacort®	(der′ ma kort)
DermiCort®	(der′ meh kort)

Drug Name	Pronunciation
Dermatop®	(der′ ma top)
DermiCort®	(der′ meh kort)
Dermatop®	(der′ ma top)
Dimetapp®	(dime′ tap)
DermiCort®	(der′ meh kort)
Dermacort®	(der′ ma kort)
DermiCort®	(der′ meh kort)
Dermatop®	(der′ ma top)
deserpidine	(de ser′ pi deen)
desipramine	(dess ip′ ra meen)
Desferal®	(des′ fer al)
Disophrol®	(dye′ so frol)
Desferal®	(des′ fer al)
desflurane	(des flu′ rane)
desflurane	(des flu′ rane)
Desferal®	(des′ fer al)
desipramine	(dess ip′ ra meen)
deserpidine	(de ser′ pi deen)
desoximetasone	(des ox i met′ a sone)
dexamethasone	(deks a meth′ a sone)
Desoxyn®	(de soks′ in)
digoxin	(di joks′ in)
Devrom®	(dev′ rom)
Darvon®	(dar′ von)
dexamethasone	(deks a meth′ a sone)
desoximetasone	(des ox i met′ a sone)
Diaβeta®	(dye a bay′ tah)
Diabinese®	(dye ab′ beh neese)
Diaβeta®	(dye a bay′ tah)
Zebeta®	(ze′ bay tah)
Diabinese®	(dye ab′ beh neese)
Diaβeta®	(dye a bay′ tah)
Dialume®	(dy′ a lume)
Dalmane®	(dal′ mane)
Diamox®	(dye′ a moks)
Trimox®	(trye′ moks)
diazoxide	(dye a soks′ ide)
Dyazide®	(dye′ a zide)
Dicarbosil®	(dye kar′ bow sil)
dacarbazine	(da kar′ ba zeen)
diclofenac	(dye kloe′ fen ak)
Diflucan®	(dye flu′ can)
dicumarol	(dye koo′ ma role)
Demerol®	(dem′ eh rol)
Diflucan®	(dye flu′ can)
diclofenac	(dye kloe′ fen ak)
Diflucan®	(dye flu′ can)
Diprivan®	(dye′ pri van)

Drug Name	Pronunciation
digitoxin	(di ji tox′ in)
digoxin	(di jox′ in)
digoxin	(di joks′ in)
Desoxyn®	(de soks′ in)
digoxin	(di jox′ in)
digitoxin	(di ji tox′ in)
Dilantin®	(dye lan′ tin)
Dilaudid®	(dye law′ did)
Dilantin®	(dye lan′ tin)
diltiazem	(dil tye′ a zem)
Dilantin®	(dye lan′ tin)
Dipentum®	(dye pen′ tum)
Dilaudid®	(dye law′ did)
Dilantin®	(dye lan′ tin)
diltiazem	(dil tye′ a zem)
Dilantin®	(dye lan′ tin)
dimenhydrinate	(dye men hye′ dri nate)
diphenhydramine	(dye fen hye′ dra meen)
Dimetabs®	(dime′ tabs)
Dimetapp®	(dime′ tap)
Dimetapp®	(dime′ tap)
Dermatop®	(der′ ma top)
Dimetapp®	(dime′ tap)
Dimetabs®	(dime′ tabs)
Diovan®	(dye oh′ van)
Darvon®	(dar′ von)
Dipentum®	(dye pen′ tum)
Dilantin®	(dye lan′ tin)
diphenhydramine	(dye fen hye′ dra meen)
dimenhydrinate	(dye men hye′ dri nate)
Diphenatol®	(dye fen′ ah tol)
diphenidiol	(dye fen′ i dole)
diphenidiol	(dye fen′ i dole)
Diphenatol®	(dye fen′ ah tol)
Diphenylan®	(dye fen′ eh lan)
dyphenylan	(dye fen′ eh lan)
Diprivan®	(dye′ pri van)
Diflucan®	(dye flu′ can)
Diprivan®	(dip′ riv an)
Ditropan®	(di troe′ pan)
Diprosone®	(dip′ ro sone)
dapsone	(dap′ sone)
dipyridamole	(dye peer id′ a mole)
disopyramide	(dye soe peer′ a mide)
Disophrol®	(dye′ so frol)
Desferal®	(des′ fer al)
disopyramide	(dye soe peer′ a mide)
dipyridamole	(dye peer id′ a mole)

Drug Name	Pronunciation
Ditropan®	(di troe′ pan)
Diprivan®	(dip′ riv an)
Ditropan®	(di troe′ pan)
Intropin®	(in troe′ pin)
Diutensin®	(dye yu ten′ sin)
Salutensin®	(sal yu ten′ sin)
dobutamine	(doe byoo′ ta meen)
dopamine	(doe′ pa meen)
docusate	(dok′ yoo sate)
Doxinate®	(dox′ eh nate)
Dolobid®	(dol′ ah bid)
Slo-Bid®	(slo′ bid)
Donnapine®	(don′ a peen)
Donnazyme®	(don′ a zime)
Donnazyme®	(don′ a zime)
Donnapine®	(don′ a peen)
dopamine	(doe′ pa meen)
dobutamine	(doe byoo′ ta meen)
dopamine	(doe′ pa meen)
Dopram®	(doe′ pram)
Dopar®	(doe′ par)
Dopram®	(doe′ pram)
Dopram®	(doe′ pram)
dopamine	(doe′ pa meen)
Dopram®	(doe′ pram)
Dopar®	(doe′ par)
doxepin	(dox′ e pin)
Doxidan®	(dox′ e dan)
Doxidan®	(dox′ e dan)
doxepin	(dox′ e pin)
Doxil®	(doks′ il)
Paxil®	(paks′ il)
Doxinate®	(dox′ eh nate)
docusate	(dok′ yoo sate)
doxorubicin	(dox o roo′ bi sin)
daunorubicin	(daw noe roo′ bi sin)
Duo-Cyp®	(du′ o sip)
DuoCet™	(du′ o set)
DuoCet™	(du′ o set)
Duo-Cyp®	(du′ o sep)
Dura-Gest®	(dur′ a gest)
Duragen®	(dur′ a gen)
Duragen®	(dur′ a gen)
Dura-Gest®	(dur′ a gest)
Dyazide®	(dye′ a zide)
diazoxide	(dye a soks′ ide)
Dyazide®	(dye′ a zide)
Dynacin®	(dye′ na sin)

Drug Name	Pronunciation
Dymelor®	(dye′ meh lo)
Demerol®	(dem′ eh rol)
Dymelor®	(dye′ meh lor)
Pamelor®	(pam′ meh lor)
Dynabac®	(dye′ na bac)
Dynapen®	(dye′ na pen)
Dynacin®	(dye′ na sin)
DynaCirc®	(dye′ na sirk)
Dynacin®	(dye′ na sin)
Dyazide®	(dye′ a zide)
Dynacin®	(dye′ na sin)
Dynapen®	(dye′ ne pen)
DynaCirc®	(dye′ na sirk)
Dynacin®	(dye′ na sin)
Dynapen®	(dye′ na pen)
Dynabac®	(dye′ na bac)
Dynapen®	(dye′ ne pen)
Dynacin®	(dye′ na sin)
dyphenylan	(dye fen′ eh lan)
Diphenylan®	(dye fen′ eh lan)
Dyrenium®	(dye ren′ e um)
Pyridium®	(pye rid′ dee um)
Dwelle®	(dwell)
Kwell®	(kwell)
Ecotrin®	(eh′ ko trin)
Edecrin®	(ed′ eh crin)
Edecrin®	(ed′ eh crin)
Ecotrin®	(eh′ ko trin)
Edecrin®	(ed′ eh crin)
Ethaquin®	(eth′ a kwin)
Elase®	(e′ lase)
Ellence®	(el′ lens)
Elavil®	(el′ a vil)
Aldoril®	(al′ doe ril)
Elavil®	(el′ a vil)
Eldepryl®	(el′ de pril)
Elavil®	(el′ a vil)
Equanil®	(eh′ kwa nil)
Elavil®	(el′ a vil)
Mellaril®	(mel′ la ril)
Elavil®	(el′ a vil)
Oruvail®	(or′ yu vale)
Eldepryl®	(el′ de pril)
Elavil®	(el′ a vil)
Eldepryl®	(el de pril)
enalapril	(e nal′ a pril)
Elixicon®	(eh lix′ i con)
Elocon®	(ee′ lo con)

Drug Name	Pronunciation
Ellence®	(el′ lens)
Elase®	(e′ lase)
Elocon®	(ee′ lo con)
Elixicon®	(eh lix′ i con)
emetine	(em′ eh teen)
Emetrol®	(em′ eh trol)
Emetrol®	(em′ eh trol)
emetine	(em′ eh teen)
enalapril	(e nal′ a pril)
Anafranil®	(a naf′ ra nil)
enalapril	(e nal′ a pril)
Eldepryl®	(el de pril)
Endal®	(en′ dal)
Intal®	(in′ tal)
Enduron®	(en′ du ron)
Imuran®	(im′ yu ran)
Enduron®	(en′ du ron)
Inderal®	(in′ der al)
Enduronyl®	(en dur′ o nil)
Inderal®	(in′ der al)
Enduronyl® Forte	(en dur′ o nil for′ tay)
Inderal® 40	(in′ der al for′ tee)
enflurane	(en′ floo rane)
isoflurane	(eye soe flure′ ane)
Enkaid®	(enn′ kaid)
Cankaid®	(kan′ kaid)
Entex®	(en′ teks)
Tenex®	(ten′ eks)
ephedrine	(e fed′ rin)
Epifrin®	(ep′ eh frin)
EpiPen®	(ep′ eh pen)
Epifrin®	(ep′ eh frin)
Epifrin®	(ep′ eh frin)
ephedrine	(e fed′ rin)
Epifrin®	(ep′ eh frin)
EpiPen®	(ep′ eh pen)
Epinal®	(ep′ eh nal)
Epitol®	(ep′ eh tol)
Epitol®	(ep′ eh tol)
Epinal®	(ep′ eh nal)
Equanil®	(eh′ kwa nil)
Elavil®	(el′ a vil)
erythromycin	(er ith roe mye′ sin)
clarithromycin	(kla rith′ roe mye sin)
Esimil®	(es′ eh mil)
Estinyl®	(es′ teh nil)
Esimil®	(es′ eh mil)
Ismelin®	(is′ meh lin)

Drug Name	Pronunciation
Esimil®	(es′ eh mil)
F.M.L.®	(ef′ em el)
Estinyl®	(es′ teh nil)
Esimil®	(es′ eh mil)
Estratab®	(es′ tra tab)
Ethatab®	(eth′ a tab)
Eskalith®	(es′ ka lith)
Estratest®	(es′ tra test)
Estratest®	(es′ tra test)
Eskalith®	(es′ ka lith)
ethanol	(eth′ e nol)
Ethyol®	(eth′ e ole)
Ethaquin®	(eth′ a kwin)
Edecrin®	(ed′ eh crin)
Ethatab®	(eth′ a tab)
Estratab®	(es′ tra tab)
ethosuximide	(eth o sux′ i mide)
methsuximide	(meth sux′ i mide)
Ethyol®	(eth′ e ole)
ethanol	(eth′ e nol)
etidocaine	(e ti′ doe kane)
etidronate	(e ti droe′ nate)
etidronate	(e ti droe′ nate)
etidocaine	(e ti′ doe kane)
etidronate	(e ti droe′ nate)
etretinate	(e tret′ i nate)
etretinate	(e tret′ i nate)
etidronate	(e ti droe′ nate)
Eurax®	(yoor′ aks)
Serax®	(sear′ aks)
Eurax®	(yoor′ aks)
Urex®	(yu′ eks)
Factrel®	(fak′ trel)
Sectral®	(sek′ tral)
Feldene®	(fel′ deen)
Seldane®	(sel′ dane)
fenoprofen	(fen o proe′ fen)
flurbiprofen	(flure bi′ proe fen)
Feosol®	(fee′ o sol)
Fer-In-Sol®	(fehr′ in sol)
Feosol®	(fee′ o sol)
Festal®	(fes′ tal)
Feosol®	(fee′ o sol)
Fluosol®	(flu′ o sol)
Fer-In-Sol®	(fehr′ in sol)
Feosol®	(fee′ o sol)
Ferralet®	(fer′ a let)
Ferrlecit®	(fer′ le set)

Drug Name	Pronunciation
Ferrlecit®	(fer′ le set)
Ferralet®	(fer′ a let)
Festal®	(fes′ tal)
Feosol®	(fee′ o sol)
Feverall™	(fee′ ver all)
Fiberall®	(fye′ ber all)
Fiberall®	(fye′ ber all)
Feverall™	(fee′ ver all)
Fioricet®	(fee oh′ reh set)
Lorcet®	(lor′ set)
Fiorinal®	(fee or′ reh nal)
Florinef®	(flor′ eh nef)
Flaxedil®	(flaks′ eh dil)
Flexeril®	(fleks′ eh ril)
Flexeril®	(fleks′ eh ril)
Flaxedil®	(flaks′ eh dil)
Flexeril®	(fleks′ eh ril)
Hectoral™	(hek′ to ral)
Flexon®	(fleks′ on)
Floxin®	(floks′ in)
Flomax™	(flo′ maks)
Fosamax®	(fos′ a maks)
Flomax®	(flo′ maks)
Volmax®	(vol′ maks)
Florinef®	(flor′ eh nef)
Fiorinal®	(fee or′ reh nal)
Floxin®	(floks′ in)
Flexon®	(fleks′ on)
flunisolide	(floo nis′ o lide)
fluocinonide	(floo o sin′ o nide)
fluocinolone	(floo o sin′ o lone)
fluocinonide	(floo o sin′ o nide)
fluocinonide	(floo o sin′ o nide)
flunisolide	(floo nis′ o lide)
fluocinonide	(floo o sin′ o nide)
fluocinolone	(floo o sin′ o lone)
Fluosol®	(flu′ o sol)
Feosol®	(fee′ o sol)
flurbiprofen	(flure bi′ proe fen)
fenoprofen	(fen o proe′ fen)
F.M.L.®	(ef′ em el)
Esimil®	(es′ eh mil)
Fosamax®	(fos′ a maks)
Flomax™	(flo′ maks)
Fostex®	(fos′ teks)
pHisoHex®	(fye′ so heks)
Fulvicin®	(ful′ vi sin)
Furacin®	(fur′ a sin)
Furacin®	(fur′ a sin)
Fulvicin®	(ful′ vi sin)
Gamastan®	(gam′ a stan)
Garamycin®	(gar a mye′ sin)
Gantanol®	(gan′ ta nol)
Gantrisin®	(gan′ tri sin)
Gantrisin®	(gan′ tri sin)
Gantanol®	(gan′ ta nol)
Gantrisin®	(gan′ tri sin)
Gastrosed™	(gas′ troe sed)
Garamycin®	(gar a mye′ sin)
Gamastan®	(gam′ a stan)
Garamycin®	(gar a mye′ sin)
kanamycin	(kan a mye′ sin)
Garamycin®	(gar a mye′ sin)
Terramycin®	(tehr a mye′ sin)
Gastrosed™	(gas′ troe sed)
Gantrisin®	(gan′ tri sin)
Genapap®	(gen′ a pap)
Genapax®	(gen′ a paks)
Genapap®	(gen′ a pap)
Genatap®	(gen′ a tap)
Genapax®	(gen′ a paks)
Genapap®	(gen′ a pap)
Genatap®	(gen′ a tap)
Genapap®	(gen′ a pap)
gentamicin	(jen ta mye′ sin)
kanamycin	(kan a mye′ sin)
Glucophage®	(glue′ co faagsch)
Glucotrol®	(glue′ co trol)
Glucotrol®	(glue′ co trol)
Glucophage®	(glue′ co faagsch)
Glycotuss®	(glye′ co tuss)
Glytuss®	(glye′ tuss)
Glytuss®	(glye′ tuss)
Glycotuss®	(glye′ co tuss)
gonadorelin	(goe nad o rell′ in)
guanadrel	(gwahn′ a drel)
Gonak™	(gon′ ak)
Gonic®	(gon′ ik)
Gonic®	(gon′ ik)
Gonak™	(gon′ ak)
Granulex®	(gran′ u lecks)
Regranex®	(re gra′ neks)
guaifenesin	(gwye fen′ e sin)
guanfacine	(gwahn′ fa seen)
guanadrel	(gwahn′ a drel)
gonadorelin	(goe nad o rell′ in)

Drug Name	Pronunciation
guanethidine	(gwahn eth′ i deen)
guanidine	(gwahn′ i deen)
guanfacine	(gwahn′ fa seen)
guaifenesin	(gwye fen′ e sin)
guanidine	(gwahn′ i deen)
guanethidine	(gwahn eth′ i deen)
Haldol®	(hal′ dol)
Halenol®	(hal′ e nol)
Haldol®	(hal′ dol)
Halog®	(hay′ log)
Halenol®	(hal′ e nol)
Haldol®	(hal′ dol)
Halfan®	(hal′ fan)
Halfprin®	(half′ prin)
Halfprin®	(half′ prin)
Halfan®	(hal′ fan)
Halfprin®	(half′ prin)
Haltran®	(hal′ tran)
Halog®	(hay′ log)
Haldol®	(hal′ dol)
Halotestin®	(hay lo tes′ tin)
Halotex®	(hay′ lo teks)
Halotestin®	(hay lo tes′ tin)
Halotussin®	(hay lo tus′ sin)
Halotex®	(hay′ lo teks)
Halotestin®	(hay lo tes′ tin)
Halotussin®	(hay lo tus′ sin)
Halotestin®	(hay lo tes′ tin)
Haltran®	(hal′ tran)
Halfprin®	(half′ prin)
Hectoral™	(hek′ to ral)
Flexeril®	(fleks′ eh ril)
Herplex®	(her′ pleks)
Hiprex®	(hi′ preks)
Hespan®	(hes′ pan)
Histaspan®	(his′ ta span)
Hexadrol®	(heks′ a drol)
Hexalol®	(heks′ a drol)
Hexalol®	(heks′ a drol)
Hexadrol®	(heks′ a drol)
Hiprex®	(hi′ preks)
Herplex®	(her′ pleks)
Histaspan®	(his′ ta span)
Hespan®	(hes′ pan)
Hycamtin®	(hye cam′ tin)
Hycomine®	(hye′ co meen)
Hycodan®	(hye′ co dan)
Hycomine®	(hye′ co meen)
Hycodan®	(hye′ co dan)
Vicodin®	(vye′ co din)
Hycomine®	(hye′ coe meen)
Byclomine®	(bye′ clo meen)
Hycomine®	(hye′ co meen)
Hycamtin®	(hye cam′ tin)
Hycomine®	(hye′ co meen)
Hycodan®	(hye′ co dan)
Hydergine®	(hye′ der geen)
Hydramyn®	(hye′ dra min)
hydralazine	(hye dral′ a zeen)
hydroxyzine	(hye drox′ i zeen)
Hydramyn®	(hye′ dra min)
Hydergine®	(hye′ der geen)
Hydramyn®	(hye′ dra min)
Bydramine®	(bye′ dra meen)
Hydrocet®	(hye′ dro set)
Hydrocil®	(hye′ dro sil)
Hydrocil®	(hye′ dro sil)
Hydrocet®	(hye′ dro set)
hydroxyurea	(hye drox ee yoor ee′ a)
hydroxyzine	(hye drox′ i zeen)
hydroxyzine	(hye drox′ i zeen)
hydralazine	(hye dral′ a zeen)
hydroxyzine	(hye drox′ i zeen)
hydroxyurea	(hye drox ee yoor ee′ a)
Hygroton®	(hye gro′ ton)
Regroton®	(reg′ ro ton)
Hyperab®	(hye′ per ab)
HyperHep®	(hye′ per hep)
Hyperstat®	(hye′ per stat)
Hyper-Tet®	(hye′ per tet)
Hyperstat®	(hye′ per stat)
Nitrostat®	(nye′ troe stat)
Hyper-Tet®	(hye′ per tet)
HyperHep®	(hye′ per hep)
Hyper-Tet®	(hye′ per tet)
Hyperstat®	(hye′ per stat)
HyperHep®	(hye′ per hep)
Hyperab®	(hye′ per ab)
HyperHep®	(hye′ per hep)
Hyper-Tet®	(hye′ per tet)
Hytone®	(hye′ tone)
Vytone®	(vye′ tone)
Idamycin®	(eye da mye′ sin)
Adriamycin™	(ade rya mye′ sin)
Imferon®	(im′ fer on)
interferon	(in ter fer′ on)

Drug Name	Pronunciation
imipramine	(im ip′ ra meen)
amitriptyline	(a mee trip′ ti leen)
imipramine	(im ip′ ra meen)
Norpramin®	(nor pray′ min)
Imuran®	(im′ yu ran)
Enduron®	(en′ du ron)
Inapsine®	(i nap′ seen)
Nebcin®	(neb′ sin)
Inderal®	(in′ der al)
Adderall®	(ad′ der all)
Inderal®	(in′ der al)
Enduron®	(en′ du ron)
Inderal®	(in′ der al)
Enduronyl®	(en dur′ o nil)
Inderal®	(in′ der al)
Isordil®	(eye′ sor dil)
Inderal®	(in′ der al)
Medrol®	(meh′ drol)
Inderal® 40	(in′ der al for′ tee)
Enduronyl® Forte	(en dur′ o nil for′ tay)
Indocin®	(in′ doe sin)
Lincocin®	(lin′ coe sin)
Indocin®	(in′ doe sin)
Minocin®	(min′ o sin)
Intal®	(in′ tal)
Endal®	(en′ dal)
interferon	(in ter fer′ on)
Imferon®	(im′ fer on)
Intropin®	(in tro′ pin)
Isoptin®	(eye sop′ tin)
Intropin®	(in troe′ pin)
Ditropan®	(di troe′ pan)
Ismelin®	(is′ meh lin)
Esimil®	(es′ eh mil)
Ismelin®	(is′ meh lin)
Ritalin®	(ri′ ta lin)
isoflurane	(eye soe flure′ ane)
enflurane	(en′ floo rane)
isoflurane	(eye soe flure′ ane)
isoflurophate	(eye soe flure′ o fate)
isoflurophate	(eye soe flure′ o fate)
isoflurane	(eye soe flure′ ane)
Isoptin®	(eye sop′ tin)
Intropin®	(in tro′ pin)
Isoptin®	(eye sop′ tin)
Isopto® Tears	(eye sop′ tow tears)
Isopto® Tears	(eye sop′ tow tears)
Isoptin®	(eye sop′ tin)

Drug Name	Pronunciation
Isordil®	(eye′ sor dil)
Inderal®	(in′ der al)
Isordil®	(eye′ sor dil)
Isuprel®	(eye′ sue prel)
Isuprel®	(eye′ sue prel)
Isordil®	(eye′ sor dil)
K-Lor™	(kay′ lor)
Kaochlor®	(kay′ o klor)
kanamycin	(kan a mye′ sin)
Garamycin®	(gar a mye′ sin)
kanamycin	(kan a mye′ sin)
gentamicin	(jen ta mye′ sin)
Kaochlor®	(kay′ o klor)
K-Lor™	(kay′ lor)
kaolin	(kay′ oh lin)
Kaon®	(kay′ on)
Kaon®	(kay′ on)
kaolin	(kay′ oh lin)
Kaopectate®	(kay oh pek′ tate)
Kayexelate®	(kay eks′ e late)
Kayexelate®	(kay eks′ e late)
Kaopectate®	(kay oh pek′ tate)
Keflex®	(keh′ fleks)
Keflin®	(keh′ flin)
Keflin®	(keh′ flin)
Keflex®	(keh′ fleks)
Kefzol®	(kef′ zol)
Cefzil®	(sef′ zil)
Kemadrin®	(kem′ a drin)
Coumadin®	(ku′ ma din)
Klonopin™	(klon′ o pin)
clonidine	(kloe′ ni deen)
Komex®	(koe′ meks)
Koromex®	(kor′ o meks)
Koromex®	(kor′ o meks)
Komex®	(koe′ meks)
Kwell®	(kwell)
Dwelle®	(dwell)
lactose	(lak′ tose)
lactulose	(lak′ tu lose)
lactulose	(lak′ tu lose)
lactose	(lak′ tose)
Lamictal®	(la mic′ tal)
Lamisil®	(lam′ eh sil)
Lamictal®	(la mic′ tal)
Lomotil®	(lo′ mo til)
Lamisil®	(lam′ eh sil)
Lamictal®	(la mic′ tal)

Drug Name	Pronunciation
lamotrigine	(la moe′ tri jeen)
lamivudine	(la mi′ vyoo deen)
lamivudine	(la mi′ vyoo deen)
lamotrigine	(la moe′ tri jeen)
Lanoxin®	(lan ox′ in)
Levoxine®	(lev ox een)
Lanoxin®	(lan ox′ in)
Levsinex®	(lev′ si neks)
Lanoxin®	(lan ox′ in)
Mefoxin®	(me fox′ in)
Larylgan®	(la ril′ gan)
Auralgan®	(a ral′ gan)
Lasix®	(lay′ siks)
Lidex®	(lye′ deks)
Lasix®	(lay′ siks)
Luvox®	(lu′ voks)
leucovorin	(loo koe vor′ in)
Leukeran®	(lu′ keh ran)
Leukeran®	(lu′ keh ran)
leucovorin	(loo koe vor′ in)
levodopa	(lee voe doe′ pa)
methyldopa	(meth ill doe′ pa)
levothyroxine	(lee voe thye rox′ een)
liothyronine	(lye o thye′ roe neen)
Levoxine®	(lev ox een)
Lanoxin®	(lan ox′ in)
Levsinex®	(lev′ si neks)
Lanoxin®	(lan ox′ in)
Lidex®	(ly′ decks)
Cidex®	(sy′ tecks)
Lidex®	(lye′ deks)
Lasix®	(lay′ siks)
Lidex®	(lye′ deks)
Lidox®	(lye′ dox)
Lidex®	(lye′ deks)
Videx®	(vye′ deks)
Lidex®	(lye′ deks)
Wydase®	(wye′ dase)
Lidox®	(lye′ dox)
Lidex®	(lye′ deks)
Lincocin®	(link′ o sin)
Cleocin®	(klee′ o sin)
Lincocin®	(lin′ coe sin)
Indocin®	(in′ doe sin)
Lincocin®	(link′ o sin)
Minocin®	(min′ o sin)
Lioresal®	(lye or′ reh sal)
lisinopril	(lyse in′ o pril)

Drug Name	Pronunciation
liothyronine	(lye o thye′ roe neen)
levothyroxine	(lee voe thye rox′ een)
lisinopril	(lyse in′ o pril)
Lioresal®	(lye or′ reh sal)
Lithane®	(lith′ ane)
Lithonate®	(lith′ o nate)
Lithonate®	(lith′ o nate)
Lithane®	(lith′ ane)
Lithostat®	(lith′ o stat)
Lithotabs®	(lith′ o tabs)
Lithotabs®	(lith′ o tabs)
Lithostat®	(lith′ o stat)
Lodine®	(low′ deen)
codeine	(koe′ deen)
Lomodix®	(lo′ mo dix)
Lovenox®	(lo′ ve nox)
Lomotil®	(lo′ mo til)
Lamictal®	(la mic′ tal)
Loniten®	(lon′ eh ten)
clonidine	(kloe′ ni deen)
Lopressor®	(lo pres′ sor)
Lopurin®	(lo pure′ in)
Lopurin®	(lo pure′ in)
Lopressor®	(lo pres′ sor)
Lopurin®	(lo pure′ in)
Lupron®	(lu′ pron)
Lorcet®	(lor′ set)
Fioricet®	(fee oh′ reh set)
Lotrimin®	(low′ tri min)
Otrivin®	(oh′ tri vin)
Lovenox®	(lo′ ve nox)
Lomodix®	(lo′ mo dix)
Loxitane®	(loks′ e tane)
Soriatane®	(sor′ e ah tane)
Luminal®	(lu′ mi nal)
Tuinal®	(tu′ i nal)
Lupron®	(lu′ pron)
Lopurin®	(lo pure′ in)
Lupron®	(lu′ pron)
Nuprin®	(nu′ prin)
Luvox®	(lu′ voks)
Lasix®	(lay′ siks)
Maalox®	(may′ loks)
Maox®	(may′ oks)
Maalox®	(may′ loks)
Marax®	(mare′ aks)
Maalox®	(may′ loks)
Monodox®	(mon′ o doks)

Drug Name	Pronunciation
Maltsupex®	(malt′ su peks)
Manoplax®	(man′ o laks)
Mandol®	(man′ dole)
nadolol	(nay doe′ lole)
Manoplax®	(man′ o laks)
Maltsupex®	(malt′ su peks)
Maox®	(may′ oks)
Maalox®	(may′ loks)
Maox®	(may′ oks)
Marax®	(may′ raks)
Marax®	(mare′ aks)
Maalox®	(may′ loks)
Marax®	(may′ raks)
Atarax®	(at′ a raks)
Marax®	(may′ raks)
Maox®	(may′ oks)
Marcaine®	(mar′ kane)
Narcan®	(nar′ kan)
Marinol®	(mare′ i nole)
Marnal®	(mar′ nal)
Marnal®	(mar′ nal)
Marinol®	(mare′ i nole)
Matulane®	(mat′ chu lane)
Modane®	(moe′ dane)
Maxidex®	(maks′ i deks)
Maxzide®	(maks′ zide)
Maxzide®	(maks′ zide)
Maxidex®	(maks′ i deks)
Mebaral®	(meb′ a ral)
Medrol®	(med′ role)
Mebaral®	(meb′ a ral)
Mellaril®	(mel′ a ril)
Mebaral®	(meb′ a ral)
Tegretol®	(teg′ ree tol)
mecamylamine	(mek a mill′ a meen)
mesalamine	(me sal′ a meen)
Meclan®	(me′ klan)
Meclomen®	(meh′ klo men)
Meclan®	(me′ klan)
Mezlin®	(mes′ lin)
Meclomen®	(meh′ klo men)
Meclan®	(me′ klan)
Medrol®	(med′ role)
Mebaral®	(meb′ a ral)
Medrol®	(meh′ drol)
Inderal®	(in′ der al)
Mefoxin®	(me fox′ in)
Lanoxin®	(lan ox′ in)

Drug Name	Pronunciation
Mellaril®	(mel′ la ril)
Elavil®	(el′ a vil)
Mellaril®	(mel′ a ril)
Mebaral®	(meb′ a ral)
melphalan	(mel′ fa lan)
Mephyton®	(meh fye′ ton)
mephenytoin	(me fen′ i toyn)
Mephyton®	(meh fye′ ton)
mephenytoin	(me fen′ i toyn)
Mesantoin®	(meh san′ toyn)
mephenytoin	(me fen′ i toyn)
phenytoin	(fen′ i toyn)
mephobarbital	(me foe bar′ bi tal)
methocarbamol	(meth o kar′ ba mole)
Mephyton®	(meh fye′ ton)
melphalan	(mel′ fa lan)
Mephyton®	(meh fye′ ton)
mephenytoin	(me fen′ i toyn)
Mephyton®	(meh fye′ ton)
methadone	(meth′ a done)
mepivacaine	(me piv′ a kane)
bupivacaine	(byoo piv′ a kane)
Meprospan®	(meh′ pro span)
Naprosyn®	(na′ pro sin)
mesalamine	(me sal′ a meen)
mecamylamine	(mek a mill′ a meen)
Mesantoin®	(meh san′ toyn)
mephenytoin	(me fen′ i toyn)
Mesantoin®	(meh san′ toyn)
Mestinon®	(meh′ sti non)
Mestinon®	(meh′ sti non)
Mesantoin®	(meh san′ toyn)
Metahydrin®	(me ta hye′ drin)
Metandren®	(me tan′ dren)
Metandren®	(me tan′ dren)
Metahydrin®	(me ta hye′ drin)
metaproterenol	(met a proe ter′ e nol)
metoprolol	(me toe′ proe lole)
metaxalone	(me taks′ a lone)
metolazone	(me tole′ a zone)
methadone	(meth′ a done)
Mephyton®	(meh fye′ ton)
methazolamide	(meth a zoe′ la mide)
metolazone	(me tole′ a zone)
methenamine	(meth en′ a meen)
methionine	(me thye′ o neen)
methicillin	(meth i sill′ in)
mezlocillin	(mez loe sill′ in)

Drug Name	Pronunciation
methionine	(me thye′ o neen)
methenamine	(meth en′ a meen)
methocarbamol	(meth o kar′ ba mole)
mephobarbital	(me foe bar′ bi tal)
methsuximide	(meth sux′ i mide)
ethosuximide	(eth o sux′ i mide)
methyldopa	(meth ill doe′ pa)
levodopa	(lee voe doe′ pa)
metolazone	(me tole′ a zone)
metaxalone	(me taks′ a lone)
metolazone	(me tole′ a zone)
methazolamide	(meth a zoe′ la mide)
metolazone	(me tole′ a zone)
minoxidil	(mi nox′ i dill)
metoprolol	(me toe′ proe lole)
metaproterenol	(met a proe ter′ e nol)
metyrapone	(me teer′ a pone)
metyrosine	(me tye′ roe seen)
metyrosine	(me tye′ roe seen)
metyrapone	(me teer′ a pone)
Mevacor®	(me′ va cor)
Mivacron®	(mi′ va cron)
Mexitil®	(meks′ i til)
Mezlin®	(mes′ lin)
Mezlin®	(mes′ lin)
Meclan®	(me′ klan)
Mezlin®	(mes′ lin)
Mexitil®	(meks′ i til)
mezlocillin	(mez loe sill′ in)
methicillin	(meth i sill′ in)
miconazole	(mi kon′ a zole)
Micronase®	(mye′ croe nase)
Micro-K®	(mye′ cro kay)
Micronase®	(mye′ croe nase)
Micronase®	(mye′ croe nase)
Micro-K®	(mye′ cro kay)
Micronase®	(mye′ croe nase)
Micronor®	(mye′ croe nor)
Micronase®	(mye′ croe nase)
miconazole	(mi kon′ a zole)
Micronor®	(mye′ croe nor)
Micronase®	(mye′ croe nase)
Midrin®	(mid′ rin)
Mydfrin®	(mid′ frin)
Milontin®	(mi lon′ tin)
Miltown®	(mil′ town)
Milontin®	(mi lon′ tin)
Mylanta®	(mye lan′ tah)
Miltown®	(mil′ town)
Milontin®	(mi lon′ tin)
Minizide®	(min′ i zide)
Minocin®	(min′ o sin)
Minocin®	(min′ o sin)
Indocin®	(in′ doe sin)
Minocin®	(min′ o sin)
Lincocin®	(link′ o sin)
Minocin®	(min′ o sin)
Minizide®	(min′ i zide)
Minocin®	(min′ o sin)
Mithracin®	(mith′ ra sin)
Minocin®	(min′ o sin)
niacin	(nye′ a sin)
minoxidil	(mi nox′ i dill)
metolazone	(me tole′ a zone)
Mithracin®	(mith′ ra sin)
Minocin®	(min′ o sin)
mitomycin	(mye toe mye′ sin)
Mutamycin®	(mute a mye′ sin)
Mivacron®	(mi′ va cron)
Mevacor®	(me′ va cor)
Moban®	(moe′ ban)
Modane®	(moe′ dane)
Modane®	(moe′ dane)
Matulane®	(mat′ chu lane)
Modane®	(moe′ dane)
Moban®	(moe′ ban)
Modicon®	(mod′ i kon)
Mylicon®	(mye′ li kon)
moexipril	(mo ex′ i pril)
Monopril®	(mon′ oh pril)
Monodox®	(mon′ o doks)
Maalox®	(may′ loks)
Monopril®	(mon′ oh pril)
moexipril	(mo ex′ i pril)
Mutamycin®	(mute a mye′ sin)
mitomycin	(mye toe mye′ sin)
Myambutol®	(mya am′ byoo tol)
Nembutal®	(nem′ byoo tal)
Mycelex®	(mye′ si leks)
Myoflex®	(mye′ o fleks)
Mycifradin®	(mye ce fray′ din)
Mycitracin®	(mye ce tray′ sin)
Mycitracin®	(mye ce tray′ sin)
Mycifradin®	(mye ce fray′ din)
Mydfrin®	(mid′ frin)
Midrin®	(mid′ rin)

Drug Name	Pronunciation
Mylanta®	(mye lan′ tah)
Milontin®	(mi lon′ tin)
Myleran®	(mye′ leh ran)
Mylicon®	(mye′ li kon)
Mylicon®	(mye′ li kon)
Modicon®	(mod′ i kon)
Mylicon®	(mye′ li kon)
Myleran®	(mye′ leh ran)
Myochrysine®	(mye o kris′ seen)
vincristine	(vin kris′ teen)
Myoflex®	(mye′ o fleks)
Mycelex®	(mye′ si leks)
nadolol	(nay doe′ lole)
Mandol®	(man′ dole)
Naldecon®	(nal′ dee kon)
Nalfon®	(nal′ fon)
Nalfon®	(nal′ fon)
Naldecon®	(nal′ dee kon)
Nallpen®	(nall′ pen)
Nalspan®	(nal′ span)
naloxone	(nal ox′ one)
naltrexone	(nal treks′ one)
Nalspan®	(nal′ span)
Nallpen®	(nall′ pen)
naltrexone	(nal treks′ one)
naloxone	(nal ox′ one)
Naprosyn®	(na′ pro sin)
Meprospan®	(meh′ pro span)
Naprosyn®	(na′ pro sin)
naproxen	(na prox′ en)
Naprosyn®	(na′ pro sin)
Natacyn®	(na′ ta sin)
Naprosyn®	(na′ pro sin)
Nebcin®	(neb′ sin)
naproxen	(na prox′ en)
Naprosyn®	(na′ pro sin)
Narcan®	(nar′ kan)
Marcaine®	(mar′ kane)
Narcan®	(nar′ kan)
Norcuron®	(nor′ ku ron)
Nardil®	(nar′ dil)
Norinyl®	(nor′ eh nil)
Nasacort®	(nay′ sa cort)
Nasalcrom®	(nay′ sal crome)
Nasalcrom®	(nay′ sal crome)
Nasacort®	(nay′ sa cort)
Natacyn®	(na′ ta sin)
Naprosyn®	(na′ pro sin)

Drug Name	Pronunciation
Navane®	(nav′ ane)
Norvasc®	(nor′ vask)
Nebcin®	(neb′ sin)
Inapsine®	(i nap′ seen)
Nebcin®	(neb′ sin)
Naprosyn®	(na′ pro sin)
nelfinavir	(nel fin′ a vir)
nevirapine	(ne vir′ a peen)
Nembutal®	(nem′ byoo tal)
Myambutol®	(mya am′ byoo tol)
Neptazane®	(nep′ ta zane)
Nesacaine®	(nes′ a kane)
Nesacaine®	(nes′ a kane)
Neptazane®	(nep′ ta zane)
Neupogen®	(nu′ po gen)
Nutramigen®	(nu′ tra gen)
nevirapine	(ne vir′ a peen)
nelfinavir	(nel fin′ a vir)
niacin	(nye′ a sin)
Minocin®	(min′ o sin)
nicardipine	(nye kar′ de peen)
nifedipine	(nye fed′ i peen)
Nicobid®	(nye′ ko bid)
Nitro-Bid®	(nye′ troe bid)
Nicoderm®	(nye′ co derm)
Nitroderm®	(nye′ tro derm)
Nicorette®	(nik′ o ret)
Nordette®	(nor det′)
nifedipine	(nye fed′ i peen)
nicardipine	(nye kar′ de peen)
nifedipine	(nye fed′ i peen)
nimodipine	(nye moe′ di peen)
nifedipine	(nye fed′ i peen)
nisoldipine	(nye′ sole di peen)
Nilstat®	(nil′ stat)
Nitrostat®	(nye′ troe stat)
Nimodipine	(nye moe′ di peen)
nifedipine	(nye fed′ i peen)
nisoldipine	(nye′ sole di peen)
nifedipine	(nye fed′ i peen)
Nitro-Bid®	(nye′ troe bid)
Nicobid®	(nye′ ko bid)
Nitroderm®	(nye′ tro derm)
Nicoderm®	(nye′ co derm)
Nitroglycerin	(nye troe gli′ ser in)
Nitroglyn®	(nye′ troe glin)
Nitroglyn®	(nye′ troe glin)
nitroglycerin	(nye troe gli′ ser in)

Drug Name	Pronunciation
Nitrostat®	(nye′ troe stat)
Hyperstat®	(hye′ per stat)
Nitrostat®	(nye′ troe stat)
Nilstat®	(nil′ stat)
Norcuron®	(nor′ ku ron)
Narcan®	(nar′ can)
Nordette®	(nor det′)
Nicorette®	(nik′ o ret)
Norinyl®	(nor′ eh nil)
Nardil®	(nar′ dil)
Norlutate®	(nor′ lu tate)
Norlutin®	(nor lu′ tin)
Norlutin®	(nor lu′ tin)
Norlutate®	(nor′ lu tate)
Norpramin®	(nor pray′ min)
imipramine	(im ip′ ra meen)
Norvasc®	(nor′ vask)
Navane®	(nav′ ane)
Norvasc®	(nor′ vask)
Norvir®	(nor′ vir)
Norvir®	(nor′ vir)
Norvasc®	(nor′ vask)
Novacet®	(no′ va set)
NovaSeven®	(no′ va se ven)
Novafed®	(nove′ a fed)
Nucofed®	(nu′ co fed)
NovaSeven®	(no′ va se ven)
Novacet®	(no′ va set)
Nucofed®	(nu′ co fed)
Novafed®	(nove′ a fed)
Nuprin®	(nu′ prin)
Lupron®	(lu′ pron)
Nutramigen®	(nu′ tra gen)
Neupogen®	(nu′ po gen)
olanzapine	(oh lan′ za peen)
olsalazine sodium	(ole sal′ a zeen)
olsalazine sodium	(ole sal′ a zeen)
olanzapine	(oh lan′ za peen)
Omnipaque®	(om′ ne pak)
Amnipaque®	(am′ ne pak)
Omnipaque®	(om′ ni pak)
Omnipen®	(om′ ni pen)
Omnipen®	(om′ ni pen)
Omnipaque®	(om′ ni pak)
Omnipen®	(om′ ni pen)
Unipen®	(yu′ ni pen)
Oncet®	(on′ set)
Ontak®	(on′ tak)

Drug Name	Pronunciation
Oncovin®	(on′ coe vin)
Ancobon®	(an′ coe bon)
Ontak®	(on′ tak)
Oncet®	(on′ set)
Ophthaine®	(op′ thane)
Ophthetic®	(op thet′ ik)
Ophthalgan®	(opp thal′ gan)
Auralgan®	(a ral′ gan)
Ophthetic®	(op thet′ ik)
Ophthaine®	(op′ thane)
Ophthochlor®	(op′ tho klor)
Ophthocort®	(op′ tho kort)
Ophthocort®	(op′ tho kort)
Ophthochlor®	(op′ tho klor)
oprelvekin	(op rel′ ve kin)
Proleukin®	(pro lu′ kin)
Orabase®	(or′ a base)
Orinase®	(or′ in ase)
Orasol®	(or′ a sol)
Orasone®	(or′ a sone)
Orasone®	(or′ a sone)
Orasol®	(or′ a sol)
Oretic®	(or et′ ik)
Oreton®	(or′ eh ton)
Oreton®	(or′ eh ton)
Oretic®	(or et′ ik)
Orex®	(or′ ecks)
Urex®	(yur′ ecks)
Orinase®	(or′ in ase)
Orabase®	(or′ a base)
Orinase®	(or′ in ase)
Ornade®	(or′ nade)
Orinase®	(or′ in ase)
Tolinase®	(tole′ i nase)
Ornade®	(or′ nade)
Orinase®	(or′ in ase)
Oruvail®	(or′ yu vale)
Elavil®	(el′ a vil)
Os-Cal®	(os′ cal)
Asacol®	(as′ a col)
Otrivin®	(oh′ tri vin)
Lotrimin®	(low′ tri min)
oxymetazoline	(ox i met az′ o leen)
oxymetholone	(ox i meth′ o lone)
oxymetholone	(ox i meth′ o lone)
oxymetazoline	(ox i met az′ o leen)
oxymetholone	(ox i meth′ o lone)
oxymorphone	(ox i mor′ fone)

Drug Name	Pronunciation
oxymorphone	(ox i mor′ fone)
oxymetholone	(ox i meth′ o lone)
Pamelor®	(pam′ meh lor)
Dymelor®	(dye′ meh lor)
pancreatin	(pan kre′ a tine)
Panretin®	(pan ree′ tin)
Panretin®	(pan ree′ tin)
pancreatin	(pan kre′ a tine)
Patanol®	(pa′ ta nol)
Platinol®	(pla′ ti nol)
Pathilon®	(path′ i lon)
Pathocil®	(path′ o sil)
Pathocil®	(path′ o sil)
Pathilon®	(path′ i lon)
Pathocil®	(path′ o sil)
Placidyl®	(pla′ ce dil)
Pathocil®	(path′ o sill)
Bactocill®	(bak′ tow sill)
Pavabid®	(pav′ a bid)
Pavased®	(pav′ a sed)
Pavased®	(pav′ a sed)
Pavabid®	(pav′ a bid)
Paxil®	(paks′ il)
Doxil®	(doks′ il)
Paxil®	(packs′ ol)
Taxol®	(tacks′ ol)
pentobarbital	(pen toe bar′ bi tal)
phenobarbital	(fee noe bar′ bi tal)
Percodan®	(per′ coe dan)
Decadron®	(dek′ a dron)
Perdiem®	(per dee′ em)
Pyridium®	(pye rid′ dee um)
Persantine®	(per san′ teen)
Pertofrane®	(per′ toe frane)
Pertofrane®	(per′ toe frane)
Persantine®	(per san′ teen)
Phazyme®	(fay′ zeem)
Pherazine®	(fer′ a zeen)
Phenergan®	(fen′ er gan)
Phrenilin®	(fren′ ni lin)
Phenergan®	(fen′ er gan)
Theragran®	(ther′ a gran)
phenobarbital	(fee noe bar′ bi tal)
pentobarbital	(pen toe bar′ bi tal)
phentermine	(fen′ ter meen)
phentolamine	(fen tole′ a meen)
phentolamine	(fen tole′ a meen)
phentermine	(fen′ ter meen)
phentolamine	(fen tole′ a meen)
Ventolin®	(ven′ to lin)
phenytoin	(fen′ i toyn)
mephenytoin	(me fen′ i toyn)
Pherazine®	(fer′ a zeen)
Phazyme®	(fay′ zeem)
pHisoHex®	(fye′ so heks)
Fostex®	(fos′ teks)
Phos-Flur®	(fos′ flur)
PhosLo®	(fos′ lo)
PhosLo®	(fos′ lo)
Phos-Flur®	(fos′ flur)
PhosLo®	(fos′ lo)
ProSom™	(pro′ som)
Phosphaljel®	(fos′ fal gel)
Phospholine®	(fos′ fo leen)
Phospholine®	(fos′ fo leen)
Phosphaljel®	(fos′ fal gel)
Phrenilin®	(fren′ ni lin)
Phenergan®	(fen′ er gan)
Phrenilin®	(fren′ ni lin)
Trinalin®	(tri′ na lin)
physostigmine	(fye zoe stig′ meen)
Prostigmin®	(pro stig′ min)
physostigmine	(fye zoe stig′ meen)
pyridostigmine	(peer id o stig′ meen)
Pitocin®	(pi toe′ sin)
Pitressin®	(ph tres′ sin)
Pitressin®	(ph tres′ sin)
Pitocin®	(ph toe′ sin)
Placidyl®	(pla′ ce dil)
Pathocil®	(path′ o sil)
Plaquenil®	(pla′ kwe nil)
Platinol®	(pla′ tee nol)
Platinol®	(pla′ ti nol)
Patanol®	(pa′ ta nol)
Platinol®	(pla′ tee nol)
Plaquenil®	(pla′ kwe nil)
Plendil®	(plen′ dill)
Isordil®	(eye′ sor dil)
Plendil®	(plen′ dil)
Pletal®	(ple′ tal)
Pletal®	(ple′ tal)
Plendil®	(plen′ dil)
Ponstel®	(pon′ stel)
Pronestyl®	(pro nes′ til)
Posicor®	(pos′ e cor)
Proscar®	(pros′ car)

Drug Name	Pronunciation
pralidoxime	(pra li dox' eem)
pramoxine	(pra moks' een)
pralidoxime	(pra li dox' eem)
pyridoxine	(peer i dox' een)
Pramosone®	(pra' mo sone)
prednisone	(pred' ni sone)
pramoxine	(pra moks' een)
pralidoxime	(pra li dox' eem)
prazepam	(pra' ze pam)
prazosin	(pra' zoe sin)
prazosin	(pra' zoe sin)
prazepam	(pra' ze pam)
Precare®	(pre' kare)
Precose®	(pre' kose)
Precose®	(pre' kose)
Precare®	(pre' kare)
Predalone®	(pred' a lone)
prednisone	(pred' ni sone)
prednisolone	(pred nis' o lone)
prednisone	(pred' ni sone)
prednisone	(pred' ni sone)
Pramosone®	(pra' mo sone)
prednisone	(pred' ni sone)
Predalone®	(pred' a lone)
prednisone	(pred' ni sone)
prednisolone	(pred nis' o lone)
prednisone	(pred' ni sone)
primidone	(pri' mi done)
Premarin®	(prem' a rin)
Primaxin®	(pri maks' in)
Prepidil®	(pre' pi dil)
Bepridil®	(be' pri dil)
prilocaine	(pril' o kane)
Prilosec™	(pre' lo sek)
Prilosec™	(pre' lo sek)
Prozac®	(proe' zak)
Prilosec™	(pre' lo sek)
prilocaine	(pril' o kane)
Primaxin®	(pri maks' in)
Premarin®	(prem' a rin)
primidone	(pri' mi done)
prednisone	(pred' ni sone)
Priscoline®	(pris' coe leen)
Apresoline®	(aye press' sow leen)
Pro-Banthine®	(pro ban' theen)
Banthine®	(ban' theen)
procaine	(pro' cane)
Prokine®	(pro' keen)

Drug Name	Pronunciation
procarbazine	(proe kar' ba zeen)
dacarbazine	(da kar' ba zeen)
Prokine®	(pro' keen)
procaine	(pro' cane)
Proleukin®	(pro lu' kin)
oprelvekin	(op rel' ve kin)
promazine	(proe' ma zeen)
promethazine	(proe meth' a zeen)
Prometh®	(proe' meth)
Promit®	(proe' mit)
promethazine	(proe meth' a zeen)
promazine	(proe' ma zeen)
Promit®	(proe' mit)
Prometh®	(proe' meth)
Pronestyl®	(pro nes' til)
Ponstel®	(pon' stel)
Propacet®	(proe' pa set)
Propagest®	(proe' pa gest)
Propagest®	(proe' pa gest)
Propacet®	(proe' pa set)
Proscar®	(pros' car)
Posicor®	(pos' e cor)
Pro-Sof®	(proe' sof)
ProSom™	(pro' som)
ProSom™	(pro' som)
PhosLo®	(fos' lo)
ProSom™	(pro' som)
Pro-Sof® Plus	(proe' sof)
ProStep®	(proe' step)
Prozac®	(proe' zak)
Prostigmin®	(pro stig' min)
physostigmine	(fye zoe stig' meen)
protamine	(proe' ta meen)
Protopam®	(proe' toe pam)
Protopam®	(proe' toe pam)
protamine	(proe' ta meen)
Protopam®	(proe' toe pam)
Protropin®	(proe tro' pin)
Protropin®	(proe tro' pin)
Protopam®	(proe' toe pam)
Prozac®	(proe' zak)
Prilosec™	(pre' lo sek)
Prozac®	(proe' zak)
ProStep®	(proe' step)
Pyridium®	(pye rid' dee um)
Dyrenium®	(dye ren' e um)
Pyridium®	(pye rid' dee um)
Perdiem®	(per dee' em)

Drug Name	Pronunciation
Pyridium®	(pye rid′ dee um)
pyridoxine	(peer i dox′ een)
Pyridium®	(pye rid′ dee um)
pyrithione	(peer i thye′ one)
pyridostigmine	(peer id o stig′ meen)
physostigmine	(fye zoe stig′ meen)
pyridoxine	(peer i dox′ een)
Pyridium®	(pye rid′ dee um)
pyridoxine	(peer i dox′ een)
pralidoxime	(pra li dox′ eem)
pyrithione	(peer i thye′ one)
Pyridium®	(pye rid′ dee um)
quinidine	(kwin′ i deen)
clonidine	(kloe′ ni deen)
quinidine	(kwin′ i deen)
quinine	(kwye′ nine)
quinine	(kwye′ nine)
quinidine	(kwin′ i deen)
Reglan®	(reg′ lan)
Regonol®	(reg′ o nol)
Regonol®	(reg′ o nol)
Reglan®	(reg′ lan)
Regonol®	(reg′ o nol)
Regutol®	(reg′ yu tol)
Regranex®	(re gra′ neks)
Granulex®	(gran′ u lecks)
Regroton®	(reg′ ro ton)
Hygroton®	(hye gro′ ton)
Regutol®	(reg′ yu tol)
Regonol®	(reg′ o nol)
remifentanil	(rem i fen′ ta nil)
alfentanil	(al fen′ ta nil)
Repan®	(ree′ pan)
Riopan®	(rye′ o pan)
Restore®	(res tore′)
Restoril®	(res′ tor ril)
Restoril®	(res′ tor ril)
Restore®	(res tore′)
Restoril®	(res′ tor ril)
Vistaril®	(vis′ tar ril)
Retrovir®	(re′ tro vir)
ritonavir	(ri ton′ o vir)
Revex®	(rev′ ex)
Revia®	(rev′ ve ah)
Revia®	(rev′ ve ah)
Revex®	(rev′ ex)
Rhythmin®	(rith′ min)
Rythmol®	(rith′ mol)
ribavirin	(rye ba vye′ rin)
riboflavin	(rye′ boe flay vin)
riboflavin	(rye′ boe flay vin)
ribavirin	(rye ba vye′ rin)
Rifadin®	(rif′ a din)
Ritalin®	(ri′ ta lin)
Rimactane®	(ri mak′ tane)
rimantadine	(ri man′ to deen)
rimantadine	(ri man′ to deen)
Rimactane®	(ri mak′ tane)
rimantadine	(ri man′ to deen)
amantadine	(a man′ ta deen)
Riobin®	(rye′ o bin)
Riopan®	(rye′ o pan)
Riopan®	(rye′ o pan)
Repan	(ree′ pan)
Riopan®	(rye′ o pan)
Riobin®	(rye′ o bin)
Ritalin®	(ri′ ta lin)
Ismelin®	(is′ meh lin)
Ritalin®	(ri′ ta lin)
Rifadin®	(rif′ a din)
Ritalin®	(ri′ ta lin)
ritodrine	(ri′ toe dreen)
ritodrine	(ri′ toe dreen)
Ritalin®	(ri′ ta lin)
ritonavir	ri ton′ o vir)
Retrovir®	(re′ tro vir)
Rocephin®	(roe sef′ fen)
Roferon®	(roe fer′ on)
Roferon®	(roe fer′ on)
Rocephin®	(roe sef′ fen)
Rynatan®	(rye′ na tan)
Rynatuss®	(rye′ na tuss)
Rynatuss®	(rye′ na tuss)
Rynatan®	(rye′ na tan)
Rythmol®	(rith′ mol)
Rhythmin®	(rith′ min)
Salacid®	(sal as′ sid)
Salagen®	(sal′ a gen)
Salagen®	(sal′ a gen)
Salacid®	(sal as′ sid)
Salutensin®	(sal yu ten′ sin)
Diutensin®	(dye yu ten′ sin)
saquinavir	(sa kwin′ a veer)
Sinequan®	(si′ ne kwan)
Seconal™	(sek′ o nal)
Sectral®	(sek′ tral)

Drug Name	Pronunciation
Sectral®	(sek′ tral)
Factrel®	(fak′ trel)
Sectral®	(sek′ tral)
Seconal™	(sek′ o nal)
Seldane®	(sel′ dane)
Feldene®	(fel′ deen)
Senexon®	(sen′ e son)
Cenestin®	(se nes′ tin)
Septa®	(sep′ tah)
Septra®	(sep′ trah)
Septra®	(sep′ trah)
Septa®	(sep′ tah)
Ser-Ap-Es®	(ser ap′ ess)
Catapres®	(kat′ a pres)
Serax®	(sear′ aks)
Eurax®	(yoor′ aks)
Serax®	(sear′ aks)
Urex®	(yu′ eks)
Serax®	(sear′ aks)
Zyrtec®	(zir′ tec)
Serentil®	(su ren′ til)
Surital®	(su′ ri tal)
Seroquel®	(seer′ oh kwel
Sinequan®	(si′ ne kwan)
Silace®	(sye′ lace)
Silain®	(sye′ lain)
Silain®	(sye′ lain)
Silace®	(sye′ lace)
Sinequan®	(si′ ne kwan)
saquinavir	(sa kwin′ a veer)
Sinequan®	(si′ ne kwan)
Seroquel®	(seer′ oh kwel
Slo-Bid®	(slo′ bid)
Dolobid®	(dol′ ah bid)
Solarcaine®	(sole′ ar kane)
Solatene®	(sole′ a teen)
Solatene®	(sole′ a teen)
Solarcaine®	(sole′ ar kane)
Soriatane®	(sor′ e ah tane)
Loxitane®	(loks′ e tane)
Staphcillin®	(staf sil′ lin)
Staticin®	(stat′ i sin)
Staticin®	(stat′ i sin)
Staphcillin®	(staf sil′ lin)
streptomycin	(strep toe mye′ sin)
streptozocin	(strep toe zoe′ sin)
streptozocin	(strep toe zoe′ sin)
streptomycin	(strep toe mye′ sin)

Drug Name	Pronunciation
Sudafed®	(sue′ da fed)
Sufenta®	(sue fen′ tah)
Sufenta®	(sue fen′ tah)
Alfenta®	(al fen′ tah)
Sufenta®	(sue fen′ tah)
Sudafed®	(sue′ da fed)
sufentanil	(sue fen′ ta nil)
alfentanil	(al fen′ ta nil)
sulfasalazine	(sul fa sal′ a zeen)
sulfisoxazole	(sul fi sox′ a zole)
sulfisoxazole	(sul fi sox′ a zole)
sulfasalazine	(sul fa sal′ a zeen)
sumatriptan	(soo ma trip′ tan)
zolmitriptan	(zohl mi trip′ tan)
Suprax®	(su′ prax)
Surbex®	(sur′ beks)
Surbex®	(sur′ beks)
Suprax®	(su′ prax)
Surbex®	(sur′ beks)
Surfak®	(sur′ fak)
Surfak®	(sur′ fak)
Surbex®	(sur′ beks)
Surital®	(su′ ri tal)
Serentil®	(su ren′ til)
Sytobex®	(sye′ toe beks)
Cytotec®	(sye′ toe tek)
Tacaryl®	(tak′ a ril)
tacrine	(tak′ reen)
tacrine	(tak′ reen)
Tacaryl®	(tak′ a ril)
Tagamet®	(tag′ a met)
Tegopen®	(teg′ o pen)
Talacen®	(tal′ a sen)
Tegison®	(teg′ i son)
Talacen®	(tal′ a sen)
Tinactin®	(tin ak′ tin)
Taxol®	(tacks′ ol)
Paxil®	(packs′ ol)
Tedral®	(ted′ ral)
Teldrin®	(tel′ drin)
Tegison®	(teg′ i son)
Talacen®	(tal′ a sen)
Tegopen®	(teg′ o pen)
Tagamet®	(tag′ a met)
Tegopen®	(teg′ o pen)
Tegretol®	(teg′ ree tol)
Tegopen®	(teg′ o pen)
Tegrin®	(teg′ rin)

Drug Name	Pronunciation
Tegretol®	(teg′ ree tol)
Mebaral®	(meb′ a ral)
Tegretol®	(teg′ ree tol)
Tegopen®	(teg′ o pen)
Tegrin®	(teg′ rin)
Tegopen®	(teg′ o pen)
Teldrin®	(tel′ drin)
Tedral®	(ted′ ral)
Temaril®	(tem′ a ril)
Demerol®	(dem′ eh rol)
Temaril®	(tem′ a ril)
Tepanil®	(tep′ a nil)
Tenex®	(ten′ eks)
Entex®	(en′ teks)
Tenex®	(ten′ eks)
Xanax®	(zan′ aks)
Tepanil®	(tep′ a nil)
Temaril®	(tem′ a ril)
Tepanil®	(tep′ a nil)
Tofranil®	(toe fray′ nil)
terbinafine	(ter′ bin a feen)
terfenadine	(ter fen′ na deen)
terbinafine	(ter′ bin a feen)
terbutaline	(ter byoo′ ta leen)
terbutaline	(ter byoo′ ta leen)
terbinafine	(ter′ bin a feen)
terbutaline	(ter byoo′ ta leen)
tolbutamide	(tole byoo′ ta mide)
terconazole	(ter kone′ a zole)
tioconazole	(tye o kone′ a zole)
terfenadine	(ter fen′ na deen)
terbinafine	(ter′ bin a feen)
Terramycin®	(tehr a mye′ sin)
Garamycin®	(gar a mye′ sin)
testolactone	(tess toe lak′ tone)
testosterone	(tess toss′ ter one)
testosterone	(tess toss′ ter one)
testolactone	(tess toe lak′ tone)
Theelin®	(thee′ lin)
Theolair™	(thee′ o lare)
Theoclear®	(thee′ o clear)
Theolair™	(thee′ o lare)
Theolair™	(thee′ o lare)
Theelin®	(thee′ lin)
Theolair™	(thee′ o lare)
Theoclear®	(thee′ o clear)
Theolair™	(thee′ o lare)
Thiola™	(thye oh′ la)

Drug Name	Pronunciation
Theolair™	(thee′ o lare)
Thyrolar®	(thye′ roe lar)
Theragran®	(ther′ a gran)
Phenergan®	(fen′ er gan)
Theramin®	(there′ a min)
thiamine	(thye′ a min)
thiamine	(thye′ a min)
Theramin®	(there′ a min)
Thiola™	(thye oh′ la)
Theolair™	(thee′ o lare)
thioridazine	(thye o rid′ a zeen)
thiothixene	(thye o thix′ een)
thiothixene	(thye o thix′ een)
thioridazine	(thye o rid′ a zeen)
Thyrar®	(thyer′ are)
Thyrolar®	(thye′ roe lar)
Thyrar®	(thyer′ are)
Ticar®	(tye′ kar)
Thyrolar®	(thye′ roe lar)
Theolair™	(thee′ o lare)
Thyrolar®	(thye′ roe lar)
Thyrar®	(thyer′ are)
Thyrolar®	(thye′ roe lar)
Thytropar®	(thye′ troe par)
Thytropar®	(thye′ troe par)
Thyrolar®	(thye′ roe lar)
Ticar®	(tye′ kar)
Thyrar®	(thyer′ are)
Ticar®	(tye′ kar)
Tigan®	(tye′ gan)
Ticon®	(tye′ kon)
Tigan®	(tye′ gan)
Tigan®	(tye′ gan)
Ticar®	(tye′ kar)
Tigan®	(tye′ gan)
Ticon®	(tye′ kon)
timolol	(tye′ moe lole)
Tylenol®	(tye′ le nole)
Timoptic®	(tim op′ tik)
Viroptic®	(vir op′ tik)
Tinactin®	(tin ak′ tin)
Talacen®	(tal′ a sen)
Tindal®	(tin′ dal)
Trental®	(tren′ tal)
tioconazole	(tye o kone′ a zole)
terconazole	(ter kone′ a zole)
TobraDex®	(toe′ bra deks)
Tobrex®	(toe′ breks)

Drug Name	Pronunciation
tobramycin	(toe bra mye′ sin)
Trobicin®	(troe′ bi sin)
Tobrex®	(toe′ breks)
TobraDex®	(toe′ bra deks)
Tofranil®	(toe fray′ nil)
Tepanil®	(tep′ a nil)
tolazamide	(tole az′ a mide)
tolazoline	(tole az′ o leen)
tolazamide	(tole az′ a mide)
tolbutamide	(tole byoo′ ta mide)
tolazoline	(tole az′ o leen)
tolazamide	(tole az′ a mide)
tolbutamide	(tole byoo′ ta mide)
terbutaline	(ter byoo′ ta leen)
tolbutamide	(tole byoo′ ta mide)
tolazamide	(tole az′ a mide)
Tolinase®	(tole′ i nase)
Orinase®	(or′ in ase)
tolnaftate	(tole naf′ tate)
Tornalate®	(tor′ na late)
Tonocard®	(ton′ o kard)
Torecan®	(tor′ e kan)
Torecan®	(tor′ e kan)
Tonocard®	(ton′ o kard)
Tornalate®	(tor′ na late)
tolnaftate	(tole naf′ tate)
Trandate®	(tran′ date)
Trendar®	(tren′ dar)
Trandate®	(tran′ date)
Trental®	(tren′ tal)
Trendar®	(tren′ dar)
Trandate®	(tran′ date)
Trental®	(tren′ tal)
Bentyl®	(ben′ til)
Trental®	(tren′ tal)
Tindal®	(tin′ dal)
Trental®	(tren′ tal)
Trandate®	(tran′ date)
tretinoin	(tret′ i noyn)
trientine	(trye′ en teen)
Tri-Levlen®	(trye′ lev len)
Trilafon®	(tri′ la fon)
triacetin	(trye a see′ tin)
Triacin®	(trye′ a sin)
Triacin®	(trye′ a sin)
triacetin	(trye a see′ tin)
triamterene	(trye am′ ter een)
trimipramine	(trye mi′ pra meen)

Drug Name	Pronunciation
Triapin®	(trye a pin)
Triban®	(trye′ ban)
triazolam	(trye ay′ zoe lam)
alprazolam	(al pray′ zoe lam)
Triban®	(trye′ ban)
Triapin®	(trye a pin)
trientine	(trye′ en teen)
tretinoin	(tret′ i noyn)
Trilafon®	(tri′ la fon)
Tri-Levlen®	(trye′ lev len)
trimeprazine	(trye mep′ ra zeen)
trimipramine	(trye mi′ pra meen)
trimethaphan	(trye meth′ a fan)
trimethoprim	(trye meth′ o prim)
trimethoprim	(trye meth′ o prim)
trimethaphan	(trye meth′ a fan)
trimipramine	(trye mi′ pra meen)
triamterene	(trye am′ ter een)
trimipramine	(trye mi′ pra meen)
trimeprazine	(trye mep′ ra zeen)
Trimox®	(trye′ moks)
Diamox®	(dye′ a moks)
Trimox®	(trye′ moks)
Tylox®	(tye′ loks)
Trinalin®	(tri′ na lin)
Phrenilin®	(fren′ ni lin)
Triofed®	(trye′ o fed)
Triostat™	(tree′ o stat)
Triostat™	(tree′ o stat)
Triofed®	(trye′ o fed)
Trisoralen®	(trye sore′ a len)
Trysul®	(trye′ sul)
Trobicin®	(troe′ bi sin)
tobramycin	(toe bra mye′ sin)
Tronolane®	(tron′ o lane)
Tronothane®	(tron′ o thane)
Tronothane®	(tron′ o thane)
Tronolane®	(tron′ o lane)
Trysul®	(trye′ sul)
Trisoralen®	(trye sore′ a len)
Tuinal®	(tu′ i nal)
Luminal®	(lu′ mi nal)
Tuinal®	(tu′ i nal)
Tylenol®	(tye′ le nole)
Tussafed®	(tus′ a fed)
Tussafin®	(tus′ a fin)
Tussafin®	(tus′ a fin)
Tussafed®	(tus′ a fed)

Drug Name	Pronunciation
Tylenol®	(tye' le nole)
atenolol	(a ten' oh lole)
Tylenol®	(tye' le nole)
timolol	(tye' moe lole)
Tylenol®	(tye' le nole)
Tuinal®	(tu' i nal)
Tylenol®	(tye' le nole)
Tylox®	(tye' loks)
Tylox®	(tye' loks)
Trimox®	(trye' moks)
Tylox®	(tye' loks)
Tylenol®	(tye' le nole)
Tylox®	(tye' loks)
Wymox®	(wye' moks)
Uni-Bent®	(yu' ni bent)
Unipen®	(yu' ni pen)
Unipen®	(yu' ni pen)
Uni-Bent®	(yu' ni bent)
Unipen®	(yu' ni pen)
Omnipen®	(om' ni pen)
Urex®	(yu' eks)
Eurax®	(yoor' aks)
Urex®	(yur' ecks)
Orex®	(or' ecks)
Urex®	(yu' eks)
Serax®	(sear' aks)
V-Cillin K®	(vee sil' lin kay)
Bicillin®	(bye sil' lin)
V-Cillin K®	(vee' sil lin kay)
Wycillin®	(wye sil' lin)
Vamate®	(vam' ate)
Vancenase®	(van' sen ase)
Vancenase®	(van' sen ase)
Vamate®	(vam' ate)
Vanceril®	(van' ser il)
Vansil™	(van' sil)
Vansil™	(van' sil)
Vanceril®	(van' ser il)
Vasocidin®	(vay so sye' din)
Vasodilan®	(vay so di' lan)
Vasodilan®	(vay so di' lan)
Vasocidin®	(vay so sye' din)
Vasosulf®	(vay' so sulf)
Velosef®	(vel' o sef)
VePesid®	(veh' pe sid)
Versed®	(ver' sed)
Velosef®	(vel' o sef)
Vasosulf®	(vay' so sulf)

Drug Name	Pronunciation
Ventolin®	(ven' tow lin)
Benylin®	(ben' eh lin)
Ventolin®	(ven' to lin)
phentolamine	(fen tole' a meen)
Verelan®	(ver' e lan)
Voltaren®	(vo tare' en)
Versed®	(ver' sed)
VePesid®	(veh' pe sid)
Viagra®	(vye ag' ra)
Allegra®	(al leg' ra)
Vicodin®	(vye' co din)
Hycodan®	(hye' co dan)
vidarabine	(vye dare' a been)
cytarabine	(sye tare' a been)
Videx®	(vye' deks)
Lidex®	(lye' deks)
vinblastine	(vin blas' teen)
vincristine	(vin kris' teen)
vincristine	(vin kris' teen)
Myochrysine®	(mye o kris' seen)
vincristine	(vin kris' teen)
vinblastine	(vin blas' teen)
Viroptic®	(vir op' tik)
Timoptic®	(tim op' tik)
Visine®	(vye' seen)
Visken®	(vis' ken)
Visken®	(vis' ken)
Visine®	(vye' seen)
Vistaril®	(vis' tar ril)
Restoril®	(res' tor ril)
Volmax®	(vol' maks)
Flomax®	(flo' maks)
Voltaren®	(vo tare' en)
Verelan®	(ver' e lan)
Voltaren®	(vo tare' en)
Vontrol®	(von' trole)
Vontrol®	(von' trole)
Voltaren®	(vo tare' en)
Vytone®	(vye' tone)
Hytone®	(hye' tone)
Vytone®	(vye' tone)
Zydone®	(zye' doan)
Wycillin®	(wye sil' lin)
Bicillin®	(bye sil' lin)
Wycillin®	(wye sil' lin)
V-Cillin K®	(vee' sil lin kay)
Wydase®	(wye' dase)
Lidex®	(lye' deks)

Drug Name	Pronunciation
Wymox®	(wye′ moks)
Tylox®	(tye′ loks)
Xanax®	(zan′ aks)
Tenex®	(ten′ eks)
Xanax®	(zan′ aks)
Zantac®	(zan′ tak)
Xalatan®	(za lan′ tan)
Zarontin®	(za ron′ tin)
Xylo-Pfan®	(zye′ lo fan)
Zyloprim®	(zye′ lo prim)
Yocon®	(yo′ con)
Zocor®	(zoe′ cor)
Zantac®	(zan′ tak)
Xanax®	(zan′ aks)
Zarontin®	(za ron′ tin)
Xalatan®	(za lan′ tan)
Zarontin®	(za ron′ tin)
Zaroxolyn®	(za roks′ o lin)
Zaroxolyn®	(za roks′ o lin)
Zarontin®	(za ron′ tin)
Zebeta®	(ze′ bay tah)
Diaβeta®	(dye a bay′ tah)

Drug Name	Pronunciation
Zerit®	(zer′ it)
Ziac™	(zye′ ak)
Ziac™	(zye′ ak)
Zerit®	(zer′ it)
Zocor®	(zoe′ cor)
Cozaar®	(koe′ zar)
Zocor®	(zoe′ cor)
Yocon®	(yo′ con)
Zofran®	(zoe′ fran)
Zosyn™	(zoe′ sin)
zolmitriptan	(zohl mi trip′ tan)
sumatriptan	(soo ma trip′ tan)
Zosyn™	(zoe′ sin)
Zofran®	(zoe′ fran)
Zydone®	(zye′ doan)
Vytone®	(vye′ tone)
Zyloprim®	(zye′ lo prim)
Xylo-Pfan®	(zye′ lo fan)
Zyprexa®	(zye preks′ a)
Celexa®	(se lex′ a)
Zyrtec®	(zir′ tec)
Serax®	(sear′ aks)

NEW DRUGS INTRODUCED OR APPROVED BY THE FDA IN 1999

Brand Name	Generic Name	Use
Aciphex™	rabeprazole	Reflux ulcer and duodenal ulcer
Actos®	pioglitazone	Type II diabetes
Agenerase™	amprenavir	HIV
Alamast®	pemirolast	Allergic conjunctivitis
Antagon™	ganirelix	Prevent premature LH surges
Avandia®	rosiglitazone	Type II diabetes
Busulfex®	busalfan	Chronic myelogenous leukemia
Cenestin®	synthetic conj. estrogens, A	Symptoms of menopause
Chirocaine®	levobupivacaine	Local or regional anesthesia
DepoCyt®	cytarabine liposome	Lymphomatous meningitis
Ellence™	epirubicin	Antineoplastic
Ferrlecit®	sodium ferric gluconate complex	Iron deficiency in dialysis patient
Hectoral™	doxercalciferol	Hyperparathyroidism
Nabi-HB®	hepatitis B immune globulin	Hepatitis B
NovoSeven®	recombinant factor VIIa	Hemophilia A or B
Ontak®	denileukin dititox	Cutaneous T-cell lymphoma (CTCL)
Panretin™	alitretinoin	AIDS-related Kaposi's sarcoma
Pletal®	cilostazol	Intermittent claudication
Rapamune™	sirolimus	Immunosuppressant
Raplan®	rapacuronium	Neuromuscular blocking agent
Relenza®	zanamivir	Influenza
Sonata®	Zaleplan	Hypnotic agent
Synercid®	quinupristin/dalfopristin	Antibiotic (vancomycin-resistant bacteria)
Tamiflu™	oseltamivir	Type A & B influenza
Temodar®	temozolomide	Alkylating agent
Vioxx®	rofecoxib	Osteoarthritis, pain, dysmenorrhea
Xenical®	orlistat	Obesity
Xopenex®	levalbuterol	Bronchospasm
Zaditor®	ketotifen fumarate	Allergic conjunctivitis

PENDING DRUGS OR DRUGS IN CLINICAL TRIALS

Brand Name	Generic Name	Use
Aggrenox®	dipyridamole & aspirin	Reduce risk of nonfatal stroke
Alredase®	tolrestat	Controlling late complications of diabetes
Arkin-Z®	vesnarinone	Congestive heart failure agent
Baypress®	nitrendipine	Calcium channel blocker for hypertension
Berotec®	fenoterol	Beta-2 agonist for asthma
Catatrol®	viloxazine	Bicyclic antidepressant
Cipralan®	cifenline succinate	Antiarrhythmic agent
Cytolex®	pexiganan	Diabetic foot ulcers
Decabid®	indecainide hydrochloride	Antiarrhythmic agent
Delaprem®	hexoprenaline sulfate	Tocolytic agent
Dirame®	propiram	Opioid analgesic
Enable®	tenidap sodium	Arthritis
Exelom®	rivastigmine	Alzheimer's disease
Fareston®	toremifene citrate	Antiestrogen for breast cancer
Freedox®	triliazad mesylate	Prevents progressive neuronal degeneration
Frisium®	clobazam	Benzodiazepine
Gastrozepine®	pirenzepine	Antiulcer drug
Inhibace®	cilazapril	ACE inhibitor
Isoprinosine®	inosiplex	Immunomodulating drug
Lacipil®	lacidipine	Hypertension
Malarone®	atavaquone/proguanil	Malaria
Maxicam®	isoxicam	NSAID
Mentane®	velnacrine	Alzheimer's disease agent
Micturin®	terodiline hydrochloride	Agent for urinary incontinence
Mogadon®	nitrazepam	Benzodiazepine
Motilium®	domperidone	Antiemetic
Napa®	acecainide	Antiarrhythmic agent
Natrecor®	nesiritide	Congestive heart failure
Pindac®	pinacidil	Antihypertensive
Prothiaden®	dothiepin hydrochloride	Tricyclic antidepressant
Protonix®	pantopraxole	Proton pump inhibitor
Rimadyl®	caprofen	NSAID
Roxiam®	remoxipride	Antipsychotic agent
Selecor®	celiprolol hydrochloride	Beta-adrenergic blocker
Spexil®	trospectomycin	Antibiotic, a spectinomycin analog
Targocoid®	teicoplanin	Antibiotic, similar to vancomycin
Tikosyn®	dofetilide	Antiarrhythmic agent
Unicard®	dilevalol	Beta-adrenergic blocker
Zaditen®	ketotifen	Antiasthmatic

DRUG PRODUCTS NO LONGER AVAILABLE

Brand Name	Generic Name
Achromycin® Parenteral	tetracycline
Achromycin® V Capsule	tetracycline
Achromycin® V Oral Suspension	tetracycline
ACTH-40®	corticotropin
Actidil®	triprolidine
Actifed® Syrup	triprolidine and pseudoephedrine
Actifed® With Codeine	triprolidine, pseudoephedrine, and codeine
Adipex-P®	phentermine (all products)
Adipost®	phendimetrazine tartrate
Adphen®	phendimetrazine tartrate
Adrin®	nylidrin hydrochloride
Aerolate® Oral Solution	theophylline
Aerosporin® Injection	polymyxin B
Agoral® Plain	mineral oil
Akoline® C.B. Tablet	vitamin
AK-Zol® Tablet	acetazolamide
Ala-Tet®	tetracycline
Amin-Aid®	amino acid
Amonidrin® Tablet	guaifenesin
Anacin-3® (all products)	acetaminophen
Anaids® Tablet	alginic acid and sodium bicarbonate
Anergan® 25 Injection	promethazine hydrochloride
Anoxine-AM® Capsule	phentermine hydrochloride
Antinea® Cream	benzoic acid and salicylic acid
Antivert® Chewable Tablet	meclizine hydrochloride
Antrocol® Capsule & Tablet	atropine and belladonna
Apomorphine	apomorphine (now available as an orphan drug only)
Arcotinic® Tablet	iron and liver combination
Argyrol® S.S.	silver protein, mild
Arlidin®	nylidrin (all products)
Arthritis Foundation® Ibuprofen	ibuprofen
Arthritis Foundation® Nighttime	acetaminophen and diphenhydramine
Arthritis Foundation® Pain Reliever, Aspirin Free	acetaminophen
Arthritis Strength Bufferin®	aspirin (buffered)
Articulose-50® Injection	prednisolone
Asbron-G® Elixir	theophylline and guaifenesin
Asbron-G® Tablet	theophylline and guaifenesin
Asproject®	sodium thiosalicylate
Atabrine® Tablet	quinacrine hydrochloride
Atropine Soluble Tablet	atropine soluble tablet
Aureomycin®	chlortetracycline
Axotal®	butalbital compound and aspirin
Azlin® Injection	azlocillin
Azo Gantanol®	sulfamethoxazole and phenazopyridine
Azo Gantrisin®	sulfisoxazole and phenazopyridine
Azulfidine® Suspension	sulfasalazine
B-A-C®	butalbital compound with aspirin
Bactocill®	oxacillin
Bancap®	butalbital compound with acetaminophen
Banesin®	acetaminophen
Bantron®	lobeline (all products)
Baypress®	nitrendipine
Becomject-100®	vitamin B complex
Beesix®	pyridoxine hydrochloride

(continued)

Brand Name	Generic Name
Bellafoline®	levorotatory alkaloids of belladonna (all products)
Bemote®	dicyclomine
Bena-D®	diphenhydramine
Benadryl® 50 mg Capsule	diphenhydramine hydrochloride
Benadryl® Cold/Flu	acetaminophen, diphenhydramine, and pseudoephedrine
Benahist® Injection	diphenhydramine hydrochloride
Benoject®	diphenhydramine hydrochloride
Betapen-VK®	penicillin V potassium
Beta-Val® Ointment	betamethasone
Biamine® Injection	thiamine hydrochloride
Bilezyme® Tablet	pancrelipase
Biomox®	amoxicillin
Biphetamine®	amphetamine and dextroamphetamine
Blanex® Capsule	chloroxazone and acetaminophen
Bretylol®	bretylium
Bronkephrine®	ethylnorepinephrine hydrochloride
Buffered®, Tri-buffered	aspirin
Bufferin® Arthritis Strength	aspirin
Bufferin® Extra Strength	aspirin
Buf-Puf® Acne Cleansing Bar	salicylic acid
Butace®	butalbital compound
Caladryl® Spray	diphenhydramine and calamine
Calciparine® Injection	heparin calcium
Camalox® Suspension & Tablet	aluminum hydroxide, calcium carbonate, and magnesium hydroxide
Cantharone®	cantharidin
Cantharone Plus®	cantharidin
Caroid®	cascara sagrada and phenolphthalein
Catarase® 1:5000	chymotrypsin (all products)
Cedilanid-D® Injection	deslanoside
Cenocort® A-40	triamcinolone
Cenocort® Forte	triamcinolone
Centrax® Capsule & Tablet	prazepam
Cerespan®	papaverine hydrochloride
Cetane®	ascorbic acid
Chenix® Tablet	chenodiol
Chlorgest-HD® Elixir	chlorpheniramine, phenylephrine, and hydrocodone
Chlorofon-A® Tablet	chlorzoxazone
Chloromycetin® Cream	chloramphenicol
Chloromycetin® Kapseals®	chloramphenicol
Chloromycetin® Ophthalmic	chloramphenicol
Chloromycetin® Otic	chloramphenicol
Chloromycetin® Palmitate Oral Suspension	chloramphenicol
Chloroserpine®	reserpine and hydrochorothiazide
Chlortab®	chlorpheniramine maleate
Choledyl®	oxtriphylline
Chymex®	bentiromide (all products)
Cipralan®	cifenline
Cithalith-S® Syrup	lithium citrate
Citro-Nesia® Solution	magnesium citrate
Clistin® Tablet	carbinoxamine maleate
Clorpactin® XCB Powder	oxychlorosene sodium
Cobalasine® Injection	adenosine phosphate
Codimal-A® Injection	brompheniramine maleate
Codimal® Expectorant	guaifenesin and phenylpropanolamine
Coly-Mycin® S Oral	colistin sulfate
Constant-T® Tablet	theophylline

(continued)

Brand Name	Generic Name
Control-L®	pyrethrins
Cortaid® Ointment	hydrocortisone
Cortrophin-Zinc®	corticotropin
Crysticillin® 300 A.S.	penicillin G procaine
Crysticillin® 600 A.S.	penicillin G procaine
Crystodigin® 0.05 mg & 0.15 mg Tablet	digitoxin
Cyclospasmol®	cyclandelate (all products)
Cycrin® 10 mg Tablet	medroxyprogesterone acetate
D-Amp®	ampicillin
Danex® Shampoo	pyrithione zinc
Dapex-37.5®	phentermine hydrochloride
Darbid® Tablet	isopropamide iodide (all products)
Daricon®	oxyphencyclimine (all products)
Darvon® 32 mg Capsule	propoxyphene hydrochloride
Darvon-N® Oral Suspension	propoxyphene napsylate
Datril® Extra Strength	acetaminophen
Decadron® 0.25 mg & 6 mg Tablets	dexamethasone
Decaspray®	dexamethasone
Dehist®	brompheniramine maleate
Deltalin® Capsule	ergocalciferol
Depo-Provera® 100 mg/mL	medroxyprogesterone
Deprol®	meprobamate and benactyzine hydrochloride
Dermoxyl® Gel	benzoyl peroxide
Despec® Liquid	guaifenesin, phenylpropanolamine, and phenylephrine
Dexacen-4®	dexamethasone
Dexacen® LA-8	dexamethasone
Dexedrine® Elixir	dextroamphetamine sulfate
Dialose® Capsule	docusate sodium
Diaparene® Cradol®	methylbenzethonium
Dilantin-30® Pediatric Suspension	phenytoin
Dilantin® With Phenobarbital	phenytoin with phenobarbital
Dilaudid® 1 mg & 3 mg Tablet	hydromorphone hydrochloride
Dimetane®	brompheniramine maleate
Dispos-a-Med® Isoproterenol	isoproterenol
Diupress®	chlorothiazide and reserpine
Dizymes® Tablet	pancreatin
Dommanate® Injection	dimenhydrinate
Donphen® Tablet	hyoscyamine, atropine, scopolamine, and phenobarbital
Dopastat® Injection	dopamine hydrochloride
Doriden® Tablet	glutethimide
Doxinate® Capsule	docusate sodium
Dramamine® Injection	dimenhydrinate
Dramocen®	dimenhydrinate
Dramoject®	dimenhydramine
D-S-S Plus®	docusate and casanthranol
Duo-Medihaler®	isoproterenol and phenylephrine
Duracid®	aluminum hydroxide, magnesium carbonate, and calcium carbonate
Duract®	bromfenac (all products)
Dyflex-400® Tablet	dyphylline
Elase® Ointment	fibrinolysin and desoxyribonuclease (all products)
Elase®-Chloromycetin® Ointment	fibrinolysin and desoxyribonuclease
Eldepryl® Tablet	selegiline
Eldoquin® Lotion	hydroquinone
Elixophyllin SR®	theophylline

(continued)

Brand Name	Generic Name
E-Lor® Tablet	propoxyphene and acetaminophen
Emete-Con® Injection	benzquinamide
Emetine Hydrochloride	emetine hydrochloride
Endep® 25 mg, 50 mg, 100 mg	amitriptyline hydrochloride
Enduron® 2.5 mg Tablet	methyclothiazide
Enkaid®	encainide
Enovid®	mestranol and norethynodrel
E.N.T.®	brompheniramine and phenylpropanolamine
Entozyme®	pancreatin
E.P. Mycin® Capsule	oxytetracycline
Ergostat®	ergotamine
Ergotrate® Maleate	ergonovine maleate
Eridium®	phenazopyridine hydrochloride
Ery-Sol® Topical Solution	erythromycin, topical
Esidrix® 100 mg Tablet	hydrochlorothiazide
Estradurin® Injection	polyestradiol phosphate
Estroject-2® Injection	estradiol
Estroject-L.A.® Injection	estradiol
Estronol® Injection	estrone
Estrovis®	quinestrol
Ethaquin®	ethaverine hydrochloride
Ethatab®	ethaverine hydrochloride
Ethavex-100®	ethaverine hydrochloride
Euthroid® Tablet	liotrix
Fansidar®	sulfadoxine and pyrimethamine
Fastin®	phentermine (all products)
FemCare®	clotrimazole
Femstat®	butoconazole nitrate
Fergon Plus®	iron with vitamin B
Fer-In-Sol® Capsule	ferrous sulfate
Fermalox®	ferrous sulfate, magnesium hydroxide, and docusate
Ferndex	dextroamphetamine sulfate
Flonase® 9 g	fluticasone
Folex® Injection	methotrexate
Gamastan®	immune globulin, intramuscular
Gammagard® Injection	immune globulin, intravenous
Gammar®	immune globulin, intramuscular
Gantrisin® Ophthalmic	sulfisoxazole
Gantrisin® Tablet	sulfisoxazole
Gelusil® Liquid	aluminum hydroxide, magnesium hydroxide, and simethicone
Gen-D-phen®	diphenhydramine hydrochloride
Grisactin®	griseofulvin
Gynogen® Injection	estradiol
Halazone Tablet	halazone
Halenol® Tablet	acetaminophen
Harmonyl®	deserpidine
HemFe®	iron with vitamins
Hep-B-Gammagee®	hepatitis B immune globulin
Herplex®	idoxuridine
Hetrazan®	diethylcarbamazine citrate
Hismanal®	astemizole
Histaject®	brompheniramine maleate
Histamine Phosphate Injection	histamine phosphate
Hydeltra-T.B.A.®	prednisolone
Hydramine®	diphenhydramine hydrochloride
Hydrobexan® Injection	hydroxocobalamin
Hydropres® 25 mg Tablet	hydrochlorothiazide and reserpine

(continued)

Brand Name	Generic Name
Hydroxacen®	hydroxyzine
Intal® Inhalation Capsule	cromolyn sodium
Intercept®	nonoxynol 9
Iodo-Niacin® Tablet	potassium iodide and niacinamide hydroiodide
Ionamin®	phentermine (all products)
Iophen®	iodinated glycerol
Iophen-C®	iodinated glycerol and codeine
Iophen-DM®	iodinated glycerol and dextromethorphan (all products)
Iophylline®	iodinated glycerol and theophylline
Iotuss®	iodinated glycerol and codeine
Iotuss-DM®	iodinated glycerol and dextromethorphan (all products)
Iso-Bid®	isosorbide dinitrate
Isopto® P-ES	pilocarpine and physostigmine
Isovex®	ethaverine hydrochloride
Isuprel® Glossets®	isoproterenol
Kaopectate® Children's Tablet	attapulgite
Kato® Powder	potassium chloride
Keflin®	cephalothin sodium
Kestrin® Injection	estrone
Koate®-HS Injection	antihemophilic factor (human)
Koate®-HT Injection	antihemophilic factor (human)
Kolyum® Powder	potassium chloride and potassium gluconate
Konyne-HT® Injection	factor IX complex (human)
Kwell®	lindane
Lamprene® 100 mg	clofazimine
Laniazid® Tablet	isoniazid
Lasan® Topical	anthralin
Lasan® HP-1 Topical	anthralin
Ledercillin VK®	penicillin V potassium
Libritabs® 5 mg	chlordiazepoxide
Listerex® Scrub	salicylic acid
Lorcet®	hydrocodone and acetaminophen
Lorelco®	probucol
Malatal®	hyoscyamine, atropine, scopolamine, and phenobarbital
Malotuss® Syrup	guaifenesin
Mandelamine® Tablet	methenamine
Mantadil® Cream	chlorcyclizine
Marezine® Injection	cyclizine hydrochloride
Marplan®	isocarboxazid
Materna®	prenatal vitamin
Max-Caro®	beta-carotene
Meclomen®	meclofenamate sodium
Medihaler-Epi®	epinephrine
Medihaler Ergotamine®	ergotamine
Medrapred®	prednisolone and atropine
Medrol® Acetate Topical	methylprednisolone
Melfiat® Tablet	phendimetrazine tartrate
Meprospan®	meprobamate
Metaprel® Aerosol	metaproterenol sulfate
Metaprel® Inhalation Solution	metaproterenol sulfate
Metaprel® Tablet	metaproterenol sulfate
Metizol® Tablet	metronidazole
Metopirone® Tablet	metyrapone tartrate
Metra®	phendimetrazine tartrate
Miflex® Tablet	chlorzoxazone and acetaminophen
Milprem®	meprobamate and conjugated estrogens
Minocin® Tablet	minocycline

(continued)

Brand Name	Generic Name
Miochol®	acetylcholine
Moisturel® Lotion	dimethicone
Monocete® Topical Liquid	monochloroacetic acid
Moxam® Injection	moxalactam
Mus-Lax®	chlorzoxazone
Mylaxen® Injection	hexafluorenium bromide
Myochrysine®	gold sodium thiomalate
Nafcil®	nafcillin
Nalfon® Tablet	fenoprofen calcium
Nandrobolic® Injection	nandrolone phenpropionate
Narcan® 1 mg/mL Injection	naloxone hydrochloride
Navane® Concentrate & Injection	thiothixene
N-B-P® Ointment	bacitracin, neomycin, and polymyxin B
Neo-Castaderm®	resorcinol, boric acid, acetone
Neo-Cortef® Topical	neomycin and hydrocortisone
NeoDecadron® Topical	neomycin and dexamethasone
Neo-Medrol® Acetate Topical	methylprednisolone and neomycin
Neoquess® Injection	dicyclomine hydrochloride
Neoquess® Tablet	hyoscyamine sulfate
Neo-Synalar® Topical	neomycin and fluocinolone
Neo-Synephrine® 12 Hour Nasal Solution	oxymetazoline hydrochloride
Neutra-Phos® Capsule	potassium phosphate and sodium phosphate
Niac®	niacin
Niacels®	niacin
Niclocide®	niclosamide
Nidryl®	diphenhydramine hydrochloride
Niferex Forte®	iron with vitamins
Niloric®	ergoloid mesylates
Nipride® Injection	nitroprusside sodium
Nisaval®	pyrilamine maleate
Nitro-Bid® Oral	nitroglycerin
Nitrocine® Oral	nitroglycerin
Nitrostat® 0.15 mg Tablet	nitroglycerin
Noctec®	chloral hydrate
Noludar®	methyprylon
Norlutate®	norethindrone
Norlutin®	norethindrone
Novafed®	pseudoephedrine
Novahistine DH® Liquid	chlorpheniramine, pseudoephedrine, and codeine
Novahistine DMX® Liquid	guaifenesin, pseudoephedrine, and dextromethorphan
Novahistine® Elixir	chlorpheniramine and phenylephrine
Novahistine® Expectorant	guaifenesin, pseudoephedrine, and codeine
Nursoy®	enteral nutritional therapy
Nydrazid® Injection	isoniazid
Obe-Nix® 30	phentermine (all products)
Obephen®	phentermine (all products)
Obermine®	phentermine (all products)
Obestin-30®	phentermine (all products)
Ophthaine®	proparacaine
Ophthocort®	chloramphenicol, polymyxin B, and hydrocortisone
Oradex-C®	dyclonine
Oratect®	benzocaine
Oreticyl®	deserpidine and hydrochlorothiazide
Organidin®	iodinated glycerol
Otic Tridesilon®	desonide and acetic acid
Oxsoralen® Oral	methoxsalen

(continued)

Brand Name	Generic Name
Panwarfin®	warfarin sodium
Paplex®	salicylic acid
Paradione®	paramethadione
Para-Hist AT®	promethazine, phenylephrine, and codeine
Pargen Fortified®	chlorzoxazone
Par Glycerol®	iodinated glycerol
Parmine®	phentermine hydrochloride
Parsidol®	ethopropazine (all products)
Pavabid HP®	papaverine hydrochloride
Pavasule®	papaverine hydrochloride
Pavatym®	papaverine hydrochloride
Pavesed®	papaverine hydrochloride
PBZ® Elixir	tripelennamine
Pentids®	penicillin G potassium, oral (all products)
Pfizerpen-AS®	penicillin G procaine
Phenaphen®	acetaminophen
Phenaphen®/Codeine #4	acetaminophen and codeine
Phenaseptic®	phenol
Phencen-50®	promethazine
Phenetron®	chlorpheniramine
Phentrol®	phentermine (all products)
Phenurone®	phenacemide
Phos-Ex® 62.5	calcium acetate
Phos-Ex® 125	calcium acetate
Phos-Ex® 167	calcium acetate
Phos-Ex® 250	calcium acetate
pHos-pHaid®	ammonium biphosphate, sodium biphosphate, and sodium acid pyrophosphate
Phosphaljel®	aluminum phosphate
Pindac®	pinacidil
Polargen®	dexchlorpheniramine maleate
Poliovax® Injection	poliovirus vaccine, inactivated
Polycillin® Oral	ampicillin
Polycillin-N® Injection	ampicillin
Polycillin-PRB®	ampicillin and probenecid (all products)
Polyflex® Tablet	chlorzoxazone
Polygam® Injection	immune globulin, intravenous
Polymox®	amoxicillin
Pondimin®	fenfluramine
Posicor®	mibefradil (all products)
Predaject-50®	prednisolone
Predalone®	prednisolone
Predicort-50®	prednisolone
Preludin®	phenmetrazine hydrochloride
Premarin® Vaginal Cream	conjugated estrogens
Proampacin®	ampicillin and probenecid (all products)
Procan SR®	procainamide
Profilate-HP®	antihemophilic factor (human)
Projestaject® Injection	progesterone
Prokine® Injection	sargramostim
Prolamine®	phenylpropanolamine
Proloid®	thyroglobulin
Prometh®	promethazine
Proplex® SX-T Injection	factor IX complex (human)
Pro-Sof®	docusate sodium
Prostaphlin®	oxacillin
Protopam® Tablet	pralidoxime chloride

(continued)

Brand Name	Generic Name
Provatene®	beta-carotene
Pyridium Plus®	phenazopyridine, hyoscyamine, and butabarbital
Questran® Tablet	cholestyramine resin
Quinamm®	quinine sulfate
Quiphile®	quinine sulfate
Q-vel®	quinine sulfate
Rectacort® Suppository	hydrocortisone
Redux®	dexfenfluramine
Regutol®	docusate
Rep-Pred®	methylprednisolone
R-Gen®	iodinated glycerol
Rhesonativ® Injection	Rh_0(D) immune globulin
Rhindecon®	phenylpropanolamine
Rhinolar®	chlorpheniramine, phenylpropanolamine, and methscopolamine
Rhuli® Cream	benzocaine, calamine, and camphor
Robicillin® Tablet	penicillin V potassium
Robitet®	tetracycline
Romycin® Solution	erythromycin, topical
Rondomycin® Capsule	methacycline hydrochloride (all products)
Rufen®	ibuprofen
Scabene®	lindane
Sclavo - PPD® Solution	tuberculin purified protein derivative
Sclavo Test - PPD®	tuberculin purified protein derivative
Sebulex®	sulfur and salicylic acid
Sebulon®	pyrithione zinc
Seconal™ Oral	secobarbital sodium
Seldane®	terfenadine
Seldane-D®	terfenadine and pseudoephedrine
Selecor®	celiprolol
Selestoject®	betamethasone
Senolax®	senna
Serpasil®	reserpine
Siblin®	psyllium
Skelex®	chlorzoxazone
Slo-Salt®	salt substitute
Sodium P.A.S.®	aminosalicylate sodium
Sofarin®	warfarin sodium
Solatene®	beta-carotene
Spasmoject®	dicyclomine
Spectrobid® Oral Suspension	bacampicillin
Staphcillin®	methicillin (all products)
Statobex®	phendimetrazine tartrate
Sterapred®	prednisone
Streptomycin	streptomycin
Sucostrin®	succinylcholine chloride
Sudafed® Children	pseudoephedrine
Sudafed® Cough	guaifenesin, pseudoephedrine, and dextromethorphan
Sudafed Plus® Liquid	chlorpheniramine and pseudoephedrine
Superchar®	charcoal
Superchar® With Sorbitol	charcoal
Surital®	thiamylal sodium
Symmetrel® Capsule	amantadine hydrochloride
Synkayvite®	menadiol sodium
Syntocinon® Nasal	oxytocin
Tabron®	vitamins, multiple
Tacaryl®	methdilazine hydrochloride (all products)
Taractan®	chlorprothixene

(continued)

Brand Name	Generic Name
T-Caine® Lozenge	benzocaine
Tegopen®	cloxacillin
Teline®	tetracycline
Temaril®	trimeprazine tartrate
Tepanil®	diethylpropion hydrochloride
Tepanil® TenTabs®	diethylpropion hydrochloride
Tes-Tape®	diagnostic aids (*in vitro*), urine
Tetralan®	tetracycline
Tetram®	tetracycline
Theelin® Aqueous Injection	estrone
Theobid® Jr Duracaps®	theophylline
Theo-Dur® Sprinkle®	theophylline
Theo-Organidin®	iodinated glycerol and theophylline
Theramin® Expectorant	guaifenesin and phenylpropanolamine
Thiacide®	methenamine and potassium acid phosphate
Tiject-20®	trimethobenzamide
Tindal®	acetophenazine maleate
Torecan® Suppository	thiethylperazine
Totacillin-N®	ampicillin
Tral®	hexocyclium methylsulfate
Travase®	sutilains
Tridione® Suppository	trimethadione
Trimox® 500 mg	amoxicillin
Trofan®	L-tryptophan
Trofan DS®	L-tryptophan
Tryptacin®	L-tryptophan
Tucks® Cream	witch hazel
Tusal®	sodium thiosalicylate
Tussi-Organidin®	iodinated glycerol and codeine
Tussi-Organidin® DM	iodinated glycerol and dextromethorphan (all products)
Tusso-DM®	iodinated glycerol and dextromethorphan (all products)
Tuss-Ornade®	caramiphen and phenylpropanolamine
Ultralente® U	insulin zinc suspension, extended
Ultrase® MT24	pancrelipase
Unipen®	nafcillin
Unipres®	hydralazine, hydrochlorothiazide, and reserpine
Ureacin®-40 Topical	urea
Uri-Tet®	oxytetracycline
Urobiotic-25®	oxytetracycline and sulfamethizole
Uticort®	betamethasone (all products)
Valadol®	acetaminophen
Valergen® Injection	estradiol
Valmid® Capsule	ethinamate
Valpin® 50	anisotropine methylbromide
Valrelease®	diazepam
Vanex-LA®	guaifenesin and phenylpropanolamine
Vanseb-T® Shampoo	coal tar, sulfur, and salicylic acid
V-Cillin K®	penicillin V potassium
Velsar® Injection	vinblastine sulfate
Vercyte®	pipobroman
Verr-Canth®	cantharidin
Verrex®	podophyllin and salicylic acid
Verrusol®	salicylic acid, podophyllin, and cantharidin
V-Gan® Injection	promethazine hydrochloride
Vicks® Vatronol®	ephedrine
Vioform®-Hydrocortisone Topical	clioquinol and hydrocortisone

(continued)

Brand Name	**Generic Name**
Visine®	tetrahydrozoline hydrochloride
Vistaject-25®	hydroxyzine
Vistaject-50®	hydroxyzine
Vontrol®	diphenidol
Wehamine® Injection	dimenhydrinate
Wehdryl®	diphenhydramine
Wesprin® Buffered	aspirin
Wyamycin S®	erythromycin
Zebrax®	clidinium and chlordiazepoxide
Zetran®	diazepam
Zolyse®	chymotrypsin alpha (all products)
Zyban® 100 mg	bupropion

PHARMACEUTICAL MANUFACTURERS AND DISTRIBUTORS

Abbott Laboratories
(Abbott Diagnostic Division)
One Abbott Park Road
Abbott Park, IL 60064-3500
www.abbott.com

Abbott Laboratories
(Hospital Products Division)
200 Abbott Park Road
Abbott Park, IL 60064-3537

Abbott Laboratories
(Pharmaceutical Product Division)
100 Abbott Park Road
Abbott Park, IL 60064-3500
www.abbott.com

Able Laboratories
6 Hollywood Court
South Plainfield, NJ 07080

Adams (see Medeva)

Adria (see Pharmacia)

Agouron Pharmaceuticals, Inc
10350 N Torrey Pines Road
La Jolla, CA 92037
www.agouron.com

Akorn, Inc
2500 Millbrook Drive
Buffalo Grove, IL 60089
www.akorn.com

Alcon Laboratories, Inc
6201 South Freeway
Ft Worth, TX 76134-2099
www.alconlabs.com

Allerderm Laboratories
PO Box 2070
Petaluma, CA 94953-2070

Allergan Herbert (see Allergan)

Allergan Pharmaceuticals
PO Box 19534
Irvine, CA 92623-9534
www.allergan.com

Alpha Therapeutic Corp
5555 Valley Boulevard
Los Angeles, CA 90032

Alpharma
(U.S. Pharmaceuticals Division)
7205 Windsor Boulevard
Baltimore, MD 21244

Alra Labs, Inc
3850 Clearview Court
Gurnee, IL 60031

Alto Pharmaceuticals, Inc
PO Box 1910
Land O'Lakes, FL 34639-1910
altopharm@aol.com

Alza Pharmaceuticals
950 Page Mill Road
Palo Alto, CA 94303-0802
www.alza.com

Ambix Labs, Inc
210 Orchard Street
East Rutherford, NJ 07073

American Drug Industries, Inc
5810 South Perry Avenue
Chicago, IL 60621

American Pharmaceutical, Co
12 Dwight Place
Fairfield, NJ 07004-3434

American Regent Laboratories Inc
1 Luitpold Drive
Shirley, NY 11967

Ames (see Miles Biological Products)

Amgen Inc
One Amgen Center Drive
Thousand Oaks, CA 91320-1789
www.ext.amgen.com

Amide Pharmaceuticals, Inc
101 East Main Street
Little Falls, NJ 07424

Anaquest (see Ohmeda)

ANDRX Pharmaceuticals, Inc
4001 South West 47th Avenue
Fort Lauderdale, FL 33314

Angelini Pharmaceuticals, Inc
70 Grand Avenue
River Edge, NJ 07661
dapp@nac.net

Apotex Corp
50 Lakeview Parkway
Suite 127
Vernon Hills, IL 60061

Apothecary Products, Inc
11531 Rupp Drive
Burnsville, MN 55337-1295
pillminder@aol.com

Apothecon Products
(A Bristol-Myers Squibb Company)
PO Box 4500
Princeton, NJ 08543-4500
www.apothecon.com

Applied Genetics Inc
205 Buffalo Avenue
Freeport, NY 11520
www.agiderm.com

Arcola Laboratories
500 Arcola Road
Collegeville, PA 19426-0107
www.rpr.rpna.com

Astra Pharmaceuticals, L.P.
725 Chesterbrook Blvd
Wayne, PA 19087-5677
information.center@astramerck.com
www.astramerck.com

Baker Norton Pharmaceuticals, Inc
4400 Biscayne Boulevard
Miami, FL 33137

Banner Pharmacaps, Inc
PO Box 2210
4125 Premier Drive
High Point, NC 27261-2210

Barr Laboratories, Inc
Box 2900
Pomona, NY 10970-0519
www.barrlabs.com

Bausch & Lomb Pharmaceuticals, Inc
8500 Hidden River Parkway
Tampa, FL 33637
www.bausch.com

Bausch & Lomb Surgical
555 W Arrow Highway
Claremont, CA 91711
www.blsurgical.com

Baxter Healthcare Corporation
Corporate Headquarters
One Baxter Parkway
Deerfield, IL 60015-4833
www.baxter.com

Baxter Healthcare Corporation
(I.V. Systems Division)
One Baxter Parkway
Deerfield, IL 60015
www.baxter.com

Bayer Corporation
N 3525 Regal Street
Box 3145
Spokane, WA 99220

Bayer Corporation
(Diagnostic Division)
430 South Beiger Street
PO Box 2004
Mishawaka, IN 46544-2004
www.bayerdiag.com

Bayer Corporation
(Pharmaceutical Division)
400 Morgan Lane
West Haven, CT 06516-4175
www.bayer.com

Bayer, Inc
77 Belfield Road
Toronto, Ontario, Canada M9W 1G6
www.bayerdiag.com

Becton Dickinson Microbiology Systems (Division of Becton Dickinson and Company)
PO Box 999
7 Loveton Circle
Sparks, MD 21152
www.ms.bd.com

Bedford Laboratories
(Division of Ben Venue Laboratories)
300 Northfield Road
PO Box 46568
Bedford, OH 44146
www.boehringer-ingelheim.com

Beecham (see SmithKline Beecham)

Beiersdorf
PO Box 5529
Norwalk, CT 06856-5529

Beiersdorf Inc
187 Danbury Road
Wilton, CT 06897

Berlex Laboratories
15049 San Pablo Avenue
Richmond, CA 94804-0099
www.betaseron.com
www.fludara.com

Berna Products, Corp
4216 Ponce de Leon Blvd
Coral Gables, FL 33146
www.bernaproducts.com

Beta Dermaceuticals, Inc
PO Box 691106
San Antonio, TX 78216-1106

Beutlich Pharmaceuticals
1541 Shields Drive
Waukegan, IL 60085-8304
www.beutlich.com

Biocraft (see Teva USA)

Biogen Inc
14 Cambridge Center
Cambridge, MA 02142
www.biogen.com

Biopharmaceutics, Inc
990 Station Road
Bellport, NY 11713
www.feminique.com

Bio-Technology General Corp
70 Wood Avenue South
Iselin, NJ 08830

Blaine Company, Inc
1515 Production Drive
Burlington, KY 41005
www.blainepharma.com

Bock (see Sanofi Winthrop)

Boehringer Ingelheim Pharmaceuticals, Inc
900 Ridgebury Road
PO Box 368
Ridgefield, CT 06877-0368
www.boehringer-ingelheim.com

Boots (see Knoll)

Braintree Laboratories, Inc
PO Box 850929
Braintree, MA 02185-0929

Brightstone Pharma
109 MacKenan Drive
Cary, NC 27511
www.brightstonepharma.com

Bristol-Myers Squibb
(Oncology/Immunology Division)
PO Box 4500
Princeton, NJ 08543-4500
www.bms.com

Bristol-Myers Squibb
(OTC Products)
225 High Ridge Road
Stanford, CT 06905
www.bms.com

Bristol-Myers Squibb Company
(Pharmaceutical Division)
PO Box 4500
Princeton, NJ 08543-4500

BTG (see Bio-Technology General Corp)

Burroughs Wellcome (see Glaxo Wellcome)

C&M Pharmacal, Inc
1721 Maple Lane Avenue
Hazel Park, MI 48030-2696
www.glytone.com

Caraco Pharmaceutical Laboratories Ltd
1150 Elijah McCoy Drive
Detroit, MI 48202
www.caraco.com

Celgene Corporation
7 Powder Horn Drive
Warren, NJ 07059

Centeon
1020 First Avenue
King of Prussia, PA 19406-1310
www.centeon.com/na

Center Labs
35 Channel Drive
Port Washington, NY 11050
www.centerpharm.com

Century Pharmaceuticals, Inc
10377 Hague Road
Indianapolis, IN 46256

Chemrich Laboratories
5211 Telegraph Road
Los Angeles, CA 90022

Cheshire Drugs
6225 Shiloh Road, Suite D
Alpharetta, GA 30005
www.cpsrx.com

Circa Pharmaceuticals, Inc
33 Ralph Avenue
PO Box 30
Copiague, NY 11726-0030
www.circapharm.com

Clay-Park Labs, Inc
Bathgate Industrial Park
1700 Bathgate Avenue
Bronx, NY 10457

Coast Labs, Inc
521 West 17th Street
Long Beach, CA 90813-1513

Copley Labs, Inc
25 John Road
Canton, MA 02021

Danbury Pharmacal, Inc
131 West Street
Danbury, CT 06810

Del-Ray Laboratories, Inc
22-20th Avenue North West
Birmingham, AL 35215

Denison Pharmaceuticals, Inc
60 Dunnell Lane
PO Box 1305
Pawtucket, RI 02862

Dermik Labs, Inc
500 Arcola Road
PO Box 1200
Collegeville, PA 19426-0107
www.rpr.rpna.com

Dey Laboratories
2751 Napa Valley Corporate Drive
Napa, CA 94558
www.deyinc.com

Duramed Pharmaceuticals, Inc
5040 Duramed Drive
Cincinnati, OH 45213
www.duramed.com

Emrex/Economed Pharmaceuticals, Inc
4305 Sartin Road
PO Box 3303
Burlington, NC 27217

Endo Generic Products
223 Wilmington West Chester Pike
Chadds Ford, PA 19317
www.endo.com

Eon Labs Manufacturing, Inc
227-15 North Conduit Avenue
Laurelton, NY 11413

ESI Lederle
PO Box 41502
Philadelphia, PA 19101
www.AHP.com

Ethex Corp
10888 Metro Court
St Louis, MO 63043-2413
www.ethex.com

Falcon Opthalmics, Inc
6201 South Freeway
Fort Worth, TX 76134
Parent Company: Alcon Laboratories
www.alconlabs.com

Faulding/Purepac Pharmaceutical Co
200 Elmora Avenue
Elizabeth, NJ 07207
www.faulding.com.au

Ferndale Laboratories, Inc
780 West Eight Mile Road
Ferndale, MI 48220

Fisons (see Medeva)

Fisons (see Rhone-Poulenc Rorer)

C.B. Fleet Co, Inc
4615 Murray Place
P0 Box 11349
Lynchburg, VA 24506-1349

Forest/Inwood Laboratories, Inc
500 Commack Road
Commack, NY 11725-5000

Forest Pharmaceuticals, Inc
13600 Shoreline Drive
St Louis, MO 63045
www.tiazac.com

Fougera
(Division of Altana Inc)
60 Baylis Road
Melville, NY 11747
www.fougera.com

Fujisawa Healthcare, Inc
Parkway North Center
Three Parkway North
Deerfield, IL 60015-2548
www.fujisawa.com

Galderma Laboratories, Inc
PO Box 331329
Fort Worth, TX 76163-1329
www.galderma.com

Gebauer Company
9410 St Catherine Avenue
Cleveland, OH 44104
www.gebauerco.com

GenDerm Corporation
600 Knightsbridge Parkway
Lincolnshire, IL 60069
www.genderm.com

Genentech, Inc
1 DNA Way
South San Francisco, CA 94080
www.gene.com

Genetco, Inc
711 Union Parkway
Ronkonkoma, NY 11779

Geneva Pharmaceuticals, Inc
2655 W Midway Boulevard
PO Box 446
Broomfield, CO 80038-0446
www.genevarx.com

Gensia Automedics, Inc
9360 Town Center Drive
San Diego, CA 92121
www.gensia.com

GensiaSicor Pharmaceuticals, Inc
19 Hughes
Irvine, CA 92618-1902
www.gensiasicor.com

Genzyme Corp
One Kendall Square
Cambridge, MA 02139
www.genzyme.com

Genzyme Genetics
5 Mountain Road
Framingham, MA 01701

Genzyme Tissue Repair
64 Sidney Street
Cambridge, MA 02139

Genzyme Transgenics
5 Mountain Road
Framingham, MA 01701

Gilead Sciences, Inc
333 Lakeside Drive
Foster City, CA 94404
www.gilead.com

Glades Pharmaceuticals, Inc
500 Satellite Boulevard
Suwanee, GA 30024
www.glades.com

Glaxo Wellcome, Inc
Five Moore Drive
Research Triangle Park, NC 27709
www.glaxowellcome.com

Glenwood, LLC
83 North Summit Street
Tenafly, NJ 07670
www.glenwood-llc.com

Glenwood-Palisades
One New England Avenue
Piscataway, NJ 08855

Global Pharmaceutical Corp
Castor & Kensington Avenues
Philadelphia, PA 19124
www.globalphar.com

Gray Pharmaceutical Company
100 Connecticut Avenue
Norwalk, CT 06856

Great Southern Laboratories
10863 Rockley Road
Houston, TX 77099

Guardian Drug Co
72 Prince Street
Trenton, NJ 08638

G&W Laboratories, Inc
111 Coolidge Street
South Plainfield, NJ 07080-3895

Gynex (see BTG)

Halsey Drug Company, Inc
695 North Perryville Road
Rockford, IL 61107
www.halseydrug.com

The Harvard Drug Group
31778 Enterprise Drive
Lovonia, MI 48150

Healthpoint
2600 Airport Freeway
Forth Worth, TX 76111
www.healthpoint.com

Heartland Healthcare Services
4755 South Avenue
Toledo, OH 43615

H&H Laboratories
4701 25 Mile Road
Shelby Township, MI 48316

Hi-Tech Pharmacal Co, Inc
369 Bayview Avenue
Amityville, NY 11701
www.diabeticproducts.com

Hoechst Marion Roussel, Inc
PO Box 9627
Kansas City, MO 64134-0627
www.hmri.com

Hoechst-Roussel (see Hoechst Marion Roussel)

ICI Pharma (see Zeneca)

ICN Pharmaceuticals, Inc
3300 Hyland Avenue
Costa Mesa, CA 92626

Immunex Corporation
51 University Street
Seattle, WA 98101
www.immunex.com

ImmunoGen, Inc
148 Sidney Street
Cambridge, MA 02139

Immuno-U.S., Inc
1200 Parkdale Road
Rochester, MI 48307-1744

International Ethical Labs
Avenue America Miranda #1021
Reparto Metropolitano
Rio Piedras, Puerto Rico 00921

International Medication Systems, Ltd (IMS)
1886 Santa Anita Avenue
S El Monte, CA 91733

Interpharm, Inc
3 Fairchild Avenue
Plainview, NY 11803

Invamed, Inc
2400 Route 130 North
Dayton, NJ 08810

Ion Laboratories
7431 Pebble Drive
Fort Worth, TX 76118-6416

Janssen Pharmaceutica
1125 Trenton-Harbourton Road
P0 Box 200
Titusville, NJ 08560-0200

Jerome Stevens Pharmaceuticals, Inc
60 Da Vinci Drive
Bohemia, NY 11716

Jones Pharma
1945 Craig Road
PO Box 46903
St Louis, MO 63146
www.jmedpharma.com

Kabi (see Pharmacia)

Kenwood Laboratories
383 Route 46 West
Fairfield, NJ 07004-2402
www.bradpharm.com

Key Pharmaceutical
2000 Galloping Hill Road
Kenilworth, NJ 07033

King Pharmaceuticals, Inc
501 Fifth Street
Bristol, TN 37620
www.kingpharm.com

The Knoll Pharmaceutical Company
30 North Jefferson Road
Whippany, NJ 07981

Konsyl Pharmaceuticals, Inc
4200 South Hulen
Fort Worth, TX 76109
www.konsyl.com

Kremers Urban
PO Box 427
Mequon, WI 53092

Lannett Co, Inc
9000 State Road
Philadelphia, PA 19136-1615
www.lannett.com

Lederle (see Wyeth-Ayerst)

Lemmon (see Teva USA)

Eli Lilly and Company
Lilly Corporate Center
Indianapolis, IN 46285
www.lilly.com

The Liposome Company, Inc
One Research Way
Princeton, NJ 08540-6619
www.lipo.com

Liquipharm, Inc
PO Box D-3700
Pomona, NY 10970
www.liquipharm.com

L. Perrigo Company
515 Eastern Avenue
Allegan, MI 49010
www.perrigo.com

Lyphomed (see Fujisawa)

3M Pharmaceuticals
3M Center, 275-2E-13
P0 Box 33275
St Paul, MN 55133-3275
www.mmm.com/pharma/

Mallinckrodt
675 McDonnell Boulevard
P0 Box 5840
St Louis, MO 63134
www.mkg.com
www.mallinckrodt.com

Marion Merrell Dow (see Hoechst Marion Roussel)

Marlop Pharmaceuticals, Inc
5704 Mosholu Avenue
Bronx, NY 10471-0536

Marsam Pharmaceuticals Inc
(Subsidiary of Schein Pharmaceutical, Inc)
P0 Box 1022
24 Olney Avenue, Bldg 31
Cherry Hill, NJ 08003
www.schein-rx.com

Martec Pharmaceutical, Inc
1800 North Topping Avenue
PO Box 33510
Kansas City, MO 64120-3510
Parent Company: Ratiopharm, GmbH
www.martec-kc.com

Mason Pharmaceuticals, Inc
4425 Jamboree Road
Suite 250
Newport Beach, CA 92660

McGaw, Inc
P0 Box 19791
Irvine, CA 92713-9791

McNeil Pharmaceutical
Route 202, PO Box 300
Raritan, NJ 08869-0602
www.ortho-mcneil.com

Mead Johnson (see Bristol-Myers Squibb)

Med-Derm Pharmaceuticals
PO Box 5193
Kingsport, TN 37663

Medeva Pharmaceuticals, Inc
PO Box 1710
755 Jefferson Road
Rochester, NY 14603-1710
www.medeva.com

Medirex, Inc
20 Chapin Road
PO Box 731
Pine Brook, NJ 07058
Parent Company: Sidmak Laboratories

Merck Human Health Division
P0 Box 4, WP39-207
West Point, PA 19486-0004
www.merck.com

Meridian Medical Technologies, Inc
10240 Old Columbia Road
Columbia, MD 21046
info@meridianmt.com
www.meridianmeds.com

Merrell Dow (see Hoechst Marion Roussel)

Merz Pharmaceuticals, Inc
4215 Tudor Lane
Greensboro, NC 27410

MGI Pharma, Inc
9900 Bren Road East
Suite 300E, Opus Center
Minnetonka, MN 55343-9667

Mikart, Inc
1750 Chattahoochee Avenue
Atlanta, GA 30318
www.mikart.com

Miles (see Bayer)

Miles Allergy (see Bayer)

Monarch (see King Pharm)

Monarch Pharmaceuticals, Inc
355 Beecham Street
Bristol, TN 37620
www.monarchpharm.com

Moore Medical
389 John Downey Drive
New Britain, CT 06050
www.mooremedical.com

Morton Grove Pharmaceuticals, Inc
6451 West Main Street
Morton Grove, IL 60053
www.mgp-online.com

Mova Pharmaceutical Corp
214 Carnegie Center
Suite 106
Princeton, NJ 08540

Muro Pharmaceuticals, Inc
890 East Street
Tewksbury, MA 01876

Mutual Pharmaceutical Co, Inc/United Research Laboratories
1100 Orthodox Street
Philadelphia, PA 19124
www.mutual.com

Mylan Pharmaceuticals, Inc
781 Chestnut Ridge Rd
P0 Box 4310
Morgantown, WV 26504-4310
www.mylan.com

Nephron Pharmaceuticals Corporation
4121 - 34th Street SW
Orlando, FL 32811-6458
www.hephronpharm.com
rwilburn@pharmacy.com

Nestle Clinical Nutrition
3 Parkway North, Suite 500
P0 Box 760
Deerfield, IL 60015

Norwich Eaton (see Proctor & Gamble)

Novartis Pharmaceuticals
59 Route 10
East Hanover, NJ 07939
www.novartis.com

Novo Nordisk Pharmaceuticals Inc
100 Overlook Center
Suite 200
Princeton, NJ 08540
www.novo-nordisk.com

Novopharm USA, Inc
165 East Commerce Drive
Schaumburg, IL 60173-5326
www.novopharmusa.com

Ohm Laboratories, Inc
PO Box 7397
North Brunswick, NJ 08902
Parent Company: Ranbaxy Pharmaceuticals
www.ranbaxy.com

Ohmeda (see Baxter Pharmaceutical Products)

OMJ Pharmaceuticals, Inc
PO Box 367
San German, Puerto Rico 00683

Organon Inc
375 Mt Pleasant Avenue
West Orange, NJ 07052
shapsed@am.father.umc.akzonobel.nl

Ortho Biotech Inc
700 Route 202 South
P0 Box 670
Raritan, NJ 08869-0670
www.procrit.com

Ortho-McNeil Pharmaceutical, Inc
PO Box 300
Route 202
Raritan, NJ 08869-06O2
www.ortho-mcneil.com

Otsuka America Pharmaceutical Inc
2440 Research Boulevard
Rockville, MD 20850

Paddock Laboratories
P0 Box 27286
3940 Quebec Avenue North
Minneapolis, MN 55427
www.paddocklabs.com

PAR Pharmaceutical, Inc
One Ram Ridge Road
Spring Valley, NY 10977
Parent Company: Pharmaceutical Resources, Inc
www.parpharm.com

Parkedale Pharmaceuticals, Inc
(Subsidiary of King Pharmaceuticals, Inc)
501 Fifth Street
Bristol, TN 37620
www.kingpharm.com

Parke-Davis
(Division of Warner-Lambert Company)
201 Tabor Road
Morris Plains, NJ 07950
www.warner-lambert.com

Parmed Pharmaceuticals, Inc
4220 Hyde Park Boulevard
Niagra Falls, NY 14305-6714
Parent Company: Alpharma

Parnell Pharmaceuticals, Inc
1525 Francisco Blvd
San Rafael, CA 94901
www.parnellpharm.com

Pasteur Merieux Connaught
Discovery Drive
Swiftwater, PA 18370-0187
www.us.pmc-vacc.com

PD-RX Pharmaceuticals
72 North Ann Arbor
Oklahoma City, OK 73127
www.pdrx.com

Pecos Pharmaceutical
25301 Cabot Road
Suites 212-213
Laguna Hills, CA 92653

Pedinol Pharmacal Inc
30 Banfi Plaza North
Farmingdale, NY 11735
www.pedinol.com

Person & Covey
616 Allen Avenue
Glendale, CA 91201

Pfizer First Connect Information Network
Pfizer Inc
U.S. Pharmaceuticals Group
235 East 42nd Street
New York, NY 10017-5755
www.pfizer.com

Pharma Tek, Inc
PO Box 1920
Huntington, NY 11743
www.pharma-tek.com

Pharmaceutical Formulations, Inc
460 Plainfield Avenue
Edison, NJ 08818

Pharmaceutical Laboratories
1170 W Corporate Drive
Suite 102
Arlington, TX 76006

Pharmaceutical Specialties, Inc
P0 Box 6298
2112 15th Street NW
Rochester, MN 55901
www.psico.com

Pharmacia & Upjohn Company (Ophthalmics Division)
701 E Milham Road
Kalamazoo, MI 49001
pnu.com

Pharmacia & Upjohn, Inc
7000 Portage Road
Kalamazoo, MI 49001
pnu.com

Pharmacy Division of Bayer
400 Morgan Lane
Westhaven, Conneticut 06516-4175
www.bayer.com

Pharmakon Labs, Inc
6050 Jet Port Industrial Boulevard
Tampa, FL 33634

Pharmics, Inc
PO Box 27554
Salt Lake City, UT 84127
www.pharmics.com

Physician's Total Care
5415 South 125th East Avenue
Suite 205
Tulsa, OK 74146

Plantex USA, Inc
482 Hudson Terrace
Englewood Cliffs, NJ 07632

Pratt Pharmaceuticals Division
Pfizer Inc
U.S. Pharmaceuticals Group
235 East 42nd Street
New York, NY 10017-5755

Procter & Gamble Pharmaceuticals
P0 Box 231
Norwich, NY 13815-0231

Procter & Gamble Pharmaceuticals
11450 Grooms Road
Cincinnati, OH 45242-1434

The Purdue Frederick Company
100 Connecticut Avenue
Norwalk, CT 06850-3590

PUREPAC Pharmaceutical Co
200 Elmora Avenue
Elizabeth, NJ 07207
Parent Company: F.H. Faulding and Company
www.Faulding.com

Qualitest Pharmaceuticals, Inc
1236 Jordan Road
Huntsville, AL 35811

Quality Research Pharmaceuticals, Inc
1117 Third Avenue South West
Carmel, IN 46032

Ranbaxy Pharmaceuticals, Inc
600 College Road East
Princeton, NJ 08540

Reed & Carnrick (see Schwarz Pharma)

Rhone-Poulenc Rorer Pharmaceuticals, Inc
500 Arcola Road
PO Box 5094
Collegeville, PA 19426-0998
www.rp-rorer.com

Richwood Pharmaceutical Company, Inc
7900 Tanners Gate Drive
Suite 200
Florence, KY 41042

R.I.D. Inc
609 North Mednik Avenue
Los Angeles, CA 90022

Roberts Pharmaceutical Corp
4 Industrial Way West
Eatontown, NJ 07724
www.robertspharm.com

Robins (see Wyeth-Ayerst)

Roche Laboratories
340 Kingsland Street
Nutley, NJ 07110
www.roche.com

Roerig Division
Pfizer Inc
U.S. Pharmaceuticals Group
235 East 42nd Street
New York, NY 10017-5755

Rorer (see Rhone-Poulenc Rorer)

Rosemont Pharmaceutical Corp
301 South Cherokee Street
Denver, CO 80223
Parent Company: Akzo Nobel

Roxane Laboratories, Inc
1809 Wilson Road
Columbus, OH 43228
PO Box 16532
Columbus, OH 43216
www.roxane.com

Rugby Laboratories, Inc
2725 Northwoods Parkway
Norcross, GA 30071
Parent Company: Watson Laboratories

Sandoz Pharmaceuticals Corp
59 Route 10
East Hanover, NJ 07936
www.sandoz.com

Sanofi Pharmaceuticals
90 Park Avenue
New York, NY 10016

Savage Laboratories
(Division of Altana Inc)
60 Baylis Road
Melville, NY 11747
www.savagelabs.com

Scandipharm, Inc
22 Inverness Center Parkway
Suite 310
Birmingham, AL 35242
www.scandipharm.com

Schaffer Laboratories
1058 North Allen Avenue
Pasadina, CA 91104

Schein Pharmaceutical, Inc
100 Campus Drive
Florham Park, NJ 07932
www.schein-rx.com

Schering Laboratories
2000 Galloping Hill Road
Kenilworth, NJ 07033
www.myhealth.com

Schwarz Pharma
5600 West County Line Road
Mequon, WI 53092
www.schwarzusa.com
www.schwarzpharma.com

G.D. Searle & Company
5200 Old Orchard Road
Skokie, IL 60077
www.searlehealthnet.com

Seneca Pharmaceutical, Inc
PO Box 25021
8621 Barefoot Industrial Road
Raleigh, NC 27613

Sequus Pharmaceuticals, Inc
980 Hamilton Court
Mento Park, CA 94025
www.sequus.com

Serono Laboratories, Inc
100 Longwater Circle
Norwell, MA 02061
www.seronousa.com

Sheffield Laboratories
170 Broad Street
New London, CT 06320
www.sheffield-labs.com

Shire Richwood, Inc
7900 Tanners Gate Drive
Suite 200
Florence, KY 41042
www.shiregroup.com

Sidmak Laboratories, Inc
17 West Street
PO Box 371
East Hanover, NJ 07936-0371
www.sidmaklab.com

Sigma-Tau Pharmaceuticals, Inc
800 South Frederick Avenue
Suite 300
Gaithersburg, MD 20877
www.sigmatau.com/na

SmithKline Beecham
P0 Box 7929
One Franklin Plaza
Philadelphia, PA 19101-7920
charles.depew@sb.com
www.sb.com

SmithKline Beecham Consumer Healthcare
P0 Box 1467
Pittsburgh, PA 15230
www.sb.com

Sola/Barnes (see Pilkington Barnes Hind)

SoloPak Pharmaceuticals Inc
6001 Broken Sound Parkway
Suite 600
Boca Raton, FL 33487

Solvay Pharmaceuticals, Inc
901 Sawyer Road
Marietta, GA 30062
www.solvay.com

Somerset Pharmaceuticals, Inc
P0 Box 30706
Tampa, FL 33630-3706

Southward Pharmaceuticals, Inc
33 Hammond Street
Suite 201
Irvine, CA 92718

Squibb (see Bristol-Myers Squibb)

Steris Laboratories, Inc
620 N 51st Avenue
Phoenix, AZ 85043-4705
Parent Company: Schein Pharmaceutical
www.schein-rx.com

Sterling (see Sanofi Winthrop)

Stratus Pharmaceuticals
14377 South West 142nd Street
Miami, FL 33186
www.stratuspharmaceuticals.com

Stuart (see Zeneca)

Superior Pharmaceutical Co
1385 Kemper Meadow Drive
Cincinnati, OH 45240-1635
www.superiorpharm.com

Survival (see Meridian Medical)

Syncor Pharmaceuticals, Inc
1313 Washington Avenue
Golden, CO 80401

Syntex (see Roche)

TAP Pharmaceuticals, Inc
2355 Waukegan Road
Deerfield, IL 60015

Taro Pharmaceuticals USA, Inc
5 Skyline Drive
Hawthorne, NY 10532
www.taropharma.com

Taylor Pharmaceuticals
1222 West Grand
Decatur, IL 62526

Teva Pharmaceuticals USA
151 Domorah Drive
Montgomeryville, PA 18936
www.tevapharmusa.com

Teva Pharmaceuticals USA
650 Cathill Road
Sellersville, PA 18960
www.tevapharmusa.com

Thames Pharmacal Co
2100 Fifth Avenue
Ronkonkoma, NY 11779

Triton (see Berlex)

UCB Pharma, Inc
1950 Lake Park Drive
Smyrna, GA 30080
suzan.leake@ucb-group.com

UDL Laboratories, Inc
P0 Box 2629
Loves Park, IL 61132-2629

Upjohn (see Pharmacia & Upjohn)

Upsher-Smith Laboratories, Inc
14905 23rd Avenue North
Minneapolis, MN 55447
www.upsher-smith.com

U.S. Pharmaceutical Corp
2401 Mellon Court
Suite C
Decatur, GA 30035

Value in Pharmaceuticals (VIP)
3000 Alt Boulevard
Grand Island, NY 14702
www.vippharm.com

Wallace Laboratories
(Division of Carter-Wallace, Inc)
Half Acre Road
Cranbury, NJ 08512-0181

Warner Chilcott Laboratories
Rockaway 80 Corporate Center
100 Enterprise Drive
Suite 280
Rockaway, NJ 07866
www.wclabs.com

Warrick Pharmaceuticals
1095 Morris Avenue
Union, NJ 07083-7137

Watson Laboratories, Inc
311 Bonnie Circle
Corona, CA 91720
www.watsonpharm.com

West-Ward
465 Industrial Way West
Eatontown, NJ 07724
Parent Company: Hikma Pharmaceuticals

Westwood-Squibb
(Dermatologic Division)
100 Forest Avenue
Buffalo, NY 14213
www.westwood-squibb.com

Whitby (see UCB Pharma)

Winthrop (see Sanofi Winthrop)

Wyeth-Ayerst Laboratories
P0 Box 8299
Philadelphia, PA 19101-1245
www.ahp.com

Zeneca Pharmaceuticals
1800 Concord Pike
Wilmington, DE 19803
www.zeneca.com

Zenith Goldline Pharmaceuticals
4400 Biscayne Boulevard
Miami, FL 33137
Parent Company: Ivax Corp
www.ivax.com

Zila Pharmaceuticals, Inc
5227 North 7th Street
Phoenix, AZ 85014-2800
www.zila.com

INDICATION/THERAPEUTIC CATEGORY INDEX

Antibiotic, Topical

Antiseborrheic Agent, Topical

Keratolytic Agent

Retinoic Acid Derivative

Tetracycline Derivative

(Continued)

Adrenal Corticosteroid (Mineralocorticoid)

ALCOHOL WITHDRAWAL

Alpha-Adrenergic Agonist

Antihistamine

Benzodiazepine

(Continued)

Adrenergic Agonist Agent

Antihistamine

(Continued)

(Continued)

Vasodilator

ANGIOEDEMA (HEREDITARY)

Anabolic Steroid

Androgen

ANGIOGRAPHY (OPHTHALMIC)

Diagnostic Agent

ANTICHOLINERGIC DRUG POISONING

Cholinesterase Inhibitor

ANTIFREEZE POISONING

Antidote

ANXIETY

Antianxiety Agent

Antianxiety Agent, Miscellaneous

(Continued)

(Continued)

(Continued)

Antihistamine *(Continued)*

Corticosteroid, Topical

(Continued)

(Continued)

(Continued)

Androgen *(Continued)*

Antiandrogen

Antineoplastic Agent

(Continued)

(Continued)

(Continued)

Antitussive

Antitussive/Analgesic

Antitussive/Decongestant

Antitussive/Decongestant/Expectorant

Antitussive/Expectorant

(Continued)

Antitussive/Expectorant *(Continued)*

Cold Preparation

Cough and Cold Combination

Expectorant

(Continued)

Adrenal Corticosteroid *(Continued)*

DERMATOMYCOSIS

Antifungal Agent

DERMATOSIS

Anesthetic/Corticosteroid

Corticosteroid, Topical

(Continued)

(Continued)

DIVERTICULITIS

Aminoglycoside (Antibiotic)

Antibiotic, Miscellaneous

(Continued)

(Continued)

Nonsteroidal Anti-inflammatory Drug (NSAID) *(Continued)*

Selective Cyclooxygenase-2 Inhibitor

DYSURIA

Analgesic, Urinary

Antispasmodic Agent, Urinary

Sulfonamide

EAR INFECTION *see* OTITIS MEDIA

EAR WAX

Otic Agent, Cerumenolytic

EATON-LAMBERT SYNDROME

Cholinergic Agent

ECLAMPSIA

Barbiturate

Benzodiazepine

ECZEMA

Antifungal/Corticosteroid

Corticosteroid, Topical

(Continued)

(Continued)

(Continued)

ESSENTIAL THROMBOCYTHEMIA (ET)

Platelet Aggregation Inhibitor

ETHYLENE GLYCOL POISONING

Pharmaceutical Aid

EXTRAPYRAMIDAL SYMPTOMS

Anticholinergic Agent

EXTRAVASATION

Alpha-Adrenergic Blocking Agent

Antidote

EYE INFECTION

Antibiotic/Corticosteroid, Ophthalmic

Antibiotic, Ophthalmic

(Continued)

(Continued)

Cephalosporin (Second Generation)

Cephalosporin (Third Generation)

Cephalosporin (Fourth Generation)

Genitourinary Irrigant

Macrolide (Antibiotic)

Penicillin

(Continued)

HEMOLYTIC DISEASE OF THE NEWBORN

Immune Globulin

HEMOPHILIA

Antihemophilic Agent

Vasopressin Analog, Synthetic

HEMOPHILIA A

Antihemophilic Agent

Blood Product Derivative

HEMOPHILIA B

Antihemophilic Agent

(Continued)

(Continued)

HOMOCYSTINURIA

Urinary Tract Product

HOOKWORMS

Anthelmintic

HORMONAL IMBALANCE (FEMALE)

Progestin

H. PYLORI INFECTION

Antidiarrheal

HUNTINGTON'S CHOREA

Monoamine Depleting Agent

HYDATIDIFORM MOLE (BENIGN)

Prostaglandin

HYPERACIDITY

Antacid

(Continued)

(Continued)

HYPERPLASIA, VULVAR SQUAMOUS

Estrogen Derivative

HYPERPROLACTINEMIA

Ergot Alkaloid and Derivative

Ergot-like Derivative

HYPERSENSITIVITY SKIN TESTING (DIAGNOSTIC)

Diagnostic Agent

HYPERTENSION

Adrenergic Agonist Agent

Alpha-Adrenergic Agonist

Alpha-Adrenergic Blocking Agent

Alpha-/Beta- Adrenergic Blocker

Angiotensin-Converting Enzyme (ACE) Inhibitor

(Continued)

Angiotensin-Converting Enzyme (ACE) Inhibitor *(Continued)*

Angiotensin II Antagonist

Antihypertensive Agent, Combination

Beta-Adrenergic Blocker

Calcium Channel Blocker

Diuretic, Combination

Diuretic, Loop

Diuretic, Miscellaneous

Diuretic, Potassium Sparing

Diuretic, Thiazide

(Continued)

HYPERTHYROIDISM

Antithyroid Agent

Beta-Adrenergic Blocker

HYPERTRIGLYCERIDEMIA

Antihyperlipidemic Agent, Miscellaneous

HMG-CoA Reductase Inhibitor

Vitamin, Water Soluble

HYPERTROPHIC CARDIOMYOPATHY

Calcium Channel Blocker

HYPERURICEMIA

Uricosuric Agent

Xanthine Oxidase Inhibitor

HYPOALDOSTERONISM

Diuretic, Potassium Sparing

HYPOCALCEMIA

Electrolyte Supplement, Oral

Vitamin D Analog

(Continued)

INFERTILITY (FEMALE)

Ergot Alkaloid and Derivative

Gonadotropin

Ovulation Stimulator

Progestin

INFERTILITY (MALE)

Gonadotropin

INFLAMMATION (NONRHEUMATIC)

Adrenal Corticosteroid

(Continued)

(Continued)

(Continued)

MIGRAINE

Analgesic, Non-narcotic

Antidepressant, Tricyclic (Tertiary Amine)

Antimigraine Agent

Beta-Adrenergic Blocker

Decongestant/Analgesic

Ergot Alkaloid and Derivative

(Continued)

(Continued)

Anticoagulant *(Continued)*

Antiplatelet Agent

Beta-Adrenergic Blocker

Thrombolytic Agent

MYOCARDIAL REINFARCTION

Antiplatelet Agent

Beta-Adrenergic Blocker

(Continued)

Adrenal Corticosteroid *(Continued)*

NEPHROLITHIASIS

Alkalinizing Agent

NEPHROPATHIC CYSTINOSIS

Urinary Tract Product

NEPHROTIC SYNDROME

Adrenal Corticosteroid

Antihypertensive Agent, Combination

(Continued)

OBESITY

Adrenergic Agonist Agent

Amphetamine

Anorexiant

Lipase Inhibitor

OBSESSIVE-COMPULSIVE DISORDER (OCD)

Antidepressant, Selective Serotonin Reuptake Inhibitor

Antidepressant, Tricyclic (Tertiary Amine)

OCULAR INJURY

Nonsteroidal Anti-inflammatory Drug (NSAID)

OILY SKIN

Antiseborrheic Agent, Topical

ONYCHOMYCOSIS

Antifungal Agent

OPHTHALMIC DISORDERS

Adrenal Corticosteroid

(Continued)

(Continued)

(Continued)

(Continued)

Analgesic, Non-narcotic

(Continued)

Analgesic, Non-narcotic *(Continued)*

(Continued)

(Continued)

(Continued)

PLAGUE

Antibiotic, Aminoglycoside

PLANTAR WARTS

Keratolytic Agent

Topical Skin Product

PLANTARIS

Keratolytic Agent

PLATELET AGGREGATION (PROPHYLAXIS)

Antiplatelet Agent

(Continued)

Antiplatelet Agent *(Continued)*

PNEUMOCYSTIS CARINII

Antibiotic, Miscellaneous

Antiprotozoal

Sulfonamide

Sulfone

PNEUMONIA

Aminoglycoside (Antibiotic)

Antibiotic, Miscellaneous

Antibiotic, Penicillin

Antibiotic, Quinolone

Carbapenem (Antibiotic)

Cephalosporin (First Generation)

(Continued)

(Continued)

(Continued)

Corticosteroid, Topical *(Continued)*

Keratolytic Agent

Psoralen

Retinoid-like Compound

PSYCHOSES

Antipsychotic Agent

Antipsychotic Agent, Benzisoxazole

Antipsychotic Agent, Butyrophenone

Antipsychotic Agent, Dibenzoxazepine

Antipsychotic Agent, Dihydroindoline

Phenothiazine Derivative

RAYNAUD'S DISEASE

Vasodilator

REGIONAL ENTERITIS *see* GASTROINTESTINAL DISORDERS

RENAL ALLOGRAFT REJECTION

Immunosuppressant Agent

RENAL COLIC

Analgesic, Non-narcotic

Anticholinergic Agent

RESPIRATORY DISORDERS

Adrenal Corticosteroid

RESPIRATORY DISTRESS SYNDROME (RDS)

Lung Surfactant

RESPIRATORY SYNCYTIAL VIRUS (RSV)

Antiviral Agent

Monoclonal Antibody

RESPIRATORY TRACT INFECTION

Aminoglycoside (Antibiotic)

Antibiotic, Carbacephem

Antibiotic, Macrolide

Antibiotic, Miscellaneous

Antibiotic, Penicillin

Cephalosporin (First Generation)

Cephalosporin (Second Generation)

Cephalosporin (Third Generation)

Cephalosporin (Fourth Generation)

Macrolide (Antibiotic)

(Continued)

(Continued)

(Continued)

SEBORRHEIC DERMATITIS

Antiseborrheic Agent, Topical

Keratolytic Agent

SEIZURE *see* EPILEPSY

SERUM THYROGLOBULIN (TG) TESTING

Diagnostic Agent

SEVERE ERYTHEMA MULTIFORME *see* DERMATOLOGIC DISORDERS

SHOCK

Adrenal Corticosteroid

Tetracycline Derivative

SKELETAL MUSCLE RELAXANT (SURGICAL)

Skeletal Muscle Relaxant

SKIN INFECTION (TOPICAL THERAPY)

Antibacterial, Topical

Antibiotic/Corticosteroid, Topical

Antibiotic, Topical

Intravenous Nutritional Therapy

Topical Skin Product

TINEA

Antifungal Agent

Antifungal/Corticosteroid

Antiseborrheic Agent, Topical

Disinfectant

TISSUE GRAFT

Immunosuppressant Agent

(Continued)

Antibiotic, Miscellaneous

Antibiotic, Penicillin

Cephalosporin (First Generation)

Cephalosporin (Second Generation)

Cephalosporin (Third Generation)

Cephalosporin (Fourth Generation)

Genitourinary Irrigant

Irrigating Solution

Penicillin

(Continued)

VITAMIN B DEFICIENCY

Vitamin, Water Soluble

VITAMIN B_5 DEFICIENCY

Vitamin, Water Soluble

VITAMIN B_6 DEFICIENCY

Vitamin, Water Soluble

VITAMIN B_{12} DEFICIENCY

Vitamin, Water Soluble

VITAMIN C DEFICIENCY

Vitamin, Water Soluble

VITAMIN D DEFICIENCY

Vitamin D Analog

VITAMIN E DEFICIENCY

Vitamin, Fat Soluble

VITAMIN K DEFICIENCY

Vitamin, Fat Soluble

VITILIGO

Psoralen

Topical Skin Product

VOMITING

Anticholinergic Agent

Antiemetic

Antihistamine

Phenothiazine Derivative

VOMITING, CHEMOTHERAPY-RELATED

Selective 5-HT_3 Receptor Antagonist

WHIPWORMS

Anthelmintic

WILSON'S DISEASE

Chelating Agent

WORMS

Anthelmintic

XEROPHTHALMIA

Ophthalmic Agent, Miscellaneous

XEROSTOMIA

Cholinergic Agent

ZOLLINGER-ELLISON SYNDROME (DIAGNOSTIC)

Diagnostic Agent

ZOLLINGER-ELLISON SYNDROME

Antacid

Antineoplastic Agent